HAND SURGERY
SECOND EDITION

HAND SURGERY

SECOND EDITION

J. EDWARD FLYNN, M.D.

THE WILLIAMS & WILKINS COMPANY

BALTIMORE

Made in the United States of America

Reprinted 1976

Library of Congress Cataloging in Publication Data

Flynn, Joseph Edward, 1905   ed.
    Hand surgery.

    1. Hand—Surgery. 1. Title.   [DNLM: 1. Hand—Sur-
gery, WE830 F648h]
RD559.F59 1974
ISBN 0-683-03267-4   617'.575   74-17274

Composed and printed at the
Waverly Press, Inc.
Mt. Royal and Guilford Aves.
Baltimore, Md. 21202, U.S.A.

Foreword

In the preface to the second edition of his *Medical Essays*, recompiled in 1882, Dr. Oliver Wendell Holmes said, "These *Essays* are now old enough to go on alone without staff or crutch in the shape of Prefaces. A very few words may be a convenience to the reader who takes up the book and wishes to know what he is likely to find in it." Similarly, the first edition of Dr. Flynn's *Hand Surgery*, published in 1966, is now so well known and universally accepted by the profession that it would be surplusage to dwell at length on the text of the second edition.

This book is a welcome reconfirmation to those who practice the healing arts that when, in the evolutionary process of learning, new techniques, new names, and new ideas emerge, they will be brought to us in strikingly intelligible and usable form through the dedication of men like Dr. Flynn and the other eminently qualified surgeons and physicians who have collaborated to produce this excellent work.

In the second edition the demonstrable improvements in hand surgery since 1966, whether revisions of established procedures or the creation of new methods, are clearly presented. Illustrative of what the reader will find, but by no means all that he will discover, are anatomical guidelines for more easily reaching the deep important structures, an expansive discussion of the appropriate methodology to deal with congenital abnormalities, and a fine description of the team effort required between anesthetist and surgeon in the use of the new and the not so new anesthetic agents.

The treatment of open wounds of the hand is re-evaluated in a framework of the physiology of wound healing. Crushing, compactor, mangle, and wringer injuries are considered with meaningful emphasis in the problem of obviating complications by adequate initial evaluation and care. Special wounds, including new injuries occasioned by recently developed instrumentalities and substances, are skillfully delineated. All this and a great deal more which is equally meaningful will be found in the second edition of *Hand Surgery*.

To have been in on the ground floor when at first six and later nine hand centers were developed by Dr. Sterling Bunnell in World War II was a privilege. To read new authors in hand surgery and to see the evolution of new and advancing techniques from Dr. Bunnell's time to now is exhilarating and stimulating. The continuous quest for knowledge in this field of surgery and the ongoing development of teaching facilities and microsurgical centers will bring further improvements in surgery of the hand. Flynn and those who with him contributed so much to the second edition merit the highest praise.

W. Brandon Macomber, M.D.
Albany, New York

Preface

World War II presented the stimulus for a concentrated and universal interest in surgery of the hand. Hand Surgical Societies have been established in the United States, Australia, England, France, Germany, Sweden, South America, and Japan. With such universal interest, it is important that foreign and American writers contribute to this text.

Hand surgery has developed many subspecialties. The surgical treatment of the arthritic hand and wrist have improved. Investigations of tendon transfers with median, ulnar, and radial nerve palsies with trauma and leprosy still progress. Vasomotor and trophic disorders present the most difficult problems and studies in these problems are multiple. Investigations in anesthesia, congenital anomalies, wounds, fractures, skin grafts and skin flaps, island pedicle flaps, tendon repair, tendon transplants, joint contractures, pyogenic infections, and tetanus persist.

Studies in tests for sensation, a most perplexing problem, electromyography, primary and delayed nerve sutures, nerve grafts, and compression of nerves present controversial problems.

The nuclear age has increased the number and severity of irradiation burns. The treatment of electric burns, thermal burns, chemical burns, and frostbites is still controversial.

Studies in arterial, venous, and lymphatic surgery have made great progress. Much knowledge was gained in arterial suturing and arterial grafting in the Korean and Vietnam Wars.

Clinical and laboratory investigations on the etiology of Dupuytren's contracture continue. Much has been learned in the universal clinical studies on Volkmann's and local ischemic contractures.

The use of the operating microscope has increased universally and has aided the exactness of the repair of nerves and small blood vessels. Limb reimplantation is still controversial.

Laboratory investigations continue on the healing of tendons and tendon transplants and controversy still persists. The biochemistry of collagen synthesis in tendon healing aids in understanding tendon healing. In this age of organ transplants, tendon offers an ideal organ for autogenous, homologous, and heterogenous studies.

Studies of artificial sheaths with silicone are widely performed and are encouraging.

Surgery of the hand has really developed into many subspecialties. Thus it is important that investigators in special phases expound their special interests. It was with this thought that 59 authors were asked to contribute to the Second Edition of *Hand Surgery*. Of these authors, 21 are new contributors. The other authors have brought up to date the chapters of their special interest.

I wish to express my appreciation to all the authors who have contributed to this book. I wish to thank my wife, Alice, for her patience and assistance, and also Miss Margaret Mahoney for her secretarial aid.

J. Edward Flynn, M.D.

vii

Contributors

Franklin L. Ashley, M.D., Professor of Surgery and Chief of Division of Plastic Surgery, U.C.L.A. School of Medicine. Attending Plastic Surgeon, U.C.L.A. Hospital and Clinics.

George J. Baibak, M.D., Clinical Associate, Department of Surgery, Medical College of Ohio at Toledo. Director of Burn Unit, St. Vincent Hospital and Medical Center, Toledo, Ohio.

John L. Bell, M.D., Associate Professor of Surgery, Northwestern University Medical School, Attending Surgeon, Northwestern Memorial Hospital, Passavant Pavilion, Chicago.

Charles H. Bradford, M.D., Consultant Surgeon, Orthopedic Service, Boston City Hospital.

Paul W. Brand, C.B.E., F.R.C.S. (London), Chief Rehabilitation Branch, U. S. Public Service Hospital, Carville, Louisiana.

Henry Brown, M.D., Assistant Clinical Professor of Surgery, Harvard Medical School, Visiting Surgeon, Boston City Hospital. Member, Sears Laboratory, Surgeon, Massachusetts Institute of Technology.

Paul W. Brown, M.D., Professor of Orthopedic Surgery, Chief Division of Hand Surgery Service, University of Miami, Miami, Florida.

John J. Byrne, M.D., Professor of Surgery, Boston University, School of Medicine. Director of Boston University Surgical Service and Research Laboratory, Boston City Hospital.

John M. Cahill, M.D., Associate Professor of Surgery, Boston University School of Medicine. Visiting Surgeon, University Hospital and Boston City Hospital.

Bradford Cannon, M.D., Clinical Professor of Surgery, Harvard Medical School. Visiting Surgeon, Massachusetts General Hospital.

Robert E. Carroll, M.D., Professor, Orthopedic Surgery, Columbia Physicians and Surgeons, New York. Surgeon in Charge of Hand Surgery, New York Orthopedic Hospital and Columbia Presbyterian Medical Center. Attending Orthopedic Surgeon, Columbia-Presbyterian Medical Center.

Robert A. Chase, M.D., Professor and Director, Department of Surgery, Stanford University Medical School, Palo Alto, California.

John H. Crandon, M.D., Associate Clinical Professor of Surgery, Tufts University Medical School. Visiting Surgeon, Mount Auburn Hospital, Cambridge. Surgeon-in-Chief, Winthrop Community Hospital.

Raymond M. Curtis, M.D., Associate Professor of Plastic Surgery, Johns Hopkins University Medical School. Visiting Staff, Johns Hopkins Hospital. Consultant in Hand Surgery, Union Memorial Hospital and Childrens Hospital. Consultant in Hand Surgery to Surgeon General of the Army.

Robert K. Dean, M.D., Clinical Associate, Medical College of Ohio at Toledo. Active Staff, St. Vincent's Hospital and Medical Center, Toledo, Ohio.

Ralph A. Deterling, Jr., M.D., Professor and Chairman, Department of Surgery, Tufts University School of Medicine; Surgeon-in-Chief, New England Medical Center Hospital, Boston.

James A. Dolphin, M.D., Clinical Instructor, Orthopedic Surgery, Boston University School of Medicine. Visiting Orthopedic Surgeon, Carney Hospital, Lakeville State Hospital; Canton Massachusetts Hospital School.

Milton T. Edgerton, Jr. M.D., Professor and Chairman, Department of Plastic Surgery, University of Virginia Medical Center, Charlottesville, Virginia.

Martin A. Entin, M.D., C.M., M.Sc., F.A.C.S., Associate Professor of Surgery, McGill University Medical School. Plastic Surgeon-in-Chief, Royal Victoria Hospital, Montreal. Consultant in Plastic and Hand Surgery, Shriners Hospital for Crippled Children, Montreal.

J. Edward Flynn, M.D., Clinical Professor of Surgery, Tufts University School of Medicine, Visiting Surgeon, Tufts Surgical Service, and Chief of Hand Surgical Service, Boston City Hospital. Visiting Surgeon and Chief of Hand Surgical Service, Boston V.A. Hospital. Consultant Surgeon, St. Elizabeth's Hospital, Chelsea Naval Hospital, Brighton U.S.P.H.S. Hospital, Morton (Taunton) Hospital, Norwood Hospital.

William F. Flynn, M.D., Assistant Clinical Professor of Surgery, Harvard Medical School, Visiting Surgeon, Harvard Surgical Service, Boston City Hospital, Visiting Surgeon and Chief of Hand Surgical Service, Carney Hospital

J. Leonard Goldner, M.D., Professor and Chairman, Division of Orthopedic Surgery, Duke University Medical Center. Chief of Orthopedic Hand Service, Duke University School of Medicine.

Frederik C. Hensen, M.D., Assistant Professor of Plastic Surgery, Johns Hopkins University and School of Medicine, Surgeon, Johns Hopkins Hospital, Baltimore.

James M. Hunter, M.D., Associate Professor of Orthopedic Surgery and Chief of the Division of Hand Surgery, Jefferson Medical College of the Thomas Jefferson University, Philadelphia. Chief of Orthopedic Surgery, State Hospital for Crippled Children, Elizabethtown, Pennsylvania. Consultant in Hand Surgery, Naval Regional Medical Center, Philadelphia, and Valley Forge General Hospital.

Stanley L. James, M.D., Senior Clinical Instructor of Orthopedics, University of Oregon Medical School, Adjunct Associate Professor, Center of Research for Human Performance, and Orthopedic Consultant, University of Oregon Athletic Department, Orthopedic Staff, Sacred Heart General Hospital.

Emanuel B. Kaplan, M.D., Clinical Professor of Orthopedic Surgery, New Jersey School of Medicine and Dentistry, Newark. Emeritus Associate Professor of Anatomy, College of Physicians and Surgeons, Columbia University, New York City, Consultant Orthopedic Surgeon, Hospital for Joint Diseases and Medical Center, New York City.

John C. Kelleher, M.D., Assistant Clinical Professor, Department of Surgery, Medical College of Ohio at Toledo. Director of Surgery, St. Vincent's Hospital Medical Center, Toledo.

David G. Kline, M.D., Professor of Surgery, Chairman of Neurosurgery, Louisiana State University Medical Center, New Orleans.

Robert D. Larsen, M.D., Clinical Associate Professor of Surgery, Wayne State University, Detroit.

Robert D. Leffert, M.D, Assistant Professor of Orthopedic Surgery, Harvard Medical School. Chief of The Surgical Upper Extremity Rehabilitation Unit and the Department of Rehabilitation Medicine, Massachusetts General Hospital.

Robert B. Linberg, Ph.D., Chief of Microbiology, U.S. Army Institute of Surgical Research, Brooke Army Medical Center, Fort Sam Houston, Texas.

Paul R. Lipscomb, M.D., Professor and Chairman, Department of Orthopedic Surgery, University of California, Davis, California.

Henry C. Marble, M.D., Consultant Surgeon, Massachusetts General Hospital, deceased.

Frank H. Mayfield, M.D., Clinical Professor of Surgery (Neurosurgery), University of Cincinnati College of Medicine. Director, Department of Neurosurgery, The Christ Hospital and Good Samaritan Hospital, Cincinnati.

William F. McManus, M.D., Assistant Professor of Surgery, The Medical College of Wisconsin, Milwaukee. Associate Attending Surgeon, Milwaukee County General Hospital, Wood V.A. Hospital, Wood, Wisconsin.

Stephen W. Meagher, M.D., Senior Clinical Instructor in Surgery, Tufts University Medical School. Attending Surgeon, Hand Surgical Service, Boston V.A. Hospital, St. Elizabeth's Hospital. Consultant in Hand Surgery, Holy Ghost Hospital and Cardinal Cushing Rehabilitation Unit.

Erik Moberg, M.D., Professor Emeritus Orthopaedic and Hand Surgery, University of Göteborg, Sweden. Former Chief of Orthopaedic and Hand Surgery, Sahlgren Hospital, Göteborg.

John C. Molloy, M.D., Clinical Instructor of Orthopedic Surgery, Tufts Medical School. Assistant Orthopedic Surgeon, St. Elizabeth's Hospital, Faulkner Hospital, and Hahnemann Hospital.

Joseph E. Murray, M.D., Professor of Surgery, Harvard Medical School. Chief, Plastic Surgery, Peter Bent Brigham Hospital and The Children's Medical Center.

Donald A. Nagel, M.D., Associate Professor and Head, Division of Orthopedic Surgery, Stanford University School of Medicine.

H. Minor Nichols, M.D., Clinical Associate of Surgery, University of Oregon Medical School, Surgeon, Good Samariton Hospital, Portland, Oregon.

Frank E. Nulsen, M.D., Harvey Hunting Brown, Jr. Professor of Neurosurgery, Western Reserve University School of Medicine, Cleveland, Ohio.

George S. Phalen, M.D., Director of Orthopedic Section, Dallas Medical and Surgical Clinic. Former Associate Professor, Frank E. Bunts Educational Institute, Cleveland, Ohio, and Orthopedic Surgeon, Cleveland Clinic Foundation.

Joseph L. Posch, M.D., F.A.C.S., Clinical Professor of Surgery, College of Medicine, Wayne State University. Director, Hand Surgery Program, Grace Hospital Division, United Hospitals of the Detroit Medical Center

Austin D. Potenza, M.D., Director Division of Orthopedic Surgery, Professor of Clinical Surgery, School of Medicine, Health Sciences Center, SUNY, Stonybrook, New York.

Basil A. Pruitt, Jr., M.D., Colonel, M. C., Commander and Director, U. S. Army Institute of Surgical Research, Brooke Army Medical Center, Fort Sam Houston, Texas.

R. Guy Pulvertaft, C.B.E., M.D. (Hon.) M.Chir., F.R.C.S., (England), Orthopedic Surgeon Emeritus, Derbyshire Royal Infirmary. Honorary Civil Consultant Royal Air Force. Fellow British Association of Plastic Surgeons.

Harris B. Shumacker, Jr., M.D., Professor of Surgery, Indiana University-Purdue University Medical Center at Indianapolis.

Donald B. Slocum, M.D., Associate Clinical Professor of Orthopedic Surgery, Oregon Medical School, Orthopedic Surgeon, Sacred Heart Hospital, Eugene, Oregon.

James W. Smith, M.D., Assistant Clinical Professor of Surgery (Plastic), The New York Hospital-Cornell Medical Center, Assistant Attending (Plastic Surgery), The New York Hospital, New York.

Richard J. Smith, M.D., Assistant Clinical Professor of Orthopedic Surgery, Harvard Medical School, Chief of Hand Surgical Service (Orthopedic), Massachusetts General Hospital.

James G. Sullivan, M.D., Clinical Associate Department of Surgery, Medical College of Ohio at Toledo, Director, Plastic Surgical Service, St. Vincent's Hospital and Medical Center, Toledo, Ohio.

Alfred B. Swanson, M.D., Clinical Professor of Orthopedic Surgery, Michigan State University, Lansing, Michigan. Chief, Orthopedic Surgery and Orthopedic Research, Blodgett Memorial Hospital, Chief, Orthopedic Training Program, Blodgett Memorial Hospital and Buttersworth Hospital.

G. de Groot Swanson, M.D., Orthopedic Research Department, Blodgett Memorial Hospital, and Plastic Surgery Department, Blodgett Memorial Hospital.

Radford C. Tanzer, M.D., Associate Professor of Plastic Surgery, Dartmouth Medical School. Plastic Surgeon, Hitchcock Clinic.

Dennis P. Thompson, M.D., Staff, St. John's Hospital, Santa Monica and Beverly Glen Hospital, Los Angeles, Instructor, Beverly Glen Hospital.

Dr. Raoul Tubiana, Directeur Scientifique de l'Institute de la Main-27, bd Victor Hugo-Neuilly/Seine. Directeur d'enseignement associé, Faculté de Médecine de Cochin-Port-Royal, 24 rue du faubourg Saint-Jacques, Paris-14e. Attending surgeon of the American Hospital of Paris-63, bd Vcitor Hugo Neuilly/Seine.

Leroy D. Vandam, M.D., Professor of Anesthesia, Harvard Medical School. Anesthesiologist-in-Chief, Peter Bent Brigham Hospital.

Claude E. Verdan, M.D., Professor Ordinaire (Full Professor) of Surgery and Dean of Faculty, University of Lausanne, Switzerland, Chief of Surgical Polyclinic University of Lausanne, Switzerland.

George V. Webster, M.D., Clinical Professor of Surgery (Plastic) U.C.L.A. School of Medicine, Los Angeles, California.

Elden C. Weckesser, M.D., Clinical Professor of Surgery, Case Western Reserve University Medical School. Associate Surgeon, University Hospital, Highland View Hospital, V.A. Hospital, Cleveland.

Louis Weinstein, M.D., Professor of Medicine, Tufts University School of Medicine, Boston.

Contents

chapter one

History of Hand Surgery

Henry C. Marble, M.D.

J. Edward Flynn, M.D.

Surgery today is quite different from the surgery of 60 years ago. The senior author's career began soon after the turn of the century, and he therefore had the rather special privilege of watching the transition from the old era to the new. When he began as a surgical intern at the Massachusetts General Hospital in 1910, there were still active a few old surgeons who had received their basic training before the era of antisepsis, and who in their declining years tended to have little slips of their aseptic conscience. He recalls very well one master surgeon who in the midst of an operation would take off his rubber gloves and hurl them on the floor with the words "I can't operate with those damn things on." The same surgeon refused to wear a mask, and the nurses on duty in the operating room had to be constantly alert for his unconscious breaks in surgical technique. The professor of surgery disliked wearing the surgical mask and would at times wander afield and lean against the rail in front of the spectators' seats. All these breaks in aseptic technique were promptly noted by the long suffering nurse in the operating room who would quietly superintend repairs. This the surgeon accepted much as a little boy does when found with his fingers in the cookie jar. These few surgeons marked the end of one and the beginning of a new surgical era.

The hospital services were then set up very simply. There were the Medical Service and the Surgical Service, but no Neurosurgical Gynecologic, Pediatric, or other special services. Thus all surgery was done by general surgeons. There were nine senior surgeons, nine junior surgeons, and a dozen or so surgeons to out-patients, who occupied the lowest rung in the surgical ladder. There were three surgical services, the senior surgeon and a junior service surgeon being on duty on each service for a four-month period each year. These surgeons did all kinds of surgery. Division into special assignments came some years later. If the senior surgeon saw fit to invite one of the surgeons or assistant surgeons not on duty to do a special case, he might do it.

At that time only one surgeon, Dr. C. Allen Porter, was greatly interested in the surgery of the hand. This interest grew out of his studies of x-ray burns on the hands of the early radiologists, all of which he published in a well known article in 1907, describing his method of excision of carcinomas following x-ray dermatitis. I do not recall any other surgeon on the staff of the hospital caring for any surgical conditions of the hand. The care of infections, injuries, and fractures of the hand fell to the surgical interns who, one or two years after their graduation from medical school, did the greater part of all hand surgery.

At about the same time that my teacher, Dr. Porter, published his work, Dr. Allen Buckner Kanavel[53] published his masterpiece on infections of the hand. This was the true beginning of the modern era. However, before we discuss modern surgery of the hand, it might be interesting to study the history of general surgery, because even as far back as the fourth century, B.C., doctors were recording observations about the human body that would interest doctors today.

In the history of surgery the conventional place to begin is with Hippocrates,[61] who lived from 460 to 377 B.C. Hippocrates was, if not the father, at least the patron saint of surgery. The procedure which he advocated for operating on a patient was:

"We must turn the parts to be operated upon to that which is most brilliant and convenient to light."

"The operator is sitting conveniently for himself."

"When sitting the knee should be a little higher than the groins and the elbows rest upon them."

(now on a table).

"The nails should be neither longer nor shorter than the points of the fingers. The surgeon should practice with the extremities of the fingers, the index finger being usually turned to the thumb. This promotes dexterous use of the fingers. He should practice all sorts of work with them, endeavoring to do things well, elegantly, quickly without trouble, neatly and promptly. The instruments should be prepared so as not to impede the work. If another gives them he must be ready a little beforehand and do so directly."

(Could we offer any better advice to young surgeons even today?) Hippocrates had other advice for aspiring doctors.

"It is the business of the phsyician to know in the first place, things similar and things dissimilar."

"In all cases of accident it was the practice of the ancient surgeons to compare carefully the injured part with its fellow or corresponding part on the opposite side."

"It should be kept in mind that exercise strengthens and inactivity wastes."

"It will be found that the natural position is that which suits best with the instrument that is used and the work to be performed."

This is the position of function.

"All mechanical contrivances should either be properly done or not be had recourse to at all, for it is a disgraceful and awkward thing to use mechanical means in an unmechanical way."

(A splint that fits everyone fits no one.)

After this Hippocrates described very accurately the proper method of reduction of a fracture of the wrist, which is to my mind the same method as that used now. He also pointed out that the bandage should be inspected carefully on the day after the injury to make certain that it was neither too loose nor too tight. All of this, in accordance with good modern teaching, was 300 years B.C.

We find another interesting note by Heliodorus,[61] written about the end of the first century. He described the amputation of a finger as follows:

"A circular incision is made around the digit. Two vertical incisions are made opposite one another and the flap so formed is dissected upward. The bone is lain bare. The digit is removed by cutting forceps and the flaps are brought together and sutured."

Who could do better today?

After the Greek School, which was essentially the school of Hippocrates, the center of medicine and medical teaching moved to Alexandria, Egypt. Here surgery was taught as well as anatomy. "Wounds were sutured *after refreshing the wound edges* and a dressing was applied of lint or linen soaked in honey," wrote one Egyptian doctor. The Alexandrian School had needles, sounds, in fact most of the instruments that we use today. They also had special forceps for removing foreign bodies.

It is said[17] that St. Luke was a student in this school. In connection with his studies of anatomy St. Luke is said to have painted very beautiful pictures of his subjects. The professor of art saw these pictures and urged him to give up the thought of studying medicine and become an artist because he felt that there was a greater field for him in art than there was in medicine. To this St. Luke replied, "Master, I am a physician from my birth, I can conceive of nothing else." To this I can only add that even today many surgeons use the brush nearly as well as they use the scalpel.

Historians have shown us that the Hindus in India were exceedingly adept at surgery in both the pre-Christian and Christian eras. The semilegendary Hindu surgeon Susruta, who may have lived about the first century A.D., wrote the following note:

"Cutting instruments must split a hair longitudinally; the surgeons must have short beards, close cut and clean nails, fresh operating garments for each operation, and the operating room should be fumigated before and after each operation."

This is good advice. The only problem might be — how does a master surgeon split a hair longitudinally?

Susruta also described an operation for the reconstruction of the nose, which was in every way similar to our modern flap graft. (The penalty for adultery in ancient India was the cutting off of the nose.) Here is the description of the operation:

"The physician should take the leaf of a tree the same size as the nose and apply it to the cheek, cut a piece out of the cheek in such a way that a stem is still adherent. Then he stitches the cheek with needle and thread, scarifies the stump of the nose and quickly but carefully places the flap in the nose. After the transplanted piece has grown, the stem is cut off." "In like manner the flap might be turned up from the upper or lower arm and attached to the nose — with the arm over the head."

In 1210, Roger of Salerno wrote, "A nerve with a clean transverse cut and well aligned heals better than a diagonal cut."[61]

We must not pass over the medieval period without mentioning the anatomical drawings (Figs. 1.1 and 1.2) of Leonardo da Vinci, who was born in 1450. Over 700 of these drawings have been published.[110] Da Vinci was an artist and his work represented the relation of art to anatomy. He showed the problems of muscle leverage and muscle action, in labor, pushing, running, restraining, and resting. How many cadavers he was able to dissect is not known, but probably very few. In those days such material was rare.

In the 16th century another Italian, Paracelsus, wrote:[91]

"It is necessary to know in the first place what is the efficient cause of the curing of wounds, because this may of itself indicate the proper treatment. Know then that the human body contains in itself its own proper radical balsam, born in it and with it, and not only the body as a whole contains it, but all its parts, such as flesh, bones and nerves have there own peculiar juice competent to cure wounds . . . It is not the surgeon who cures wounds, it is the natural balsam in the part itself." ". . . the wound needs nothing so much as to be left alone."

(This is the first note that I find on wound healing.)

Another surgeon of the 16th century was the Frenchman Ambroise Paré, who lived from 1510 to 1590.

Paré trained as an Army doctor and such was his experience and his tenacity that he became accepted all over Europe as one of the leading surgeons of the time. His judgment was excellent, his mortality rate was unusually low, his patients were made comfortable, and his results in operations were good. Some of his most important teachings were: to enlarge the wound for drainage; to remove bone splinters and foreign bodies from wounds; to control hemorrhage with liga-tures; not to encourage suppuration; and to amputate through sound tissues.

Paré was very interested in orthopedic devices and even developed one for the upper extremity (Fig. 1.3). His great knowledge of the principles and practice of surgery made him immortal. Von Hilden devised a mechanism to correct deformity in the hand (Fig. 1.4).

During the 17th century the use of the tourniquet to control hemmorrhage became common.

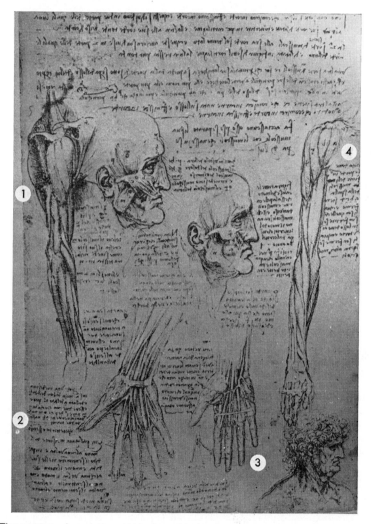

Figure 1.1. The centenarian pictured is believed to be the subject of most of these sketches. *Sketch 1.* The superficial muscles of the arm and forearm (lateral aspect). *Sketch 2.* The distribution of the median and ulnar nerves in the hand. (This splendid figure of the digital distribution of the median and ulnar nerves shows the great attention paid by Leonardo to the mechanism of the hand, and his simple experiment recounted below, how great his insight.) Leonardo writes, "Here, following a cut in the hand, sometimes the sensation and not the motion of the fingers is blocked, and sometimes the motion and not the sensation. Sometimes it is both sensation and motion." *Sketch 3.* A dissection of the blood vessels of the hand showing the superficial palmar arch and the distribution of its branches to the muscles and to the skin of the fingers. *Sketch 4.* Superficial muscles of the arm and forearm (anterior aspect). In this beautiful dissection the shoulder and upper arm are shown in the anterior aspect. The forearm and hand are shown in the posterior aspect in full pronation.

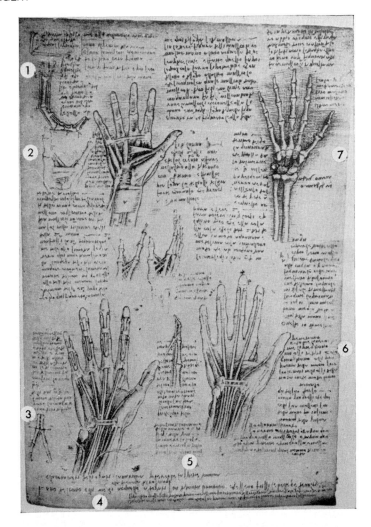

Figure 1.2. Sketch 1. This small sketch I believe demonstrates the mechanism of flexion of the finger. The long flexor tendon is shown, as well as the pulleys. Leonardo was interested in the mechanics of motion. *Sketch 2*. This dissection is interesting. Let us presume that the subject here was the centenarian whose face is shown in Figure 1.1. This is a superficial dissection of the palm. The heavy bands that we see must be the palmar fascia, which clearly must be hypertrophied. These bands go to the little and ring fingers and also to the thumb. They are connected at the base and then a structure is shown which is pulled to the radial side of the wrist above the transcarpal ligament. This must be the palmaris longus tendon. (Could it be that the palmar fascia of this centenarian in 1500 may have had that which was described 300 years later by Dupuytren?) *Sketch 3*. This drawing with the arrow we believe demonstrates that the metacarpophalangeal joints are capable of lateral as well as anterior motion. *Sketch 4*. In this beautiful dissection the median and ulnar nerves are reflected. The superficial and the deep tendons are demonstrated, together with their insertion, and the pulleys of the fingers. The four lumbrical muscles are indicated. In the hypothenar eminence, the abductor, flexor and opponens digiti quinti may be identified. *Sketch 5*. This tiny sketch demonstrates the insertions of the two flexor tendons of the finger. *Sketch 6*. A deeper dissection of the hand showing the deep tendons. The abductor muscle of the thumb is here shown. *Sketch 7*. This is a very careful sketch of the bones of the hand, wrist, and forearm. The other small sketches on this page we believe are to demonstrate the function of the interossei muscles. Leonardo says, "Note how the muscles which arise from the bones of the palm of the hand are attached to the first bone of the digits, how they flex them and how the nerves are distributed there."

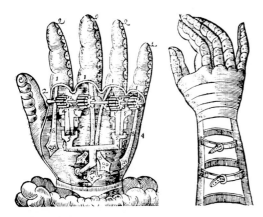

Figure 1.3. Artifical articulated hand designed by Ambroise Paré (1510-1590), most celebrated Renaissance surgeon, could be tied to arm or sleeve. Reproduced from *Great Ideas in the History of Surgery*[110] by permission of the Williams and Wilkins Company.

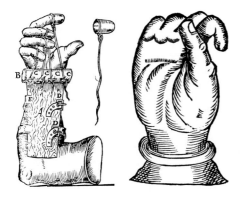

Figure 1.4. Deformity of the hand *(right)* and method of correcting it *(left)* appear in *Wund-Artzney* by German surgeon, Wilhelm von Hilden. Reproduced from *Great Ideas in the History of Surgery*,[110] by permission of the Williams and Wilkins Company.

Then in 1800 appeared two men whose names are still inscribed in the literature of the hand surgeon. The first was Abraham Colles, an Irishman, the second Guillaume Dupuytren, a Frenchman.

Abraham Colles was a broadly and well trained general surgeon. He was Professor of Surgery at the Royal College of Surgeons in Dublin, Ireland, and his lecture notes[70A] are still in existence and can be read in the library there. He wrote one small article, ''Treatment of Fractures of the Distal End of the Radius,'' in which he accurately described what is now called a Colles fracture and outlined its treatment very thoroughly. Of his many surgical articles there were only two others published that remotely might be associated with hand

surgery. In the first article he describes a student and a professor who dissected a body in the anatomical laboratory. They both chanced, unfortunately, to cut their fingers. He describes the ascending infection in both of them, the streaks running up the arm, the shoulder, and the extensive abscess formation, the high temperature — clearly a generalized lymphatic infection. The professor died but the student, after being sick for many days, survived. Following this, Dr. Colles, directed that in the future students working in the anatomical laboratory, if they should cut themselves, should wash the wound with turpentine.

The second article described his operation for suture of the subclavian artery for aneurysm.

Across the channel in Paris at about the same time, Guillaume Dupuytren[70B] was leading his busy surgical life. He was the Professor of Surgery in Paris and was the Chief Surgeon at the Hotel Dieu. He published many articles on surgical subjects, sometimes 50 in 1 year. In one of these clinical lectures, he described the contraction of the fingers as the result of hyperplasia of the palmar fascia, seen in an anatomical dissection on the cadaver of a man who had suffered from this condition. Before this, it was believed that the condition was due to contraction of the tendons but Dupuytren's anatomical and clinical work showed that it was all an *overgrowth* plus a *contraction* of the palmar fascia. Since then it has been called Dupuytren's contracture. As nearly as we can find, that is the only article related to hand surgery that this tremendously busy surgeon wrote.[70B]

Dupuytren was famous in surgery, not only for his description of this contracture of the hand, but also for his interest in pathology. When he died he left money to establish an institute of pathology which bears his name. It is in the Musée Dupuytren that many of the great pathologists of modern time were trained.

Following Colles and Dupuytren came the great French physician, William Duchenne, who lived from 1806 to 1875. Duchenne discovered in 1835 that the faradic current could be applied by electrodes to the skin and thus safely produce muscular contraction. He wrote a book called *The Physiology of Motion*,[32] based on his lifetime of study and clinical experience, which showed the true actions of the living muscles. This book, when added to other anatomical knowledge, is of great help to contemporary surgeons in their reconstructions, particularly in the upper extremity. One paragraph will indicate the quality of the work which this man did in the matter of physiology of motion:

''Muscles of the Forearm''

''The muscular forces which act on flexion of the forearm, on pronation and supination are so distributed that one muscle only produces each of these movements independently of the other movements, or that one muscle only produces simultaneous flexion and supination, or flexion and pronation.

Thus, the brachialis is an independent flexor, the brachial biceps is the flexor supinator, the muscle called long supinator (brachioradialis) is a flexor pronator and the three muscles: the supinator, pronator teres and pronator quadratus are independently supinator and pronators.

No one will fail to recognize the usefulness of this mixed flexion, supination, or pronation produced by the same muscle. These movements produced without special effort are very frequent in the activities of the upper extremity.

But it was also important for the skillful use of the hand that pronation and supination be made independent of flexion and extension of the forearm.

Only on very strong effort all the muscles participating in these movements contract synergistically.''

Thus far we have said nothing about anesthesia. Opium was known from the early days, as was alcohol, and it is probably true that many of the patients operated upon were given large doses of wine or laudanum. Despite all this, they surely must have had severe pain. They had to be strapped to the table and the surgeons tried to reduce the agony by working rapidly and skillfully, getting the ordeal over as quickly as possible. Some of the writings refer to a pain-killer called a soporific sponge. This sponge was wet with hyoscyamus, poppy, mandratoro, mulberry, hemlock, and lettuce. This was put over the patient's nose but we cannot believe there was any real relief.

In 1846 William Thomas Green Morton, a dentist, found that he could extract teeth painlessly when his patient inhaled the fumes of sulfuric ether. On October 16, 1846, John Collins Warren at the Massachusetts General Hospital performed the first surgical operation using sulfuric ether, with Dr. Morton serving as the anesthetist, and another great step was taken in the world of surgery.

In the 1920's the senior author recalls a patient who came under his care. She was a tiny old lady who had been struck by an automobile, receiving a fracture of the upper arm. During her convalescence she asked him to walk with her out onto the Bullfinch Building lawn. She pointed up at the Ether Dome, and turning to him said, ''My father was Dr. William Morton who gave the first ether in that Dome.''

In 1862 Louis Pasteur, a Frenchman, found that the fermentation of wine could be stopped by the application of heat; he maintained that there were tiny organisms growing that caused the fermentation, and which could be killed by heat. Pasteur became the father of bacteriology.

For centuries surgeons knew that better results were obtained in surgery following the use of soap and water, cleanliness, and the use of clean linen. This was proven further as the result of the work of Ignaz Semmelweis of Vienna. He noted that in two of the obstetrical wards in the Vienna General Hospital only one ward was frequented by medical students who came directly from the dissecting rooms. In this ward the mortality rate for puerperal fever was very high. The second ward was a clean ward and was attended by midwives, graduate doctors, and doctors in training. In this ward the mortality rate was infinitely lower. Semmelweis then directed that the students carefully wash their hands when leaving the dissecting room and that they further immerse them in chlorinated lime. As the result of this the mortality rate in the first ward, the student's ward, fell to equal the rate in the second ward.

Joseph Lister, a young English surgeon, knew about this work. He also knew of Pasteur's work. Further, he knew of the power of carbolic acid, which had been used for the disinfection of sewers. He combined the principles of Semmelweis, plus the teachings of Pasteur, adding to this the power of carbolic acid which he used in a weak solution on the gauze dressings and as a spray in the operating room. Thus, the work of Pasteur, plus the observations of Semmelweis and the genius of Lister, in 1865 gave birth to antiseptic surgery.

Now the field of surgery was wide open. Many surgeons were slow in accepting and adopting the work of Lister, but slowly and surely, decade by decade, the surgeons adopted his principles, adding the use of high pressure steam for sterilizing as well as boiling. The world of aseptic surgery then came into existence and was fully accepted in the last part of the 19th century. As stated before, an accident of time and birth made it possible to see and observe the last surgeons who had had at least a part of their training before the teachings of Lister had been fully developed and accepted.

At almost the same time that Lister and Pasteur were working in the field of asepsis, an American neurologist, Dr. S. Weir Mitchell, working in Civil War hospitals noted a condition which he named ''causalgia.'' It was characterized by severe and burning pain, usually in the arm and hand. This condition was also studied by Raynaud and Berger and gradually Mitchell's observations opened the way for extensive studies on the sympathetic system.

In 1881 Richard von Volkmann published the first of three articles describing contraction of the hand, which condition still bears his name, Volkmann's contracture. Volkmann was Professor of Surgery at Halle and is well known for his studies on tar and paraffin to cancer and the description of his operation for rectal cancer. He was the foremost champion advocating Listerian antisepsis, as well as one of the editors of the *Zentralblatt für Chirurgie*. He published a specific account of the rapid post-traumatic muscle contraction and the progressive relentless destruction of the muscles together with contracture of the hand. This condition he described as ''ischemic.'' At that time he believed the condition to be due to the stoppage of arterial blood and reported that the changes in the muscle were not inflammatory.

This condition, which is feared and dreaded by every surgeon, has been the object of much study and research since Volkmann (Griffith in 1910, Clark and Hildebrandt in 1920, and Black in 1922). We now believe that any patient, following injury to the upper extremity, having no sign of pulse, a pale, anesthetic hand, and a boardlike swelling about the site of the injury has the beginning of Volkmann's contracture. Further, we believe that the treatment indicated to prevent Volkmann's contracture is immediate surgical intervention — incision of fascial roof of the anticubital space with the release of blood clots and exposing the brachial artery, releasing it if it is impaled on bone fragments.

We have observed Volkmann's contracture following elbow fractures in which no splints or casts have been applied, and we have seen a full blown Volkmann's contracture in a case of hemophilia, and again a threatened case in a patient having myelogenous leukemia following a very slight injury. It is still a much feared calamity following injuries of the forearm and elbow.

World War I marked a milestone in the surgery of trauma. Up to then few if any surgeons had had extensive training in such surgery, but during the war under the guidance of French surgeons we learned to do debridement, now meaning enlargement of the wound and removal of all contamination and all injured tissue. The entire wound area was excised down to bleeding contracting tissue. Block excision was rarely done. No effort was made to do primary closure. Small Dakin tubes were put into the wound and the patient was evacuated to a permanent hospital. It was in the permanent hospital that for the first time true bacteriology of the wound was practiced. Careful cultures were taken of the wound and if these showed that all of the infected material in the wound had been removed and that it contained no streptococci or gas-forming bacilli a second debridement was done and the wound was closed. This was the beginning of proper management of the wound.

Methods of blood typing became known and transfusion became a reality. Somewhat later physicians learned to use sodium citrate to prevent coagulation of the blood, and transfusions became even easier and more useful.

In the postwar period, with coming of the automobile and greater industries, the picture changed and the wards filled up with injury patients.

Passage of the Workmen's Compensation laws, which aimed to protect the working man and to ensure that he received adequate medical care, was another step forward. Adequate medical care of the hand came to mean that if the working man received an injury to his hand he should be put in such a condition that he could return to do the work that he had done prior to his injury, and the responsibility for carrying this out was thrown directly upon the shoulders of the surgical profession. Little by little the public demanded that the surgeon be so equipped that he could care for a wound of the hand in such a way that the patient should end up with a useful functioning member.

Industrial leaders also gradually began to see that it was in their own interest to have good medical care for their workers until they were cured. Among other things, industries discovered that they were the ones who were paying the bills and would continue to pay until their injured workers were restored to their jobs. Surgical techniques moved ahead to keep pace, and eventually the need for more skilled hand surgeons became apparent.

In all these years, however, it is difficult to find much literature on the surgery of the hand. Two French surgeons touched briefly on the problem at the end of the 19th century. One described the extension of infections of the hand as coming through the tendon sheaths and the other described the extension of infections as coming through the lymphatics. We can now see that both these gentlemen were correct. We also find an article written in 1885 in the *Journal of the American Surgical Society* in which a surgeon described the care of hand injuries in railroad employees. It was an interesting article but little or nothing was said about the end results of the treatments. (Even at this relatively advanced date one surgeon discussing this presentation said that the "teachings of Lister had not been completely accepted by his community.")

The senior author's own experience in World War I is a further case in point. Although he had in his wards in France a large number of bone and joint cases, he recalls only a few injuries of the hand. Presumably this was because the hand presents such a small target to rifle fire and further the hand grenade was only then beginning to be extensively used. Surgery of the hand seemed to be almost completely neglected until the advent of Dr. Allen B. Kanavel of Chicago.

Dr. Kanavel was a general surgeon, and as a young man working in the dispensary, was appalled at the great number of infections of the hand that passed through his clinic and he was shocked at the crippling effect that followed these badly treated infections. Determined to do something about it, he went into the laboratory, there injected the tendon sheaths, and with the aid of the x-ray found the extent of each tendon sheath, including the radial and ulnar bursas. In like manner he studied the spaces; he studied the midpalmar, the lumbrical, and the thenar spaces and he obtained radiographs. With this knowledge he went back to his clinic and applied what he had found. Finally he wrote his book showing the methods of extension of infection in the tendon sheath. At the same time he observed those infections which were extended by the lymphatics, followed their course, and published the results of these studies of lymphatic infections. He then knew which cases required watchful waiting. He pointed out what measures and operations were proper for draining the infections without leaving a crippled and mangled hand. This and a great deal more he published in *Infections of the Hand,*[53] the first great monograph on the hand.

In the second and third decade of this century infections of the hand were so common in the Massachusetts General Hospital that the senior author was able to demonstrate to each resident every type of infection of the hand, and every resident under his direction during his term of service had an opportunity to treat each type of infection as described in the Kanavel book. (Early in their training the House Staff complained that Kanavel's book was intricate and complex but as greater knowledge of these infections unfolded during their term of service they found that it was much easier to digest. At one time the senior author told this to Dr. Kanavel, saying, "My House Staff finds your book hard to read." To this Dr. Kanavel replied, "You tell your House Staff that I found it a much harder book to write.")

There is one other matter that we must not forget. Dr. Kanavel taught that patients with infections of the hand should be hospitalized, and that patients be made comfortable, given ample fluids, and visited daily. He further recommended that the ailing hand should be put at rest. All of this was even more important in the case of lymphatic infection, which often advances with tremendous rapidity forming abscesses anywhere in the arm or axilla.

At the end of the senior author's third year in medical school he had a practical examination in surgery and he happened to be questioned by a senior surgeon. He asked, "What is a felon?" The senior author doesn't recall his answer but I do distinctly recall the answer he gave, correcting his humble effort. He said "A felon is an exostosis of the terminal phalanx of the thumb." This was the accepted teaching concerning infections of the hand in 1909.

This brings us to the modern era. Dr. Kanavel has taught us how to care for the infections of the hand. The bacteriologists have come to our help by identifying the infecting organisms. We have learned about contamination and debridement during the first world war, and the sum of it all is what we know today about proper care of a wound. But let us not forget that until World War II there were no antibiotics to help. The fear of sepsis was still with us, as was the danger of tetanus.

The discovery of antibiotics has changed the situation radically. They are unquestionably useful but they are not substitutes for good surgery or good surgical care. We believe that we must still treat infections and injuries with the same fine careful surgery that was the practice before the days of antibiotics. These new drugs should be used not as a substitute, but as an *aid to supplement* surgery and tender medical care.

With these tools now in his hands a modern surgeon can safely graft tendons and nerves, and graft skin to cover denuded areas. Many books have lately been written about tendon and nerve repair, and the physiology of healing is now well understood.

The most valuable contribution in this field came from Dr. Sterling Bunnell,[15] a well trained general surgeon in California. Dr. Bunnell turned his great talents and long experience to the reconstruction of mangled hands. He insisted on all of the teachings of the past masters, stressing particularly the gentle handling of the tissues. He called this atraumatic surgery. He exercised his skill also in plastic, bone, tendon, nerve, blood vessel, and muscle surgery to reconstruct crippled hands. He showed that tendons could be grafted to substitute for lost ones, and could be transferred to give function to useless digits or joints. He taught that nerves could be grafted and that whole fingers could be moved about for better function. Thus he opened the door for the complete reconstruction of the injured hand.

Doctors Kanavel and Bunnell, with their associates, have built a solid foundation upon which the future care of the hand — long neglected — now rests. They have shown the world that a serious infection or a massive mutilation of the hand may be cared for in such a way that a useful member may result.

In the past decade there have been advances in most phases of hand surgery. Chase has reviewed recent advances in hand surgery (111).

ANATOMY

Anatomy and function of the extensor apparatus have been described by Landsmeer[56] and later by Stack.[99] The details include: (1) the tendon of the extensor; (2) central slip and its point of insertion; (3) interosseous tendon; (4) tendon of lumbrical; (5) dorsal hood or superficial intertendinous sheet; (6) oblique fibers; (7) lateral tendinous band; (8) common terminal tendon; (9) triangular sheet; (10) transverse part of the retinacular ligament (Landsmeer); (11) oblique part of retinacular ligament.

WOUND HEALING

Illingsworth,[51] Dunphy and Van Winkle,[33] and Warren report on dynamic changes in wound healing. The research in wound healing, particularly that of Madden and Peacock[67] and others in collagen synthesis, intermolecular banding and remodeling seems to be near the solving of problems in general healing. Preservation of gliding with end-to-end healing of tendons remains the challenge.

Dr. R. Smith in his chapter on "Open Wound" reports in detail on wound healing (Chapter 5A).

DUPUYTREN'S CONTRACTURE

A comprehensive monograph on Dupuytren's contracture was presented by Hueston[49] in 1963. The deformity is more severe in males than females but no association to occupation can be established statistically. Hyperplasia of palmar fascia increases when diseased fascia is subjected to linear forces. Dupuytrens hypertrophy frequently diminishes when stress forces are released by incision of the fascial bands supports this notion. Gonzales[43] suggests that with Dupuytren's contracture in a digit, an incision in skin and fascia, and the insertion of a skin graft results in resolution of the hypertrophied fascial nodes.

The Dupuytren's diathesis is described by

Skoog[93] — the knuckle pads, plantar lesions, penile lesions (Peyronie's disease), and general proliferative nodular fasciitis.

In surgical treatment, band fasciectomy has proven to have less morbidity and fewer complications than radical fasciectomy. However, radical fasciectomy is necessary with widespread disease. Z-shaped or W-shaped incisions as suggested by Deming[30] along the longitudinal fibers continuous onto the palmar surface of the digit allows excision without wide undermining.

Bassot[9] has reviewed injection therapy. He presents evidence of correction in 34 patients by injection of trypsin, alphachymotrypsin, hyaluronidase, thiomucase, and lidocain (lognocaine) in several points in the fascia followed by forceful extension of the fingers and splinting in extension of two to five days.

CARPAL-TUNNEL SYNDROME

Carpal tunnel syndrome was rarely recognized by surgeons in 1950. Phalen[84] in 1970 reported on 21 years experience with this disorder.

There is usually a positive Tinel's sign, hypesthesia, positive wrist-flexion test, and occasionally thenar atrophy. Median nerve conduction time tests are valuable.

Steroid injection may give temporary relief. Surgery with complete transection of the volar carpal ligament give the best results.

Phalen dilates on this problem in his chapter.

ULNAR-TUNNEL

Recently compression of the ulnar nerve beneath a portion of the volar carpal ligament (Guyon's canal) in the wrist has been noted by Dupont[34] in 1965, and Kleinert[54] in 1971. Surgical release of the roof gives relief.

POSTERIOR INTEROSSEOUS NERVE COMPRESSION

Spontaneous paralysis of the posterior interosseous branch of the radial nerve, described in 1930, has been reviewed by Bryan, Miller, and Panijayanond.[13] The arcade of Frohse[40] is the usual site of the nerve compression. Electromyograph locates the lesion. The extensor carpi radialis longus and brevis and the brachioradialis are unaffected, whereas the extensor digitorum communis, extensor pollicis longus, extensor carpi ulnaris, extensor indicis proprius, the extensor minimi digiti, and the oblique muscles of the thumb are paralyzed.

Early surgical release of the offending anatomic structures is indicated.

RHEUMATOID ARTHRITIS

The merits of surgical arthroplasty for rheumatoid arthritis were thoroughly reviewed in the International Workshop on Artificial Finger Joints by Calnan[18] and Holt, et al. Smith and Kaplan[96] have investigated the causes of rheumatoid deformity of the metacarpophalangeal joint. Lipscomb in Chapter 8C in this book reviews the basis for ulnar drift and palmar subluxation of the metacarpophalangeal joints and these agree with others — Zancoli,[109] Backhouse,[7] Stack[100] Vaughan-Jackson,[103] Kuczynski,[55] Hakstian and Tubiana[44] and Flatt.[37]

The surgical procedures are reviewed by Lipscomb. Lipscomb also raises doubts concerning early synovectomy for multiple small joints.

ARTHROPLASTY

Vaughan-Jackson[103] has recently reviewed excisional arthroplasty at the metacarpophalangeal joint and has suggested that with modifications added by Riordan and Fowler and Vainio the procedure has an important place. The tendency today is to have excision arthroplasty replaced by implant arthroplasty.

IMPLANT ARTHROPLASTY

The Metacarpophalangeal Joint

In 1964 Flatt developed digital joint prostheses and discussed indications. Since then many implantable devices have been developed. Most notable are the silicone prosthesis of Swanson, the silicone-dacron prosthesis of Niebauer and the polypropylene prosthesis of Reis-Calnan.

Swanson presents a chapter in detail later on silastic joint spacers (Chapter 8E).

THE PROXIMAL INTERPHALANGEAL JOINT

Harrison believes that synovectomy of the proximal interphalangeal joint is useful and advocates early silastic prostheses.

THE WRIST JOINT

Synovectomy at the wrist is more successful in arresting destruction than in the finger joints. Ranamot et al. report that wrist arthrography helps on deciding on the indications of early synovectomy. Brown has outlined the technique for diagnostic arthrography.

Lipscomb in Chapter 8C discusses the surgery of the wrist joint.

TENDON SURGERY

The debate of primary versus secondary repair of flexor tendons within the digital theca continues.

Verdan's[105] statistics suggest better results with primary repair and his experience is presented in detail in Chapter 7D.

Bassett and Carroll[8] introduced in 1963 the use of silicone rod tendon spacers in preparation for tendon grafting. Promising results are reported after insertion of a tendon graft by Gaisford et al. and Hunter and Salisbury;[50] Hunter presents his experience in Chapter 7H.

PERIPHERAL NERVE SURGERY

Current opinions on peripheral nerve surgery are presented in Sunderland's volume.

The contributions of Moberg, Önne, and Omer are notable in the assessment of nerve recovery. Moberg elucidates in length in a later chapter.

Sunderland[102] believes that a severed nerve should be repaired immediately if local conditions are favorable.

Smith[94] has demonstrated microsurgical techniques for nerve repair and will elaborate on this procedure in Chapter 13B.

THE PROXIMAL INTERPHALANGEAL JOINT

The pathology of the proximal-interphalangeal-joint stiffness and methods of treatment have been advanced by Curtis[26] and he presents his investigations in Chapter 8B.

VASCULAR PROBLEMS

Trauma

Darling[27] has reviewed vascular trauma of the upper extremity. Morton *et al.*[76] have stressed that conservative treatment of arterial injuries can no longer be justified. Indications for operations are sensory or motor loss, pallor, coolness and lack of pulses, with arteriography in the operating room as indicated. Adar *et al*[3] have stressed the high priority of vascular injuries in the multiply injured patient.

In World War II, in which major vessels were ligated, the amputation rate was 49 per cent. Salvage rate has increased to an amputation rate of 13 per cent in the Korean and Vietnam wars in which arteries were sutured or repaired by a saphenous or cephalic vein graft. Rich[87] reports amputation rates of 5 to 6 per cent for injuries to axillary and brachial arteries. A Fogarty[38,39] catheter and heparin distal to the injury ensure no distal thrombosis. Deterling and J. W. Smith describe gross and microsurgical techniques in Chapters 13A and B.

Occlusive Disease

One quarter of all limb emboli lodge in upper extremity arteries: 5 per cent in the subclavian, 30 per cent in the axillary, and 65 per cent brachial arteries, according to Darling.[27]

Fogarty[38] reported 100 operations using catheter embolectomy, with 84.6 per cent survival rate and 96 per cent limb salvage. Deterling dilates on occlusive disease in Chapter 13A.

Inadvertent Intra-Arterial Injections

Reverse arterial flow has been reported in monitoring arterial pressures in cardiac surgery. With increase in intravenous drugs by addicts, serious tissue loss has been reported with amphetamine and other drugs by Engler *et al.*[36]

Bypass Grafting in Arterial Occlusion

Arterial occlusion may be arteriosclerotic or traumatic in origin. Garret *et al.*[41] have reported 13 cases of occlusive disease in the brachial artery successfully treated by venous bypass graft.

Vasomotor Disorders

Controvery over the indications and technique of dorsal sympathectomy continues. Conley[25] reported on 117 patients with resection of the second through the fourth thoracic ganglia, and the second and third intercostal nerves by a posterior extrapleural approach. Haxton has reviewed various techniques and prefers the anterior supraclavicular approach, a modified Telford technique without ganglionectomy.

Mayfield has reviewed this problem in detail in Chapter 13C.

Frostbite

Martinez et al.[69] have studied specific arterial lesions in frostbite by angiography. In first degree injuries, there is a distal arterial spasm and arteriovenous shunting. In severe or fourth degree frostbite, spasm and shunting are present in addition to thrombosis.

Washburn[106] has outlined first-aid care for frostbite.

Shumacher has reviewed this problem in detail in Chapter 12C.

Replantation of Limbs

Eiken, *et al.*[35] have shown replantation after complete amputation to be experimentally feasible. Malt and McKhann[68] reported a successful replantation in 1962. Since then Herbsman et al.,[47] Williams *et al.*,[108] Inoue *et al.*,[52] Rosenkranz *et al.*, White,[107] and Komatsu *et al.*, have reported successes.

Replantation of a complete amputation above the elbow in an adult usually results in a functional failure. There are reports by Rosenkrantz *et al.*, and White of replantation of the arm amputated through the humerus in children with recovery of useful function. The ideal for replantation is a sharp, clean amputation just proximal to the wrist.

Digit replantation with vessels less than 1 mm. in diameter is feasible with microsurgical technique.

Engler and Hardin have a complete review of extremity replantation.

Neurovascular Island Pedicle

Littler[64] described a composite transfer of a digit for a thumb on neurovascular bundles. This prompted Moberg to suggest islands of skin and neurovascular bundles to be transferred to anesthetic areas of the hand. Littler,[64] Peacock, Chase, Tubiana, and Winsten have reported successes with this technique.

Chase has suggested the neurovascular flap as an

excellent method for salvage of digits rendered ischemic by trauma.

SPECIAL INJURIES

Airless-Spray-Gun Injuries

Stark et al[101] report on the dangers of spray gun for painting, with paint spreading widely in soft tissues.

Tear Gas Pen

Adams et al.[2] report on tear gas, a combination of chloroacetophenone and silica anhydride, 1:1. When the pen is held at close range, the material penetrates the hand. The material is toxic to peripheral nerves and skeletal muscle.

Rucksack Paralysis

Daube[28] has reported that the paralysis is due to the heavy backpack which causes traction on the upper trunk of the brachial plexus.

Snowblower Injury

Crush injuries from the large worm gear that pushes snow to the blower or lacerations from the blower fan by reaching into the throwing nozzle to clear it of snow are common.

Meagher[72] reports on special injuries in Chapter 5C.

Prosthesis

Bonner[11] has noted that prosthetic devices were greatly improved with lightweight laminated plastic and the ability to fit any amputation stump.

Glanville,[42] Montgomery,[75] Epps, et al. and McKenzie report on powered prostheses. Hartman et al., and Chandler et al. report that myoelectric control of powered prostheses is applicable to the functional powered end device in the upper extremity.

Burns

Sulfamyalon, early motions in a saline bath, and splinting in a position of function are indicated for deep burns. Cannon and Murray report on thermal burns in detail in Chapter 12B.

Infections

With major infections, early incision and drainage is indicated. Local antibiotics seem logical. Carter[19] uses polyethelene tubes through which an antibiotic is injected for irrigation.

Nichols[79] recently reported that, in a study of 91 purulent hand infections, 62 per cent of cultures grew bacteria resistant to penicillin, while only 7 per cent grew bacteria resistant to tetracycline. Thus when an antibiotic is indicated, before culture reports are available, tetracycline is preferable to penicillin.

REFERENCES

1. Adams, F. The Genuine Works of Hippocrates. Baltimore, Williams & Wilkins, 1939.
2. Adams, J. P., Fee, N., and Kenmore, P.I. Tear-gas injuries: a clinical study of hand injuries and an experimental study of its effects on peripheral nerves and skeletal muscles in rabbits. J. Bone, Joint Surg. (Am.), 48: 436-442, 1966.
3. Adar, R., Nerubay, J., Katznelson, A. et al. Management of acute vascular injuries. J. Cardiovasc. Surg., 11: 435-439, 1970.
4. Alexander, J. W. Host defense mechanism against infection. Surg. Clin. North Am., 52: 1367-1378, 1972.
5. Backhouse, K. M. Mechanical factors influencing normal and rheumatoid metacarpophalangeal joints. Ann. Rheum. Dis., 28 (5): 15-19, 1969.
6. Backhouse, K. M. The mechanics of digital control in the hand and an analysis of the ulnar drift of rheumatoid arthritis. Ann. R. Coll. Surg., Engl., 43: 154-173, 1968.
7. Backhouse, K. M., Kay, A., Kates, A. et al. Tendon involvement in rheumatoid arthritis. Ann. R. Coll. Surg. Engl., 43: 154-173, 1968.
8. Basset, C. A. L., and Carroll, R. E. Formation of tendon sheath by silicone-rod implants. J. Bone Joint Surg. (Am.), 45: 884-885, 1963.
9. Bassot, J. Traitment de la maladie de Dupuytren par exerese, pharmacodynamique bases, physiobiologiques technique. Gaz. Hop., No. 16, June 10, 1969, p. 557.
10. Blue, A. L., and Dirstine, M. J. Grease-gun damage: subcutaneous injection of paint, grease and other materials by pressure guns. Northwest Med., 64: 342-344, 1965.
11. Bonner, C. D. Physical medicine and rehabilitation. N. Engl. J. Med., 271: 189-195, 1964.
12. Brooks, L. A., Sachatello, C. R., Dyer, W. C., Jr. et al. Gangrene of the hand following intra-arterial drug injection. J. Bone Joint Surg. (Am.), 49: 579, 1967.
13. Bryan, F. S., Miller, L. S., and Panijayanond, P. Spontaneous paralysis of the posterior interosseous nerve: a case report and review of the literature. Clin. Orthop., 80: 9-12, 1971.
14. Buncke, H. J., Jr., and Schulz, W. P. Experimental digital amputation and reimplantation. Plast. Reconstr. Surg., 36: 62-70, 1965.
15. Bunnell, S. Surgery of the Hand, Ed. 4. Philadelphia, Lippincott, 1964.
16. Bywatwaters, D. G. L. Pathogenesis of finger joint lesions in rheumatoid arthritis. Ann. Rheum. Dis., 28 (5): 5-10, 1969.
17. Caldwell, T. Dear and Glorious Physician. New York, Doubleday, 1959.
18. Calnan, J. S.. Operative technique for joint replacement. Ann. Rheum. Dis., 28 (5): 81-88, 1969.
19. Carter, S. J., and Mersheimer, W. L. Infections of the Hand Orthop. Clin. North Am. 1: No. 2, November 1970.
20. Chandler, S. A. G., and Sedgwick, S. R. Functional stimulation of disabled limbs. Hand, 3: 15-19, 1971.
21. Chase, R. A. Salvage in acute hand injuries by reintroduction of blood supply using the island pedicle technique. Plast. Reconstr. Surg., in press.
22. Childress, D. S., Hampton, F. L., Lambert, C. N. et

al. Myoelectric immediate postsurgical procedure: a concept for fitting the upper-extremity amputee. Artif. Limbs, *13 (2):* 55-60, 1969.

23. Coffman, J. D., and Cohen, A. S. Total and capillary fingertip flow in Reynaud's phenomenon. N. Engl. J. Med., *285:* 259-263, 1971.

24. Collins, D. W. Some new thoughts on hand prostheses. Hand, *3:* 9-11, 1971.

25. Conley, J. E., and Endeloff, G. L. M. Sympathectomy for upper extremity vasomotor disorders. J. Cardiovasc. Surg., *10:* 436-439, 1970.

26. Curtis, R. M. Joints of the hand. See *Hand Surgery,* edited by J. E. Flynn. Baltimore, Williams & Wilkins, 1966, pp 350-376.

27. Darling, R. C. Peripheral arterial surgery. N. Engl. J. Med., *280:* 26-30, 84-91, 141-146, 1969.

28. Daube, J. R. Rucksack paralysis. J.A.M.A., *208:* 2447-2452, 1969.

29. deJong, P., Golding, M. R., Sawyer, P. N. *et al*. The role of sympathectomy in the early management of cold injury. Surg. Gynecol. Obstet., *115:* 45-48, 1962.

30. Deming, E. G. Y-V advancement pedicles in surgery for Dupuytren's contracture. Plast. Reconstr. Surg., *29:* 581-586, 1962.

31. Dibbell, D. G., and Chase, R. A. Small blast injuries. Plast. Reconstr. Surg., *37:* 304-313, 1966.

32. Duchenne, W. *The Physiology of Motion*. Translated and edited by E. B. Kaplan. Philadelphia, Lippincott, 1949.

33. Dunphy, J. E., and Van Winkle, W., Jr. *Repair and Regeneration. The Scientific Basis for Surgical Practice*. New York, McGraw-Hill, 1969.

34. Dupont, C., Cloutier, G. E., Provost, Y. *et al*. Ulnar-tunnel syndrome at the wrist: a report of four cases of ulnar-nerve compression at the wrist. J. Bone Joint Surg. (Am.) *47:* 757, 1965.

35. Eiken, O., Nabseth, D. C., Mayer, R. F. *et al*. Extremity replantation. Arch. Surg., *88:* 54-56, 1964.

36. Engler, H. S., Purvis, J. G., Kanavage, C. B. *et al*. Gangrenous extremities resulting from intra-arterial injections. Arch. Surg., *94:* 644-651, 1967.

37. Flatt, A. E., *The Care of the Rheumatoid Hand*, Ed. 2. St. Louis, Mosby, 1969.

38. Fogarty, T. J. Catheter technic for arterial embolectomy. J. Cardiovasc. Surg., *8:* 22-28, 1967.

39. Fogarty, T. J., and Cranley, J. J. Catheter technic for arterial embolectomy. Ann. Surg., *161:* 325-330, 1965.

40. Frohse, F., and Frankel, M. Diemuskein des menschlichen armes. Jena G. Fisher, 1908.

41. Garret, H. E., Morris, G. C., Howell, J. F. *et al*. Revascularization of upper extremity with autogenous vein bypass graft. Arch. Surg., *91:* 751-759, 1965.

42. Glanville, H. The future of powered hand prosthesis. Hand, *3:* 20, 1971.

43. Gonzales, R. I. A simplified surgical approach in the treatment of Dupuytren's contracture. In *Symposium on the Hand*. Vol. 3, edited by L. M. Cramer and R. A. Chase. St. Louis, Mosby, pp 123-131, 1971.

44. Hakstian, R. W., and Tubiana, R. Ulnar deviation of the fingers: the role of joint structure and function. J. Bone Joint Surg. (Am)., *49:* 299-316, 1967.

45. Harrison, S. H. Rheumatoid deformities of the proximal interphalangeal joints of the hand. Ann.

Rheum. Dis., *28 (5):* 20-22, 1969.

46. Haxton, H. The technique and results of upper limb sympathectomy. J. Cardiovasc. Surg., *11:* 27-34, 1970.

47. Herbsman, H., Lafer, D. J., and Shaftan, G. W. Successful replantation of an amputated hand. Ann. Surg., *163:* 137-143, 1966.

48. Horn, J. S. The reattachment of severed extremities. In *Recent Advances in Orthopaedics*, edited by A. G. Apley. Baltimore, Williams & Wilkins, 1969, pp. 49-78.

49. Hueston, J. T. *Dupuytren's Contracture*, Baltimore, Williams & Wilkins, 1963.

50. Hunter, J. M., and Salisbury, R. E. Use of gliding artifical implants to produce tendon sheaths: technique and results in children. Plast. Reconstr. Surg., *45:* 564-572, 1970.

51. Illingsworth, *Wound Healing*, Boston, Little Brown, 1966.

52. Inoue, T., Toyoshima, Y., Kukusumi, H. *et al*. Factors necessary for successful replantation of upper extremities. Ann. Surg., *165:* 225-238, 1967.

53. Kanavel, A. B. *Infections of the Hand*, Ed. 7. Philadelphia, Lea & Febiger, 1939.

54. Kleinert, H. E., and Hayes, J. E. The ulnar-tunnel syndrome. Plast. Reconstr. Surg., *47:* 21-24, 1971.

55. Kuczynski, K. The synovial structure of the normal and rheumatoid distal joints. Hand, *3:* 41-54, 1971.

56. Landsmeer, J. M. F. Anatomical and functional investigations on articulation of human fingers. Acta. Anat. (Suppl. 24), *25:* 1, 1955.

57. Landsmeer, J. M. F. Observations on the joints of the human finger. Ann. Rheum. Dis., *28 (5):* 11-14, 1969.

58. Landsmeer, J. M. F. The coordination of finger-joint movement. J. Bone Joint Surg. (Am.), *45:* 1654-1662, 1963.

59. Lang, E. K. Neurovascular compression syndromes. Dis. Chest, *50:* 572-580, 1966.

60. Leblanc, M. A. Clinical evaluation of externally powered prosthetic elbows. Artif. Limbs, 15 (1): 14-16, 1968.

61. Leonardo, R. *History of Surgery*. New York, Froben Press, 1959.

62. Lipscomb, P. R. Is early synovectomy of the small joints of the hand worthwhile? In *Symposium of the Hand*, Vol. 3, edited by L. M. Cramer and R. A. Chase. St. Louis, Mosby, pp 29-31, 1971.

63. Lipscomb, P. R. Surgery of rheumatoid arthritis — timing and techniques: summary. J. Bone Joint Surg. (Am.), *50:* 614-617, 1968.

64. Littler, J. W. The neurovascular pedicle transfer of tissue in reconstructive surgery of the hand. J. Bone Joint Surg. (Am.), 38: 917, 1956.

65. Littler, J. W., and Cooley, S.G.E. Restoration of the retinacular system in hyperextension deformity of the proximal interphalangeal joint. J. Bone Joint Surg. (Am.), *47:* 637, 1965.

66. Littler, J. W., and Eaton, R. G. Redistribution of forces in the correction of the boutonniere deformity. J. Bone Joint Surg. (Am.), *49:* 1267-1274, 1967.

67. Madden, J., and Peacock, E. Studies on the biology of collagen during wound healing. Surgery, *64:* 288-293, 1969.

68. Malt, R. A., McKhann, C. F. Replantation of severed

arms. J.A.M.A., *189:* 716-722, 1962.

69. Martinez, A. *et al.* The specific arterial lesions in mild and severe frostbite: effect of sympathectomy. J. Cardiovasc. Surg., *7:* 495-503, 1966.

70A. McDonnell R. *The Works of Abraham Colles.* London, New Sydenham Society, 1935.

70B. McDonnell, R. *Guillaume Dupuytren,* London, Sydenham Society, 1935.

71. McWilliams, R., and Montgomery, S. R. Artificial arms — are they practical? Med. Biol. Illus., *19:* 200-201, 1969.

72. Meagher, S. W. Special wounds. In *Hand Surgery,* edited by J. E. Flynn, Baltimore, Williams & Wilkins, pp. 106-117, 1966.

73. Mettler, C. C. *History of Medicine.* Toronto, Blakiston, 1947.

74. Moberg, E. Evaluation of sensibility in the hand. Surg. Clin. North Am., *40:* 357-362, 1960.

75. Montgomery, S. R. Powered upper-limb prosthesis. Med. Biol. Illus. *19:* 207-215, 1969.

76. Morton, J. H., Southgate, W. A., and Deweese, J. A. Arterial injuries of the extremities. Surg. Gynecol. Obstet., *123:* 611-627, 1966.

77. Murray, J. F., Ord, J. V. R., and Gavelin, G. E. The neurovascular island pedicle flap: an assessment of late results in sixteen cases. J. Bone Joint Surg. (Am.), *49:* 1285-1297, 1967.

78. Nahigian, S. H. Airless spray gun; a new hazard. J.A.M.A., *195:* 688-691, 1966.

79. Nichols, R. J. Initial choice of antibiotic treatment for pyogenic hand infections. Lancet, *1:* 7797, 225-226, 1973.

80. Onne, L. Recovery of sensibility and sudomotor activity in the hand after nerve suture. Acta. Chir. Scand. (Suppl.), *300:* 1-69, 1962.

81. Ortner, A.B., Berg, H. F., and Lebendiger, A. Limb salvage through small-vessel surgery. Arch. Surg., *83:* 414-421, 1961.

82. Paletta, F. X. Replantation of the amputated extremity. Ann. Surg., *168:* 720-727, 1968.

83. Peacock, E. E., Jr., and Van Winkle, W., Jr. *Surgery and Biology of Wound Repair.* Philadelpha, Saunders, 1970.

84. Phalen, G. S. Reflections on 21 years experience with carpal-tunnel syndrome. J.A.M.A., *212:* 1365-1367, 1970.

85. Potenza, A. D. Prevention of adhesions to healing digital flexor tendons. J.A.MA., 187, 187±191, 1964.

86. Reynard, D. Rucksack paralysis. J.A.M.A., *210:* 1102, 1969.

87. Rich, N. M. Vascular trauma in Vietnam. J. Cardiovasc. Surg., *11:* 368-377, 1970.

88. Rich, N. M., and Hughes, C. W. Vietnam vascular registry: a preliminary report. Surgery, *65:* 218-226, 1969.

89. Roos, D. B., and Owens, J. C. Thoracic outlet syndrome. Arch. Surg., *93:* 71–74, 1966.

90. Schreiber, S. N., Liebowitz, M. R., Bernstein, L. H. *et al.* Limb compression and renal impairment (crush syndrome) complicating narcotic overdose. N. Engl. J. Med., *284:* 368-369, 1971.

91. Schurman, H. *Leonardo da Vinci on the Human Body.* Philadelphia, Saunders, 1952.

92. Simpson, D. C. Gripping surfaces for artificial hands. Hand, *3:* 12-14, 1971.

93. Skoog, T. Dupuytren's contracture; with special reference to aetiology and improved surgical treatment; its occurrence in epileptics: note on knuckle-pads. Acta Chir. Scand. (suppl. 1), *139:* 1-190, 1948.

94. Smith, J. W. Microsurgery of peripheral nerves. Plast. Reconstr. Surg., *33:* 317-329, 1964.

95. Smith, J. W. Microsurgery: review of the literature and discussion of microtechniques. Plast. Reconstr. Surg., *37:* 227-245, 1966.

96. Smith, R. J., and Kaplan, E. B. Rheumatoid deformities at the metacarpophalangeal joints of the fingers: a correlative study of anatomy and pathology. J. Bone Joint Surg. (Am.), *49:* 31-47, 1967.

97. Snyder, C. C., Knowles, R. P., Mayer, P. W. *et al.* Extremity replantation. Plast. Reconstr. Surg., *26:* 251-263, 1960.

98. Spinner, M. The arcade of Frohse and its relationship to posterior interosseous nerve paralysis. J. Bone Joint Surg. (Br.), *50:* 809-812, 1968.

99. Stack, H. G. Some details of the anatomy of the terminal segment of the finger. Acta Orthop. Belg. *24:* 113, 1958.

100. Stack, H. G., and Vaughan-Jackson, O. J. The zig-zag deformity of the rheumatoid hand. Hand, *3:* 62-67, 1971.

101. Stark, H. H., Ashworth, C. R., and Boyes, J. H. Paint-gun injuries of the hand. J. Bone Joint Surg. (Am.), *49:* 637-647, 1967.

102. Sunderland, S. *Nerves and Nerve Injuries.* Baltimore, Williams & Wilkins, 1968.

103. Vaughan-Jackson, O. J. Excisional arthroplasty. Ann. Rheum. Dis., *28 (5):* 43-46, 1969.

104. Vellar, I. D. A., and Doyle, J. C. The use of the cephalic or basilic veins as peripheral vascular grafts. Aust. N. Z. J. Surg., *40:* 52-57, 1970.

105. Verdan, C. E. Half century of flexor-tendon surgery. Sterling Bunnell Memorial Lecture. J. Bone Joint Surg. (Am.), *54 (A) 3:* 472-491, 1972.

106. Washburn, B. Frostbite: what it is — how to prevent it — emergency treatment. N. Engl. J. Med., *266:* 974-989, 1962.

107. White, J. C. Nerve regeneration after replantation of severed arms. Ann. Surg., *170:* 715-719, 1969.

108. Williams, G. R., Carter, D. R., Frank, G. R. *et al.* Replantation of amputated extremities. Ann. Surg., *163:* 788-794, 1966.

109. Zancolli, E. Correction of arthritic ulna before cartilage destruction — an operation to rebalance the metacarpophalangeal forces. *Symposium on the Hand,* Vol. 3, edited by L. M. Cramer and R. A. Chase St. Louis, Mosby, 1971, pp 73-93.

110. Zimmerman, L. M., and Veith, I. *Great Ideas in the History of Surgery.* Baltimore, Williams & Wilkins, 1961.

111. Chase, R. A. Surgery of hand. Parts 1 and 2. N. Engl. J. Med., *287:* no. 23, 1174 and no. 24, 1227, 1972.

chapter two

Anatomy and Kinesiology of the Hand

Emanuel B. Kaplan, M.D.

A limited review of the anatomy and the function of the hand includes the most essential structures, their relationship and interaction, as applied to clinical evaluation and surgical use. Most of the terminology is based on the Nomina Anatomica Parisiencia.[15]

If the wrist is taken as a foundation upon which the hand is built, the trapezium (multangulum major) becomes significant as a base for the mobile thumb, the trapezoid as a partly mobile factor, the capitate as a factor of stability, and the hamate as a gliding base for the fourth and especially the fifth metacarpals. The scaphoid bone presents a gliding surface for the trapezium and trapezoid but the motion in this articulation is of limited range.

The articulation between the trapezium and the first metacarpal is built like a saddle joint. This arrangement permits flexion and extension, abduction, adduction, and opposition of the metacarpocarpal of the thumb. A fairly similar articulation is presented by the ulnar half of the hamate and the fifth metacarpal base, permitting more motion and rotation of the fifth metacarpal than observed in the metacarpocarpal joints of the index, middle and ring fingers.

The joints of the wrist consisting of the articulation between the eight carpal bones and between the distal end of the radius and the ulna with the proximal row of the carpal bones are of particular significance.

The distal row articulating with the bases of the metacarpals, with the exception of the first and fifth metacarpals, presents only slight movement. The proximal row consisting of the scaphoid, lunate, triquetrum, and pisiform articulating with the trapezium, trapezoid, capitate, and hamate has a definite pattern of movement, which together with the joint formed by the radius and triangular fibrocartilage of the ulna, contribute to all movements of the wrist joint. The most important ligaments located on the volar and dorsal surfaces connect the radius with both rows of the carpal bones. The interosseous ligaments connect the carpal bones of the proximal and distal row between individual bones. The radial and ulnar collateral ligaments connect the radial styloid on the radial side with the navicular and trapezium, the ulnar styloid

with the triquetrum, pisiform, and the triangular fibrocartilage.

The movements of the wrist may be summarized as follows.

Volar flexion takes place primarily in the radiocarpal articulation and secondarily in the midcarpal joint. Dorsal flexion occurs primarily in the midcarpal joint and secondarily in the radiocarpal. Radial deviation is produced in the midcarpal joint and ulnar deviation in the radiocarpal articulation. It was calculated that about 65 to 75 per cent of volar flexion and 55 to 60 per cent of ulnar deviation takes place in the radiocarpal part of the wrist. Dorsal flexion is accounted for 75 to 85 per cent in the midcarpal joint. About 60 to 65 per cent of radial deviation also occurs in the midcarpal joint.[9]

The metacarpophalangeal joints of the fingers with the exception of the thumb are diarthrodial joints permitting movement in all directions.

The capsular and ligamentous apparatus of the metacarpophalangeal joints consists of the capsule, the lateral ligaments, and the anterior fibrocartilage.

The lateral or collateral ligaments reinforce the capsule on each side of the joint. These ligaments run from the laterodorsal side of the metacarpal head to the laterovolar side of the proximal phalanx. They form two bundles, of which one runs to the lateral side of the proximal phalanx and the other joins the fibrocartilage — the plate of the anterior aspect of the metacarpophalangeal joint.

The fibrocartilaginous plate over the anterior aspect of the joint is a quadrilateral structure firmly attached to the volar base of the proximal phalanx and loosely attached to the anterior surface of the neck of the metacarpal by means of the capsule proximal to the hyalin cartilaginous cover of the head of the metararpal. The deep transverse intermetacarpal ligament (ligamentum metacarpum transversum profundum) connects the fibrocartilaginous plates from the index to the fifth metacarpal head.

The metacarpophalangeal joint of the thumb differs from the other metacarpophalangeal joints in the configuration of the head of the first metacarpal and in the presence of two constant sesamoid bones. The head of the first metacarpal is flatter; the cartilaginous surface does not extend laterally or posteriorly. Anteriorly, there are two small facets on each side of the head for the two sesamoids.

A capsule encloses the joint from the articular borders of the base of the phalanx to below the sesmoids volarly, and dorsal border dorsally around the metacarpal head. A cartilaginous plate covers the palmar aspect of the joint. It encloses the two sesamoids. The cartilaginous plate is firmly attached to the volar base of the proximal phalanx. At the metacarpal side, it is attached through the capsule loosely. This permits normal extension of the proximal phalanx. The flexor pollicis longus tendon passes over the anterior aspect of the fibrocartilaginous plate in a fibrous sheath between the two sesamoid bones and their tendons of insertion. The capsule is reinforced by collateral ligaments. The collateral ligament runs from the lateral tubercle of the head of the first metacarpal toward the latervolar side of the proximal phalanx. Of its two parts, one is directed toward the lateral side of the phalanx and the other to the sesamoid. The part directed to the radial sesamoid is blended with the insertion of the flexor pollicis brevis. The part directed to the ulnar sesamoid is intimately connected with the whole of the insertion of the adductor pollicis.

The anterior surfaces of the tendons of the extensor pollicis longus and brevis are attached loosely but functionally with the dorsal capsule of the metacarpophalangeal joint similarly to the attachment of the other extensor tendons.

The interphalangeal joints are hinge joints with a capsule enclosing the joints around the articular borders of the contiguous surfaces. The capsule is reinforced by collateral ligaments. The articular surface of the head of the phalanx is convex in the anteroposterior direction. It presents a depression in the middle in the same direction forming two condyles that articulate with the base of the phalanx distal to it. The base presents a concave surface divided by an elevated ridge into two concave depressions. On the dorsum of the base of each phalanx, the dorsal end of the ridge forms a tubercle which stands out posteriorly. This tubercle serves as an insertion area for the midband of the extensor tendon on the middle phalanx and an insertion area for the combined lateral bands on the distal phalanx.

The fibrocartilaginous plate is similar to the fibrocartilaginous plate of the metacarpophalangeal joint.

The dorsal capsule of the proximal interphalangeal joint is intimately connected with the midband of the extensor tendon which is inserted into the tubercle located just distal to the articular line. The dorsal capsule of the distal interphalangeal joint is similarly related to the combined insertion of the two lateral bands of the extensor tendon.

The interphalangeal joint of the thumb is similar to the metacarpophalangeal joint of the thumb. The col-

lateral bands of the metacarpophalangeal joint in their thickest portion are so placed that they are loose in extension; however, when the proximal phalanx moves over to the volar articular bulge of the head of the metacarpal the collateral bands become tense because of the increase of the distance produced by the bulge of the metacarpal head. When the colateral bands are loose, the movements at the metacarpophalangeal joint are possible in all directions. A recent study[12] challenges the contention that the collateral ligaments are loose in extension. According to this study the "oblique ligaments are under constant tension, thus contributing largely to the stability of the joint . . . since rotation and abduction are actually linked movements there is no slackening of the oblique lateral band."

THE MUSCLES OF THE FINGERS AND WRIST

The long flexors, the flexor digitorum profundus, and superficialis are the most important flexors; however, without the synergistic action of the other muscles, their action is inefficient. The flexor pollicis longus depends on the synergistic action of the thenar muscles, the extensors of the thumb, and the ulnar extensor of the wrist.

The flexor digitorum profundus originates deep to other muscles of the forearm from the proximal two-thirds of the ulna on its volar and medial side. On the ulnar side the muscle originates from the septum of the flexor carpi ulnaris. On the radial side the muscle originates from the interosseous membrane. The common fleshy mass of the muscle divides into four parts. The part to the index divides more proximally. The fleshy fibers descend distally to the carpal canal where they end on tendons corresponding to each finger.

The flexor superficialis is superficial to the flexor profundus. The flexor superficialis originates from the medial epicondyle of the humerus, from the ulnar collateral ligament of the elbow, and from the medial aspect of the coronoid process. The muscle originates medial to the origin of the pronator teres and also medial to the insertion of the brachialis. From here the line of origin is directed distally toward the supinator line of the radius. The oblique line of the supinator runs from the ulnar border of the radius obliquely and distally toward the lateral border of the radius. The supinator line separates the supinator which is proximal to this line from the origin of the flexor pollicis longus which is distal to this line. The line itself represents the area of origin of the lateral part of the flexor superficialis. Superficial to the line of the flexor superficialis and parallel to it runs the proximal border of the pronator teres which has practically the same direction of its fibers as the flexor superficialis from the medial humeral epicondyle to the lateral border of the radius.

The flexor pollicis longus originates from the entire middle third of the volar surface of the radius proximal to the supinator, and also from the radial third of the interosseous membrane. The muscle also has a frequent additional muscular slip originating from the coronoid process and the medial condyle of the humerus. This is known as the accessory muscle of Gantzer. The flexor pollicis muscle may be united with the flexor indicis of the flexor profundus. In this case flexion of the distal phalanx of the thumb is accompanied by simultaneous flexion of the index fingers or vice versa. It also occurs that the flexor pollicis longus may be completely absent.

The flexor carpi radialis originates from the medial epicondyle together with the pronator teres which is lateral to the origin, the palmaris longus which is medial, and the humeral head of the flexor carpi ulnaris which is most medial.

The muscular bodies of these muscles running toward the wrist are arranged so that the pronator teres, the flexor carpi radialis, the palmaris longus, and the flexor carpi ulnaris form the most superficial layer. On the radial side of the forearm they are limited by the brachioradialis muscle which descends from the lateral humeral epicondyle toward the wrist. Deep to these muscles is the layer of the flexor supericialis which overlies the flexor profundus. The deepest layer is found in the distal volar part of the forearm and is represented by the pronator quadratus.

The extensor digitorum originates in common with the other muscles from the lateral epicondyle of the humerus and from a small area posterior to the radial notch of the ulna. The extensor digiti minimi originates from the posterior aspect of the radial epicondyle of the humerus from a common tendon medial to the extensor digitorum and radial to the extensor carpi ulnaris, posterior to the supinator. The brachioradialis originates from the epicondylar line proximal to the radial epicondyle. Although it is not a muscle belonging to the wrist or finger group, it is a useful muscle for transplantations because it is located in an area where it can be easily transferred in the desired direction and also because it has a sufficient functional length.

The extensor carpi radialis longus originates from the epicondylar line between the insertion of the brachioradialis and the lateral epicondyle.

The extensor carpi radialis brevis originates from the anterior aspect of the lateral epicondyle between the extensor carpi radialis longus proximally and the extensor digitorum and extensor digiti minimi distally. The extensor carpi ulnaris originates from the posteroinferior part of the lateral epicondyle from the common extensor mass in front and the anconeus muscle posterior, also from the crest of the posterior border of the ulna, distal to the anconeus muscle.

The extensor digiti minimi originates from the common tendon. The origin is medial to the extensor digitorum and radial to the origin of the extensor carpi ulnaris.

The extensor indicis originates from the distal third of the posterior aspect of the ulna and from the contiguous part of the interosseous membrane distal and posterior to the origin of the long extensor of the thumb. The direction of the tendon of the extensor indicis almost parallels the direction of the tendon of the extensor pollicis longus. This position of the extensor indicis in its course through a retinacular tunnel on the dorsum of the wrist makes it a very useful tendon for transplantation in case of loss of the extensor pollicis longus.

The extensor pollicis longus has its origin on the middle third of the posterior aspect of the ulna and the interrosseous membrane, distal and posterior to the origin of the extensor pollicis brevis, proximal and anterior to the origin of the extensor indicis.

The extensor pollicis brevis originates just proximal and anterior to the extensor pollicis longus and the abductor pollicis longus originates from the same area but proximal and anterior to the extensor pollicis brevis.

The short muscles are divided into four groups: the interossei, the lumbrical, the hypothenar, and the thenar muscles. The interossei muscles originate between the metacarpals.[2,6,7]

The dorsal originates by means of two muscular bellies. The larger belly arises from the entire anterolateral surface of the metacarpal which faces away from the long axis of the long finger. The smaller body originates from the anterolateral third of the shaft of the metacarpal which faces the axis of the long finger.

The palmar interosseous originates by a single belly from the palmar two-thirds of the metacarpal shaft facing the axis of the middle finger.

There are four dorsal interossei. The first dorsal interosseous originates from the first and second metacarpals; the second dorsal interosseous originates between the second and third; the third, between the long and ring metacarpals; and the fourth, between the fourth and fifth metacarpals.

The insertions of the interossei follow a definite pattern. The tendon of insertion usually has two heads. One head is inserted into the lateral tubercle of the base of the proximal phalanx, volar to the center of flexion-extension of the metacarpophalangeal joint. This insertion is usually not attached to the collateral ligament of the joint. It is covered by transverse fibers connecting the extensor tendon with the dorsal side of the deep transverse intermetacarpal ligament. The transverse fibers of the extensor digitorum tendon are responsible for maintaining the tendon of the extensor digitorum over the center of the metacarpophalangeal joint.

The other head of the dorsal interosseous is inserted into the expansion of the extensor tendon. Some of the fibers of this insertion run directly across the midband of the extensor tendon to join similar fibers from the other side of the proximal phalanx. Other fibers continue distally into the lateral bands of the extensor tendon. On the radial side these fibers join the insertion of the tendon of the lumbrical muscle.[13]

There are three volar interossei; the first volar interosseous is between the second and third metacarpal, the second between the third and fourth, and the third is found between the fourth and fifth metacarpals. The insertion of the volar or palmar interossei is very similar to the insertion of the dorsal interosseus. Sometimes, however, the volar interosseous has no insertion into the lateral tubercle of the base of the proximal phalanx. The insertion then is totally into the lateral band of the extensor digitorum tendon. The volar interossei are inserted into the proximal phalangeal sides which are away from the middle finger. Thus, the first volar interosseus is running along the ulnar side of the proximal phalanx of the index. The second volar interosseus along the radial side of the proximal phalanx of the ring, and the third volar interosseous along the radial side of the fifth.[6,7,13]

THENAR MUSCLES

On the radial side of the hand, there are four intrinsic muscles. Three of these are thenar; one occupies the midportion of the hand.

The three thenar muscles are the abductor pollicis brevis, the flexor pollicis brevis, and the opponens pollicis. The muscle originating in the midhand is the adductor pollicis.

The abductor pollicis brevis originates from the lateral half and the distal border of the volar carpal ligament (flexor retinaculum). The insertion of the muscle is on the radial tubercle of the proximal phalanx of the thumb by a tendon which is about 6 to 8 mm wide. Some fibers of the tendon join the tendon of the flexor pollicis brevis at the radial sesamoid, some other fibers run toward the tendon of the extensor pollicis brevis and longus to the dorsal expansion.

Flexor Pollicis Brevis

The muscle is located under the abductor brevis. It originates by two heads: one from the distal lateral border of the volar carpal ligament and from the volar surface of the tunnel of the flexor carpi radialis near the insertion of the tendon into the base of the second metacarpal, also from the crest of the trapezium covered by the carpal ligament; the other head which is deeper and originates from the volar surface of the trapezoid and from the capitate bone, proximal and radial to the origin of the adductor pollicis. The insertion is by a tendon into the radial sesamoid and also into the radial tubercle of the proximal phalanx. An expansion of the insertion runs into the expansion of the extensor tendons.[3,6,7]

Opponens Pollicis

The muscle originates under the abductor brevis from the volar carpal ligament and the crest of the trapezium and is widely inserted into the volar aspect of the first metacarpal and the volar aspect of the metacarpophalangeal joint.

Adductor Pollicis

The muscle originates in two parts, transverse and oblique. The transverse head originates from the volar crest of the middle metacarpal from under the head to the base, from the ligaments of the base, the proximal part of the capsule of the metacarpophalangeal joint of the middle finger, and from the interosseous fascia covering the volar surface of the second dorsal interosseous muscle. The oblique head originates from the ligaments uniting the capitate, the trapezoid, and the tunnel near the insertion of the flexor carpi radialis. The two heads insert separately or together into the tubercle on the ulnar side of the base of the proximal phalanx and into the expansion of the extensor tendons of the thumb.

HYPOTHENAR MUSCLES

The muscles of the hypothenar eminence are: abductor digiti minimi, flexor brevis digiti minimi, the opponens digiti minimi, and palmaris brevis.

The abductor digiti minimi originates from the distal part of the pisiform, the pisiform hamate ligament, and from the nearest part of the volar carpal ligament. The muscle is frequently divided into two longitudinal parts. The flexor carpi ulnaris tendon appears to continue into the fibers of origin of the abductor digiti minimi, but the action of either muscle is not transmitted to either. The contraction of the abductor digiti minimi produces simultaneous contraction of the palmaris brevis. The insertion of the abductor digiti minimi runs into the lateral ulnar tubercle of the base of the proximal phalanx and also into the expansion of the extensor tendons.

The Flexor Brevis Digiti Minimi

The muscle originates from the volar carpal ligament, the hamulus of the hamate bone and from the pisiform hamate ligament. The flexor brevis is inserted on the tubercle of the ulnar side of the base of the proximal phalanx volar to the insertion of the abductor brevis.

The Opponens Digiti Minimi

The muscle is located deep to the flexor brevis. It originates from the hamulus of the hamate bone and the pisiform hamate ligament and inserts into the ulnar side of the shaft of the fifth metacarpal.

There are normally four lumbrical muscles. They all originate from the tendons of the flexor digitorum profundus. The first lumbrical originates from the volar and radial aspect of the flexor profundus tendon to the index. The second originates in a similar manner from the flexor profundus tendons of the long finger. The third originates from the flexor profundus tendons of the long and ring fingers and the fourth originates from the flexor profundus tendon of the ring and little fingers. The area of origin on each tendon varies according to the finger between 3.5 cm to 4 cm with the fingers extended, the proximal end of the origin of the lumbrical reaches the level of the distal end of the pisiform bone. When the fingers are flexed the lumbricals are pulled into the carpal canal and may reach the distal end of the radius. The lumbrical muscles run between the heads of the metacarpals, except the first lumbrical which is located on the radial side of the metacarpophalangeal joint of the index finger. The lumbrical is placed normally volar to the axis of flexion and extension of the metacarpophalangeal joint and cannot normally become an extensor of the metacarpophalangeal joint. The insertion of the lumbrical tendon is usually found on the radial side of the lateral band of each extensor expansion. It is situated more distally than the insertion of the interosseous into the same lateral band.

INSERTION OF THE LONG FLEXORS AND EXTENSORS OF THE FINGERS AND WRIST

The long flexors of the fingers: the flexor digitorum profundus and superficialis run into the carpal canal and then into the palm of the hand. Proximal to the metacarpophalangeal joint the flexors enter the fibrous sheath, the profundus being on a deeper plane than the superficialis. Over the metacarpophalangeal joint a line of longitudinal division appears on the superficials tendon. This line splits approximately over the volar surface of the proximal phalanx. The flexor profundus passes through this line of division which spreads wider as the tendon of the superficialis advances toward the middle phalanx. The flexor profundus becomes more superficial. The tendon of the superficialis divides into two halves. Each half covers the corresponding side of the flexor profundus. Thus, the half that covers the anterior aspect of the profundus moves toward the corresponding side of the profundus then turns behind the profundus and crosses to the other side where it inserts into the lateral volar crest of the middle phalanx. A similar relationship is found on the other side. The two halves cross each other on the surface of the middle phalanx and form the chiasma tendinum of Camper dorsal to the tendon of the flexor profundus.

The flexor profundus tendon emerges from the opening in the tendon of the flexor superficialis and moves on the chiasma bound only by the vincula. The flexor profundus tendon spreads out over the distal interphalangeal joint adhering to the capsule of the joint. The tendon is frequently split longitudinally into two parts and then inserts widely to the base and to the volar aspect of the distal phalanx. The division of the flexor profundus into two parts starts immediately distal to the perforation of the flexor superficialis tendon.

The flexor pollicis longus has a long tendon which descends on the radial side of the flexor profundus of the index finger in the forearm, crosses the pronator quadratus, then enters the carpal canal deep to the tendon of the flexor carpi radialis. Under the cover of the thenar muscles, the tendon progresses toward the metacarpophalangeal joint where it is enclosed in a fibrous tunnel between the two sesamoids. It further progresses toward the distal phalanx, where it inserts into the base and more distally by a doubled wide tendon.

The Flexor Carpi Radialis

The muscle is superficial in the forearm to the flexor superficialis. At the wrist it enters a special tunnel under the crest of the trapezium. The tendon of the flexor pollicis longus then crosses the tendon of the flexor carpi radialis from the ulnar to the radial side to enter the thumb. The flexor carpi radialis tendon emerges from the tunnel and inserts into the base of the second metacarpal. A slip to the base of the third metacarpal is frequently present at this level.

Palmaris Longus

The tendon runs toward the wrist where it inserts into the apex of the midpalmar fascia.

Flexor Carpi Ulnaris

The muscle follows a straight line from its origin to its insertion into the pisiform. The muscular fibers follow the tendon on the ulnar and posterior side almost to the pisiform. A fascial extension of the tendon to the volar base of the fourth and fifth metacarpals and to the hamulus of the hamate appears. Another extension to the volar carpal ligament forms a roof for passage of the ulnar nerve and artery. This passage is known as Guyon's tunnel.

LONG EXTENSORS OF THE FINGERS AND WRIST

The tubercle of Lister on the dorsum of the distal radius is an important point of reference. On the ulnar side of the tubercle the tendon of the extensor pollicis longus runs from the forearm to the hand. On the radial side of the tubercle runs the tendon of the extensor carpi radialis brevis. Immediately distal to the tubercle the two tendons cross, the extensor pollicis longus running radialward crosses the tendon of the extensor carpi radialis brevis, running ulnarward toward the dorsal base of the third metacarpal. The tendon of the extensor pollicis longus is crossed again more distally by the tendon of the extensor carpi radialis longus which passes dorsally to the extensor pollicis longus. To the ulnar side of the tendon of the extensor pollicis longus runs the common group of the extensor digitorum and the extensor indicis. Ulnar to the extensor digitorum runs the almost constantly double tendon of the extensor digiti minimi and medial to the extensor digiti minimi runs the extensor carpi ulnaris in its special tunnel over the ulnar head. On the radial side, the extensor pollicis brevis and the abductor pollicis longus run in their common tunnel. All the extensors of the fingers arrive to the dorsum of the metacarpophalangeal joint. At the level of the joint the extensor tendons from the index to the little finger form an expansion over the dorsum of each finger. The expansion extends on each side of the metacarpophalangeal joint and inserts on the deep transverse intermetacarpal ligament and, thus, to the volar fibrocartilage of the joint. The extensor tendon then continues its course toward the distal parts of the finger. In this course it divides into three bands, one middle and two lateral, which are interconnected. The midpart, or midband, inserts into the posterior tubercle of the middle phalanx; it adheres to the dorsal capsule of the proximal phalanx. The two lateral bands run along the sides of the proximal phalanx, then toward the dorsum

of the middle phalanx, where they run separately until they come to the distal interphalangeal joint, where they form a single band which is inserted into the base of the distal phalanx. The lateral bands are located dorsally in reference to the axis of the proximal and distal interphalangeal joints. Over the middle phalanx the lateral bands are held by spiral fibers fixing the lateral bands to the sides of the proximal interphalangeal joint, so that normally the bands cannot descend volarly below the axis of the joint. The interosseous tendon on each side of the finger is inserted into the lateral base of the proximal phalanx and also into the lateral bands by a winglike expansion. The lumbrical tendon is inserted on the radial side of the lateral band slightly more distally. The extensor tendon in its passage over the dorsum of the metacarpophalangeal joint is also attached loosely to the capsule of this joint (Fig. 2.1).

The extensor expansion of the finger (Fig. 2.1) which covers the dorsum of each digit, extends from the metacarpophalangeal joint to the distal phalanx, crossing the proximal and distal interphalangeal joints. It includes the extensor tendon with its divi-

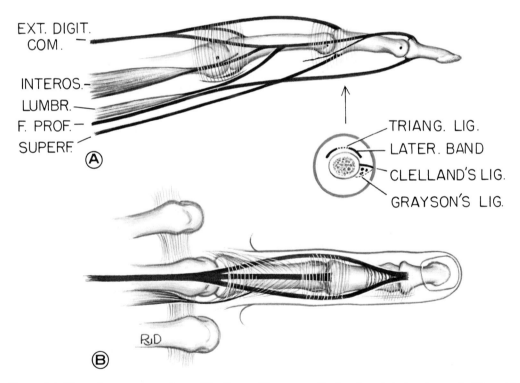

EXT. DIGIT. COM.

INTEROS.
LUMBR.
F. PROF.
SUPERF.

Ⓐ

TRIANG. LIG.
LATER. BAND
CLELLAND'S LIG.
GRAYSON'S LIG.

RjD

Ⓑ

Figure 2.1. The extensor expansions of the finger. Diagrammatic drawing. *A.* Lateral aspect of the middle finger of the left hand with a transverse section at the level of the proximal third of the middle phalanx demonstrating the oblique retinacular ligament of Landsmeer and the transverse ligament over the proximal interphalangeal joint. The extensor expansion is observed over the metacarpophalangeal joint. The relationship of the tendons is shown. There is also a capsular attachment of the extensor tendon to the capsule of the m.p. joint.

The transverse section of the middle phalanx shows the relationship of Clelland's and Grayson's ligaments. *B.* Dorsal view of the expansion.

sion, the terminal tendons of the interossei and the lumbricals and also the two important retinacular ligaments of Landsmeer[11,12] and the cutaneous ligaments of Cleland and Grayson.[14] The transverse retinacular ligament of Landsmeer crosses over the extensor expansion at the proximal interphalangeal joint stabilizing it. The oblique retinacular ligament of Landsmeer unites the lateral band of the extensor tendon near the distal interphalangeal joint and the lateral aspect of the distal end of the proximal phalanx, proximal to the proximal interphalangeal joint. This ligament passes volar to the axis of rotation of the proximal interphalangeal joint. It prevents passive or active flexion of the distal interphalangeal joint when the proximal interphalangeal joint is in extension.

The cutaneous ligament of Cleland actually consists of bundles of fibers connecting the skin with the flexor tunnels dorsal to the neurovascular bundle on each side of the finger, acting as stabilizers of the skin.

The cutaneous ligament of Grayson is similar to the ligament of Cleland but runs volar to the neurovascular bundle of the finger. Its function also consists of stabilization of the skin.

Thus the intrinsic action of the interossei and lumbrical produce simultaneous flexion at the metacarpophalangeal joints and extension of the two distal phalanges. The dorsal expansion over the metacarpophalangeal joint forms transverse fibers similar to the transverse retinacular ligament of Landsmeer over the proximal interphalangeal joint. The transverse fibers at this joint are known as the sagital fibers; they transfix the extensor apparatus to the deep intermetacarpal ligament on each side of the finger at the metacarpophalangeal joint. The rated participation of all the different motor factors is responsible for the complex action of the finger. The various retinacular structures are participating in the regulatory combination. The elimination of either motor or retinacular factors in injury or disease creates some of the well-known deformities or disabilities.

The arrangement is somewhat different over the metacarpophalangeal joint of the thumb. The long and short extensors of the thumb are also fixed by transverse fibers to the sides of the joint and mostly to the area of insertion of the adductor pollicis on the ulnar side, with the flexor brevis and abductor brevis on the radial side. In addition, the adductor sends a winglike expansion into the extensor expansion. A similar winglike structure joins the expansion of the extensor tendons on the radial side. There is no doubt that in ordinary cases with paralysis of the radial nerve, extension of the distal phalanx is possible by electric stimulation of the thenar muscles.

The abductor pollicis longus inserts into the radial base of the first metacarpal. The extensor pollicis brevis inserts into the lateral base of the proximal phalanx. The extensor carpi radialis longus is inserted into the dorsal base of the second metacarpal. The extensor carpi radialis brevis is inserted into the base of the middle metacarpal. The extensor carpi ulnaris is inserted into the ulnar tubercle of the base of the fifth metacarpal.

THE BLOOD SUPPLY OF THE HAND[7,9]

The blood supply to the hand is carried by the radial and ulnar arteries and their multiple branches. The artery of the median nerve, which normally is very small, may infrequently become very large and participate notably in the arterial system of the hand. This artery, arteria mediana, is a branch of the palmar interosseous artery. When enlarged it joins the deep palmar arch and forms a large arterial trunk.

The radial artery supplies muscular branches in the forearm:

The metacarpal arteries supply the dorsum of the fingers and communicate freely with the palmar digital arteries from the superficial palmar arch.

The superficial palmar arch is formed by the superficial branch of the radial artery which arises near the abductor pollicis brevis and runs either superficially or deep to the abductor brevis. It anastomoses with the end branch of the ulnar artery under the midpalmar fascia. It rarely assumes the form of an arch and varies in the supply of the common digital arteries. The common digital arteries supply the digital arteries. The deep palmar arch is located dorsal to the flexor tendons on the palmar interosseous fascia. It is formed by the end of the radial artery which perforates the space between the two heads of the first dorsal interosseous.

As soon as it passes into the palmar aspect of the hand it supplies a branch to the thumb — the princeps pollicis — and the volar indicis radialis arteries.

The venous system of the hand consists of deep and superficial veins. The deep veins run as venae comitantes of the arteries: the deep palmar and superficial palmar arches, the palmar and volar carpal arches, and the volar metacarpal arteries. There is no evidence available that the proper volar digital arteries have venae comitantes. All the deep veins intercommunicate with the dorsal veins. The superficial veins are mostly dorsal and consist of the digital dorsal, metacarpal veins which drain into the basilic vein on the ulnar side, and cephalic veins on the radial side.

The lymphatic system consists of two or three vessels which accompany the corresponding proper digital arteries and form a superficial volar system which is very dense and a dorsal system which is less condensed. The deep arteries are also accompanied by lymph channels. The ulnar collectors communicate with the ulnar artery collectors, the posterior with the posterior interosseous trunk of the forearm.

NERVE SUPPLY OF THE HAND AND WRIST[17, 20]

This description of the nerve supply is limited to the hand and wrist, although it is somewhat artificial because of direct and important connections with the entire brachial plexus.[19]

The median, radial, ulnar, and musculocutaneous nerves in their terminal course are responsible for sensory and motor transmissions. The autonomic nerve system plays an important role in the control of blood supply and also in certain perceptions carried from the joints of the wrist and fingers.

The superficial sensory distribution is usually shared by the median, radial, and ulnar nerves. It is well known that, although there is a definite pattern of this distribution, variations are fairly frequent. The description will include the most frequent distribution only. The volar side of the hand, the midline passed longitudinally from the tip of the ring finger, through the length of the finger to the wrist, indicates the distribution of the median nerve on the radial side of this line and of the ulnar nerve, on the ulnar side of the line. On the dorsal side, the line of division between the distribution of nerves is different. A longitudinal line along the middle of the ring finger runs from the tip to the proximal interphalangeal joint; from this point a horizontal line passing over the dorsum of the proximal interphalangeal joints of the long and index finger, indicates the area of the median nerve distribution. It is located to the radial side opf the longitudinal line on the ring finger, and distal to the horizontal line passing over the proximal interphalangeal joints of the long and index fingers. Another line drawn from the middle of the horizontal line of the proximal interphalangeal joint of the long finger to the wrist indicates the line of separation between the ulnar nerve on the ulnar side and the radial nerve on the radial side of this line. Thus, the dorsum of the little finger, the ulnar half of the two distal phalanges, and the entire proximal phalanx of the ring finger and the ulnar half of the proximal phalanx of the long finger as well as the dorsum of the hand on this side are supplied by the ulnar nerve. The radial half of the two distal phalanges of the ring finger, the two distal phalanges of the long and of the index fingers are supplied by the median nerve. The radial side of the proximal phalanx of the middle and the entire proximal phalanx of the index finger as well as the dorsum of the thumb are supplied by the radial nerve. The area around the dorsum of the thumb over the metacarpocarpal joint is supplied frequently by the end branches of the musculocutaneous nerve.

The motor nerves of the hand are supplied by the three nerves: median, ulnar, and radial. The long hand flexors, with the exception of the two ulnar heads of the flexor profundus, are supplied by the median nerve. The flexor carpi radiali and the pronators of the forearm are also supplied by the median nerve. The muscles of the thenar eminence, with the exception of the deep part of the flexor pollicis brevis, which is occasionally supplied by the ulnar nerve, and the adductor are supplied by the median nerve. All the muscles of the hypothenar and fourth lumbrical muscles, the flexor carpi ulnaris, and the flexor profundus to the ring and little fingers are supplied by the ulnar nerve. The radial nerve supplies all the long extensors of the hand and wrist and the long abductor as well as the short extensor of the thumb.

KINESIOLOGY OF THE HAND AND WRIST[2,4,18]

It is well known that any active movement produced by contraction of muscles involves the participation of a group of muscles and cannot be produced by contraction of one individual muscle. Action of muscles deduced on traction of tendons in the cadaver must be considered as limited actions. Electromyography also has definite limitations.[1] Electric stimulation of individual muscles or even groups of muscles is also only helpful.

Contraction of the muscles produces shortening which is transmitted to the point corresponding to the insertion of the muscle. Measurements of this contraction is important because it indicates the range of motion between maximal relaxation and maximal contraction. This is called functional length of the muscle. When measured in the living, when the muscle is surgically exposed, especially under local anesthesia, and then compared with the length obtained in fresh anatomical material, the measurements have a definite value. This is of significance when transplantation or substitution of muscles is contemplated.

These measurements were previously reported by different investigators and by the author on the basis of personal investigations. They should be considered only as guides.[2,9]

THE FUNCTIONAL LENGTH OF THE MUSCLES OF THE FINGERS (EXCURSION)

Flexors

The flexor profundus for the: index *(a)* at the wrist, 3 cm, *(b)* at the m.p. joint, 2.5 to 2.7 cm; long *(a)* at the wrist, 4 cm, *(b)* at the m.p. joint, 3 to 3.5 cm; ring *(a)* at the wrist, 4.5 cm, *(b)* at the m.p. joint, 4 cm; little *(a)* at the wrist, 3.5 cm, *(b)* at the m.p. joint, 3 to 3.5 cm; flexor pollicis longus of the thumb, 5.5 to 6 cm at the wrist; flexor pollicis brevis of the thumb, approximately 1 cm at the wrist. Flexor superficialis has generally about 0.75 to 0.5 cm less than the profundus.

Extensors

The extensor digitorum for the: index, about 3 cm at the wrist and m.p. joint; long, about 4 cm at the wrist and m.p. joint; ring, about the same; little, about 3 cm at the wrist and m.p. joint. Extensor indicis proprius is slightly less effective and is shorter than the extensor digitorum. Extensor digiti minimi is slightly more effective and longer than the extensor digitorum. Extensor pollicis longus, 5.5 to 6 cm at the wrist; extensor pollicis brevis, 3 cm at the wrist; abductor pollicis longus, 3 cm at the wrist; abductor pollicis brevis, 0.5

cm at the m.p. joint; adductor pollicis, 1.5 to 2 cm at the m.p. joint.

It was difficult to estimate the functional length of the interossei. The lumbricals, however, showed a considerable length, considering the size of the muscles. The functional length varied between 3 and 4 cm, according to the finger of the individual.

THE FUNCTIONAL LENGTH OF THE MUSCLES OF THE WRIST

Flexors

Flexor carpi radialis, 5 cm; flexor carpi ulnaris, 3 to 3.5 cm.

Extensors

Extensor carpi radialis longus, 4 cm; extensor carpi radialis brevis, 3.5 to 4 cm; extensor carpi ulnaris, 2.5 to 3 cm.

FUNCTION OF THE HAND PRODUCED BY ACTIVITY OF THE MUSCLES[1,3,4]

Fundamental principles only will be presented in this review in view of the extent and complexities of the problems.

It is well known that even a simple act of flexion of the fingers requires the direct and indirect participation of the following muscles — the flexor digitorum profundus and superficialis with the interossei and lumbricals acting directly. Additionally, the two radial extensors and the ulnar extensor of the wrist act indirectly.

Flexion of the thumb involves the action of the flexor pollicis longus and the thenar muscles and indirect participation of the long abductor and even extensors of the thumb. The distal phalanx of the thumb is flexed by the flexor pollicis longus independently.

Extension of the fingers is produced by direct action of the extensor digitorum, the extensor indicis proprius and extensor digiti minimi with the palmar and dorsal interossei and indirect action of the palmaris longus, flexor carpi radialis, and flexor carpi ulnaris. Extension of the thumb in all joints and, especially, the interphalangeal joint is produced by the extensor pollicis longus. The extensor pollicis brevis, the thenar muscles, and the abductor longus also participate in this action. Abduction of the fingers is produced by action of the abductor pollicis brevis, the dorsal interossei, and additional help of the long extensors. Adduction is produced by the adductor pollicis, the volar interossei, and, in flexion, by the long flexors, additionally.

Flexion of the wrist requires the action of the flexor carpi radialis and ulnaris, palmaris longus, directly, and the long flexors of the fingers and abductor pollicis longus, indirectly.

Extension of the wrist is produced by the extensor carpi radialis longus and brevis, extensor carpi ulnaris, directly, and the extensor digitorum, extensor indicis proprius, extensor digiti minimi, and extensor pollicis longus indirectly.

Radial deviation is produced by the abductor pollicis longus, extensor carpi radialis longus, and flexor carpi radialis.

Ulnar deviation is produced directly by the extensor and the flexor carpi ulnaris.

The flexor profundus is primarily a flexor of the distal phalanx and of the proimal interphalangeal joint. The flexor superficialis is acting mostly on the middle phalanx but it may also act on the proximal phalanx, when the hand is in dorsiflexion. Normally, the two muscles contract simultaneously producing flexion of the distal and proximal interphalangeal joints, but under certain circumstances, the flexor profundus can produce flexion of the distal phalanx without action on the proximal interphalangeal joint.

The interossei produce flexion of the metacarpophalangeal joint with simultaneous extension of the two distal interphalangeal joints. They also contribute to the preservation of the normal width of the hand. In addition, the dorsal interossei act as abductors of the extended fingers and the palmar interossei act as adductors of the fingers considering the long finger as the central line.

The lumbrical muscles are very important because they act in several ways. They contribute with the interossei to flexion of the fingers at the metacarpophalangeal joint and extension of the two distal phalanges. They also act as moderators between the extensors and flexors of the fingers and also produce slight radial deviation of the fingers.

In normal extension of the fingers from the position of a fist, the extensor digitorum produces extension of the proximal and partial extension of the middle and distal phalanges. The lumbricals and interossei intervene after a varying angle of extension at the distal and proximal interphalangeal joints completing the extension.

In the thumb, the flexor pollicis longus produces flexion of the distal phalanx; however, it is not capable of producing efficient simultaneous flexion at the metacarpophalangeal and carpometacarpal joints. The extensor pollicis longus, on the other hand, produces full extension of the distal and proximal phalanges and also adduction of the thumb. Its efficiency is enhanced by simultaneous contraction of the extensor carpi ulnaris.

The extensor pollicis brevis is responsible for extension at the metacarpophalangeal joint but it is mostly an efficient abductor of the thumb.

The abductor pollicis longus extends and abducts the first metacarpal and is a secondary flexor and abductor of the wrist.

The important action of opposition of the thumb is due to the action of the thenar muscles. The abductor brevis and the flexor brevis together with the opponens are the primary muscles responsible for this action. The opponens muscle is apparently the least important. The adductor, abductor longus, and extensor brevis are important muscles, indirectly. The extension of the distal phalanx of the thumb in opposition is due to the action of the adductor and abductor brevis which is transmitted through the extensor expansion of the thumb to the distal phalanx.

The hypothenar muscles play an important role in the action of the little finger which has a sufficient mobility on the hamate to permit a slight rotation, which is significant in approximation of the thumb to the little finger in opposition.

Flexion of the fingers produces synergistic contraction of the extensor carpi radialis longus and brevis. Extension of the fingers produces a strong contraction of the extensor carpi radialis longus and brevis and also of the extensor carpi ulnaris.

The flexor carpi radialis is a strong flexor of the wrist; when maximally contracted, it also produces a slight radial inclination of the wrist.

The flexor carpi ulnaris produces strong flexion of the ulnar side of the hand with slight supination and very slight ulnar deviation.

The extensors carpi radialis longus and brevis produce extension of the wrist with radial deviation. When the extensor longus alone is stimulated there is definite radial deviation. The extensor carpi radialis brevis, inserted into the third metacarpal base, produces straight extension. The extensor carpi ulnaris contracts strongly with the long and short radial extensors when extension is produced against resistance.

GUIDE LINES TO STRUCTURES OF THE HAND

For practical purposes, especially for surgical application, it may be useful to follow a few lines which facilitate exposure of anatomical structures. They are based on personal experience and are presented here. A few lines can be drawn on the palm of the hand (Fig. 2.2A) and also on the dorsum (Fig. 2.2B).

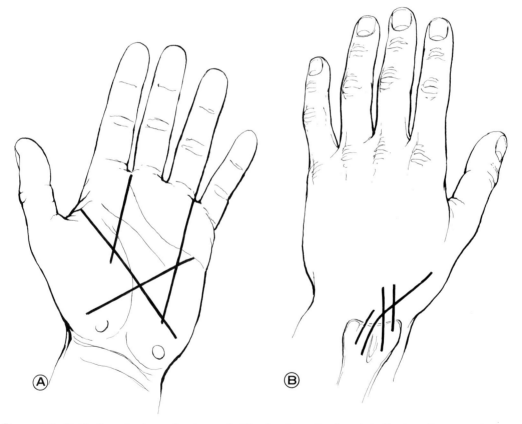

Figure 2.2. Guide lines to deep structures. A. The line from the thumb to the hypothenar eminence shows the location of the recurrent branch of the median nerve to thenar muscles at the index line crossing. The ring finger crossing indicates the apex of the hook of the hamate bone. The line from the little finger to the thenar eminence indicates the direction of the metacarpophalangeal joint of the thumb at the thenar eminence. B. Dorsal aspect of the hand shows the guide lines around Lister's tubercle. On the ulnar side of the tubercle the line indicates the direction of the extensor pol. long. and ulnar to it, the extensor indic. propr. On the radial side of the tubercle the first is the tendon of the extensor carpi radialis brevis and the second is the extensor carpi radialis longus.

REFERENCES

1. Basmajian, J. V. *Muscles Alive. Their Function Revealed by Electromyography,* Ed. 2. Baltimore, Williams & Wilkins, 1967.

2. Boyes, J. *Bunnel's Surgery of the Hand,* Ed. 5, Philadelphia, Lippincott, 1970.

3. Day, M. H. and Napier, J. R. The two heads of the flexor pollicis brevis. J. H. Anat., *95:* 123, 1961.

4. Duchenne, G. B. *Physiology of Motion,* translated and edited by E. B. Kaplan. Philadelphia, Lippincott, 1949.

5. Flatt, A. E. *The Pathomechanics of Ulnar Drift.* Social and Rehabilitation Services, Grant # R.D. 2226 M. 1971.

6. Grant, J. C. B. *Atlas of Anatomy,* Ed. 6. Baltimore, Williams & Wilkins, 1972.

7. Gray, H. *Anatomy of the Human Body,* Ed. 27, edited by C.M. Goss, Philadelphia, Lea and Febiger, 1959.

8. Kanavel, A. *Infections of the Hand.* Philadelphia, Lea and Febiger, 1933.

9. Kaplan, E. B. *Functional and Surgical Anatomy of the Hand,* Ed. 2. Philadelphia, Lippincott, 1965.

10. Kaplan, E. B. Guide lines to deep structures and dynamics of intrinsic muscles of the hand. Surg. Clin. North Am., *48-5:* 993, 1968.

11. Landsmeer, J. M. F. The anatomy of the "dorsal" aponeurosis of the human finger and its functional significance. Anat. Rec., *104:* 31, 1949.

12. Landsmeer, J. M. F. Anatomical and functional investigations on articulation of human fingers. Acta Anat. (Suppl. 24), *25:* 1, 1955.

13. Last, R. J. *Anatomy Regional and Applied,* Ed. 4. London, Churchill, 1967.

14. Milford, L. W. *Retaining Ligaments of Digits of the Hand.* Philadelphia, Saunders, 1968.

15. Nomina Anatomica (Revised by the International Anatomical Nomenclature Committee in 1950 and approved in 1956), Baltimore, Williams & Wilkins, 1956.

16. O'Rahilly, R. The developmental anatomy of the extensor assembly Acta Anat., *47:* 363, 1961.

17. Spinner, M. *Injuries to the Major Branches of Peripheral Nerves of the Forearm.* Philadelphia, Saunders, 1972.

18. Steindler, A. *Kinesiology of the Human Body.* Springfield, Charles C Thomas, 1955.

19. Stookey, B. *Surgical and Mechanical Treatment of Peripheral Nerves.* Philadelphia, Saunders, 1922.

20. Sunderland, S. *Nerves and Nerve Injuries.* Baltimore, Williams & Wilkins, 1968.

21. Tubiana R., and Valentin, P.: L'extension des doigts. Rev. Chir-Orth., *49:* 543, 1963.

22. Zantolli, E.: *Structural and Dynamic Bases of Hand Surgery.* Philadelphia, Lippincott, 1968.

chapter three

Congenital Anomalies

Martin A. Entin,
M.D., C.M., M.Sc., F.A.C.S.

Congenital deformities pose a real challenge to the surgeon and stimulate continuous search for newer concepts and methods for restoration of function. The complexity of the entire field of congenital anomalies is compounded by the fact that there is no categorical information regarding the causation of most of the deformities, nor accurate data about the frequency of their occurrence on this continent. In addition to the challenge that the primary deformities pose to reconstructive surgeons from the architectural and functional aspects, there are continuous changes which occur with growth that impose secondary alterations and imbalances.

Because of the dynamic nature of these deformities, even if successful reconstruction is attained, constant vigilance is required to detect early changes of recurrence or of new derangement. The goal of reconstruction for the congenital deformities is provision of a normal hand in appearance and function. However, for complex deformities it is more practical to attain useful function of hand and limb by provision of good skin cover, adequate sensation, satisfactory prehension, and the ability to place the hand in strategically useful positions.

ETIOLOGY

The causes of malformations are traditionally divided into *endogenous* type, implying some defect of the germ plasm which may be hereditary, and *exogenous,* which are associated with intra-uterine conditions. While these criteria of causation of congenital anomalies have been used by some authors as the basis of etiologic classification,[1,3,7] these are often difficult to establish from the sketchy history of the pedigree or from the examination of the patient and his anomaly. The hereditary nature of any deformity can be established by observation of the obvious similarity between the siblings and their parents, but if there had been no previous occurrence in the family, its subsequent transmission to future progeny is uncertain.

The establishment of the teratogenic action of thalidomide in man has re-emphasized the susceptibility of the developing fetus to the vagaries of the environment and to various chemical and physical agents.[46] The anlage of a given organ in the fetus is more susceptible to environmental stress during the period of most rapid development.[24,49] On the basis of experimental work and careful analysis of congenital malformation under the influence of known teratogenic agents, certain anomalies of the upper limb are more likely to occur in the following period of gestation: absence of limb in the third and fourth week; absence of hand at the fifth and sixth week; digital absence in the seventh week; digital stunting in the eighth week.[28]

The various teratogenic agents that can affect the developing fetus are drugs, chemicals, hormones, physical agents, viruses, nutritional deficiencies, and many others. They may be directly toxic to the fetus or may interfere with metabolic processes, or act as anti-metabolites, or upset the endocrine balance.

Some congenital deformities have been established as hereditary, and recur in subsequent generations: certain types of syndactyly, symphalangism, and supranumerary digits are some of the examples.[1,14,24] However, because of variation of penetrance, occasionally a generation may be skipped. Frequently, information available from the parents is not reliable or incomplete; it is obvious that, considering the complexity of human genetics, lengthy consideration of etiologic factors based on incomplete data is not justified.

CLASSIFICATION

It is apparent from the preceding discussion, that while a classification based on etiologic factors would be very helpful, in most of the deformities the causative agent is not known. Moreover, similar causative agents frequently produce widely different manifestations.[14] Consequently, most of the classifications that were accepted in the past offered a cavalcade of polyglot, polysyllabic items that did not materially help to establish order in this very complicated field.

Seeking to introduce some semblance of order, Entin published in the early fifties, an iconoclastic classification which attempted to get away from the traditional approach.[14] It attempted to oversimplify what was a complex problem, but it provided a stimulus for re-assessment and led to establishment of a committee by the American Society for Surgery of the Hand whose recommendation was adopted for trial by the International Federation of Hand Societies.[18]

This classification evolved from the morphologic patterns of the anomalies proposed by several authors,[23,44] and grouped the different entities into a system according to the parts that have been affected by specific embryologic failures.[45] Six major groups are used by this classification:

I. Failure of Differentiation of parts

II. Arrest of Development

III. Focal Defects

IV. Duplications

V. Overgrowth

VI. General Conditions

The major groups are subdivided further into subgroups, but while this classification is not all-inclusive, it is sufficiently broad to permit adaptation of greater breakdown. Table 3.1 presents the details of classification.

The adaptation of uniform classification throughout the world is mandatory for monitoring research and for valid comparision of methods of management. While it is not a perfect classification, it warrants adaptation for testing.[22] The consideration of various anomalies in this chapter will follow the grouping and subdivisions as outlined in this classification.

INCIDENCE

It is difficult to collect meaningful statistics on the incidence of congenital anomalies without establishing state or provincial registries for recording of birth anomalies. Because of relative lack of these facilities on this continent, it is impossible to get significant data on the incidence of any specific type of anomaly. Although there have been published reports in the United States and Canada regarding the frequency of occurrence of congenital deformities in a specific locality, one has to extrapolate the figures in order to get some idea what the actual incidence might be in one's own community.

Birch-Jensen published an important monograph in 1949 in which he recorded all living patients with congenital anomalies of upper extremity in Denmark.[5] Although the study did not include some of the very common types of deformity, it is valuable since it gives the incidence for the entire population of about 4 million. We shall allude to these figures throughout this chapter; the monograph records the pedigrees of a number of anomalies and should be consulted for further details.

MANAGEMENT OF THE ANOMALIES

Failure of Differentiation of Parts

This division spans the entire limb from shoulder to the fingertips and has a variety of entities, some rare, others fairly common (e.g., syndactyly). The consideration of the different entities includes a description

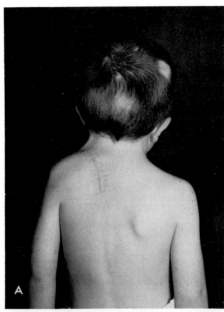

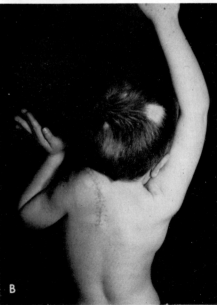

Figure 3.1. Undescended scapula. *A.* Posterior view following operation shows reasonably good correction of deformity. *B.* Limitation of function of right upper limb.

of the anomaly, and the method of management that we found useful in our series of cases; limitation of space permits discussion of only the more common deformities.

Shoulder

Congenital Elevation, Sprengel's Deformity. The deformity of an undescended scapula is one that has taxed the ingenuity of the reconstructive surgeon. It is often associated with skeletal anomalies of the cervical and thoracic spine. This anomaly is characterized by obvious elevation of one shoulder and a highly placed scapula which may be tilted toward the spine, and there is limitation of the function of the affected limb.

The correction of this deformity is difficult and recurrences are likely with growth. The technique described by Schrock[53] is generally followed; it entails stripping of the scapula subperiosteally, moving it down, and attaching by suture to the appropriate rib. It is recommended to cut the superior border of the spine if there is tethering of the scapula. The results are predicated upon the severity of the deformity; but improvement in function does not always follow the improved appearance (Fig. 3.1).

Absence of Pectoral Muscles. This is found in association with a number of other congenital deformities. The association of pectoral absence with syndactyly has been reported to vary in its frequency.[21,39]

Sometimes it is associated with absence of nipple and aplasia of the breast; this is fairly disturbing in the female patients (Fig. 3.2). Its relationship to syndactyly is not understood. No treatment for pectoral muscle absence has been available.[8,11]

Arm

Synostosis of the elbow is usually associated with arrest of the development of the ulnar component and will be discussed under that heading.

Forearm

Proximal synostosis of the radius and ulna with or without radial head dislocation has been observed more frequently in patients who have hypoplasia of the radius, whereas the dislocation of the radio-humeral joint in our series of cases was present in patients who had arrest of the development of the ulna, especially the proximal portion (Fig. 3.22). This too will be considered below.

Hand

Carpal. Carpal deformities and carpal synostosis rarely cause problems by themselves, when the rest of the digital configuration is normal.

Metacarpal. Short metacarpals are occasionally found in some patients on the ulnar side of the hand, but apart from that have no dysfunction and require no treatment (Fig. 3.3). Fusion of the bases of the adja-

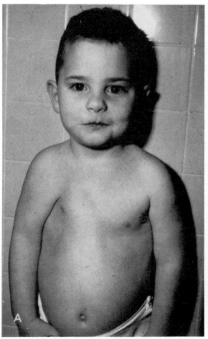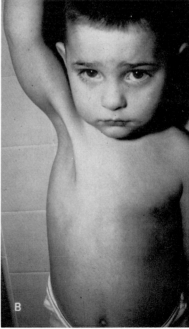

Figure 3.2. Congenital phalangeal malformation of right hand associated with absence of pectoralis major. *A.* Position in repose (note flatness of right lateral chest). *B.* With right arm raised: some fibers of the upper portion of pectoralis muscles persist.

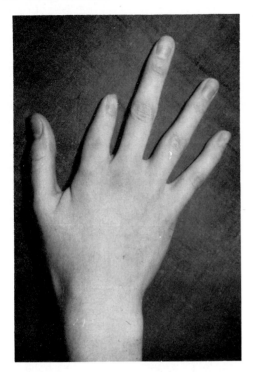

Figure 3.3. Right hand of 14-year-old girl showing the shortening of metacarpal of index finger. The pinch is good and there is no need for functional improvement.

cent metacarpals may restrict some mobility of the fingers. Occasionally, nondivision of two neighboring metacarpals results in the phalanges of two fingers articulating with the same metacarpal. This gives rise to deformities and may require ablation of a digit (Fig. 3.20A).

Digital Anomalies. Syndactyly.

Simple syndactyly between fingers usually involves only the soft tissue (Fig. 3.4). The most frequent type is between long and ring fingers and this anomaly is usually bilateral: this is a familial type of syndactyly which is frequently dominant and repeats itself from one generation to the next.[14] There is little interference with function and treatment can be delayed until the child is older, provided one can allay the pressure from the parents for surgical intervention.

The treatment of simple syndactyly requires creation of a proximally based dorsal or volar flap to reconstitute the "floor" of the web space, and division of the common skin envelope by a wavy line to avoid straight line contracture (Fig. 3.5). The skin envelope is always too short to completely cover the finger and additional skin grafting is usually required.[4,14,15]

Complicated syndactyly may affect only the soft tissue, but the nails may be joined. If skeletal elements are also affected, there might be side to side fusion of the phalanges or even confluence of several digits crowned by one common semicircular nail, as occurs in Apert's syndrome.

Acrosyndactyly is included into the classification by some experts.[22] This anomaly is called "secondary syndactyly",[7,32] "ectosyndactyly" or "fenestrated syndactyly."[35] It is usually unilateral and the webs have proximal tunnels. Ring constriction may be present and distal parts may be completely amputated and found floating *in utero.*[47] It does not not appear to be hereditary. The treatment is the same as for simple syndactyly, but is complicated by the fact that that parts of digits are missing, and soft tissue may be invaded by fibrous tissue, the result of attempted healing[32] (Fig. 3.6).

In Apert's syndrome there is symphalangism between the proximal and middle phalanges and synostosis of the terminal phalanges and often the thumb is involved. This is associated with malformation of the skull and facial bones (acrocephalosyndactyly). Several stages are required in reconstruction: the border fingers are freed first, preferably before one year of age; six months later, the remaining fingers are separated. If one finger is discarded, there is sufficient skin to cover the remainder with good sensation.[27] This regime provides an adequately functioning three-fingered hand.

Contractures. This group of anomalies involves the soft tissues, namely, skin, facia, ligaments and muscles. The simplest form is *contracture of thumb* web space without bony anomalies. This can be corrected by shifting of skin as in Z-plasty, or may require addition of skin grafts.

Trigger digit is due to constriction of the peritendinous structures, such as proximal pulleys or a band of fascia causing the tendons to be blocked in flexion. This anomaly is more common for the thumb and may be bilateral. Since it restricts efficient use of the hand function, it should be corrected early. The simple division of the constricting band or of the tight pulley may suffice. Occasionally, lenthening of a shortened muscle may be necessary.

Camptodactyly is a hereditary condition caused by painless progressive bilateral flexion contracture of the little fingers and occasionally of neighboring fingers. When long-standing, there is secondary contracture of ligaments and skin. It is thought by some authors to be caused by shortening of the flexor digitorum superficialis and lengthening of this tendon in the palm or wrist helps,[40] but we could not correct this deformity by this procedure alone: in some patients correction of bony alignment and addition of skin was needed. Mild cases without serious interference with function should be left alone.

Flexion and adduction contracture of the thumb appears to be asociated with a sex-linked recessive gene, is more common in males, and frequently is bilateral. Weckesser attributed the condition to congenital ab-

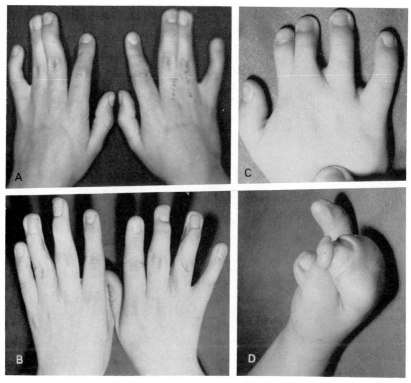

Figure 3.4. Syndactyly. *A.* Bilateral syndactyly between long and ring fingers is usually familial and dominant. *B.* Same as *A,* after separation with aid of rectangular flap and skin graft. *C.* Simple syndactyly of index and long fingers with partial syndactyly of third web. *D.* Complicated syndactyly of Apert's syndrome.

sence of the extensor pollicis brevis and sometimes even longus.[51] The deformity can be corrected in mild cases by splinting and stretching. In more severe cases, a cast may be applied after a few months of age to prevent contracture. In severe or fixed deformities, release of the joint capsule and of the adductor muscle as well as skin grafts may be necessary before muscle transfer to provide extension is carried out. The extensor indicis proprius is used to provide extension of the thumb. The flexor digitorum superficialis can be used as an alternative.[31]

Arthrogryposis is a congenital anomaly of unknown etiology. It comprises a syndrome involving multiple joints in rigid flexion contracture, associated with hypoplastic muscles and increased amount of subcutaneous fat. The incidence of arthrogryposis is unknown.

Weeks divided arthrogryposis of upper extremities into three groups and reported the results of treatment.[52] In the first group with limited localized deformities the pronation contracture was released by detaching the insertion of pronator muscle and tendon transfer to restore digital extension. Correction of the adducted thumb requires application of abdominal

pedicle and lengthening of flexor pollicis longus. We have used a similar program of treatment for our own cases (Fig. 3.7*A*.)

In the second group wrist flexion was corrected by shortening the forearm bones, proximal to pronator quadratus, removal of forearm fascia and of contracted wrist joint capsule. The results were satisfactory in the second group, provided the wrist was held in extension with splints up to six weeks. Spontaneous recovery of digital extensors frequently takes place.

The third group has no functional muscle mass and, while the joints may be rigid or flaccid, there is no available surgical treatment (Fig. 3.7*B*).

Skeletal Deformities. The specific anomalies that are grouped together in this subdivision result from failure of development of a part of the bone, resulting in inequality of growth or in fusion of neighboring bones.

Clindactyly is a condition due to lateral deviation of the digits and is caused by some malalignment of the joint due to the wedge-shape of the bone or to the inequality of the rate of growth of the two sides of the epiphysis (Fig.3.8). It may be bilateral and symmetrical. The use of casts and splints does not correct this

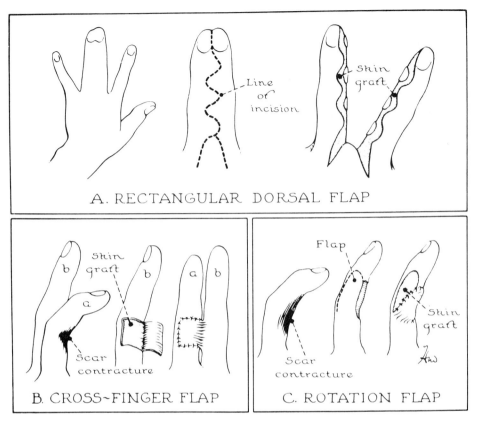

Figure 3.5. Graphic illustration of management of simple webbed fingers (syndactyly). *A.* Dorsal rectangular flap and wavy lateral incisions along the margin are used. The defects are filled with skin grafts. *B.* Secondary deformity due to scar formation result. Correction may require cross-finger flaps to provide skin and subcutaneous tissue to area of contracture. *C.* Shifting of lateral flap to bring normal supple skin to replace deep scar. (Reproduced from Journal of Bone and Joint Surgery, *41: A,* 681, 1959.)

anomaly. The surgical treatment requires resection of a wedge of bone and may have to be repeated. If there is no serious interference with function, the surgical treatment may be delayed until school-age since there are recurrences of deviation with growth.

If lateral deviation is associated with absence of a metacarpal so that two digits articulate with the same metacarpals, it may be simpler to amputate the lateral digit.

Delta phalanx is a deformity considered a variant of duplication of a digit and, if supernumerary fragments are present, these should be removed. The correction of a deformity is done by removing the abnormal epiphysis and correcting the alignment of the finger by osteotomy and insertion of a wedge-shaped bone graft.[29,50]

Symphalangism is an anomaly caused by the end-to-end fusion of adjacent phalanges of a finger. It occurs in a number of conditions and may be associated with complex syndactyly such as Apert's syndrome.

This condition may be an isolated finding and is in-

herited. One family in England traced the recurrence of this anomaly through 14 generations to John Talbot, the first Earl of Shrewsburg.[12]

For patients with other associated anomalies the correction is concentrated on provision of essential function to the hand and symphalangism may not need to be treated. However, judicious change of the alignment of the involved digits by an osteotomy is sometimes useful.

Arrest of Development

This group of anomalies comprises three major divisions, transverse, intermediate, and longitudinal. These have been referred to in other classifications as "terminal transverse", "intercalary", and "paraxial".

Transverse

This group of anomalies varies from absence of terminal phalanges to complete absence of the entire limb (Amelia) and is referred to by some authors as

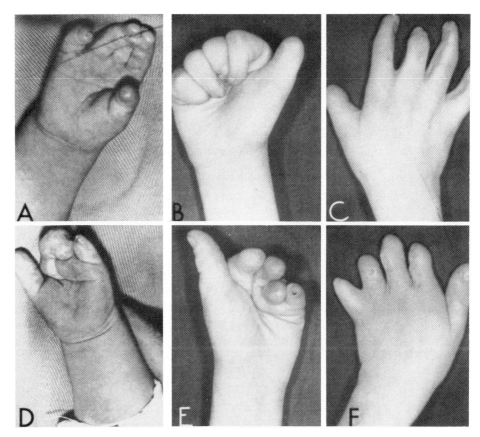

Figure 3.6. Secondary syndactyly with loss of portion of terminal phalanges. *A* and *D.* Right and left hands prior to reconstruction at three years of age (note incomplete skin fusion at bases of fingers). *B* and *C.* Right hand following reconstruction at the age of seven. *E* and *F.* Left hand following reconstruction at the age of seven. The grasp was limited due to absence of distal phalanges, but the general function was adequate. (Reproduced from Journal of Bone and Joint Surgery, *41-A:* 681, 1959.)

"congenital amputations" (Table 3.1). In the transverse arrest the stump is usually well padded and may have dimpling or remnants of rudimentary digits (Fig. 3.9).

There is little that can be done surgically for most of these anomalies: most patients that have these deficiencies are fitted with conventional upper limb prosthesis or its variants.

For patients with bilateral absence of hands (Acheiria) that require the use of bilateral prostheses, Krukenberg operation done on one side provides an organ with normal sensation and efficient prehension that does not interfere with fitting of a prosthesis. This procedure makes these patients independent even without putting on a prosthesis. It is an essential requirement for a bilateral amputee, and avoids putting on the prosthesis in the middle of the night which is a distinct nuisance.

Adactylia. For patients who have bilateral absence of digits (adactylia), we found that provision of post-like thumb by a bony elongation of the scaphoid-trapezial complex, removal of the capitate, and a similar elongation of the hamate bone on one limb, provides a pincer-like organ with sensation that is especially valuable in combination with a contralateral prosthesis devoid of sensibility.

However, if all digits are absent, even in the presence of normal carpal components with good motion, it is not always practical to construct digital elements (Fig. 3.9). On one occasion when we did attempt to reconstruct a moveable thumb by shifting available skin and carpal bone, we failed to provide efficient prehension. Thus it would be practical to fit a prosthesis to these children as early as possible, by overcoming the adamancy of the parents.

In a bilateral absence of digits instead of fitting two prostheses it may be more practical to carry out a Krukenberg procedure on the dominant side. Conventional prosthesis can be fitted over the Krukenberg if desired.

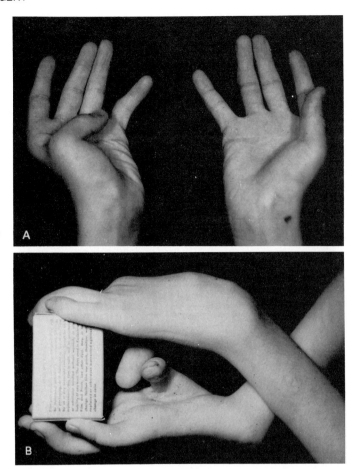

Figure 3.7. Arthrogryposis. *A.* Right and left hands of 11-year-old male showing typical deformities with ulnar deviation and adduction contracture of thumbs, worse on the left. *B.* Severe bilateral arthrogryposis without prehension in 12-year-old girl. The patient uses hands pincer-fashion for holding objects.

Aphalangia. Considerable improvement of function can be attained for patients with phalangial deficiencies (aphalangia). There is a tremendous amount of variation in the level of deficiency among these deformities.

While the absence of phalangeal elements is a relatively small deformity in relation to the whole upper limb, which frequently is entirely normal; nevertheless it interferes with the basic prehensile function.

The provision of ability to pinch and grasp may require deepening of webs, construction of bony framework, shifting of local or distant skin. The reconstructive procedures which we found useful for this group of patients fall into the following groups:

1. Separation of parts by phalangization.

2. Deepening of web spaces and shifting of bony elements (Fig. 3.10).

3. Pollicization of a finger and ablation of parts to create web space (Fig. 3.10).

4. Lengthening of digital components by shifting of local skin and by bone grafting (Fig. 3.11).

For any specific type of anomaly one should select the procedures which would permit attainment of the best function with the minimum number of surgical procedures. Since there is the likelihood of interference with growth of the transferred part of bone, constant vigilance is needed to detect and correct the new deformities.

Intermediate

Arrest of development of the intermediate segment of a limb is a confirmation of the concept that any region of the limb anlage can be affected during the embryonic period of development. This congenital anomaly became especially common with the introduction of thalidomide [17] but was recognized even in ancient times and was inaccurately referred to as a "seal-hand" (phocomelia) because of its superficial resemblance. The seal has all elements present, but they are foreshortened.

Several types occur: (1) *The classical phocomelia* has a *complete* arrest of the intermediate part of a limb,

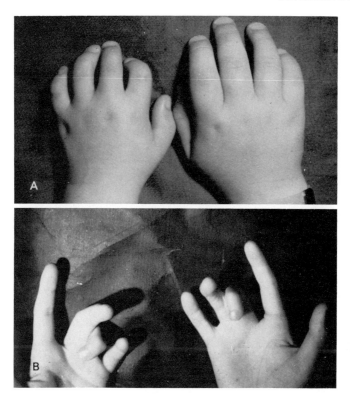

Figure 3.8. *A.* Clinodactyly of left index finger in four-year-old boy. Correction was carried out by wedge osteotomies of the middle phalanx in stages. *B.* Clinodactyly of right long and left ring fingers associated with severe tissue contracture. These deformities can only be corrected by combined wedge osteotomy and addition of all elements of skin.

so that the hand is attached directly to the trunk (Fig. 3.12*A*). (2) *Proximal phocomelia* is due to the arrest of the upper arm; the forearm (with a normal hand) is attached to the trunk (Fig. 3.12*B*). (3) *Distal phocomelia* in which the hand is attached to the upper arm at the elbow with the absence of the forearm (Fig. 3.12*C*).

The management of these anomalies requires primarily the fitting of prostheses. A number of complex sophisticated devices have been developed which require manipulation of some levers. These are especially suitable for patients with complete phocomelia since the rudimentary hand has sufficient function to control them.

Surgical reconstruction is confined to incomplete phocomelias which have an associated malformation of the hand or forearm.

The management of one patient with such a problem as well as other associated anomalies may serve as an illustration of handling several simultaneous problems of limb placement as well as lack of prehension.

This young girl was born with absent ulna on the left, radio-humeral synostosis, and fusion of the only two digits she had in her hand. Her right upper limb had an intermediate arrest of development with the tiny bit of appendage, representing the hand, attached to the distal humerous (distal

phocomelia). Thus she had no prehensile organ and, until she presented herself for treatment at our hospital at the age of 12, used her teeth and mouth for handling small objects. In addition, she had internal rotation of her left humerus so that the back of her elbow faced anteriorly, and hypersupination deformity of her left forearm (Fig. 3.13).

Reconstruction was carried out in several stages: the first procedure entailed a derotation osteotomy of the distal humerus. A few months later osteotomy of the proximal radius permitted placing the hand in neutral position. Finally, a complex separation of the two webbed digits with the aid of abdominal flap to provide a wide web space, provided her with a prehensile organ with normal sensibility, with satisfactory pinch and reasonable grasp. The right upper limb was fitted with a conventional prosthesis (Fig. 3.13).

Longitudinal

The forearm and hand are divided into three distinct developmental areas. These are: the *radial* component which forms the radius; the thumb, and the intervening carpal bones; the *central* component, consisting of the central carpal bones and the index and middle fingers; and the *ulnar* component which consists of the ulna and the three ulnar fingers with their carpal bones. Each of these anatomic areas can be adversely affected during embryonic development, producing deformities confined primarily to the area involved (Fig. 3.14). These abnormalities are referred to as

TABLE 3.1
Classification of congenital anomalies*

I. Failure of Differentiation of Parts	II. Arrest of Development

I. Failure of Differentiation of Parts

  A. *Shoulder*
    1. Undescended scapula
    2. Absence of pectoral muscle

  B. *Arm*
    1. Synostosis of elbow

  C. *Forearm*
    1. Soft tissue anomalies
    2. Synostosis of radius and ulna
    3. Radio-humeral dislocation

  D. *Hand*
    1. Carpal anomalies
    2. Metacarpal anomalies
    3. Digital anomalies[†*]

    a. Syndactyly
      1. Simple
      2. Complicated
        a. Soft tissue and nails
        b. Skeletal
          i. Fusion: phalangeal;
            Apert's syndrome
            acrosyndactyly[††]
          ii. Brachysyndactyly
          iii. Disarray

    b. Contractures
      i. Thumb web space
      ii. Trigger digits
      iii. Campodactyly
      iv. Arthrogryposis

    c. Skeletal deformities
      i. Clinodactyly
      ii. Delta phalanx
      iii. Symphalangism

II. Arrest of Development

  A. *Transverse* (terminal transverse)
    1. At shoulder (amelia)
    2. At arm
    3. At elbow
    4. At forearm
    5. At wrist (acheiria)
    6. At carpo-metacarpal
      level (adactylia)
    7. At phalangeal level
      (aphalangia)
  B. *Intermediate* (intercalary)
    1. Complete
      i. Classical (hand to trunk)
      ii. Proximal (hand and
        forearm to trunk)
      iii. Distal (hand to arm)
    2. Incomplete

  C. *Longitudinal*
    1. Complete
      a. Radial
        i. Radius and thumb
        ii. Radius only
        iii. Thumb only
      b. Central
        i. Soft tissue cleft
        ii. Absence of one or more
          central digits
      c. Ulnar
        i. Ulna and fingers
        ii. Ulna only
        iii. Ulnar fingers only
    2. Incomplete
      1. Radial
      2. Central
      3. Ulnar

III. Focal Defects
    1. Soft tissue
      A. Annular constriction bands
    2. Skeletal

IV. Duplication
    1. Digital
      A. Polydactyly
    2. Whole Hnad or Limb
      A. Mirror Hand

V. Overgrowth (Gigantism)
    1. Arm
    2. Forearm
    3. Hand
    4. Digit

VI. Generalized Skeletal Defects
    (affecting the Upper Limb also)

*This Classification is after Swanson, Barsky, and Entin[45] and recommended for trial by International Federation of Societies for Surgery of the Hand.

†As suggested by A. E. Flatt.[22]

††This is considered as "Secondary syndactyly" by some authors.[7,32,35]

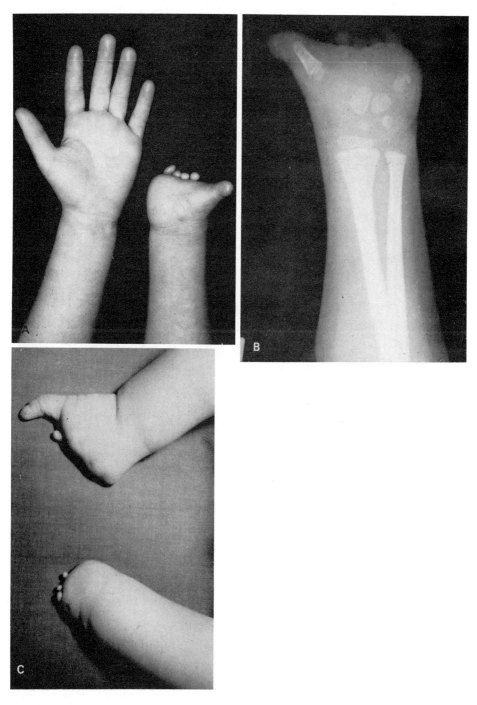

Figure 3.9. Transverse arrest of development. *A.* Absence of all digits with exception of first metacarpal of right hand. Note the spherical remnants of fingers. *B.* X-ray of right hand shown in *A* at age of six years. *C.* Complete absence of digits of the left hand of four-year-old female (adactylia). Note the spherical remnants of fingers.

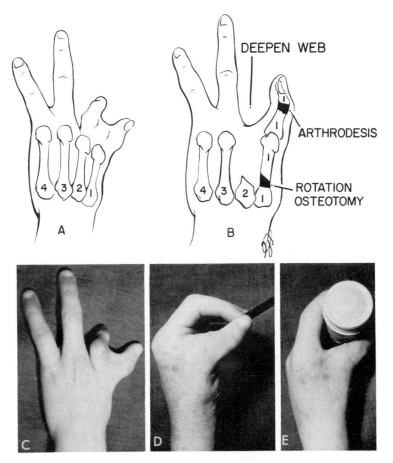

Figure 3.10. Transverse arrest of development: aphalangia *A* and *B.* Diagram of left hand of six-year-old boy with aplasia of phalanges. Reconstruction was carried out by re-alignment of radial digit, rotation osteotomy at base and arthrodesis of terminal joint. *B.* Removal of second digit and deepening of cleft improved prehension. *C.* Left hand shows preoperative condition. Prehension was difficult. *D.* Same hand as *C* after reconstruction. *E.* Same as *C* showing satisfactory grasp. (Reproduced from Surgical Clinics of North America, *48:* 1155, 1968.)

longitudinal absences and vary from complete absence of the part to abnormalities in which only a portion of the long bone or of the digits is lacking.

Radial. The etiology of these malformations is not certain: they appear in families without previous history of similar conditions. Partial absence of the thumb was reported in one of monozygotic twins, the other twin being entirely normal.[33] On the other hand, Fanconi anemia which occasionally occurs in association with arrest of development of the radial component is familial and is transmitted as a recessive trait.[25]

The radial component consists of the radius, the multangular bones, and the scaphoid, the bones of the thumb, the muscles, ligaments, and neurovascular structures associated with these parts. The deformities may be due to the absence of the entire component or to any part of it, depending on the severity of the deformity (Fig. 3.15). The radius forms the main support of the hand; when this bony buttress is absent, the muscles exert their pull on the unsupported hand, angulating it in relation to the long axis of the forearm.[14,38] The arrest of the development of the radial component is generally classified as complete and partial aplasia and hypoplasia of the radius and of the thumb ray with its associated carpal bones (Fig. 3.16). Complete arrest of development of the radial component is associated with absence of the thumb and this forms a severe handicap since in addition to the deformity there is absence of prehension.

The objective of reconstruction is to align the limb in a correct position, provide stabilization by bony support, and construct a thumb for efficient prehen-

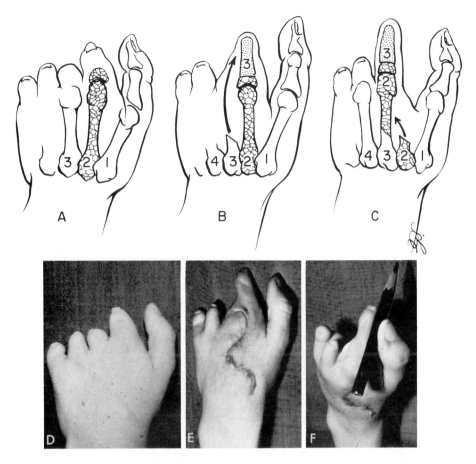

Figure 3.11. Transverse arrest of development: aphalangia. *A.* Diagram of left hand of six-year-old boy showing aplasia of phalanges. Thumb is normal. *B.* First stage of reconstruction. Remnant of proximal phalanx of index is lengthened by distal half of third metacarpal. *C.* Second stage of reconstruction. The index finger is shifted on to the remaining proximal portion of the third metacarpal. This widens the first web. *D.* Photograph of the hand (same as *A*). *E.* Same as *D* after reconstruction. The lengthening of the index finger was attained by the shifting of dorsal skin. *F.* Same as *E* showing pinch. (Reproduced from Surgical Clinics of North America, *48:* 1155, 1968.)

sion. Obviously, this cannot be accomplished in one sitting and requires several procedures extending over a period of time.

Correction of Alignment. The angulation of the hand in relation to the axis of the forearm which is characteristic of radial absence is not difficult to correct in the infant. However, some patients have fixed deformities due to shortening of the muscles and skin. Surgical lengthening of the muscles, severance of the ligamentous bands, and Z-plasty of the skin may be necessary before corrected alignment is achieved.[13]

The alignment is maintained in corrected position with the aid of a light dynamic splint (Fig 3.17). This splint has evolved after many trials: it is made from a thin steel wire coiled in the center to provide the dynamic force for correction of deviation; the portions of splint around the limb are padded with leather. An important advantage of this splint is that it is easily adjustable: the parents are instructed to watch for signs of irritation, and make suitable adjustment themselves with the aid of pliers as required with growth of the child. Wearing of the splint for at least 12 hours a day is usually sufficient to maintain the hand in correct alignment.

Bony Stabilization. In the preceding years the procedure introduced by Starr[41] was used by many clinics. This entailed the use of the proximal half of the autogenous fibula. The head was abbutted against the carpus, while the proximal end was wedged into the ulna. We have used this procedure in about a dozen patients, but usually after 3 or 4 years of age. This method has several disadvantages: fibular epiphysis

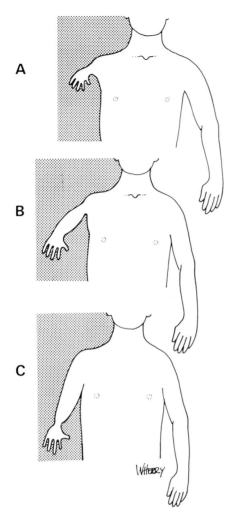

Figure 3.12. Diagram of intermediate arrest of development. *A.* Complete phocomelia. *B.* Proximal phocomelia. *C.* Distal phocomelia.

does not survive and there is recurrence of the deformity with growth of the ulna; there is some deformity in the donor site. In several of our patients; fairly satisfactory stabilization has been attained (Fig. 3.18).

There is no agreement among authorities on the correct age of bony stabilization. Some recommend that stabilization should be done within a few months after birth.[6,37] This became practical since the introduction of "centralization" of the hand over the distal end of the ulna, preserving the epiphysis. This method is now enjoying widespread popularity (Fig. 3.19).

The procedure of centralization is carried out through the dorsal bayonet incision. The distal ulna is freed and advanced between muscles toward the lunate bone. A nest is created in the carpus by removing the lunate and capitate bones. If the ulnar end is unusu-

ally wide, some longitudinal trimming has to be done, but the epiphysis is preserved. The stabilization is maintained with the hand in a neutral position by passing a stout Kirschner wire through the ring or long metacarpal into the ulna. We like to keep this wire in permanently; some surgeons prefer to remove it after a few weeks and maintain support with splints for an indefinite period.

In addition to bony stabilization, it is necessary to provide muscle support. This is done by advancing the insertion of the extensor carpi ulnaris distally on to the fifth metacarpal and the origin of the hypothenar muscles proximally, on to the radius.[37,43] Other muscles were also used to maintain the alignment by overcoming the predominant flexor forces.[6] This management results in satisfactory stabilization of the hand over the period of *follow-up* of several years; none of our patients has reached adolescence yet.

Reconstruction of Absent Thumb. Provision of efficient thumb is considered a more difficult undertaking than the stabilization of the hand, since special skills, precision, and delicacy are required. Pollicization of the index finger is the procedure of choice when the thumb is absent, since it provides all the necessary components; neurovascular supply, and the long tendons. The technical aspects of this procedure have evolved in the last 20 years through the contributions of several surgeons in different countries.[9,10,26,30,31,36] The principle is to create a shorter digit with stability and optimum placement for opposing the other fingers. The index finger is shortened by removing the middle two-thirds of its metacarpal, maintaining neurovascular bundles, pronating the finger, and wedging the distal portion of metacarpal into the proximal part. Thus the metacarpophalangeal joint of the index becomes the carpometacarpal joint of the reconstructed thumb, now positioned in abduction for efficient prehension (Fig. 3.19 and 3.20). There are a number of specific techniques that have been described regarding the positioning and stabilization of the head of the metacarpal, the shortening of the tendons, transfer of the interossei muscles of the index for balance, and others.

Recently, Buck-Gramcko published his experience with 100 pollicizations in congenital deformities and assessed critically the principles and available techniques. He introduced a number of refinements that should prove to be valuable in this procedure.[9] Because of the ready adaptation to function and growth, he recommends that this procedure should be done early. Our own experience tends to support this view.

Hypoplasia of the Thumb (Pouce Flottant). The typical deformity consists of a vestigial thumb, having a nail, good sensation, and two phalanges; a portion or the entire metacarpal may be absent and so are the greater multangulars. In two of our patients, the scaphoid was also absent so that the vestigial thumb remains immobile and consequently quite useless.

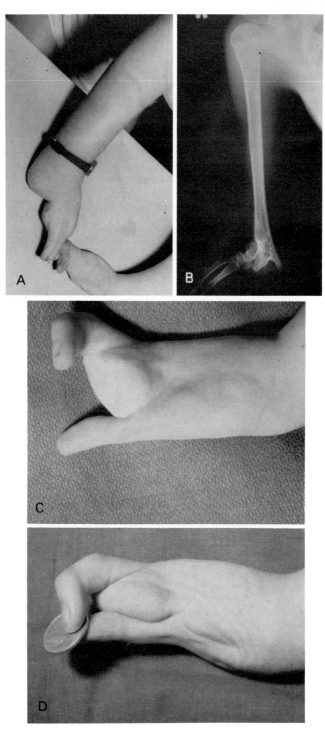

Figure 3.13. Intermediate arrest of development. *A.* Right upper limb shows attachment of the hand to the lower end of humerus (see x-ray at *B*). The two digits of left hand are fused. *B*. X-rays of the right limb shown at *A*. *C*. Left hand after separation of the two digits by osteotomy and addition of abdominal pedicle. *D*. Same as *C,* showing strong pinch.

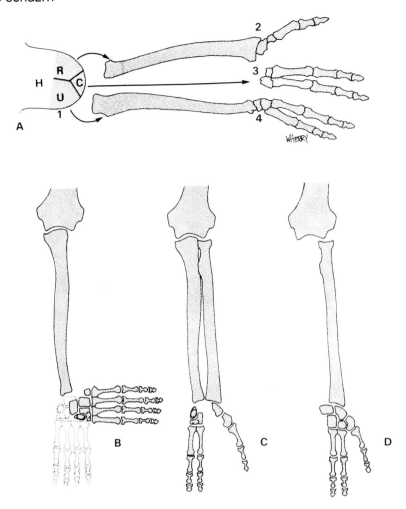

Figure 3.14. The three developmental areas of the embryonic upper limb. *A.* Radial *(R)*, Central *(C)* and Ulnar *(U)* components of developing limb bud (1). *B.* Absence of radial component results in radial deviation of unsupported wrist. *C.* Absence of contral component. *D.* Absence of ulnar component.

We feel that it is more practical, ordinarily, to discard the floating thumb and to provide efficient pinch-and-grasp by pollicization of the index finger. Many parents, however, are reluctant to discard the hypoplastic thumb since they consider that, although pollicization does provide efficient grasping motion, it deforms the hand even further cosmetically. In recent years, free autogenous joint transfer has been tried for various conditions and this procedure was used for reconstruction in several patients with hypoplasia of the thumb.[1,19]

The deformity of the thumb is characterized by the absence of the proximal half or of the entire first metacarpal (Fig. 3.19*C*). In addition, there are no greater multangular bones and no scaphoid, and usually, no tendons attached to the thumb. Several stages of reconstruction are thus required. First is the transfer of the metatarsophalangeal joint from the toe in order to establish bony continuity between the hand and the vestigial thumb, and to provide a movable joint at the carpometacarpal level. By making a semicircular incision on the dorsal aspect of the second metacarpal, it is possible to advance the thumb and the flap of dorsal skin radially. The dorsal skin defect is covered with skin graft (Fig. 3.19*C*).

Although we have carried out this procedure in several patients in the past, because of the consistent degenerative changes which occur in the free transferred joint resulting in the disintegration of the architecture, it is not recommended.[16]

Central. Arrest of development of the medial or central component is also known as *lobster* or *cleft* hand. In a typical case, one or more central digits are absent forming a metacarpal cleft which may extend into the carpus. These patients can develop an amaz-

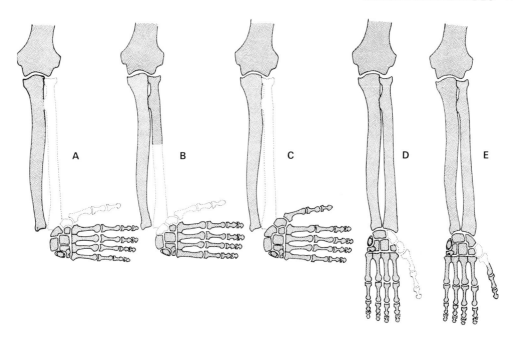

Figure 3.15. Longitudinal arrest of development: variation of radial absence (missing parts are shown in white). *A.* Total aplasia of radial component. *B.* Partial aplasia of radius. *C.* Total aplasia of radius, thumb is normal. *D.* Radius normal, thumb ray is absent. *E.* Hypoplasia of proximal part of thumb .pouce flottant).

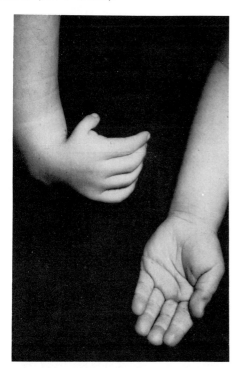

Figure 3.16. Photograph of both hands of five-year-old boy showing total aplasia of radius and partial aplasia of the thumb (pouce flottant). Note radial dislocation of the hand.

ing degree of dexterity; one of our patients was a rapid and accurate typist. One should not obliterate the cleft of the palm simply to improve appearance, because this may interfere with the efficiency of function (Fig. 3.21*A* and *B*).

A few of our patients with cleft hand, especially those who had syndactyly between ulnar digits of unequal size, developed deformities of subluxation at metacarpophalangeal joints which interfered with pinching and grasping. Separation of webbed digits and osteotomy to correct alignment improved pinch and prehension (Fig. 3.21*C*).

"Atypical" cleft hand has only the two lateral digits and, not unfrequently, the thumb is short-changed also. Barsky [2] recommended releasing the web by means of a Z-plasty. Some of our patients with these deformities had only the metacarpal present in the thumb and required elongation of the thumb to provide minimum prehensile function.

Ulnar. The arrest of development of the ulna is less frequent than either the central or radial absence. [14,34] The thumb and one or two radial fingers are usually present; the radius is usually foreshortened and may be fused with the humerus, or there may be a radio-humeral dislocation. The hand is frequently deviated ulnarward and this is due to the bowing of the radius whose growing potential has been impaired in the area adjacent to the ulna; there is often a fibrocartilagenous band which also may cause some deviation of the hand.

In correcting the deformity, it is necessary to excise

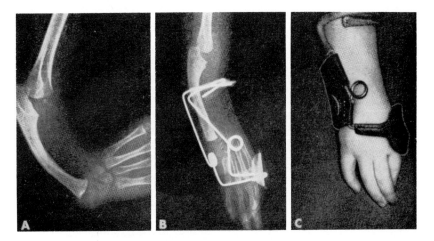

Figure 3.17. Early management of radial absence. *A.* X-ray of forearm showing typical position of hand in a moderately severe case before treatment. *B.* Same as *A,* but with dynamic splint maintaining alignment of hand with forearm. *C.* Photograph of dynamic splint which is made with steel wire and is covered with leather. Its use reduces the progression of the deformity with growth until stabilization of the hand is attained. (Reproduced from Surgical Clinics of North America, *40:* 497, 1960.)

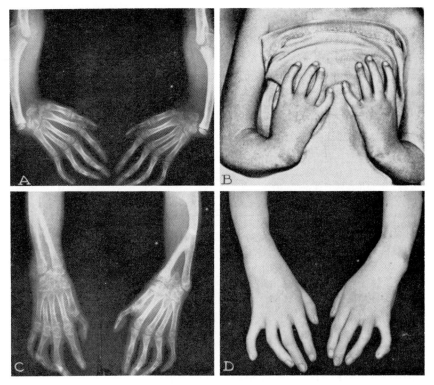

Figure 3.18. Reconstruction of bilateral absence of the radius. *A.* X-rays of both arms of six-year-old girl before treatment. *B.* Photograph of the arms of this patient before treatment. *C.* X-rays of both forearms after completion of treatment with the aid of bilateral fibular grafts. Right hand one year after grafting; left hand two years after grafting. *D.* Photograph of both hands at age 11. Right hand, three years, and left hand, four years after fibular graft. (Reproduced from Surgical Clinics of North America, *48:* 1155, 1968.)

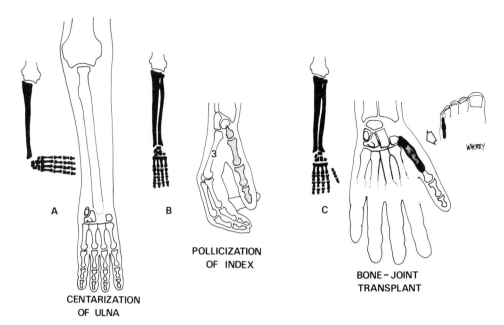

Figure 3.19. Reconstruction of radial absence. A. Centralization of ulna into the carpal nest produced by removal of lunate and capitate bones. (The pre-operative condition is shown in black silhouette.) B. Pollicization of thumb corrected by free transfer of autogenous metatarso-phalangeal joint. Subsequent degenerative changes, which lead to disintegration of the transferred joint, make this procedure impractical.

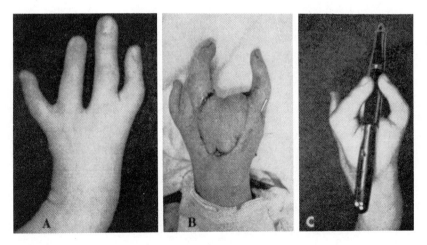

Figure 3.20. Reconstruction of absent thumb. A. The left hand of an eight-year-old boy with complete absence of the thumb and bent little finger. The ring and little fingers articulate with a common metacarpal. B. Pollicization of the index finger was begun four weeks before this photograph was taken. The new web space between the index and middle finger was covered with an abdominal flap. Rotation osteotomy at the base of the index finger and stabilization with the aid of an iliac bone graft between second and third metacarpals provided good position for the pinch and grasp. C. Efficient prehension was possible as shown one year after reconstruction. (Reproduced from Surgical Clinics of North America, 40: 497, 1960.)

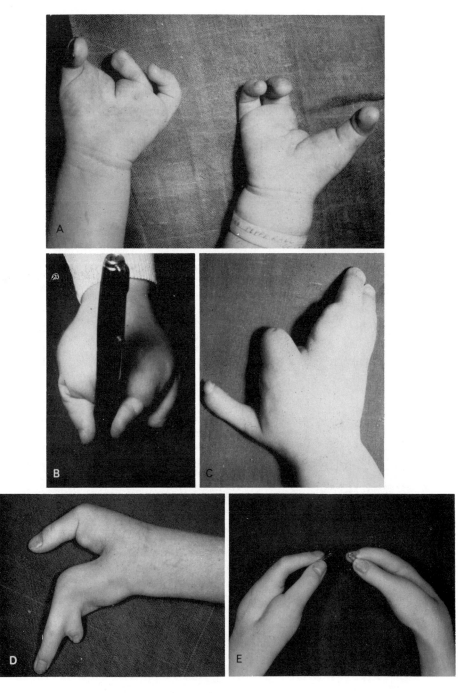

Figure 3.21. Arrest of central component. *A.* Right and left hands of four-year-old girl. Left hand reconstructed by deepening of first web space (Shown in *B*). *B.* Improved pinch of left hand shown in *A* after deepening of web space. *C.* Variation of central absence associated with syndactyly of ring and little fingers. *D.* Typical "cleft" or "lobster" hand with syndactyly between ring and little fingers with subluxation of the ring finger caused by tethering to the little finger. The pinch was poor. *E.* Same as *D* after separation and discarding of the little finger. Better pinch restored.

the fibrocartilagenous band. If the radial bowing is marked, it can be corrected by osteotomy. Proximal radial dislocation has not been a problem since there is sufficient soft tissue fixation for relative stability at the elbow with moderate range of movement. If a proximal portion of the ulna is present and is articulating with the humerus, Straub suggested fusion of the proximal radius, after excision of the radial head, to the ulnar remnant; this gives a stable elbow and forearm.[42]

If the thumb and at least two fingers are present and functioning well, no further reconstruction is required. However frequently there are other associated deformities of the digits which require reconstruction.

There is a recurrent characteristic pattern of anomalies associated with arrest of development of various components. In complete radial absence there may be *limitation of elbow movement* due to fibrous tissue, *curving of the ulna* and *radial dislocation of the wrist*. In partial radial absence *proximal radio-ulnar synostosis* occurs. In unlar absence there may be *internal rotation of the humerous, radio-humeral dislocation, radio-humeral fusion, hypersupination of the forearm* and *ulnar deviation of the wrist* (Fig. 3.22).

All these associated deformities at various levels interfere primarily with the placement of the hand and often have to be corrected before reconstruction of the hand; otherwise it cannot be properly positioned for efficient use.

The management of some of these entitles has been included in the discussion of *Intermediate and Lon-*

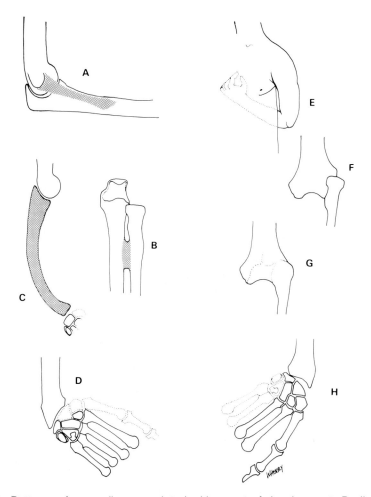

Figure 3.22. Patterns of anomalies associated with arrest of development. *Radial absence or hypoplasia: A.* Persistent ligamentous bands about the elbow cause limitation of elbow motion. *B.* Radio-ulnar synostosis. *C.* Bowing of ulna, probably caused interference with growth on the side adjacent to radial absence. *D.* Radial deviation of unsupported hand. *Ulnar Absence or Hypoplasia: E.* Internal rotation of the humerus associated with hypersupination of the forearm. *F.* Radio-humeral dislocation. *G.* Radio-humeral synostosis. *H.* Ulnar deviation of the wrist.

gitudinal Absences. Discussion of correction of all of the deformities of placement are beyond the scope of this chapter, but the interested reader is referred to other sources.[7,20,42]

Focal Defects

There is still a controversy regarding the mechanism of formation of the focal defects. Some consider these a sequela of necrosis of the fetal mesenchyma tissue which develops into annular constricting bands or rings. If these constrictions are very deep, intra-uterine gangrene and true fetal amputation may take place. Subsequent "healing" results in fusion of the remaining parts forming acrosyndactyly or "secondary syndactyly."

Annular Constriction Bands, Grooves, or Rings

This anomaly consists of a circular band or groove in the skin of the limb or digit. The depth of the groove may vary from a rather superficial level or may interfere with circulation of the affected distal part of the limb. The presence of annular grooves alone does occur, but frequently there are associated anomalies involving the skeletal elements of the digits such as absence of distal phalanges, syndactyly, and fusion of adjacent bony elements (Fig. 3.23).

In shallow constriction, the correction is carried out primarily for appearance. In deeper grooves with interference of circulation, it is mandatory to remove the constriction and interdigitate the skin by multiple Z-plasty to prevent secondary scar contractures. It is less risky to treat only one half of the constriction, leaving the rest for another stage.

Duplications

Experimentally, duplication of a limb can be produced by cutting off part of the fetal limb bud and replacing it with 90 degrees of rotation. In man it is

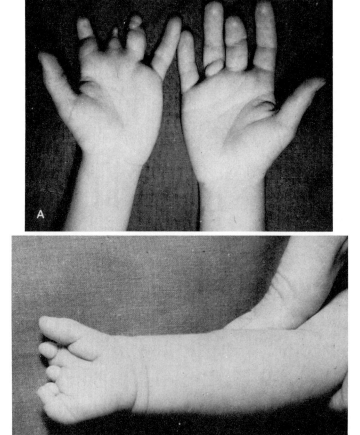

Figure 3.23. Annular constriction bands and grooves. *A.* Bilateral grooving in fingers of 10-year-old girl. Left long finger appears to be "amputated." *B.* Annular rings on four fingers of the right hand of one-year-old male.

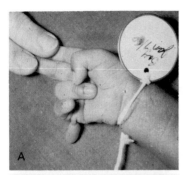

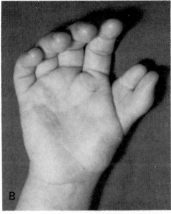

Figure 3.24. Polydactyly. *A*. Right hand of newborn boy showing a supranumerary appendage. *B*. Right hand of four-year-old girl with duplication of some elements of the thumb. There is only one metacarpal. The ulnar thumb was amputated.

thought to be caused by some insult to the fetal limb bud in the very early stages of development.

Polydactyly

This anomaly is inherited, but may appear as part of complex congenital deformities. It is often referred to as duplication of parts of digits or of an entire digit. The supranumerary digit frequently occurs on either the ulnar or radial side of the hand and may have independent tendons. The supranumerary fingers may articulate with the metacarpal of the normal finger or thumb, and it is sometimes difficult to decide which of the components is to be discarded. The condition may be bilateral.

Surgical correction is relatively simple if a digit is anatomically distinct (Fig. 3.24). In polydactyly where a common metacarpal is shared or where there is intermingling of vessels and tendons, careful judgment has to be exercised in order to give good function to the remaining part without imbalance. In some of our patients secondary wedging of bones in the "normal" remaining finger was required to attain correct alignment.

Mirror Hand (Ulnar Duplication)

This type of deformity is associated with seven or eight digits in addition to duplication of carpal elements and the presence of two complete ulnas (Fig. 3.26).In spite of multiplicity of fingers, these patients have no pinch or grasp since none of the fingers can oppose each other. The reconstruction in this case in our series was carried out when the child, then eight years of age, presented himself for treatment, but it should be started earlier. The second digit of the ulnar component on the radial side was selected for "pol-

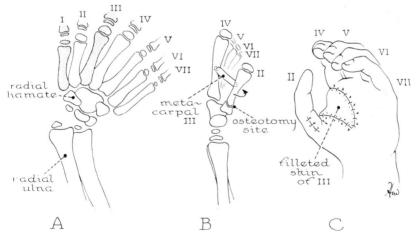

Figure 3.25. Ulnar duplication. *A*. Diagrammatic representation of the x-ray of ulnar duplication showing the seven digits and fusion of the two capitate and two lunate bones. In reconstruction, digits I and III were discarded. The second digit was retained for pollicization. *B*. Pollicization of the second digit. The proper position was attained through osteotomy at the base and stabilization of the pollicized finger with the bone graft utilizing the metacarpal of the ablated third finger. *C*. The filleted skin of the third digit was used as a flap to cover the space created by pollicization. The fourth, fifth, sixth, and seventh digits were retained. (Modified after Entin: Journal of Bone and Joint Surgery, *41-A:* 692, 1958.)

licization''; the two fingers on either side of it were discarded, but filleted skin of one of these fingers was utilized as a flap to cover the newly created web space (Fig. 3.25). This procedure permitted efficient pinching and grasping but did not correct the radial deviation of the hand (Fig. 3.26). Arthrodesis of the wrist was deferred until 12 years of age, and improved the alignment.

Overgrowth

The gigantism may affect the entire limb and involves the skeletal elements as well as all the soft tissue. The digital overgrowth (macrodactyly) may affect any digit but is usually associated with excess of fat or excessive development of neural elements, vessels, and lymphatics.

The correction of the gigantism is by two methods: one is destruction of the epiphyses to check growth;

the other is by ablation of parts of the skeletal, soft tissue, and skin elements.[3,48] Several stages are required and some deformities may defy reconstruction and end up in amputation of the part in order to salvage the rest of the limb. One of our patients whose gigantic thumb brought him in for treatment showed at operation skeletal gigantism as well as massive ''hypertrophy'' of the neurovascular elements which defied excision. The correction was done in stages (Fig. 3.27).

General Disorders

This group includes congenital malformations of the upper limb in association with systemic or generalized skeletal defects. This group includes a number of conditions such as *dyschondroplasia; achondroplasia, arochnodactyly;* and numerous others. Consideration of these conditions is beyond

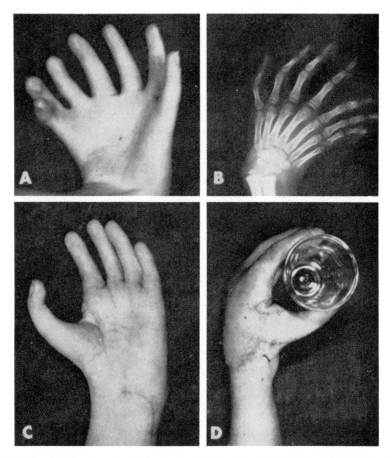

Figure 3.26. Ulnar duplication. *A.* Photograph of the left hand of eight-year-old boy showing seven digits. The central digit corresponds to the index finger. Two sets of ulnar components are present on either side of the central index finger. *B.* X-ray of the hand shown in *A. C.* Photograph of the same hand shown six months after reconstruction by the procedures illustrated in Figure 3.25. Muscle transfer of flexor carpi ulnaris to the common extensors of the digits improved extension. *D.* Same hand showing grasping motion. (Reproduced from Surgical Clinics of North America, *40:* 497, 1960.)

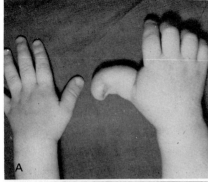
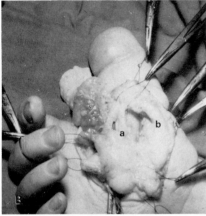

Figure 3.27. Overgrowth. *A.* Right thumb of three-year-old boy showing moderate gigantism. *B.* Same as *A,* showing the large size of neurovascular elements. The proper digital nerves (*a* and *b*) come out of a large mass of nerve tissue.

the scope of this subject, but they are simply enumerated for completion.

SUMMARY

In order to crystallize the reconstructive needs, the congenital absences and deformities were classified on the basis of the developmental and anatomic manifestation. In complex deformities, the reconstructive procedures entailed stabilization of parts by bone graft and bone fusion, grafting of the free joints, shifting of local and distal skin, and muscle transfer to give motion to newly constructed parts. In several patients, the specific procedures were described in detail in order to illustrate the complexities of the reconstructive phases and to stress the individual needs.

Because of the dynamic alteration with continuous growth, even if successful reconstruction is achieved in the patient's early years, subsequent recurrence of the deformity may take place. Consequently, constant vigilance is required during the growth period to correct recurrence of the deformity owing to unequal

growth of parts or to inherent imbalance of muscle action.

The complexities of many of the congenital anomalies make it impractical to attempt the restoration of normal appearance and function of the limb which, ordinarily, is the ideal aim of reconstruction. Consequently the practical goal is to attain the relatively greatest function with the least number of surgical procedures.

Although many new procedures have been developed which have found ready application in reconstruction of these congenital anomalies, certain of them still defy the ingenuity of the surgeon. This difficult field of reconstructive surgery still poses a challenge to the skill, patience, and imagination of the surgeon.

REFERENCES

1. Barsky, A. J. *Congenital Anomalies of the Hand and Their Surgical Treatment.* Springfield, Charles C Thomas, 1958.
2. Barsky, A. J. Cleft Hand: Classification, incidence and treatment. Review of literature and report of 19 cases. J. Bone Joint Surg., *46-A:* 1707, 1964.
3. Barsky, A. J. Macrodactyly. J. Bone Joint Surg., *49-A:* 1255, 1967.
4. Bauer, T. B., Tondra, J. M., and Trusler, H. M. Technical modification in repair of syndactylism. Plast. Reconstr. Surg., *17:* 385, 1956.
5. Birch-Jensen, A. *Congenital Deformities of the Upper Extremities.* Copenhagen, Munksgaard, 1950.
6. Bora, F. W., Jr., Nicholson, J. T., and Cheema, H. M. Radial meromelia: The deformity and its treatment. J. Bone Joint Surg., *52-A:* 966, 1970.
7. Boyes, J. H. *Bunnell's Surgery of the Hand,* Ed. 5. Philadelphia, Lippincott, 1970.
8. Brown, J. B., and McDowell, F. Syndactylism with absence of the pectoralis major. Surgery, *7:* 599, 1940.
9. Buck-Gramcko, D. Pollicization of the index finger: Method and results in aplasia and hypoplasia of the thumb. J. Bone Joint Surg., *53-A:* 1605, 1971.
10. Bunnell, S. Digital transfer by neurovascular pedicle. J. Bone Joint Surg., *34-A:* 772, 1952. (Also see Boyes, J. H.)
11. Clarkson, P. Poland's syndactyly. Guy's Hosp. Rep., *111:* 335, 1962.
12. Drinkwater, H. Phalangeal anarthrosis (synostosis ankylosis) transmitted through fourteen generations. Proc. R. Soc. Med., *10:* 60, 1916-17.
13. Entin, M. A., and Petrie, J. G. Reconstruction of congenital absence of the radius. In *Transactious International Society of* Plastic Surgeons. Baltimore, Williams & Wilkins, 1957, p. 448.
14. Entin, M. A. Reconstruction of congenital abnormalities of the upper extremities. J. Bone Joint Surg., *41-A:* 681, 1959.
15. Entin, M. A. Congenital anomalies of the upper extremity. Surg. Clin. North Am., *40:* 497, 1960.
16. Entin, M. A. Reconstruction of congenital aplasia of radial component. Surg. Clin. North Am., *44:* 1091, 1964.
17. Entin, M. A. Reconstruction of congenital aplasia of

phalanges in the hand. Surg. Clin. North Am., *48:* 1155, 1968.

18. Entin, M. A., Barsky, A. J., and Swanson, A. B. Report of the Committee of American Society for Surgery of the Hand on Classification of Congenital Malformations of Hand and Upper Extremities.

19. Entin, M. A., Daniel, G., and Kahn, D. Transplantation of autogenous half-joints. Arch. Surg., *96:* 359, 1968.

20. Entin, M. A. Malformation of the hand associated with the elbow, forearm and wrist. In *The hand,* Edited by R. Tubiana. Philadelphia, Saunders, to be published.

21. Epstein, L. I., and Bennett, J. E. Syndactyly with ipsilateral chest deformity. Plast. Reconstr. Surg., *46:* 236, 1970.

22. Flatt, A.E. A test of classification of congenital anomalies of the upper extremity. Surg. Clin. North Am., *50:* 509, 1970.

23. Frantz, C. H., and O'Rahilly, R. Congenital skeletal limb deficiencies. J. Bone Joint Surg., *43-A:* 1202, 1961.

24. Fraser, F. C. Causes of congenital malformations in human beings. J. Chronic Dis., *10:* 97, 1959.

25. Goldstein, R. Hypoplastic anaemia with multiple congenital anomalies. Am. J. Dis. Child., *89:* 618, 1955.

26. Gosset, J. La pollicisation de l'index (technique chirurgicale). J. Chir., *65:* 403, 1949.

27. Hoover, G. H., Flatt, A. E., and Weiss, M. W. The hand and Apert's syndrome. J. Bone Joint Surg., *52-A:* 878, 1970.

28. Ingalls, T. H. Mechanisms of congenital malformations. In *Proceedings Second Scientific Conference of the Association for the Aid of Crippled Children.* New York, 1954.

29. Jones, G. B. Delta phalanx. J. Bone Joint Surg., *46-B:* 226, 1964.

30. Littler, J. W. The neurovascular pedicle method of digital transposition for reconstruction of the thumb. Plast. Reconstr. Surg., *12:* 303, 1953.

31. Littler, J. W. Principle of reconstructive surgery of the hand. In *Reconstructive Plastic Surgery,* edited by J. M. Converse, Philadelphia, Saunders, 1964, p. 54.

32. Losch, G. M., and Duncker, H-S. Anatomy and surgical treatment of syndactylism. Plast. Reconstr. Surg., *50:* 167, 1972.

33. Nitsche, F., and Armknecht, P. Orthopodische Leiden bei Zeillingen. Z. Orthop. Chir., *58:* 518, 1933.

34. Patterson, I. J. S. Congenital deformities of the hand. Ann. R. Coll. Surg. Engl., *25:* 306, 1959.

35. Patterson, T. J. S. Congenital deformities. Postgrad.

Med. J., *40:* 275, 1964.

36. Riordan, D. C. Congenital absence of the radius. J. Bone Joint Surg., *37-A:* 1129, 1955.

37. Riordan, D. C. Congenital absence of the radius. A fifteen-year follow-up. Proceedings of the American Orthopaedic Association. J. Bone Joint Surg., *45-A:* 1783, 1963.

38. Skerik, S., and Flatt, A. E. The anatomy of congenital radial dysplasia. Clin. Orthop., *66:* 125, 1969.

39. Skoog, T. Syndactyly: A clinical report on repair. Acta Chir. Scand., *130:* 537, 1965.

40. Smith, R. J., and Kaplan, E. Camptodactyly and similar atraumatic flexion deformities of the proximal interphalangeal joints of the fingers. J. Bone Joint Surg., *50-A:* 1187, 1968.

41. Starr, D. E. Congenital absence of the radius: A method of surgical correction. J. Bone Joint Surg., *27:* 527, 1945.

42. Straub, L. R. Congenital absence of the ulna. Am. J. Surg., *109:* 300, 1965.

43. Straub, L. R. Personal communication (Orthopaedic Travelling Club, 1969, Montreal, Canada).

44. Swanson, A. B. A classification for congenital malformations of the hand. N. J. Bull. Acad. Med., *10:* 166, 1964.

45. Swanson, A. B., Barsky, A. J., and Entin, M. A. Classification of limb malformations on the basis of embryological failures. Surg. Clin. North Am., *48:* 1169, 1968.

46. Sullivan, F. M. Mechanism of action of teratogenic drugs. Proc. R. Soc. Med., *63:* 1252, 1970.

47. Torpin, R., and Faulkner, A. Intrauterine amputation with the missing member found in the fetal membranes. J.A.M.A., *198:* 185, 1966.

48. Tsuge, K. Treatment of macrodactyly. Plast. Reconstr. Surg., *39:* 590, 1967.

49. Warkany, J. Factors in etiology of congenital malformations. Am. J. Ment. Defic., *50:* 231, 1945.

50. Watson, H. K., and Boyes, J. H. Congenital angular deformity of the digits: Delta phalanx. J. Bone Joint Surg., *49-A:* 333, 1967.

51. Weckesser, E. C., Reed, J. R., and Heiple, K. G. Congenital clasped thumb (congenital flexion adduction deformity of the thumb). J. Bone Joint Surg., *50-A:* 1417, 1968.

52. Weeks, P. M. Surgical correction of upper extremity deformities in arthrogryposis. Plast. Reconstr. Surg., *36:* 459, 1965.

53. Woodward, J. W. Congenital elevation of scapula and paralysis of serratus magnus muscle. J. Bone Joint Surg., *43-A:* 219, 1961.

chapter four

Anesthesia for Hand Surgery

Leroy D. Vandam, M.D.

The general principles of anesthesia for operation on the hand differ in no way from those involving other areas of the body. A basic tenet in anesthesia, however, is that the best anesthetic is given only when problems of patient and surgeon are clearly in mind. From this standpoint, therefore, anesthesia for hand surgery is specialized, and the inexperienced anesthetist should attempt to gain some knowledge of surgical problems met in this area. This discussion is directed both toward the surgeon and anesthetist so that each may understand the other's problems.

THE PATIENT AND THE PROBLEM

Compared to surgery on the leg, operations on the arm are more exacting and the outcome probably of greater consequence to the patient. Hand surgery is more often an emergency than most any other kind, owing to trauma, burns, or infection. This brings to the operating room an apprehensive patient, often with a full stomach or in a state of shock brought on by pain, blood loss, and realization of the consequences of his injury. It is said that approximately 70 per cent of all injuries result in some kind of permanent disability of the hand.

Other areas of the body may be involved either as part of the initial trauma or in the use of skin and bone grafts. When general anesthesia is used, it must be remembered that a secure dressing or plaster cast may be needed at the termination of the procedure to protect suture lines or structures under tension. The patient must lie still and emerge from anesthesia without excitement. This aspect alone speaks highly in favor of regional anesthesia.

Use of electric cautery calls for selection of nonflammable anesthetics. On the other hand, flammable anesthetics may be used if the patient's condition or the limited experience of the anesthetist requires such use. It is considered safe to give a flammable anesthetic with a tight seal about the face, beyond a two-foot radius of the source of ignition.[12]

GENERAL ANESTHESIA

The longer the time involved and the more complex a procedure, the more the indication for general anes-

thesia. General anesthesia is given whenever regional anesthesia is unsuitable for the patient: the very young; the agitated psychotic or alcoholic; the spastic; or in the presence of extreme anxiety. Simultaneous operation on other parts of the body is an additional indication for general anesthesia.

The ambulatory patient may be given a brief general anesthetic if he appears at the hospital having fasted for at least six hours, in time for a physical examination, laboratory work, and preanesthetic medication. Recovery should take place under supervision.

The inpatient is brought into the best possible condition for anesthesia. If general anesthesia is elected, therefore, a tracheal tube with an inflatable cuff is introduced beforehand under topical anesthesia. When the patient cannot cooperate, rapid induction of general anesthesia with intravenous agents is utilized.

REGIONAL ANESTHESIA

Regional anesthesia is economical and the equipment required minimal. In complicated tendon and nerve injury an important feature of regional anesthesia is the patient's ability to move a particular muscle and its tendon so that it may be matched with the severed distal portion.

Reasons why regional anesthesia is not more widely used are as follows: (1) lack of patient acceptance and the wish to be unconscious during operations; (2) it is impractical to anesthetize some areas of the body, radical mastectomy for example. This reservation need not apply to operations on the arm or hand but a factor when other areas of the body must be anesthetized simultaneously; (3) insufficient duration of anesthesia feared by patient and surgeon alike; (4) previous unsatisfactory local anesthesia or sensitivity reaction is often a deterrent.

PHARMACOLOGY OF LOCAL ANESTHETICS

Theories of Action

Local anesthetics interfere with the initiation and transmission of the nerve impulse. Theory holds that the local anesthetics prevent depolarization of the nerve membrane that results in propagation of the impulse, through interference with exchange of sodium and potassium ions across the nerve membrane. As a consequence, a negative electrical potential necessary for a propagated discharge does not develop.

The Local Anesthetics

Although many local anesthetics are available, the surgeon or anesthetist need be familiar with only a few, using only those drugs that have passed the test of time. Criteria of an acceptable local anesthetic are: complete reversibility of action, freedom from local irritation and systemic toxicity in the therapeutic range, appropriate onset and duration of action, ease of sterilization without loss of activity, a readily synthesized compound, and low cost.

Ester Compounds.

Procaine hydrochloride (Novocain), an ester of diethylaminoethanol and p-aminobenzoic acid, lacks topical activity but is still a widely used local anesthetic. The basic portion of the ester is a tertiary amino-alcohol that combines with hydrochloric acid to form a soluble salt with a weakly acidic reaction. Procaine is injected in concentration from 0.5 to 5 per cent for any kind of anesthetic procedure ranging from infiltration of skin to spinal subarachnoid block.

Halogen substitution in the aromatic portion of the procaine molecule yields substances that are rapidly hydrolyzed in plasma, therefore less toxic than the parent compound. Chloroprocaine (Nesacaine), one such compound, is not topically active but more potent and shorter in duration of action than procaine. It is probably the safest local anesthetic from the standpoint of systemic toxicity. Concentrations employed for injection range from 0.5 to 1 per cent in doses not exceeding 1 gm.

Tetracaine (Pontocaine) has a potency and duration of action greater than the other anesthetics mentioned, but systemic toxicity is correspondingly higher. Tetracaine is used in 0.1 per cent concentration for injection when the duration of anesthesia required is longer than several hours.

Nonester Compounds

Lidocaine hydrochloride (Xylocaine), an acetanilide derivative, has achieved widespread acceptance since its introduction in 1948. Major advantages are rapid onset of anesthesia and freedom from local irritation. Lidocaine because of its nonester structure is detoxified in the circulating plasma slowly, if at all. For this reason, the drug is considered twice as toxic as procaine, and dosages larger than 0.5 gm should not be used when the recommended 0.5 to 2 per cent concentrations are employed for injection.

Mepivacaine hydrochloride (Carbocaine) is an amide with the amide radical linked to a saturated heterocyclic ring in a piperidine group. Concentrations used range from 0.5 to 4 per cent for injection or topical anesthesia. Untoward reactions reported thus far have been few.

Bupivacaine (Marcaine) hydrochloride was synthesized in 1957 by Ekenstam, since used extensively abroad. The compound, an anilide derivative, differs from mepivacaine in that a butyl group is substituted for a methyl in the molecule. More potent and with a markedly longer action than lidocaine or mepivacaine, probably as a result of increased protein-binding, the drug is used in concentrations ranging from 0.25 to 0.75 per cent for the complete span of regional nerve blocks. Epinephrine in 1:200,000 concentration is added to the solution when indicated; total amount of drug injected at a time should not exceed 200 to 500 mg, as toxicity approximates that of tetracaine.

Long Acting Local Anesthetics

In the treatment of postoperative pain and management of intractable pain, there is need for a local anesthetic with a duration of action longer than six to eight hours, the maximum obtainable with currently available substances. The long lasting effects of certain compounds do not represent true anesthesia; histologic examination after injection of these compounds has revealed destruction of fine nerve fibers.[5]

Suspensions of local anesthetics in oil are thought to act as repositories from which the anesthetic is gradually released, thereby prolonging the effect. Prolongation of anesthesia, however, has not been demonstrated by such means.

Reactions to Local Anesthetics

Untoward reaction to local anesthetics are categorized as follows: (1) those owing to absorption of the anesthetic into the circulation; (2) those due to local tissue destruction; (3) true allergic reactions. Reactions are often erroneously ascribed to sensitivity or idiosyncrasy whereas they can be explained on pharmacologic grounds, even though exceedingly small doses may have been responsible for the effects observed.

Systemic Reactions

Systemic reactions result from absorption of drug into the blood stream in sufficient quantity to produce convulsions or loss of consciousness. The depressant effect on the medullary centers may lead to apnea and vascular collapse. It is not generally appreciated that local anesthetics can depress the myocardium directly by a quinidine like effect on conduction, contractility, and irritability. For this reason procaine and lidocaine have been employed as anti-arrhythmic agents. The effect on the myocardium resulting in hypotension or cardiac standstill, is enhanced by the peripheral vasodilating actions of these drugs. All these untoward effects can occur rapidly in response to injection of much less than the expected toxic dose. The most feared outcome is cardiac arrest.

As the blood level of local anesthetic is the primary factor in systemic reactions, site of injection is important in rapidity of absorption. The intravenous route is the most dangerous but absorption from pharyngeal, tracheal, and bronchial mucosa produces high blood concentrations almost as rapidly. Rapid absorption from the lungs and direct circulation of drug to the myocardium result in depression. Thus most reported cases of sudden cardiovascular collapse have involved topical application of anesthetics to the respiratory tract. Other hazardous sites are the head, neck, and paravertebral region. Least dangerous are subcutaneous tissues of the trunk and limbs.

A second factor in causation of reactions is the rapidity of hydrolysis, once an anesthetic reaches the circulation. The enzymes responsible for hydrolysis are pseudocholinesterases formed in the liver.

Prevention of Systemic Reactions.

In view of the causative factors noted, the least quantity of anesthetic should be utilized for a procedure. Total amount of drug injected is more significant than cocentration or volume.

Rate of absorption should be slowed as much as possible. This can be accomplished by slow injection and repeated aspiration for blood to avoid intravascular injection. However, the vascoconstrictive property of epinephrine added to the anesthetic provides greater assurance against rapid absorption. Additional benefits are prolongation of anesthesia and decrease in bleeding. Peak prolongation of anesthesia and maximal decrease in absorption are achieved with 1:200,000 to 1:300,000 concentrations, 0.5 and 0.3 mg of epinephrine per 100 ml, respectively.[9] These quantities should be measured with a calibrated syringe rather than added to the anesthetic solution according to the number of drops.

Only the most effective and least harmful concentrations of epinephrine should be employed, as the drug is toxic in its own right.

Pre-anesthetic administration of a short acting barbiturate, secobarbital (Seconal), or pentobarbital (Nembutal) in sedative doses is generally believed to protect against the central stimulating or convulsive properties of local anesthetics. Experimental evidence suggests that full narcotic rather than sedative doses of the barbiturate are required to prevent convulsions. This is not meant to imply that the barbiturates should not be used in the treatment of this kind of reaction. A more useful drug as a preventive is diazepam (Valium) in 5 to 10 mg dosage intravenously or intramuscularly.

Treatment of Systemic Reactions.

Intravenous injection of a short acting barbiturate, thiopental sodium (Pentothal Sodium) or thiamylal (Surital), is the treatment of choice for incipient or fully developed convulsions. Some suggest that succinylcholine (Anectine) be used because of its paralyzing effect, but artificial respiration must be employed until spontaneous respiration resumes. Hazards of a convulsion are: cerebral hypoxia, body injury, aspiration of vomitus, and postictal respiratory and circulatory arrest consequent to anoxia. Therefore, oxygen should be administered by mask simultaneously with injection of a barbiturate or diazepam.

Circulatory depression is treated with a vasopressor

drug intravenously or intramuscularly as the situation warrants. For this purpose single dose ampuls of ephedrine or phenylephrine (Neosynephrine) are used. If cardiac arrest is suspected external manual cardiac systole may restore the circulation.

It is obvious that treatment of cardiovascular and respiratory depression requires knowledge of the principles of resuscitation. Every physician should be able to perform mouth-to-mouth breathing.

Local Irritation and Tissue Destruction.

A number of local anesthetics have been introduced to practice before appropriate tests were made to detect tissue destructive properties. Anesthetics mentioned in this chapter are safe from this standpoint.

Allergic Reactions.

True allergic reactions to the local anesthetics have been reported from time to time. Dermatitis after repeated exposure to local anesthetics occurs not uncommonly in professional personnel.

REGIONAL NERVE BLOCK

The Brachial Plexus

Surgery of the hand extends from the elbow downward, occasionally in reconstructive surgery involving the entire arm. The unique aspect of regional anesthesia for the arm is that only the nerves of the brachial plexus are involved and these nerves are readily accessible to local anesthetic injection. In addition to the performance of nerve block, knowledge of the brachial plexus carries additional significance. Tourniquet injury usually results from application of excessive pressure.[6, 10]

General Anatomy

Arising from several roots, the nerves of the brachial plexus join briefly, and are ultimately reformed and routed to their respective end organs. A further impediment is the overlapping of dermatomes as five spinal nerves have sensory representation in the hand (Fig. 4.1).[7] The plexus of the upper extremity differs

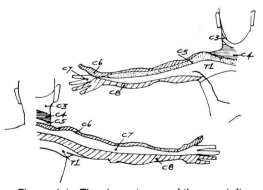

Figure 4.1. The dermatomes of the arm (after Keegan[7]).

from that of the lower extremity in that it innervates an extremely mobile limb and participates in movements of the shoulder. This mobility and relatively superficial location account for the vulnerability as well as the accessibility of the plexus to nerve block.

Anatomic Relationships

The brachial plexus is formed chiefly from the anterior rami of the lower four cervical and the first thoracic nerves (Fig. 4.2). At the base of the transverse processes of the cervical vertebrae, the nerves lie posterior to the vertebral artery coursing through the cervical foramina. The nerves are invested in meningeal sheaths which extend the subarachnoid space beyond the foramina. Therefore, bleeding may take place or subarachnoid puncture occur when injections are made at the transverse processes.

Beyond the transverse processes, the nerves lie between the anterior and middle scalene muscles. It is necessary, therefore, in the differential diagnosis of neurovascular syndromes of the arm to consider the possibility of herniated intervertebral disc, cervical rib, cervical osteoarthritis, or cord tumor.

The nerves of the plexus divide between the scalene muscles into trunks, cords, and divisions, receive fascial investment and are in proximity to pleura, second portion of the subclavian artery and first rib. The fascia surrounding the plexus is formed by condensation of connective tissue. Thus the brachial plexus with the subclavian artery is enveloped in fascia which extends toward the axilla forming a compartment into which anesthetic solution may be injected.

The cupola of the pleura rises amidst the scalene muscles to the level of the neck of the first rib posteriorly. Since the first rib slants downward, forward and medially, the pleura protrudes from 3 to 6 cm above the rib anteriorly, and from 1 to 4 cm above the clavicle. In the supraclavicular approach to injection of the brachial plexus where the first rib is sought as a landmark, pneumothorax is a not infrequent complication. The subclavian artery and vein course over the first rib, the artery lying between the scalene muscles in the subclavian groove close to the lower nerves of the brachial plexus, the vein anteriorly, separated from the other structures by the anterior scalene muscle. Puncture of the artery is not uncommon in supraclavicular block.

Formation of the Plexus

A schema of the plexus without reference to trunks and divisions is presented here. The cords of the plexus are designated according to their relationship to the axial artery of the limb (Fig. 4.3). The term "medial" implies a position anteromedial to the axillary artery, "lateral" means anterolateral to the artery, and posterior is self explanatory.

1. The anterior primary divisions are derived from the fifth, sixth, seventh, and eighth cervical and the first thoracic nerves.

2. All five nerves contribute to formation of the posterior cord and the terminations of the posterior cord are the axillary and radial nerves.

3. Cervical nerves five, six, and seven, the upper three, contribute to the lateral cord, and the terminals are the musculocutaneous nerve and lateral division of the median nerve. The musculocutaneous nerve supplies muscles in the arm and cutaneous structures of the forearm.

4. Cervical nerve eight and thoracic one, the lower two, contribute to the medial cord, the terminals being the ulnar nerve and the medial component of the median nerve. The medial component crosses the axillary artery to join the lateral component; ultimately the median nerve lies medial to the brachial artery at the elbow.

A number of nonplexiform nerves are associated wit the brachial plexus.

1. Sympathetic nerves. An important relationship is the proximity of the cervical sympathetic chain to the anterior tubercles of the transverse processes, with

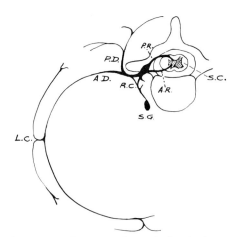

Figure 4.2. Diagram of a typical spinal nerve. *S.C.*, spinal cord; *A.D.*, anterior division; *P.D.*, posterior division; *R.C.*, rami communicantes; *S.G.*, sympathetic ganglion; *L.C.*, lateral cutaneous nerve; *A.R.*, anterior root; *P.R.*, posterior root.

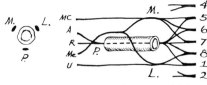

Figure 4.3. Formation of the brachial plexus. The lateral *(L.)*, medial *(M.)*, and posterior *(P.)*, cords of the plexus are shown in relation to the axillary artery of the limb. The contributing nerves are indicated by *numerals*. *M.C.*, musculocutaneos nerve; *A.*, axillary nerve; *R.*, radial nerve; *Me.*, median nerve; and *U.*, ulnar nerve.

gray rami communicants from sympathetic ganglia passing to each cervical nerve. Block of cervical nerves therefore interrupts sympathetic impulses; thus brachial plexus block results in sympathetic block.

2. The phrenic nerve receives its chief fibers from the fourth cervical with lesser contributions from the third and fifth cervical nerves. Occasionally, the phrenic nerve is given off by the nerve to the subclavius muscle. Because of its origin and course, phrenic nerve paralysis is not uncommon during brachial plexus block performed via the supraclavicular route.[14]

3. The suprascapular nerve with contributions from the fifth and sixth cervical nerves is of importance in shoulder pain supplying structures in and about the shoulder joint. Suprascapular nerve block for relief of pain is performed with relative ease.

Function and Innervation of Brachial Musculature

In Table 4.1 a classification according to function of the arm with their innervation is presented.

APPROACH TO REGIONAL ANESTHESIA

A patient scheduled for nerve block should refrain from eating or take an easily digestible meal at least four hours before the procedure to avoid vomiting. An anesthesia machine with oxygen and other resuscitative equipment is at hand for emergency use and for supplementary general anesthesia when necessary. For major procedures, an intravenous infusion is started.

The patient is recumbent at the time of injection, the skin prepared with an antiseptic that does not stain clothing or bedding. Although freshly prepared solutions of local anesthetics are the most reliable, the physician does best to employ sterilized single dose ampuls of drugs. The quantity of anesthetic injected is calculated in advance, keeping below the toxic dose. This is done by selecting the minimal effective concentration and injecting at a point where maximal anesthetic effect is obtained.

Upon completion of a procedure performed under local anesthesia the patient is observed for some time to detect delayed complications. If an untoward reaction to the anesthetic has been observed, the patient is fully informed so that repetition can be avoided. Finally, a record of the procedure must be kept as protection both for patient and physician.

Some of the equipment required for nerve block is shown diagrammatically in Figure 4.4. A tray containing this equipment, suitably wrapped, is autoclaved and stored before use, without possibility of contami-

TABLE 4.1
*The muscles of the upper extremity**

The brachial plexus supplies all the muscles that move the upper extremity except the levator scapulae, the trapezius, and sternomastoid. Muscles of the upper extremity may be classified into two functional groups.

Flexors	Extensors
Flexors (strict sense)	Extensors (strict sense)
Adductors	Abductors
Pronators	Supinators

Exceptions: Adduction and abduction in the hand refer to movement away from and toward a midaxis. This runs from the head of the radius through the middle digit. Therefore, at the wrist there is both radial and ulnar abduction (also true for the middle digit).

Wrist abduction is accomplished by synergistic action of flexors and extensors, while finer finger movements are largely accomplished by intrinsic hand muscles.

The biceps muscle (fundamentally a flexor) is a powerful supinator. The brachioradialis in man, although in relation to and supplied by extensor nerves, brings the forearm into a position midway between pronation and supination, either by partially supinating or by partially pronating, then acting as a weak flexor of the elbow.

Motor Nerve Supply of the Upper Extremeity

All muscles of the flexor group are supplied by the lateral and medial cords of the brachial plexus (anterolateral and anteromedial to the artery).

All muscles of the extensor group are supplied by the posterior cord of the brachial plexus (posterior to the artery).

All long muscles arising from the ulnar epicondyle of the humerus or immediately distally (ulnar-volar group, i.e., flexors), are supplied by the median nerve.

Exception: the flexor carpi ulnaris and those portions of the flexor digitorum profundus going to digits (three), four and five.

All long muscles arising from the radial epicondyle of the humerus or immediately distally (the radiodorsal group, i.e., extensors), are supplied by the radial (musculospiral) nerve. There are no short extensor muscles in the hand.

In the hand the nerve supply does not follow the general rule. All short muscles of the ball of the thumb are activated by the median nerve. All remaining short muscles of the hand are activated by the ulnar nerve.

Exceptions: the lumbrical muscles (actually parts of the deep flexor muscle) have the same nerve supply as the flexor profundus, *i.e.,* for digits two, (three), median nerve, for digits (three), four, and five ulnar nerve. The nerve supply of the flexor pollicis brevis may be either from the median nerve or from ulnar nerve or both.

*Courtesy of Oscar V. Batson, M.D.

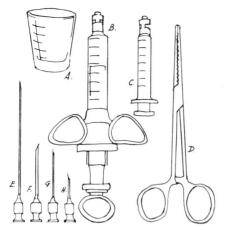

Figure 4.4. Some of the equipment required for nerve block. *A*, medicine glass; *B*, 10-ml Luer-Lok syringe; *C*, 2-ml syinge; *D*, Kelly forceps for sponges and skin preparation; *E, F, G,* and *H,* needles of various size.

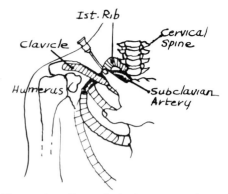

Figure 4.5. Supraclavicular approach to the brachial plexus. Index finger on the subslavian artery. (Reproduced with permission from R.D. Dripps, J. E. Eckenhoff, and L. D. Vandam. *Introduction to Anesthesia*. Philadelphia, Saunders, 1972.)

nation. Disposable nerve block trays are now commercially available.

NERVE BLOCKS OF THE ARM

Supraclavicular Block of the Brachial Plexus

Until resurgence of interest in the axillary approach to the brachial plexus block, the supraclavicular approach had been considered the least complicated and most reliable technique.

Supraclavicular block is made possible because of concentration of the nerves of the plexus within a circumscribed area, their relation to the first rib, and the site immediately posterior to the anterior scalene muscle. In a thin patient, muscle and rib are easily felt and pressure on the nerves produces paresthesias in the arm. The general direction of the plexus is envisioned as passing from the transverse processes of the lower four cervical vertebrae toward apex of the axilla. Usually the prominent pulsation of the second portion of the subclavian artery as it crosses the first rib can be used as a guide to the neurovascular bundle (Fig. 4.5). Additional landmarks are the midpoint of the clavicle or the external jugular vein.

The anesthetist stands at the side of the recumbent patient whose head is turned away, shoulder drawn downward. The area is prepared and draped so that all landmarks are visible. Depending upon dexterity, either hand may be employed for insertion of the needle, the shortest possible compatible with reaching the plexus; a 3/4-inch 23-gauge needle is usually satisfactory. A skin wheal is raised at a point 1 cm above the midpoint of the clavicle between acromial tip and sternoclavicular articulation, marking the lateral border of the first rib. To avoid puncturing the subclavian artery, the artery is depressed with the index finger of one hand while inserting the needle with the other just

above the fiingertip (Fig. 4.5). Direction of the needle is backward, inward, and downward. When paresthesias are elicited in the fingers, the anesthetic is injected slowly, usually 20 to 25 ml of a 1.5 to 2 per cent solution.

An important detail of this technique is instruction of the patient in reporting of paresthesias; these are described as "electric shock" or striking the "funny bone." If the rib is not reached at the expected depth, anywhere from 0.5 to 5 cm beneath the skin depending upon habitus of the patient, the needle is withdrawn to avoid entering pleura and direction altered. If the rib is touched, the plexus has already been passed. When contact is made with rib without paresthesias, the needle is reinserted and "walked" up and down the rib until paresthesias are obtained. If the latter cannot be elicited after repeated attempts, the zone between skin and rib is infiltrated in several planes: behind the artery, down to the first rib, and toward the transverse process of the sixth cervical vertebra.

An intracutaneous and subcutaneous wheal is then made in bracelet fashion about the upper arm to interrupt sensory fibers of the second and third thoracic nerves carried in the intercostobrachial nerve.

The most serious complication of supraclavicular nerve block is tension pneumothorax occurring in 1 to 3 per cent of blocks.[11] That pneumothorax develops gradually suggests slow escape of air from the lung rather than entrainment during injection. Symptoms comprise dyspnea and chest pain diagnosis made by physical examination, and x-ray of the chest. If the collection of air is small, it is allowed to absorb spontaneously; otherwise, closed underwater chest drainage is instituted. Phrenic nerve paralysis is found in approximately 25 per cent of cases, although causing no difficulty.[14] However, bilateral supraclavicular block should be avoided, particularly in the patient with serious pulmonary or cardiac disease. Horner's syndrome, recurrent laryngeal nerve paralysis, and hematoma may develop. In a small number of cases persistent subjective paresthesias and sensory deficit have been noted.[16]

Axillary Block of the Brachial Plexus

Principles of axillary block are the same as for supraclavicular injection. Either block suffices for anesthesia of hand, forearm, and distal two-thirds of the arm. Because of ease and accuracy of placement of the needle as well as minimal incidence of complications, axillary approach to the brachial plexus has largely replaced the supraclavicular approach. Additional advantages are that the block may be repeated during the course of a lengthy operation and a technique easily applied to the child or uncooperative patient.

The skin of the axilla is shaved and the arm abducted to 90° with the forearm flexed at a right angle, lying flat (Fig. 4.6). A tourniquet is placed just below the axilla to direct the local anesthetic toward the supraclavicular region. The operator stands at the patient's side with the axillary artery fixed between index and middle fingers of one hand. A skin wheal is raised high in the axilla, usually 1 to 3 cm above the insertion of the pectoralis major muscle. At this point the terminal nerves of the plexus have not yet begun to diverge from the artery. A 3/4-inch 23-gauge needle is inserted at a 45°-angle in the direction of the artery to enter the neurovascular sheath. A distinct impression of penetration of fascia may be experienced as well as production of paresthesias or perforation of the artery. The latter is of little moment when a small needle is used and immediately withdrawn. Pulsations transmitted to the needle are a good sign. In the original technique, injection of local anesthetic concentrations

of 1.5 to 2.0 per cent was made as follows: superior and lateral to the artery to anesthetize musculocutaneous and median nerves; superiorly and medially for ulnar nerve; and inferiorly and laterally for radial nerve. From 5 to 10 ml are injected in each area for a total volume of 30 to 40 ml. Recent observations suggest that mere injection of this volume of solution into the neurovascular sheath without repositioning of the needle results in successful block.

Complications of axillary block are limited essentially to minimal extravasation of blood in a small percentage of cases.

NERVE BLOCK AT THE ELBOW

There is usually little need to block radial, median, or ulnar nerve at the elbow because of ease of performance of axillary block, but occasionally elbow block may be necessary. Block at the elbow does not prevent pain when a forearm tourniquet is used. The techniques of Labat described here are commonly employed.[8]

Proper use of local anesthetics for peripheral nerve block entails precepts set forth by Burnham:[1-3] (1) complete anesthesia for more than the operative site to ensure that no part of the procedure shall cause pain; (2) painless injection as effected by small gauge needles and slow infiltration; (3) a bacteriologically safe site of injection; (4) use of minimal amount of solution to avoid compression of vascular and lymphatic tissue; and (5) avoidance of injection into nerves.

Median Nerve

Both median and radial nerves are approached on the arm where the crease is formed when the supinated forearm is held at a right angle (Fig. 4.7). The tendon of the biceps is palpated, pulsation of the brachial artery identified, and a skin wheal raised just medial to the artery for block of the median nerve. This point is

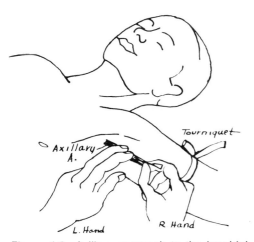

Figure 4.6. Axillary approach to the brachial plexus. The position of the hands and the axillary artery are shown. (Reproduced with permission from R. D. Dripps, J. E. Eckenhoff, and L. D. Vandam. *Introduction to Anesthesia.* Philadelphia, Saunders, 1972.)

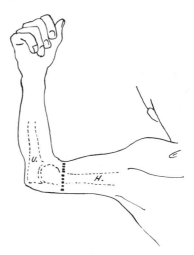

Figure 4.7. Site of injection for the median and radial nerves shown by the *dotted line H.,* humerus; *U,* ulna.

midway between the medial condyle of the humerus and medial border of the biceps. Occasionally the median nerve can be rolled beneath the finger. A 1-1/2-inch 23-gauge needle is inserted perpendicular to skin through deep fascia where a paresthesia may be produced. From 2 to 3 ml of a 2 per cent solution of anesthetic are injected or 5 ml introduced fanwise in the absence of paresthesia.

Radial Nerve

At the same level as for median nerve the needle for block of the radial nerve is inserted 1 cm lateral to the biceps tendon through deep fascia, in a direction toward the operator's index finger as it is held against the posterior surface of the lateral condyle of the humerus. The intermuscular septum is thereby penetrated between brachioradialis and brachialis muscles, about 10 cm above the lateral condyle in the axis of the humerus. The needle is advanced to bone, where 10 to 20 ml of solution are injected fanwise over a distance of 6 to 7 cm. It should be recalled that once the radial nerve has supplied the muscles arising from the lateral condyle, extensors, external rotators, and supinators, it is purely sensory to forearm and hand.

Ulnar Nerve

Block of the ulnar nerve at the elbow is easily performed because the nerve can be rolled beneath the fingers as it lies in the groove between medial condyle of the humerus and olecranon process of the ulna. The patient is positioned to lie on the opposite side with forearm extended, or supine with forearm flexed and the arm held across the chest. Injection is made about the nerve with a 3/4-inch 25-gauge needle inserted from above downward into the groove, the nerve held immobile between two fingers. Paresthesias are easily produced, and 1 to 2 ml of 2 per cent anesthetic solution injected.

For operation on the forearm, a bracelet injection of local anesthetic is made at the elbow to anesthetize the cutaneous nerves of the forearm.

NERVE BLOCK AT THE WRIST

Median Nerve

Satisfactory anesthesia for operation on the hand is had by block of nerves at the wrist. Block of the median nerve is made at a level corresponding to the tip of the styloid process of the ulna at a point between the tendons of the palmaris longus and flexor carpi radialis muscles (Fig. 4.8). The main part of the nerve lies beneath the volar fascia, either beneath or just to the radial side of the palmaris longus tendon. To identify the latter. the patient flexes his wrist against counterpressure, with fingers and thumb straight. A ⅝-inch 25-gauge needle is directed perpendicularly to a depth 0.5 cm below deep fascia where 1 to 2 ml of a 2 per cent solution of anesthetic are injected, when a paresthesia is obtained; if not, an additional 2 ml are injected fanwise.

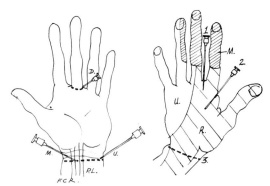

Figure 4.8. *Left*. Palmar surface of the hand. Needes at *M*. and *U*. show points of injection for the median and ulnar nerves, respectively. The *dotted line* is at the level of the styloid process of the ulna. Needle at *D*. shows site of injection for field block of finger. *F.C.R.*, flexor carpi radialis tendon; *P.L.*, palmaris longus tendon.
Right. Dorsum of the hand showing cutaneous distribution of the radial (*R*), ulnar (*U*), and median (*M*) nerves. Needles 1 and 2 indicate approaches to the interosseous spaces. The *dotted line* indicates bracelet injection for cutaneous nerves.

Ulnar Nerve

Ulnar nerve block at the wrist is performed at the same level as for median nerve (Fig. 4.8). With the hand supine, and the tendon of the flexor carpi ulnaris held between the fingers, the needle is inserted perpendicularly, tangential to the tendon beneath deep fascia, where injection is made as for median nerve. A good landmark is the ulnar artery with injection beneath fascia just lateral to it, then dorsally and subcutaneously with injection into subcutaneous fat to secure small branches of the nerve.

Radial Nerve

At the wrist, the radial nerve, now purely sensory, has diverged from the radial artery at the lower third of the forearm, turned dorsally and pierced deep fascia to supply cutaneous branches to wrist, dorsum of the hand and dorsum of the first, second, and third fingers (Fig. 4.8). Here at the same level as for block of median and ulnar nerves, a subcutaneous and intracutaneous bracelet will anesthetize not only the radial branches but other cutaneous nerves of the forearm extending into the proximal part of the palm. Specifically for radial nerve fibers, the radial artery is identified, skin penetrated over it, the needle then angled dorsally and parallel to skin with injection subcutaneously for the length of the needle.

HAND AND DIGITAL BLOCK

Commonly employed nerve blocks of the hand are largely of the field and infiltrative variety. It is best to inject via the dorsum of the hand rather than through the skin of the palm (Fig. 4.8). Injection should not be made into an infected area. It is important to avoid excessive distention of tissues and use of epinephrine, either of which may compromise circulation to the fingers.

The digits are anesthetized by subcutaneous infiltration bilaterally at the base of the finger (Fig. 4.8). Operations on the fifth finger, involving palm and metacarpal bone, can be performed with ulnar nerve block at the elbow or block at the wrist.

INTRAVENOUS REGIONAL ANESTHESIA

Intravenous injection of a local anesthetic to produce anesthesia in an extremity was introduced by Bier in 1908, reintroduced by Holmes in 1963. The method entails bloodless exsanguination of an extremity and injection of a finite amount of local anesthetic which is confined to the area by use of a tourniquet. Onset of anesthesia is prompt, probably relating to diffusion of the anesthetic to sensory nerve endings, in part to pressure of the tourniquet on large nerve fibers.

For operations on the hand or wrist a pneumatic tourniquet is applied to the forearm; for operations above this level the tourniquet is applied to the arm. Initially the tourniquet is inflated just above venous pressure to permit venipuncture close to the site of operation, with a small scalp vein needle or catheter, small syringe attached. The tourniquet is released to permit exsanguination of the part by elevation above venous pressure, by use of an Esmarch bandage. The tourniquet is then inflated about 100 mm Hg above the level of systolic blood pressure. With the part positioned for operation, injection of local anesthetic is made, usually a 0.5 per cent solution, after prior flushing of plastic tubing and needle with saline. Lidocaine is the current choice, a 0.5 per cent solution in a dose range from 1.5 to 3.0 mg/kg. For a 60 kg subject, the volume ranges from 20 to 40 ml, the amount adjusted for muscle mass. While a larger dose affords effective anesthesia more consistently, the incidence of toxic reactions is higher upon termination of anesthesia.

Intravenous regional anesthesia is employed largely for minor operations on the arm where the procedure lasts less than an hour or two at most. The time limitation is imposed by onset of tourniquet pain and concern over damage to nerves after prolonged application of the tourniquet. At termination of anesthesia, toxic reactions to the local anesthetic run the gamut from lightheadiness, mild degrees of hypotension and syncope through muscle twitching, generalized seizures, and cardiac arrest. Although largely preventable, the anesthetist must be prepared to treat those occurrances by the recommended means.

SYMPATHETIC NERVE BLOCK

Stellate Ganglion Block

Stellate ganglion block is beneficial in treatment of peripheral vascular disease, sympathetic dystrophy, perhaps as an adjunct to operation on the hand when vessel, nerve, or bone healing are in jeopardy.

The sympathetic fibers that course through the ganglion supply blood vessels, sweat glands, and pilomotor fibers of the skin of the head, arm, and upper chest wall, as well as deeper blood vessels, pupils, salivary glands, and heart and lungs.

The stellate ganglion usually comprises the conjoint ganglia of the inferior cervical and first thoracic sympathetic ganglia. It is a discrete more or less encapsulated structure with its own blood supply, lying upon the seventh cervical vertebral transverse process and neck of the first rib. Posteromedially situated is the longus colli muscle; posterolaterally, scalenus muscles; and anteriorly the cupula of the pleura. Adjacent structures include carotid sheath, first portion of the subclavian artery, thyrocervical and vertebral arteries, phrenic and recurrent laryngeal nerves, esophagus, the vertebrae, and spinal nerves. Major complications resulting from stellate ganglion injection are: pneumothorax, perforation of blood vessels, and subarachnoid injection.

Many approaches to stellate ganglion block have been described, classified according to point of entry in the neck and the relation to sternocleidomastoid muscle: anterior, anterolateral, lateral, or posterior paravertebral approach.

A safe technique is that described by de Sousa Pereira,[13] utilizing the anterior tubercle of the sixth cervical transverse process (Chassaignac's or carotid tubercle) as a landmark. With the patient semi-erect, sternomastoid muscle and carotid sheath displaced medially, the tubercle is felt just beneath skin easily reached with a short small gauge needle. Infiltration of 15 to 20 ml of a 0.5 per cent anesthetic solution and downward diffusion produce effective block with little likelihood of major complications.

The simplest approach is a median paratracheal injection just beside the cricoid cartilage, corresponding to the level of the sixth cervical vertebra (Fig. 4.9). With the patient supine in semi-erect position, the sternomastoid muscle is displaced laterally. A pillow is placed beneath the shoulders so that the neck is hyperextended. A 1½-inch 23-gauge uncapped needle is inserted perpendicular to skin tangential to trachea until bone is met at a depth from 1 to 1½ inches. This may be either the sixth vertebral body or base of the transverse process. The cervical sympathetic chain lies laterally at a distance no greater than 1.5 cm from the point of contact. After slight withdrawal of the needle to avoid injection into longus colli muscle, 10 to 20 ml of 0.5 per cent anesthetic are injected slowly, with intermittent aspiration. The patient is then tilted upright to faciliate diffusion downward to the ganglion.

The first sign of successful stellate ganglion block usually is ptosis of the eylid on the blocked side, followed by miosis. Enophthalmos is an illusion seemingly produced by paralysis of the sympathetic component to the levator palpebrae superioris muscle.

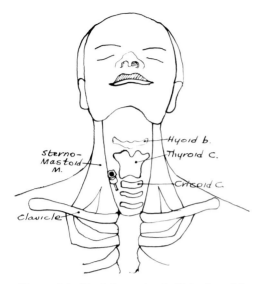

Figure 4.9. Medial, paratrachal injection of the stellate ganglion. (Reproduced with permission from R. D. Dripps, J. E. Eckenhoff, and L. D. Vandam. *Introduction to Anesthesia*. Philadelphia, Saunders, 1972.)

Scleral injection, warmth, and dryness of the face follow. Appearance of Horner's syndrome indicates interruption of cervical sympathetic impulses to the head. To be certain of a satisfactory effect in arm and hand, warmth, anthydrosis, and vasodilatation should be apparent.

For sustained block of six to eight hours' duration, tetracaine in 0.1 per cent concentration (1 mg per ml), is added to the 0.5 per cent solution of local anesthetic, containing, in addition, epinephrine in 1:200,000 concentration. Continuous ganglion block by injection through an indwelling catheter seems too traumatic a procedure.

Notes on Anesthesia Relative to Protection of the Hand during General Surgery

During operation, the arm is positioned carefully to avoid pressure on nerves and prevent stretch of the brachial plexus. Intravenous needles are placed strategically to prevent extravasation of blood and fluids as well as vasoconstrictive drugs. Peripheral neuritis and extensive slough of tissue have occurred after extravasation of thiopental and levarterenol (Levophed).

In prevention of postanesthetic brachial palsy, certain anatomic relationships must be borne in mind. Injury to the plexus is probably the result of stretch, the nerves fixed by fascia to the vertebrae and distally at axilla. Distraction between these points stretches the nerves. If the patient is suspended by wrist restraints in the head-down position, the brachial plexus may be stretched over the first rib. When the arm is hyperab-

ducted and a brace immobilizes the shoulder the plexus may not only be stretched but pinched between clavicle and first rib.

Tourniquet paralysis probably is the result of local ischemia of nerve and follows a pattern involving larger nerve fibers.[10] Muscle paralysis, loss of touch and position sense, and some obtundation of deep pain sensation may ensue. Smaller nerve fibers carrying pinprick sensation, heat, and cold, as well as autonomic function are spared. Complete recovery following such injury usually occurs, but palsy may last up to six months.

Accidental intra-arterial injection of drugs may result in disaster. Arteries are often anomalous in their course and it is comparatively easy to inject a drug under the misconception that an intravenous injection has been made. Thiopental has been the frequent offender.[4,15] If awake, the patient experiences a diffuse scalding type of pain. Vasoconstriction follows the intra-arterial spread of the alkaline barbiturate solution. This accident has not been noted with the use of 2.5 per cent thiopental or lesser concentrations. Experimental work suggests that levarterenol may be released from the blood vessel wall. Ischemia, gangrene, and loss of part or all of an extremity have resulted in such cases.

REFERENCES

1. Burnham, P. J. Regional block at the wrist of the great nerves of the hand. J.A.M.A., *167:* 847, 1958.
2. Burnham, P. J. Regional block anesthesia for surgery of fingers and thumb. Industr. Med., *27:* 67, 1958.
3. Burnham, P. J. Simple regional nerve block for surgery of the hand and forearm. J.A.M.A., *169:* 941, 1959.
4. Cohen, S. M. Accidental intra-arterial injection of drugs. Lancet, *2:* 409, 1948.
5. Duncan, D., and Jarvis, W. H. A comparison of the action on nerve fibers of certain anesthetic mixtures and substances in oil. Anesthesiology, *4:* 465, 1943.
6. Flatt, A.E. Tourniquet time in hand surgery. Arch. Surg., *104:* 190, 1972.
7. Keegan, J.J., and Garrett, F.D. The segmental distribution of the cutaneous nerves in the limbs of man. Anat. Rec., *102:* 409, 1948.
8. Labat, G. *In Regional Anesthesia,* Ed. 3, edited by John Adriani. Philadelphia, Saunders, 1967.
9. Leser, A. J. Duration of local anesthesia in relation to concentrations of procaine and epinephrine. Anesthesiology, *1:* 205, 1940.
10. Moldaver, J. Tourniquet paralysis syndrome. Arch. Surg., *68:* 136, 1954.
11. Moore, D. C., and Bridenbaugh, L. D. Pneumothorax — its incidence following brachial plexus block analgesia. Anesthesiology, *15:* 475, 1954.
12. National Fire Protection Association. *Standard for the Use of Inhalation Anesthetics.* Boston, 1970.
13. Pereira, de S. A. Blocking of the middle cervical and stellate ganglion by descending infiltration anesthesia: technique, accidents and thereapeutic indications. Arch. Surg., *50:* 152, 1945.

14. Shaw, W. M. Paralysis of phrenic nerve during brachial plexus anesthesia. Anesthesiology, *10:* 627, 1949.
15. Stone, H. H., and Donnelly, C. C. The accidental intra-arterial injection of thiopental. Anesthesiology, *22:* 995, 1961.
16. Wooley, E. J., and Vandam, L. D. Neurological sequelae of brachial plexus nerve block. Ann. Surg., *149:* 53, 1959.

chapter five
Injuries

A.

Open Wounds

Richard J. Smith, M.D.
Robert D. Leffert, M.D.

The decisions of the surgeon who first treats the injured hand are often decisive in influencing the nature of future reconstructive surgical procedures, the duration and severity of disability, and the ultimate function of the limb. That this responsibility is borne so frequently in any busy emergency area in no way lessens its importance. The principles and techniques of judicious wound care are based upon an understanding of the histological and chemical processes involved in wound healing.

PHYSIOLOGY OF WOUND HEALING

The dynamic changes of wound healing begin within moments of an open injury. Skin edges retract. Blood collects within the wound cavities and dissects soft tissue plains causing swelling and capillary stasis. Increased capillary permeability secondary both to stasis and to the release of histamine about the perimeter of the wound results in increased fluid exudate and edema. Soon, polynuclear and monocytic leukocytes migrate through the endothelial walls of the capillaries to the wound edges, there to release phosphatase, nuclease, lactic dehydrogenase, and proteolytic enzymes. These enzymes begin the destruction of damaged epithelial cells within two or three hours of injury. Much of the necrotic debris in cleaner wounds will be destroyed and phagocytized within two to three days.

Within the first 24 to 48 hours, thin budding capillaries begin to bridge the wound defect, fibroblasts at the wound borders are stimulated to secrete an amorphous acid mucopolysaccharide ground substance, and the blood clot at the base of the wound has started to contract. the edges of the wound are thickened with dilated vessels and edema fluid. This period is known as *the inflammatory phase* of wound healing.

Early fibroblastic activity occurs at this time. Within three hours of injury marked metabolic changes are noted at the basal layers of the dermis and epidermis in the region of the wound edges. Within 12 to 24 hours, the fibroblasts actively synthesize DNA. Fibroblastic proliferation and evidence of frequent mitoses are first noted within 24 to 36 hours of injury.

For many years it had been thought that a wound hormone is released from dead or damaged cells at the time of injury to initiate fibroblastic mitotic activity. Much experimental evidence still tends to support this theory. More recent studies, however, would suggest that under normal quiescent conditions, in undamaged tissue, an internal tissue secretion called *epidermal chalone* inhibits the mitotic activity of the fibroblasts. Chalone is a glycoprotein with a molecular weight of 30,000 and may well require epinephrine or glucocorticoid hormones as cofactors. When it is lost from the wounded tissues (perhaps due to increased cell wall permeability), the mitotic genes of the fibroblasts become activated at the basal layers of the epidermis. Keratin production ceases in these germinating layers and the fibroblastic proliferation accelerates at the wound borders.

The *proliferative* or *fibroblastic phase* of wound healing occurs between the second and fifth days at which time fibroblastic proliferation is at its maximum. The wound defect is not bridged solely by regenerating fibroblasts, however. Migration of fibroblasts along the loose fibrin strands of the clot may proceed at the rate of 2 to 3 mm per day and is most rapid during the second to fifth day following injury. The migrating fibroblasts do not proliferate until they reach their final positions at which time there is a sudden resurgence of active mitotic activity. Thus, mitosis and migration are alternative activities in the basal cells adjacent to the wound. As the migrating fibroblasts align themselves on fibrin strands within the wound, clot contraction and wound retraction may impose a longitudinal orientation upon them. When a fibroblast contacts another fibroblast its movement stops through "contact inhibition." Cell migration is therefore directed across the open spaces of the wound.

Within five days of injury, in the uncomplicated coapted wound, the wound margins are bridged and the fibroblasts have reached a "saturation density." Mucopolysaccharide production peaks at about five days, later to decline. The tensile strength of the wound at this point is extremely poor and is dependent largely upon adhesions between the fibroblasts and upon the viscosity of the mucopolysaccharide ground substance. Dehiscence is prevented almost entirely by the sutures. As the mucopolysaccharide secretion and the fibroblastic migration and proliferation ebbs, elaboration of their subcellular components necessary for collagen synthesis accelerates and the collagen production phase of wound healing begins.

The *collagen production phase* of wound healing begins five days after injury. Collagen molecules are first formed and secreted by the fibrocytes at the borders of the wound within 48 hours of injury. It is not until the fifth day, however, when *intramolecular cross-links* are added to the triple helix configuration. These intramolecular cross-links do not add significantly to tensile strength. The relatively poor tensile strength of the wound which does exist is due mainly to cohesion of the ground substance with the collagen fibrils. The diameter and the orientation of the newly formed collagen fibril varies with the mucopolysaccharide composition of the ground substance in which they lie. Whether the character of the collagen is influenced by the ground substance, or whether both collagen and ground substance reflect differences in the wound fibroblasts, is still uncertain.

By the end of two weeks the wound consists of a network of collagen fibrils, elastic fibrils, blood vessels, nerve fibrils, and lymphatics suspended in a gel of mucopolysaccharide ground substance and covered by keratinized epithelium. Although the synthesis of collagen within a wound may continue for up to six months, its rate of production is markedly decreased after the first one to two months.

The tensile strength of a wound continues to rise even after collagen production has virtually ceased. This is due to continued *intermolecular collagen cross-bonding,* remodeling and reorientation of the collagen fibrils and wound involution. This is known as the *remodeling phase* of wound healing and develops six months after injury. Collagenase is formed and aids in the resorption of many of the collagen fibrils; fibroblasts contract; water is lost from the wounds; the number of fibroblasts and the degree of vascularization decreases, and the entire wound shrinks. The ultimate tensile strength of the wound is dependent not only upon the number of collagen fibrils but their orientation, the quantity of extramolecular cross-links, and the cohesive force between the fibrils and the ground substance. The normal pre-wound state is probably never reached. In this regard it is interesting to note that British sailors of centuries past suffered a breakdown of wounds which had been healed for many years when they developed scurvy.

Interference with Wound Healing

Many factors may interfere with the normal process of wound healing. Excessive contamination with surface bacteria may result in an immune reaction and retarded fibrinogenesis, collagen formation, and mucopolysaccharide metabolism.

Excessive necrosis about the wound prolongs the inflammatory stage of wound healing, increases the edema and leukocytic migration, and delays fibroblastic bridging of the wound gap. Dead tissue also serves as a nidus for infection which may further delay wound healing.

Increased glucocorticoids and adrenalin, both of which may be cofactors of chalone, inhibit mitosis of the fibroblasts. Diabetes results in decreased glucose metabolism and lipogenesis with a decrease in peptide and protein synthesis.

Oxygen is necessary for protein synthesis and if oxygen tension in the advancing edge of granulation tissue is insufficient for normal metabolism, growth is retarded. Any decrease in vascular supply to the wound edges will therefore slow healing. As infection and necrosis cause edema, compression of capillary walls and vascular sludging with reduced oxygen tension at the wound edges will interfere with the wound healing. The administration of hyperbaric oxygen, however, may cause vasoconstriction and thus, paradoxically decrease the oxygen available in the granulating tissue.

Adequate nutrition is, of course, essential for wound healing and marked deficiencies in Vitamin C and protein may prolong the collagen phases of healing.

EVALUATION OF THE WOUNDED HAND

History

To evaluate and treat the wounded hand properly an adequate history must be obtained. Information regarding drug and antibiotic allergies and recent tetanus immunizations is essential if one is to plan antibacterial therapy. The anesthetist must know when the patient has eaten last and his cardiac, pulmonary, and metabolic status. Has the patient sustained injuries elsewhere? The victim of a stabbing attack may be mainly concerned with his bleeding palm and may well have sustained a nick in the chest wall which is rapidly developing into a pneumothorax.

The treatment of hand injuries is often influenced by the occupation and the handedness of the patient.

The mechanism of the injury should be carefully determined. If the hand has been cut by glass, what kind of glass? Tinted bottles and fine glassware contain lead which is usually visible on x-ray. If a hand was crushed in a press at work, was the press hot? Did it "repeat" after the initial injury, and if so how many times? With what foreign material was the wound in contact at or subsequent to the injury? Machine oil at the edges of the wound may give a filthy appearance but be rather innocuous. By contrast, the innocent-looking lacerations of the dorsum of the fourth and fifth metacarpals, which are often said to result from a fall, may well harbor the anaerobic streptococci, spirochetes, staphylococci, and the clostridia of a friend's tooth.

Examination

The main purposes of the emergency room examination of the injured hand are to assess the nature and severity of the wound in order to determine whether definitive care should be carried out, and to determine the anatomic diagnosis of deep tissue injury *without probing the depths of the wound.*

Prior to the examination of the wound, the entire limb must be checked for self-applied tourniquets or constricting articles. All rings and jewelry must be removed from the hand regardless of the patient's sentiments to the contrary. Rings and bracelets even in areas not directly affected by trauma may soon act as a tourniquet as the limb becomes swollen. Particularly if a dressing is to be applied about the hand, an area of ring constriction may result in disastrous consequences.

Assesment of the Wound

Severe crush or explosion injuries and burns need not be exposed in the emergency room, as undressing and redressing the wound prior to surgery will be painful and will cause unnecessary contamination. Less severe wounds may be examined under optimum conditions. The patient should be calmed and preferably lying supine. The surgeon should wear a mask and sterile gloves. The injured hand should be placed on a sterile field. All dressings may then be cut down to the bottom layer which, if adherent to the wound, may be soaked loose in a pan of sterile saline. The deepest layer should then be gently peeled from the wound rather than pulled. The wound should be observed and not probed. If the skin adjacent to the wound cannot be adequately evaluated because of contamination, it may require cleansing. Coagulated blood may be gently removed with a hydrogen peroxide sponge. Benzene, ether, and acetone are excellent solvents for many types of grease, ink, or paint, although it is not necessary to remove all the ingrained dirt or grease on the calloused hands of a laborer. After the wound is observed, it should be gently lavaged with sterile electrolyte solution and a sterile sponge placed over it until definitive care can be rendered.

Diagnosis of Deep Tissue Injury

Inspection of the cleansed hand lying at rest is probably the most valuable part of the hand examination. With the wrist in mild dorsiflexion any deviation of the gradual slope of the semiflexed fingers will be apparent at once and will call attention to a flexor tendon injury. With the forearm turned into pronation, the wrist falls into palmar flexion and a droop or lag of one or more digits will signal evidence of an extensor tendon injury. Do the fingernails line up or is one rotated, indicating a fracture of a tubular bone? Can all the metacarpal heads be seen or is one depressed due to a metacarpal neck fracture? The color, the temperature, and the moisture of the fingertips are noted. With laceration of the sensory nerve the perspiration to the corresponding part of the finger stops at once. Although a finger can survive if both of its neurovascular bundles are severed, it is likely to be blue and cool and its vi-

ability may be tenuous. With a suspected median nerve injury, observe the thumb. Although thenar atrophy will not occur for some time, the immediately paralyzed thenar muscles will not support the thumb in abduction and the digit will lie supinated and adducted against the index finger. With ulnar nerve injury the ring and little fingers will be flexed more acutely at the interphalangeal joints than the adjacent fingers.

Alternate flexion and extension of the fingers, thumb, and wrist; active abduction of the thumb and of the index finger; and a brief sensory test will often provide all the information required for a neuromuscular evaluation.

Allow a child to watch, as he is asked to differentiate the sharp from the dull end of the pin. The skin should be touched not jabbed with a pin point. After a while, his fingertip may be masked with the examiner's other hand so as to prevent the visual clues. For a finer and less frightening test ask the child or adult to differentiate the edge of a milled quarter dollar from that of a smooth nickel. Again the fingertips may be masked after the first few attempts.

All wounds about the hand, save for the most trivial lacerations, should be x-rayed. The value of these films in diagnosing fractures and dislocations, in locating foreign bodies, and occasionally in detecting soft tissue gas shadows is obvious. Their forensic value is well known. If the x-ray can be taken rapidly and the patient is not in shock it is usually advisable to take the films prior to examination of the hand.

The anatomic diagnosis and the extent of all injuries is carefully noted, preferably with a sketch of the hand wounds. Photographs are taken. A decision is then made whether treatment is to be rendered in the emergency room or in the operating room. Either definitive care is then carried out or the patient is prepared for surgery.

While awaiting surgery, the limb should be splinted and elevated. The surgeon should have some idea as to his general plan of treatment. The patient and his family should be told at this point what the general plan of treatment will be.

WHEN SHOULD A HAND WOUND BE CLOSED?

Should wounds about the hand be treated in the emergency room or office, or should they be dealt with in the operating room? Sterility, light, assistance, instruments, suture material, and usually the patience and attitude of the surgeon and his assistants may be far superior in the operating room than in an outpatient area. Weighed against these obvious advantages, are the exigencies of time, expense, and convenience.

The decision depends upon the patient and his wound, the facilities available in the emergency room, and the operating room delay time. Open reduction of fractures, flexor tendon repairs, nerve repairs, swinging skin flaps, and extensive debridement of crush or explosive injuries can rarely be justified in the emergency room. Split thickness skin grafts to small dermal wounds, the repair of a solitary extensor tendon both ends of which are visible in the wound, and closure of "tidy" skin wounds usually can be performed safely in a clean and efficient emergency room.

WOUND LAVAGE AND DEBRIDEMENT

Thorough cleansing of a wound is among the most important tasks in the treatment of the injured hand. The uninjured portion of the hand may be washed and shaved in the emergency room to permit proper examination. Careful cleansing of the depth of a complex wound, however, should not be performed without appropriate anesthesia and unless there are sterile operating conditions. Most bleeding vessels can be controlled in the emergency room with gentle pressure. Major vessels are clamped and tied or coagulated. It is unnecessary and inadvisable to attempt to achieve complete hemostasis prior to debridement and lavage.

After the patient has been brought to the sterile area of definitive care (treatment room or operating room), the limb is elevated, a pneumatic tourniquet padded with sheet cotton is applied to the upper arm, the limb is exsanguinated, and the tourniquet cuff is inflated to 250 to 300 mm of pressure. The use of a rubber-band tourniquet about the base of a finger, or a tightly wrapped rubber tourniquet about the wrist or forearm is dangerous. Rarely does one encounter a patient who cannot tolerate a properly applied pneumatic tourniquet for 20 to 30 minutes if the limb has been exsanguinated.

The skin about the wound is thoroughly washed and the hand is gently sponged with soapy water using sterile technique. Coagulated blood is removed. The wound is lavaged with four liters of sterile saline and placed on a sterile towel. The surgeon is then regloved, and the limb is prepared with an antiseptic solution (we prefer Providone-Iodine) and draped for surgery.

The depths of the wound may now be explored. Foreign bodies are extracted. Splinters of bone lying freely about the wound and not attached to soft tissue are removed. Dark muscle is excised. Blunt rakes fold back flaps for thorough exposure and debridement. The surgical findings are correlated with the preoperative diagnosis and appropriate surgical reconstruction of the deeper tissues is preformed. (Details of reconstruction are covered elsewhere throughout this volume.)

After the surgery is completed, the wound is again copiously irrigated, the limb is elevated, and the tourniquet is released and removed from the arm. Gentle pressure is applied for about four to five minutes. Tissues of doubtful viability are excised and hemostasis is secured. The use of coagulation for hemostasis is usually quicker and less traumatic than the use of larger amounts of catgut.

With the exception of wounds requiring remote pedicle flaps, most emergency hand surgery can be performed under local anesthesia or with regional blocks. The details of local infiltration, digital, regional, and intravenous anesthesia are described elsewhere in this volume. As no child has an empty stomach, the use of Ketamine and Fentanyl Citrate may be used in calming an injured child sufficiently to instill local anesthetics.

WHEN SHOULD A HAND WOUND BE CLOSED

Appropriate primary closure of the hand wound will prevent continued contamination and mechanical injury to the deep tissues and will therefore minimize edema, scar, and joint stiffness. Injudicious wound closure, however, may jeopardize the ultimate function of the hand. If all necrotic tissues are not excised, if skin sutures serve as instruments of tissue strangulation because of progressive edema, or if a grossly contaminated wound cannot be lavaged thoroughly, primary wound closure may only retard proper wound healing. The decision as to whether a wound may be safely closed primarily is dependent upon several factors:

Degree and Type of Contamination at the Time of Injury

The quantity and virulence of the bacteria which enter certain types of wounds are notoriously dangerous. Only if all other wound factors are ideal should the surgeon risk closing these most serious injuries. A smear and gram stain of the organisms at the wound edges may be of value in evaluating the extent and type of wound contamination.

Time Since Injury

For the first six hours after wound contamination with staphylococci, bacterial growth is slow. Thereafter, the bacterial count increases geometrically and the risk of infection with wound closure similarly increases. For this reason, the first six hours following injury have been termed "the golden period." The time since injury is but one factor which must be considered in making this decision.

Type of Wound

Formerly, wounds were classified into those caused by puncture, abrasion, incision, and laceration. Other classifications have proven useful as a guide to treatment. Perhaps the simplest is "tidy" and "untidy" as suggested by Rank and Wakefield. The tidy wound is one where a sharp instrument such as a knife, a glass edge, or a razor has opened the skin of the hand, often to have severed important soft tissue structures below. In the tidy wound, edema is minimal; only local tissues are injured and the viability of the skin can usually be determined with accuracy. The untidy wound is one in which the hand has been crushed, torn,

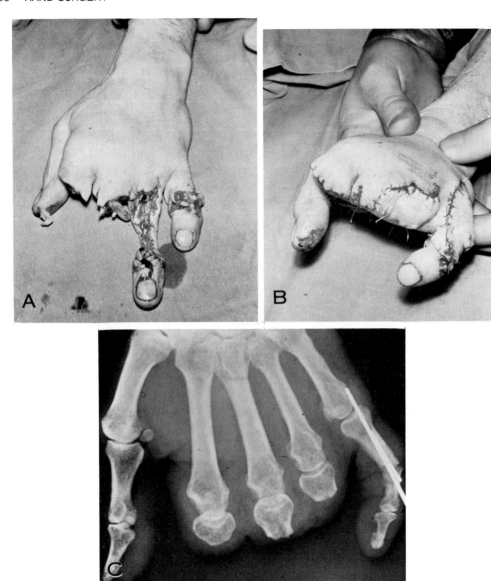

Figure 5.1.1A. A young carpenter sustained this severe wound to his left hand with a wood-cutting power tool at work two hours previously. Should primary closure be performed?

Figure 5.1.1B. The wound was fresh, contamination was minimal, and tissue viability could be easily judged. Primary closure was therefore performed. The partially amputated ring finger was used as a fillet flap and as the source of a free graft to the little finger.

Figure 5.1.1C. To provide better thumb to little finger pinch, the proximal interphalangeal joint of the little finger was arthrodesed in supination. No further reconstructive surgery was required and the patient returned to work within a few weeks.

burned, or ripped by explosion such as may occur with machines, high-pressure injection devices, or war missiles. After such injuries, the extent of venous thrombosis, edema, undetected bleeding, deep tissue injury, necrosis, and contamination are often impossible to assess at first examination. The goals of *primary treatment* in these patients are therefore to prevent infection, to minimize swelling, and to perform only those reconstructive procedures that, if delayed, would permanently jeopardize hand function. Skeletal stabilization may often be essential in these injuries.

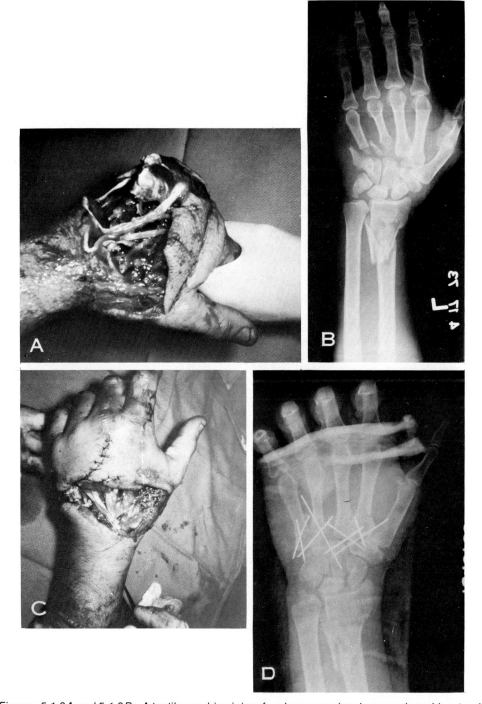

Figures 5.1.2A and 5.1.2B. A textile machine injury four hours previously caused crushing, tearing, and avulsion of the skin, the subcutaneous tissues, and the extensor tendons of the left hand in this young worker. There were multiple fractures and dislocations about the carpometacarpal joints as well as fractures of the distal end of the radius and of the ulnar styloid. The skin about the fingers was blue.

Figures 5.1.2C and 5.1.2D. The fracture-dislocations of the metacarpal bases were reduced and held with multiple Kirschner wires to maintain skeletal support. No primary treatment was rendered to the fractured radius and it was conceded that radial settling would later necessitate resection of the ulnar head. Avulsed tendons were not repaired in order to avoid forearm dissection. Where the skin could be brought together without tension it was closed. The more proximal portion of the wound was left open and wet packs applied. When nonviable tissues had demarcated, they were debrided, and a groin flap was applied. Tendon reconstruction is performed only after good skin coverage has been obtained.

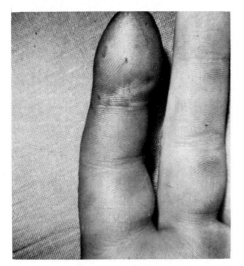

Figure 5.1.3. A small, barely visible punctate wound at the tip of the index finger caused by a paint gun injury several days previously had been treated with a small adhesive bandage. Often small, innocent looking wounds caused by high-pressure injection tools are most dangerous. They should be opened widely at once and debrided. This patient ultimately required amputation of the distal segment of the finger.

Other Factors

There are many additional factors that must be evaluated in determining whether a wound should be closed primarily. The hand may be but one of many sites of injury, particularly in cases of explosion injuries, war wounds, or burns. There may thus be life-saving procedures which take precedence over definitive treatment of the hand. In these instances, closure and repair may be delayed. At times, the available facilities or the experience of the personnel may be limited. There should be no hesitancy or embarrassment in electing delayed closure of a complex wound until the patient can be transferred to a large clinical center. Under such circumstances, repair of deep tissues similarly should be deferred.

The experience of many surgeons has indicated that if a hand wound is properly cleaned, debrided, packed, and splinted soon after injury, deferred closure does not necessarily doom the function of the hand or the digits. Indeed, deferred closure may often be the treatment of choice.

CLOSURE TECHNIQUES

Retraction of the wound edges due to the natural elasticity of the skin and subcutaneous tissues often gives the appearance of skin loss. This is particularly true of wounds at the dorsum of the hand. Gentle traction of the skin edges with skin hooks may often permit the closure of the wound that is gaping widely.

If skin has been lost, closure may require advancement or rotation of adjacent skin as is the use of a skin graft or pedicle flap.

With "tidy" lacerated wounds treated early, a scar crossing a flexion crease may be altered by means of a Z-plasty or local flap to avoid flexion contractures. Sharp angles often may be closed with an apical suture that passes from skin edge transversely across the subcutaneous tissues of the flap apex and then back to the other skin edge. Vertical mattress sutures are valuable to evert the edges of thick palmar skin. If thorough hemostasis cannot be secured, a drain may be allowed to remain in the wound for one or two days. Suction drainage is occasionally, but infrequently, required.

DRESSINGS

The purposes of the surgical dressings are to protect the wound from contamination, to absorb any discharge, to provide even compression so as to minimize the development of a hematoma or edema, and to close potential "dead spaces." Most dressings also serve as a splint.

A wide mesh gauze, petrolatum gauze, or plastic-covered sponges will prevent granulation tissue from sticking to the dressings. Loosely packed fluffs may then be used to cover the wound and the natural concavities of the hand. Sheet cotton or loose, springy gauze roll may then provide further bulk finally to be covered with an outer layer of crepe bandage. If the fingers need not be immobilized, they should not be. If the fingers must be included within the dressings, they should be separated by just one thin gauze sponge in each web space to prevent maceration. The assistant who is holding the hand that is being dressed should grasp it by the tips of the index and middle fingers only. This will preserve the width and the concavity of the palm and will prevent the mobile first, fourth, and fifth metacarpals from being uncomfortably squeezed together.

PREVENTION OF POSTWOUND EDEMA OF THE HAND

The hands of many patients who have suffered severe crushing injuries show borderline viability as a result of edema, capillary sludging, and poor venous backflow. The fingers are cool and blue. One may attempt to improve the circulation of these hands by the use of low molecular weight Dextran and cervical sympathetic blocks. We have used three units of Dextran daily for four successive days in order to expand the plasma volume, to decrease the fluid transudate into the tissues, and thus to improve peripheral blood flow. One should be cautious in the use of Dextran in patients suffering from pulmonary edema or from renal or cardiac disease.

Improved circulation to the injured limb may be obtained by a continuous sympathetic block. A number 16-gauge polyethylene catheter, approxi-

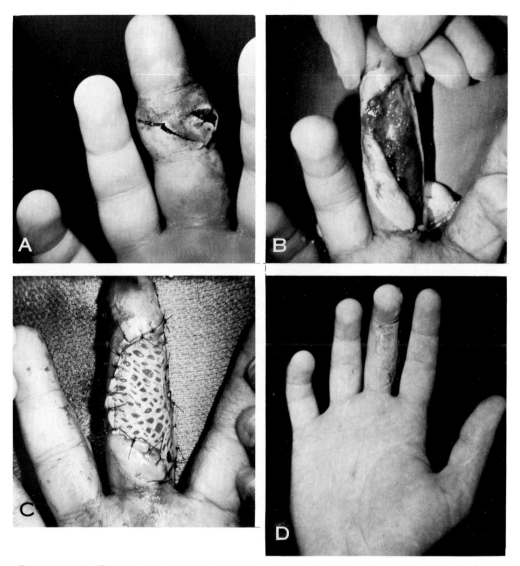

Figure 5.1.4A. This boy lacerated his middle finger when he fell upon a rock in a city park several days previously. The wound was dirty and tender. The finger was red.

Figure 5.1.4B. Closure of an old, dirty wound is certainly contraindicated. The wound was debrided and wet soaks applied. Four days later erythema has subsided and the wound borders and base appear clean.

Figure 5.1.4C. A split thickness skin graft is applied with generous interstices cut for easy drainage. Wet dressings are applied to the graft.

Figure 5.1.4D. Three weeks later the wound is completely healed with no further signs of infection.

mately five inches in length is inserted under local anesthesia to the cervical sympathetic chain at the level of the cricoid cartilage. A 10=cc syringe is left attached to the tubing and taped to the neck. Ten cc of 1 per cent Xylocaine with 1/200,000 epinephrine and 10 mg of pontocaine are injected into the tubing every four hours. This continuous block will frequently relieve limb pain and may help to prevent small vessel shutdown in the injured edematous hand.

Postoperatively the wounded limb should be elevated higher than the level of the heart. The limb should be elevated immediately upon the completion of the surgery and, particularly with more severe wounds, suspended from an intravenous pole so that the arm, the elbow, the fore arm, and the hand are all virtually vertical. Dependency for even 10 minutes

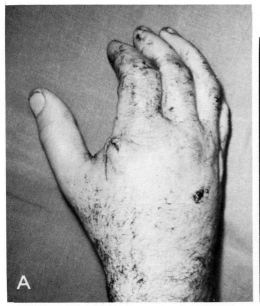
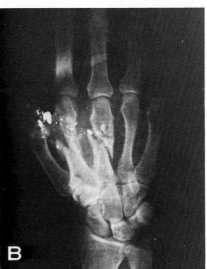

Figure 5.1.5A. This shopkeeper was shot at close range three days previously. Attention has been directed towards chest wounds and the hand had been treated merely with irrigation of the wound and a volar pancake splint for the hand and wrist. There was diffuse edema and metacarpophalangeal joint stiffness.

Figure 5.1.5B. X-rays revealed comminuted fractures of the second and third metacarpals and multiple opaque foreign bodies from the fragmented bullet.

per hour may cause significant edema. A simple and effective means of suspending the limb is to spray a skin adherent about the upper arm and then to roll a three or four-inch stockinette about the hand, forearm, and up to the axilla. The stockinette is partially opened so that the hand may be seen and its distal end knotted for intravenous pole suspension.

Proper splinting will also help prevent edema. The position in which a hand should be splinted is not always the "position of function." For example, after flexor tendon repairs, the wrist should be palmar flexed. If, however, tendon, nerve, and/or bone repair does not dicate the position of immobilization, the wrist should be placed in mild dorsiflexion and the metacarpophalangeal joints of the fingers (if they require immobilization) in moderate flexion. If the thumb requires immobilization it is best splinted in a position of abduction and opposition. If possible, one should avoid the use of a circular cast following wound closure.

ANTIBIOTICS AND TETANUS PROPHYLAXIS

A full discussion of antibiotics is reviewed in detail in Chapter 14. Antibiotic therapy is indicated in the presence of severely contaminated, deep, and contused wounds of the hand. The selection of the antibi-

otic to be used initially is determined by the circumstances of the injury, the appearance of the wound, and the patient's history of drug sensitivity or previous hepatic, renal, or auditory pathology. Special wounds, such as those caused by potentially rabid animals, by laboratory accidents with bacterial cultures, or those showing evidence of clostridial myonecrosis demand specific antibiotic treatment.

In a 1969 report of hand infections seen in a municipal hospital, 59 per cent were due to staphylococci, 12 per cent to beta hemolytic streptococci, 8 per cent to *Escherichia coli,* 4 per cent to alpha hemolytic streptococci and 4 per cent to *Aerobacter aerogenes.* Seventy-eight per cent of the organisms were gram positive; 22 per cent were gram negative. The (gram positive) staphylococci and streptococci are usually sensitive to methicillin, oxycillin, lincomycin or cloxacillin, erythromycin, cephalothin, chloramphenicol, and a lesser percentage to penicillin, ampicillin, and nafcillin. The (gram negative) *E. coli* and *A. aerogenes* were most susceptible to kanamycin, chloramphenicol, colistin, polymyxin B (for *E. coli*), ampicillin (for *E. coli*), cephalothin, and gentamycin. The antibiotic sensitivity and resistance of these organisms is most variable. In all severe wounds culture and sensitivity studies should be performed.

Antibiotic toxicity may take many forms. The most

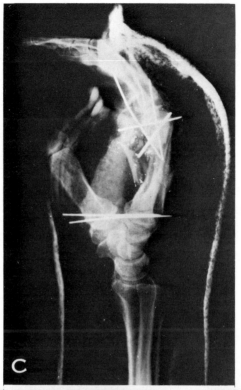

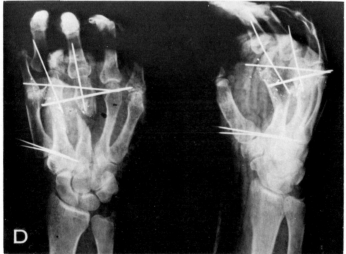

Figures 5.1.5C and 5.1.5D. Maximum length of the second and third metacarpals is preserved with transverse Kirschner wires. Flexion at the second and third MP joints is maintained with longitudinal Kirschner wires. An adduction contracture of the thumb is prevented by holding the first metacarpal in abduction and pronation with two Kirschner wires. The wound is debrided and splinted, and antibiotics are administered.

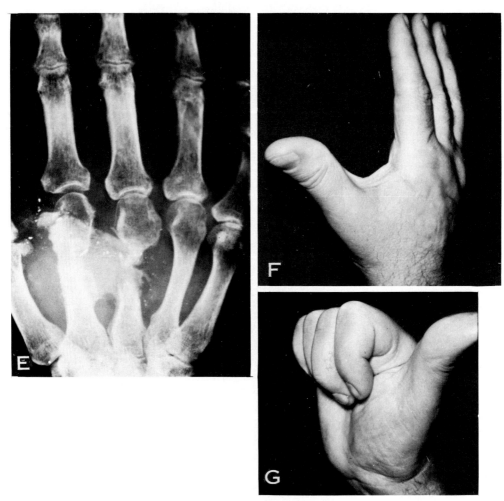

Figure 5.1.5E. Two months later, an iliac bone graft is inserted to restore skeletal integrity to the second and third metacarpals. Within three months it is solidly united.

Figures 5.1.5F and 5.1.5G. Motion and function are restored.

TABLE 5.1

History of Tetanus Immu- nization Doses	Clean Minor Wounds		Dirty Wounds	
	Give toxoid	Give immune globulin	Give toxoid	Give immune globulin
Uncertain, 0 or 1	Yes	No	Yes	Yes
2	Yes	No	Yes	Yes, if wound over 24 hours old
3 or more	No, unless greater than 10 years since last dose	No	No, unless greater than 10 years since last dose	No

frequent site of toxic reaction for several antibiotics is listed:

Penicillin: Anaphylaxis and skin reaction
Methicillin: Anaphylaxis and skin reaction
Erythromycin: Rare
Lincomycin: Hepatic, anaphylaxis, skin, and cardiovascular
Cephalothin: Anaphylaxis, skin, phlebitis with intravenous
Ampicillin: Anaphylaxis, skin, CNS
Gentamicin: Renal, auditory
Chloramphenicol: Blood dyscrasia, CNS, GI
Tetracycline: Hepatic, phlebitis with IV, GI
Kanamycin: Renal, auditory
Colymycin: Renal, auditory, phlebitis with IV
Amphotericin B: Renal, hepatic, blood, skin, CNS, phlebitis with IV, GI

Our preference for the treatment of street wounds has been the use of intravenous methicillin, cephalothin, or lincomycin for four days with all patients requiring hand surgery and admission. Thereafter, if the patient remains afebrile and the wound appears innocent, the intravenous antibiotics are stopped and the patient is given oral antibiotics. Outpatients with dirty or edematous hand wounds are treated with oral oxycillin, cephalexin, or lincomycin. In each case, however, the choice of antibiotics is influenced by the wound, the patient, and ultimately the response to the antibiotic being used.

Local antibiotic irrigation is used for more severe wounds and for those wounds entering the joints. We have noticed no untoward effect from the use of bacitracin and neomycin as irrigating solutions.

Decisions regarding the advisability of *tetanus prophylaxis* arise in the treatment of all hand wounds. The problem is greatly simplified if the wound is treated promptly and if there is a reliable history of complete primary tetanus immunization. For several years in the United States, there has been no documented case of tetanus in a patient who has had adequate primary tetanus immunization. Protective levels of antitoxin persist for at least five years after four doses of toxoid. Up to 10 years after having received primary immunization, the patient will elicit a prompt reaction to a booster dose. In cases of older untreated wounds, or when prior immunization was incomplete, Human Tetanus Immune Globulin (TIG) is preferable to equine or bovine antitoxin, both of which are prone to provoke an antiphylactic response or serum sickness in sensitized patients. The guide to *tetanus prophylaxis* given in Table 5.1 has been suggested by the Center for Disease Control, United States Department of Health, Education, and Welfare.

CONCLUSIONS

The proper primary care of the hand wound is the foundation of the restoration of hand function. The results of tendon, nerve, joint, and bone repair and reconstruction may be hopelessly jeopardized if an ap-parently trivial wound becomes purulent, if crushed fingers become nonviable, or if the slough of skin and subcutaneous fat leaves scar and a contracted mass of granulation tissue about the wrist. The judicious care of a hand wound is based upon an understanding of the dynamics of wound healing, an intelligent evaluation of the wound, and the proper selection of surgical techniques, medications, and postoperative management that are available.

BIBLIOGRAPHY

1. Alexander, J. W. Host defense mechanisms against infection. Surg. Clin. North Am., *52:* 1367-1378, 1972.
2. Allen, H. S. Crushing wounds of the hand. Am. J. Surg., *80:* 780-783, 1950.
3. Baxter, C. R. Surgical management of soft tissue infections. Surg. Clin. North Am., *52:* 1483-1499, 1972.
4. Boyes, J. H. A philosophy of care of the injured hand. Bull. Am. Coll. Surg., *50:* 341, 1965.
5. Burkhalter, W. E. Thoughts on delayed closure of hand wounds. In *Symposium on the Hand,* Vol. 3, edited by L. M. Cramer and R. A. Chase. St. Louis, Mosby, 1971, pp. 168-173.
6. Burkhalter, W. E., Butler, B., Metz, W., and Omer, G. Experiences with delayed primary closure of war wounds of the hand in Viet Nam. J. Bone Joint Surg., *50A:* 945-954, 1968.
7. Center for Disease Control; Morbidity and Mortality. Supplement-Collected Recommendations of the Public Health Service Advisory Committee on Immunization Practices, *21:* #25: 4-6, 1972.
8. Dittrich, H. Wundheilungsstorungen (Disturbances of Wound Healing). Chirurgurie, *42:* 289, 1971.
9. Dunphy, J. E., and Jackson, D. S. Practical applications of experimental studies in the care of the primarily closed wound. Am. J. Surg., *104:* 273-282, 1962.
10. Dunphy, J. E., and Van Winkle, Jr., W. *Repair and Regeneration. The Scientific Basis for Surgical Practice.* New York, McGraw Hill, 1969.
11. Farmer, C. B., and Mann, R. J. Human bite infections of the hand. South. Med. J., *59:* 515-518, 1966.
12. Flatt, A. E. *The Care of Minor Hand Injuries,* Ed. 3. St. Louis, Mosby, 1972.
13. Flynn, J. E. Open wounds of the hand. In *Hand Surgery.* Baltimore, Williams & Wilkins, 1966, pp. 75-84.
14. Illingsworth, *Wound Healing.* Boston, Little, Brown, 1966.
15. Jabaley, M. E., and Peterson, H. D. Early treatment of war wounds of the hand and forearm in Viet Nam. Ann. Surg., *177:* 167-173, 1973.
16. Kaplan, E. B. *Functional and Surgical Anatomy of the Hand,* Ed. 2. Philadelphia, Lippincott, 1965.
17. Longacre, J. J. *Scar Tissue, Its Use and Abuse.* Springfield, Charles C Thomas, 1972, pp. 10-19.
18. Lowry, K. F., and Curtis, G. M. Delayed suture in the management of wounds: Analysis of 721 traumatic wounds illustrating the influence of time interval in wound repair. Am. J. Surg., *80:* 280, 1950.
19. Madden, J., and Peacock, E. Studies on the biology of collagen during wound healing. Surgery, *64:* 288-293, 1968.
20. Mason, M. L., and Bell, J. L. The crushed hand. Clin. Orthop., *13:* 84-96, 1959.

21. Moberg, E. *Emergency Surgery of the Hand.* Edinburgh, Livingstone, 1967.
22. Rank, B. K., and Wakefield, A. R. *Surgery of Repair as Applied to Hand Injuries.* Baltimore, Williams & Wilkins, 1960.
23. Smith, R. J. Principles of skin coverage for the hand. Bull. Hosp. Joint Dis., *24:* 48-55, 1963.
24. Stark, H. H., Wilson, J. N., and Boyes, J. H. Grease gun injuries of the hand. J. Bone Joint Surg., *43A:* 485-491, 1961.
25. Stone, N. H., Hursch, H., Humphrey, C. R., and Boswick, J. A. Empirical selection of antibiotics for hand infections. J. Bone Joint Surg., *51A:* 899-903, 1969.

B.

Crush, Cornpicker, Mangle, and Wringer Injuries

John L. Bell, M.D.

The injuries under consideration in this chapter vary from closed contusions or simple lacerations and abrasions to extensive mutilating injuries of the hand and forearm. The severity of the injury is determined not only by the degree of compression but by the duration of application of the force.

In some cases the temptation is to attempt excessive reconstructive procedures aimed at anatomic restoration, utilizing tissues badly damaged and destined to necrosis or those whose powers of survival depend upon the avoidance of further trauma. On the other hand, one should not take a completely pessimistic attitude and assume that nothing can be saved and thereby proceed with radical amputation without considering the basic principles of modern wound surgery. The basic hand functions of grasp, pinch, and sensibility must be kept in mind throughout the entire course of treatment. A fundamental concept is to salvage function rather than form.

The main objectives of early treatment are to attain: (1) Prompt healing of wounds without infection, and (2) sufficient alignment and reduction of fractures and dislocations to obviate further operations to stabilize the skeletal framework of the hand. Infection and prolonged wound healing usually follow tissue necrosis, and malunion or nonunion of fractures are usually avoidable complications of treatment. When infection supervenes, any amount of additional surgery may not suffice to restore appreciable function, and if the skeletal framework is not reestablished at the earliest possible time, the chance for a return of active motion is significantly reduced.

INITIAL APPRAISAL OF THE SEVERE INJURY

In the severely mutilated hand, the need for urgent surgical intervention should be apparent after a quick glance. The history provides information essential to estimate the degrees of contamination as well as to anticipate the severity of tissue damage. Injuries contaminated by barn yard soil, street dirt, or those that occur in the meat packing industry should be suspect and regarded with a proper awareness of the danger of developing a severe infection in spite of early thorough wound care. In such severely contaminated cases, closure of the wound must be purposely delayed until the danger of infection has passed.

A consideration of the patient's age, occupation, and general physical and mental status are of invaluable aid in planning treatment.

Pain or emotional disturbances accompanying injury may prevent the patient from being able to cooperate in an extended examination of the hand. Preoperative examination of the severely crushed hand usually has to be limited to observation of wounds, carefully noting the posture of the hand and attempting a few simple tests to try to establish the integrity of sensation. Tendon injuries and fractures or dislocations should be suspected by observing any abnormal posture of the hand or digits. During examination and observation of the hand, the vascular status of its various parts can be cursorily assessed. In the crush injury, extensive damage to bones and joints may be in areas remote from obvious external wounds.

Roentgenographic examination is an essential supplement to the initial history and physical examination.

After weighing the evidence obtained from the preliminary history and examination, the primary surgical procedure can be more intelligently outlined.

OPERATIVE CARE

Operative care of any open hand injury consists of four phases: (1) exploration and assessment of tissue damage, (2) debridement or wound excision, (3) deep repair, and (4) wound closure. Whether all phases should be carried out at the time of the initial operative procedure is a matter for careful consideration. Exploration and debridement are the essential parts of the primary operative procedure, but under certain circumstances, deep repair and even wound closure should be purposely delayed. Other important factors are the patient's age and general condition. If, at the time of the primary operation, nothing other than thorough cleansing and adequate debridement were done the most important step toward salvaging function of the severely injured hand would have been accomplished.

Axillary brachial plexus block anesthesia is the safest and most effective kind of anesthesia for managing the severely crushed hand or forearm in the adult patient. In children, general anesthesia has to be used.

After anesthesia has become effective, a pneumatic

cuff on the arm is inflated to the appropriate pressure which will provide a satisfactory bloodless field. The preparation of the operative field and the wounds should be carried out under a bloodless field.

Exploration and Assessment of Tissue Damage

The first formal step in the operative procedure is assessment of damage to the various tissues. Severely displaced fractures should be placed into better alignment to relieve tension or distortion on adjacent blood vessels, nerves, or skin flaps. Blood clots and any foreign material should be removed. Tissues shredded beyond recognition or use may be trimmed or excised at this time, but excision of large tissue flaps or segments which might possibly be viable should be deferred until exploration has been completed. Any major vessels encountered should be secured with atraumatic vascular clamps if repair is contemplated. With a bloodless field there is less risk of operative injury to nerves or blood vessels and operative trauma can be minimized.

Following thorough exploration of the wounds with identification of normal as well as injured structures, the second part of the primary operative procedure can be contemplated. Before commencing debridement or wound excision, the tourniquet pressure should be released in order to allow blood to recirculate in the extremity. It should be remembered that anoxia is such a critical factor in crushing injuries that tissues should not be subjected to tourniquet ischemia any longer than is absolutely necessary.

Debridement

Debridement is the keystone of all acute wound surgery. The main objective is to convert an accidental wound into one that is surgically clean and contains only viable tissue.

Skin frequently is the most difficult tissue to evaluate as to its viabilty. In crushing injuries it may have been damaged beyond salvation by the compressive force applied at the time of the accident. Degloved skin cannot be replaced with any degree of assurance that it will survive, and necrosis of a major portion of skin so replaced is almost a certainty. Many distally based avulsion flaps or other traumatic pedicles have a precarious blood supply and may fail to survive. Survival of skin flaps depends upon adequate circulation of both arterial and venous elements. A pale flap which does not bleed at the cut edge indicates a deficient arterial supply. A skin pedicle that is dusky or purple indicates impaired venous circulation, and careful inspection usually reveals that the veins of the flap are thrombosed (Fig. 5.2.1).

In many cases, the tourniquet blush test aids in determining viability of skin flaps. The rate and quality of the return of circulation to the skin of the hand is observed after release of the pressure in the tourniquet. Because of an intense active hyperemia resulting from the sudden inflow of arterial blood, viable skin turns pink but areas deprived completely of arterial supply remain pale. In some instances, however, blanched skin flaps may change gradually to a pink color after a few minutes. When viability is doubtful, it is well to wait for about five minutes before excising the skin in question. A flap that appears dusky or has a purple hue indicates impaired venous circulation. In some cases, return to normal color may occur, but if the skin flap remains dusky it should be excised.

Palmar skin is thick and superficial layers may be avulsed, leaving the dermis exposed. If there is bleeding from the cut edge of a pink dermis it is likely that the damaged skin will survive.

There is usually no difficulty in determining viability of muscles. Viable muscle is red, its cut surface bleeds actively, and contractions occur with external stimulation. Devitalized muscle is discolored, does not bleed actively, and fails to contract when touched. Damaged muscle has to be thoroughly excised.

In crushing injuries, nerves frequently escape disruption even though accompanying blood vessels are torn or avulsed and adjacent bones are fractured. When a division is encountered, nerve ends should not be debrided. Nerve tissue should not be excised unless the nerve leads to a digit already amputated or crushed beyond recall.

Tendons and joint tissues are subjected to minimal excision. Bone fragments with soft tissue attachments usually survive and should not be excised.

Amputations

In mutilating injuries involving multiple digits, the only absolute indication for primary amputation of a part is a complete lack of blood supply without a possible of its restoration. Besides the wound conditions, the patient's age, occupation, and other personal factors have to be weighed.

In order to determine the functional potential and value of an injured but vascularized digit, it is necessary to appraise the damage to the skin, tendons, nerves, bones, and joints. If three or more of the tissues are so severely damaged that reparative procedures are required, then amputation should be considered. Where several fingers are about equally damaged, every effort should be made to save as much as possible from each, since even a finger with limited motion but good sensibility far surpasses any prosthesis.

When digital amputation is carried out, there must be adequate soft tissue covering over the bone end, and digital nerves have to be resected sufficiently to avoid a painful stump.

Fractures and Joint Injuries

Many fractures encountered in the severely crushed hand are not only unstable but are markedly comminuted. Experience has shown that it was difficult and almost impossible to attain either a satisfactory reduction or to maintain the reduction by splinting alone.

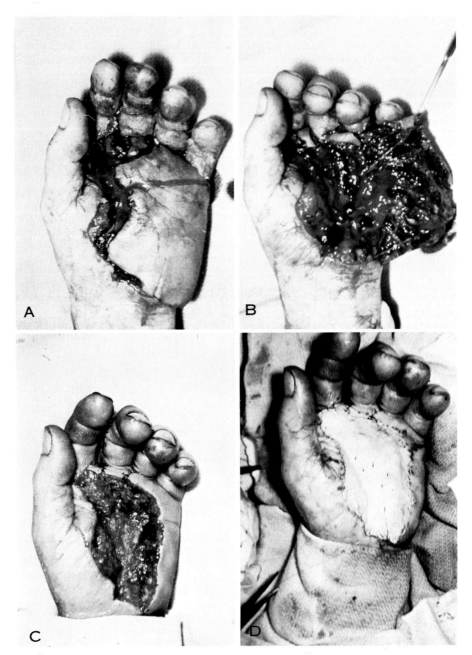

Figure 5.2.1. A. Acute avulsion flap of palm. *B.* Flap has deficient arterial supply and thrombosed viens. *C.* 72 hours following primary debridement the wound is clean, viable, and there is no bleeding problem. *D.* Partial thickness skin graft used to close wound at 72 hours.

The use of Kirschner wire fixation has supplanted the former method of maintaining reduction of the fractured bones of the hand as encountered in the severe crush.

Direct visualization of the fracture site is frequently necessary to align the displaced comminuted fragments into satisfactory position. In some instances the commonly advocated crossed wire technique cannot be accomplished without causing either undue operative trauma or distraction of the fracture.

An important advantage of using Kirschner wire fixation to maintain reduction is that the wounds can be inspected and cared for during the postoperative period without disturbing the position of the fracture.

Other parts of the hand also may be mobilized without jeopardizing reduction of the fractures.

Most joint injuries of the hand result in some loss of motion. In crushing injuries of the hand, joints remote from obvious surface wounds may be damaged or dislocated. Open and closed joint injuries require careful attention to minimize the loss of function. Dislocations have to be accurately reduced and maintained in position during the healing process. All open joint injuries should be irrigated thoroughly to remove loose tissue debris and foreign material. Displaced intra-articular fractures have to be reduced into anatomic position and usually require Kirschner wire fixation to maintain reduction.

Tendon Injuries

In crushing injuries it is seldom advisable to repair flexor tendons in the distal palmar region or within the digits. Occasionally, if overlying skin and soft tissue coverage is adequate, repair of flexor tendons at the forearm and wrist levels can be considered. There are many reasons for not repairing flexor tendon injuries in the severe crush injury. Generally, multiple tissue damage about the site of the flexor tendon injuries results in excessive scarring and prevents a return of satisfactory active flexion following repair. Fractures and flexor tendon injuries at the same level commonly result in marked scarring. Furthermore, accessory or wound enlarging incisions necessary for securing retracted flexor tendons may jeopardize the circulation of skin flaps whose viability may already be doubtful.

In contrast to flexor tendons, the extensors often can be approximated over metacarpal or phalangeal areas even in the presence of an underlying fracture. On the digits and dorsum of the hand, divided extensor tendons do not retract to great lengths and are more easily exposed than flexor tendons.

Nerve Injuries

In many crushing injuries, nerves escape division but are commonly contused and at times avulsed. When a nerve is severed in a crush injury, the nerve ends are usually damaged over a considerable but undetermined length from the site of the injury. Primary repair should not be undertaken when such circumstances prevail.

Wound Closure

If possible, closure of a hand wound should be accomplished with local skin. In crush injuries, however, skin loss is common and frequently is the greatest problem in the early treatment. There must be no tension on approximated tissues, particularly on the skin edges.

When direct suture is not possible, the wounds may be closed by one or a combination of methods. Free skin grafting, local shifting of adjacent tissue, and applying of distant pedicle flaps are the procedures that have to be considered.

If a recipient site is composed of viable subcutaneous or well-vascularized areolar tissue, free skin grafting is preferable. A partial thickness skin graft should be used in preference to a free full thickness skin graft.

Although a free skin graft may not survive on large areas of exposed cortical bone, joints, or tendons stripped of areolar covering, it may take over small avascular areas. Occasionally, it may be possible to shift adjacent areolar tissue to cover large areas of avascular tissue and then apply a skin graft. Experience has shown that a partial thickness skin graft may provide a permanent functional cover in many instances (Fig. 5.2.2).

Transposition flaps of adjacent skin and subcutaneous tissue may be used in some instances to cover fracture sites, bared joints, or tendons. Over the dorsal surfaces of the hand and fingers such rotation flaps can be fashioned without difficulty. Following application of the flap over the bared structures, the donor area is closed with a partial thickness skin graft.

When use of local flaps or free grafts is not possible, distant pedicle flaps may be considered. They need not be applied primarily and, in fact, primary distant pedicle flap application is becoming a rarity. It is only safe to contemplate a distant pedicle flap when there is no question regarding the likelihood of developing an infection or the possibility of applying the flap on a part containing nonviable tissue. If after three days, the wound is clean and vascular it may be permissible to apply a pedicle flap from a distance. Another advantage of purposeful delay is less risk of bleeding beneath the pedicle. As a primary procedure, temporary coverage of a large defect with a partial thickness graft is a safer method to protect deep structures.

Degloving injuries are difficult to manage. Generally, circumferential avulsion of skin and subcutaneous tissue of a single finger is best treated by amputation, but a degloved thumb may be worth the time and effort necessary to save it. Some avulsing injuries of the thumb can be covered by a pedicle flap raised from the dorsum of the hand. Larger areas of degloving, especially when multiple digits are involved, may require eventual application of a distant pedicle from either the chest, abdomen, or even the opposite extremity.

Staged Wound Management

Staged wound management is a term used by Burkhalter in discussing the advantages of a second look procedure and primary delayed closure in managing certain extensive mutilating injuries that occur as a result of civilian accidents. As with most military and all combat injuries it is advocated that initial debridement be followed by reevaluation of the wounds in from 72 to 96 hours. If at that time, wounds contain only viable tissue and there are no signs of infection, fracture stabilization and wound closure can be carried out safely with an expectation of healing with minimal reaction. If the wound is clean and vascular, it is permissible to cover the exposed deep structures by rota-

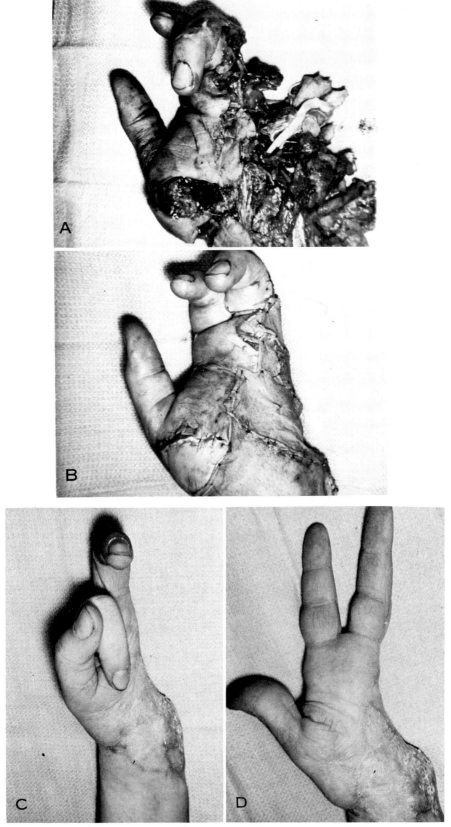

Figure 5.2.2. A. Severely crushed hand with ring and little fingers damaged beyond recall. *B.* Skin loss replaced with partial thickness skin graft. *C.* Free skin graft served as permanent cover. View of hand in flexion. *D.* View of hand in extension.

tion flaps, or in some instances a direct pedicle from a distance may be applied (Fig. 5.2.3).

Experience has shown that under proper conditions exposure of tendon or bone for three to four days does not necessarily threaten the viability of these tissues. If the dressing is not removed between the time of primary surgery and the second look, sufficient tissue fluid protects these structures from desiccation and necrosis.

Some surgeons advocate a modification of the aforementioned staged management, particularly in respect to initial management of unstable fractures. The majority of industrial injuries treated within the first few hours are seldom severely contaminated by pathogenic bacteria in spite of gross staining of tissues with carbon or grease. Following proper cleansing and thorough debridement, it is usually permissible to stabilize fractures primarily with Kirschner wires, but complete closure may be wisely delayed if there is doubt about the adequacy of debridement or concern that difficulty with control of minute bleeding could result in loss of skin grafts or jeopardizing skin flaps. Having carried out a thorough primary debridement coupled with stabilization of the skeletal framework,

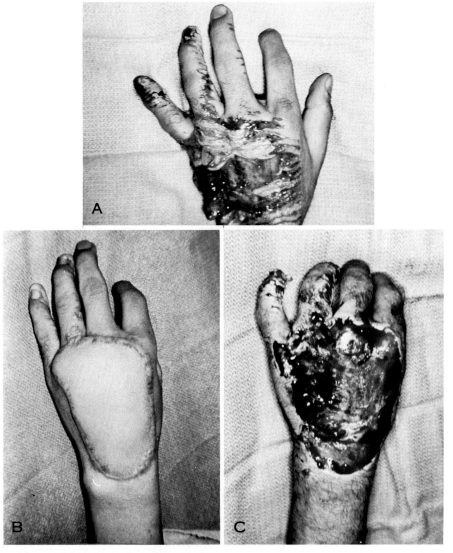

Figure 5.2.3. A. Meat cubing machine injury of dorsum of hand involving skin loss and avulsion of extensor tendons of all fingers. *B.* A pedicle flap was used to cover the skin loss because later tendon grafting to replace avulsed tendons was anticipated from onset of treatment. *C.* 72 hours following initial debridement the wounds are clean and vascular and can be closed with either a partial thickness skin graft or a distant pedicle flap.

it is usually possible at the time of the second look procedure to close completely the remaining wounds of the hand.

CORNPICKER INJURIES

Some of the most destructive injuries of the upper extremity are caused by the machine used to pick and husk corn. The roller and conveyer portion of the machine are prone to become clogged with corn stalks and other debris. Accidents most commonly occur when a worker tries manually to clear an obstruction without turning off the machine. Immediately upon removal of the obstructing piece, the machine suddenly resumes its activities, entrapping that hand or at times the forearm between the rollers. Many of the injuries crush the fingers but spare the thumb. In some instances the hand passes between the rollers and the wrist and forearm are caught and compressed. The hand or extremity may be trapped in the machine for a considerable period of time before its release.

Soft tissue damage is extensive and characterized by crushing, avulsing, and burning of the tissues. Wounds are heavily contaminated by pieces of soil and corn roughage. Grease, oil, and dirt are ground into the tissues. Traumatic amputations of the digits and hand are common. Wrist and forearm injuries have a high incidence of open fractures and dislocations of the carpal and forearm bones.

For cornpicker and other crushing injuries occurring on the farm, the essence of the primary treatment should be a thorough and meticulous debridement with alignment of displaced fractures. Because of the known danger of infection, primary wound closure should not be done, but a second look should be planned in 72 hours after the primary surgery. The dressings should be changed in the operating room. If the wounds are then clean and vascular, unstable fractures of the hand may be reduced and held with Kirschner wires, and wounds can be closed.

In some cases it may be necessary to carry out further debridement to remove additional devitalized tissues. A partial thickness skin graft is the safest type of coverage to replace a skin loss. It may be designed to serve only as a temporary cover, but in many instances may function as permanent coverage. Distant pedicle flap application should be reserved for the reconstructive phases following healing of the initial wounds and not for the purpose of wound closure.

MANGLE INJURIES

The mangle is a machine used commonly in the home for ironing and pressing laundry. It consists of a mechanically driven roller and a metal shoe which supplies the heat. The main feature of a mangle injury is a deep thermal burn, usually on the dorsal surface of the hand. In severe cases, amputation of the digits may result from the burning. Compression also may be a factor but laceration, fractures, and dislocations are rarely encountered. Unfortunately, many of the victims in the home are children. In commercial laundries deep burns occur when a worker's hand is compressed by the hot head of a shirt press. The thermal injury frequently involves the extensor tendons and the metacarpals and phalanges. These injuries may also result in complete necrosis of the digits from the effects of the heat and compression.

Usually it is not difficult to assess accurately the depth and extent of the burn within the first few days following injury. By the third to fifth day after injury, the area of full thickness skin loss is well delineated. As soon as this loss can be determined, an operative procedure to remove surgically the devitalized tissues should be planned before liquefaction necrosis and infection occur.

The devitalized skin is removed by sharp dissection. In the more severe injuries, it will be found that the underlying extensor tendons may have been partially burned or completely destroyed by the heat. The nonviable tendon has to be removed. When the bone has been burned its outer surface appears dry and is usually discolored. An efficient way of removing devitalized bone is by means of a high speed rotating burr. When fresh bleeding bone is encountered the debridement can be considered adequate, but it is usually advisable to wait for another 48 hours before applying partial thickness skin grafts to close the wound (Fig. 5.2.4). This purposeful delay will lessen the chance for loss of the graft by oozing and will make certain that the recipient area contains only viable tissues.

Distant pedicle flap application may play a part in reconstructive procedures following these deep burns, but the application of a primary pedicle flap in the presence of burned bone carries a risk of a deep infection and also the possibility of loss of the pedicle flap. The goal of early management in mangle and hot press injuries is to obtain wound closure without infection at the earliest possible moment. With an aggressive plan to remove devitalized tissues surgically followed by early application of partial thickness skin grafts as soon as the recipient site is clean and vascular, it will be possible to obtain closure and healing within the first week to 10 days following injury in the majority of cases.

WRINGER INJURIES

Injuries from the wringer-type washing machine are an existing but, fortunately, an ever decreasing problem. The accidents most commonly involve children under the age of five years. The size of the child's extremity usually determines whether the location of the injury will be at the arm and axilla, the forearm and elbow, or at the hand and wrist. The younger and smaller child suffers the more proximal injury.

The majority of injuries consist of contusions, superficial abrasions, or friction burns, and simple lacerations. Associated complex injuries are uncommon and only about 5 per cent of the accident victims sustain injuries involving nerves or tendons, amputations, or

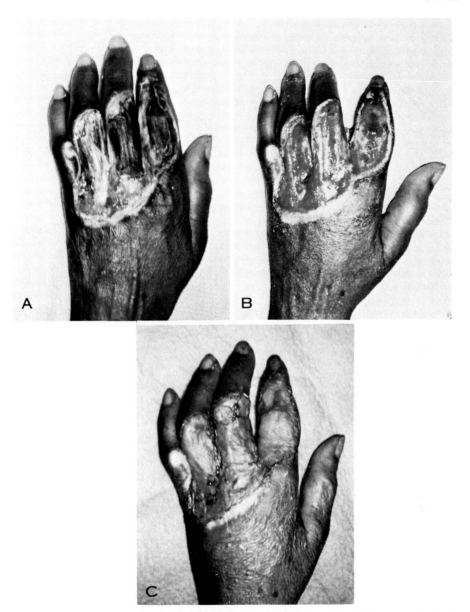

Figure 5.2.4. A. Hot press burn in middle-aged diabetic woman on admission to hospital 15 days after injury. Bone and tendon burned. *B.* 48 hours following debridement of necrotic tendon and bone. Rotatory burr used to decorticate nonviable bone. *C.* 5 days following application of partial thickness skin graft to hand. Complete take of graft over exposed but vascular bone.

major skin losses. Fractures are rarely encountered, and the incidence has been reported to be as low as 3 per cent. Transient nerve palsies involving either the median, ulnar, or radial nerves have been reported on rare occasions. Serious vascular complications or development of ischemic contractures are rarely encountered following washing machine wringer injuries.

Various reports show that about 25 per cent of the patients need delayed surgical procedures. Several days after the injury, hematomas may need drainage.

Areas of full thickness skin loss may require surgical excision and application of partial thickness skin grafts. Pedicle flap application is rarely necessary as a method for obtaining early wound closure, but pedicle flaps may be needed during reconstructive phases.

The primary treatment for the majority of injuries need not be complicated. The injured extremity is carefully cleansed and vesicles are removed. Simple lacerations may be debrided and closed under local anesthesia. Skin injuries should be covered with a single layer of fine mesh gauze followed by application of a resilient bulky dressing to the entire upper extremity. Fingertips should remain exposed in order to assess distal circulation. The limb should be elevated as well as put at rest.

In complex injuries, the need for restorative surgery can be anticipated from the onset. Surgical removal of devitalized tissues should not be delayed more than a few days following injury. Closure by partial thickness skin grafts is usually possible before the end of the first week.

BIBLIOGRAPHY

1. Burkhalter, W. E. Thoughts on delayed closure of hand wounds. In *Symposium on the Hand*. Vol. 3, edited by L. M. Cramer and R. A. Chase. St. Louis, Mosby, 1971, p. 168.
2. Burkhalter, W. E., Butler, B., Metz, W., Omer, G. Experiences with delayed primary closure of war wounds of the hand in Viet Nam. J. Bone Joint Surg., *50A:* 945, 1968.
3. Butler, B. Initial management of hand wounds. Milit. Med., *134:* 1, 1969.
4. Chase, R. A. The severely injured upper limb. Arch. Surg., *100:* 382, 1970.
5. McCulloch, J. H., Boswick, J. A., Jr., and Jonas, R. Household wringer injuries: A three-year review. J. Trauma, *13:* 1, 1973.
6. Melvin, P. M. Corn picker injuries of the hand. Arch. Surg., *104:* 26, 1972.
7. Posch, J. L., and Weller, C. N. Mangle and severe injuries of the hand in children. J. Bone Joint Surg., *36A:* 57, 1954.
8. Rank, B., Wakefield, A., and Hueston, J. *Surgery of Repair as Applied to Hand Injuries,* Ed. 3. Baltimore, Williams & Wilkins, 1968.

C.

Special Wounds

Stephen W. Meagher, M.D.

GUNSHOT WOUNDS

Gunshot wounds were first encountered during the Hundred Years War;[36] the first description of therapy was published in 1497 by Hieronymus Brunschwig.[23] The present day practice of debridement of gunshot wounds was advocated by Thomas Gale in 1563.[6]

In 1941 Black and associates[7] reported a series of ingenious experiments in which gelatin blocks and rabbit soft tissues were used. In these experiments a gun fired a 3/32-inch steel ball weighing 53 mg at ve-

locities ranging from 500 to 5,000 feet per sec. The ball pushed a head cone before it as it emerged from the block but caused no other distortion in its passage. As soon as the block was completely perforated, it expanded to three to four times its original volume. In spite of the great distortion the block returned to its original size and shape. It was concluded that particles of matter in the path of the missile were thrown radially with great violence, creating a cavity.

Krauss[31] discovered additional information about the cavitation effect in soft tissues by inflicting gunshot wounds into animal organs. He established that the cavity appears and attains its maximal size within 3 to 5 msec. after passage of a small steel ball at velocities up to about 3,300 feet per sec.

In Krauss's studies, a liquid plastic was poured into the cavity through the wound of entrance. After the plastic had hardened, the surrounding soft tissues were removed. These molds demonstrated conclusively that the size of the cavity is determined by the velocity of the missile and increases as the velocity increases.

Puckett[38] and associates have pointed out that nerve damage may be inflicted when the missile passes through the vicinity of the nerve without striking it directly, provided the velocity is high enough.

Low velocity missiles do not cause comparable destruction. When the velocity is low it is possible for a small caliber bullet to pass through the palm without leaving behind any tendon, nerve, or skeletal injury; when injuries are produced, they occur by direct hit and not by the cavitation effect.

Adams[2] published a brilliant paper on small caliber missile blast wounds of the hand in which eight cases of self-inflicted palmar wounds were reported. The pattern was the same in every case. The wound of entrance was neat and small; the wound of exit in the dorsum of the hand was characterized by large stellate tears in every case. Adams found that within 24 hours the hand had attained a thickness of three times normal; at seven to 10 days wrinkling and subsidence of the edema were present. On the eighth day, a delayed primary closure of the dorsal wound of exit was carried out; the palmar wound was allowed to remain open. Tetanus prophylaxis and antibiotics were given at the outset of treatment and the antibiotics were continued.

Milford[33] emphasized the widespread destruction to all tissues encountered in the treatment of shotgun wounds. The need for reconstruction is much greater in this type of wound which frequently requires new skin cover, tendon transplants, transfers, and fracture management. Shotguns cause severe wounds at short range only.[17]

Nail gun injuries of the hand result in small skin lesions and more serious damage in deeper structures. The nail gun is powered by a 22-caliber long rifle cartridge developing a velocity of 1,000 meters per sec.[9]

The Korean War provided one of the most significant advances in the treatment of missile wounds.

Inui's[28] report spans the two periods of arterial Ligation and arterial repair. In his series, the amputation rate was 50 per cent in six patients who underwent ligation of the brachial artery; the amputation rate was 0 per cent in 25 patients who underwent repair of the brachial artery.

In the series reported by Jahnke and Seeley[29] relating the Korean War experience, amputation was not required. Thirty-two patients with arterial wounds in the upper extremity underwent arterial repair by end-to-end anastomosis, transverse closure, or vein graft.

Treatment

The extremity is shaved and scrubbed for 10 minutes with an agent containing hexachlorophene or a suitable substitute after a regional block has been administered. Irrigation of the wound is performed with a few to many liters of sterile Ringer's solution or isotonic saline, depending on the characteristics of the wound. When hemorrhage is a factor the pneumatic tourniquet may be inflated before the period of preparation. A thorough excision of nonviable tissues is done; the contaminated wound margins are excised. Reconstruction of tendons is delayed in all patients with gunshot wounds. Arterial wounds of significant vessels are repaired as soon as possible because the patency rate following arteriorrhaphy falls sharply when primary repair is performed more than eight hours after injury. Nerves made surgically clean should be repaired primarily.

Skeletal fragments that have been stripped of tissue attachments should be removed. Internal fixation of fractures is carried out as required to provide stability during the anticipated period of immobilization.

It is inappropriate to close gunshot wounds primarily; there is no support in the literature for doing so.

Since gas gangrene is not an expected complication, prophylaxis is confined to the administration of human hyperimmune globulin, tetanus toxoid, and antibiotic coverage with a broad spectrum drug.

A compression dressing and elevation of the hand are mechanical measures which assure the best possible control over the edema of the hand that is certain to follow within the first 24 hours, as stressed by Adams.[2]

After the first week has passed, the gunshot hand falls into the broad category of traumatic injury. Reconstruction may be planned so that a maximal return of function can be provided.

Grease Gun Injuries

The grease gun operated by compressed air is used by all modern service centers for vehicles and aircraft. In addition, the emission of fuel oil under pressure in diesel engines[21] [40] duplicates the mechanism of a grease gun and provides a similar opportunity for injury.

In most recorded cases, the injection of the hand was sustained by the inadvertent slipping of the needle from the nipple.

The presence and intensity of pain in the digit and hand are determined by the location and volume of the injection, because when a large volume of lubricant is injected into the digit there is immediate compression of the neurovascular bundles with resultant blanching and numbness of the digit.

The wound of entrance measures from one to several mm in diameter. Grease or diesel fuel may exude from this minute wound. The foreign material follows the tissue planes; it has been known to reach the region of the epitrochlear gland.[27]

The lubricant acts as an irritant and evokes an inflammatory response characterized by loculating fibrosis with an infiltration of lymphocytes and foreign body giant cells. When these sites become well organized they are called oleomas.

With one exception, all authors[10, 20, 25, 27, 37, 39 40, 43, 44, 46] advocate immediate incision and evacuation of as much material as possible as the best method of preserving the digit and minimizing the loss of function. Byrne[12] feels that longitudinal incisions may compromise viability and that surgery should be reserved for the removal of sloughing tissues and incision of fluctuant areas when abscesses develop.

Despite all efforts to remove the grease at the original procedure, there is general agreement that it cannot be done completely. Most patients develop chronic oleomas which require drainage or excision.

The low incidence of injuries is remarkable when we consider the widespread use of grease guns. Stark and associates[44] collected 14 cases and added five of their own in their 1961 report.

PUNCTURE WOUNDS

The puncture wound is one of the most common hand injuries, being inflicted by such objects as wooden splinters, tacks, pins, needles, staples, pencils, knives, awls, screwdrivers; chisels, glass, metal, plastic, grease guns, etc. It is frequently associated with the problems of a retained foreign body, divided tendons and nerves, infection and, rarely, false aneurysms, arteriovenous fistulas, and hematomas of a tendon sheath.[20]

When the patient is first seen, a thorough examination of sensation and function must be carried out systematically to detect unsuspected injuries. For this reason, the function of each long flexor and extensor tendon must be tested in all cooperative patients. Motor nerves in the hand must be evaluated by observing the patient's ability to abduct the thumb and remaining digits. In addition, the bilateral digital nerves to every finger must be tested for sensation with a pin to avoid the embarrassment of overlooking an important injury.

In the absence of evidence of functional or sensory impairment or positive x-ray findings, it is frequently satisfactory to prescribe a cleansing of the wound and hot water soaks to control contaminating organisms.

If the surgeon has reason to believe that a nerve or

tendon has been injured, operative exploration to debride and repair injured tissues is advisable.

When it is decided to attempt a removal of a foreign body, a reasonable time limit should be set and adhered to by the surgeon, and x-rays in at least two planes of the hand or arm should be taken before operating. The value of the Berman locator in finding suitable objects should not be overlooked.

POWER MOWER INJURIES

When the rotary power mower obtained recognition as a status symbol, there was an enormous increase in its production to meet a nationwide demand.

The extremely dangerous aspects of power mowers have been stressed by all authors.[11,14,24,26,47] It has been estimated that more than 50,000 injuries are sustained annually through the use of power mowers.[11] Direct contact injuries and missile injuries are the two basic methods of injury. The blades of a rotary mower revolve at a rate of 2,400 to 3,600 revolutions per min at a force that may reach 10,000 lb per square in.[47] Missiles that are cast by the mower may attain a speed of 300 ft per sec[47] (near the speed of a low velocity missile).

The operator usually sustains a partial or complete amputation of one or more toes; rarely the heel may be involved. The hand is injured when the operator attempts to clear away weeds trapped by the blade; in this instance, digits are badly lacerated or amputated.

The treatment of patients with hand injuries sustained on a power mower or snow blower usually consists of cleansing and debridement of lacerations and traumatic amputation stumps, followed by procedures that complete the amputation and provide skin cover. The most important late morbidity is provided by inadequate skin cover of the stump and improper disposition of the severed digital nerves (Fig. 5.3.1).

The amputation stump must be well padded beyond the tip of the underlying bone. In lieu of primary closure, this can best be accomplished by a cross-finger pedicle or abdominal pedicle flap.

SNOW BLOWER INJURIES

The snow blower has attained prominence in the same manner as the power mower among home owners who regard the snow blower as a new symbol of personal wealth (Fig. 5.3.2).

Snow blowers can produce an injury to the hand in three basic ways. First, the fingers may be crushed, lacerated, or amputated by the slowly turning escalating auger that seizes and feeds snow to the blower for ejection through a chute at high speed (Fig. 5.3.3). Second, the fingers may be lacerated or amputated by inadvertently introducing them into the high speed fan which can be reached by placing the hand in the chute to clear away snow, or to change the direction of the chute (Fig. 5.3.4). Third, missiles ejected by the blower from the chute at a moderate rate of speed constitute a definite percentage of the injuries produced by this machine.

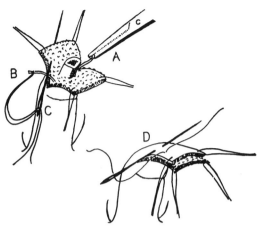

Figure 5.3.1. A correct method of procedure in disposing of the severed ends of the digital nerves following a traumatic amputation. The nerve should be crushed (A), ligated (B), and, with a needle (C), transposed into the dorsal tissues (D) away from the working surface of the digit and the terminal scar.

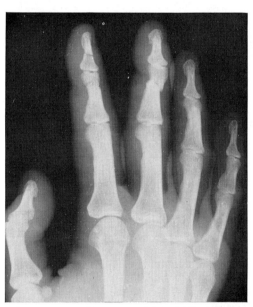

Figure 5.3.2. Fractures of the middle and distal phalanges of the index finger and the middle phalanx of the long finger of the right hand sustained by placing the hand into the chute of a snowblower. The unstable fracture of the middle finger required internal fixation with crossed Kirschner wires to maintain satisfactory alignment.

COMPRESSED AIR INJURIES

Compressed air tools are most widely known among physicians for their effect on the peripheral ar-

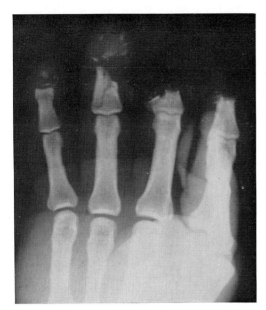

Figure 5.3.3. Partial amputation of the index, long, ring, and small fingers of the hand sustained by placing the hand into the chute of a snowblower.

teries which is attributed to their vibratory action. These tools are used in great quantity by riveters, pneumatic shisellers, and drillers.

Less well known is the use of compressed air as a tool coolant and blowing device for the removal of dust, chips, and turnings during the machining of metals and other materials. The air leaves the nozzle of a tube with a force of 70 to 90 lb per square in; this force can dent the soft tissues of the hand.[48] Desmond[19] and Whitwell[48] have independently reported instances of emphysema of the hand sustained by compressed air injection through minor preexisting puncture wounds and lacerations.

MOLTEN PLASTIC INJURIES

The plastics industry has introduced the molten plastic injury. Molten plastic, heated to 500°F, is injected under a pressure of 4,000 lb per square in into molds, according to Baker.[5] He reported two cases of hand injection when the hands inadvertently were placed over the injector nozzle. In both cases the plastic hardened immediately and caused extensive damage to adjacent tissues. Desjacques and Cognat[18] reported a similar injury; in their case x-ray showed the plastic clearly.

The pressure and heat destroy tissues and cause thrombosis of vessels. This feature was responsible for gangrene of the distal pads of two fingers in the case of Desjacques and Cognat.

The plastic solidifies into a single, easily removable mass. Debridement is the essential step in primary treatment.

The fact that Baker had to treat a gas infection due to *Bacillus welchii* in one patient and Desjacques and Cognat's patient had gangrenous areas should clearly discourage attempts at primary reconstruction.

PORCELAIN FAUCET INJURIES

The term "porcelain faucet injury" was coined by Boyes and Melone[8] for their 1952 report of 74 consecutive cases of this type of injury. The straight bar type of porcelain faucet handle was responsible for the injuries in 73 patients.

The mechanism of injury in the majority was thought to be the added force required to close a leaking faucet with a handle that had been cracked beforehand.

They concluded that the wound was usually small and located in the midpalm. All but one patient had a nerve or tendon injury or both; 73 per cent had flexor tendon damage and 85 per cent had nerve damage. Nerve and tendon involvement was usually confined to the thumb and index rays.

WELDERS' INJURIES

In welding, metal parts are joined by a combination of mechanical pressure and the heat generated in the metal by passage of an electric current. During this process, "splashing" of sparks of red hot metallic particles may occur, causing the small superficial scars seen on the hands and arms of welders.

Reynard[42] reported 12 patients with welders' injuries. He stressed that the injuries seldom keep the welders from their work. Occasionally, it is necessary to drain a small abscess or excise a sinus tract; electromagnets were useful in removing some of the metallic foreign bodies.

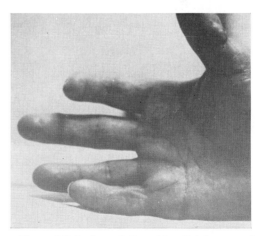

Figure 5.3.4. Amputation of the distal segment of the right index finger and lacerations of the distal segment of the right long finger involving the lateral digital nerve. These injuries were sustained when the hand grasped the chute of a snowblower to change its direction.

Protective gloves and clothing are of first importance in preventing injuries.

AEROSOL BOMB INJURIES

Metzler[32] related an incident that underscores one of the dangerous aspects of the aerosol bomb. A man was holding a DDT bomb. He opened the needle valve a three-quarter turn; in doing so the valve was blown out, allowing a mixture of phrethrum, DDT, and Freon to escape. He placed his hand over the opening to stop the spray and rushed from the building. When he dropped the bomb outside, his hand was frozen in the shape in which it had been cupped over the bomb. The injuries sustained were equivalent to a third degree burn. Every aerosol bomb and pressure can is capable of inflicting blast wounds and missile injuries.

TEAR-GAS PEN

Sociologic changes have caused some to carry a tear-gas pen for self defense. Tear-gas powder combines chloracetophenone and silica anhydride, 1:1. At short range the material will penetrate the hand. The powder is toxic to pheripheral nerves. Necrosis may occur in skeletal muscle. Complete debridement is necessary for best results.[1]

RUCKSACK PARALYSIS

Daube[15] has reported this condition in some Army personel in Vietnam. Traction injury of the upper trunk of the brachial plexus has been caused by the heavy backpack. This problem is increasing with the current enthusiam in camping and hiking. Renard[41] has taken issue with Daube on certain features, particularly the importance of the hip belt. It seems logical that a properly fastened hip belt results in loose shoulder straps and little shoulder pressure.

REFERENCES

1. Adams, J. P., Fee, N., Liebowitz, Bernstein, L. H. Tear-gas injuries: a clinical study of hand injuries and an experimental study of its effects on peripheral nerves and skeletal muscle in rabbits. J. Bone Joint Surg., 48A: 436-442, 1966.
2. Adams, R. W. Small caliber missile blast wounds of the hand. Am. J. Surg., 82: 219, 1951.
3. Aids to the investigation of peripheral nerve injuries. Medical Research Council, War Memorandum, No. 7. London, Her Majesty's Stationery Office, 1943.
4. Amato, J. J. Vascular injuries. Arch. Surg., 101: 167, 1970.
5. Baker, J. M. Molten plastic injuries of the hand. Plast. Reconstr. Surg., 15: 233, 1955.
6. Berry, F. P. Editorial. U. S. Armed Forces Med. J., 5: iv, 1954.
7. Black, A. N., Burns, B. D., and Zuckerman, S. An experimental study of the wounding mechanism of high velocity missiles. Br. Med. J., 2: 872, 1946.
8. Boyes, J. H., and Melone, F. C. Injuries to the hand from broken porcelain faucet handles. West. J. Surg., 60: 59, 1952.
9. Braun, R. M. Nail-gun injury of the hand. J. Bone Joint Surg., 53A: 383, 1971.
10. Brooke, R., and Rooke, C. J. Two cases of grease-gun finger. Br. J. Med., 2: 1186, 1939.
11. Butterworth, T. R. Rotary lawn mower injuries. Am. J. Surg., 23: 815, 1957.
12. Byrne, J. J. Grease-gun injuries. J.A.M.A., 125: 405, 1944.
13. Byrne, J. J. The Hand, Springfield, Charles C Thomas, 1959, p. 189
14. Chazen, E. M., and Chamberlain, J. L., 3rd. Hazards to health. Missile injuries due to power lawn mowers. N. Engl. J. Med., 266: 822, 1962.
15. Daube, J. R. Rucksack paralysis. J.A.M.A., 208: 2447-2452, 1969.
16. DeBakey, M. E., and Simeone, F. A. Battle injuries of the arteries in World War 11. Ann. Surg., 123: 534, 1946.
17. De Muth, W. E., Jr. The mechanism of shot gun wounds. J. Trauma, 11: 219, 1971.
18. Desjacques, R., and Cognat, M. Injection accidentella a chaud de matière plastique dans la main. Presse Med., 67: 1878, 1959.
19. Desmond, A. M. Surgical emphysema due to compressed air. Br. Med. J., 1: 842, 1947.
20. Devenish, E. A. Haematoma of the flexor tendon sheaths of the hand following penetrating wounds. Lancet, 1: 447, 1939.
21. Dial, D. E. Hand injuries due to injection of oil at high pressures. J.A.M.A., 110: 1747, 1938.
22. Dimond, F. C., Jr., et al. M-16 rifle wounds in Vietnam. J. Trauma, 7: 619, 1967.
23. Garrison, F. H.: An Introduction to History of Medicine, Ed. 3. Philadelphia, Saunders, 1921, p. 276.
24. Grosfeld, J. L. et al. Lawn mower injuries in children. Arch. Surg., 100: 582. 1970.
25. Harrison, R. Grease-gun injury. Br. J. Surg., 46: 514, 1959.
26. Henley, T. H.: Rotary lawn mower injuries. J. Okla. State Med. Assn., 54: 97, 1961.
27. Innes, C. B. Grease-gun finger. N. Z. Med. J., 58: 177, 1959.
28. Inui, F. K., Shannon, J., and Howard, J. M. Arterial injuries in the Korean conflict. Surgery, 37: 850, 1955.
29. Jahnke, E. J., Jr., and Seeley, S. F. Acute vascular injuries in Korean war: An analysis of 77 consecutive cases. Ann. Surg., 138: 158, 1953.
30. Kenny, N. J. et al. Motor mower injuries. Med. J. Aust., 2: 547, 1966.
31. Krauss, M. Studies in wound ballistics: Temporary cavity effects in soft tissues. Milit. Med., 121: 221, 1957.
32. Metzler, D. F. Injury resulting from use of aerosol bomb. Pub. Health Rep., 61: 546, 1946.
33. Milford, L. Shotgun wounds of the hand and wrist. South. Med. J., 52: 403, 1959.
34. Ogilvie, H. Shot-gun wounds. Practitioner, 175: 304, 1955.
35. Oglesby, J. E. Twenty-two months war surgery in Vietnam. Arch. Surg., 102: 607, 1971.
36. Omer, G. E., Jr. The early management of gunshot wounds of the extremities. S. D. J. Med., 9: 340, 1956.
37. Osborne, J. C. Grease-gun injury. Can. J. Surg., 3: 339, 1960.
38. Puckett, W. D., Grundfest, H., McElroy, W. D., and

McMillan, J. H. Damage to peripheral nerves by high velocity missiles without a direct hit. J. Neurosurg., *3:* 294, 1946.

39. Raines, A. J. H. Grease-gun injury to the hand. Br. J. Med., *1:* 625, 1958.

40. Rees, C. E. Penetration of tissue by fuel oil under high pressure from Diesel engine. J.A.M.A., *109:* 866. 1937.

41. Reynard, D., Rucksack paralysis. J.A.M.A., *210:* 1102, 1969.

42. Reynard, W. A. B. Digital foreign bodies in spot welders. Br. Med. J., *1:* 843, 1947.

43. Smith, H. F. Penetration of tissue by grease under pressure of 7000 pounds J.A.M.A., *112:* 907, 1939.

44. Stark, H. H., Wilson, J. N., and Boyes, J. H. Grease-gun injuries of the hand. J. Bone Joint Surg., *43A:* 485, 1961.

45. Symonds, F. C., and Graves, A. L. Tear gas gun injury of the hand. Plast. Reconstr. Surg., *39:* 175, 1967.

46. Vivian, D. N., and Christian, S. G. Grease-gun injury. Ind. Med. Surg., *25:* 282, 1956.

47. White, W. L. Menace of rotary lawn mower. Am. J. Surg., *93:* 674, 1957.

48. Whitwell, G. P. B. Subcutaneous emphysema due to compressed air. Br. J. Ind. Med., *1:* 129, 1944.

49. Woodruff, C. E. The causes of the explosive effect of modern small caliber bullets. N. Y. J. Med., *67:* 593, 1898.

chapter six

Fractures of the Hand and Wrist

Charles H. Bradford, M.D.

James A. Dolphin, M.D.

HAND FRACTURES

The remarkable effectiveness of the human hand as a mechanical tool and as a precision instrument depends on many characteristics, but from the standpoint of fracture treatment the characteristic of greatest concern lies in a proper alignment of the struts and lever arms furnished by the skeletal structures. The *mobility* of these structures is as important as their positioning. Thus, in dealing with the broken down mechanism that confronts us after trauma, we are faced with the double problem of replacing the struts in their optimal functional position and also of restoring the fullest possible movement to the joints. Healing of broken bones requires immobilization and time, but if this is pursued too insistently rigid immobilization for a prolonged interval will cause irreversible stiffness in the joints. The corollary is equally true, for if movement of the fractures is carried out too soon the essential efficiency of the lever arms will be lost through nonunion or malalignment.

With these thoughts in mind the fracture surgeon should never forget that his primary objective is to obtain the best possible functioning hand that can be salvaged from the injuries with which he is dealing. He must adapt general principles to individual cases, as there is hardly any single case that conforms to an academic pattern. Some fractures will require prolonged and patient immobilization, and still others will call for open surgery, some authorities reporting better results from one routine and some from another. The surgeon, therefore, must keep an open mind on all these questions and must recognize that there is no single or isolated solution to the more difficult problems.

In this chapter, emphasis will be centered on the various types of fractures that deserve to be recognized, as it is felt that too little attention has been devoted to this aspect of the problem. For each category, or type of fracture, we will present those considerations that we feel to be most significant; but where other successful methods are in use, the relative advantages and disadvantages will be discussed. Attention will also be called to prevalent common errors and to the methods by which these errors can be avoided. The source from which our experience has been drawn originated with a closely supervised series of over 700 cases studied on the Hand Service at the Boston City Hospital.

Distal Phalanx

Simple Fractures of Distal Phalanx

The simplest type of fracture that we may encounter is perhaps that of the distal phalanx. This is almost invariably the result of a crushing injury. In most of these cases the mechanical pull of the tendons is not exerted on the bony fragments and hence there is practically no complicating factor to consider. The position of the fragmented spicules seldom offers any serious threat of future disability. Hence these fractures may usually be treated by a malleable metal padded splint curved to place the fingers in slight flexion or with a simple "gutter splint" of light plaster.

The accumulating hematoma in these cases compresses the mesh of nerve tissue in the pulp of the finger. Thus, the first step in treatment should be to release this tension by evacuating the attendant subungual hematoma. Small holes rapidly fill up with blood clot and the better practice is to drill three or four holes through the nail, in a triangular or a rectangular pattern close enough together to lift up the central portion and thus provide a sizable outlet. The skin and nail are first carefully washed with antiseptic and the open wound is then covered with an antiseptic dressing. As soon as the digit ceases to be tender all protection may be removed.

A practical note on the technique for drilling holes through the fingernail may be helpful. An ordinary paper clip is straightened out so as to present the round, free end of the wire. This is held in a hemostat and is heated red hot in an alcohol flame or Bunsen burner. The tip of the wire is then pressed against the finger nail and with three or four such applications it will burn a neat hole through the nail. This is usually painless because the nail is elevated from its bed by the hematoma.

Compound Fractures of the Distal Phalanx

The usual cleaning, lavage, and debridement will, of course, be necessary, followed by some procedure that will cover the bare wound. Often the skin flaps left by the wound will suffice but if these fail to do so a free, full thickness graft, taken from the forearm or thigh, should be applied. A convenient donor area is the skin of the antecubital fossa. An elliptical incision just distal and parallel to the elbow crease yields an adequate size graft of good quality and an easily closed wound. The graft should be thoroughly and carefully defatted. Alternative methods of split thickness grafts and pedicle flaps do not seem to us to work as well. The full thickness graft may have poorer chances of survival than those of split thickness but its chances are still reasonably good and it leaves a better stump when it heals.

In cases where the fracture is grossly comminuted and where the finger nail and its bed are seriously damaged the possible need for removing the finger nail *in toto* deserves consideration. However, it is preferable to leave the intact segment of the nail and merely remove the avulsed portion. A common accompanying injury with distal phalangeal fractures is avulsion of the nail bed. It is impossible to predict the degree of nail damage at the time of injury and therefore attempts at eradicating the matrix and nail bed are not part of the initial wound care. A deformed, troublesome nail following a finger injury can be corrected later.

Avulsion Fractures of Distal Phalanx

Many fractures of the distal phalanx involve an avulsion of the common extensor attachment. This may carry a thin fragment of the base of the phalanx (Fig. 6.1) with it as it is torn away, or it may more frequently tear the tendinous fibers themselves without disturbing the bone. The result in either case is the familiar "baseball" or "mallet" finger which, if untreated, leaves a partially flexed distal phalanx lacking the power of extension. This injury, of course, requires a splint which will maintain hyperextension of the distal joint while it also holds the interphalangeal joint in moderate flexion. The old method of splinting with a throat stick which holds the finger fully extended has generally been discarded on the grounds that this position stretches the lumbricales and interossei, thereby increasing the tension at the site of injury.

In our own practice we have followed the technique of Bohler,[4] which is also accepted by most of the leading authorities. This involves application of plaster to maintain hyperextension of the distal joint and flexion of the interphalangeal joint. The plaster splint is carried from the midpalm to the tip of the finger and is then folded back over the dorsum to extend to the midportion of the metacarpal. The metacarpophalangeal joint is flexed to about 30°, the proximal interphalangeal joint to about 60° and the distal joint is hyperextended about 10° (Fig. 6.2). The plaster splint should be the same width as the breadth of the finger and must be moderately thick. It can be applied moist enough to mold and then be bound around the finger with gauze or elastic bandage. Then the patient can be supervised in holding it with the proper position with his other hand while the plaster sets, a period of fully 5 to 10 min. The splint should be retained for it least six weeks, after which the finger tip should be protected from undue flexion strain for another two weeks with a light splint. An alternative method of treating this injury has recently been reviewed by Stark *et al.*[33]

Perhaps more important than the type of splint is the cooperation of the patient in providing uninterrupted rest to the distal finger joint. Callus must form between the bone segments or fibrosis between the tendon ends to restore the extension continuity. The patient who removes his splint to wash or the surgeon who tests the finger weekly is courting failure.

Weekly inspection of the splint is recommended with changes being done only while extension of the distal phalanx is maintained by the surgeon.

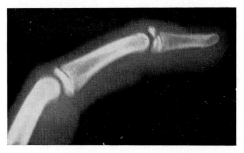

Figure 6.1. Avulsion fracture of distal phalanx, showing fragment of base of phalanx torn away.

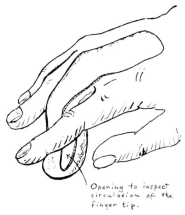

Figure 6.2. "Baseball" finger injury. Flexion at proximal interphalangeal joint and hyperextension at distal joint.

Frequently these cases are not brought to the surgeon until some time after they occur, which greatly affects the prognosis. The best results come from immediate treatment, and after one week it is rare to obtain success with this closed treatment, although it might be worth trying up to two weeks. If the patient is first seen with a "mallet finger" later than two weeks after injury, surgical correction must be considered. In arriving at a decision, several points must be borne in mind. The most important thing to remember is that a mallet finger is frequently not disabling. If, after a trial of several months, the patient does find the deformity a handicap, arthrodesis of the distal finger joint can be performed. This gives a cosmetically suitable finger that functions quite well.

Should the patient feel that his or her job requirement is such that hyperflexion of the distal phalanx is incapacitating, surgical correction may be attempted without this "trial period." Surgeons should not be overoptimistic in recommending it, for, although the flail character of the joint can be corrected, this is apt to be accompanied by stiffness which patients sometimes find very disappointing.

The pullout technique of Bunnell, with No. 34ss wire suture, is satisfactory if the extensor tendon can be advanced to its normal insertion. This is especially applicable when an avulsed bone chip is present. If the extensor tendon cannot be mobilized and advanced distalward, a suture graft as described by Nichols[25] has given satisfactory results. The graft source is either the palmaris longus tendon or a two inch "shaving" from the flexor carpi radialis tendon.

Alternative methods for the primary treatment of these avulsion fractures include the use of a Kirschner wire as described by Pratt.[28] This is inserted through the finger tip, transfixing the distal and proximal phalanges, the distal joint being held in hyperextension and the proximal interphalangeal joint in slight flexion. Such a technique might be justified in skilled hands but it involves risk of damage to the tactile end of the finger and damage to the joint. In unskilled hands it also involves risk from infection and in one case where it was used this complication led to amputation of the finger. A second alternative lies in primary rather than secondary operation to bind the avulsed fragment back into place. This also might be justified in skilled hands but it does not seem necessary in treating fresh injuries and it offers its own risk of surgical disappointments. Mich would depend on the size of the avulsed fragment, the time interval after injury and the age of the patient in deciding on such a procedure but it is certainly well worth bearing in mind.

Common Errors in Treating Distal Phalanx

1. Neglect of an extensor-avulsion injury ("mallet" finger) may be due to the patient's own indifference in seeking treatment, or to advice of an inexperienced surgeon who tells him that splinting is useless. Lack of early treatment of this injury is a common cause of the permanent disability that results.

2. Improper splinting of an extensor-avulsion injury is still far too commonly practiced.

3. Removal of a splint too early after an extensor-avulsion injury is equivalent to neglect of splinting altogether. At least six weeks of full splinting and a week of protection are required.

Fractures of the Proximal and Middle Phalanges

Analysis of Fracture Mechanics

It is impossible to discuss the intricacies of phalangeal fractures without becoming involved in the confusing topic of tendinous insertions and muscular pulls. Our simple diagram (Fig. 6.3) illustrates that the attachment of the extensor tendon pulls the proximal fragment up, while the sublimus tendon pulls the distal fragment down. When the fracture occurs more distally, however, the extensor pull is neutralized and the proximal fragment is directed downward, rather than upward, by the sublimus tendon which acts upon it. The true problem, however, it not by any means as simple as this since the fracture line is often comminuted or oblique, without clear demarcation. In addition, the capsular ligaments and the retinacular expansions of the tendons affect the muscular pull to a degree that could not be represented in simple diagrammatic form. The common displacement of middle phalanx fractures is volar angulation. Manipulation is performed to reverse this deformity and the finger immobilized in partial flexion. We have not seen cases with the base of the phalanx held in extension, but when this occurs, it is probably best handled by manipulative correction and immobilization in the slightly flexed neutral position.

The muscle pulls applied to the proxmial phalanx are somewhat less complicated than those of the middle phalanx, as they are also less specific. Here the governing mechanism is that of the lumbrical pull, which tightens down on the fracture, producing angulation that invariably displaces the fracture with its apex toward the palm, as illustrated in Figure 6.4. It is more apparent here than in the middle phalanx, that treatment requires flexion to release the tension of the lumbrical pull and to allow the extensor tendons to help stabilize the fracture.

In addition to our analysis of muscle pull, we must devote attention to the traumatic mechanism of the fracture itself. This can be judged to some extent by

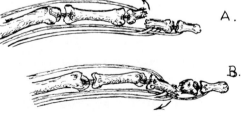

Figure 6.3. Mechanisms of tendons pulling on midphalangeal fractures at different levels.

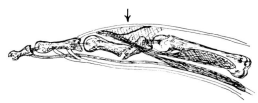

Figure 6.4. Schematic drawing of the pull of the interosseus and lumbrical muscles on a proximal phalangeal fracture.

x-ray interpretation, traumatic history, and theoretical analysis. In industry there are, of course, many instances of direct trauma; by learning the details of the accident, their mechanical forces can be reconstructed. Shattering and comminuted fractures are apt to be due to this cause and the deformity will take the pattern of the precipitating force rather than following an anatomic pattern. In the absence of such direct trauma, a great number of phalangeal fractures occur from indirect strain as the finger is violently hyperextended. These forces have been well described by O'Donoghue[27] in his excellent textbook on athletic injuries. Under forcible hyperextension, the proximal phalanx tends to displace backward on the metacarpal, but its movement is resisted by the capsule. This may tear off a fragment of the proximal phalanx by ligamentous pull on the palmar side, or there may be impaction and displacement of a lip of the phalanx on the dorsal side (Fig. 6.5). In the case of dorsal impaction close to the joint with displacement, the fracture should be immobilized in extension; whereas avulsion fractures, where the phalangeal fragment has been torn off on the palmar side, require flexion.

A little more distally, the same application of mechanical force in hyperextension will account for fractures of the midportion of the proximal phalanx. As the finger is suddenly hyperextended, the pull of the joint capsule refuses to "let go," which is perhaps aided by pull of the flexor tendons. The bone gives way under the compression of the lumbrical expansion, causing a fracture of the type we have already discussed in analyzing the muscle pulls.

Still another, rather infrequent form of indirect trauma in the opposite direction may be found at the distal end of the proximal phalanx where the finger is violently pulled into flexion and the head of the phalanx is pulled downward, breaking off at its neck. Here it is a little hard to explain the resistive force that causes angulation, other than the mechanical pull itself and the localized downward pressure of the lumbricals exerted on the distal fragment. O'Donoghue[27] has aptly described this action by saying that "the distal end of the phalanx is snubbed downward toward the palm." As he notes, it produces a displacement similar to the familiar type in fractures of the distal end of the metacarpal, which it closely resembles. Quite obviously, it requires manipulation to replace it in proper alignment; and it may be held in a neutral position.

Our mechanical analysis of phalangeal fractures should be carried one step further in attempting to draw a distinction between stable and unstable types. This distinction is basically important for deciding whether traction is or is not needed to maintain alignment. On this point a certain amount of disagreement exists, and Howard,[16] in an excellent, unpublished instructional course has expressed opposition to the use of traction. He employs two very sound arguments — the first being that a pull on the capsular ligaments of the phalangeal joints tends to stiffen them, and the second, that as it is generally applied, the traction is apt to compress the palmar surface of the finger against the splint, perhaps injuring circulation. He also points out that a true pull cannot be exerted around a corner — which must be done when the finger is bent in a flexed position. It might also be added that unless traction is very carefully calibrated, it has a tendency to separate bone ends, and thus delay fracture healing. In justification of these observations, it should be admitted that traction has been greatly abused in the past; that it is perhaps seldom necessary; and that when applied it should be used with no more than a realtively light pull, more to stabilize the fracture than to draw it into place. Nevertheless, the great preponderance of authoritative opinion favors the use of some traction in selected cases, and the real problem is to decide which fractures are too unstable to be treated without such a safeguard.

The recognition of "an unstable fracture" is largely a matter of judgment, but this will be governed by some factors that can be defined under three headings. First, there are fractures with such extensive comminution that they are likely to be pulled into malalignment unless a stabilizing degree of traction is applied. Second, there are fractures with such oblique surfaces that they are likely to slip past each other and override when any muscle pull is exerted. Third, there are fractures where the bone ends lack stabilizing support and where they seem too "wobbly" to hold themselves without help. From our own experience, we

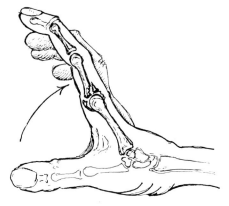

Figure 6.5. Hyperextension causing impaction of the dorsal fragment and avulsion of the volar fragment at the base of the first phalanx.

feel that traction definitely has a place in treating phalangeal fractures, although we are glad to have the dangers and the abuses of traction brought to notice.

Techniques of Treatment

We begin with the displaced fracture of the proximal phalanx, augulated with its apex downward in the usual position of deformity (Fig. 6.6). This, according to Marble, ''may become the most incapacitating injury of the hand'' since defective treatment proves so damaging to the entire complex mechanism of the flexor tendon and associated lumbricals and interossei. These fractures of the proximal phalanx incidentally occur twice as often as either of the other phalanges,[6] indicating the proportionate degree of leverage and stress that is exerted at this level. Under appropriate anesthesia, the fracture should first be manipulated to obtain as nearly anatomic alignment as possible. It is a serious mistake to rely on traction to align the fragments, for at the most traction aims at stabilization, not correction, of the position. In order not to lose position after the reduction, a plaster half-splint should be prepared in advance, extending under the forearm from just below the elbow, and under the whole hand to the proximal interphalangeal joints. This splint is best applied while it is still partially moist and while it lends some support, but can still be molded to fit the exact contours of the hand — that is, within 10 to 15 min after its first preparation (Fig. 6.7). As a preliminary, the surgeon can first mold the splint to his own hand, allowing for the difference in size of the patient, and can then fit it on the patient as soon as the fracture has been manipulated and reduced. This half-cast should be dorsiflexed about 35° at the wrist and should be palmar-flexed about 40° at the metacarpal level. If the fracture is felt to be stable, the plaster should be extended under the affected finger. The interphalangeal joint should be flexed about 45°. Separate consideration will be given to the thumb. This palmar splinting should be securely attached to the forearm. The volar, plaster splint, as mentioned above, should be secured to the hand and forearm with a well applied elastic bandage and adhesive. The end of the finger should be left free for inspection at the finger tip. If the fracture is felt to be potentially unstable, traction applied to the finger may

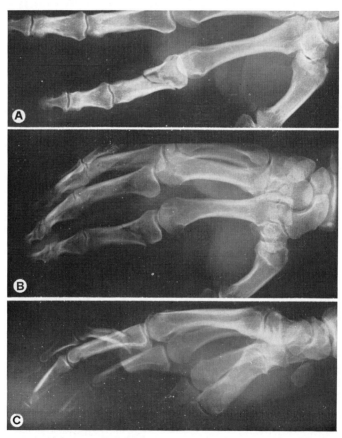

Figure 6.6. A. Anteroposterior view of fractured base first phalanx (index finger) showing what appears to be *no* serious displacement. *B.* Oblique view; suggests only slight angulation. *C.* True lateral view shows disastrous deformity.

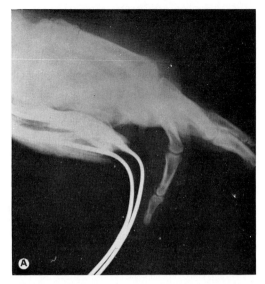 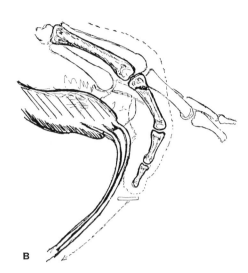

Figure 6.7. (Same case as Fig. 6.6*A*.) *A*. Fracture of base of first phalanx (index finger) under treatment with traction splint. *B*. Tracing of x-ray gives clearer view of position of fragments. Traction should be maintained two and a half to three weeks; then a simple supporting splint substituted from palm to finger tip, and gentle movement started for a week; then index and middle finger loosely bound together for protection and more active movement allowed; and all apparatus removed at end of six weeks from fracture.

be used as described in the next section.

In the follow-up care, there will usually be adequate fibrous healing in two to four weeks (depending on the security of the fracture), and at this time, the patient should begin guarded, active (unassisted) exercise. No specific length of immobilization can be stated, except to say that motion should be begun *as early as possible* to prevent stiffness of the phalangeal joints. On the other hand, splinting will be required long enough to protect against displacement; thus there may be an interval of two to three weeks when the patient performs active movements while still retaining the supportive protection of plaster splints. In the latter week or two, the splint may be discarded. *Early* movement and *prolonged* protection are the two governing principles throughout convalescence.

Other phalangeal fractures do not call for much additional comment, as the routine of treatment is essentially the same: (1) anesthesia; (2) manipulative reduction if displaced; (3) adequate splinting; (4) and traction if the fracture seems unstable; followed by similar rules of *early* movement and *prolonged* protection. Local consideration will alter the specific method of immobilization, but the underlying principles will still apply.

Longitudinal or Splintered Fractures

Another type of phalangeal fracture occurs so commonly that it deserves a separate category, even though few of the authoritative writers place much emphasis upon it. Instead of oblique, transverse, or comminuted separation of the bone fragments, frac-

ture lines run longitudinally, quite often without serious displacement (Fig. 6.8). They may be compared to the fascist symbol of a bundle of sticks bound together, representing the strength of mutual support, their chief characteristic. Usually these fractures will not need manipulation; or if they do, this will seldom have to be more than a molding or pinching together of the "staves." Treatment consists of support extend-

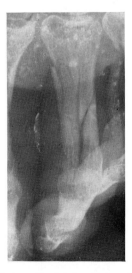

Figure 6.8. Longitudinal, splintered fracture of phalanx.

ing above the wrist and including the neighboring finger for two weeks.

Open Reduction and Pin Fixation

In recent years there has been a tremendous increase in the use of pin fixation for phalangeal fractures. In discussing this technique, a sharp distinction should be drawn between surgeons who are skilled in its use and cognizant of its complications; and those who merely find it appeals to them as an easy way to treat a fracture. The latter group will discover that this method carries with it a distinct risk that should never be overlooked. The wire is introduced through joints that are themselves very complex as well as being relatively minute. It does not require massive infection to damage these joints; low grade irritation can do it, bringing on disastrous results. In some cases not one, but two, or even three joints are trespassed upon with distinctly increased risk. Adhesions may form between the joint capsules and the gliding ligaments that invest them; the articular surface of the joint may be damaged severely enough to respond with traumatic arthritis; adjoining tendons may be involved if the point of the wire "goes wrong;" and surgical infection can always develop. Notwithstanding these objections, it must be conceded that there are cases where wire fixation proves extremely helpful, offering a form of treatment that nothing else would supply. In cases where there are multiple proximal phalangeal fractures, Clarkson[9] observes that they "should be treated by intramedullary fixation; control is better, immobilization is easier and more rapid, and the functional results are superior to those of conventional splinting." This is sound advice, but in following it the surgeon should remember the dangers involved and should look for safer methods first.

The technique of pinning does not require much discussion. The interphalangeal joint is flexed to a right angle and a fine Kirschner wire is inserted through the head of the phalanx and up the shaft of the bone to lodge at its base. Use of the smallest caliber wire that will hold the bone adequately will reduce the tendency toward irritation. The wire is left projecting ¼ inch from the joint and the skin may or may not be allowed to close over it.

Other forms of open surgery on phalangeal fractures may sometimes be advisable, but in general, they are not recommended as the results tend to prove disappointing. This is an area where we have not yet achieved much that improves on nature, although a great deal can be accomplished by employing the healing forces of nature to their best advantage.

Phalangeal Fractures into Joints

Among the more perplexing problems of phalangeal fractures are those involving the joints. These may be produced by the mechanism already indicated in our earlier discussion. Hyperextension of the proximal phalanx may cause an avulsion of a fragment at its base on the palmar side or impaction of the base on the dorsal aspect. Similarly, lateral movement of the second phalanx may avulse or impact the base of this bone or the head of the proximal bone. Fragments of different sizes will break off, involving a condyle or condyles of the phalanx and entering the joint or forming a T. No specific rule can be laid down as to treatment of these variable injuries, and in the end, the decision is likely to be based on the surgeon's point of view. Certainly if the fragment is small or but slightly displaced, all would agree that a minimum of immobilization should be carried out and movement of the joint should be started as soon as possible. Sometimes either traction or pinning will give a good result if properly applied as illustrated in Figures 6.9 and 6.10. A great deal of skilled technique has developed in the application of wires for this purpose and even conservative surgeons should not decry their use when indicated. On the other hand, there is much to be said in favor of leaving a fracture alone just long enough for some fibrous healing to "gum" the fragments together—possibly 10 days—and then beginning early, active motion. Although this is neither as dramatic nor as "positive" as implanting a wire, it will often lead to a better result in the long run. Unfortunately, there are no reliable criteria that can be laid down between the operative or nonoperative cases. The size of the fragment alone is not a decisive factor. It has been said that if the fracture involves more than a third of the articular surface, the case deserves surgery, but we cannot agree with this if the fragments seem stable or but little displaced. Perhaps our decision should rest on asking ourselves the following questions: (1) is the fracture-displacement great enough to destroy the function of the joint, or can it be tolerated; (2) is there an associated subluxation of the joint that requires mechanical fixation, or is the joint itself intact; (3) is the fracture fragment large enough to tolerate a wire for fixation, or is it too small a "crumb" for such treatment; (4) is the fracture basically unstable, or does it appear secure in its reduced position; (5) are there multiple fractures or complications, making it impossible to stabilize the fracture without fixation, or is the problem limited to this one injury alone? Obviously, where the answer to the first of these alternatives is *yes,* some type of fixation will be indicated; whereas *yes* to the second of the alternatives would favor conservative treatment with splint and early movement. At least we have come to realize that these fractures will not tolerate prolonged immobilization, especially with traction; and if wire implantation is used too promiscuously, it will teach us that this method also has its serious complications and disappointments. A review of this type of injury has recently been presented by Eaton.[12]

Techniques of Plaster Splinting and Traction

Splinting and Positioning

At this point, some general observations should be offered regarding the application of plaster splints and

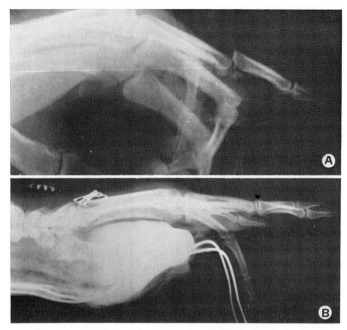

Figure 6.9. Patient was injured practicing karate. *A.* Hyperextension fractured base of second phalanx had been neglected for one week before treatment with manipulative reduction under anesthesia and traction splint. *B.* Traction splint applied showing anatomical maintenance of fracture, which had slipped persistently until elastic skin traction was used. Follow-up: Traction splint was maintained continuously for three weeks, and movements allowed for two weeks. At end of two months full, normal function regained — but no more karate!

the techniques of traction. The point of primary importance to begin the discussion is that the hand is essentially rounded in contour, as is well expressed by the familiar phrase, "the hollow of the hand." Consequently any form of immobilization that ignores both the longitudinal and the transverse arches of the hand, and binds these structures to a flat surface is unphysiologic: better to support it on an orange or a baseball than on a wooden splint! There are many commercial hand splints ingeniously designed for general use, but as a basic rule we feel that molded plaster of Paris provides the best "universal splint" available. With a minimum of inconvenience, it can be prepared to fit the exact size and needs of every patient. Very often the surgeon will find it helpful to shape the splint on his own hand before applying it, making adequate allowance for differences of size. This is particularly useful when the fingers must be bent to special angles. In 4 or 5 min plaster begins to solidify enough to hold its form; but in the next 10 to 15 min it can still be readily molded to new contours, and unless it is continually bent back and forth, the plaster will retain its shape and will harden properly. In preparing such a splint, the first rule is to *remember the dome of the hand* and support its arched structure.

A second thought to bear in mind is that the normal position of rest, or neutral position of the hand, is not in extension but in semiflexion of the fingers. No diagram is needed to illustrate the point as anyone can demonstrate it by noting the position of the fingers when the hand hangs idly at the side. The middle finger is flexed to about 30 to 35° at the metacarpophalangeal joint and almost 40° at the first phalangeal joint. The head of the middle knuckle is about one-half inch higher than that of the index finger and the palm is rounded enough to fit over a tennis ball.

Still a third rule is easily overlooked, although all the standard texts emphasize it and from a practical standpoint it is of extreme importance. In splinting the fingers or when applying traction to them, the pull must not draw them straight down, but rather obliquely, aiming at the thenar muscles, or more specifically, at the location of the navicular bone.

Our fourth rule of position relates to the thumb. In earlier days of practice there was a strong tendency to splint or apply traction with the thumb extended and abducted. Actually, the neutral position is with the thumb held almost directly in front of the index finger and about one and one-half inches from it, tip to tip. From this position it can function best and if any of its joints stiffen, the others can regain activity far better from this base. Putting the thumb backward in extension flattens the whole palm and can be rather disabling. Certain conditions, such as a nerve paralysis, tend to promote adduction contracture of the thumb, which must be guarded against. This can be counteracted by the simple use of a saddle of plaster over the web that joins the thumb and index finger; but here, also, the

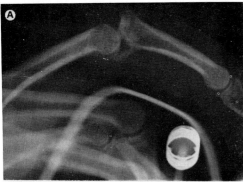
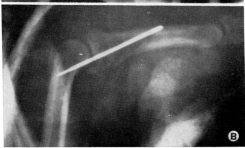

Figure 6.10. A. Lateral x-ray of the long finger, showing dorsal dislocation of the proximal interphalangeal joint with a chip fracture on the volar aspect of the base of the middle phalanx. This is an unstable fracture. *B.* Treatment consisted of reduction and immobilization with a transfixing pin. This was removed after three weeks and motions of the finger joint were encouraged.

thumb should be allowed to ride forward rather than in backward extension.

In brief, the four rules of splinting offered here may be summarized: (1) splinting of the hand must conform to the dome-shaped contour of the palm; (2) splinting should allow for the normal flexion of the fingers in neutral position, unless some special consideration makes extension necessary; (3) the line of obliquity and rotation that fingers assume on flexion must be remembered when they are splinted; (4) the neutral position of the thumb should be recognized, holding it in front of the index finger with about one to two inches separating tip from tip.

Padding, Circulation, and Pressure Sores

It is hardly necessary to emphasize the risks of splinting a hand too tightly, as these are obvious to all; but the safeguard here will not lie solely in careful application of the plaster so much as in close follow-up observation of the patient. As already noted, we have been impressed with the advantages of applying a half cast and binding it on with elastic bandage, rather than using a full circular cast. With the elastic bandage compression can be made as tight as needed, whereas a circular cast cannot allow adequately for subsidence

of swelling, which may end up with a hand that will "rattle around" inside its encasement. It is also relatively easy, without much risk of losing position, to take down an elastic bandage and examine the hand, should this become advisable.

Traction

There have been numerous methods for applying traction to the fingers, many of which deserve mention in order to present a complete survey of the topic. (1) The basket finger-trap is a woven basket which tightens under tension and permits the use of heavy traction. The drawback to this method would be the danger from pressure necrosis if applied for too long a time. (2) Fingernail traction is a somewhat primitive, but very simple procedure. (3) Skeletal traction is often recommended with a Kirschner wire passed through the base of the distal phalanx. This is a wholly reliable method and is favored by many of the best authorities. The risk of introducing infection is minimal if simple precautions are taken, but the to-and-fro motion of the wire can produce irritation at the wounds of entrance and exit and would offer very slight, potential hazard. (4) In our experience pulp traction, as advocated by Böhler,[4] is somewhat easier to apply. Instead of drilling through the bone, a commercially available yoke, or a Kirschner wire that will not bow, is pushed through the soft tissue just under the tip of the distal phalanx and actually scraping against the edge of the bone when it is inserted (Fig. 6.11). The pulp contains tough fibrous septa that will not give way or produce pain under traction. (5) Skin traction is now less popular than the use of wire, but we have found it equally effective and thoroughly safe if applied with proper technique. It is particularly applicable to the thumb, where the pull is safely exerted in a straight line with the axis of the digit. All finger traction should be exerted in the posture of partial flexion: *i.e.*, the position of function. Application of traction begins by painting the finger with compound tincture of benzoin, over which four adhesive skin straps are applied. These are prepared with far greater simplicity than is needed to describe them in detail. Two ½-inch wide straps of adhesive, 8 inches long, are laid on a table, crossing each other at right angles with their adhesive surfaces facing up. A slightly larger square of wood, (⅝ inch or ¾ inch) cut from a throat stick is placed on top of the adhesive straps at the point of their intersection. This acts as a "spreader" with four "tails" of adhesive that can be glued to the two sides, front, and back of the finger. A gauze bandage can be bound very lightly over this strapping and the tip of the finger left visible between the straps for a circulation check. Elastic bands can then be passed between the adhesive straps and under the wooden "spreader" and these bands can then be attached to the traction bar of the plaster splint. In applying this or any other form of traction, it is to be remembered that the purpose is merely to stabilize and *retain* the fracture in position.

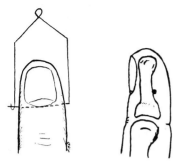

Figure 6.11. Pulp-periosteum yolk traction.

This type of traction should, of course, *never* be used to "drag" fragments into alignment, for unless the fracture has already been reduced by manipulation, elastic traction alone will fail to carry out this objective. There is always some risk to any form of traction and whatever technique is employed will require close supervision.

One form of traction we have seen employed deserves to be condemned. This consists in application of a small stockinette to the finger with skin glue. The projecting end of the stockinette is then drawn together with a purse string tied to elastic traction bands. This method lacks any "spreader" and will cause pressure necrosis as the stockinette pulls over the finger tip, as we have seen. Another defect in the technique is that it hides the finger tip from follow-up observation, thus preventing a check on the circulation.

The three alternative methods of finger traction that can be recommended are skeletal, pulp, and skin traction. Each has its hazards and all require careful technique in their application and constant follow-up observation. In our own hands, for general purposes, we find skin traction more convenient than the other two, although all three are completely acceptable.

Metacarpal Fractures

Fractures of the metacarpals involve somewhat different mechanical problems from those of the phalanges. In the first place, except at the metacarpophalangeal joint, they contribute far less to the accurate and precise movements of the fingers and consequently even a moderate amount of displacement can be tolerated without any serious functional impairment. The second distinction applying to metacarpals lies in the degree of mutual support they gain from each other, which greatly limits their rotational, as well as their lateral displacement, and which lessens the tendency toward increased shortening.

We feel that the literature on this subject pays too little attention to the differentiation of metacarpal fractures into characteristic types, for each of which the problems of treatment vary. Five distinct categories can be suggested for separate discussion; those of the neck, oblique fractures of the shaft, transverse fractures of the shaft, multiple and comminuted fractures of the shaft, and fractures at the base.

Metacarpal Neck Fractures

Injuries of the neck of the metacarpal constitute the commonest of all hand fractures due in part to the weakness of the bone at this point, and due also to the belligerent tendencies of *Homo sapiens.*

The pull of the interosseus muscles together with the bowstring effect of the flexors, combined with the impact of a blow, will almost invariably drive the broken off head downward toward the palm, angulating the fracture in the direction of flexion. If the head is fully displaced it assumes a position completely beneath the metacarpal shaft which is not only extremely disabling to the mechanism of the metacarpophalangeal joint but is also damaging to the pull of the flexor tendons which it displaces downward into the palm. Such a position is obviously very destructive to the function of the finger and, in addition, the prominence of the rounded head pressing against the palm incapacitates the grip of the hand on any heavy tool such as a shovel or wrench. This degree of displacement, however, is not often reached. More frequently the head is merely bent downward 15 to 20°, in which case function may be only insignificantly affected. One of the first decisions the surgeon must make is whether the degree of displacement is great enough to interfere materially with the use of the hand or whether it can be accepted in its displaced position with no treatment except the splinting necessary for protection against further slipping. More important than the degree of angulation of the metacarpal head and neck is the metacarpal involved. The second and third rays have practically no carpometacarpal motion and therefore tolerate head displacement poorly. The fourth metacarpal has approximately 20° of motion at its base and the fifth about 30° of carpometacarpal motion. These two, therefore, can compensate by this motion for palmar displacement of their heads with no interference in gripping. Happily, the majority of metacarpal fractures involve the fifth ray and frequently need no reduction. If the fracture displacement involving the second and third rays exceeds 15°, reduction is recommended. In the fourth and fifth metacarpals angulation to 30° can be accepted with no reduction. We have seen many patients whose only disability after 30° angulation of a fifth metacarpal head is loss of the terminal 10 to 15° of finger extension (Figs. 6.12 and 6.13). We agree with Eichenholtz and Rizzo[13] that these fractures, when over one week old, are generally better left untouched.

The manipulative technique is relatively simple on an early case and follows the long observed standard practice (Fig. 6.14). The metacarpophalangeal joint is flexed 90° and likewise the first interphalangeal joint. This will bring the phalanx directly under the angulated metacarpal head to which it is attached, while flexion of the second joint makes it possible to press

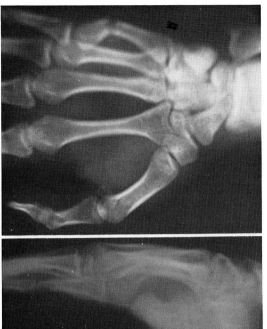

Figure 6.12. Oblique and lateral x-rays showing displaced, healing fracture of distal shaft of fifth metacarpal. This was sustained in a fight four weeks earlier. Reduction had been attempted but not maintained.

upward with great force on the distal end of the first phalanx; this pressure will be transmitted through the proximal end of the phalanx to elevate the metacarpal head. The head displacement can also be reduced by combining direct, accurate pressure on the palmar side beneath the head, while an opposite force is directed downward on the metacarpal shaft. Many of these fractures are rather firmly impacted and if any difficulty is encountered it may be necessary to apply strong traction to the finger before the upward force is exerted. Heavy downward, counter pressure must be applied at the same time, on the dorsum of the metacarpal shaft, to complete the manipulation. If the fracture is fresh the reduction can be accomplished without difficulty but unfortunately many of these cases do not turn up until the third or fourth day, which adds to the difficulties of treating them. Late fractures of the second or third metacarpal neck (two weeks or so after injury) might necessitate open surgery if its head is displaced into the palm. The fourth or fifth, however, should never require open reduction, short of a fully displaced metacarpal head.

Although we have mentioned that this manipulative technique follows the standard practice, we should at this point protest against the standard rules for immobilization presented in most of the older text books. The hazardous technique of applying a closely fitting

plaster in the position of 90° flexion of the metacarpophalangeal joint is sometimes taught, as it was said that without this the fracture would lose its position. Where such a technique has been employed we have seen extremely serious complications from (1) pressure necrosis over the metacarpophalangeal joint, or (2) over the first interphalangeal joint (Fig. 6.15), or (3) even from the tip of the finger pressing against the palm. Also, the maintenance of flexion at both joints, in conjunction with the trauma, exercises a strong tendency to produce intractable flexion contractures. We would therefore advocate complete abandonment of this technique, recommending instead that the hand be placed on a plaster splint with the first phalanx resting in semiflexed position but fully supported to the end of the finger. A special piece of felt or a mold in the plaster should be designed to maintain upward pressure under the head of the metacarpal, and a strap of adhesive should be passed over the dorsum, where it should compress sponge rubber or felt downward against the shaft of the metacarpal. The fracture is not too unstable to be immobilized in such a splint if it is prepared with a little ingenuity and applied with care. Close follow-up supervision will, of course, be required. At the end of two weeks, fairly firm fibrous union should develop so that a simple palmar splint in neutral position can be substituted and this continued as long as the fracture needs support—another one to two weeks in most cases. Thereafter it might be wise to limit the activity of the hand to some degree as a precaution against trauma, but guarded active motion of the joint should be encouraged as early as possible, perhaps even at the end of the first two weeks when the splint could be removed and replaced. Some loss of position after reduction is common but the end results confirm earlier observations on disability in these injuries.

Oblique Fractures of the Metacarpals

The mechanism that produces oblique fractures of the shafts of bones usually involves some rotational torque but we are not familiar with any studies of this principle applied to the hand. Wherever such fractures exist, two considerations come to mind. The sloping surfaces of bone that oppose each other afford moderately good opportunity for stabilizing them against further displacement, except for the tendency they will have to slide by each other and produce overriding and shortening. Fortunately, the neighboring metacarpals will help to counteract this tendency to a very significant degree and it will therefore seldom prove necessary to utilize traction as a means of treatment. The second characteristic of oblique fractures is that they offer an extensive area of bone surface for the healing process to occur. They are, therefore, decidedly less prone to develop delays in union or to end in nonunion. From both of these considerations the outlook for these fractures is extremely good and we feel that here a warning should be expressed against the excesses of overtreatment that are too often rec-

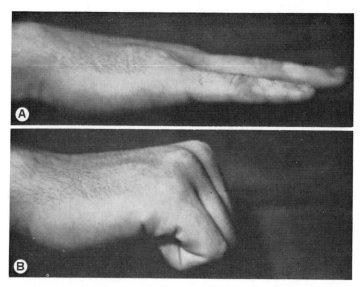

Figure 6.13. Extension (*A*) and flexion (*B*) views of hand shown in x-ray views in Figure 6.12. Note prominence on dorsum of hand over fracture site and almost normal range of motion one month after injury.

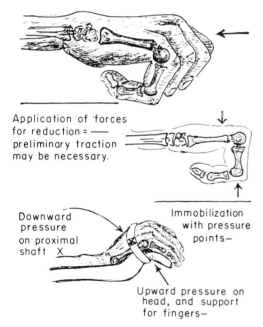

Application of forces for reduction = —
preliminary traction may be necessary.

Downward pressure on proximal shaft X

Immobilization with pressure points—

Upward pressure on head, and support for fingers—

Figure 6.14. Mechanical analysis of knuckle fracture.

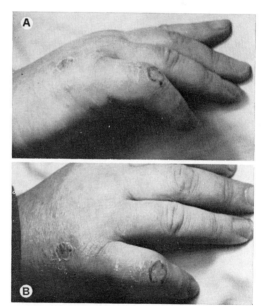

Figure 6.15. Pressure sores and flexion contractures from "classic" treatment of fifth metacarpal neck fracture. Errors: (1) flexion of both joints continued too long; (2) exposed joint surfaces inadequately padded; (3) too much pressure maintained.

ommended in this regard. We like to follow the point of view that most of these fractures, when uncomplicated, will require only very simple treatment. This is not true, of course, where multiple fractures have occurred, destroying the mutual support of the other bones, nor does it apply when the original traumatizing force has produced gross displacement, or where compound or soft tissue injuries have created complications. On the other hand, for the more simple types that are frequently seen this basic observation should guide our treatment. A palmar cast will generally prove adequate for immobilization but the two adjoining metacarpals should be given full support, as well as the injured bone and corresponding finger. If the fifth metacarpal alone is involved, the index finger and thumb may still be allowed active movement outside the molded plaster splint, and this will also be true of the fourth, although not of the third metacarpal.

If the tendency to shortening seems greater than the surgeon feels should be accepted, it can readily be overcome by a manipulative pull under anesthesia, followed by traction upon the finger involved. Skin traction, as described, is adequate and the pull need not be more than moderate in force. Furthermore, it need not be maintained, as a rule, for more than 10 days to two weeks, by which time some fibrous healing will have occurred. This, we feel, is preferable to pin fixation, although the latter technique is recommended by many highly competent authorities and seems to be in general use among experts. Another technique that may occasionally prove useful consists of running two wires transversely through the injured metacarpal and through the neighboring uninjured bone. This would seldom be called for and is not generally recommended, but where special considerations apply it could be useful. Although it does not offer any risk to the metacarpophalangeal joint, surgeons not experienced in its use may be surprised to find how far the point of a needle can go astray. Damage to the interosseous muscles frequently follows the use of these pins. In the palm of the hand, filled with so many important structures, this is not good and, what is more important, this technique is seldom necessary.

Transverse Fractures of the Shaft

Where a fracture is transverse, the force of a direct blow has usually been applied, or there has been a very sudden, forcible angulation. The hand is so exposed to trauma in industry of athletics that such injuries are relatively frequent, although not as common as the oblique types. These transverse fractures differ from the oblique because of their greater tendency toward overriding and the more deforming displacement of the fracture ends that accompanies them. Inasmuch as the two fracture ends impact on one another after they have been reduced, the danger of subsequent slipping is not great but the fracture surfaces themselves are so small that strong healing is not likely to develop until much later than would be the case with oblique fractures.

If a transverse fracture is fresh, manipulative reduction under anesthesia may be carried out simply by pulling heavily on the finger to correct overriding, accompanied by angulating the fragments and applying upward and downward pressure to work them back into place. If they are once fully corrected retention depends largely on avoiding any jarring movement that would joggle the opposing ends off each other. Such movements can be eliminated by a molded platform splint which should extend to the finger tips and

should include the two adjoining fingers. As an extra security it is wise to include the whole palm on the volar splint and to utilize a dorsal splint that will provide a compressive, downward force on the back of the hand. Inasmuch as the diameter of the metacarpal shaft is small the actual fracture surfaces that have to be held in approximation require fairly close splinting. No time rule can be set for the length of immobilization but it should be remembered that these fractures do not form strong fibrous healing as early as the oblique types; consequently their active motion cannot be started until somewhat later. Clinical testing of the fracture at the end of three to four weeks may very likely show subsidence of local tenderness and firm resistance to any displacement and when these findings are present, cautious, active motion may be started while still continuing with the splints, except for the exercise periods (Fig. 6.16).

These fractures give much more trouble if they are seen by the surgeon several days later, when overriding has tightened into a fixed deformity. Closed reduction at this stage becomes increasingly difficult and the surgeon is often faced with the choice of accepting a slight deformity without correction or recommending open surgery. Although in general operative techniques add considerably to the risks of fracture treatment, the metacarpal shafts are so accessible and they can be surgically reduced with so little risk to other tissues that open treatment of these injuries is often the more conservative choice. The bone lies in an almost subcutaneous position and once it has been exposed the fragments can usually be levered back into position with only minimal difficulty. Once this has been accomplished it may be wiser to use internal splinting with Kirschner wires rather than risk the possibility of the fracture displacing again after the operative wound is closed or while the splint is applied. Leading authors seem to favor introducing the wire through the metacarpophalangeal joint and passing it up the medullary canal, but as an alternative method there is much to say in favor of extending the operative incision as far as the carpometacarpal joint and then introducing the wire from this end (Fig. 6.17). Such a procedure involves somewhat greater technical skill and may prove difficult for the inexperienced operator, but it is a more favorable position mechanically, eliminating any risk to the metacarpophalangeal joint, which is of vital importance to the function of the hand.

Multiple and Comminuted Fractures of the Shaft

The considerations outlined in the two preceding sections must be adapted to the more complex problem of multiple fractures. These can be placed in two general categories. Some of them present marked angulation and deformity that would be very damaging if left untreated and that would yield very readily to open surgery with wire fixation. In these cases, furthermore, the advantage normally provided by mutual

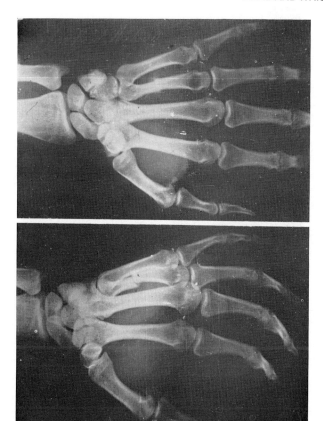

Figure 6.16. Transverse fracture, midshaft of fourth metacarpal showing slight displacement, but functionally serviceable position. Treated conservatively with molded plaster splint, including wrist to tips of middle, ring, and little fingers. Some callus beginning to show at five weeks. Ring and middle fingers then bound together loosely, in order to limit activity for another two weeks, then very guarded, unprotected activity for another two weeks before unrestricted use.

splinting of the neighboring metacarpals has been destroyed. Therefore the wisdom of resorting to operative treatment at the very start becomes apparent. On the other hand, some cases involve marked comminution of the shafts with splintering fractures that cannot be much improved by surgery of any type. Their one hope for functional survival seems to lie in their being left alone so that every crumb of bone can contribute its share to healing. Mere splinting of these fractures may not be adequate, as there may be a strong tendency for them to shorten and angulate. In these cases, therefore, a palmar platform splint should be supplemented with a traction bar and adhesive traction with a light pull should be applied to each finger requiring it. This may have to be maintained 10 days to two weeks or perhaps up to three weeks but at the earliest possible date the traction should be removed and cautious movement should be begun. Should internal fixation be the method elected, we prefer, if at all possible, separate medullary wires for each metacarpal, rather than transverse, multiple transfixing wires.

Fractures of the Base of the Metacarpals

In dealing with fractures at the carpometacarpal joint the surgeon should recognize that the problems are far less complex than in any other region of the hand (Fig. 6.18). This is partly because these joints are very strongly supported by ligamentous reinforcement both anteriorly and posteriorly. Furthermore, movements of these joints contribute so little to the over-all function of the hand that they can be allowed to fuse in many cases without significant disability. Finally, these fractures, as a rule, occur from direct trauma in industry, or in athletics by indirect trauma transmitted from a blow on the knuckles, as O'Donoghue[27] reports. In either case there is a strong tendency to impaction which leads to relatively early healing. In addition, the area is rather easy to splint, being extremely stable as compared to the fingers, and there is an ample surrounding blood supply with good tendency to healing. Cotton,[11] who wrote years ago, on the basis of great experience and keen observation, reported "certain

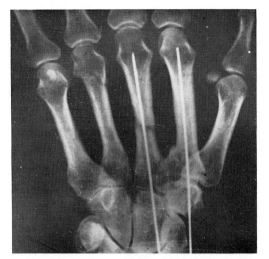

Figure 6.17. Oblique fractures second and third metacarpals treated with intramedullary Kirschner wires which were introduced under open surgery. Single incision exposed both fractures adequately. Wires inserted through proximal fragments to eliminate any risk to metacarpophalangeal joint. Follow-up: Ends of wires cut off subcutaneously and left *in situ* eight weeks. Hand splinted for three weeks, then active movement encouraged. No residual disability after four months.

ones of them remain persistently tender after injury." This we have not confirmed in our own experience, as the fractures we have seen have involved no serious complications.

One point that several authors bring out deserves a word of caution. The area of the base of the metacarpals is difficult to project on lateral or even oblique x-ray films and even in A.P. views, some fogging or overlapping occurs where the bones meet. It is easy to miss the diagnosis in these cases. Sometimes the original fracture lines may be too insignificant to notice at the start, although they may become visible in the healing stage, as sometimes happens with the carpal scaphoid and is routinely the case with march fractures of the metatarsals. For this reason surgeons should be warned, when clinical signs indicate acute trauma in this area, to look closely at the films and to make guarded statements. The signs themselves may not be outstanding, since there is not likely to be any easily visible deformity, and the strong ligamentous binding lessens the tendency to crepitus. There will, however, be rather sharply localized bony tenderness, which remains the one most reliable sign if the surgeon tries to elicit it carefully and accurately.

In treating these fractures it is usually adequate to rest them on a palmar splint for two to three weeks, allowing finger movement from the start and beginning full hand movement as early as it can be tolerated.

In some cases the fracture may be overriding to such an extent that traction will be needed to reduce the deformity. Once reduced, if the fracture proves unstable, wire fixation rather than finger traction is recommended for maintenance of position. There does not seem to be any justification in tying up a whole finger ray for a prolonged time just to treat a fracture at its base.

These considerations apply far less to the fifth metacarpal than to the other three. Since this joint has no collateral support on its outer side, it is apt to prove more of a problem than the others and may even offer some of the complications of a Bennett fracture. However, its treatment must be governed by the individual considerations of each case and, in the main, the principles stated above still apply.

Thumb Fractures

Fractures of the base of the first metacarpal constitute a group by themselves and deserve specific con-

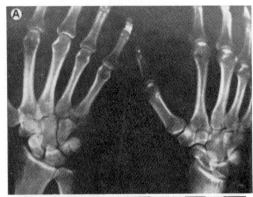

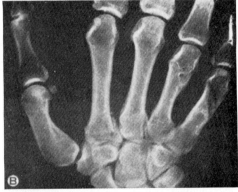

Figure 6.18. A. Fractured base of fifth metacarpal treated by molded, palmar splint (plaster of Paris) and elastic bandage for two weeks of continuous immobilization; followed by 10 days of protective splinting with hot soaks and active movement twice a day; then free but guarded use of hand for another week, ending with full activity five weeks after fracture. *B.* Fractured bases of second and third metacarpals; similar treatment.

sideration. The name of Bennett has been applied so commonly to all fractures of the thumb that its specific meaning has been lost in the more generalized usage. Surgeons today often forget that when Bennett[2] published his description of these cases in 1882, he referred to an "oblique fracture through the base of the bone, detaching the greater part of the articular facet with that piece of the bone supporting it which projects into the palm." Although honor is still due Bennett for his splendid contribution in the field of hand fractures, the time has come to discontinue use of his name in favor of a more descriptive classification. There are two important types of fractures in this region which should be distinguished.

Fractures across the Shaft of the Metacarpal at Its Base

Fractures across the shaft of the metacarpal at its base are relatively common (Fig. 6.19). If no displacement is involved, treatment will offer no problem except for the simple requirement of immobilization sufficient to protect it from slipping and to guard against further injury. The position of function should, of course, be utilized in applying whatever cast may be necessary; and in any case where there is danger of slipping the plaster should be carried to the interphalangeal joint. Not infrequently when the shaft is broken transversely, the distal fragment may be forced outward until partial or complete displacement has occurred. In such a case, manipulation under anes-

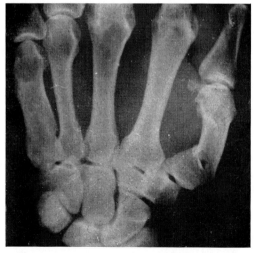

Figure 6.19. Fractured shaft of first metacarpal (not a true Bennett's fracture). Treatment: Closed reduction under Xylocaine anesthesia. Plaster cast from well above wrist to thumb tip for four weeks. Traction is not necessary but plaster must be molded to prevent lateral bowing. After removal of cast, protective splinting and guarded motion for two to three weeks more before full activity.

thesia will often be necessary. Overriding must be corrected before reduction is possible; and this can best be accomplished by strong manual traction on the thumb. As an aid in obtaining traction, it may be helpful to apply adhesive to the skin in the manner already described. The operator can often exert a stronger pull in this way than with his bare hands. Once shortening has been overcome, the fragment can be pushed back into place by lateral compression at the fracture site. A special grip is useful for this purpose. The operator grasps the patient's injured thumb with his own contralateral hand — diagonally opposite — and holds the proximal and distal phalanges between his own flexed fingers and palm, while his thumb extends down the side of the injured metacarpal to its base. He can then pull, circumduct, or angulate the thumb by the grip of his clenched fingers, while he is free to press strongly in on the fracture site with the ball of this thumb.

Many of these fractures are stable enough to maintain themselves if a well fitted plaster gauntlet is applied. This should include firm immobilization of the lower half of the forearm and should extend to include the first phalanx of the thumb. The more oblique fractures and the comminuted ones will require traction to maintain their position. Here the choice of skin, pulp, or skeletal traction should be optional with the operator. The tendency for the fragment to slip laterally should be offset when the cast is applied, by padding the fracture area with felt and applying lateral compression to the plaster while it is setting. Follow-up care will be governed on the usual principles covering metacarpal shaft fractures, making allowance for each individual case. Inasmuch as the carpometacarpal joint itself has not been damaged, there is not likely to be any unusual danger of stiffness here and certainly none of dislocation. The plaster cast, or later splint, will probably be needed for four to six weeks.

Fracture-Dislocation of the Base of the First Metacarpal

The fracture that Bennett actually described differs from those we have just discussed because of the factor of subluxation; in fact, the brilliance of Bennett's original discovery lay in his recognition that an injury which all others were attributing to dislocation was in fact a fracture, with the dislocation complicating it. This results from the antomic weakness of this articulation, where the base of the metacarpal is seated in the "saddle" of the multangular, where it holds itself through the projection, sometimes called a "hook" that comprises its base. As Gedda[15] has shown in his careful studies, this "hook" is only very moderate, and may not be present at all. In fact, he states that there is nothing in the metacarpocarpal joint that inherently prevents potential dislocation. When longitudinal force is driven downward along the shaft, the base of the metacarpal is sheared off, leaving the proximal or volar fragment in its original contact with the multangular, while the broken shaft angles out, dorsally and laterally, and overrides to a considerable extent. The metacarpal shaft then becomes subluxed, or at least "simulates a subluxation" as Bennett described the overriding. The proximal fragment may be rotated or comminuted, or may not be greatly injured (Fig. 6.20).

Closed Treatment. There may be said to be three principal techniques of treatment, each of which has so much to offer that separate descriptions are needed for all. The first is carried out with closed reduction under local or general anesthesia. In our practice we begin this procedure by first preparing the wrist and thumb for traction by applying a firm and closely fitting gauntlet cast with a traction strut made of coat hanger wire. The cast is not fully completed, however, as the space over the base of the metacarpus is not filled in. The wire strut is bent to the side so that nothing will interfere with manual traction on the thumb itself. The skin is painted with compound tincture of benzoin and adhesive traction straps are made ready to apply in the manner already described. The next step is then carried out by pulling very hard on the thumb while at the same time pressing in on the base of the metacarpal from a dorsolateral direction. The pull will reduce overriding, and the lateral compression will correct the bowing and sideward displacement of the shaft, thus snugging it back against the proximal fragment from which it had been split away. The final step involves immobilizing the fracture in its corrected position by applying the skin traction and connecting this with the traction strut which is now bent directly into place. A heavy pull should not be required, as it only needs to overcome the counterpull of the thenar muscles. If the cast and traction apparatus have not been made ready ahead of time, as described here, there is likely to be loss of position at the fracture site. For this reason it is important to follow the order of procedure outlined above. The base of the metacarpal is then covered with sheet wadding and a thick piece of sponge rubber, over

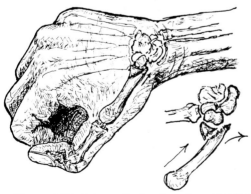

Figure 6.20. Schematic drawing of mechanics of fractured base of first metacarpal with volar fragment split off, and shaft subluxed and overriding.

which a splint of plaster is laid and then dented in moderately firmly in order to apply persisting lateral compression. The plaster must be held until it hardens; and there will, of course, be need for care to avoid too great a pressure that would produce a local slough. However, if carried out by anyone familiar with plaster work, the technique is reasonably simple and is perfectly safe, provided good follow-up observation is maintained. Furthermore, the reduction of the fracture can be maintained by this method, and when properly handled we have good confidence in it (Fig. 6.21).

Some authors have felt that traction is not necessary in this type of closed treatment, provided adequate lateral pressure is maintained. Böhler,[4] for example, who formerly advocated pulp traction, discontinued it in favor of a simple, unpadded cast. We do not doubt that this is often sufficient, but in such cases, the cast must be carefully and well applied and the lateral pressure must be skillfully localized and calibrated to meet the exact need for maintenance. Blum,[3] who reported earlier on this technique at an outpatient department where it may not have been well applied, found that *all* the cases slipped out of place very shortly. Because of the added security it affords, we feel that traction is an important aid in closed treatment. It need not be maintained more than about four weeks and never needs to be very heavy. The cast itself should be continued six weeks, and then governed by x-ray appearances (Fig. 6.22).

Open Reduction. The popular tendency today, in dealing with these fractures, is to resort to open surgery. This could be in part due to the finality of an operative technique as compared with the delays of closed plaster. It might also be because many surgeons today are unfamiliar or unskilled in the use of plaster, although adept with a knife. Finally, it is very largely influenced by the decreasing risks of surgery now as compared to 25 or 30 years ago. None of these influences are likely to be reversed, so that we may say that open reduction of these cases, wherever they present serious displacement, is becoming the standard, orthodox treatment, even though we feel it is not necessary in more than a very few cases. There can be no denying that it has distinct advantages from the standpoint of accuracy, stability, and simplification of the follow-up. However, as fully recognized by Gedda,[15] one of its advocates, "the open method is not technically altogether easy," and there is still much to say in favor of closed treatment. Our feeling would be that if closed treatment has failed, open reduction should be resorted to.

There are numerous techniques of open surgery available, but we may do best by referring to that described by Moberg and Gedda, as summarized in Gedda's study of the subject. Briefly, this is done under brachial plexus block and with a tourniquet. An oblique incision is made over the carpometacarpal joint on the palmar aspect of the thumb. This affords a good view of the fracture. A wire is introduced through the volar fragment, while the metacarpal itself

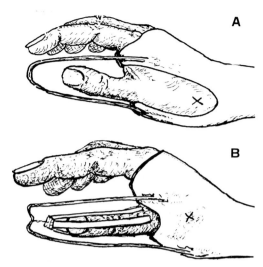

A

B

Figure 6.21. A. Preliminary cast. Ready for manipulation with open space over metacarpal head (×) for pressure when reduction is carried out. *B.* Completed cast. Note: Base of metacarpal has been padded and plaster compressed at this point (×). Gauze bandage will be used to encircle thumb. Only light elastic pull is required.

is pulled down to offset its displacement and to reduce the fracture. Aided by a wire sling, the Kirschner wire is then driven through the oblique end of the shaft, belonging to the distal fragment, where it is firmly implanted. The volar fragment is then pressed closely to the metacarpal bed from which it has been split away. If necessary, a second wire may be used for greater security. These wires are cut off just below the skin which is sewed up over them. A plaster gauntlet is applied, including all but the tip of the thumb, and this is retained for six to eight weeks. The results from this treatment, as followed at the Sahlgren Hospital, were far superior to closed reduction methods.

Treatment by Supervised Neglect. It may seem odd that any surgeons should advocate "supervised neglect" as a method of treatment for this fracture, but on more careful consideration there are strong arguments in favor of such a practice in selected cases. Most theoretic studies tend to neglect the ugly, practical facts of life, which in the case of Bennett fractures show that a great majority of these are incurred by alcoholics who are too undisciplined to submit to any regimented form of treatment, and who are incapable of disciplined routines. On these patients, it is a total waste of time to apply even the simplest form of traction; and since patients of this character cannot be relied upon to attend follow-up visits, increased risk is involved in tight casts. For them, also, the danger of sepsis from open surgery would be greater. Blum[3] advocates treating these patients with minimal immobilization consisting of elastic bandage support for a few weeks, and early return to activity, which very soon becomes "not particularly painful." From cases

of this type that we have seen (but not treated), it is surprising how good the functional result may be. Blum rationalizes this on the ground that as the fracture heals it incorporates its volar component, providing a broader base to the metacarpal, which now becomes an enarthrodial, or ball and socket joint, rather than the normal diarthrodial joint that existed before the fracture. Blum describes the functional results as "excellent;" and Gedda's follow-up studies, which were very thoroughly carried out, would tend to give this some occasional support: as one case, 12 years later, that had "no pain;" and other "comparatively satisfactory" after 11 years. On the whole, however, arthritis develops, pain increases with time, and work capacity is increasingly diminished. For this reason, treatment by neglect is not to be recommended except where the patient's general outlook is extremely unfavorable. In such cases, it is perhaps a more realistic approach to the problem; and on a temporary basis it offers, as Blum claims, a "shorter, simpler, and perhaps better method of treatment."

Late Treatment. Numerous methods have been suggested for treatment of late cases, where the carpometacarpal joint becomes disabled with arthritis or instability or both. No large follow-up series is available, and therefore it seems reasonable to be satisfied with the simplest of these procedures as advocated by Bunnell.[6] This consists in opening the joint through incision along the dorsum of the base of the metacarpal, swinging around to the volar side as it follows the flexion crease at the wrist. After stripping off the muscles, good exposure of the multangular bone and the fracture is obtained. The multangular can then be fused to the metacarpal, still allowing plenty of functional movement for the thumb through its other joints. If the position of the metacarpal is angulated by the fracture, this can be corrected by an osteotomy at the same time. Wires through the multangular and through the osteotomy will retain position until the bone heals. From very slight experience on our part, these operations have offered better results than the alternative of a tendon graft to stabilize the carpometacarpal joint as sometimes suggested.

Common Errors in Treatment of Thumb Fractures

Although the commonest errors, in these cases, are due to the patient's irresponsibility, sloth, and lack of cooperation, some warnings may be listed for the doctors: (1) Inadequate reduction of fracture' dislocation — surgeons often lack a clear conception of the mechanics of the fracture, or they are unfamiliar with manipulative technique, or they rely on traction to accomplish the reduction without attempting manipulation. Adequate manipulative reduction is essential for this type of fracture. (2) Inadequate traction — poorly applied adhesive traction or careless supervision of traction follow-up often leads to relaxation of the pull and loss of position. (3) Inadequate lateral compression at the fracture site sometimes permits the subluxation to persist even while traction is in force. (4) Inadequate follow-up observation — these cases call for close supervision. (5) Application of cast with thumb fully abducted and extended is still a common error instead of the correct, physiologic position with the thumb partially flexed, partially opposed, and partially abducted.

CARPAL AND WRIST FRACTURES

Carpal Fractures

Carpal Navicular

Fractures of the navicular impose two problems on the surgeon and if these are correctly handled, the prospects of success are extremely good. The first problem is diagnosis, for the injury is often and easily misjudged as a minor sprain. The patient himself is likely to neglect seeing a doctor at the start and may very often minimize the symptoms when he describes his complaint. This provides the surgeon with a strong inducement to let the patient ''work it off'' and also to ''save the expense'' of an x-ray at the first visit. However, the clinical signs should provide warning of possible bone injury, particularly if a careful test is made for localized tenderness. Here palpation over the dorsum of the wrist, with the examiner's finger tip applied just beyond the lower end of the radius, should encounter the navicular bone, where the patient will wince a little when pressure is applied. Another fairly reliable sign is to have the patient dorsiflex the wrist and then press against resistance with the heel of the hand. This will refer pain to the navicular area if dorsiflexion has not already produced the same complaint. Even without these two tests, it is a good rule for a surgeon to x-ray every sprained wrist at the first consultation. If pain is severe enough to bring the patient to the doctor's office, it deserves this study, and without this, the diagnosis cannot be made.

X-ray interpretation also requires careful analysis since the usual A.P. and lateral films often fail to reveal the fracture even when it is clearly present. This is due, of course, to the curved projection of the bone which can only be thrown into profile by an oblique view. Most roentgenologists accomplish this by rotating the wrist, although Böhler[4] states ''it can be best demonstrated by the x-rays in an anterior-posterior view of the wrist joint slightly dorsiflexed with the· fingers bent.'' Our routine includes a lateral, an oblique, and an A.P. view with the wrist in ulnar deviation. Another misleading factor will occur in the occasional case where an old, unrecognized fracture was already prsent, pre-existing the trauma that brings the patient to his doctor. The fracture may be demonstrated by x-ray; but it is important to recognize the fact that this is an old, and therefore untreatable condition, rather than a fresh injury. The age of the fracture is sometimes difficult to judge, but old cases usually show some evidence of an attempt at bone healing and there is apt to be some density or sclerosis along the fracture edges which will probably be smoother than in a fresh case. There also may be more cavitation than would be expected in a fresh fracture, or possibly some extraneous calcification. Also, an x-ray taken immediately after injury cannot be relied upon in cases where the fracture is of minimal extent (Fig. 6.23). Not uncommonly it appears normal, even under careful scrutiny, whereas 10 days or two weeks later, bone will have absorbed around the fracture line, making it clearly visible. Therefore, it is advisable from the start to apply a gauntlet cast including the thumb in the functional position, even though the patient seems to have sustained only a sprain. At the end of two weeks if there is the slightest ground for suspicion, x-rays should be repeated, at which time the definitive diagnosis can be made.

On making the diagnosis, the surgeon must form some judgment as to the type of fracture he is dealing with, since there is considerable variation in the rate of healing at various locations. Böhler pointed out, as long ago as 1932, that there are significant levels governed by their blood supply, much like intracapsular fractures of the hip. Fractures of the tubercle are essentially extra-articular and ''heal by bony union under any treatment,'' as he states, often taking only three or four weeks. Fractures of the waist or midsection heal by ''vessels growing from the peripheral to the central fragment'' in cases where the latter happens to be lacking in its own blood supply. Such a process requires absolute immobilization and, if interrupted by mobility, may be obstructed altogether, causing nonunion. Fractures of the proximal quarter will, of course, be the hardest to heal because this section is furthest from the reparative source of blood and usually has no circulation of its own.

From this point on, the surgeon meets the second problem of navicular fractures, which consists in providing adequate immobilization. The word *adequate* bears two important connotations. Obviously the plaster must be well applied, *i.e.,* well padded and then rolled very firmly and as tight as possible, short of endangering the circulation. A cast that ''bells outward'' at its proximal end around the forearm muscles only serves to add leverage to any stress that may come to the wrist; therefore care is needed to pull plaster tight here; this cannot be done safely unless moderately heavy padding has been applied. In addition, it is helpful to secure the upper end of the cast with elastic bandage, rolling this above the elbow as well. We have not found it necessary to bind the plaster itself above the elbow, however, and some freedom of movement of this joint is beneficial. The lower end of the cast must be equally well fitted as far as the metacarpophalangeal joints. The cast should include the thumb as far as the interphalangeal joint and it should be pressed against the palm and held here long enough to harden in the dome-shaped mold of the hand. The fingers may be allowed free movement to give the patient a fair amount of functional use of the hand in spite

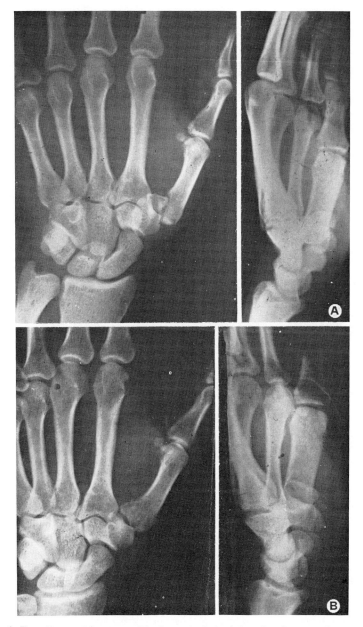

Figure 6.22. A. True Bennett fracture with characteristic deformity. Seen and treated the day after it occurred. *B.* Result at end of eight weeks. Treatment followed method outlined in the text. Patient was extremely cooperative and regained normal function.

of the restrictions of the cast. Unless all these precautions are taken, a cast is likely to become unstable and thus it will invite nonunion.

In our experience, Castex has proven a better material than plaster of Paris because it is more durable, much lighter, completely waterproof, and fully penetrated by x-ray (Fig. 6.23). Follow-up films, therefore, can be taken through the cast with no obstructing shadow, which is a great help in observing progress. Castex requires care in its application and cannot be used successfully by the inexperienced surgeon. It will not harden for half an hour and does not become actually solid for half a day or more. However, it will hold its form adequately in 20 minutes. During this time care must be taken to maintain its mold over the hand. A simple roll (10 yards by three inches) is usu-

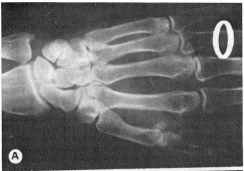

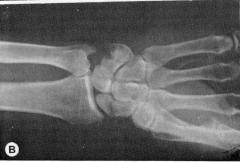

Figure 6.23. A. Fractured navicular scaphoid. X-ray taken the day after injury. Patient's age, 60 years. *B.* Same case. X-rays taken two weeks after injury. This film was taken through Castex cast, indicating the permeability of this material for follow-up x-ray studies. Treatment consisted of 11 weeks of full immobilization in cast, followed by 3 weeks of protective splinting, hot soaks, and active mobilization. Patient has returned to playing tennis.

ally adequate for the entire cast and thus protected, a patient is able to engage in minor use of his hand with a minimum handicap. We have, for example, treated truck drivers who were able to continue working while wearing such a cast.

The second connotation of "adequate immobilization" is that it must be continued until full time for bone healing has been allowed. Here the surgeon will be under much pressure, since the hand is the source of a patient's livelihood, and to be deprived of its use for three months or longer becomes both costly and monotonous. Nevertheless, nonunion is likely to ensue unless the fracture is allowed time to repair itself with full bony union, which commonly takes 12 to 16 weeks. Very often it will be noticed that x-rays may look much worse after four weeks than at the start, and what begins as an innocent appearing "impacted" fracture becomes an extensive cystlike defect in the bone. The first three or four weeks of "healing" are therefore largely occupied with absorption; in such cases the date of true healing in the sense of reconstruction does not begin until at least a month after the injury. It then progresses rather slowly and successive

x-rays, if taken every 10 days, may simply discourage the patient. It is best to space them not more often than every two weeks, or better every three weeks, although the patient should be seen more often than this for inspection of the cast. If this becomes loose, it should be reapplied to maintain constant snugness.

Since it is so important to maintain firm and secure immobilization, we would advise against the use of dorsal and palmar plaster splints, and even less a ready-made metal or plastic splint. Splints tend to work loose, and the prepared splints seldom fit snugly or hold the hand in the desired position of rest. There has been a certain amount of disagreement as to what the optimum position may be. Some authors advocate putting the wrist in mild supination. Such a recommendation will be nullified unless the cast is carried above the elbow, for quite obviously rotation of the wrist cannot be prevented if the elbow is free. Nevertheless, from a practical standpoint, we have not found it necessary to immobilize higher than the antecubital space; nor do other writers advise going proximal to this, for the loss of elbow movement would detract from whatever use the patient may still retain in his cast, and it would also run some risk of stiffening the elbow joint from such prolonged fixation. In our own practice, we simply place the wrist in neutral position with some 15 to 20° of dorsiflexion and take comfort in O'Donoghue's[27] statement, "No bizarre position of the wrist is either necessary or desirable."

If all these precautions are taken, and if treatment is begun at the time of fracture or reasonably soon thereafter, we feel that there is every reason to *expect* good bony healing. Most of the nonunions on which this fracture earned its bad reputation are the result of nontreatment until too late a date, inadequate treatment from too short a time of immobilization, or improper treatment through the use of poorly applied splints. There will, of course, still be some nonunions under the best of care, but the prospects of success through the conservative measures outlined above seem to us far too bright to justify primary surgical procedures. Although O'Donoghue disagrees with the opinion just stated, his experience and judgment carry so much weight that they should not be ignored. He believes that the fracture should be tested by manipulation, and if it seems to be unstable, a primary operation and screw fixation should be performed. McLaughlin[21] has voiced a somewhat similar opinion; but where we have tried it on fresh cases, the results have been less, rather than more, favorable than closed treatment. We feel very strongly that surgery should be reserved for *late* cases.

If healing does not develop by the end of 12 weeks, the question arises whether it can be expected from further immobilization. The answer would depend somewhat on the circumstances. A fracture that has suffered from neglectful or inadequate immobilization during the first three months certainly deserves a try at gaining union under full immobilization. It must be recognized, however, that the chances of good healing are diminished by allowing movement in the fracture area for so long a time, thereby promoting growth of chondral rather than osteal cells with the proliferation of nonossifying connective tissue. If the fracture has received adequate immobilization from the start, simple delay in healing may be the cause of apparent nonunion and it is worthwhile to prolong immobilization at least another month, or possibly even two months. One roentgenographic sign to watch for at this stage is the development of a heavily sclerosed layer at the fracture site. If this is present, further possibility of union becomes extremely unlikely. Although some authors recommend continuing a cast for as long as a year, Böhler[4] points out that "the treatment of nonunion and necrosis of the navicular by long fixation is useless, because it cannot effect recovery, as the growth of the vessels from one fragment to another has become impossible by the sealing off of the fractured surfaces."

There comes a time when frank nonunion must be acknowledged, and at this stage alternate choices deserve consideration. The simplest course is to allow the patient to accept the minor inconvenience that may be caused by his injury without attempting further treatment. This method could be recommended for a patient who does not engage in very active manual work, especially if the fracture does not involve his dominant hand. As is well known, great numbers of unsuspected cases were brought to light when men were drafted for the army in World War II and widespread x-ray diagnosis became available. These men had been using their wrists freely, without enough disability to require treatment. On the other hand, there is a strong tendency for chronic irritation to develop under these circumstances, with increasing disability over the years as traumatic arthritis develops. Consequently, for younger patients at least, a more definitive course of treatment is advisable.

For a time it became popular to remove the bone altogether in cases of nonunion; but Böhler[4] showed very convincingly that this increased the disability rather than correcting it. He stated emphatically, "I have never seen a case in which the usefulness of the hand has returned to normal after removal of the navicular....I have heard the same from all expert insurance assessors." Our own observation would confirm Böhler's findings in the few cases we have seen where surgeons resorted to this method as a measure of desperation. We should even question whether removal of a small fragment is often necessary or advisable.

In active adults, especially of the younger age groups, the presence of a frank nonunion causing disabling pain makes the indication for surgical interference almost mandatory. A great number of procedures have been proposed. Böhler advocated Beck's dirlling, under x-ray control, as the procedure of choice; followed by 12 weeks of plaster immobilization. Others have recommended fixation with stainless steel screws. A special type of screw was designed by McLaughlin[21] for this purpose, but in a short series of cases we found it technically difficult to use and unfavorable in the final results. Fett[14] designed a metal ball, to substitute for the navicular; but this, too, proved unsatisfactory in our hands. From our own experience, we strongly favor the operative technique of Burnett,[7] from which we have seen a very high percentage of successful results.

This operative procedure begins with an incision originating in the anatomical snuff box just below (palmarward) the long extensor tendon of the thumb. The incision extends longitudinally, with slight dorsal inclination, to a point about one and one-half inches above the radial styloid. Care is taken to avoid the superficial sensory nerve. Bleeding can be controlled without a tourniquet if care is used, although a tourniquet may simplify the operation. By retracting the skin dorsally, and by opening the radiocarpal joint, a good view of the navicular can be obtained. It is easy to make the error of identifying the wrong bone; but this can be avoided in three ways. First, the dissection should afford an adequate view so that the navicular can be clearly recognized in its usual profile, articulating with the distal radius. Second, the fracture itself should be visible in this dissection. Third, an x-ray should be made available and used in case any doubt persists. With the hand deviated toward the ulna and in slight flexion, the distal end of the navicular projects prominently enough to permit drilling with a ¼-inch bit and as this is done under direct vision, the alignment of the drill can be readily controlled. It is, of course, aimed at the fracture surface of the proximal fragment in its reduced position. When the fracture line is reached, a smaller bit — ⅛-inch or 3/16-inch — is substituted so that the proximal drill hole will be of a slightly smaller bore. A 1⅛-inch splinter of bone is cut from the radial shaft just above the styloid and whittled down and sharpened enough to fit the drill hole precisely. This bone, if it is properly taken from the cortex, will be hard enough to permit gentle hammering by which means it can be tapped securely through the tunnel made by the drill holes. The drilling is carried to, but not through, the cortex of the proximal fragment. The use of a smaller hole in the proximal fragment helps the bone graft to fit more snugly. Any bone projecting at the distal entrance of the tunnel can be rongeured off. There are those who feel that the use of a graft adds nothing to actual drilling and that a screw would do as well. Without a very large series of cases and controls, it would be difficult to prove this, but in our experience, the bone peg procedure has proven extremely successful and the technique does not offer any excessive difficulties for an experienced surgeon. After the operation, the wrist must be immobilized as carefully as for a fresh fracture. Again a period of at least 10 to 12 weeks is required. Full immobilization is necessary until good evidence of healing appears and then partial protection with a half-splint will be advisable for another month or so (Fig. 6.24).

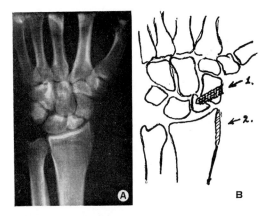

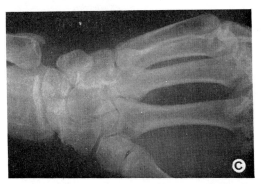

Figure 6.24. A. Postoperative x-ray of navicular fracture (one year old) that has had Burnett pegging procedure. *B.* Tracing of same x-ray to point out the location of the bone peg (*1*), and the radial site from which it had been taken (*2*). *C.* Full healing of same fracture at end of 12 weeks. Patient resumed college hockey. No further complaints.

One final problem arises in navicular fractures at the late stage when disabling arthritis has developed in the wrist joint. Such cases deserve surgical interference if the pain is severe enough to provide a major handicap. The operation of choice is that of wrist fusion, which may be carried out by any method the surgeon elects. We prefer bone grafting with a piece of the iliac crest, although in the past we have followed Brittain's[5] excellent technique with a carefully fitted graft from the tibia. The disadvantage of the latter procedure is that it weakens the tibia, producing a serious risk of fracture for the next four months.

The technique we advocate for such a fusion begins with a dorsal, Z-shaped incision extending from the base of the third metacarpal to the distal end of the radius. The carpal bones are exposed and a channel about ⅜- to ½-inch wide is cut. This is extended into the base of the metacarpus and also into the articular end of the radius. Often the graft can be shaped to be countersunk at the two ends. The curve of the iliac crest makes it a favorable bone site to allow for the

necessary 15° dorsiflexion of the wrist. The hand should be centered so that the thumb, when held in opposition, will represent a straight prolongation of the line of the radius. Well molded plaster is required for 11 to 12 weeks, or again, Castex may be used in preference. For the first six weeks the cast should extend above the elbow, and thereafter may be cut down to just below the elbow. The results from this procedure are likely to be extremely good and, despite the loss of wrist movements, an ambitious worker can return to active manual function if all goes well. The absence of pain and the strength and stability of the wrist offer every advantage over the previous weak and painful joint that was associated with the original injury and the traumatic arthritis that followed.

Errors in Treatment

These are the common errors that may occur in the care of navicular fractures. (1) The fracture may be missed through the patient's own carelessness or indifference, and the doctor who treats him may be misled into diagnosing the injury as a sprain. (2) X-rays may be too hazy to recognize the fracture, the oblique x-ray view may be neglectfully omitted so that the fracture is not seen, or the first x-ray may be essentially negative and subsequent, confirmatory x-rays may not be taken, thus losing the chance to see the fracture after absorption has made it clearly visible. (3) Treatment may prove inadequate through use of ill fitting splints that allow movement, or through too short a period of immobilization. (4) When operative treatment is carried out, improper techniques, such as removal of the bone, will aggravate the condition, ill conceived surgical techniques, such as impractical types of screws or the use of balls or ''prostheses,'' will lead to failure, except in the hands of these especially trained in their use; inadequate immobilization during the postoperative stage will also nullify the surgical benefits. From all of this, it becomes apparent that success with navicular fractures requires a crafty, skillful, meticulous, and persistent surgeon, and a cooperative patient.

Other Carpal Fractures

As a rule, fractures of the carpal bones, unassociated with dislocations, do not offer very serious problems except with the navicular. Cotton[11] once observed, ''No bone of the carpus is exempt from fracture, but save for those noted (navicular) there are no *type* fractures.'' Although surgeons who treat them often feel that their carpal fracture cases are great rarities, Böhler[4] has shown statistically that this is not the case, even though the fractures are not common. Treatment consists of application of a palmar splint to support the wrist until the ligamentous strain, which may be severe, has subsided, a matter of 10 days to 3 weeks. As in all other fractures involving joints, it is important to *mobilize* the wrist as early as movement can be tolerated safely. This can usually be done after five or six days by allowing the patient to remove the splint temporarily for hot soaks; but the splint should be replaced and worn as long as pain is present.

O'Donoghue[27] has pointed out that the prolonged symptoms following wrist "sprains" may be due to unrecognized compression fractures, not discernible in x-rays because of overlapping of the bones and because of their minimal character. He considers the cystic degeneration of the lunate bone, known as Kienbock's disease, to be of this type. He also feels that prolonged pain after wrist trauma may be due to chondral fractures which, of course, could not be recognized roentgenographically except, perhaps, where small flakes of bone are visible. Such injuries, if inadequately immobilized, would have a greater tendency to give late arthritic changes and pain.

COLLES' FRACTURE

Abraham Colles[10] of Dublin first described one of the most common fractures about the hand and wrist. The characteristic "dinner fork" deformity of the injury is familiar to all. In the obese and in the aged with osteoporosis this typical physical appearance may be missing but the roentgenogram will disclose the dorsal displacement and tilting of the distal fragment of the radius. The term "Colles' " fracture is here applied to all fractures with dorsal displacement involving the distal 1½ inches of the radius.

Indications for Reduction

Not all Colles' fractures require reduction. In the elderly, moderate radial shortening and dorsal displacement may be accepted with little or no disability. Commonly, after reduction and immobilization, absorption of the osteoporotic bone occurs, producing radial shortening regardless of the position of the fragments immediately following reduction. In the middle-aged or young person, nearly complete restoration of the normal radiocarpal joint should be sought. In children, the closer the fracture to the epiphysial plate the less the chance of permanent deformity.

The judgment of each surgeon decides the course when he asks himself, "Can I improve and maintain the position of this fracture and will the function of the wrist and hand be helped?"

Technique of Reduction

General anesthesia is an excellent agent to reduce Colles' fractures. Unfortunately, conditions are not always ideal for this, particularly in one who has recently eaten or in a poor risk patient. Axillary nerve block is an excellent method when performed by one skilled in this technique. Local infiltration, in our opinion, is a safe and efficient procedure, especially in a fresh fracture seen within 24 hours after injury. We have never seen infection with this method, although the risk is always present. The skin should be surgically prepared prior to injection. Introducing the nee-

dle above the fracture site and directing the needle volarward and distally will place its point into the fracture site (Fig. 6.25). Aspiration yields gross red blood and confirms the position of the needle. Between 5 and 10 cc of anesthetic solution (usually 1 per cent or 2 per cent Xylocaine without ephedrine) are injected. A time lapse of 5 to 10 min should occur between injection and reduction.

The first step in reduction of a simple Colles' fracture is to correct the overriding of the distal fragment. This is achieved by muscular relaxation and traction. With the patient recumbent, an upward steady pull on the thumb and a downward pressure on the arm above the flexed elbow will separate the fragments (Fig. 6.26). Next, the deformity is increased and the dorsal cortex used as a hinge to reduce the distal fragment into position. During this maneuver the assistant maintains traction by holding the thumb with one hand and the arm with the other. With experience the surgeon readily recognizes by feel the smooth contour of the dorsum of the radius after reduction.

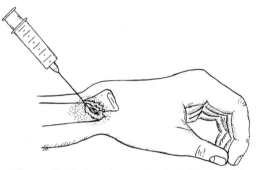

Figure 6.25. Local anesthesia infiltration into hematoma and fracture site.

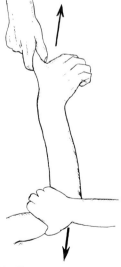

Figure 6.26. Traction-countertraction in ulnar deviation.

Care must be used while applying the cast to prevent slipping of the fragments and loss of reduction. The assistant is directed to hold the fingers firmly and place the hand in ulnar deviation and slight flexion. This will permit the ulna to serve as a buttress and help preserve the reduction.

In our opinion, comminuted fractures of the distal radius are best treated by molding the fragments into as normal a position as possible and applying the cast while the hand and wrist are held in full ulnar deviation and slight flexion. We believe this positioning is an important point in technique for, in this way, the ulna serves as a buttress to abnormal shortening of the radius as the fracture heals and absorption occurs. If this principle is followed, skeletal traction will rarely be required. We oppose the use of the "Cotton-Loder," or "bell-hop" position of immobilization of a Colles' fracture. This can cause vascular compression and abnormal swelling. Lynch and Lipscomb[20] have recently drawn attention to the carpal tunnel syndrome following use of this position.

Apart from the already open Colles' fracture, open reduction is almost never indicated. The poor results following adequate closed or open treatment of this injury appear to be determined by the degree of involvement of the radiocarpal joint, a feature uninfluenced by surgery.

Occasionally a Colles' fracture, unreduced, is seen two or three weeks after injury. One closed attempt at this late reduction may be made, but open reduction and prying of the fragment into position is usually required. Internal fixation is not ordinarily necessary.

Many techniques are used to immobilize a Colles' fracture. These must retain the reduction but not cause swelling of the hand or jeopardize the circulation. The surgeon should master the method that serves him best.

We have found that these fractures do not require above-elbow immobilization. Anteroposterior splints, if properly applied with the wrist in ulnar deviation and slight flexion, are adequate. The plaster should include the radial side of the second metacarpal head, the distal ulna, and the proximal radial forearm, thus giving the three point fixation so necessary to maintain position of any fracture. If roller gauze is applied to hold the plaster while it sets, the gauze should be subsequently cut.

A safe, efficient, simple method used by the authors is a circular forearm cast applied in the position as outlined above (Fig. 6.27A). While the plaster is setting, it is gently and smoothly molded to the distal radius. While the postreduction x-ray develops, a one-inch strip of the cast is excised from its dorsal surface (Fig. 6.27B). The sheet wadding is divided down to the skin. The sides of the cast can then be sprung wider at that time; or subsequently, without risking loss of reduction. The plaster should never extend beyond the distal palmar crease, except in children. The thumb must be free.

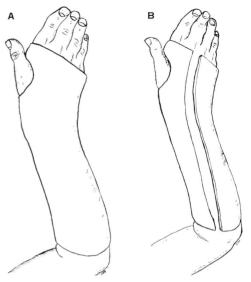

Figure 6.27. A. Cast applied in ulnar deviation and slight flexion. B. Dorsal segment of cast removed as circulation precaution.

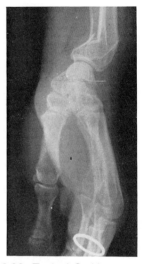

Figure 6.28. Typical Smith or reverse Colles fracture with volar displacement of distal fragment and deformity opposite of "silver-fork" of Colles fracture.

Aftercare

The patient must be warned about swelling, numbness, and discoloration of the fingers upon application of the cast and dismissal from the fracture room. A circulation check is performed by the surgeon on the following day. Elevation, sling and rest are urged for the first few days. The need for finger exercises and active shoulder motions is impressed upon the patient. This warning must be repeated frequently throughout the period of treatment.

It is wise to see the patient and repeat the x-ray of the wrist in one week. Ordinarily, the initial cast may remain for three to four weeks, providing the "fit" remains and the wrist is in the described position of maximum ulnar deviation and slight flexion. At the end of this time the cast is changed and a new circular one applied with the wrist in neutral position and some ulnar deviation. The second cast remains two weeks. After its removal, the volar half can be used while working and at night for the next two weeks. During this period frequent soaks in warm soapy water, self-massage, and active motions are prescribed.

Ordinarily, one year passes before the wrist feels "normal" or has reached its final stage. The patient should be warned of this lengthy convalescence.

On completion of treatment and dismissal of the un-complicated Colles' fracture, it is a good habit for the surgeon to ask his patient to return one year after injury. Thus the surgeon will have many happy and, oc-casionally, humbling experiences with this interesting fracture.

Complications

Immediate injury to the median nerve is sometimes seen with Colles' fracture and should be looked for in all cases. We have not observed, however, any per-manent motor or sensory damage to this nerve.

Vascular impairment of the forearm with Volk-mann's contracture or ischemia of the intrinsic mus-cles of the hand are disasters avoided by proper casting and careful check of the circulation after reduction.

Despite all measures to minimize vascular complica-tions there are certain persons who tolerate trauma poorly. These patients are prone to develop trophic skin changes, osteoporosis, and pain after trauma and immobilization.

Every effort must be made to prevent stiff fingers. The hand should be elevated on a pillow at night and a sling worn by day for one or two weeks after reduc-tion. The cast must be properly applied with its end not beyond the distal palmar crease and the thumb free. Constant urging and instruction for finger motion is necessary, particularly in the individual with a low pain threshold.

Shoulder pain is a rather common complication fol-lowing wrist immobilization. It is prevented by active exercises of the shoulder throughout the period of treatment.

An unusual complication of Colles' fracture is rup-ture of the extensor pollicis longus tendon. We have seen this following an undisplaced fracture of the dis-tal radius, so that it need not follow only the incom-

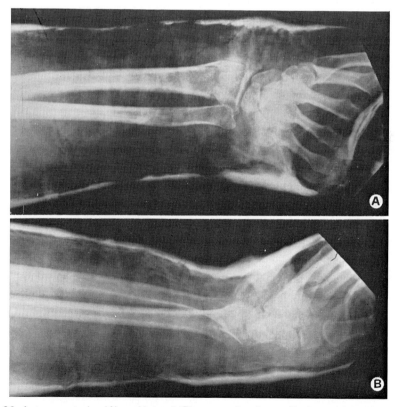

Figure 6.29. Anteroposterior (A) and lateral (B) x-rays showing reduction and cast immobilization in ulnar deviation, dorsiflexion, and supination.

pletely reduced or malunited fractures. Although usually a late complication, we have seen this occur as early as the fifth week after injury. Transfer of the extensor indicis proprius tendon to the extensor pollicis longus distal to the dorsal carpal ligament is a simple and efficient corrective procedure for this condition.

Malunion, with either much shortening or residual dorsal tilt of the radial fragment, occurs occasionally. Frequently function of the wrist is satisfactory and no treatment is necessary. The Darrach procedure, or resection of the distal ulna, is sometimes necessary for the symptomatic wrist with radial shortening and restricted pronation-supination motions. Osteotomy of the radius with bone graft to correct the dorsal tilt can be performed if the symptoms warrant.

A complication easily missed in the early phase of treatment of a Colles' fracture is an accompanying fracture of the carpal navicular bone. The wise surgeon will cast an eye on this bone on the initial and the final roentgenogram.

SMITH FRACTURE

A reverse Colles', or a Smith fracture,[32] is not an uncommon injury. It is opposite both in appearance and on x-ray to the Colles' fracture. The distal radial fragment is displaced volarward and usually shortened, while the distal ulna is very prominent on the dorsum of the wrist (Fig. 6.28). The surgeon should be alert to this injury and not confuse it with the much more common Colles' fracture.

Reduction is obtained by reversing the maneuvers of the Colles' fracture, i.e., traction, pressure on the flexor aspect of the radius, and supination. We agree with Thomas[35] that casting in supination is important. A long-arm cast with the forearm in ulnar deviation and supination is applied (Fig. 6.29 A and B). This position is maintained for six to eight weeks.

We feel open reduction or skeletal traction is rarely indicated if the principles of reduction and immobilization are carried out as described here and in the section on Colles' fracture.

Common Errors

1. Failure to distinguish a reverse Colles', or a Smith fracture, from a Colles' fracture.

2. Immobilization in too much flexion and too little ulnar deviation. This results in stiffness of the wrist and fingers and a greater likelihood of neurovascular complications.

3. Lack of finger and shoulder exercises during convalescence.

4. Failure to inspect the hand for circulatory complications the day after reduction.

5. Failure to appreciate the frequent discrepancy between the appearance of an old malunited Colles' fracture on the roentgenogram and the function of the wrist. Not all malunions require surgical correction.

REFERENCES

1. Barr, J. S. *et al.* Fractures of carpal navicular bone. J. Bone Joint Surg., *35A:* 609, 1953.
2. Bennett, E. H. Fracture of the metacarpal bone of the thumb. Bri. Md. J., *12:* 2, 1886; Trans. R. Acad. Med. Ireland, *15:* 309, 1897; Dublin J. M. Sc. *73:* 1882.
3. Blum, L. Treatment of Bennett's fracture-dislocation of first metacarpal bone. J. Bone Joint Surg., *23:* 578-580, 1941.
4. Böhler, L. *Treatment of Fractures* (Hey Groves transl.) Baltimore, Williams & Wilkins, 1935.
5. Brittain, T. *Arthrodesis.* Baltimore, Williams & Wilkins, 1949.
6. Bunnell, S. *Surgery of the Hand.* Philadelphia, Lippincott, 1944.
7. Burnett, J. H. Treatment fractured carpal scaphoid. J. Bone Joint Surg., *19:* 1099, 1937.
8. Charnley, J. *Closed Treatment of Common Fractures.* Baltimore, Williams & Wilkins, 1958.
9. Clarkson, P., and Pelly, A. *General and Plastic Surgery of the Hand.* Oxford, Blackwell, 1962.
10. Colles, A. On the fracture of the carpal extremity of the radius. Edinburgh Med. Surg. J., 1814.
11. Cotton, F. J. *Dislocations and Fractures.* Philadelphia, Saunders, 1924.
12. Eaton, R. G. *Joint Injuries of the Hand.* Springfield, Charles C Thomas, 1971.
13. Eichenholtz, S. U., and Rizzo, P. C. Fracture of the neck of the fifth metacarpal bone. J.A.M.A., *178:* 151, 1961.
14. Fett, H. C. Management of carpal fractures. Compens. Med., *4:* 15, 1952.
15. Gedda, K. O. Studies of Bennett's fracture. Acta Chir. Scand., 1954.
16. Howard, L. D., Jr. Unpublished instructional course — hand fractures. Am. Acad. Orthop. Surgeons, Lect. 1960.
17. Howland, W. S. Gunshot fractures in civilian practice. An evaluation of the results of limited surgical treatment. J. Bone Joint Surg., *53A:* 47-55, 1971.
18. Johnson, J. F. Tendon and nerve injuries in fractures and dislocations. Nebraska Med. J., *23:* 4, 1938.
19. Laskin, R. S. Simple splint for finger injuries. Postgrad. Med., *48:* 174-175, 1970.
20. Lynch, A. C., and Lipscomb, P. R. The carpal tunnel syndrome and Colles' fractures. J.A.M.A., *185:* 363, 1963.
21. McLaughlin, H. L. Fracture of carpal navicular. J. Bone Joint Surg., *36-A:* 765, 1954.
22. McNealy, R. W., and Lichtenstein, M. E. Fractures of bones of the hand. Am. J. Surg., *50:* 563-570, 1940.
23. Milch, H. Recurrent dislocation of thumb: Capsulorrhaphy. Am. J. Surg., *6:* 237-239, 1929.
24. Mondry, F. Surgical therapy of post-traumatic functional disturbance of proximal joint of the thumb. Zentralbl. Chir., *67:* 1532-1535, 1940.
25. Nichols, H. M. *Manual of Hand Injuries.* Chicago, Year Book Publishers, 1957.
26. Nutter, P. D. Interposition of sesamoids in metacarpophalangeal dislocations. J. Bone Joint Surg., *22:* 730-734, 1940.
27. O'Donoghue, D. H. *Treatment of Injuries to Athletes.* Philadelphia, Saunders, 1962.
28. Pratt, D. R. Internal splint for closed and open treatment

of injuries of the extensor tendon. J. Bone Joint Surg., *34A:* 785, 1952.

29. Rider, D. L. Fractures of the metacarpals, metatarsals, and phalanges. Am. J. Surg., *38:* 549, 1937.

30. Rued, T. P., *et al.* Staple internal fixation of fractures of the hand. J. Trauma, *11:* 381-389, 1971.

31. Scudder, C. L. *Treatment of Fractures.* Philadelphia, Saunders, 1958.

32. Smith, R. W. A *Treatise on Fractures in the Vicinity of Joints and on Certain Forms of Accidents and Congenital Dislocations.* Dublin, Hodges and Smith, 1847.

33. Stark, H. H., Boyes, J. H., and Wilson, J. N. Mallet finger. J. Bone Joint Surg., *44A:* 1061, 1962.

34. Swanson, A. B. Silicone rubber implants for replacement of arthritic or destroyed joints in the hand. Surg. Clin. North Am., *48:* 5, 1968.

35. Thomas, F. B. Reduction of Smith's fracture. J. Bone Joint Surg., *39B:* 463, 1957.

36. Wise, R. A. Unusual fracture of the terminal phalanx of the finger. J. Bone Joint Surg., *21:* 467-469, 1939.

chapter seven

Injuries to Tendons

A.

Technique of Tendon Repair

Elden C. Weckesser, M.D.

The most successful solution to the problems of tendon repair lies in the observance of the following basic principles.

I. Employment of an atraumatic surgical technique: (1) gentleness, fine instruments and the judicious use of magnification; (2) bloodless field — pneumatic tourniquet; (3) adequate physiologic incisions; (4) nonreactive suture material; (5) special sutures and techniques to hold tendons.

II. Performance by or under direct supervision of a surgeon interested and skilled in the techniques required.

III. Use of the main operating room.

IV. Avoidance of infection by: (1) liberal cleansing, irrigation, and limited debridement; (2) definitive repair of early, clean cases only; (3) soft tissue closure only after cleansing and limited debridement of late, contaminated, or severely traumatized cases (tendon repair through a fresh incision three to six weeks later); (4) antibiotics and specific immunizations.

V. Postoperative supervision: (1) elevation; (2) aseptic wound care; (3) immobilization; (4) prophylactic antibiotics.

ATRAUMATIC SURGICAL TECHNIQUE

Surgical technique in tendon repair should be most careful and gentle. No repair should be undertaken without a bloodless field, which minimizes operative trauma. Incisions should be adequate according to sound physiologic principles (Fig. 7.1.), usually with little regard to the traumatic wound, in order to give good exposure. Instruments should be small and the cutting instruments sharp. The more gentle the surgical technique, the fewer adhesions produced and the better the results will be. Magnification of five diameters supplied by a head loop has been found very helpful in obtaining accurate tendon approximation. The best in aseptic, atraumatic technique, with the best light and assistance is required to produce primary healing and a good result.

THE TOURNIQUET

A bloodless field, provided by a pneumatic cuff tourniquet about the upper arm, is indispensable in tendon repair.

When the instrument has a broad cuff, and is inflated to no more than 250 mm Hg, it can be left in place for 90 min with safety. If a longer time is required, it is safest to deflate the cuff for 10 min and then reinflate it.

The extremity is most effectively emptied of blood by wrapping with a rubber Esmarch bandage prior to inflating the cuff. Many types of good apparatus are available. One with a broad cuff should be chosen.

INCISIONS FOR TENDON REPAIR

Figure 7.1.1 illustrates useful physiologic incisions for tendon repair. In the palm, these are parallel to the skin creases or parallel to Langer's lines.

In the finger, the midlateral incision gives excellent exposure of the volar or dorsal mechanism depending

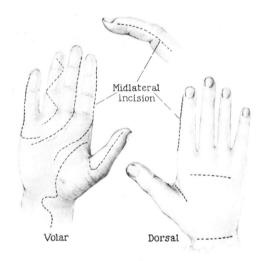

Midlateral incision

Volar   Dorsal

Figure 7.1.1. Proper incisions for tendon repair. The midlateral incision of the finger may be made with or without a palmar incision, with or without cutting the web space: the digital nerves and vessels are carefully protected. The zig-zag incision gives excellent volar exposure when early postoperative motion is not to be employed. Incisions which follow skin lines or creases are highly desirable.

on which flap is elevated. In elevation of the volar flap, the digital nerve and vascular pedicle are elevated with it. The midlateral finger incision and palmar incision may be made with or without cutting the web space, as diagrammed. This gives good exposure at the base of the digit particularly for the flexor tendon. The digital nerve and vessel should be carefully preserved when the flaps are elevated.

The zig-zag incision advocated by Bruner[3] (Fig. 7.1.1.) gives excellent exposure of the flexor surface of the finger. It requires more dissection and is not well suited for early postoperative motion. It is fine for tendon grafting. The angles should be carried well to each side to spare the volar flexion creases.

The extensor tendons on the dorsum of the hand are best approached through transverse incisions parallel with the folds of skin. The extensor mechanism in the finger is well visualized through a midlateral incision when the dorsal flap is elevated.

SUTURE MATERIALS

The ideal suture material should have little or no tissue reaction and remain at least three to four weeks while the slow processes of tendon repair take place.

Silk or stainless steel wire have many of the desired qualities. They have been popular for many years and are still two of the best. The pullout suture of Bunnell or the gig pullout suture (Fig. 7.1.3, *A* and *B*) have the added advantage of complete removal of the stitch after several weeks when it is no longer needed. If wire is used as a permanent buried stitch, it should be of very fine caliber. Nylon and some of the new plasticized nonabsorbable materials are quite suitable on the basis of their lack of tissue reaction. Some do not hold knots well. Chromic cat gut is not considered to have the desired qualities of a tendon suture.

METHODS OF UNITING TENDONS
Silk Suture Techniques

Since tendon is made up of many longitudinal fibers, simple sutures tend to pull out. For this reason, special sutures which have a lateral purchase on the tendon are important. Figure 7.1.2 shows some of the more common types of stitches used which have a good purchase on the tendon and are less apt to pull free.

So that less strain is put on the site of repair it is wise to relax the tendon in question by flexing or extending the involved joint, as the case may be, and holding it in position by means of a plaster splint for three to four weeks.

For most flexor and extensor tendons of the finger, 4-0 silk is suitable. For the larger wrist flexors, 3-0 or stronger is desirable.

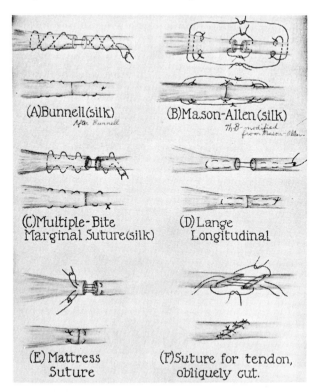

(A) Bunnell (silk)
After Bunnell

(B) Mason-Allen (silk)
Th.B. modified from Mason-Allen.

(C) Multiple-Bite Marginal Suture (silk)

(D) Lange Longitudinal

(E) Mattress Suture

(F) Suture for tendon, obliquely cut.

Figure 7.1.2. Types of silk for tendons. Simple stitches *(F)* tend to pull free. The other types shown have more secure purchase on the tendon.

Wire Suture Techniques

If wire is used for buried stitches, similar to silk, it should be quite fine, gauge 38 or 40. I prefer not to bury wire permanently but to use it as a pullout stitch after the method of Bunnell (Fig. 7.1.3, A and B). By this method, the suture is withdrawn at the end of three to four weeks when it has served its purpose.

For most finger flexors, gauge 34 stainless steel wire is suitable. This is threaded onto a small, flexible, striaght needle at either end, criss-crossed through the tendon once before being brought out through the proximal cut end of the tendon, and threaded through the distal cut end for a centimeter or so, then brought out through the skin and tied over a button as diagramed in Figure 7.1.3, A and B. The pullout strand, previously looped under the stitch, is then brought out with both free ends in a single needle so that a straight line of pull exists when the stitch is to be removed. For ensurance of free removal with the pullout wire, it is wise to use only one or two zig-zags in the stitch and to avoid all kinks, which weaken the wire and also prevent free removal.

In the suture at a distance technique (Fig. 7.1.3C), the pullout stitch is applied at some area proximal to the tendon laceration to prevent the pull of the muscle from separating the two cut ends of the tendon. The cut ends of the tendon are then accurately united with small stitches of 6-0 silk.

The gig pullout stitch (Fig. 7.1.3B) uses the same principle as the pullout suture just described. The wire stitch is threaded through two holes in a small piece of metal 6 mm thick. This "gig" prevents the suture from advancing through the tendon when tension is applied. This pullout stitch is more quickly applied and requires fewer perforations of the tendon. The double wire strands are again tied over a button to hold the proximal cut end of the tendon advanced against the distal cut end. The pullout strands looped through the proximal end of the gig are allowed to project from the skin until removal time at the end of three or four weeks. A this time, all wire along with the gig is removed.

Barb stitches are also available which work on the same principle as the gig pullout. Some of these are hard to pull out but otherwise work well.

Transfixation Techniques

Nicoladoni[16] first advocated the introduction of needles through the skin to hold tendons at rest during the process of repair. Linnartz[11] applied traction to a wire suture passed through an extensor tendon to relieve the tension on the area of tendon repair. Salomon[23] in 1924 reported the use of a straight needle through the skin and flexor tendon of the finger to hold it at rest. Montant[15] transfixed the flexor tendon with safety pins. Bove[1] transfixed it with straight pins incorporated in plaster of Paris. Iselin[9, 10] transfixed the flexor tendon with through and through wire sutures tied over buttons.

Transfixation during the process of healing of digital flexor tendons has been most highly developed in recent years by Verdan[25] (Fig. 7.1.4).

Uniting Tendons of Unequal Size and The Lateral Union of Tendons

Fig. 7.1.5. outlines the methods of joining tendons of unequal size (A and B). The objective is to avoid raw areas of cut tendon which are most prone to produce adhesions. Figure 7.1.5C depicts the method of joining adjacent tendons by weaving and mattress sutures of silk. Again raw areas are covered.

Uniting Tendon to Bone

This is most readily done by elevating the periosteum with an elevator, making a small drill hole through the bone and threading the two strands of a pullout wire through this hole and out through the soft tissues on the opposite side where the strands are tied over a button.

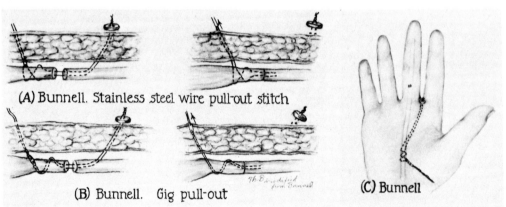

(A) Bunnell. Stainless steel wire pull-out stitch

(B) Bunnell.   Gig pull-out

(C) Bunnell

Figure 7.1.3. A. Bunnell pullout technique. *B.* Gig pullout technique. In both of these the suture is removed completely in three or four weeks. *C* is a method of removing muscle tension from the site of repair in the finger.

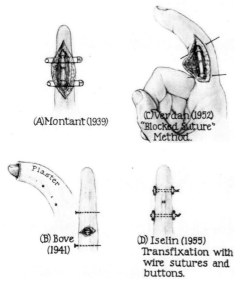

(A)Montant (1939)

(C)Verdan (1952) "Blocked Suture" Method.

(B) Bove (1941)

(D) Iselin (1955) Transfixation with wire sutures and buttons.

Figure 7.1.4. Transfixation techniques for primary repair of flexor tendons in the flexor tunnel area. Tension on the site of repair is prevented by the pins or wires traversing the tendons. Only fine sutures are utilized at the site of repair. Fixation is only moderately secure by these techniques. External splinting should also be employed.

If a short segment of tendon stump remains, the pullout strands can be threaded through this and out through the soft tissues without traversing the bone. This simple technique has been most satisfactory in the experience of the author. Care is taken to use a short distal stump so that the union is distal to the distal joint.

Wagner[26] splits the distal stump of the flexor profundus tendon longitudinally and draws the proximal segment into the cleft thus produced. When a wedge shaped portion of the distal stump is removed from the cut end, the union is less bulky fig. 7.1.6.

REPAIR IN THE DIGITAL FLEXOR TUNNEL

The digital flexor tunnel area of the fingers (Fig. 7.1.7, *Zone II*) where the sublimis and profundus tendons glide, one on the other in close quarters, offers the greatest challenge in tendon repair. It has been named "No Man's Land" by Bunnell, "critical area" (Boyes[2]) and described as "the death bed of many a stout profundus" (McCash[14]).

The following are some generalizations regarding tendon repair in this area.

1. It should be performed only by, or under the direct supervision of, a surgeon experienced in dealing with the problem.

2. Primary repair should be limited to the most favorable cases.

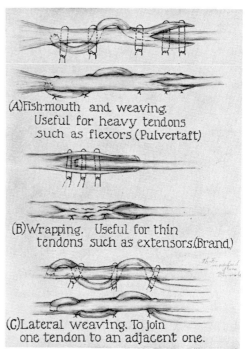

(A)Fishmouth and weaving. Useful for heavy tendons such as flexors (Pulvertaft)

(B)Wrapping. Useful for thin tendons such as extensors.(Brand)

(C)Lateral weaving. To join one tendon to an adjacent one.

Figure 7.1.5. The union of tendons of unequal size and of an adjacent tendon. These techniques should be utilized only when sufficient space allows free movement of the rather bulky union.

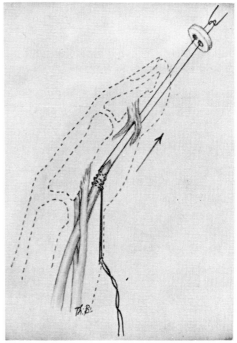

Figure 7.1.6. Method of advancement of the profundus tendon .Wagner). The distal stump is split and the proximal end pulled into it.

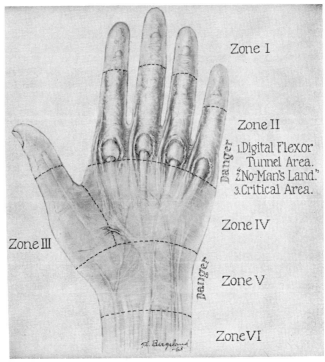

Figure 7.1.7. Zones of the hand in which results of flexor tendon repair are variable. Poorest results are in *Zone II* ("No Man's Land," critical area).

3. Debridement, wound irrigation, and primary wound closure followed by tendon grafting three to four weeks later is advocated by some as the safest procedure after primary healing has occurred, but this is controversial.

4. When both tendons are severed in this area, only the profundus is restored.

5. An intact sublimis tendon should not be sacrificed.

6. Restoration of profundus function by tendon graft is justifiable when only the profundus is divided, in some circumstances.

7. The tendon tunnel should be partially removed leaving pulleys at the proximal and middle phalangeal levels.

8. When primary repair is undertaken, special technique is necessary in view of many poor results in this area.

TENSION FOR SUTURING TENDONS

It is important to restore tension to as near normal as possible so that the excursion of muscle contracture will be adequate to produce a full range of motion in the joint served. In performing an acute tendon repair, one can judge usually by the tension of an adjacent tendon. However, one can best judge the proper tension by bringing joints served by the tendon to the normal position of rest for that digit.

In performing a delayed repair the situation is more

difficult, particularly when the proximal end of the tendon has been allowed to remain retracted over a period of time, for, in this case, the muscle will have shortened to some extent. But even here, in the experience of the author, it is best to restore the normal position of rest to the fingers.

REPAIR BY ADVANCEMENT

Sponsel[24] has advocated advancement of the flexor profundus tendon to its insertion for any laceration less than 2 cm from its distal extremity. Holm and Embick[7] recommend advancement to 1.5 cm. Wagner[26] advocates late repair by advancement. McCash[14] states that advancement works well in patients up to middle age.

In my experience, advancements up to 1.5 cm for the profundus flexor of the adult finger will be adequately compensated for. Greater advancements are not recommended.

MAKING PULLEYS

As the digits are flexed by the long flexor tendons, the latter are normally held close to the phalanges and prevented from bowing volarward by strong fibrous tunnels or pulleys at the level of the proximal and the middle phalanges. Bunnell advised repair of the annular ligament or pulley by a removable stainless steel wire tied over to bolster (Fig. 7.1.8 A).

When the tendon tunnels are destroyed, or lost for any reason, their pulley effect should be restored by encircling tendon grafts as shown in Figure 7.1.8B or C. These grafts, made preferably of flat tendon, may pass superficially to the extensor tendon as they encircle the phalanx. These are best restored at the time of tendon repair or tendon graft so that they are healed at the time flexor tendon motion is begun. Posch[19] (Fig. 7.1.8C) places the graft through a transverse drill hole through the phalanx and about the flexor tendon. Either of these two methods works satisfactorily.

EXTENSOR TENDON REPAIR

Exposure of lacerated extensor tendons can usually be made through transverse skin incisions due to their more superficial location and the fact that they retract less than flexor tendons. In the finger, vertical extensions at either end of the transverse incision, bayonet fashion, aid the exposure.

Acute boutonniere deformity from laceration of the central slip of the extensor hood should be repaired primarily with nonreactive mattress sutures when the case is clean and seen early. With this injury be sure the lateral bands of the hood are restored back to their normal position since they frequently slip volarward. Mattress sutures are also excellent for extensor tendons over the back of the hand. The same sutures employed for flexor tendons are best for the large wrist extensors and the extensors of the thumb and fingers in the forearm.

The extensor tendons, with the exception of the distal insertion as noted above, should be splinted in a relaxed position for four weeks after repair to relieve tension and prevent separation.

POSTOPERATIVE TREATMENT

Systemically the patient should be on a well balanced diet, have adequate fluids, electrolytes, vitamins, and rest. The hemoglobin should be within

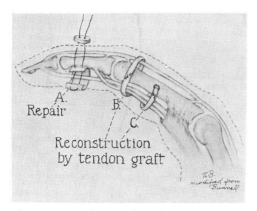

Figure 7.1.8. Repair of tendon pulley (A) and methods of replacement (B and C). These pulleys prevent bowing of the tendons on flexion of the digit.

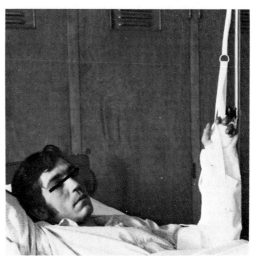

Figure 7.1.9. Method of postoperative elevation to diminish swelling of the hand.

normal limits. Special care should be taken to prevent infection and this should include prophylactic antibiotics since infection is so destructive to the delicate gliding surfaces of the tendon required for a successful result. Special immunizations for tetanus and gas gangrene should be considered and used if contamination has been severe.

Local treatment should include aseptic wound care with loose gauze dressings covered by a lightly applied elastic bandage. The dressing should be applied to allow evaporation and the wound should be kept dry. The arm should be elevated in the early postoperative period to further diminish edema (Fig. 7.1.9).

Plaster splint immobilization with the repaired tendon in relaxed position should be employed for approximately three weeks for flexor tendons and four to five weeks for extensor tendons.

On removal of the splint at the end of three to four weeks, active motions are started and usually one week later hot soaks in soapy water are begun for one-half hour three times a day. Active exercises are done during the soaks with the patient squeezing a sponge.

Passive assistive motions are begun in a graded manner the fifth or sixth week after repair.

A trained physical therapist is most valuable during this phase of treatment. The surgeon should see the patient at frequent intervals to follow the progress, give added encouragement and direct necessary changes in treatment, to determine the date for return to work, and to estimate the percentage of disability due to injury.

REFERENCES

1. Bove, C. Suturing of flexor tendons of the hand (Transfixation). Med. Rec. Ann., *153:* 94, 1941.

2. Boyes, J. H. Flexor-tendon grafts in the fingers and thumb. An evaluation of end results. J. Bone Joint Surg., *32A:* 489-499, 531, 1950.

3. Bruner, J. M. The zig-zag volar digital incision for flexor-tendon surgery. Plast. Reconstr. Surg., *40:* 571-574, 1967.

4. Bsteh, O. Sehnentransfixation (Sehnendurchspiessung) eine Operationsmethode bei Sehnendurchtrennung. Chirurg, *26:* 460-461, 1955.

5. Bunnell, S. *Surgery of the Hand,* Ed. 3. Philadelphia, Lippincott, 1956.

6. Fowler, S. B. A Discussion of Eyler, D. L.: The anatomy and function of the intrinsic musculature of the fingers. J. Bone Joint Surg., *36A:* 18, 1954.

7. Holm, C. L., and Embick, R. P.: Anatomical considerations in the primary treatment of tendon injuries of the hand. J. Bone Joint Surg., *41 A:* 599-608, 1959.

8. Howard, L. D., Jr. Personal communication.

9. Iselin, M. *Chirurgie de la Main,* Ed. 2. Paris, Masson, 1955, p. 248.

10. Iselin, M., *et al. Atlas de Technique en Chirurgie de la Main,* Vol. 1. Paris, Flammarion, 1958, p. 57.

11. Linnartz, M. Wie lasst sich die Spannung der Sehnenstupfe bei der Naht Alter Sehnenverletzunger Ausschalten? Zentralbl. Chir., *48:* 225-226, 1921.

12. Littler, J. W. Free tendon grafts in secondary flexor tendon repair. Am. J. Surg., *74:* 315-321, 1947.

13. Littler, J. W. The severed flexor tendon. Surg. Clin. North Am., *39:* 435-447, 1959.

14. McCash, C. R. The immediate repair of flexor tendons. Brit. J. Plast. Surg., *14:* 53-58, 1961.

15. Montant. R. Technique rèparatrice personnelle de la section des tendons fléchisseurs des doigts. J. Chir., *53:* 768-774, 1939.

16. Nicoladoni, C. Ein Vorschag zur Sehnennaht (Flexor tendon suture of the hand). Wien med. Wochenschr., *30:* 1413-1417, 1880.

17. Paletta, F. X. Circulatory studies in tourniquet ischemia. To be published. Read at Eighteenth Annual Meeting of American Society for Surgery of the Hand. Miami Beach, Fla., Jan. 18, 1963.

18. Peacock, E. E., Jr., and Hartrampf, C. R. The repair of flexor tendons in the hand. Int. Abstr. Surg., *113:* 411-432, 1961.

19. Posch, J. L. Primary tenorrhaphies and tendon grafting procedures in hand injuries. Arch. Surg., *73:* 609-624, 1956.

20. Pratt, D. R. Internal splint for closed and open treatment of injuries of the extensor tendon at the distal joint of the finger. J. Bone Joint Surg., *34 A:* 785-788, 1952.

21. Pratt, D. R., Bunnell, S., and Howard, L. D., Jr. Mallet finger. Classification and methods of treatment. Am. J. Surg., *93:* 573-579, 1957.

22. Rozov, V. I., and Lunber, A. A. Actual problems in the primary suture of the flexor tendon of the finger. Vestn. khir., *80:* 3-11, 1958.

23. Salomon, A. Klinische und experimentelle Untersuchungen über Heiling von Sehnenverletzungen insbesondere innerhalb der Sehnenschieden. Arch. klin. Chir., *129:* 397-430, 1924.

24. Sponsel, K. H. Urgent surgery for finger flexor tendon and nerve lacerations with emphasis on advancement of the divided profundus tendon distal to the level of laceration. J.A.M.A., *166:* 1567-1572, 1958.

25. Verdan, C. E. Primary repair of flexor tendons. J. Bone Joint Surg., *42 A:* 647-657, 1960.

26. Wagner, C. Delayed advancement in the repair of lacerated flexor profundus tendons. J. Bone Joint Surg., *40 A:* 1241-1244, 1958.

B.

Healing with Tendon Sutures and Tendon Transplants

Austin D. Potenza, M.D.

One of the most vexing problems confronting hand surgeons is that of severance of the flexor tendons within the fingers. The results of the surgical repair of these tendons are often uncertain and unpredictable.

A comprehensive study of flexor tendon healing was begun in May of 1959. The literature revealed no unanimity of opinion regarding the processes by which digital flexor tendons healed. Early studies were of academic interest since what little tendon surgery was performed[42] was limited to subcutaneous tenotomy[1] rather than to repair of injured tendons.

Although new experimental studies have been reported,[15,29,35,54] controversy as to the exact nature of tendon healing persists. Some[17,29,53,55] hold that tendon heals by reparative cellular growth derived directly from cut tendon ends. Others[1,21,38,54] believe tendon is repaired by the peritendinous tissues. Mason and Shearon,[35] Mason and Allen,[34] and later, Flynn and Graham,[15] believe that both processes are important.

There is no agreement regarding the fate of autogenous tendon grafts. Some investigators[15,54] believe that such grafts undergo degeneration and replacement, while others[16,28,35] believe that free tendon grafts can survive in their new locations. The fate of the collagen of autogenous tendon grafts is unresolved. In the search for better grafts and grafting techniques, investigators have used fresh[13,27,51] and preserved homografts,[11,24,37] heterografts,[14] and composite homologous grafts.[41]

Good functional results are most difficult to achieve after repair of injuried flexor tendons within the fingers,[7] where the tendons are enclosed in synovial sheaths and are held close to the underlying bone of the digit by inelastic annular ligaments. With rare exceptions[23,29] previous investigators of tendon healing and tendon grafting have used carpal flexor[31] or extensor tendons[34] of dogs and Achilles tendon in rabbits.[1,52,54] These tendons do not present the anatomic peculiarities of the flexor tendons within the fingers, nor in clinical practice do they present the severe problems of scarring and the subsequent poor functional results often seen after flexor tendon repair or grafting. It was essential that tendon healing and tendon grafts be studied within the biologic context of a synovium-lined digital flexor mechanism comparable to that of the human finger.

The flexor tendon mechanism in the canine forefoot is comparable to that in the human hand,[49] and was therefore selected as an experimental model.

FLEXOR DIGITORUM PROFUNDUS TENDON HEALING WITHIN THE FLEXOR DIGITAL SHEATH

This series of experiments[49] was designed to define the mechanisms of healing of flexor profundus tendons within the flexor sheath under as near atraumatic conditions as possible. The methods and techniques described in this part provided the common denominator for each of the experiments described later. They formed the basis for a standard wound which was consistently employed under rigidly controlled circumstances in order to achieve maximum control of surgical variables.

Adult mongrel dogs were appropriately anesthetized and one paw and foreleg of each dog was surgically prepared, draped into a sterile operative field, and operated upon aseptically under tourniquet control. The operated digits were opened by midlateral incisions. All tendons were handled atraumatically; no forceps or any device was ever used to hold them. The details of the technique have been described.[49] The vincula of the profundus tendons were left undis-

turbed. Divided profundus tendons were repaired with stainless steel pullout sutures. The sheath and skin were also closed with stainless steel. All operated parts were immobilized in reinforced padded plaster casts until sacrifice.

Seventy canine profundus tendons were studied, leaving the sublimis tendons undisturbed. The profundus tendons were divided and repaired and studied from one through 128 days postoperatively.

After profundus tendon division and repair, the repaired synovial layer of the sheath in the vicinity of the wound disrupts as its cells proliferate and gives rise to granulation tissue which grows between the ends of the severed tendon (Fig. 7.2.1) and into the suture tracts in the tendon. At one week, fine, new collagen fibers appear in this granulation tissue and by the 10th day the granulation tissue has a pronounced fibroblastic character. The fibroblasts that grow into the wound between the tendon stumps are oriented in a plain perpendicular to the long axis of the tendon and the collagen fibers which they deposit are similarly oriented. In contrast, the collagen fibers laid down by the fibroblasts in the granulation tissue on the surface of the repaired tendon are oriented parallel to that surface. By the 21st day, the fibroblasts in the early scar between the tendon ends begin to orient themselves in line with the longitudinal axis of the tendons; by the 28th postoperative day this process is complete so that all the fibroblasts and the new collagen fibers are aligned in the long axis of the tendon. The newly deposited collagen fibers in the tendon scar remain separate though parallel fibers until the 90th postoperative day, when early collagen bundle formation is seen; this pro-

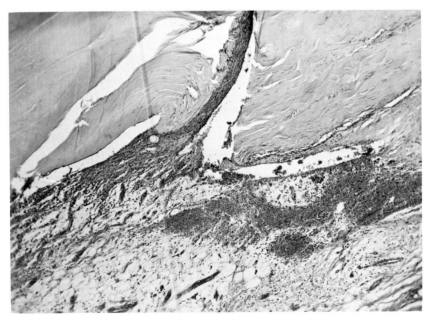

Figure 7.2.1. Longitudinal section of tendon and sheath at 9 days showing growth of fibroblasts from the sheath between the tendon stumps (hematoxylin and eosin, × 21).

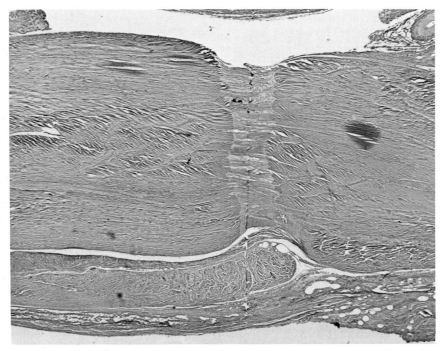

Figure 7.2.2. Longitudinal section of a tendon at 42 days showing advanced maturation of the wound with remaining filmy adhesions at the wound site (hematoxylin and eosin, × 8).

gresses so that, by 112 days, the collagen in the former scar between the tendon ends is in the form of bundles microscopically identical with those of the original tendon.

Paralleling the process of collagen maturation, the synovial layer of the flexor sheath is gradually restored, reaching completion at 21 days except for persistent filmy vascular adhesions at the line of tendon repair. Although there is ultimately complete maturation of the collagen in the tissue between the tendon ends (the tendon wound), the collagen in the persisting filmy adhesions attached to the line of tendon repair remains sparse, delicate, and loose and does not interfere with function (Fig. 7.2.2). At no point in the processes described was there any evidence of proliferation of tenocytes in either tendon stump. There was no migration of tenocytes from one stump to the other across the line of division, nor was there any collagen production by the tenocytes. Thus, flexor tendons are completely passive in regard to the processes of their own healing. The sheath tissues appear to be the sole active healing agents.

CRITICAL EVALUATION OF FLEXOR TENDON HEALING AND ADHESION FORMATION WITHIN ARTIFICIAL DIGITAL SHEATHS

Surgeons have attempted to prevent adhesions to healing flexor tendons by interposing some material between the repaired tendon and the surrounding tis-

sues in order theoretically to block the formation of restrictive adhesions. The materials used have included nylon,[9] cellophane,[12] [56] Teflon,[19] polyethylene,[18] Millipore,[4] [5] Ivalon,[22] Silastic,[36] stainless steel,[54] vil-tallium,[36] and certain naturally occurring anatomical structures.[2] [6] [12] These materials have not gained acceptance in surgical practice and their proponents often cease using them with no further comment. The results described in the first part of this section are inconsistent with the "blocking membrane" concept of tendon-adhesion prevention and conflict with reports in the literature of successful use of blocking membranes and tubes about healing flexor tendons. If such devices truly block adhesion formation and yet allow tendon healing to occur, the conclusion enunciated in the first part of this section, that the digital flexor tendons are passive in their own healing processes would be incorrect, for these tendons would have to effect their own union if all adhesions from surrounding tissues were truly "blocked out."

In new experiments,[43] the sublimis tendons were removed from the digits in order to provide room for various blocking materials. Profundus tendons were atraumatically divided and repaired and the digital sheaths and skin were closed. Fifteen profundus tendons were enclosed in ¾ inch long animal tested polyethylene tubes centered over the lines of repair and were studied from six to 56 days postoperatively. Gross and microscopic examination showed that the polyethylene proved an effective barrier between tendon and surrounding tissues, since no tissue was observed to grow through the plastic. However, longitudinal sections of all specimens demonstrated that granulation tissue formed by the healing synovial sheath grew beneath the edges of the tubing at both ends along the surface of the tendon within the tube, finally to reach tendon wounds. Only then was granulation tissue seen between the tendon ends; at no stage was there any intrinsic proliferative activity observed in the tendon ends. The entire potential for tendon union resided in the sheath-derived granulation tissue which grew beneath the tubing; there was no evidence of tendon healing until this tissue reached sites of tendon anastomosis. Healing was delayed by the time necessary for the sheath granulation tissue to grow along the surface of the tendon beneath the tubing to the lines of repair. There were two sets of thick adhesions at either end of the tubes since these adhesions provided the cellular and vascular support for the healing reaction within the tubes.

In another group, 15 profundus tendons divided and repaired within the flexor sheath and blocked from surrounding tissues by intact Millipore tubes, the exact same mechanism of tendon healing was observed. The healing granulation tissue from the sheath grew beneath the edges of the tubing (Fig. 7.2.3), along the surface of the tendon finally to reach tendon repair sites (Fig. 7.2.4). There were no adhesions between the healed tendons within the tubes and the surrounding tissues, but, instead, there were two sets of very thick tethering adhesions at either end of the tubes.

Thus, tubes or membranes placed about sites of flexor tendon repair required the healing cellular and vascular elements of the flexor digital sheath to grow beneath the tubing to reach wound sites. In every case, gross and histologic observations revealed two sets of thick adhesions at tube ends rather than the mild, filmy adhesions normally expected at wound sites when no tubing was used as in the first part of this section. Such devices either delay or prevent tendon healing and result in thicker, more restrictive adhesions than occur if they are not used.

EFFECT OF ASSOCIATED TRAUMA ON HEALING OF DIVIDED TENDONS

Thirty profundus tendons were atraumatically divided and repaired within the flexor sheath, and subjected to discrete controlled trauma of two types:[44] one group received multiple needle wounds while another group received a crush injury.

Tendons healed by the same processes observed earlier. However, adhesions formed between the repaired tendons and the surrounding tissues at each point at which the physical integrity of tendon surfaces had been disturbed by trauma, both puncture and crush. Following crush, there was an intense cellular response and the resultant adhesions were dense and thick in proportion to the area of tendon surface disturbed. Adhesions to punctured tendons formed in relation to the discrete puncture wounds.

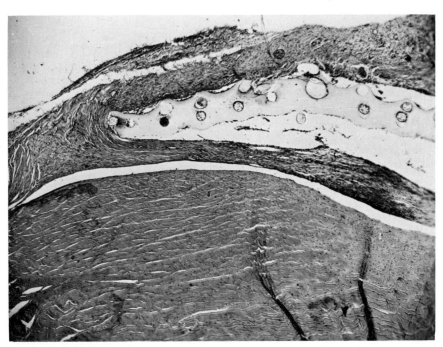

Figure 7.2.3. Longitudinal section of repaired profundus tendon within Millipore tube 14 days after surgery shows healing granulation tissue from the digital sheath growing beneath the edge of the tubing along the tendon surface (hematoxylin and eosin, × 44).

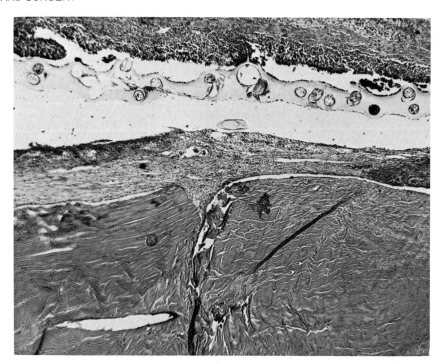

Figure 7.2.4. Longitudinal section of tendon within Millipore tube 14 days after repair shows that the healing granulation tissue from the sheath has grown beneath the tubing and has finally just reached the site of repair. Healing between the stumps is just about to begin (hematoxylin and eosin, × 44).

It was seen that adhesions occurred at each point at which the physical integrity of tendon surfaces was disturbed and were quantitatively proportional to the number of puncture wounds inflicted or the extent of crush injury.

THE RELATIONSHIP BETWEEN SURGERY ON CONTIGUOUS ANATOMIC STRUCTURES AND THE FORMATION OF ADHESIONS TO HEALING DIGITAL FLEXOR TENDONS

Here[46] I evaluated what role surgery on other structures within the flexor digital sheath might have on the healing of repaired flexor profundus tendons. At the time, it was common surgical practice to excise the sublimis tendon and flexor sheath at the time of primary flexor tendon repair or free flexor tendon grafting. It had been noted in the second part of this section, that total sublimis tendon excision resulted in a more intense cellular reaction and greater adhesions to repaired profundus tendons than in the series of experiments in which sublimis tendons were preserved. It was therefore essential to evaluate sublimis tendon excision and flexor sheath excision.

Thirty profundus tendons divided into two groups of 15 each were studied after atraumatic division and repair. In one group, the flexor sheaths were excised, while in the second or controlled group the sheaths

were closed. In both groups, the sublimis tendons and annular ligaments were left intact. Animals were sacrificed in from three to 56 days.

In the control group, as in the first part of this section, union was effected by local cellular activity of the sheath at the wound site. There was no intrinsic tendon tenoblastic response.

In the experimental group in which the digital sheaths had been excised, an intense inflammatory reaction, derived from the subcutaneous tissue, surrounded the repaired profundus tendons. Fibrin deposited by the subcutaneous tissue about the tendons formed a pseudosheath. The fibroblasts and capillary buds from the extensive granulation tissue engulfing the tendons invaded the tendon wounds, deposited new collagen between the severed segments, and ultimately effected tendon union. Concomitantly, fibroblasts also arranged themselves parallel to tendon surfaces, forming a fibroblastic layer over the precipitated layer of fibrin so that the tendons were soon surrounded by a new gliding sheath mechanism consisting of a fibroblastic layer in place of the synovial layer which had been excised. This fibroblastic layer ultimately took on the histologic appearance of synovium, so that a new smooth synoviallike sheath eventually surrounded each repaired tendon. As in the control group, adhesions to tendon surfaces became loose and gradually resolved, remaining attached to the tendons only at the immediate lines of union and at suture tracked sites.

Another experiment evaluated the role of sublimis tendon excision in the healing of profundus tendons. Sublimis tendon vincula are highly vascular structures, broadly based upon the underlying osseous floor of the osseofibrous digital canal. The two vincula, one for each sublimis tendon slip, arise from approximately one-half the total area of the volar aspect of the proximal phalanx of the digit; they represent a tissue continuum with the periosteum of the phalanx. Total sublimis excision, including the two slips of insertion of the tendon, effectively excises and destroys the integrity of the periosteal floor of the digital tunnel in the region of the proximal phalanx as well as at the insertion of the sublimis tendon slips into the base of the middle phalanx. It seemed that this disturbance of the vascular, cellular periosteal floor of the digital canal might be responsible for some of the adhesions formed to repaired profundus tendons after sublimis excision.

Forty canine digits, divided into two groups of 20 each, were studied after atraumatic division and repair of each profundus tendon. All sublimis tendons were removed by one of two techniques: in one group, the tendons were completely excised down through their slips of insertion into the bases of the middle phalanges; this included sharp division of their broadly based vincula over the proximal phalanx, the volar plate of the proximal interphalangeal joint, and the base of the middle phalanx. In the second group, sublimis tendons were excised by transverse division immediately proximal to their vincula, preserving

their vincula and slips of insertion over the distal half of the proximal phalanx, the proximal interphalangeal joint and the base of the middle phalanx; the highly vascular vincula were not disturbed and the integrity of the periosteal floor of the digital tunnel was not violated. Animals were sacrificed at intervals from three to 36 days.

The processes of profundus tendon healing remained the same. There was one important difference between the two groups of repaired tendons.

In the second group, in which the sublimis tendons had been excised by sharp division proximal to their vincula, the healing granulation tissue arose only from the repaired digital sheaths; the periosteal floor of the digital canal, having been preserved, remained intact, and did not give rise to granulation tissue. No adhesions formed between the healing tendons and the osseous floor of the digital canal in this group (Fig. 7.2.5). No adhesions arose from the cut ends of the sublimis tendons.

In the first group with total sublimis excision, not only did the digital sheath give rise to a healing granulation tissue, but in addition there was a profound and florid cellular and vascular reaction from the disturbed periosteal floor of the flexor tunnel; this proliferative periosteal cellular reaction contributed to the healing of the profundus tendons as did, of course, the cellular response of the digital sheaths. Since total excision of the sublimis tendon with its vincula involved the vascular-osseous bed of the digital tunnel over the distal half of the proximal phalanx and the base of the middle phalanx, the granulation tissue arising from

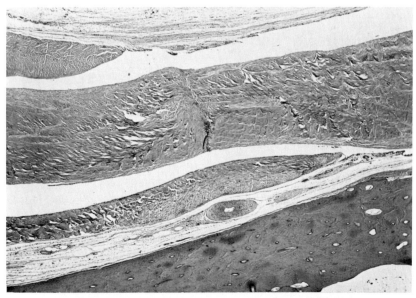

Figure 7.2.5. Longitudinal section of repaired profundus tendon 28 days after excision of sublimis immediately proximal to its vincula. Note intact periosteal floor of the digital tunnel and complete absence of adhesions between floor and repaired profundus (hematoxylin and eosin, × 19).

this bed produced broadly based adhesions to the profundus wounds; these broad adhesions ultimately anchored the healed tendons to the underlying bone (Fig. 7.2.6).

The gross results were striking. Subtotal sublimis tendon excision by transverse division immediately proximal to the vincula resulted in only a few filmy, loose adhesions between the healing tendon and the digital sheath at wound sites and at suture tract sites (Fig. 7.2.7). Total excision of the sublimis tendon resulted in dense restrictive adhesions to the osseous floor of the digital canal (Fig. 7.2.8).

Thus the formation of adhesions to healing profundus tendons within the digits is not an inexplicable vagary of surgery. Adhesions occur at each point of trauma to tendon surfaces; so-called "atraumatic" instrument techniques result in adhesions at each point of instrument trauma to tendon surfaces. Since the flexor tendons do not manifest an intrinsic tenoblastic response when severed, they are dependent upon a vascular and cellular response from surrounding tissues for their healing. This healing granulation tissue must of necessity, therefore, form discrete adhesions to the healing tendon at wound sites and at points of tendon trauma. Trauma to tendon surfaces is a major factor in the quantity and quality of adhesions that form following surgery. The anatomic integrity of the digital tunnel is also an essential factor in adhesion formation. This is, as it were, the other side of the coin in the problem of adhesions following flexor tendon surgery. Excision of the flexor sheath after primary repair of the profundus tendon with preservation of the sublimis tendon has no adverse effect on tendon healing or the ultimate functional results, since a new glid-ing sheath mechanism forms. However, if the integrity of the osseous floor of the digital canal is violated, as in total sublimis tendon excision, a profound inflammatory response occurs which produces tendon adhesions that are broadly based upon the rigid, ungliding osseous phalanx of the digit; tendon healing is accompanied by the formation of dense, restrictive adhesions that assure an unacceptable functional result. Significantly, however, if the sublimis tendon is excised by transverse division immediately proximal to its vinculum, the integrity of the periosteal floor of the digital canal is preserved, and the healing profundus tendon remains free of any adhesions to it.

THE HEALING OF AUTOGENOUS TENDON GRAFTS WITHIN THE FLEXOR DIGITAL SHEATH

These experiments[50] were designed to determine the fate of autogenous tendon grafts within the digits. This was not the first study devoted to this problem;[15, 28] however, the experimental design incorporated features which eliminated several previously uncontrolled and ill-defined variables; it involved the study of flexor profundus tendon grafts within a synovium-line flexor digital sheath rather than in areas where tendons simply lie surrounded by loose adventitial tissue or paratenon. It preserved the anatomically specific biologic field of the profundus tendon in as unaltered a state as is possible. The study of tendon grafts in digits from which the synovial digital sheaths, the annular ligaments, and the sublimis tendons have been excised does not define normal healing processes for free flexor tendon grafts; the anatomic field has been so ir-

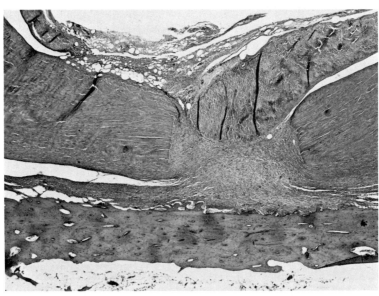

Figure 7.2.6. Longitudinal section of repaired profundus tendon 48 days after total sublimis excision. Note extensive broadly based adhesions between healing profundus and bony floor of flexor tunnel; note profund periosteal new-bone formation at base of adhesions (hematoxylin and eosin, × 19).

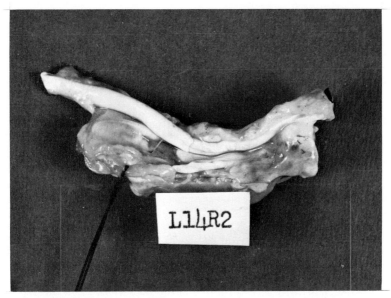

Figure 7.2.7. Gross photograph of repaired profundus tendon 28 days after subtotal sublimis excision. Note only few filmy adhesions at immediate wound site and suture-tract sites, no adhesions between profundus tendon and bony floor of digital canal or divided tendons.

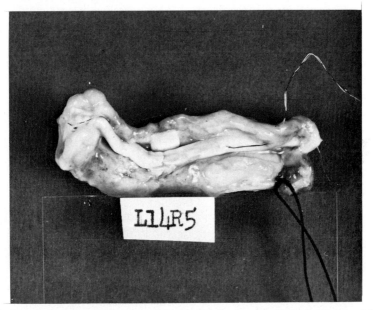

Figure 7.2.8. Gross photograph of repaired profundus tendon 28 days after total sublimis excision. Note dense restrictive adhesions between line of repair and disturbed bony floor of digital tunnel.

reparably altered as to render any allusion to a normal digit untenable.

Special (Wilder's and Rinehart's) stains used, in addition to the usual hematoxylin and eosin stain, were helpful in determining the source and status of collagen in the wounds.

Fifty-four free autogenous profundus tendon grafts were studied. A special atraumatic surgical technique[50] permitted each profundus tendon to be completely divided distally as well as proximally removed from its bed, free of all former tissue connections, and then returned to its original anatomic position within the flexor digital sheath, coursing normally through the sublimis tendon and the annular ligaments, while preserving the flexor sheath. Tendon graft surfaces were distrubed only at needle tract sites.

The digital sheath over the proximal and middle phalanges remained intact, as did the sublimis tendon and annular ligaments. "No Man's Land" was preserved as anatomically intact as possible.

Animals were sacrificed at intervals from seven to 160 days. The proximal and distal tendon graft wounds healed exclusively by the proliferative cellular activity of the surrounding tissues, namely, the paratenon in the palm and the synovial layer of the sheath distally. Adhesions formed at tendon wound sites and at points where the integrity of tendon surfaces had been broken by suture tracts or by undue suture pressure on the surface of the tendon. The tenocytes in the proximal and distal tendon stumps remained viable histologically with no evidence of karyolysis or karyorrhexis. The tenocytes of the graft appeared histologically identical with those of the adjacent tendon stumps in each wound; the collagen in both areas also had the same appearance both in H and E sections and in sections stained with special stains for collagen. There was no evidence that any graft was "dead." There was no proliferative activity in the proximal or distal tendon stumps nor in the tenocytes of the grafts. Maturation of the wounds progressed in orderly fashion paralleling the processes described for simple wounds of profundus tendons as described in the first part of this section. Adhesions gradually matured and became filmy. By 160 days, the collagen in both the proximal and distal wounds was arranged in bundles typical that of normal tendon. No intrinsic tenoblastic activity was observed in either the proximal or distal tendon stumps or in the tendon grafts. Healing was effected solely by the cellular activity of the granulation tissue derived from the tendon-investing connective tissue of paratenon in the palm and by the digital sheath at the distal anastomosis sites.

Since the sublimis tendons, annular ligaments, and digital sheaths were preserved anatomically intact, these experiments allowed evaluation of the free profundus tendon grafts in an essentially unaltered and trauma-free environment. Moreover, it was possible to compare the free grafts with the readily available sublimis tendons as normal controls at each point in the study. Any changes in the cells or collagen of a graft could be compared with those of the intact sublimis tendon within the same digital flexor sheath.

No adhesions formed between the tendon grafts and the sublimis tendons, annular ligaments or digital sheath in "No Man's Land." The grafts remained free of adhesions within the sheath. There was no change in the cellular structure or collagen of the grafts. The cells maintained all histologic evidence of viability and the collagen maintained its integrity with no evidence of swelling, degeneration, or replacement (Fig. 7.2.9). Adhesions which formed to the tendon graft wounds proximally and distally became loose and filmy. At both sites, the synovial sheath effected

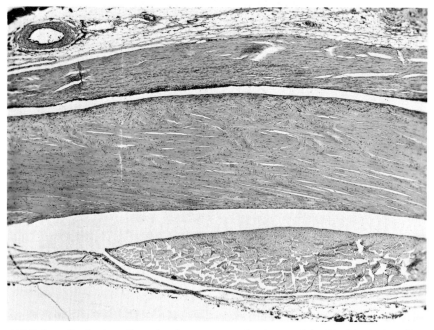

Figure 7.2.9. Longitudinal section of autogenous profundus graft in "No Man's Land" at 28 days showing normal cellular and collagenous structure of the graft when compared with the normal sublimis tendon above. Note complete absence of any adhesions between the graft, the sublimis tendon, the annular ligament, and the flexor sheath. Note absence of swelling, degeneration or replacement of the graft (hematoxylin and eosin, × 22.3).

tendon repair and restored the integrity of the flexor digital sheath.

The granulation tissue produced by the tendon-investing connective tissue in the palm also invaded those points at which tendon or tendon-graft surfaces had been broken by sutures; this increased tendon cellularity and vascularity focally; this always occurred in proximity to suture tracts. These adhesions resolved, being marked only by extremely loose adhesions at suture tract sites and by areas of increased cellularity in tendons in relation to suture tracts. *All* areas of increased tendon cellularity were directly related to suture tracts, and were not the result of intrinsic tenoblastic activity. In other areas where pressure had been exerted on tendon surfaces by the knots of buried stainless steel pullout sutures, focal tendon degeneration occurred. These areas were also invaded and recellularized by the fibroblasts from the paratenon, producing new collagen fibers in the area of tendon trauma and ultimately restoring tendon anatomy. As in all other instances adhesions to these areas resolved and became loose and filmy.

The free tendon grafts studied remained viable by all histologic criteria: the tendon cells retained their normal staining and cytologic characteristics throughout the study when compared to normal, viable, undisturbed sublimis tendons within the same sheath. There was *no* evidence of a general pattern of collagen swelling, degeneration and/or replacement of the grafts (Fig. 7.2.9); when damage to tendon caused by undue focal pressure was present, focally specific tendon degeneration occurred which was then repaired by the growth of fibroblasts from the surrounding granulation tissue into the traumatized area. The grafts did not act as tissue struts for gradual replacement by other tissue cells (Fig. 7.2.9). No adhesions occurred in "No Man's Land" between the grafts and sublimis tendons, annular ligaments or digital sheaths.

COMPARATIVE STUDY OF THE HEALING AND FATE OF PARATENON-COVERED AND NONPARATENON-COVERED TENDON GRAFTS

Sixty autogenous canine tendon grafts were studied.[47] Thirty were flexor digitorum profundus tendons, and 30 were paratenon-covered flexor carpi ulnaris tendons. In each dog, one digit received a free profundus autogenous graft while another digit in the same paw received an autogenous flexor carpi ulnaris tendon graft. Each paw represented a paired control experiment. Grafts were studied from three to 77 days. The mechanisms of healing and the rate of progress of healing were the same in the two groups of tendon grafts; these processes were identical to those described in the fifth part of this section for the healing of free autogenous profundus tendon grafts. In brief, at the proximal and distal anastomosis sites, the tendon-graft wounds were healed by the cellular activity of surrounding tissues — the digital sheath at the distal wound and the advential tissue of the palm at the proximal wound. The paratenon of the flexor carpi ulnaris grafts took part in this reaction in that it became involved in the diffuse adhesions produced by the proliferating surrounding tissue preparatory to tendon wound healing. It was not essential to the healing processes, since the profundus tendons healed at the same rate and by the same mechanisms in its absence.

As in the fifth part of this section, the tendon grafts in this series of experiments remained viable and normal by all histologic criteria upon detailed study of their cells and collagen with no evidence of graft necrosis. Adhesions to the grafts occurred as described in the fifth part; there were no adhesions to the autogenous profundus tendon grafts in "No Man's Land." The situation was quite the reverse with the autogenous flexor carpi ulnaris paratenon-covered grafts.

The flexor carpi ulnaris autografts were involved in diffuse adhesions to surrounding structures throughout their length in the palm and in the flexor digital sheath. Their surfaces were irregular with many loose tags of paratenon. The irregular and diffuse adhesions had several sources of origin; in many areas it appeared that the paratenon covering the grafts was proliferating and attaching itself to surrounding tissues, particularly the synovial layer of the sheath. In other areas the surrounding tissues in contact with the paratenon of the grafts were apparently stimulated to proliferate and form adhesions to the paratenon. This phenomenon was observed throughout the length of the synovium-lined digital sheath and was particularly noticeable in the region of the annular ligaments and the vincula breve of the untraumatized sublimis tendons. In addition to these findings, it appeared that the granulation tissue produced by the advential tissues of the palm grew along the paratenon of the flexor carpi ulnaris grafts well out into the digital sheaths; the paratenon seemed to provide a fertile and, in some way, attractive biologic bed for this proliferative tissue so that it extended itself the length of the grafts rather than simply taking part in sealing off the sheath. This tissue also occasionally attached itself to areas of the grafts microscopically denuded of paratenon although to a much lesser degree.

Adhesions to the flexor carpi ulnaris grafts, while extensive in their relative distribution, did not contain significant quantities of collagen, and would, therefore, not be expected to restrict motion of the grafts significantly under the conditions as defined; this is in keeping with the atraumatic techniques employed. However, in the presence of significant surgical trauma to the grafts or surgery on contiguous anatomic structures within the digital sheath, adhesions would be expected to be more florid and invasive and would, therefore, probably restrict graft motion significantly.

Paratenon is not essential to the survival of free autogenous tendon grafts. Its preservation results in greater adhesion formation than if it is not present. These conclusions parallel the often expressed clinical impression[30] that the preservation of paratenon on a free tendon graft often results in poorer results than if it is meticulously removed prior to transplantation.

HEALING AND FATE OF LYOPHILIZED HOMOLOGOUS TENDON GRAFTS WITHIN THE FLEXOR DIGITAL SHEATH

The series of experiments described in the fifth and sixth parts of this section strongly suggested that there was but one ideal replacement substitute for an irreparably injured profundus tendon, namely, another atraumatically obtained autogenous profundus tendon. Since there could be little of any justification for removing a normal profundus tendon from a healthy digit in order to repair a damaged one in another digit, it was decided to experiment with preserved profundus tendons.[48]

Fresh flexor digitorum profundus tendons, aseptically obtained from canine donors by atraumatic technique, were fixed by their ends at normal length on annealed, hooked Pyrex rods for atraumatic handling. All grafts were stored in a sterile nutrient medium for no longer than 45 min. and were then freeze-dried by standard technique at the Tissue Bank Department, United States Naval Medical School, Bethesda, Maryland. They were not treated chemically in any way for sterilization or for any other purpose either before or after freeze-drying.

Prior to transplantation as freeze-dry homografts, the grafts were immersed in sterile saline, without antibiotics or antiseptics for one-half hour. They were then transplanted into the flexor digital sheaths of new canine hosts, preserving host flexor digital sheaths, annular ligaments, and sublimis tendons. This was accomplished by using the host profundus tendons as guides to which the freeze-dry tendons were attached distally. They were then drawn into the normal anatomic digital bed by removal of the host profundus tendons through the palm. Proximal and distal anastomosis were accomplished. Seventeen dogs, each with two freeze-dry profundus tenodon homografts in one paw, were sacrificed at intervals from seven to 180 days.

Gross findings were remarkable; no adhesions were observed between the freeze-dry grafts and the host digital sheaths, annular ligaments, or sublimis tendons in any specimen. There was no graft degeneration or replacement at any time in this experiment. At reexploration, the freeze-dry grafts could not be distinguished from normal in situ profundus tendons by competent but unsuspecting fellow surgeon-observers (Fig. 7.2.10).

Histology revealed that the host tendon-preserved homograft junctures were healed as in all previous experiments by the cellular activity of the surrounding tissues. Fibroblasts which grew in from the surrounding tissues ultimately deposited collagen in the wounds in a manner identically paralleling those described. The freeze-dry grafts in the immediate wound areas were recellularized for a distance up to 1 cm from the immediate wound. As wound maturation progressed, the cellularity of the freeze-dry grafts and the host tendon stumps were identical in the immediate wound areas. Adhesions to wound sites became loose and filmy. In the 160- and 180-day specimens and anastomotic wounds could no longer be readily identified histologically, since the collagen in the wounds had formed bundles identical with those of

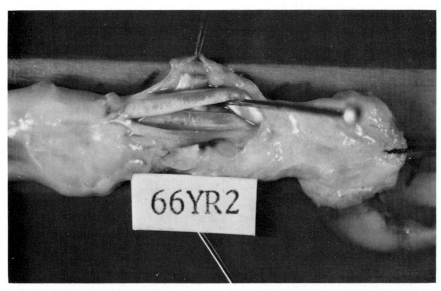

Figure 7.2.10. Gross photograph of freeze-dry profundus tendon homograft 56 days after implantation. Note normal gross appearance of tendon and complete absence of any adhesions between the graft and the sublimis tendon, annular ligament, or sheath. Note absence of any gross degeneration of graft.

tendon proper. This collagen blended perfectly with the host tendon stumps and the freeze-dry grafts. Since the cellularity of the latter was identical with that of the former in the wound areas, it was not possible to distinguish grafts from host tendons by cellular morphology.

There was no evidence of degeneration of any of the collagen in the freeze-dry grafts (Figs. 7.2.11 and 7.2.12). Staining characteristics of the grafts remained identical to those of the host tendon stumps under H and E staining as well as the staining techniques previously described. There was no graft degeneration, nor evidence of replacement of the freeze-dry collagen grafts by host tissues. It appeared that host cells recellularized the grafts, migrating along and taking their places among the collagen bundles of the grafts.

Within the flexor digital sheaths remote from the anastomotic wounds, the acellular freeze-dry grafts were carefully studied by *en bloc* histologic sections of the entire digital flexor mechanism. The experimental design provided a unique opportunity to assess critically the fate of the freeze-dry grafts since they could be accurately compared histologically to the normal untraumatized host sublimis tendons seen in longitudinal section and the normal host annular ligaments seen in cross-section in each longitudinal field. Moreover, subspecimens used for cross-sections presented the freeze-dry grafts enfolded within the normal host sublimis tendons.

The acellular freeze-dry grafts remained intact with no evidence of degeneration of their collagen from seven days postoperatively through the end point of this study at 180 days. There was no graft collagen swelling, fragmentation, or degeneration when compared with host sublimis tendons (Figs. 7.2.11 and 7.2.12). Staining characteristics of the freeze-dry grafts, except for initial acellularity, remained identical with those of the host sublimis tendons.

Cellular changes within the flexor digital sheath revealed a unique process. Areas of cellular proliferation appeared in the synovial cell layer of the sheaths apposing the freeze-dry grafts (Fig. 7.2.11). This also occurred on the apposing surfaces of the host sublimis tendons in the region of origin of their extensive, synovium-covered vincula. There was proliferation of the synovial layer of the sheath with seeding of the underlying freeze-dry tendon grafts with cells from the sheath. These proliferative cellular changes were accompanied by focal increases in the vascularity of the synovial sheaths. The areas of synovial cellular proliferation were observed to be perfectly matched by collections of similar cells opposite them on the surfaces of the otherwise acellular freeze-dry grafts (Fig. 7.2.12). These cells apparently arose from the synovium, invaded the grafts, and proceeded to recellularize them by migration from these focal areas. The seeding of the freeze-dry grafts occurred across the space between the grafts and digital sheaths. While these structures were contiguous *in situ,* the *en bloc* histologic section showed that the freeze-dry grafts remained separate from the sheaths, sublimis tendons, and annular ligaments. In some hematoxylin and eosin sections, it appeared that the sheaths and grafts were

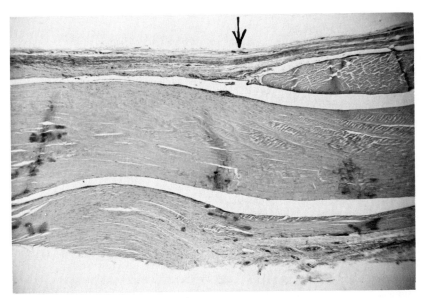

Figure 7.2.11. Longitudinal section of a freeze-dry profundus homograft 21 days after implantation. Note the normal appearance of the collagen of the graft when compared with that of the sublimis tendon seen below and the annular ligament seen above in cross-section. There is no swelling, fragmentation, or degeneration of the collagen of the graft. Note the singular area of cellularity upon the graft matched by an area of synovial proliferation on the flexor sheath opposite it (hematoxylin and eosin, × 19).

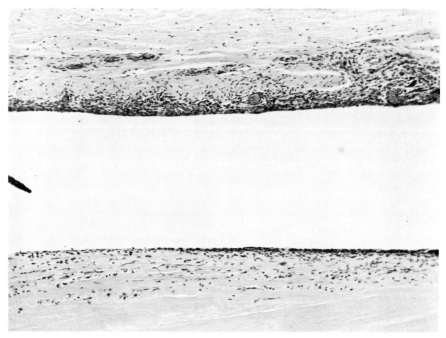

Figure 7.2.12. Longitudinal section of a freeze-dry profundus homograft 14 days after implantation. Note the increased vascularity and cellularity of the synovial sheath corresponding to a focal area of recellularization in the freeze-dry graft below. Remainder (deeper areas) of the graft is still acellular (hematoyylin and eosin, × 79).

united by intensely cellular adhesions; this apparent finding was inconsistent with gross observation that there were no adhesions to the grafts "No Man's Land." Special stains (Rinehart's and Wilder's) showed that there had been no collagen deposited in the cellular masses which arose from the sheath and seeded the grafts by bridging the sheaths space. Therefore, no adhesions were produced between the dry grafts and the other structures of the flexor mechanism.

This process of cellular seeding of the grafts from the sheath synovium progressively recellularized the grafts. By the end of the experiment at 180 days, however, all those grafts which had been immobilized throughout the postoperative period were incompletely recellularized, since they had central longitudinal cores of relative or absolute acellularity within the flexor digital sheath. The remaining peripheral graft areas had normal cellularity by 42 days. There was one exception to this; two grafts harvested at 56 days had been completely recellularized and presented the appearance of normal tendon histologically. This probably represents an instance of biologic variability in regard to the entire series of animals. Similarly, two grafts taken from an animal which had chewed off his cast and subjected his paw to functional use for eight weeks prior to sacrifice at 180 days postoperative were totally recellularized while the pair of tendons held immobile until the time had central longitudinal cores of relative acellularity.

While there was synovial sheath cellular and vascular proliferation during the process of cellular seeding of the freeze-dry grafts, no blood vessels could be detected in the freeze-dry grafts histologically and with the aid of vascular injection techniques. This supported the conclusion that the sheath synovium provided the sole basis for recellularization of the freeze-dry grafts within "No Man's Land." There was no homograft rejection phenomenon. The inflammatory cells of healing present in the wounds disappeared as normal healing progressed. They did not appear at areas remote from the wounds or about the grafts within the digital sheaths. The entire process described was one of complete host acceptance of the freeze-dry homografts.

Peacock[40] has suggested, on the basis of experiments with refrigerated and trypsin-treated tendon heterografts, that such structures may primarily represent homostatic collagen transplants. The results of the experiments presented above present no data contrary to Peacock's hypothesis.

Often, investigators have thought of nonautogenous tendons as "dead" grafts. While their cells may be dead because of processing, or may die after reimplantation, the word "dead" is meaningless in regard to the collagen of the grafts. Since collagen, a protein, is *per se* an extra cellular product of cellular activity, it can have neither "life" nor "death." The essential question concerning it in regard to transplantation is whether or not it has been denatured. If it has not been denatured and presents no clinically significant immunologic competence (as indicated by this study as well as by those of Peacock,[40] and Flynn and Graham)[14] there is no compelling reason why it should be rejected or undergo a process of necrosis and replacement.* In fact, as demonstrated in this study it may be completely accepted by the host and become an integral and apparently normal anatomic component of the host after recellularization. It appears that this favorable sequence is least likely to be adversely affected by the freeze-drying technique of preservation. Preservation of tendons in chemical disinfectants which act by denaturing essential protein complexes of microorganisms may also denature the collagen of the grafts to a degree which stimulates a prolonged host inflammatory response resulting in graft necrosis and replacement. Moreover, residual disinfectants in the grafts may cause irritation and destruction of local host tissues assuring a more profound host inflammatory response. This factor may have been responsible for the mark and persistent hyperemia about tendon homografts preserved in aqueous merthiolate by Cordrey, et al.''

CONCLUSIONS

Flexor digitorum profundus tendons repaired within the flexor digital sheath are healed by the reparative cellular response of the sheath and surrounding tissues, and not by any intrinsic response of their own.

The oft-repeated clinical impression that flexor tendons repaired within the flexor digital sheath manifest postoperative swelling and undergo necrosis unless the digital sheath and sublimis tendons are excised was not confirmed in these experiments. No such reaction or series of events was ever observed.

It is generally accepted that trauma to tendons can result in extremely poor functional results after their repair. It has not been generally appreciated, however, that adhesion formation in response to tendon trauma is a discrete and specific phenomenon. Adhesions form at each point at which the surface integrity of tendon is disrupted and in direct proportion to the degree of tendon surface trauma. This is a predictable and semiquantitative phenomenon.

Trauma to contiguous anatomic structures is also of extreme importance. When the sublimis tendon is totally excised, the disturbed periosteal floor of the digital canal gives rise to a florid, fibroblastic response which takes part in the profundus tendon healing processes. The broad, bone-based adhesions, so formed, can tether the healing profundus tendon within the digit, effectively destroying all hope of useful function. A flexor tendon requires an extrinsic source of granulation tissue for its healing. Therefore, it will become adherent to any contiguous structure which is capable of producing a fibroblastic granulation tissue response

when injured. Thus, an uninjured sublimis tendon should not be sacrificed in order to repair a damaged profundus tendon in the same finger; profundus repair in the presence of an intact sublimis tendon will not result in adhesions between the two tendons, provided the sublimis is not traumatized. If the sublimis tendon is badly damaged, it should be subtotally excised by sharp transverse division immediately proximal to its vincula. The vincula should not be injured in removing the sublimis.

The surgeon must be meticulous in the avoidance of iatrogenic injury to all structures in the fingers. It is injudicious to excise or unnecessarily disturb normal structures within the digital flexor mechanism. The price of such action is greater adhesion formation with resultant poor function.

Paratenon-covered tendons are *relatively* unsatisfactory as free tendon grafts within the digital flexor mechanism. Paratenon serves both as a source of adhesions and as an excellent recipient bed for adhesion-producing granulation tissue from other structures. Tendons normally covered by paratenon make better free tendon grafts for the digital flexor mechanism if their paratenon is first carefully removed by dissection, taking care not to injure the surface of the tendons.

However, there is no better substitute for a flexor tendon than a free graft of another flexor tendon. If an untraumatized profundus tendon is available for grafting, as in the case of amputation, it should be used as a free graft in preference to any other tendon.

The cells of the fresh tendon autografts, both profundus and flexor carpi ulnaris, survived free transplantation into the digital flexor sheath. The collagen of the grafts remained intact with no evidence of degenerative change except at sites of trauma.

Freeze-dry profundus tendon homografts are fully accepted by their new hosts and undergo a process of recellularization effected by the active cellular seeding of the grafts by the post digital sheaths. This recellularization occurs without the formation of adhesions within the area of the flexor digital sheath popularly known as ''No Man's Land.'' The excellent anatomic results following the use of these grafts are equaled only by fresh autotopic profundus grafts; remarkably, the freeze-dry profundus homografts produced better anatomic results than fresh paratenon-covered tendon autografts.

It is hoped that this chapter will provide the reader with basic information about the processes of healing of digital flexor tendons and flexor tendon grafts so that clinical flexor tendon surgery can be approached in a rational, orderly, logical, and scientific manner.

REFERENCES

1. Adams, W. *On The Reparative Process in Human Tendons after Subcutaneous Division for the Cure of Deformities. With an Account of the Appearances Presented in Fifteen Post-Mortem Examinations in the Human Subject; also a Series of Experiments on*

---

*This does not mean to imply that normal physiologic collagen turnover may not later occur in these grafts.

Rabbits, and a Resume of the English and Foreign Literature on the Subject. London, Churchill, 1860.

2. Angel, S. H., Lipscomb, P.R., and Grindlay, J.H. Construction of artificial tendon sheaths in dogs. Am. J. Surg., *101:* 355-356, 1961.

3. Ashley, F.L., Polak, T., Stone, R.S., and Marmor, L. An evaluation of the healing process in avian and mammalian digital-flexor tendons following the application of an artifical tendon sheath (silastic). In *Proceedings of the American Society for Surgery of the Hand.* J. Bone Joint Surg., *44A:* 1038, 1962.

4. Ashley, F.L., Stone, R.S., Alonso-Artieda, M., Syverud, J.M., Edwards, J.W., Sloan, R.F., and Mooney, S.A. Experimental and clinical studies on the application of monomolecular cellulose filter tubes to create artificial tendon sheaths in digits. Plast. Reconstr. Surg., *23:* 526-534, 1959.

5. Ashley, F.L., Stone, R.S., Edwards, J.W., and Sloan, R.F. Further studies on the application of monomolecular cellulose filter tubes to create artificial tendon sheaths in the hand and wrist. Western J. Surg., *68:* 156-161, 1960.

6. Benjamin, H.B., Wagner, M., Zeit, W., and Ausman, R.L. The use of an endothelial cuff in tendon repair. Med. Times, *83:* 697-699, 1955.

7. Boyes, J.H. Flexor-tendon grafts in the fingers and thumb: An evaluation of end results. J. Bone Joint Surg., *32A:* 489-499, 1950.

8. Bunnell, S. *Hand Surgery in World War II.* Washington, D.C., Dept. of the Army, 1955.

9. Burman, M.S. The use of a nylon sheath in the secondary repair of torn finger flexor tendons. Bull. Hosp. Joint Dis., *5:* 122-133, 1944.

10. Carstam, N. The effect of cortisone on the formation of tendon adhesions and on tendon healing: An experimental investigation in the rabbit. Acta Chir. Scand., Suppl. 182, 1953.

11. Cordrey, L.J., McCorkle, H., and Hilton, E. A comparative study of fresh autogenous and preserved homogenous tendon grafts in rabbits. J. Bone Joint Surg., *45B:* 182-195, 1963.

12. Davis, L, and Aries, L.J. An experimental study upon the prevention of adhesions about repaired nerves and tendons. Surgery, *2:* 877-888, 1937.

13. Fargin and Assaki. Cited by Peer.[42]

14. Flynn, J.E., and Graham, J.H. Lyophilized heterologous and autogenous tendon transplants. Surg., Gynecol. Obstet., *116:* 345-350, 1963.

15. Flynn, J.E., and Graham, J.H. Healing following tendon suture and tendon transplants. Surg. Gynecol. Obstet., *115:* 467-472, 1962.

16. Gallie, W.E., and Le Mesurier, A.B. Cited by Peer.[42]

17. Garlock, J.H. The repair processes in wounds of tendons, and in tendon grafts. Ann. Surg., *85:* 92-103, 1927.

18. Gonzalez, R.I. Experimental tendon repair within the flexor tunnels: Use of polyethylene tubes for improvement of functional results in the dog. Surgery, *26:* 181-198, 1949.

19. Gonzalez, R.I. Experimental use of Teflon in tendon surgery. Plast. Reconstr. Surg., *23:* 535-539, 1959.

20. Grant, G. The effect of cortisone on healing of tendons in rabbits. In *Proceediings of the American Society for Surgery of the Hand.* J. Bone Joint Surg., *35A:* 525, 1953.

21. Hauck, G. Über Schnenverletzungen, Sehnenregenera-tion und Sehnennaht. Arch. Klin. Chir., *128:* 568-585, 1924.

22. Hochstrasser, A.D., Broadbent, T.R., and Woolf, R. Sheath replacement in tendon repair. Rocky Mt. Med. J., *57:* 30-33, 1960.

23. Hueck, H. Über Sehnenregeneration innerhalb echter Sehnenscheiden. Arch. Klin. Chir., *127:* 137-164, 1923.

24. Iselin, M., De La Plaza, R., and Flores, A. Surgical use of homologous tendon grafts preserved in cialit. Plast. Reconstr. Surg., *32:* 401-403, 1963.

25. Kaplan, E.B. Discussion summarized. In *Proceedings of the American Society for Surgery of the Hand.* J. Bone Joint Surg., *45A:* 885, 1963.

26. Kreuz, F.P., Hyatt, G.W., Turner, T.C., and Bassett, A.L. The preservation and clinical use of freeze-dried bone. J. Bone Joint Surg., *33A:* 863-872, 1951.

27. Lewis, D., and Davis, C.B. Cited by Peer.[42]

28. Lindsay, W.K., and MacDougall, E.P. Digital flexor tendons: An experimental study. Part III: The fate of autogenous digital flexor tendon crafts. Br. J. Plast. Surg., *13:* 292-304, 1961.

29. Lindsay, W.K., and Thomson, H.G. Digital flexor tendons: An experimental study. Part I: The significance of each component of the flexor mechanism in tendon healing. Br. J. Plast. Surg., *12:* 289-316, 1960.

30. Littler, J.W. Personal communication.

31. Marchand, F. Cited by Peer.[42]

32. Mason, M.L. Primary tendon repair. J. Bone Joint Surg., *41A:* 575-577, 1959.

33. Mason, M.L. Primary versus secondary tendon repair. Q. Bull. Northwestern Med. Sch., *31 (2):* 120-123, 1957.

34. Mason, M.L., and Allen, H.S. The rate of heling of tendons: An experimental study of tensile strength. Ann. Surg., *113:* 424-459, 1941.

35. Mason, M.L., and Shearon, C.G. The process of tendon repair: An experimental study of tendon suture and tendon graft. Arch. Surg., *25:* 615-692, 1932.

36. Mc Kee, G.K. Metal anastomosis tubes in tendon suture. Lancet, *1:* 659-660, 1945.

37. Nageotte, J., and Sencert, L. Cited by Peer.[42]

38. Narvi, E.J. Cited by Skoog, Tord, and Persson.[54]

39. Neuberger, A., and Slack, H.G.B. The metabolism of collagen from liver, bone, skin and tendon in the normal rat. Biochem. J., *53:* 47-52, 1953.

40. Peacock, E.E., Jr. Morphology of homologous and heterologous tendon grafts. Surg., Gynecol. Obstet., *109:* 735-742, 1959.

41. Peacock, E.E. Some problems in flexor tendon healing. Surgery, *45:* 415-423, 1959.

42. Peer, L.A. In *Transplantation of Tissues,* Cartilage, bone, fascia, tendon and muscle. Vol. *I,* pp. 277-295. Baltimore, Williams and Wilkins, 1955.

43. Potenza, A.D. Critical evaluation of flexor tendon healing and adhesion formation within artificial digital sheaths. J. Bone Joint. Surg., *45A:* 1217-1233, 1963.

44. Potenza, A.D. Effect of associated trauma on healing of divided tendons. J. Trauma, *2:* 175-184, 1962.

45. Potenza, A.D. Flexor tendon injuries. Orthop. Clin. North Am., *1:* 355-373, 1970.

46. Potenza, A.D. Prevention of adhesions to healing digital flexor tendons. J.A.M.A., *187:* 187-191, 1964.

47. Potenza, A.D. Previously unpublished data.

48. Potenza, A.D. Previously unpublished data.

49. Potenza, A.D. Tendon healing within the flexor digital sheath in the dog: An experimental study. J. Bone Joint Surg., *44A:* 49-64, 1962.
50. Potenza, A.D. The healing of autogenous tendon grafts within the flexor digital sheath in dogs. J. Bone Joint Surg., *46A:* 1462-1484, 1964.
51. Rehn, E. Cited by Peer.[42]
52. Schwarz, E. Über die anatomischen Vorgange bei der Sehnenregeneration und dem plastischen Ersatz von Sehnendefekten durch Sehne, Fascie and Bindegewebe. Feitschr. Chir., *173:* 301-385, 1922.
53. Seggel, R. Cited by Skoog, Tord, and Persson.[54]
54. Skoog, T., and Persson, B.H. An experimental study of the early healing of tendons. Plast. Reconstr. Surg., *13:* 384-399, 1954.
55. von Ammon. Cited by Mason and Shearon.[35]
56. Wheeldon, T. The use of cellophane as a permanent tendon sheath. J. Bone Joint Surg., *21:* 393-396, 1939.
57. Wrenn, R.N., Goldner, J.L., and Markee, J.L. An experimental study of the effect of cortisone on the healing processes and tensile strength of tendons. J. Bone Joint Surg., *36A:* 588-601, 1954.

C.

Evaluation of Results of Tendon Repair

Elden C. Weckesser, M.D.

"The prick of a nerve or tendon will enduce pain and convulsion."—Galen

Although advocated by Avicenna, and practiced with increasing frequency in the 16th and 17th centuries,[28] tendon repair awaited the advent of anesthesia, aseptic surgery, and the improvement and popularization of the use of the tourniquet by Esmark.

Immediate tendon repair has the advantage of unstiffened joints at the time of surgery which is a distinct advantage if not overshadowed by other factors.

In addition, the results of tendon repair depend largely on the motivation of the patient to regain motion of the injured part.

The doctor has little control over many of these features except that encouragement and confidence can be inspired into the ofttimes bewildered patient so that he may try his greatest to regain function.

PHYSICAL THERAPY

The confidence and hope engendered by the operating surgeon should be utilized along with that engendered by the physical therapist, the two working together as a team to regain motion and use of the injured part.

RESULTS OF FLEXOR TENDON REPAIR

The flexor tendons in general offer more problems in successful repair than do the extensor tendons. The deeper location and greater excursion of the flexors make atraumatic exposure more difficult. The passage of the flexors through narrow fibroosseous tunnels at the wrist and throughout the digits creates a situation where lateral adhesions at the site of repair act as a new insertion for the tendon, and prevent the transmission of force to distal joints, a frequent cause of failure in tendon repair.

ANATOMIC ZONES

The results of tendon repair over the years have shown that the problems are much greater in certain areas than in others and this has led to the designation of anatomical zones as in the diagram in Figure 7.1.7 in "Technique of Tendon Repair". This classification is made because of the variable problems of tendon repair at the different locations and the difference in results obtained.

RESULTS IN ZONE I—VOLAR ASPECT, DISTAL PHALANX

In my experience, the results of primary or delayed suture in this zone are usually quite satisfactory, especially when the tendon can be repaired at its distal insertion.

Van't Hof and Heiple[29] obtained flexion to within 1 inch of the distal palmar crease in 89 per cent of 23 cases sutured outside the flexor tunnel and Pulvertaft[26] in 90 per cent of 28 cases. Wagner[33] reports uniformly good results by the method of delayed advancement of the profundus tendon when the latter is divided distal to the insertion of the sublimis tendon. See Figure 7.1.6, 7.1.7 in "Technique of Tendon Repair".

The intact sublimis tendon of the finger, providing complete active flexion of the middle finger joint, provides sufficiently good motion that some surgeons do not repair the isolated profundus tendon injury in this area, when seen later. In my experience, active flexion of the distal finger joint is useful, especially in the index and long fingers, and attempts should usually be made to restore it either by delayed advancement or tendon graft. An intact sublimis tendon should never be sacrificed.

In the distal thumb, the results of repair of the flexor pollicis longus tendon have usually been quite satisfactory although a full range of flexion is not always restored. When the repair is at or near the insertion, adhesions serve merely to strengthen the insertion rather than hamper gliding.

RESULTS IN ZONE II—DANGER ZONE, "NO MAN'S LAND"

This is the anatomic area of the fibroosseous tunnel of the digits, containing two tendons, where results until recent years have been notoriously poor. Both tendons are usually divided. It is the most difficult area in which to achieve satisfactory results. The advances in hand surgery which have been so great since World War II are reflected particularly in the results of repair of tendons within the fibroosseous tunnels of the digits. These tunnels are the proving ground of the surgeon. It is here that only the best techniques succeed and even these not in every case, by any means. Unless one is versed in this type of work or has strict supervision by one who is, he had best not undertake it. Instead, the wound should be carefully debrided and cleansed with copious amounts of saline and a simple soft tissue closure carried out with definitive repair done by an expert three to six weeks later, through a fresh incision. During this interval, the joints should be kept supple by passive motions. As recently as 1955, Hauge[13] reported only four successful cases of primary repair within the fibroosseous tunnels among 98 attempts, made mostly by "assistant" doctors.

When repair is carried out in the fibroosseous tunnel no attempt should be made to restore both tendons. Only the profundus tendon should be restored in this area either by primary repair or delayed graft.

PRIMARY REPAIR *VERSUS* TENDON ..GRAFTING IN ZONE II

The results of primary tendon repair in "no man's land" were notoriously disappointing in the past. This lead to the practice of delayed or secondary tendon grafting as practiced particularly by Boyes[3] and others. This technique has been a distinct favorable influence in the restoration of tendon function in Zone II. The results in 1000 cases in a recent report[4] bear out these continued good results.

In recent years favorable results from primary tendon repair in "No Man's Land," in favorable cases, have occurred with increased frequency. Posch[24] obtained satisfactory results in 86 per cent of 45 cases and Kelly[16] 66 per cent of 101 cases. Verdan[30] reported 85 per cent satisfactory results and Lindsay and McDougall[17] 89 per cent satisfactory results in children.

Favorable results with secondary tendon grafting have been reported by many authors.[4 8 11 12 13 16 17 19 23 27]

However, the successes with primary repair are usually in favorable cases treated by experienced surgeons. The more favorable cases in some series have received primary suture while the less favorable cases have had delayed tendon grafts.

Regardless of whether primary repair or delayed grafting is chosen, it is evident that "No Man's Land" is being invaded by both techniques. The danger of infection prevents the advocation of primary tendon grafting although Flynn[10] reports favorable results in selected cases.

SPECIAL TECHNIQUES FOR TENDON RE-PAIR

Paneva-Holevich Two-Stage Tenoplasty[23]

Stage I (Fig. 7.3.1)

The sublimus and profundus tendons are united in the palm at the level of lumbrical muscle after the primary wound further distal has been cleansed and closed.

Stage II (1 month later) Fig. 7.3.2A and B)

The sublimus tendon is detached from its muscle belly proximally, turned distally and inserted at the base of the distal phalanx as an extension of the profundus tendon.

This technique actually is a method of tendon grafting utilizing the sublimus tendon. Its advantage is that the proximal union between sublimus and profundus tendons has healed at the time of the second stage. This leaves only one tendon union to make at the second stage which is located at the distal insertion. Since the proximal tendon union is healed at the second stage, earlier postoperative movement is possible. A disadvantage is that the second stage requires quite extensive exposure and dissection. Doctor Paneva-Holevich reports good to excellent results (flexion to within less than 1.27 cm of the distal palmar crease) in 26 of 34 cases (76 per cent). The eight less than good results occurred in less favorable cases. Limited experience with this technique by the author has been favorable. However, it should not supplant primary repair at the site of injury in favorable cases.

Hunter[15] Silastic Rod* Technique to Produce New Tendon Sheath

This technique is particularly suited for secondary tendon repair in scarred areas where the tendon sheath has been destroyed and where the chance of adhesion formation is great. It is not advocated for acute repair in a contaminated wound due to the danger of infection. It is based on the fact that an inert foreign body becomes surrounded by a smooth layer of mesothelial cells by metaplasia which will act as new tendon sheath when a tendon graft is drawn through it several months later.

Early workers in this field include Mayer and Ransohoff,[20] Carroll and Bassett,[7] Milgrin,[21] and many others. Our early work with interposition substances showed that a new mesothelial lining of cells occurs adjacent to an inert substance placed next to a tendon.[34]

*Available from the Holter Company, Third and Mill Streets, Bridgeport, Pennsylvania.

Technique

Stage I

a. The flexor tendon area is exposed using a mid-lateral or zig-zag finger incision. A transverse

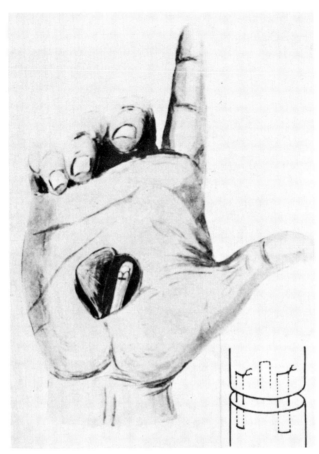

Figure 7.3.1. Stage I. Paneva-Holevich technique. The sublimus and profundus tendons are joined in the palm at the level of the lumbrical muscle. This is done at the time of primary repair but after the more distal injury has been cleansed, debrided, and closed. Reproduced with the permission of the author and *The Journal of Bone and Joint Surgery.*

palm incision and a forearm incision of operator's choice is made.

b. Scar is excised.

c. A Dacron-silastic rod prosthesis is inserted and attached to distal stump of profundus tendon at the base of the distal phalanx.

d. Portions of the tendon tunnel are reconstituted over proximal and middle phalanges as necessary.

e. Adequate space is left proximally in the palm or forearm so that the prosthesis has room to glide without buckling.

f. The wound closed.

g. Temporary postoperative splinting with wrist and finger joints in moderate flexion is used.

h. Gentle passive movement is started during the second to fourth week. This is gradually increased.

Great care must be used to insure sterility throughout the entire operation as infection is a disaster requiring removal of the prosthesis.

Stage II (Two to six months later when the finger is supple)

a. The distal insertion of the prosthesis is exposed through a short midlateral finger incision.

b. The proximal end of the prosthesis is exposed through an appropriate incision in the palm or forearm whichever it may be.

c. A tendon graft of the operator's choice of proper size is joined to the proximal end of the prosthesis and threaded distally through the new bed as the prosthesis is removed.

d. The distal union is made to the stump of the profundus tendon by means of a stainless steel suture tied over a button at the tip of the finger. The proximal union is made by interweaving and nonabsorbable, nonreactive soft sutures so that the finger at rest is held in slight flexion.

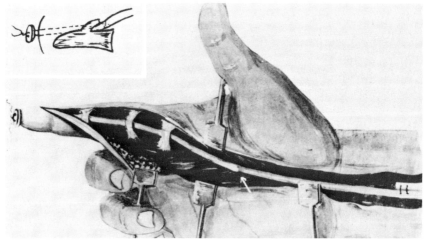

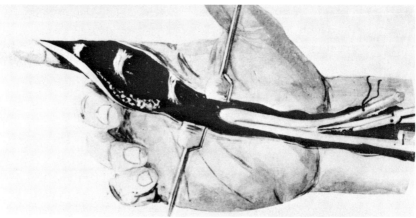

Figure 7.3.2. Stage II. Paneva-Holevich technique. A. Detachment of the sublimus tendon from its muscle belly and turning it distally. B. The sublimus tendon turned and threaded distally to act as an extension of the profundus tendon. The only union necessary at this stage is the distal insertion. Reproduced with the permission of the author and *The Journal of Bone and Joint Surgery*.

e. The finger and wrist are splinted in moderate flexion. Protected active flexion of the interphalangeal joints is allowed with the dorsal splint in place for three to four weeks.

Hunter[15] reports flexion within 1.3 cm of the distal crease of the palm in 57 per cent of 69 less than favorable fingers. 80 per cent flexed to within 2.5 cm.

Combination of Techniques

When operating on a scarred tendon in the finger it is possible to combine the Paneva-Holevich and Hunter techniques. When the finger scar has been excised, a silastic rod is inserted to the mid palmar area (lumbrical muscle area) (Stage I, Hunter technique) and at the same operation a union is made between sublimus and profundus tendon (Stage I, Paneva-Holevich technique). At the second stage, about three months later, the sublimus tendon is turned distally and threaded into the new tunnel formed around the silastic rod. The author has used this combination of

techniques successfully. It has also been reported by Chong, Cramer, and Culf.[8]

RESULTS IN ZONE III

Zone III represents the flexor tunnel of the thumb which has one tendon passing through it. This area is very apt to develop adhesions but in general is less troublesome than Zone II. This digit does not "get in the way" to the same extent as a finger when its flexion is limited. In general, results are satisfactory in this zone.

RESULTS IN ZONES IV, V, AND VI

Zone IV, the proximal area of the palm in which the lumbrical muscles take origin, is a favorable area for tendon repair as is the forearm, Zone VI. In these two areas, the tendons are surrounded by much loose tissue which moves with the tendon rather than hindering movement. Both sublimis and profundus tendons can be successfully repaired here.

Zone V, beneath the transverse carpal ligament, is a crowed area in which there is more tendency to adhere to rigid structures. Mason[19] believed that only one flexor tendon of a finger should be repaired here due to the danger of adhesions. This is wise advice, although both may be repaired in most favorable circumstances, and leaving the volar carpal ligament unsutured.

METHODS OF RECORDING RESULTS

Figures 7.3.3 through 7.3.6 show graphically four methods of recording the results of flexor tendon repair.

The Littler[18] method (Fig. 7.3.3) of angular joint measurement is without doubt the most informative. It is, however, laborious.

The Boyes[2] method (Fig. 7.3.4) of finger pulp to distal palmar crease measurement is quick and simple to use. Results lend themselves to graphic representation (Fig. 7.3.7). The method does not take into ac-

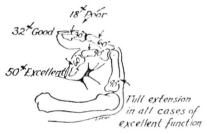

Figure 7.3.3. Method of recording results of flexor tendon grafting employed by Littler. This involves individual joint motion measurement. Reproduced by permission of the author and the American Journal of Surgery.

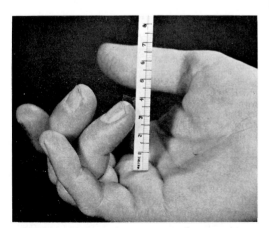

Figure 7.3.4. Method of recording results of flexor tendon grafting employed by Boyes. One measurement gives a result which can be graphically recorded as shown in Figure 7.3.5.

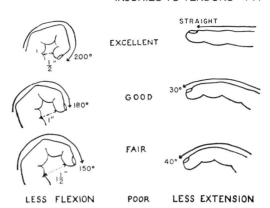

Figure 7.3.5. Method of recording results of flexor tendon grafting employed by White. This is a combination of composite angular movement and finger pulp distal palmar crease distance which also takes into account lack of extension. Reproduced by permission of the author and the American Journal of Surgery.

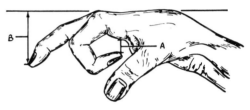

Figure 7.3.6. Method of recording results of flexor tendon grafting used by Van't Hof and Heiple which direcently takes into account lack of extension. The measurements, A and B, are added together. The sums can be recorded in graph form as shown in Figure 7.3.8. Reproduced by permission of the author and The Journal of Bone and Joint Surgery.

count, however, limitation of extension, the size of the hand, and whether or not the digit touches the palm. In spite of these features, the Boyes method is very practical for recording finger function, if limitation in finger extension is also recorded.

The method of White[35] (Fig. 7.3.5) is a combination of composite angular measurement and finger pulp to distal palmar crease measurement as shown. It does take into account lack of extension.

The method of Van't Hof and Heiple[29] (Fig. 7.3.6) is a clever method of incorporating limitation of flexion and extension into one value which can be graphically represented as shown in Figure 7.3.8. This method of evaluation gave fewer satisfactory results among their cases than the Boyes method.

Harrison's[12] method emphasizes touching the palm. It leaves something to be desired in the evaluation of those cases which do not touch the palm.

Lindsay and McDougall[17] present a three-way

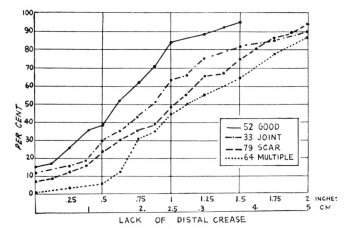

Figure 7.3.7. Finger function following tendon grafts across "no man's land" reported by Boyes.[3] It is seen that for the "good"cases, 15 per cent had complete flexion, 85 per cent flexed to within 1 inch and 95 per cent to within 1½ inches of the palm. Note that preoperative joint stiffness, scar formation, and multiple digit involvement each adversely affected results. Reproduced by permission of the author and the *American Journal of Surgery.* These reports are also borne out in a more recent report by Boyes and Stark.[4]

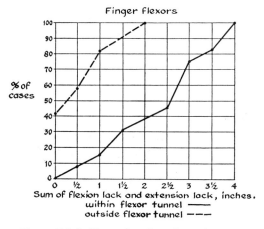

Figure 7.3.8. Finger function after primary tendon repair recorded after the method of Van't Hof and Heiple. 0 to 1 inch = good; 1 to 2 inches = fair; 2 to 3 inches = poor; over 3 inches = failure. The great difference in results within and without the flexor tunnel sheath is here shown.

evaluation based on digital pulp to distal palmar crease distance, composite flexion and functional evaluation. This is a very complete evaluation but does not take lack of extension into account directly.

The Verdan-Michon[32] method is a very good one which takes into account digital pulp distal palmar crease distance, touching the palm and deficient extension. It consists of five classes. Deficient extension is accounted for by going back one class for each 45° lack of extension. (Perhaps this latter figure should be smaller.) If the above measurements are too laborious,

the method of Van't Hof and Heiple[29] is a quick way of obtaining nearly as much information by two simple measurements.

RESULTS OF EXTENSOR TENDON REPAIR

Although results are somewhat more favorable for extensors than for flexors, here again results vary according to the location of the repair.

RESULTS OF REPAIR AT THE DISTAL IN-SERTION (MALLET FINGER, DROP PHALANGETTE)

Kelly[16] reports 78 per cent success by the internal fixation method of Pratt[25] in 14 cases. I have noted that this method has led to troublesome joint stiffness. My results have been most favorable by means of a well-padded plaster cast, if there is no fracture associated, applied with 1 inch plaster of Paris and left in place for six weeks. The middle joint of the digit is held in flexion and the distal joint in hyperextension by the cast. This has led to success in approximately three-fourths of patients, if applied early. Postimmobilization joint stiffness has constituted a minimal problem.

RESULTS OF REPAIR AT DORSUM OF FINGERS, PROXIMAL

Results of repair of lacerations are favorable near the insertion of the central slip of the extensor hood if no tendon is missing.

If a destruction of a portion of the central slip has occurred, the outlook is much less favorable and boutonniere deformity may result. This is best treated by criss-cross tendon graft after the method of Fowler.[11]

The results of extensor hood repair have been favorably reported by some authors. Kelly[16] reports 81 per cent success here in 87 cases. Adhesions frequently have been troublesome here, in my experience.

RESULTS OF REPAIR AT DORSUM OF HAND, WRIST, AND FOREARM

The dorsum of the hand and forearm have given most favorable results after tendon repair comparable to the proximal palm and forearm on the volar surface. The retinaculum should be moved over tendon repairs in this area to diminish adhesions. A portion of the retinaculum, away from the repair, should be preserved to prevent bowing on extension of the wrist.

SUMMARY

The results of tendon repair vary, depending on the extent of injury, the anatomic zone injured, the degree of contamination, associated trauma, amount of delay, the skill of the surgeon, and the will of the patient to regain function.

Results in general are good, the poorest being in the flexor tunnel area of the fingers and beneath the transverse carpal ligament. Definite indications for primary repair versus delayed tendon grafting are controversial. Primary repair with its shorter morbidity is probably indicated in clean-cut early cases in which the risk of infection is minimal and technical abilities and facilities are good.

The excellent results by delayed grafting dictate simple debridement and closure of the open wound when conditions are less than ideal. This is done with the plan that definitive repair will be performed three to six weeks later, under ideal conditions through a fresh incision.

REFERENCES

1. Bell, J. L., Mason, M. L., Koch, S. L., and Stromberg, W. B., Jr. Injuries to flexor tendons of the hand in children. J. Bone Joint Surg., 40A: 1220-1230, 1958.
2. Boyes J. H. Flexor tendon grafts in the fingers and thumb. An evaluation of end results. J. Bone Joint Surg., 32A: 489-499; 531, 1950.
3. Boyes, J. H. Evaluation of results of digital flexor tendon grafts. Am. J. Surg. 89: 1116-1119, 1955.
4. Boyes, J. H., and Stark, H. H. Flexor-tendon grafts in the fingers and thumb. J. Bone Joint Surg., 53A: 1332-1342, 1971.
5. Brand, P. Principles of free tendon grafting, including a new method of tendon suture. J. Bone Joint Surg., 41B: 208, 1959.
6. Brand, P. Tendon grafting illustrated by a new operation for intrinsic paralysis of the fingers. J. Bone Joint Surg., 43B: 444-453, 1961.
7. Carroll, R. E. and Bassett, A. L. Formation of tendon sheath by silicone rod implants. In Proceedings of the American Society for Surgery of the Hand. J. Bone Joint Surg., 45A: 884-885, 1963.
8. Chong, J. K., Cramer, L. M., and Culf, N. K. Combined two-stage tenoplasty with silicone rods for multiple flexor tendon injuries in "No Man's Land" J. Trauma, 12: 104-121, 1972.
9. Flynn, J. E., Wilson, J. T., Child, C. G., III, and Graham, J. H. Heterogenous and autogenous-tendon transplants. An experimental study of preserved bovine-tendon transplants in dogs and autogenous-tendon transplants in dogs. J. Bone Joint Surg., 42A: 91-110, 1960.
10. Flynn, J. E. Problems with trauma to the hand. J. Bone Joint Surg., 35A: 132-140 171; 251, 1953.
11. Fowler, S. B. Illustrations, pp. 548-549. In S. Bunnell, Surgery of the Hand, Ed. 3. Philadelphia, Lippincott, 1956.
12. Harrison, S. H. Repair of digital flexor tendon injuries in the hand. Br. J. Plast. Surg., 14: 211-230, 1961.
13. Hauge, M. F. Results of tendon suture of the hand. A review of 500 patients. Acta orthop. scand., 24: 258-270, 1955.
14. Huffstadt, A. J. C. Free tendon grafting in the repair of flexor tendon lesions in thumb and fingers. Arch. chir. neerl., 10: 305-317, 1958.
15. Hunter, J. M. and Salisbury, R. E. Flexor tendon reconstruction in severely damaged hands. J. Bone Joint Surg., 53A: 829-858, 1971.
16. Kelly, A. P., Jr. Primary tendon repairs. A study of 789 consecutive tendon severances. J. Bone Joint Surg., 41A: 581-598, 1959.
17. Lindsay, W. K., and McDougall, E. P. Direct digital flexor tendon repair. Plast. Reconstr. Surg., 26: 613-621, 1960.
18. Littler, J. W. Free tendon grafts in secondary flexor tendon repair. Am. J. Surg., 74: 315-321, 1947.
19. Mason, M. L. Primary tendon repair (editorial). J. Bone Joint Surg., 41A: 575-577, 1959.
20. Mayer, L. and Ransohoff, N. Reconstruction of the digital tendon sheath: A constribution to the physiological method of repair of damaged finger tendons. J. Bone Joint Surg., 18: 607-616, 1936.
21. Milgrim, J. E. Transplantation of tendons through preformed gliding channels. Bull. Hosp. Joint Dis., 21: 250-295, 1960.
22. Miller, R. C. Flexor tendon repair over the proximal phalanx. Am. J. Surg., 122: 319-324, 1971.
23. Paneva-Holevich, E. Two-stage tenoplasty in injury of the flexor tendons of the hand. J. Bone Joint Surg., 51A: 21-32, 1969.
24. Posch, J. L. Primary tenorraphies and tendon grafting procedures in hand injuries. Arch. Surg., 73: 609-624, 1956.
25. Pratt, D. R. Internal splint for closed and open treatment of injuries of extensor tendons at distal joint of fingers. J. Bone Joint Surg., 34A: 785-788, 1952.
26. Pulvertaft, R. G. Tendon grafts for flexor tendon injuries in fingers and thumb. A study of technique and results. J. Bone Joint Surg., 38B: 175-194, 1956.
27. Strandell, G. Tendon grafts in injuries of the flexor tendons in fingers and thumb. End results in a consecutive series of seventy-four cases. Acta chir. scand., 111: 124-141, 1956.
28. Unknown Author: The history of tendon suture. M. J. Rec., 127: 156-157; 213-215, 1928.
29. Van't Hof, A., and Heiple, K. G. Flexor tendon injuries of the fingers and thumb. J. Bone Joint Surg., 40A: 256-262, 1958.
30. Verdan, C. E. Primary repair of flexor tendons. J. Bone

Joint Surg., *42A:* 647-657, 1960.

31. Verdan, C. E. Half a century of flexor-tendon surgery. J. Bone Joint Surg., *54A:* 472-291, 1972.

32. Verdan, C., and Michon, J. Le traitement des plaies des tendons fléchisseurs des doigts. Rev. chir. orthop., *47:* 285-425, 1961

33. Wagner, C. J. Delayed advancement in the repair of lacerated flexor profundus tendons. J. Bone Joint Surg., *40A:* 1241-1244, 1958.

34. Weckesser, E. C., Shaw, B. W., Spears, G. N., and Shea, P. C. A comparative study of various substances for the prevention of adhesions about tendons. Surgery, *25:* 361-369, 1949.

35. White, W. L. Secondary restoration of finger flexion by digital tendon graft. An evaluation of seventy-six cases. Am. J. Surg., *91:* 662-668, 1956.

36. White, W. L. The unique, accessible and useful plantaris tendon. Plast. Reconstr. Surg., *25:* 133-141, 1960.

D.

Primary and Secondary Repair of Flexor and Extensor Tendon Injuries

Claude E. Verdan, M.D.

The detailed arrangement of the anatomy of the tendons of the hand is fundamental to its function. The two main functions of the hand are prehension and tactile sensibility. We must constantly associate the two by remembering the immense role which the proprioceptive sensations play and which arise in the special nerve endings contained in the musculotendinous complexes.

Tendofibrils consist of extremely long, linear macromolecules extending practically throughout the whole length of the tendon and are characterized by regular striation with a periodicity of 760.

Elastic fibers produce a gradual increase in tension, which absorbs the first shock of the contraction. This transmission of movement is performed quietly and progressively, as described by Schneider.[39]

METHODS OF EXAMINATION

The measurement of a healthy joint varies from subject to subject. Table 7.4.1 shows the average figures.

PERSONAL METHOD OF ASSESSING RESULTS[51]

I consider it convenient to distinguish two completely different situations to appreciate useful results. (1) The pulp touches the palm. (2) The pulp does not touch the palm. The distal segment remains in the air despite all the efforts of the patient.

When it is decided to use this method it is better to divide the cases into two categories: Category A, touching; Category B, not touching the palm. Most of the better results are included in Category A.

In my report with Jacques Michon[51] on the treatment of injuries of the flexor tendons of the fingers we proposed the following.

Fingers touching the palm: Stage 1, at 2.5 cm (1 inch) and less from the distal palmar crease; Stage 2, at more than 2.5 cm from the distal palmar crease.

Fingers not touching the palm: Stage 3, at 2.5 cm or less from the palm; Stage 4, at more than 2.5 cm from the palm; Stage 0, failures, complete blocage, ruptures, amputations.

APPRECIATION OF TENDON INJURIES — DEPENDENCE ON VASCULARIZATION

We are indebted to Brockis[6] for important anatomic studies of vascularization and to Peacock[33] for recent knowledge based on interesting animal and human investigations.

Methods of Entry for the Arterial Supply to Tendons

These are: (1) the musculotendinous junction; (2) the bony insertion; (3) the tendon structure. It is important to study the blood supply to the middle portion of the tendon itself. There, the vascular supply arrives in two fundamentally different ways, outside or inside the tendon sheaths.

THE INTRATENDINOUS VASCULAR SUPPLY

This is distributed exclusively in the interfascicular spaces, which consist of connective tissue. The bundle of collagenous fibers is a functional unit, inside which no vessels can be seen. In the interspaces, there are numerous vessels which lie parallel to the fibers, with frequent transverse anastomoses, like the rungs of a ladder, joining to each other and to the main vascular channel.

EXPERIMENTAL WORK

In the extensors, with the possible exception of the extensor longus pollicis, tendon section does not lead to devascularization because of the abundant blood supply from the paratenon network.

Peacock[33] has studied and clearly described the blood supply of the flexor tendons (Fig. 7.4.1).

Veins and Lymphatics

These closely follow the arterial supply. There are usually two satellite veins to each artery.

The Nerves

These are confined exclusively to perivascular sympathetic fibers in the body of the tendon itself. The

TABLE 7.4.1
Active flexion of joints of fingers and thumb (compared to ventral position of 180°)

Digit	Joint	Thumb	Index	Middle	Ring	Little
Five digits	MP	140° (40°)	115 (65)	110 (70)	105 (75)	95 (85)
Thumb	IP	115 (65)				
Four other fingers	PIP		70 (110)	70 (110)	75 (105)	80 (100)
Four other fingers	DIP		125 (55)	120 (60)	115 (65)	110 (70)
Sum of the angles of excurison		105°	230°	240°	245°	255°

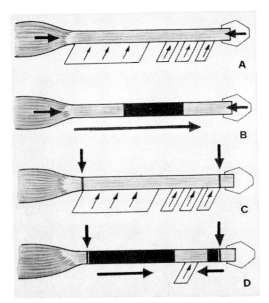

Figure 7.4.1. Diagram of Peacock's results (after Michon). Necrotic zones due to loss of vascularization are marked in *black*. Different interruptions of the blood supply are shown by *arrows*.

A. Normal routes of blood supply: musculotendinous junction; bony insertion; mesotenon at different levels; vincula (marked by *oblique arrows*).

B. Interruption of the blood supply via the mesotenon and the vinculae, causes wide necrosis of the middle section of the tendon, the extremities of the tendon survive. The vessels crossing the musculotendinous junction can support only the proximal third of the tendon, and those arriving from the bone can support the distal quarter of the tendon.

C. When the two extremities of the tendon are divided the blood supply brought by the mesotenon is sufficient to supply the whole tendon.

D. This diagram shows various combinations of vascular interruption, and the corresponding extent of the necrosis.

musculotendinous junction contains the neuromuscular corpuscles of Golgi and the neurotendinous spindles, which are clearly connected with the control of tension.

OPERATIVE INDICATIONS IN CASES OF BLOCAGE

Tenolysis

The logical treatment of blocage is tenolysis. It has a general application in many situations which have absence of sliding movement in common.

Bunnell[8] [9] has shown the relative frequency of this procedure in a general survey of the methods used after tendon repair. In 4438 tendon operations, of which the great majority were secondary and not primary, he gives the following figures (per cent): freeing (tenolysis), 41; grafting, 30: suturing, 18: transferring, 10; lengthening or shortening, 1.

Bunnell[9] writes, "Freeing tendons tops the list, because when one tendon is repaired, it is frequently necessary to free the adjoining tendons. A 41 per cent proportion of 4438 tendon operations is more than 1800 tenolyses, which puts this operation at the top of the list of operations of importance in hand surgery.

Technique and Indications for Tenolysis
Extensors

In principle, the scar of the accident should be avoided. The incision should be placed at a distance, preferable laterally, attempting to raise a flap with a lateral base and making it long enough to be able to reach healthy tissue above and below the adherent area. Proceeding from healthy tissue, the dissection approaches the adherent area, using the plane that separates the subcutaneous tissue from the tendon as a guide. When the scar is reached it is completely separated and freed. The deep surface of the tendon is then freed.

Tenolysis on the dorsum of the fingers or thumb may be valuable in cases in which suture of the tendon has been successful, as regards strength, but which leaves the finger with blocage in extension.

Flexors

Sutures in "no man's land" are followed by a certain incidence of blocage, which can be improved by tenolysis at about the third month after operation. This procedure has given us excellent results, provided that very careful technique is used.

SPECIAL PROBLEMS WITH DIFFERENT TOPOGRAPHIC ZONES

The anatomic view is not necessarily identical with the surgical viewpoint, so to distinguish all the possibilities of repair we must understand the problems of eight zones on the volar surface of the hand. We have numbered them from distal to proximal areas.

Repair of the Extensors

Recalling the character of tendon injuries on the dorsum of the digits, the hand, and the wrist, we distinguish four zones over the joints and four over the intermediate segments (Fig. 7.4.2).

The 269 cases of trauma to the extensor tendons which were observed were classified in Table 7.4.2.

Figure 7.4.3 demonstrates the details of the extensor apparatus of a digit, including the retinacular ligaments of Landsmeer, of which the functional importance has been demonstrated by Stack.[40]

TABLE 7.4.2
Distribution of injuries of extensor tendons among the 8 surgical topographic zones
(269 cases observed)

Zones	No. of Patients	No. of Tendons	Per Cent in Each Zone
1	35	37	14
2	13	14	5
3	44	48	18
4	34	37	14
5	49	52	19
6	41	60	22
7	8	19	7
8	2	2	1
Total	226	269	100

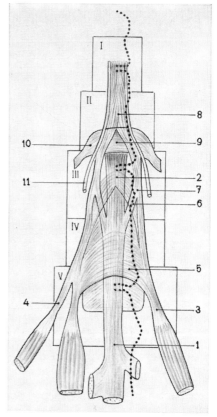

Figure 7.4.3. Details of the fasciculi of the extensor apparatus of a finger. Surgical topographic zones: *I, II, III, IV, V, 1,* tendon of the common extensor; *2,* median band near its point of insertion to the base of the middle phalanx; *3,* interosseous tendon; *4,* tendon of the lumbrical, on the radial side; *5,* superficial intertendinous sheets or dorsum; *6,* spiral fibers; *7,* lateral sheet; *8,* common terminal tendon; *9,* triangular sheet; *10,* transverse part of the retinacular ligament (Land smeer); *11,* oblique part of the retinacular ligament.

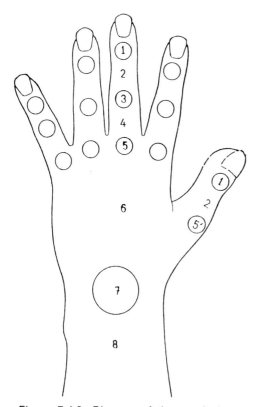

Figure 7.4.2. Diagram of the surgical topographic zones of the extensor apparatus.

ZONE 1. DORSUM OF THE DISTAL INTER-PHALANGEAL JOINT (Fig. 7.4.4)

Syndrome of Interruption

The flexion deformity of the distal phalanx is characteristic.

Treatment.

Primary Suture

In dealing with a wound of a joint, a primary repair is imperative, unless the delay is excessive. In the latter case, the finger should be immobilized in extension on a palmar splint with sterile dressings. When the wound is clean, operation is performed.

The essential in treatment is the maintenance of the joint in extension, or slight hyperextension, for at least six weeks. This may be done with a longitudinal metal wire across the joint or with two crossed wires (Fig. 7.4.5).

When the distal fragment is long enough, three buried sutures of 5-0 silk, or of fine nylon, inserted in a horizontal "U" give a satisfactory fixation. When the tendon is cut off flush with the bone, reinsertion is necessary. This is best accomplished with a removable stainless steel wire.

In wounds with loss of tendon substance, it is rare for the bone and joint to be intact. In this case, a tendon graft is performed, suturing the palmaris longus on each of the two lateral bands. When the joint is damaged it is better to perform a palliative procedure, such as arthrodesis. Fixation should be made in the following positions of flexion for the various fingers: index, 15°; middle, 20°; ring, 30°; and little, 35°.

Secondary Repair

The indications for a secondary repair depend on the disability of the flexion deformity of the distal phalanx, the presence of pain, tenderness, and awkwardness, the professional necessity, and occasionally for esthetic or cosmetic reasons. Two procedures are presented: a transverse section may be repaired by an overlapping suture, a plication of the tendon may be performed with smooth forceps, which are turned through a half "turn of the key." This technique has the advantage of not leaving any unsatisfied tendon ends, which fix themselves to the surrounding tissues and prevent movement.

Brooks recommends repair en bloc after a fusiform excision transversely of all the layers, skin and tendon on the dorsum of the distal interphalangeal joint.

ZONE 2. DORSUM OF THE MIDDLE PHALANX (Fig. 7.4.6)

The syndrome of interruption is the same as for Zone 1, but as a rule the flexion deformity of the distal phalanx is less marked because the capsule of the interphalangeal joint is intact.

Treatment

Primary repair of the extensor tendon is simple because the injury is away from the joint. The two lateral bands reunite in the middle line distal to the fine sheet that forms the triangular ligament (Fig. 7.4.6) and the transverse bands of the retinacular ligament of Landsmeer.

Operations

Simple approximating sutures are used with a horizontal loop, either of steel or 5-0 silk.

Secondary repairs offer no particular difficulties.

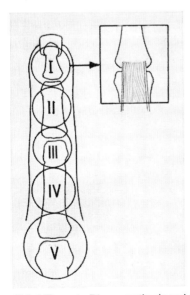

Figure 7.4.4 Zone 1. Diagramatic dorsal view

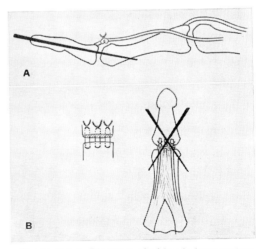

Figure 7.4.5. Diagram of wiring in hyperextension, to hold a tendon repair on the dorsum of the distal interphalangeal joint or in Zone 2. *A.* With one wire. *B.* With two wires.

ZONE 3. DORSUM OF THE PROXIMAL IN-TERPHALANGEAL JOINT (Fig. 7.4.7)

Anatomy

At this level, the extensor mechanism is complex. It is formed by the termination of the median band, corresponding to the distal insertion on the base of the middle phalanx of the proper and common extensors of the digits, and the two lateral bands which are the prolongations of the tendons of the interossei and the lumbricals. These three sheets are joined by the fine interlacements of the oblique fibers, which assure their functional interdependence while allowing some independence of movement. This central slip of the extensor tendon is in intimate contact with the capsule of the joint, so that the joint is usually opened when the tendon is divided.

Syndrome of Interruption

In fresh wounds with complete division, the whole width of the extensor apparatus is divided and also the capsule of the joint. The middle phalanx is under the influence of the flexors and is completely flexed.

A partial transection may occur. When the injury is dorsolateral, it can only involve one of the lateral bands, the symptoms will be negligible and the cut edges of the tendon will remain practically in contact, when the finger is extended at the interphalangeal joints, and flexed at the metacarpophalangeal joint.

When the section involves the median band only, the problem is more serious because it is seldom recognized. It is possible that the triangular ligament maintains the two lateral bands in position, as the axis of traction remains behind the axis of the joint.

However, if there is a longitudinal paramedian tearing of the expansion, with rupture of the triangular ligament, the two lateral bands slip anteriorly and form

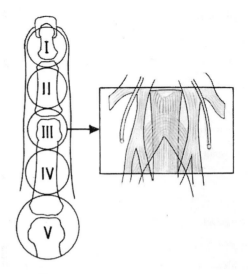

Figure 7.4.7. Diagram of Zone 3

a buttonhole, through which the joint projects, so that the proximal interphalangeal joint is flexed. At the same time, the two lateral bands exert an exaggerated traction on the distal phalanx, which becomes hyperextended. This position is characteristic of the buttonhole or boutonniere deformity.

The wounds of Zone 3 are the most important of all those of the extensor apparatus and among the most frequent.

Treatment

Injuries in this area present three therapeutic problems: coverage of the joint, prevention of arthritis, and repair of the tendon. The coverage of the joint requires a plastic repair when skin has been lost. This may be performed by using local flaps with one or two pedicles, combined often with a free graft. The prevention of arthritis is important. The closing of the joint may be preceded by careful excision of the wound and washing out of the joint with physiologic saline. It is desirable to immobilize the hand in elevation. In view of the minor degree of retraction of the cut ends of the tendon, enlargement of the wound is usually not necessary. We make one incision on one side of the finger.

In secondary operations, a longitudinal dorsolateral incision has the advantage of placing the scar not over the repair of the tendon, and thus reducing the possibility of adhesions.

In a recent clean cut, a primary repair should be performed. Failure is seldom due to the giving away of the suture line, but more often to the absence of sliding and the development of stiffness in extension.

Tenolysis after Primary Suture

Frequently, fibrous tissue fixation on the dorsum of the finger may be so firm that traction is of no value. Tenolysis gives excellent results.

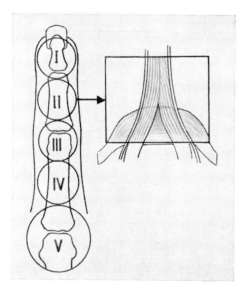

Figure 7.4.6. Zone 2. Diagramatic dorsal view

Secondary Repair

Success of secondary repair depends on the presence of full passive extension. If passive extension is not present, it may possibly be recovered by the use of a dynamic splint. After recovery of passive extension, secondary repair of the tendon may be performed. In relatively fresh cases it is possible to discover the line of demarcation between the normal tendon tissue and the newly formed bridge of scar tissue. The scar tissue is excised and the tendon sutured together, edge to edge, after separation of the different bands.

Repair of the Buttonhole

Open wounds usually involve the tendon only. Other elements of the joint are intact and capable of sliding, provided that there has been no infection.

Treatment

Excision of the central mass has also been suggested, but to bring only one-half of the lateral bands to the midline, thus forming a new median band, and at the same time conserving the lateral bands, although reduced in size.

The operation suggested by Planas[34] consists of dividing one of the lateral bands at its proximal end, transferring it to the middle of the finger, and suturing it to the distal end of the cut median band. It is possible to obtain extension of the proximal interphalangeal joint after three weeks of immobilization, but flexion of the distal interphalangeal joint takes several months.

Stack[40] has remarked that the longitudinal excursion of the median band, which is about 8 mm, is entirely absorbed on flexion of the proximal interphalangeal joint. If the lateral bands did not glide sideways over the side of this joint it would be impossible for the distal interphalangeal joint to flex.

Personal Operation for Repair of Buttonhole Deformity

The operation consists of dissecting the three principal tendon sheets from each other, over a distance of several centimeters, from the base of the middle phalanx to the distal third of the proximal phalanx. The oblique fibers which join the median and the lateral bands are divided, and the sheet is lifted carefully with fine hooks to avoid damaging the underlying periosteum.

When the lesion is relatively recent, the bridge of new fibrous tissue may be resected and the tendon repaired. If necessary, a reinsertion may be performed.

The majority of cases present problems for the resection of the new bridge of scar. With the finger in full extension, enough of the scar is resected, permitting end-to-end suture of the median band without the folding (Fig. 7.4.8). The lateral bands are then replaced in their physiologic positions and held there by a few fine catgut sutures to avoid the three bands becoming fixed together and preventing flexion of the finger (Fig. 7.4.8).

Tenotomy of the Extensor for Long-Standing Buttonhole Deformity

For old cases with marked hyperextension of the distal phalanx, Dolphin[11] has proposed that a transection of the central part of the terminal tendon is carried out at the level of the middle phalanx. As a result of this, the patient is again capable of extending and flexing the distal phalanx is usually about 45°. An explanation of this phenomenon is suggested by Stack.[40] By the division of the central part of the terminal tendon, the diamond of tendon making up the main part of the aponeurosis is allowed to move proximally, the hyperextension of the distal phalanx is relaxed, and active extension of the distal phalanx is then carried out by the oblique part of the retinacular ligament of Landsmeer, which is in a state of some contracture. The main force of extension is by means of the median band, which had previously been too long. A physiologic state is recovered and extension of the middle phalanx returns.

ZONE 4. DORSUM OF THE PROXIMAL PHALANX (Fig. 7.4.9)

What has been written about primary and secondary repairs on Zone 2 applies also to Zone 4. Partial lesions are common by reason of the curved shape of the phalanx and the consequent protection of the lateral bands. This is the area of the "dossiere" and repair is seldom performed without being complicated by adhesions (Fig. 7.4.9). Ocasionally, isolated damage to a lateral band on the radial side of the finger may justify an attempt at repair with a graft attached to the lumbrical.

ZONE 5. DORSUM OF THE METACARPOPHALANGEAL JOINT (Fig. 7.4.10)

Syndrome of Interruption

Transection of the extensor apparatus consisting of the common extensor alone in the middle and ring, and combined with the proper extensor in the index and little, causes flexion deformity of the proximal phalanx. The fragments never retract far. The diagnosis is quite simple in a fresh case but may be more difficult in an old case where there is a bridge of fibrous tissue between the ends of the tendon.

Treatment
Primary Repair

The tendon is strong. Retraction of the proximal end seldom exceeds 1 or 2 cm. The severity of the injury depends on whether or not the joint is involved. In principle, primary suture should be performed.

The tendon repair is performed with sutures in the "U" shape, passed in the thickness of the tendon in such a way as to avoid transfixion to the underlying synovial tissue. It is completed with a few simple 5-0 silk sutures in the lateral wings.

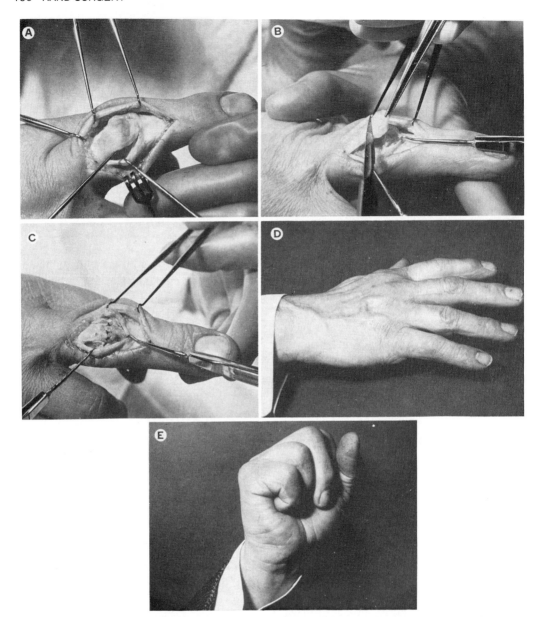

Figure 7.4.8. Personal method for repair of the buttonhole deformity. *A.* Preparation of the three tendon bands. *B.* Resection of the fibrous bridge. *C.* End-to-end suture of the shortened median band, to a small collar left at the distal point of insertion at the base of the middle phalanx (buried 5-0 silk). *D.* and *E.* Results: complete extension, flexion very slightly limited.

Secondary Repair

Secondary repair is performed when the primary suture fails or when the original injury was not recognized.

Lesions of the Lateral Wings

Luxation of the extensor tendons may occur. Besides division of the tendon proper, there are also lesions of the aponeurotic wings. The important element is the band which joins the extensor tendons from tendons of the interossei. Wounds of the bands should be repaired primarily when conditions are favorable, or secondarily when unfavorable.

When conditions prevent simple end-to-end repair, another technique is necessary. Michon[29] has devoted much thought to the repair of these conditions and recommends the following. Reconstruction of the band may be performed with a junctura tendinum (Wheeldon) or by means of a band taken off the extensor tendon itself.

ZONE 6. DORSUM OF THE HAND (Fig. 7.4.11)

Syndrome of Interruption

The symptoms are similar to those occurring with division in Zone 5 but with many variations because of the intertendinous sheets or junctura tendinum that can mask an injury. With a fresh lesion the problem is simple because the tendons can be visualized. In a late case, scarring may fix the cut ends and produce a tenodesis. This is also true in Zones 7 and 8.

Treatment
Primary Suture

When conditions are satisfactory, a primary suture should always be performed. With a small enlarge-

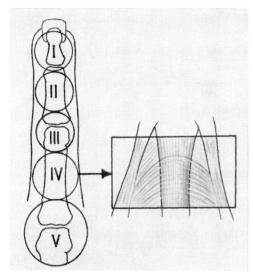

Figure 7.4.9. Zone 4. Diagrammatic dorsal view

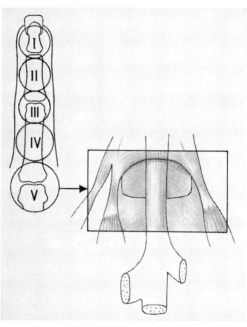

Figure 7.4.10. Diagram of Zone 5

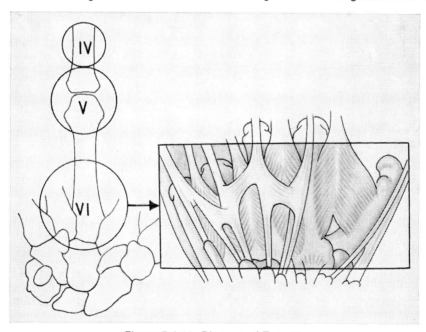

Figure 7.4.11. Diagram of Zone 6

ment of the wound and by gentle massage of the muscle belly, one can usually retrieve the proximal end of the cut tendon and repair the tendon.

Secondary Repair

Secondary repairs are necessary, with failure of a primary repair, for lesions that had not been observed, and for injuries in which the general conditions were not suitable for a primary repair.

Grafts of the Extensors. With secondary repairs, in cases with loss of substance of the tendons, it is better to use a graft rather than to attach the tendon to a neighbor, as a "Y" which leads to some disturbance of equilibrium and loss of individual function. The palmaris longus, when present, is the tendon of choice. If absent, a part of a neighboring tendon may be used. The possibility should also be kept in mind of utilizing the proper extensors of the index and little fingers for the middle and ring fingers, respectively.

When the loss is great, it is necessary to use a pedicled flap from a distance. At a later date, it is possible to insert multiple long tendon grafts. The best sources for these grafts are the plantaris and the extensors of the toes. The proximal anastomosis should be made well above the wrist and the dorsal aponeurosis of the forearm and a part of the annular ligament is resected to avoid adhesions. A short band should be left at the wrist to act as a pulley (Fig. 7.4.12).

ZONE 7. DORSUM OF THE WRIST (Fig. 7.4.13)

Syndrome of Interruption

One should systematically examine each finger individually and note the combination of flexion of the middle and ring, and also extension of the index and little, where proper extensors are independent of the common extensors.

Treatment
Primary Repair

This region is unfavorable for the repair of extensor tendons where they pass through the osseofibrous canals and are supplied with synovial sheaths. The excursion may be as much as 5.5. cm (Fig. 7.4.14). When the callus lies distal to the annular ligament, extension of the fingers is limited. To avoid these problems, resection of the dorsal annular ligament is performed.

Extensors of the Wrist

At this level, two types of tendon injury are seen. On the ulnar side of the wrist, the extensor carpi ulnaris and the extensors of the little finger may be involved. On the radial side, the two radial extensors of the wrist, the tendons of the long abductor and the long and short extensors of the thumb, are often transected. Care must be taken to suture the radial extensors, which are very deeply placed.

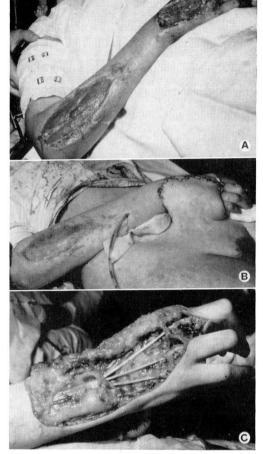

Figure 7.4.12. Multiple grafts of the extensors after repair of an extensive loss of substance on the dorsum of the right hand, in Zones 6 and 7. *A.* Auto accident, with the dorsum of the hand and the forearm scraped on a wall. Loss of the extensors of the three ulnar fingers. *B.* Application of a pedicled abdominal flap. *C.* Tendon grafts taken from the extensors of the toes.

THE THUMB

The repair of tendon injuries on the dorsum of the interphalangeal joint of the thumb is analogous to that of the other fingers and has the same indications as in Zone 1. The metacarpophalangeal joint is not quite equivalent either to the proximal interphalangeal joints or to the metacarpophalangeal joints of the fingers. This zone is designated as Zone 5 (Fig. 7.4.10).

The extensor apparatus of the thumb is complex, formed not only by the long and the short extensor tendons, but also by oblique fibers coming from elements on the palmar side, particularly the expansions of the short abductor (Fig. 7.4.14).

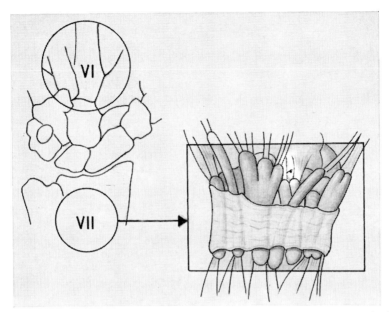

Figure 7.4.13. Diagram of Zone 7, with the synovial sheaths beneath the annular ligament

Syndrome of Interruption

This is characterized by a flexion deformity of the distal phalanx when the long extensor is divided. If only the insertion of the short extensor is damaged, the tendon injury may be overlooked, although there is some disturbance of equilibrium which gives an exaggerated dorsal extension. When both the tendons are divided, extension is lost at both the interphalangeal and metacarpophalangeal joints.

Treatment

Primary and secondary repairs do not give very different results. The sheet is large and sutures hold well. When the skin cover permits, a secondary graft of the long extensor may restore function in the thumb.

ZONES 6 AND 7 IN THE THUMB. FIRST METACARPAL-CARPAL REGION, WRIST REGION (Fig. 7.4.14)

We will study separately the two groups of tendons which diverge to form the anatomic snuffbox.

Repair of the Short Extensor and the Long Abductor of the Thumb
Syndrome of Interruption

Transection of the short extensor of the thumb is often unnoticed when the long extensor is intact because the long extensor also extends the proximal phalanx on the first metacarpal.

Transection of the long abductor is more serious. It is an important tendon, arising from a powerful muscle. Repair necessitates the excision of the sheath.

Repair of the Long Extensor of the Thumb

This tendon merits separate attention as it is most important in the function of the thumb. It forms the medial boundary of the snuffbox. This tendon is easily injured, frequently in butchers with choppers, gardeners with billhooks, and woodcutters with axes. Most of these injuries lie over the first metacarpal (Zone 6). The proximal end retracts considerably.

Primary Suture

It is better to make a separate short incision transversely on the dorsum of the wrist, and occasionally, a second proximal incision. One then constructs a tunnel subcutaneously towards the injury. The tendon is reintroduced with a guide suture which can be used for repair. Repair may be performed in the original wound. A laced suture after Cuneo, or a Bunnell steel suture, may be used. The thumb alone is immobilized in extension by means of a plaster cast. The cast maintains the thumb in hyperextension. The thumb is immobilized for five weeks.

Secondary Repair

Secondary repair of the long extensor of the thumb usually cannot be satisfactorily performed by end-to-end suture. It is often necessary to perform a tendon graft with the palmaris longus. The proximal attachment of the graft should be made near the musculotendinous junction. The distal attachment should be at the middle of the first metacarpal.

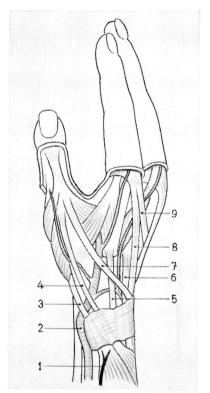

Figure 7.4.14. Radial view of the wrist, showing particularly the extensor apparatus of the thumb, and the anatomic snuffbox. *1.* Cutaneous branches of the radial nerve, interrupted to clarify the drawings. Care must be taken to preserve these branches when operating on this area. *2.* Radial artery. *3.* Abductor pollicis longus. *4.* Extensor pollicis brevis.[5] Extensor carpi radialis longus. *6.* Extensor carpi radialis brevis. *7.* Extensor pollicis longus. *8.* Extensor digitorum communis. *9.* Extensor indicis proprius.

ZONE 8. DISTAL FOURTH OF THE FOREARM (Fig. 7.4.15)

Wounds in this area involve the extensors of the fingers and also, as in Zone 7, the two radial extensors, the ulnar extensor, and occasionally the supinator longus. The fact that these injuries lie close to the musculotendinous junctions means that one can usually perform good repairs.

Primary Repair

End-to-end suture does not of itself offer any difficulty. A shoe lace, double right angle stitch with steel or silk may be used. The antebrachial fascia is thick, very strong and is the most frequent cause of blocage. It is therefore necessary to excise the antebrachial fascia, removing the whole fibrous roof which will cover the zone of movement of the tendon junction. A

plaster cast maintains immobilization with the wrist in dorsiflexion and the fingers in semiflexion.

The radial extensors and the ulnar extensors are in a muscular zone, or a musculotendinous zone, and the repair offers no difficulty. The same is true for the tendon of the supinator longus, which may also be divided and found when exploring wounds on the radial side of the forearm.

Secondary Repair

It is only after skin healing and union of the bones that repair of the tendons may be performed, usually by grafts.

FLEXOR TENDONS

The classification that we have adopted seems practical from a surgical point of view (Fig. 7.4.16). Zone 2 for the fingers and Zone 3 for the thumb correspond to the "no man's land" of Bunnell. Michon and I[51] reported 335 cases of flexor tendon injuries, the distribution of the lesions being noted in Table 7.4.3.

Syndrome of Interruption of the Flexor Tendons

In the fingers, when the two flexor tendons are sectioned, the middle and distal phalanges cannot be flexed. When the deep flexor alone is divided, the middle phalanx can be flexed at the proximal interphalangeal joint by the superficial flexor.

In a test of division of the superficial tendon, the neighboring fingers are maintained in complete extension. This draws the common muscle belly distally and prevents the deep flexor of the finger under examination from moving. This creates a syndrome which allows the examination of the function of the superficial tendon in isolation (Apley's test).

The seven topographic zones on the palmar surface will be investigated from a proximal to distal area.

ZONE 7. AT THE WRIST (Fig. 7.4.17)

The Syndrome of Interruption

This is often complicated by motor paralysis of the intrinsic muscles of the hand. In many cases, surgical exploration alone gives a complete assessment of the extent of injury. When the flexor tendons are in flexion at the time of injury, the distal tendon ends disappear, when the fingers extend, under the anterior annular ligament. In such a case one should transect the annular ligament and proceed with repair.

Primary Operations

Section of one or all of the flexors of the wrist is often encountered. The palmaris longus has little importance, whereas the flexor carpi radialis and flexor carpi ulnaris, the main stabilizers of the wrist, must be repaired. When all the flexors of the fingers are divided, it is essential to suture the flexor pollicis longus

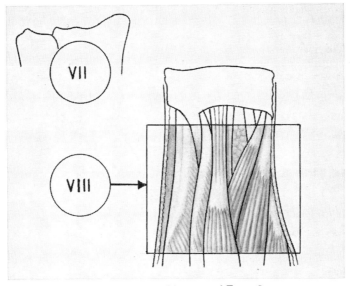

Figure 7.4.15. Diagram of Zone 8

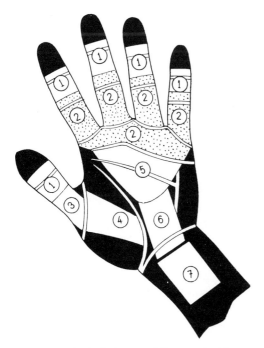

Figure 7.4.16. Scheme of the surgical topographic zones of the flexon tendons.

TABLE 7.4.3
Incidence in different zones, with 355 cases of flexor tendon injuries (Verdan and Michon)

Zone	No. of Cases	Per Cent
1	87	26
2	146	44
3	33	10
4	7	2
5	28	8
6	6	2
7	28	8
Total	335	100

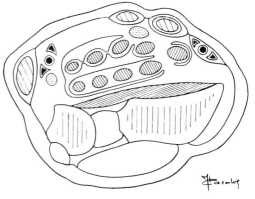

Figure 7.4.17. Cross section of wrist in Zone 7

and the four deep flexors. When the superficial flexors alone are divided, the index, middle, and ring finger tendons may be repaired and the little finger tendon abandoned, as it is small and unimportant. The ends of the nerves should be brought together and fixed with 5-0 silk sutures.

Early Secondary Operations

This method has the advantage of a single operation for both the tendons and the nerves. The tendons are well vascularized in this region and do not undergo necrosis. The cut ends when freshened readily lend themselves to suture, and there is little loss of muscular contractility at this time. The nerves may at this time be repaired with certainty as to the point of section to obtain healthy tissue. The neurilemma is sufficiently thick to allow easy suture. When after several months functional improvement ceases, one may always perform a tenolysis, combined with a neurolysis to reduce traction on the nerve and to reduce pain.

ZONE 6. CARPAL TUNNEL (Figs. 7.4.18 and 7.4.19)

Anatomic and Clinical Features

The tendons are canalized in a narrow passage, on top of each other, with the median nerve in front (Fig. 7.4.19). Wounds which penetrate the annular ligament are few in number, for to produce injury they must pass between the bony edges of the tunnel and enter the depths of this osseofibrous canal.

Syndrome of Interruption

Transection of the long flexor of the thumb and the deep flexors of the fingers are obvious. Section of the superficial flexors may pass unnoticed unless they are carefully tested.

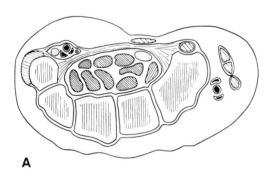

A

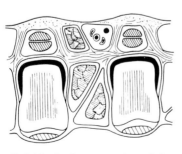

B

Figure 7.4.18. A. Cross section of the carpal tunnel. *B.* Cross section of the midpalm.

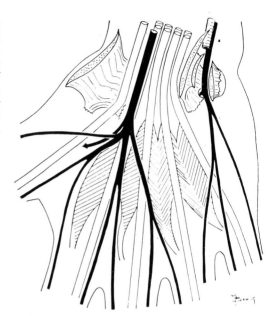

Figure 7.4.19. Topographic diagram of the carpal tunnel and the palm.

Primary or Secondary Repair

When a small penetrating wound has sectioned tendons in a deep space, with difficult surgical access, a very long palmar incision and complete division of the volar carpal ligament is required. One may two or three weeks later perform a secondary reconstruction under aseptic conditions. This procedure includes repair of the median nerve and tenorrhaphies. It is proper to perform no repair of the superficial tendons with the exception of that to the index.

For the associated section of the nerve, we proceed on the same plan as in Zone 7, as far as there are motor nerve lesions. Our principle of secondary suture applies only to mixed nerves. It does not apply to sensory branches, which are more peripheral, and where a primary nerve suture may be performed.

ZONE 5. MIDDLE OF THE PALM (Figs. 7.4.18 and 7.4.19)

Anatomic and Clinical Features

The flexor tendons make their exit from the carpal tunnel and diverge to become rearranged in groups of two superimposed tendons and are now more vulnerable. In this area tendon injuries are often associated with transection of one or more of the digital nerves.

Syndrome of Interruption

This is evident in cases of division of the deep flexors or of both the tendons. Division of the superficial tendon usually passes unnoticed in an emergency.

Treatment
Primary Repair

The rule is immediate tendon suture. A section of the superficial flexor, with an intact deep flexor, does not require repair. When the wound is clean, primary suture is performed. The tendon suture should be covered with paratenon to avoid adhesions to the palmar fascia. The deep flexor should be repaired at a primary operation because, apart from the musculotendinous junction, this is one of the most favorable sites for the repair of the flexor tendons.

Secondary Repair

In old cases, with the presence of retraction and loss of substance of the deep flexor, repair by a graft is usually necessary.

The Nerves

They are at this level purely sensory and trophic. Whether nerves should be repaired primarily or by a delayed procedure is controversial. Certainly it is desirable to allow the reestablishment of good nutrition with the least possible delay, as well as the recovery of sensation. Usually, we perform a primary repair of the tendons and a repair of nerves that are easily placed end to end.

DIGITAL CANALS

Fingers and Thumb

This region is totally different from all others. The two tendons are molded on one another. One tendon perforates another and both pass into an osteofibrous canal, like a piston into a cylinder.

In our scheme of topographic zones for the fingers (Fig. 7.4.16) we divided the digital canal into two zones. Zone 1 is the part of the canal occupied by the deep flexor tendon alone. In Zone 2 both tendons are present and are closely connected to each other.

We may further divide Zone 1 into two parts. A distal part is near the flexion crease of the distal interphalangeal joint. Here the synovial sheath is very thin beyond the pulley on the middle phalanx. A proximal part corresponds to the fibrous pulley on the middle phalanx where the deep flexor fits snugly. Our surgical experience confirms these facts: a common block of the superficial and deep flexors, provided it is free over-all, can permit very satisfactory function of the whole finger. The method of repair of Bsteh,[7] who sutures systematically the two tendons, one to the other, is an equally convincing proof.

Zones 2 for the fingers and 3 for the thumb have been numbered for the sake of simplicity.

Zone 1. The Four Fingers
Syndrome of Interruption

Wounds in Zone 1 divide the deep flexor only. There is a loss of active flexion of the distal phalanx and instability of hyperextension of the distal inter-

phalangeal joint. This latter can be the greater disability, particularly in the index and middle fingers.

Treatment

Primary and Secondary Repair. I believe that in the majority of cases primary repair should be performed. Two methods are available: (1) an end-to-end suture; (2) the reinsertion by advancement of the proximal end of the tendon. The first is preferable to the second.

A secondary end-to-end suture may be performed with excellent results, provided that the proximal end has not retracted too far.

We think that it is better to resect the tendon ends and perform a tendon suture, rather than leave the distal tendon, and shorten the tendon in the palm or at the wrist.

It is generally agreed that the advancement and reinsertion of the proximal end cannot be done unless the loss of substance is less than 2 cm. There may be marked limitation of extension with advancement. Rather than resect the small distal end which remains, we save it and perform an end-to-end suture instead of a reinsertion.

Operation. An incision is made in the midlateral line. A wide resection of the sheath and pulley on the middle phalanx is performed to assure sliding of the tendon junction. The distal phalanx is fixed in semiflexion across the distal interphalangeal joint with a stainless steel wire (0.9 mm). An exact suturing with four cardinal stiches of buried 6-0 silk is performed (Fig. 7.4.20).

Nerve suture may be performed throughout the length of the middle phalanx. The nerve breaks up into numerous small branches at the flexion creases of the distal interphalangeal joints and beyond this repair is impossible.

The Thumb
Syndrome of Interruption

This is the same for the three zones. There is a loss of active flexion of the interphalangeal joint with preservation of flexion of the metacarpophalangeal joint by the short flexor of the thumb.

In Zone 4, a division of the thenar muscles in very common. The division of a motor branch of the median nerve complicates the problem.

Treatment

Primary Repair. Wounds in Zone 1 of the thumb, at the interphalangeal crease, may be sutured primarily. Recovery is usually excellent. When the proximal end is shortened by more than 1 or 2 cm, one may lengthen the tendon at the musculotendinous junction, after the technique of Rouhier.[38] This is also recommended by Nigst and Megevand,[32] who perform it routinely with good results.

Zone 3 of the thumb is like Zone 2 in the fingers — in a "restricted area." Zone 3 may also be divided into two functionally different regions from the point of

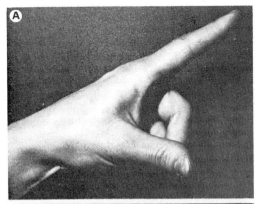

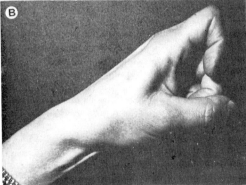

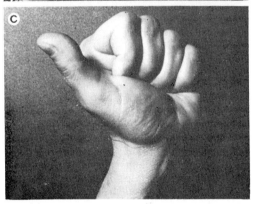

Figure 7.4.20. A, B, and *C.* Result of a primary repair of the deep flexor in Zone 1.

view of the tendon scar, the region of the pulley on the proximal phalanx, and the narrow region, corresponding to the level of the sesamoids and the metacarpal ring. The wounds of the first part will be treated by primary suture like those of the Zone 1 of the fingers, accompanied by wide resection of the fibrous sheath, up to about 1 cm proximal to the point where the tendon callus reaches, when the thumb is flexed actively at the interphalangeal joint. For wounds of the second part, a primary repair is not performed unless the metacarpal pulley is widely excised.

Secondary Repair. In Zones 1 and 3, end-to-end

sutures and reinsertions may be performed as secondary operations, with the exception of the proximal half of Zone 3. The more distal the suture line, the more is the likelihood of avoiding blocage by adhesions.

Wounds of Zone 4 involve the mass of the thenar musculature, in the middle of which the long flexor tendon is located. Tendon injuries in this region are suitable for a primary suture. Occasionally, transplantation of the superficial flexor of the ring finger to the flexor pollicis longus is a useful method. This is particularly valuable in old injuries in which there has been dengeneration of the tendon or atrophy of the muscle belly.

Zone 2. Of the Fingers (Fig. 7.4.16)

Despite the recent advances in our understanding of tendon physiology and its reparative processes, the therapeutic approach to severance of both flexor tendons in the digital canal remains controversial. The suggested solutions include primary or secondary suture with or without tenolysis, primary or secondary tendon graft (autograft or homograft), grafting of an homologous complete flexor mechanism, transfer of an adjacent sublimis, prosthetic tendon inserts, tenodesis, and arthrodesis. In more extensive injuries with both nerves and arteries sectioned in a single digit, amputation is often advised.

The area of greatest debate concerns Bunnell's "no man's land" - Zone 2 (Verdan).[48] Certainly the most common solution among experienced hand surgeons, when both tendons are cut, is a secondary graft, attached to the profundus, combined with sublimis excision. This procedure follows the injury from several weeks to several months; additionally, if, as reported by Fetrow,[12] a secondary tenolysis is required in 16 per cent of grafts (60 tenolyses out of 374 grafts performed by Pulvertaft[35]), the period of disability will range from three to six months or more. Good results from grafting as reported by Boyes[2 3] and Pulvertaft[35 36] are not easily duplicated. Such treatment remains the best solution when trained hand surgeons are not available for the initial care, or where the wound is untidy.

But under optimal conditions in the handling of freshly injured cases and for clean, fresh, tidy wounds, as is often seen with flexor tendon lacerations, we wish again to call attention to the possibility of direct tendon suture. Primary and secondary tendon suture in Zone 2, as well as tendon grafts, have been performed by Verdan[45 47 48 49 50 51] and his staff since 1951.

Progressive improvement in technique and results prompted this review of recent cases. It is our belief that skilful primary or secondary repair, even if it requires a second tenolysis,[45] gives results equal to or better than tendon grafts and shortens the period of disability.

In comparing the results of our primary sutures for section of both the flexor tendons in Zone 2 with those of secondary grafts, we have established curves on our graphs indicating the results, calculated by the simplified system of distance on flexion from the distal pulp to the distal palmar crease. We have obtained the curves shown in Graphs 7.4.1 and 7.4.2. These comparable graphs are based as separate curves on good and bad cases, and we have established a means by which we can judge the entire picture. For the two methods the results are very close, and in about 50 per cent of the cases the pulp reaches to 3 cm

or less from the distal palmar crease. However, the result for the secondary grafts is slightly below 50 per cent and that for primary sutures is a little above 50 per cent.

We have recognized other advantages in the method that we follow. They are as follows:

1. We allow for a delay of up to 12 hours and adequate preparation of the wound before intervention. This means that primary repair may be carried out on practically all cases of wounds in this region

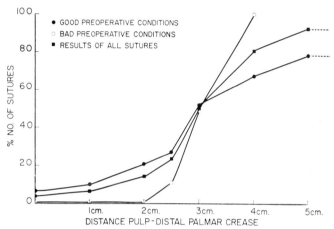

Graph 7.4.1. Primary sutures for division of both flexor tendons in Zone 2 of the fingers. Total number of fingers involved, 27 with 7 tenolyses. Good preoperative conditions, 19 (4 failures); bad preoperative conditions, 8 (0 failures (some limited extension)); number of digital nerves involved, 19; failures leading to graft, 3; failures with rupture, 1. Failures represent 15 per cent of all cases. Graph shows the results of our primary repairs in Zone 2 for transection of both flexor tendons. The results are classified according to the distance: pulp-distal palmar crease. More than 50 per cent of the cases are within 3 cm.

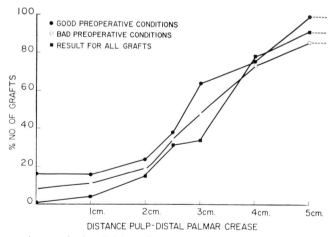

Graph 7.4.2. Secondary grafts for division of the two flexor tendons in Zone 2 (or of one alone; but with elimination of the flexor digitorum sublimis, in a bad state, at the time of the graft). Total number of fingers grafted, 45. Good preoperative conditions, 18 (no failures); bad preoperative conditions, 27 (4 failures); number with associated nerve lesion, 28. Results of secondary grafts in Zone 2, are shown. Classified according to the distance: pulp-distal palmar crease. Less than 50 per cent of the cases are within 3 cm.

that are clean, incised, or only slightly contused by a competent team.

2. The general practitioners and the general surgeons have been invited to send these cases to the center for primary repair or secondary graft, as indicated. Grujic and Buta always perform primary repair of the flexor tendons, whatever its site may be, and obtain an incidence of incapacity as low as 51 days. As many as 62 of these were situated in Zone 2, out of a total of 227 flexor tendon divisions.

3. If the nonspecialized surgeons were bold enough to perform tendon grafts, they may also attempt to perform primary sutures with a greater hope of success.

Seventy-six patients had primary or secondary flexor tendon suture in the digital canal, performed during a five-year period from 1 January 1965 to 1 January 1970 (Verdan and Crawford[49]). Sixty-six of these patients were reviewed and examined. Thirty-two of them had isolated profundus lesions anatomically occurring in Zone 1. The remaining 34 patients with 36 involved fingers, had injuries in Zone 2, "no man's land." In order to compare more easily these results with those of the tendon grafts, the system of Boyes[3] was utilized. The digits represented in the following graphs are those which extend to within 40 degrees (computed by adding the extension deficits of all joints) for the index and middle, and to within 60 degrees of full extension for the ring and little fingers. The distance between the tip and the distal palmar crease (DPC) for the middle, ring, and little fingers, and the distal portion of the midpalmar crease for the index were recorded. We recognize the limitations of this system, since a digit which touches the palm 1 cm from the distal palmar crease is clearly better than a digit which does not touch, yet is still 3 cm from the crease.[47]

TECHNIQUE

The tendon repair is usually performed through a classical midlateral incision with little regard to the wound. The nerves, if severed, are repaired at the end of the operation. Tendon sheath excision is performed so that the site of the sutured tendons can freely glide without contacting the sheath, and this sheath excision is estimated by knowing the tendon gliding amplitude at each level. The average distance for excision is approximately 3 cm. The tendons are sutured with four interrupted epitendinous simple or U-shaped sutures by use of 5-0 or 6-0 siliconized silk. Such delicate suture is sufficient once the proximal portion of the profundus has been transfixed (blocked suture) by a transverse stainless steel pin (diameter: 7/10 mm) to the adjacent skin and sheath. Occasionally, this pin is not used, the digit is held in flexion by a suture through the tip and the palm, and the adjacent fingers immobilized with the MP joint moderately flexed, and the interphalangeal joints in near full extension. The

wrist is immobilized in moderate flexion. Three weeks postoperatively the immobilization is discontinued, the pin is removed, and gentle active motion exercises are begun.

RESULTS

This series includes 34 patients with 36 fingers with Zone 2 injuries. Two patients had two fingers injured. The average age was 23 years with the range from 2 to 54 (see Table 7.4.4). There were 20 males and 14 females. Sixteen of these patients had digital nerve lacerations; and of these 16, five had both digital nerves sectioned.

Of the 36 fingers, 31 had sufficient extension to be included under the Boyes[3] evaluation system as described earlier. Of the five excluded cases, three were excluded because of extension deficits. One digit eventually required amputation (following a desperate attempt to save an index finger in a hand with a previous thumb amputation: the index damage included severance of both tendons, arteries and nerves). One patient underwent a secondary tendon graft following a poor result from primary repair and achieved an excellent result. It is of interest that of the five fingers in the complete series where both digital nerves were sectioned, three fell into this small excluded group.

Of the 31 included fingers, 15 were treated primarily and 16 secondarily. Twelve digits require secondary tenolysis to achieve the results reported. Three possibilities exist: (a) both tendons were sutured; (b) the profundus was sutured and the sublimis excised; (c) the profundus alone had been severed and was repaired.

Suture of Both the Profundus and the Sublimis

This approach to the problem of severed tendons in "no man's land" has been used only in recent years, with encouraging results. Repair of both flexor tendons is certainly new when compared with the other known techniques. Its adoption was prompted by a desire to preserve the tendon vascularity arriving through the vinculae or mesotenon. These vessels are

TABLE 7.4.4
Age of the 29 patients (31 fingers)

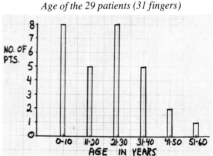

usually injured during sublimis resection (Fig. 7.4.21 A, B. C).

Fourteen fingers in 14 patients had surgical repair of both tendons in Zone 2. Ten of these were performed as primary treatment and four secondarily. The average age in this group was 24 years; five of the 14 were children, the eldest being nine years of age. Seven of these fingers had digital nerve divisions, and two of the seven had both nerves sectioned (Fig. 7.4.22 A to E).

As noted on Table 7.4.5, 90 per cent were able to flex to within 2.5 cm (1 inch) of the distal palmar crease (Fig. 7.4.23 A and B).

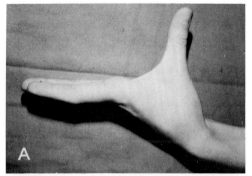
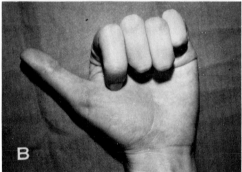
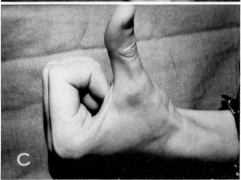

Figure 7.4.21. Primary suture of both flexor tendons without secondary tenolysis. *A.* Complete extension of index finger, 2½ years after primary repair of both flexor tendons. *B.* and *C.* Flexion of index finger to within 1 cm of distal palmar crease.

Suture of the Profundus with Sublimis Excision

Eleven digits had sublimis excision at the time of profundus repair. Two of these were performed primarily, nine secondarily. Five had associated digital nerve divisions and one of these had both nerves severed.

In this group 55 per cent (Table 7.4.25) were able to flex to within 2.5 cm of the distal palmar crease (Fig. 7.4.24 A and B).

Suture of the Profundus

Six digits involved only profundus severance although the anatomical site of the lesion was in Zone 2. Two cases were seen initially and primary repairs were performed. As expected, only one case had an associated nerve lesion. All six digits were able to flex within 2.5 cm of the distal palmar crease.

Comparison of Primary and Secondary Repair

As can be seen from the preceding tables, fresh clean lacerations of both tendons are usually treated by repair of both tendons. In secondary situations the sublimis is usually excised. Table 7.4.6 compares the results of our Zone 2 repairs with regard to primary or secondary treatment. Sixty-eight per cent of cases sutured secondary could flex to at least within 2.5 cm of the distal palmar crease, while 93 per cent of cases repaired primarily could flex to at least within 2.5 cm.

DISCUSSION

As has been long advocated by one of us,[47] flexor tendon suture in almost any region performed by experienced hand surgeons can give excellent results. We believe that primary tendon repair in cleanly cut wounds in the digital canal will produce results equal to if not better than tendon grafts. This point of view has been confirmed by other authors.[1][21] Such results, of course, are achieved much more quickly than with secondary grafts, thereby shortening the patient's period of unemployment and lessening the associated medical costs.

The previously accepted reliance on tendon grafts is undoubtedly too rigid. We know that good results may be achieved with secondary suture, but the results of primary suture are certainly better. In primary repair both tendons may be sutured, realizing that 30 to 40 per cent will require a secondary tenolysis. In this series only four cases had secondary repair of both tendons, and the results of these were no different from the primary group; but the number of secondary cases is too small for definitive statements. It should be noted (Table 7.4.5) that the results of profundus suture will sublimis excision were decidedly inferior and that this group of cases was done secondarily (nine of the 11 fingers).

In an attempt to distinguish better the results of primary from secondary treatment of severance to

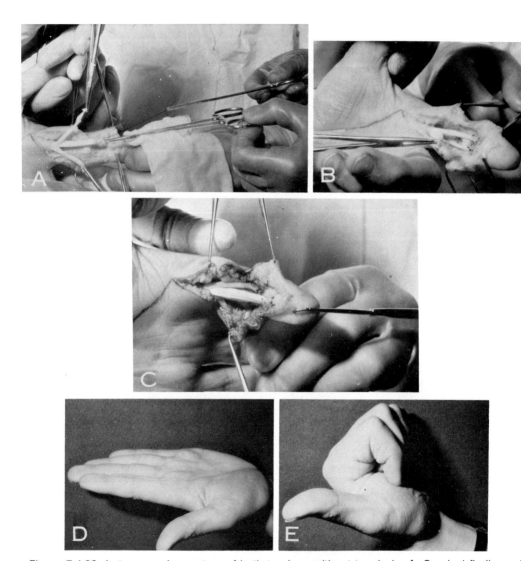

Figure 7.4.22. Late secondary suture of both tendons without tenolysis. *A.* Surgical findings six months following unrepaired transection of both flexor tendons. Good muscle mobility, despite lengthy interval. *B.* Sutures reinserted in sublimis. *C.* Sutures reinserted in profundus. *D.* Index finger extension two years postoperative. *E.* Index finger flexion two years postoperative.

TABLE 7.4.5
Comparison the flexion ability of all 31 fingers with those 10 fingers having primary suture of both tendons and with those 11 fingers having had sublimis excision

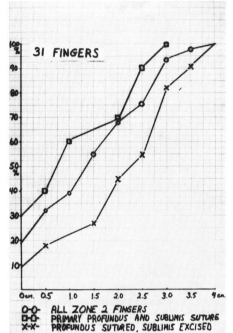

O-O ALL ZONE 2 FINGERS
□-□ PRIMARY PROFUNDUS AND SUBLIMIS SUTURE
X-X- PROFUNDUS SUTURED, SUBLIMIS EXCISED

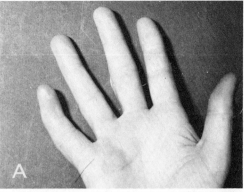

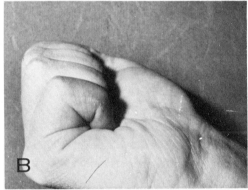

Figure 7.4.24. Early secondary suture of profundud with excision of sublimis, secondary tenolysis. *A.* Little finger extension 17 months following secondary suture of profundus with excision of sublimis. *B.* Complete little finger flexion 17 months postoperative.

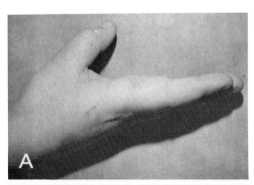

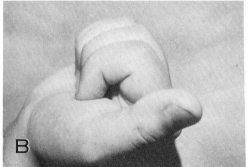

Figure 7.4.23. Secondary suture of both tendons followed by tenolysis. *A.* Index extension 13 months following secondary repair of flexor profundus and sublimis. *B.* Flexion of index finger 13 months postoperative.

both tendons, Table 7.4.7 compares primary profundus and sublimis suture with the nine cases of secondary profundus suture with sublimis excision.

Table 7.4.8 plots the results of the 25 fingers which had both tendons cut. The 14 digits with both tendons sutured are compared with the 11 fingers having had profundus repair with sublimis excision. The variable of primary or secondary treatment is therefore eliminated from this graph.

We believe that the better results from the group having had repair of both tendons, over those cases which had sublimis excision, is due to the fact that such surgery was performed primarily and to the fact that vascular damage to the profundus during sublimis excision was avoided. Possibly, a primary repair which quickly corrects or prevents tendon retraction, will in this manner avoid vascular damage through the vinculae by traction and thrombosis. This could theoretically produce fewer adhesions between the surrounding tissues and the suture site, allowing better tendon gliding and a clinically superior result.

Table 7.4.6 compares the digits treated primarily with those treated secondarily. That repair of the sublimis might actually encourage a better result is certainly an intriguing but as yet unproven idea.

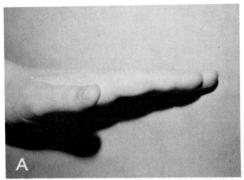

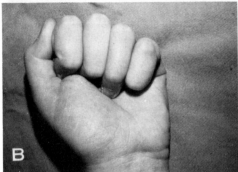

Figure 7.4.25. Primary suture of both tendons with failure: secondary tendon graft. *A* and *B*. Result of a secondary profundus graft with sublimis excision in ring finger 3½ years following injury. Both tendons were sutured primarily, and, because of extensive scarring and limited flexion, a graft was selected rather than a tenolysis.

As with most areas of hand surgery, dependence upon a single approach to these flexor tendon injuries is unrealistic. Tendon grafting plays an important and justified role in the solution of these problems. During the same period as this study, 65 tendon grafts were performed by Verdan and his staff.[45]

As demonstrated in Fig. 7.4.25 (one of the excluded five cases), a primary repair does not exclude the possibility of using a secondary graft, should the result of primary repair be unsatisfactory; and in such a situation the patient will have recovered at approximately the same date as would have occurred had secondary grafting been the original plan for treatment.

The decision as to which procedure is utilized must take into account all the well recognized variabilities: the time interval following injury, nature of the wound, the initial care administered, the age and occupation of the patient, the availability of surgeons well-trained in these techniques (as emphasized by Kleinert[21]) and proper available facilities.

FUTURE PROSPECTS

With the constant improvement of our modern organization, with the rapidity and multiplicity of the

TABLE 7.4.6
This Table eliminates the two cases of primary profundus repair with sublimis excision. In this way the primary and econdary factors may be better judged

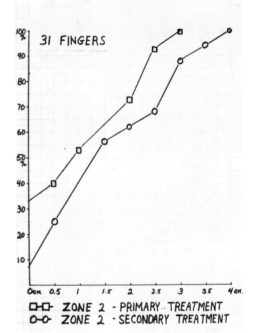

□-□ ZONE 2 - PRIMARY TREATMENT
O-O ZONE 2 - SECONDARY TREATMENT

TABLE 7.4.7
Comparison of primary suture of both tendons with secondary suture of profundus with excision of sublimis

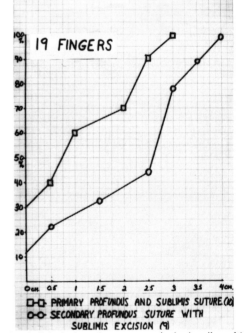

□-□ PRIMARY PROFUNDUS AND SUBLIMIS SUTURE (10)
O-O SECONDARY PROFUNDUS SUTURE WITH
      SUBLIMIS EXCISION (9)

In 10 digits both tendons were repaired primarily and in nine the profundus was repaired and the sublimis was excised secondarily.

TABLE 7.4.9
Results in 70 cases over five years

70 CASES OF PRIMARY OR SECONDARY TENDON SUTURE — ZONE 1 and 2

		Excellent	Good	Fair	Poor	Not Known
Thumb	9	1	5	3	-	---
Index	25	7	10	3	2	3
Long	11	3	3	4	-	1
Ring	8	1	3	3	-	1
Little	17	6	7	2	-	2
	70 Cases	18	28	15	2	7

TABLE 7.4.8
Comparison between suture of both tendons and suture of profundus combined with excision of sublimis

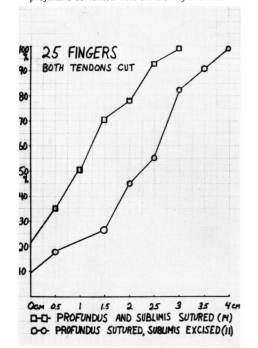

By comparing the 14 digits with both tendons sutured primarily Table 7.4.8, with 11 fingers with profundus repaired and sublimis excised, the variable of primary or secondary treatment is eliminated

means of transport, we can expect soon that an increase of accidental wounds will be seen after a very brief delay, by specialized teams, at well equipped surgical centers. Appropriate knowledge and preparation of the wounds and atraumatic technique are responsible for the low rate of sepsis in traumatized hands. One can now perform in primary repair more complex operations than those which were permissible in the past. To this new acquisition of primary suture of the flexors, we can now add the operation of primary grafting. The following authors have been the protagonists of these immediate plasties of the tendons: Lorthioir,[23] Harrison,[17] Flynn,[13,14] Torokova,[41] and Wakefield.[52]

Many favorable arguments can be invoked. There is absence of edema, the absorption of which may take several months. There is absence of scar tissue. There is good permeability of sheath and pulleys. The joints are supple. There is good muscle tone, with absence of retraction. One can measure the length required for the graft exactly by comparing it with the resected tendon. There are better biological conditions for taking the graft. There is also a reduction in the time of incapacity for work.

A comparable study of Van't Hof and Heiple[43] of primary grafts, secondary grafts, and primary repairs, shows clearly that primary grafts in Zone 2 give the best results. However, their series is small. The future will tell if we can adopt this procedure as a routine.

REFERENCES

1. Bolton, J. Primary tendon repair: the hand. J. Br. Soc. Surg. Hand, 2: 1-1970.
2. Boyes, J.H. Evaluation of results of digital flexor tendon grafts. Am. J. Surg., 89: 116, 1116-1119, 1955.
3. Boyes, J.H. Flexor tendon grafts in the fingers and thumb: An evaluation of end results. J. Bone Joint Surg., 32A: 489-499, 1950.
4. Boyes, J.H. Sixth International Congress of Sicot in Berne, Switzerland, 1954, Bruxelles Imprimerie Lilens, 1955.
5. Brand, P. Principles of free tendon grafting, including a new method of tendon suture, J. Bone Joint Surg., 41B: 208, 1959.
6. Brockis, J.G. The blood supply of the flexor and extensor tendons of the fingers in man. J. Bone Joint Surg., 35B: 131, 1953.
7. Bsteh, O. Transfixion tendineuse, methode opératoire dans les sections tendineuses. Chirug., 26: 460-462, 1955.
8. Bunnell, S. Gig pull-out suture for tendons. J. Bone Joint Surg., 36A: 850, 1954.
9. Bunnell, S. Surgery of the Hand, Ed. 3. Philadelphia, Lippincott. 1956.
10. Colson, P., Houot, R., and Gangolphe, O. Reconstitution d'un tendon fléchissour et de ses poulies de refléxion. Discussion: M. Francillon, 55: 776, 1959.
11. Dolphin, J.A. Extensor tenotomy for boutonniere deformity of the finger. American Society for Surgery of the Hand, 18th Annual Meeting, Jan. 18/19, 1963,

Miami Beach, Florida.

12. Fetrow, K.O. Tenolysis in the hand and wrist. J. Bone Joint Surg., *49A:* 667, 1967.

13. Flynn, J.E. Heterogenous and autogenous tendon transplants. J. Bone Joint Surg., *42A:* 91, 1960.

14. Flynn, J.E. Problems with trauma to hand. J. Bone Joint Surg., *35A:* 132-140, 1953.

15. Gosset, J. La réparation secondaire des tendons fléchisseurs. Essai de mécanique experimentale théorique. Ann. chir. plast. *3:* 299-31, 1958.

16. Gosset, J., Dautry, P., and Bonvallent, Jr. Le traitement des ténosynovites suppurées de la main et des doigts. Ann. chir., *31:* 562-567, 1955.

17. Harrison, S. H. Greffes primaires des tendons fléchisseurs. Br. J. Plast. Surg., *11:* 106-110, 1958.

18. Iselin, M. *Chirurgie de la Main.* Paris, Masson, 1955, p. 626.

19. Iselin, M. L'état actuel du probleme du traitement du traumatisme des tendons fléchisseurs. Arch. klin. Chir., *287:* 533-537, 1957.

20. Kaplan, E.B. *Functional and Surgical Anatomy of the Hand.* Philadelphia, Lippincott, 1953.

21. Kleinert, H.E., Kutz, J.E., Ashbell, S.T., and Martinez, E. Primary repair of lacerated flexor tendons in "no-man's land." J. Bone Joint Surg., *49A:* 577, 1967.

22. Littler, J.W. The severed flexor tendon. Surg. Clin. North Am., *39:* 435-447, 1958.

23. Lorthioir, J., Jr. La greffe immédiate dans les sections des tendons fléchisseurs. Acta chir. Belg., *56:* 386-390, 1957.

24. Lorthior, J., Evrard, J., and Vander Elst, E. Le traitement des traumatismes récents de la main. Acta orthop. Belg., *24:* 1-257, 1958.

25. Madsen, E. Delayed primary suture of flexor tendons cut in digital sheath. J. Bone Joint Surg., *52B:* No. 2, 1970.

26. Mason, L., Boyes, J., Fowler, B., and Kelly, E. P. Primary tendon repair. J. Bone Joint Surg., *41B:* 575, 1959.

27. Mayer, L. L'évolution de la chirurgie tendineuse moderne. Ann. R. Coll. Surg. Engl., *2:* 69-86, 1952.

28. Merle D'Aubigne, R., and Tubiana, R. Traumatismes anciens, généralités, Membre supérieur. 2. In *Chir. orthop. des paralyses.* Paris, Masson, 1956.

29. Michon, J., and Vichard, P. Luxations latérales des tendons extenseurs en regard de Particulation métacarpo-phalangienne. Rev. méd. Nancy, *86:* 595-601, 1961.

30. Morel-Fatio, D. Les plaies de la main. Rev. prat., *32:* 3555-3560, 1956.

31. Neiger, J. La vascularisation des tendons fléchisseurs. Z. Unfállmed. Berufsks., *48:* 69-77, 1955.

32. Nigst, H., and Megevand, R.P. La réparation du long fléichisseur du pouce. Helv. chim. acta., *23:* 456-459, 1956.

33. Peacock, E.E. A study of the circulation in normal tendons and healing grafts. Ann. Surg., *3:* 149, 1959.

34. Planas, J. Some technical modifications in tendon grafting of the hand. In *Transactions of the International Society of Plastic Surgeons.* Edinburgh, Livingstone, 212-216, 1959.

35. Pulvertaft, R. G. Experience in flexor tendon grafting in the hand. J. Bone Joint Surg., *41B:* 629, 1959.

36. Pulvertaft, R.G. The treatment of profundus division by free tendon graft. J. Bone Joint Surg., *42A:* 1363, 1960.

37. Rank, B.K., and Wakefield, A.R. *Surgery of Repair as Applied to Hand Injuries.* Edinburgh, Livingstone, 1960.

38. Rouhier, F. La restauration du tendon long fléchisseur du pouce, sans sacrifice du tendon primitif. J. chir., *8-9:* 66, 1950.

39. Schneider, H. *Die Abnützungserkrankungen der Schnen und ihre Therapie.* Stuttgart, Georg Thieme Verlag, 1959.

40. Stack, H.G. Some details of the anatomy of the terminal segment of the finger. Acta orthop. Belg., *24:* 113, 1958.

41. Torokova, A. Free tendon grafts in primary repair of injury to the flexor tendons of the hand in the area of the fibrous sheath. Acta chir. plast., *2:* 207, 1960.

42. Tubiana, R. Les voies d'abord dans la chirurgie des tendons de la main. Ann. chir. plast., *2:* 99-109, 1960.

43. Van't Hof, A., and Heiple, K.G. Flexor tendon injuries of the fingers and thumb. J. Bone Joint Surg., *39A:* 717, 1957.

44. Verdan, C. Chirurgie réparatrice et fonctionnelle des tendons de la main. Expansion Scient. Francaise, Paris, 1952.

45. Verdan, C. Half a century of flexor tendon surgery, current status and changing philosophies. J. Bone Joint Surg., *45A:* 3, 472, 1972.

46. Verdan, C. La réparation immédiate des tendons fléchisseurs dans la canal digital. Acta orthop. Belg., *24* (Supplementum 3): 1958.

47. Verdan, C. Primary and secondary repair of flexor and extensor tendon injuries. In *Hand Surgery,* edited by J. E. Flynn. Baltimore, Williams & Wilkins, 1966.

48. Verdan, C. Primary repair of flexor tendons. J. Bone Joint Surg., *42A:* 647, 1960.

49. Verdan, C., and Crawford, G.P. Flexor tendon suture in digital canal. Fifth World Congress of Plastic and Reconstructive Surgery. London, Buttersworths, 1971.

50. Verdan, C., Crawford, G.P., and Martini-Benkeddache, Y. Tenolysis in traumatic hand surgery. St. Louis, Mosby, to be published.

51. Verdan, C., and Michon, J. Le traitement des plaies des tendons fléchisseurs des doights. Revue Chir. Orthop., *47:* 285, 1961.

52. Wakefield, A.R. The management of flexor tendon injuries. Surg. Clin. North Am., *40:* 267, 399, 1960.

E.

Tendon Ruptures of the Hand and Forearm

H. Minor Nichols, M.D., M.Sc., F.A.C.S.

INTRODUCTION

The tendons of the body are susceptible to trauma from wear, stress, and direct injury. Some tendons are particularly susceptible; the story of Achilles, whose mother held him in the River Styx by his heel, shows the Achilles tendon has a well founded, long time record of weakness. Authorities differ as to the cause of tendon ruptures, the most common sites, and frequently as to the preferred method of treatment.

Etiology

McMaster's[20] experiments show that a normal flexor tendon does not rupture under stress. A 50 per cent severed tendon may rupture at times but usually, even with 75 per cent severance, normal activity will not cause rupture.

Many disruptions are associated with disease or obvious trauma. A direct blow or unusual stress placed on the muscle tendon unit is the usual cause. Unusual stress occurs during falls, athletic activities, and fights.

RUPTURE OF THE DIGITAL EXTENSORS AT THE DISTAL PHALANX

Anatomy

The insertion of the extensor tendon into the dorsal articulating lip of the distal phalanx of the fingers is a thin, easily traumatized aponeurosis.

Signs and Symptoms

At the time of injury there is usually a moderate amount of pain. Frequently the finger end is noticed to hang down almost immediately and a moderate amount of swelling occurs.

Pathology

Depending on force applied and the duration of contact, the tendon may be torn completely or incompletely, or at times the dorsal articulating lip of the distal phalanx may be fractured and separate with the tendon.

Treatment

Conservative treatment is recommended for all patients seen within a few days of the injury. Most of these can be successfully restored to normal function by splinting. The proper position is with the distal joint held in mild hyperextension and the middle joint in a mildly flexed position. This can best be maintained by plaster (Fig. 7.5.1). The patient is shown how to hold the finger in the correct position by placing the tip of the finger against the thumb of the same hand, pushing up on the finger with the thumb at the same time that the proximal interphalangeal joint is held flexed. A stockinette of Surgitube is applied to the finger and over this strips of plaster splinting 3 or 4 inches long and ¾ inch wide are laid on, a few at a time. The plaster cast is left in place for about three to four weeks; it is then removed and replaced by a simple tongue blade splint which the patient is told to

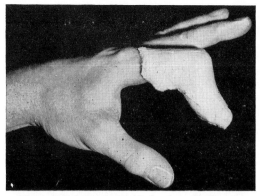

Figure 7.5.1. Cast used in fresh mallet finger injuries (Bunnell method).*

remove daily, using hot soaks and gripping exercises. Usually by the time a mallet finger of 60° or better has developed, there is a definite contracture of the flexor tendon unit and splinting will not overcome its pull. Some form of operative treatment for these patients is usually best as the disability produced by severe mallet finger is rather great.

The operative treatment for mallet finger deformity remains *sub judice*. Many orthopedists of long experience believe that arthrodesis of the distal joint in a mild degree of flexion is the best cure for this condition. Where a volar surface contracture has occurred and the tip of the finger cannot be brought up to normal extension passively, arthrodesis is unquestionably the treatment of choice.

The joint is exposed through a dorsal incision and the cartilaginous joint surfaces are rongeured away to give good apposition of the resulting contoured bony surfaces. Internal fixation is obtained by cross pinning or by a single intramedullary pin, or by a loop of 22-gauge stainless steel wire passed through horizontal drill holes in the adjacent phalanges (Fig. 7.5.2). Internal fixation must be maintained until solid bony union is established or deformity will recur.

When normal passive extension of the distal joint is present, tendon graft may be used to restore active extension to the distal joint. The tendon graft is a split off piece of the palmaris longus or a wrist flexor tendon which should be about the size of a No. 1 catgut and 5 inches in length. The tendon graft is threaded into a heavy needle and passed back and forth through the extensor tendon proximal to the defect, thence through the original insertion of the tendon, then back again, and back and forth through the extensor tendon (Fig. 7.5.3). The distal joint is hyperextended while the middle joint is flexed and the tendon graft cinched up to make it snug. A few nonabsorbable sutures fasten the graft in place. If the operator feels

*Figures 1 to 9, 11, 13 and 15 were reproduced from Nichol's Manual of Hand Injuries," by permission of Year Book Publishers, Inc.

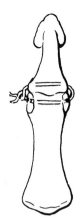

Figure 7.5.2. Arthrodesis of distal joint with fixation by buried wire loop.

that the original tendinous insertion is not adequate to hold the graft, it should be passed through a horizontal or vertical drill hole in the distal phalanx. The wound is carefully closed with a single layer of nonabsorbable sutures and the finger is dressed with a minimum of padding and placed in the plaster cast described under conservative treatment.

Splinting is maintained for about four weeks and the finger is then exercised in the daytime with the splint replaced at night.

BUTTONHOLE RUPTURE OF THE EXTENSOR TENDON AT THE MIDDLE JOINT

Rupture of the Central Slip of the Extensor Tendon at Its Insertion

Etiology

Most of the cases seen with this rather uncommon injury are due to a minute laceration occurring over the

A

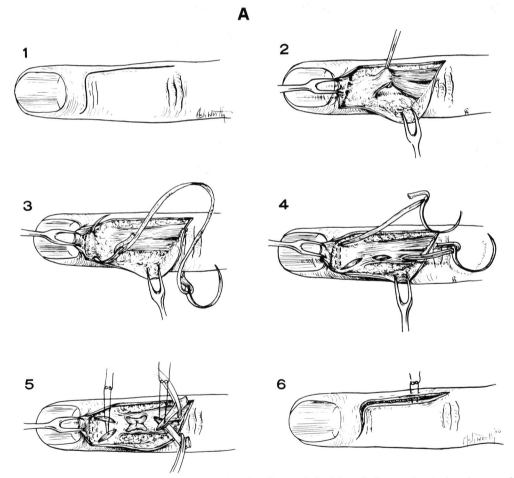

Figure 7.5.3 A. Operation for correction of mallet finger. *1,* incision; *2,* flaps retracted and scarred tendon identified; *3,* tendon graft anchored distally into dense tissue on dorsum of proximal end of phalanx; *4* and *5,* graft woven into sound tendon proximal to scar and fastened in place; *6,* half-buried mattress suture used for wound closure. (Reprinted from Nichols[23] by permission of the *Journal of Bone and Joint Surgery.) (Continued on opposite page.)*

B

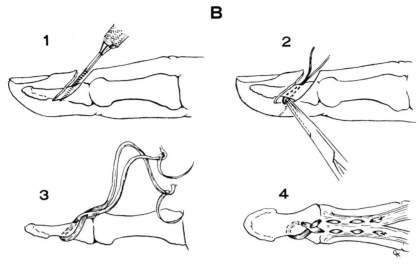

Figure 7.5.3. B. Alternative method when tendon is fastened to drill hold in bone (modification of operation shown in *A*).

dorsum of the flexed joint which penetrates and causes a partial severence of the tendon. During healing without any splinting, the tendon ruptures, and a few days after the original injury the patient finds himself unable to extend the middle joint of the finger. Some of these cases may occur from sudden, forced flexion or from a blow without any actual cutaneous wound over the flexed joint.

Treatment

Splinting for three weeks with the middle joint extended and the distal joint allowed to flex will probably prevent the development of the deformity, in cases seen early.

Late cases that show a flexion deformity of not over 30° may be treated expectantly as many of them will clear up without treatment.

Operative Treatment

A zigzag or curved incision is made extending from the distal joint to the metacarpophalangeal joint. The skin flaps should be undercut to give complete exposure of the tendon structures over the joint. The central slip must be freed from the lateral bands and advanced. A thin strip of palmaris longus or of wrist flexor tendon is used as a graft. The graft is brought back and woven into the central slip to give a firm purchase on the tendon (Fig. 7.5.4). The graft is anchored distally to a transverse drill hole in the dorsal cortex of the middle phalanx or to the scarred stump of the original insertion (Fig. 7.5.4A and B).

Tension of the graft should be strong enough to extend fully the middle joint with the wrist flexed. If the lateral bands have prolapsed around the sides of the joint, they should be released from their attachments and brought up over the dorsum of the joint as far as the center of the articulating plane. The medial edges of these lateral bands should be trimmed and sutured with one or two fine nonabsorbable sutures. The wound is closed with interrupted sutures and the finger dressed in a plaster splint, with the wrist and the metacarpophalangeal joint and the proximal interphalangeal joint extended. The splint is removed after three weeks but should be worn at night for another three weeks to prevent a recurrence of the deformity.

In a recent case it is possible to draw the central slip to its insertion and fasten it there, using a wire passed through drill holes in the middle phalanx (Fig. 7.5.5).

Normal joint excursion and radiographic evidence of a good middle joint are prerequisites for a tendon graft. If these are not present it is recommended that the joint be arthrodesed rather than be given a tendon graft. In arthrodesis, Moberg's method is preferred (Fig. 7.5.6). An intramedullary bone peg is passed down the medullary canal of the middle phalanx and through a drill hole emerging obliquely through the dorsum of the proximal phalanx. The graft is about 3 cm long and is cut square rather than round with the olecranon as a donor site. A plaster cast is kept on for six weeks. Moberg states that his healing time is much shorter, eight weeks or less, with this method, which he has used in about 60 cases.

Other Extensor Tendon Ruptures

Aside from rupture of the extensor tendon insertions over the distal and proximal interphalangeal joints, rupture of the normal finger extensor tendons is rather uncommon. Cases of rupture, occurring over the dorsum of the hand, are occasionally encountered.

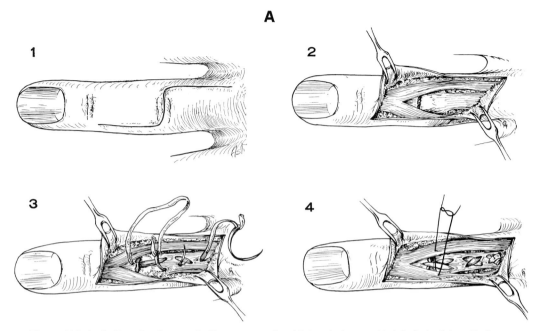

Figure 7.5.4. A. Repair of central slip over proximal interphalangeal joint. *1,* incision; *2,* flaps retracted; *3,* insertion of graft; *4,* position of tendon after grafting. A single suture line is used for triangular ligament.

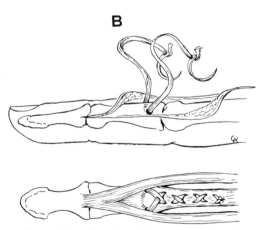

Figure 7.5.4. B. Alternative method when tendon is fastened to drill hole in bone (modification of operation shown in *A).*

Treatment

In late ruptures over the dorsum of the hand, the preferred method is a tendon transfer. The loose distal end is transferred to one of the adjacent extensor tendons and the proximal loose end is transferred to the same tendon, proximal to the dorsal carpal ligament.

Rheumatoid arthritis of the wrist accounts for most

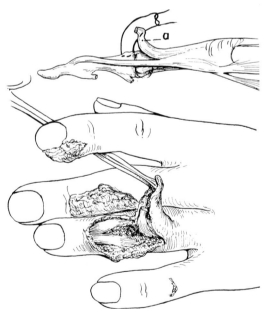

Figure 7.5.5. Multiple saw cuts of all fingers, transecting insertion of central slip of extensor tendon of ring finger with primary repair; wire is passed through tendon end and drill hole in middle phalanx to attach central slip of extensor tendon.

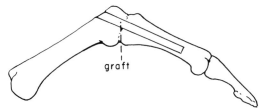

Figure 7.5.6. Arthrodesis of long finger joint. Moberg's method with bone graft.

of the cases of spontaneous rupture of tendons on the dorsum of the hand proximal to the finger joints. During the intermediate stages of rheumatoid arthritis the inferior radioulnar joint becomes eroded and the lower end of the ulna projects up under the dorsal carpal ligament to erode the involved tendons. As the process of erosion continues the tendons rupture one by one, usually starting with the little finger followed within a matter of weeks or months by rupture of the ring finger, then the long finger.

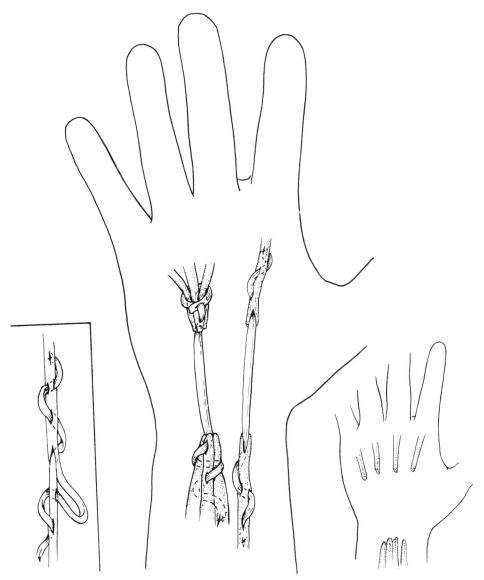

Figure 7.5.7. Graft to extensors: one tendon graft from extensor communis to third, fourth, and fifth digits; one graft from extensor indicis proprius to index finger. *Inset at left,* technique for interweaving tendon ends.

Operative Technique

Surgical reconstruction in these cases has met with failure because of progression of the disease. In inactive cases, good technique gives reasonably good results. It is better to transfer the ruptured extensors into whatever remaining normal tendons present. A single tendon graft that unites the ends of three divided tendons to their muscles is sometimes necessary (Fig. 7.5.7). Resection of the distal 1½ inches of the ulna at the same operation transplanting the carpal ligament to a position beneath the extensor digitorum tendons covers the joint and protects the tendons from further injury.

RUPTURE OF THE EXTENSOR POLLICIS LONGUS

Incidence

This condition is variously reported to occur in six in 1000 to six in 100, after Colles' fractures. A similar affection was noted in writers, sculptors, carpenters,

acrobats, and tailors. The condition is rare directly after trauma although a few cases have been reported (Fig. 7.5.8).

Direct suture of the tendon is not recommended. A tendon graft or a tendon transfer is preferred. In ten-

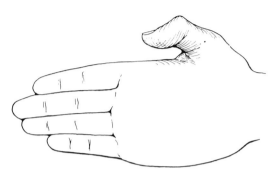

Figure 7.5.8. Long extensor tendon of thumb ruptured by fall. Such ruptures usually occur near Lister's tubercle.

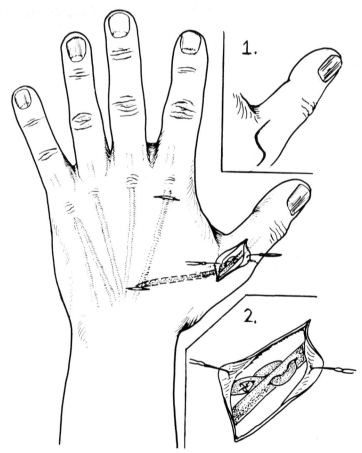

Figure 7.5.9. Technique of tendon transfer for loss of extension of thumb. Through three short incisions, made as illustrated, the extensor indicis proprius is detached at its insertion, withdrawn at the wrist, and rerouted and attached to the thumb extensor.

don grafting, the palmaris longus is used as a graft and the tendon junctures are made at the musculotendinous juncture in the forearm and over the dorsum of the metacarpal of the thumb. A better result can be obtained by using the extensor indicis proprius as a transfer. Three short transverse incisions are made and the extensor indicis proprius is detached from its insertion at the head of the index metacarpal and withdrawn through another short transverse incision just distal to the transverse carpal ligament. It is then rerouted and inserted by interweaving into the long extensor of the thumb (Fig. 7.5.9), preserving the original tension of the extensor indicis proprius. No reeducation of the patient is necessary and there is no disability to the index finger. Postoperatively, a cast should keep the wrist and thumb extended for a period of about three weeks.

FLEXOR TENDON RUPTURES

Flexor tendon ruptures are rare compared to extensor ruptures. The causes are trauma — attrition or erosion — or disease processes. The direct cause is the sudden digital hyperextension or forced flexion against resistance. Normal tendons are disinserted or avulsed from their muscles (Fig. 7.5.10). Erosion of tendons followed by rupture have occurred following Colles' fracture, Keinbock's disease, old scaphoid fracture (Fig. 7.5.11). bipartite capitate, roughening of the hamate or congenital malformations of the carpus. Disease processes which weaken tendons are tenosynovitis either rheumatoid, tuberculous or non specific, or at times weakening from infection in adjacent tissues.

Wegner[29] has recently reported four cases of avulsion of flexor profundus tendons in football players, usually in the ring finger. Gunter[12] reported 12 similar cases in football players and in each case the ring finger was involved. The most logical explanation is the lack of independent extension in the ring finger when the other digits are flexed. The injured digit usually becomes caught in an opponent's jersey.

Diagnosis

There is inability to flex the distal joint against resistance, absence of the profundus in the middle segment of the finger and some tenderness over the distal flexion crease.

Treatment

Within three weeks disinsertion of profundus tendon is not difficult to repair. Through a midlateral incision, the end of the profundus tendon is retrieved in the finger and can be brought down to its original position if the wrist is flexed. The tendon is fastened back into place with an oblique drill hole through the phalanx with a pull-out wire in the tendon and a tie down to a ½-inch piece of applicator over the dorsum of the fingernail (Fig. 7.5.12). The hand is placed in a

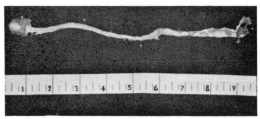

Figure 7.5.10. End of finger with flexor tendon attached, avulsed in wringer injury. Female, age 40. Case courtesy of Dr. Frank B. Packard, Portland, Oregon.

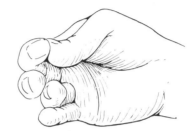

Figure 7.5.11. Injury from fall on outstretched right thumb. Patient felt severe pain in wrist and later could not flex the thumb. At operation, the long flexor was found to have been frayed by an old navicular fracture so that it broke at this point.

posterior plaster splint with the wrist flexed for three weeks and then active motions are instituted.

Old cases of disinsertion of flexor tendons are difficult due to contraction of the muscle and degeneration of the tendon.

For many of these cases arthrodesis of the distal interphalangeal joint with excision of the profundus tendon is performed. A tendon graft from the palm to the fingertip can be used as an alternative to arthrodesis or tenodesis of the distal joint.

RUPTURE OF THE FLEXOR TENDONS AT OTHER LEVELS

In most of the reported series of cases, rupture of the flexor tendons occurs at either the insertion or the musculotendinous juncture. There are, however, cases which occur in the palm or carpal tunnel, or the wrist.

Treatment

An attempt should be made to repair a flexor pollicis longus unless there are absolute contraindications such as the presence of an active rheumatoid arthritis. It is usually preferable to replace the entire tendon with a graft, using the palmaris longus with its peritenon. To uncover the site of bony roughening, make an incision along the thenar crease and across the flexion crease of the wrist, dividing the transverse carpal

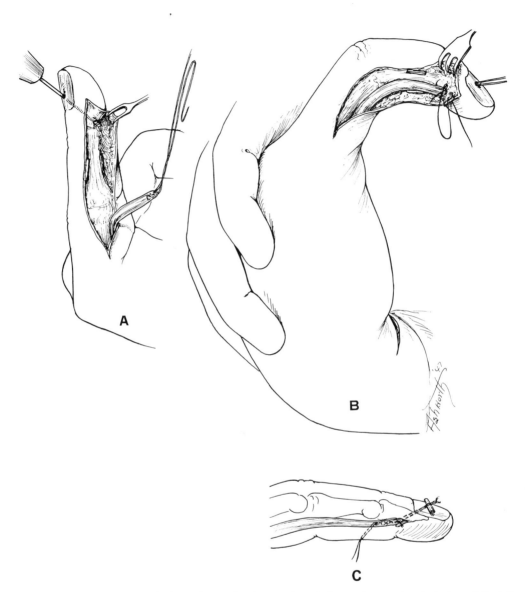

Figure 7.5.12. Technique of reinserting profundus tendon. *A.* Suture inserted and phalanx drilled. *B.* Flexing of wrist and finger to advance tendon which is then anchored to applicator on dorsum of nail. *C.* Wound closure; completed repair; pullout wire comes out through midlateral plane of finger.

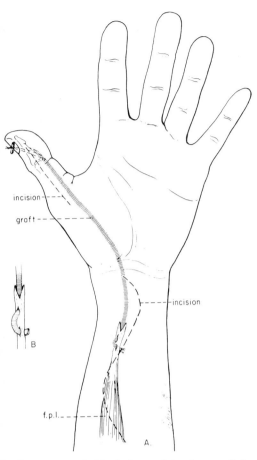

incision

graft

incision

B

f.p.l.

A.

Figure 7.5.13. Technique of tendon graft for loss of flexor pollicis longus.

ligament. Avoid injury to the median nerve and its all important thenar muscle branches. Any bony roughening is removed, and a flap of fascia pedicled over it to prevent further erosion of tendon. The palmaris longus graft is attached at the musculotendinous junction by interweaving and to the base of the distal phalanx either to bone or to the stump of the old tendon at the distal interphalangeal joint (Fig. 7.5.13). It is probably better to have this graft just a little tight as some myostatic contracture of the profundus muscle will be present but will stretch out during convalescence.

RUPTURE OF THE WRIST TENDONS

Rupture of the flexor and extensor tendons of the wrist is a comparatively rare injury. In most cases an open wound is present. Falls in which the patient catches the wrist on a sharp hook or a nail, avulsion injuries in which the wrist tendons are torn, injuries due to rollers, and extensive compound fractures can be causative.

REFERENCES

1. Anzel, S. H., Covey, K. W., Weiner, A. D., and Lipscomb, P. R., Disruption of muscles and tendons: an analysis of 1,014 cases. Surgery, *45:* 406-414, 1959.
2. Bennett, B. S. Trceps tendon rupture: Case report and a method of repair. J. Bone Joint Surg., *44A:* 741, 1956.
3. Blumel, G., and Piza, F. Subkutane Muskelund Sehnenrisse Infolge Indirekter Gewaiteinwirkung. Klin. Med. (Mosk.), *12:* 297-307, 1957.
4. Boyes, J. H. Rupture of tendons: report of four cases of latent rupture of the tendon of the extensor pollicis longus. West. J. Surg., *43:* 442-445, 1935.
5. Boyes, J. H., Wilson, J. N., and Smith, J. W. Flexor-tendon ruptures in the forearm and hand. J. Bone Joint Surg., *42A:* 637-646, 1960.
6. Brickner, W. M., and Milch, H. Ruptures of muscles and tendons. Int. Clin., *2:* 94-107, 1928.
7. Bunnell, S. *Surgery of the Hand.* Philadelphia, Lippincott, 1944.
8. Carroll, R., and Match, R. Avulsion of the flexor profundus tendon insertion. J. Trauma, *10:* 1109-1118, 1970.
9. Folmer, R. C., Nelson, C. L., and Phalen, G. S. Ruptures of flexor tendons in the hands of non-rheumatoid patients. J. Bone Joint Surg., *54A:* 579-584, 1972.
10. Fowler, S. B. In *Surgery of the Hand,* Ed. 2, edited by S. Bunnell. Philadelphia, Lippincott, 1948, p. 482.
11. Graham, W. C. Delayed tendon repairs. Am. J. Surg., *80:* 776-779, 1950.
12. Gunter, G. S. Traumatic avulsion of the insertion of flexor digitorum profundus. Aust. N. Z. J. Surg., *30:* 1-8, 1960.
13. Haldeman, K. O., and Soto-Hall, R. Injuries to muscles and tendons. J.A.M.A., *104:* 2319-2324, 1935.
14. Hunt, J. R. Paralysis of the ungual phalanx of the thumb from spontaneous rupture of the extensor pollicis longus. J.A.M.A., *64:* 1138-1140, 1915.
15. James, J. I. P. Case of rupture of flexor tendons: secondary to Kienbock's disease. J. Bone Joint Surg., *31B:* 521-523, 1949.
16. Lee, M. L. H. Rupture of the triceps tendon. Br. Med. J. *2:* 197, 1960.
17. Littler, J. W. In *Reconstructive Plastic Surgery,* edited by J. M. Converse. Philadelphia, Saunders, 1964, p. 1631.
18. Mason, M. L. Rupture of tendons of the hand: with a study of the extensor tendon insertions in the fingers. Surg. Gynecol. Obstet., *50:* 611-624, 1930.
19. Massachusetts General Hospital, Boston. *Fractures and Other Injuries,* edited by E. F. Cave. Chicago, Year Book, 1958, p. 390.
20. McMaster, P. E. Late ruptures of extensor and flexor pollicis longus tendons following Colles' fracture. J. Bone Joint Surg., *14:* 93-101, 1932.
21. Mendelaar, H. M. Post-traumatic ruptures of the tendon of the musculus extensor pollicis longus. Arch. chir. neerl., *12:* 146-156, 1960.
22. Nichols, H. M. *Manual of Hand Injuries,* Ed. 2. Chicago, Year Book, 1960.
23. Nichols, H. M. Repair of extensor-tendon insertions in the fingers. J. Bone Joint Surg., *33A:* 836-841, 1951.

24. Peacock, E. E., and Hartrampf, C. R. Repair of flexor tendons in the hand. Int. Abstr. Surg., *113:* 411-432, 1961. In: Surg. Gynecol. Obstet., 1961.
25. Platt, H. Observations on some tendon ruptures. Br. Med. J., *1:* 611-615, 1931.
26. Posch, J. L., Walker, P. J., and Miller, H. Treatment of ruptured tendons of the hand and wrist. Am. J. Surg., *91:* 669-681, 1956.
27. Spencer, W. G., and Gask, G. E. In *Practice of Surgery.* Philadelphia, Blakiston, 1910, p. 333.
28. Straub, L. R., and Wilson, E. H. Spontaneous rupture of extensor tendons in the hand associated with rheumatoid arthritis. J. Bone Joint Surg., *38A:* 1208-1217, 1334, 1345, 1956.
29. Wegner, D. R. Avulsion of profundus tendon in football players. Arch. Surg., *106:* 145-149, 1973.
30. Young, R. E. S., and Harmon, J. M. Repair of tendon injuries of the hand. Ann. Surg., *151:* 562-566, 1960.
31. Zoncalli, In *Structural and Dynamic Bases of Hand Surgery.* p. 123, 124, 125. Philadelphia, Lippincott, 1948, pp. 123-125.

F.

Flexor Tendon Grafting

R. Guy Pulvertaft, M.D. (Hon.), M. Chir., F.R.C.S.

INTRODUCTION

The repair of tendon injuries in the hand has challenged and fascinated surgeons for many years. Tendons in apposition heal sufficiently in three weeks to accept gentle strain, and the union matures rapidly until eventually there remains no trace of the original injury. No problems of delayed union or failure of union exist. It would seem, therefore, that provided an accurate suture is performed, the tendon will heal and function will be restored. Unfortunately, this does not necessarily follow and along the trail which marks the development of tendon surgery lie many failures. The reason lies in the fact that tendon heals by an ingrowth of fibroblasts from the surrounding tissue, sheath or paratenon whichever it may be. The healing process links the tendon to its surroundings and, if excessive, the tendon becomes firmly anchored. The injury caused by surgical intervention increases this reaction; unless the repair is performed with meticulous care, there is little hope of success. This challenge has been a continuing stimulus to experimental and clinical research.

HISTORY

In 1888, Robson[20] reported a successful restoration of an extensor tendon in the hand by use of a free tendon graft taken from another severely damaged finger of the same hand. This appears to be the first example of an autogenous tendon graft.

In 1918, Bunnell[5] advised that a graft should be used to replace divided tendons in the finger, "Our best method to attain this (full function) is to graft a tendon with its sheath and all ready made from some other place where it may be spared." He described one case in which this had been done with a fair measure of success. In 1922, he[6] reported five cases of grafting for thumb and finger injuries, all of which had obtained good function. He stressed the importance of the work of Biesalski and Mayer on the anatomy of tendons, the importance of the gliding mechanism, and the physiologic method of transposing tendons. Since then the operation of tendon grafting has been widely practiced and many series of results reported.

EXPERIMENTAL WORK

In the first edition,[10] a brief summary was given of the views prevailing at that time upon the healing of tendons and the biologic behaviour of tendon grafts. Since then the work of Potenza[16] upon the flexor tendons of dogs, in which the anatomy closely resembles that of man, has added to our knowledge. Potenza confirmed that tendons heal solely by cellular activity of the paratenon or the tendon sheath, and that neither the tendon nor the graft are the source of the cells which unite tendon to tendon. He showed that a graft remains viable and he could find no evidence to support the view that there is a replacement of the graft cells. He also demonstrated that adhesions along the course of the graft occur only at those points where the surface integrity of the graft has been damaged.

In the field of clinical research, the most outstanding contribution has been made by Boyes and Stark[2] in their report on a consecutive series of 700 flexor tendon grafts. This experience from a highly respected source will repay careful study and quotation of some of their conclusions will not be out of place. "Scarring from injury or additional scarring from inept previous surgery, or failed primary reparative procedures, compromised the results of secondary tendon grafting." "In the fingers with minimum scarring and only one nerve injured, the results were not impaired, but fingers with both nerves damaged had much less motion." "In flexor-tendon grafting in the thumb . . . . grafts extending from the musculotendinous juncture to the terminal phalanx gave better results than the shorter ones." Experienced surgeons will echo these words but not all, perhaps, will agree with the criticism of plantaris as a graft.

The expectation of a successful result in the difficult case has been materially improved by the use of a preformed tendon sheath. Hunter,[11] building upon the original use of Celloidin tube implants by Mayer and Ransohoff,[13] stainless steel stripes by Milgram, and flexible silicone-rubber rods by Carroll and Bassett[8] has developed a prosthesis of silicone-rubber reinforced with Dacron. A sheath forms around the prosthesis, into which the graft is later inserted after removal of the prosthesis. Reference is made later to the practical use of this method.

GENERAL INDICATIONS

A tendon divided by injury, destroyed by infection or rheumatic disease, or absent congenitally may be successfully replaced by a tendon removed from elsewhere in the body. A tendon transposed to serve a new purpose may, if necessary, be extended by a graft to reach its new attachment. These grafts are taken from the patient, and there is no occasion in normal practice for the use of homogenous or heterogenous grafts.

THE GRAFT SOURCE

The tendons to be chosen for a graft are palmaris longus, plantaris, or extensor digitorum longus (Fig. 7.6.1.). Flexor digitorum sublimis is ideal for a short bridge graft but is less suitable as a full length graft.

Palmaris longus is removed by a small transverse incision at the wrist and a second incision in the mid-forearm. It is divided at the wrist and drawn out through the proximal incision. The presence of plantaris cannot be determined until an exposure is made; if it is absent a toe extensor is used. Two incisions are needed, one on the medial border of the tendo Achillis and the other in the midcalf, three finger breadths behind the medial border of the tibia. The gastrocnemius muscle is lifted and plantaris is found on its deep surface. These tendons may be removed through a single distal incision by the use of a tendon stripper if desired. Palmaris longus is only just long enough to reach from the distal attachment in the finger to the proximal part of the palm or from the thumb attachment to above the wrist. The muscle sometimes extends down the tendon too far to leave an adequate length of normal tendon. It is present in approximately 90 per cent of persons (Wood-Jones).[23] Plantaris is sufficiently long to serve for two grafts if necessary. It is usually of suitable size but occasionally it is very thin and should not be used. It is the tendon that I prefer to use for finger grafts, palmaris being convenient for the thumb as a wrist incision is part of the necessary exposure. Plantaris has the peculiar property of opening out into a sheet-like structure when drawn apart laterally; this feature has been utilized by Brand[4] for a neat form of fixation to the proximal tendon. It is present in approximately 93 per cent of persons (Wood-Jones).[23] Extensor digitorum longus may be used if neither of the tendons mentioned are present. It can be removed cleanly only by open dissection and a long curved incision is required reaching from the base of the toes to the ankle. For a single graft, the tendon of the fourth toe is chosen, but a leash of four tendons may be removed if required. It is preferable, if possible, to avoid using the tendon of the fifth toe, as this toe has no short extensor muscle.

TREATMENT OF TENDON DIVISIONS

Flexor Digitorum Profundus

Division of profundus distal to sublimis attachment may be treated by immediate or early secondary suture with a good expectation of success. Division at a more proximal level in the finger is generally best left for secondary consideration later (Fig. 7.6.2.).

The subsequent treatment of these injuries needs careful judgment. The choice lies between acceptance of the comparatively minor disability, arthrodesis of the terminal joint, tenodesis of the profundus end, or replacement of the tendon by a free tendon graft. The decision is governed by several factors; the condition of the finger and hand generally and the age, occupation, and wishes of the patient. Not everyone is prepared to undergo an extensive operation with no certain promise of success for loss of distal joint control. There are others to whom loss of this action is more than an inconvenience and who desire that everything possible should be done to restore normal function. It is more reasonable to advise tendon grafting for the index and middle fingers than for the other fingers because of the thumb pinch. For children, it is best to advise operation for all fingers as the convalescent period is no hardship and the child's future requirements are unknown. It is necessary to emphasise that the operation of tendon grafting for profundus division in particular should be undertaken only by surgeons experienced in this work, for an unsuccessful result may make matters worse.

The technique is similar to that used for replacement of both tendons, but there are features of special interest. The ideal donor tendon is plantaris because of its small size, but if it is absent, a toe extensor may be used. Palmaris longus is not so suitable. The sublimis tendon is preserved and care is taken to avoid injury to it. The graft is drawn along the exact course of profundus (Fig. 7.6.3.).

Flexor Digitorum Sublimis and Profundus

The case for primary tendon or second tendon grafting for the acute case may be argued and no doubt will be disputed for years to come (Verdan),[21] but for the late case the only reasonable treatment is tendon grafting, by the standard method preceded by a prosthetic implant. Tendon grafting is successful only when the finger is in good over-all condition, with an adequate passive range, no severe scarring, and with at least one sensory nerve intact or successfully repaired. When the conditions are unfavorable, consideration should be given to use of a preliminary prosthesis (Hunter).[11] This method offers a reasonable expectation of success in scarred and contracted digits. The operation is performed in two stages. At the first stage the scar is removed, contractures corrected, and a new pulley system constructed if required. The flexible rod is attached to the distal phalanx and its proximal end is left free in the tissues above the wrist. After three weeks rest the finger is exercised passively to obtain the

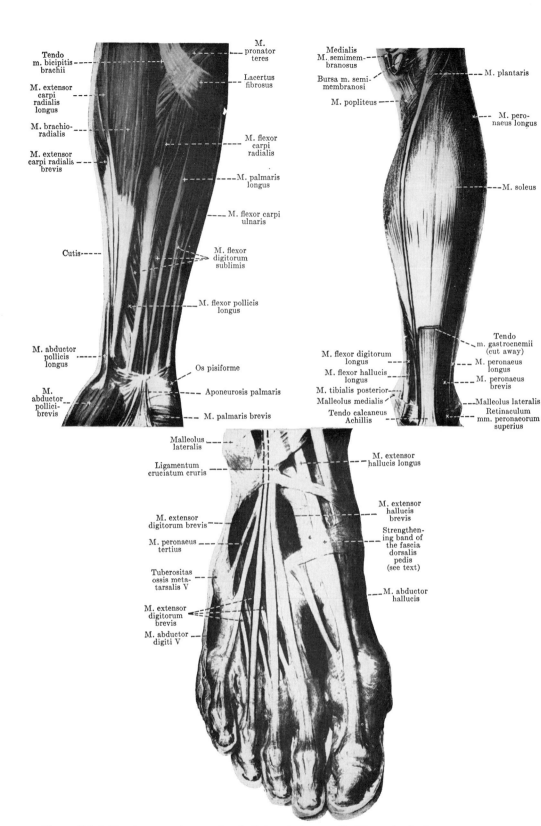

Figure 7.6.1. Tendons used as grafts. *A*. Palmaris longus. *B*. Plantaris. *C*. Extensor digitorum longus. (*From Atlas of Human Anatomy* by Spalteholz. Reproduced by courtesy of J.B. Lippincott Company, Philadelphia.)

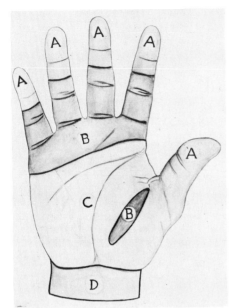

Figure 7.6.2. Recommended area methods of treatment. *A.* Primary suture when wound conditions permit. Secondary suture, arthrodesis, tenodesis or tendon graft in the fingers; secondary suture or tendon graft in the thumb. *B.* Unsuitable for primary suture as a general rule. Secondary tendon graft. *C.* Primary suture of profundus when wound conditions permit. Secondary suture or a bridge graft to close a gap in profundus. *D.* Primary suture whenever possible. Secondary suture is rarely feasible. Bridge grafts to close the gaps in the profundus and flexor pollicis longus. (From *Operative Surgery.* Reproduced by courtesy of Butterworth and Co., Ltd., London.)

incisions may be extended into the palm if exposure of the proximal section of the digit is required, but this is not always necessary (Fig. 7.6.5.). As the proximal junction of tendon and graft is made just distal to the flexor retinaculum, another small incision is required in the proximal palm for these fingers. The entire sheath is removed with the exception of the strong bands in front of the metacarpophalangeal joint, and at the midpoints of the proximal and middle phalanges. Modifications and sometimes formation of new pulleys may be needed according to circumstances. The injured tendons are completely excised and replaced by the graft (Fig. 7.6.6). The motor tendon may be either the sublimis or the profundus, depending upon their relative excursion. There is some advantage in using the sublimis for the middle and ring fingers as its individual action permits minor errors made when setting the tension to be accommodated later. In the little finger it is always better to use profundus as the sublimis muscle to this finger has insufficient power.

The proximal attachment is made by an interlacing technique which is neat and effective (Fig. 7.6.7). The distal attachment may be made by the well known Bunnell pullout stitch or by passing the graft through the profundus tag and the pulp of the finger (Fig. 7.6.8). The protruding end is held by an arterial clip while the tension of the graft is adjusted. The final tension should be such that the finger lies in slightly greater flexion than normal in relation to the other fingers. The graft is then stitched to the profundus tag and the redundant end removed.

The ideal suture material is determined by its strength, its ease of use, and the tissue response that it evokes. Synthetic materials are now available which satisfy these requirements, but I have always used stainless steel wire (British Wire Gauge 40) which is attached to 1-inch bayonet shape malleable needles.

maximum movement and to develop a sheath around the implant. Two to four months later the prosthesis is replaced by a tendon graft. Hunter has restored function to fingers which would otherwise be impossible to improve. He stresses that this method should be reserved for properly selected old injuries which are unsuitable for standard tendon grafting.

The Operation of Tendon Grafting

There are numerous variations in the operative techniques which different surgeons favor. These differences are of less significance than the gentleness and precision with which they are executed. The method to be described is the one which I have practiced for many years. A pneumatic tourniquet is used at a pressure of 220 mm Hg for adults and 180 mm Hg for children after exsanguination. The finger is exposed by a midaxial incision down to the fibrous sheath and passing posterior to the vessels and nerve. The palm is opened by extending the incision along the appropriate crease line in the case of the index and little fingers (Fig. 7.6.4.). The middle and ring finger

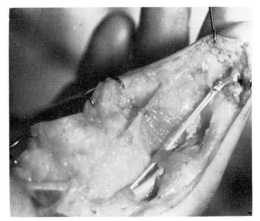

Figure 7.6.3. Exposure of the index finger to show a plantaris graft replacing the profundus tendon. The sublimis tendon is not injured. The graft in this case is attached through a transverse tunnel in the phalanx. (Reproduced by courtesy of the British Journal of Bone and Joint Surgery.)

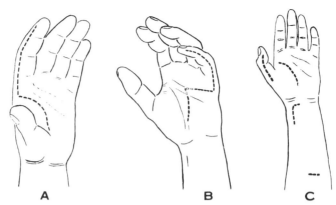

Figure 7.6.4. A. Incision for exposure of the index finger and palm. *B.* Incisions for exposure of the little finger and palm. *C.* Incisions for exposure of the thumb, palm and forearm. The proximal incision for removal of palmaris longus is also shown. (Reproduced by courtesy of the British Journal of Bone and Joint Surgery.)

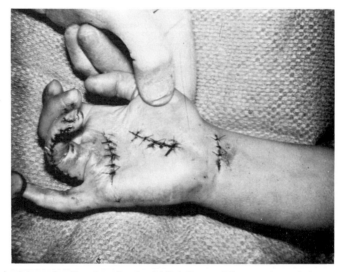

Figure 7.6.5. Incisions for the ring (and middle) finger. The tension of the graft is also shown. (Reproduced by courtesy of the American Journal of Surgery.)

After complete hemostasis has been secured, the wounds are closed and the hand dressed with all the fingers flexed over a pack of steel wool filling the palm. The limb is kept elevated for 48 hours.

Flexor Pollicis Longus

Division of flexor pollicis longus may be treated by primary suture under suitable conditions. Graft replacement offers an excellent expectation of success and it follows that it is unwise to attempt primary suture if the circumstances are difficult. There is rarely any problem in the clean-cut injury distal to the metacarpophalangeal joint and at the wrist, but between these levels a wide exposure is needed and care must be taken to avoid the hazards of severing the motor and sensory branches of the median nerve. Loss

of sensation or of opposition is a greater disability than is loss of terminal joint flexion.

Although the graft may be any one of those already mentioned, palmaris longus is generally used, as it is of suitable size, adequate length, and convenient to obtain. The thumb is exposed by a midaxial incision on the radial side, the palm along the thenar crease, and the wrist by a small straight incision. The tendon passes between the two attachments of flexor pollicis brevis and is flanked on either side by the digital nerves to the thumb (Fig. 7.6.9).

Palm Proximal to the Distal Crease, Carpal Tunnel, and Wrist.

The best results after divisions in these regions are obtained by primary suture and, unless there

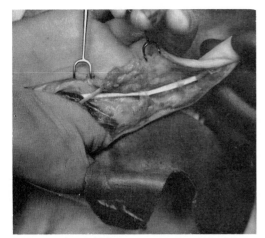

Figure 7.6.6. Exposure of the index finger showing the tendon graft, the pulleys and the digital nerve. (From Proceedings of the Sixth Congress of Société Internationale de Chirurgie Orthopédique et de Traumatologie. Reproduced by courtesy of the Secretary-General.)

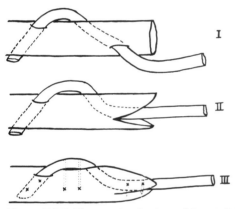

Figure 7.6.7. The proximal suture of the graft to tendon.

is a clear contraindication, this treatment is obligatory. Opinions differ as to whether both the sublimis and the profundus tendons should be repaired or whether it is better to repair profundus alone, owing to the risk of cross union. It is probably wiser to ignore or cut back sublimis in the palm, where cross union is likely to occur, and to repair both tendons at the wrist where cross union is unusual.

Those patients in whom primary repair has failed or who reach the surgeon some weeks or more after injury may have suffered a shortening of the muscle, making it difficult or impossible to secure apposition of the tendon ends. It is in these cases that a graft taken from sublimis may be used with good effect to bridge the gap in profundus. The Bunnell stitch is used and the stitch is passed through the graft (Figs. 7.6.10 and 7.6.11).

AFTERCARE

The dressing is undisturbed for three weeks. A check rein strap is then attached to the finger and forearm which permits active movement within a safe range for a further week and for two weeks in children. This strap is not suitable for the thumb which is better controlled by wool and bandage splintage, permitting slight movements. Subsequently, free movements are encouraged, assisted when necessary by a physiotherapist.

TENDON GRAFTING AFTER LONG DELAY

Patients occasionally present themselves in the hope that treatment can be given for a tendon division that occurred many years ago. Provided the digit is in good general condition, the joints mobile, and the nerves intact, treatment can offer a reasonable expectation of worthwhile improvement (Figs. 7.6.12 and 7.6.13). Tendons, when divided, retract as far as their

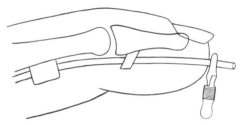

Figure 7.6.8. The distal suture of the graft. (From *Operative Surgery*. Reproduced by courtesy of Butterworth & Co., Ltd., London.)

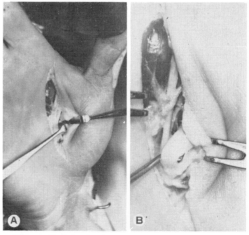

Figure 7.6.9. A. Exposure through the thenar crease to free the divided tendon of flexor pollicis longus preparatory to its replacement by a graft. *B.* The tendon is held by a hook. The digital nerves to the radial side of the index finger and to the radial side of the thumb can be seen.

natural attachments such as the vincula and the lumbricalis muscle permit. It follows, therefore, that the muscle may be continuing to work against an attachment and its integrity is preserved. There is no way of determining the quality of the muscle until the tendon

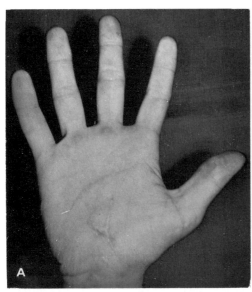

Figure 7.6.10. A graft is taken from the sublimis tendon to bridge a gap in the profundus tendon. (From *Operative Surgery*. Reproduced by courtesy of Butterworth & Co., Ltd., London.)

is exposed, but if it is deemed to be inadequate, sublimis of another finger may be used as a substitute. These facts should be explained beforehand to the patient and permission obtained for the use of a normal sublimis should it be found necessary.

A recent study (Pulvertaft)[19] of a series of grafting after long delay (average five years) revealed that in a total of 58 good preoperative cases (Table 7.6.1)— including grafting for profundus only (Table 7.6.2), profundus and sublimis (Table 7.6.3), and for flexor pollicis longus loss (Table 7.6.4) — the results were better than expected and at least equal to those obtained under normal circumstances (Pulvertaft).[17 18] This finding, which was also noted by Boyes & Stark[2] is partly explained by the fact that the preoperative state of the delay series was better than in the general series; in other words, a stricter selection for operative suitability was used. The over-all average age (15 years) was lower than in the general series (24 years). This observation influences the advice that should be given when the patient is under the age of four years. The lack of postoperative co-operation in the very young prejudices the result and it is wiser to defer surgery until the child is able to understand and practice exercises enthusiastically. The parents may be assured that no harm is caused by the deferment of treatment.

TENOLYSIS

The return of active movements after tendon grafting is often slow and much perseverance is needed by patient and surgeon. Occasionally a finger that appears unpromising at three months after operation will inexplicably improve and within the next few months

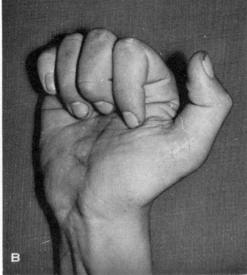

Figure 7.6.11. Result obtained by a sublimis bridge graft to restore continuity in the profundus tendon of the index finger; also a palmaris graft to replace flexor pollicis longus.

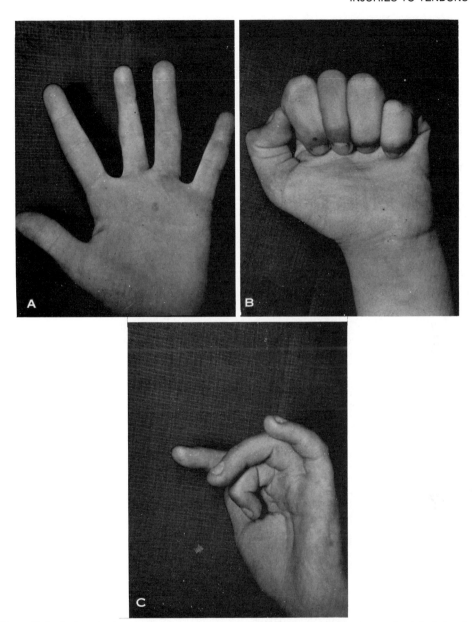

Figure 7.6.12. Result obtained by a plantaris graft to replace the profundus and sublimis tendons of the middle finger. Age at injury, two years. Age at operation, 10 years. The graft is motivated by the sublimis muscle of the injured finger.

attain a satisfactory range of movement. It is in those cases in which the active range persistently lags behind the passive range that the presence of strong adhesion bands should be suspected and the operation of tenolysis considered. Tenolysis must be deferred until it is certain that no further spontaneous improvement will occur; this, in practice, usually means at least six months from operation.

Tenolysis is no less extensive than the original operation; a limited procedure is more likely to do harm than good. A complete exposure is made, and the tendon is released throughout its full length until a pull upon the proximal end will produce complete flexion. Every effort should be made to preserve the pulleys; if a pulley is too damaged to retain, a new one may be made from a short length of tendon. Active movements are encouraged within a day or two of operation and continued until the maximum function has been obtained.

Fetrow,[9] in reviewing a series of 134 patients in

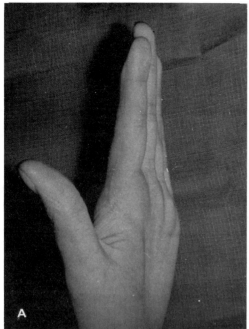

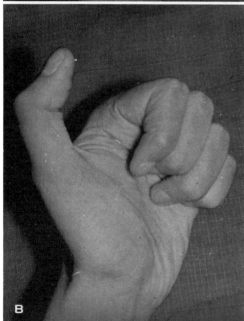

Figure 7.6.13. Result obtained by a plantaris graft to replace the profundus and sublimis tendons of the index finger. Age at injury, nine years. Age at operation 13½ years. The graft is motivated by the profundus muscle of the injured finger. (From *The Hand,* in preparation. Reproduced by courtesy of W. B. Saunders Co., Philadelphia.)

whom tenolysis had been performed, concluded that the operation is a useful procedure to improve function when the indications are correct and the technique is carefully performed. Tenolysis is unsuccessful when done in the face of poor conditions or if the tendon is not freed completely.

COMPLICATIONS

1. Immediate Postoperative

Hematoma is avoided by meticulous attention to hemostasis. The operative field must be completely dry before the wound is closed. Drainage is not, in my experience, required. Reactionary edema is equally prejudicial to a good result. Bandaging of the hand should be firm and supportive but not in any sense compressive. Elevation for 48 hours is a routine measure. Infection rarely occurs after reconstructive surgery of this kind. It is unnecessary to use prophylactic antibiotic therapy unless the operation has been unusually extensive and prolonged.

2. Rupture of the Graft

The graft may break or come adrift from its attachments if subjected to undue strain during the first few weeks of activity. Rupture is a major disaster but should rarely occur. Should it do so, the correct course is to allow time for the hand to settle completely and repeat the operation six months later.

3. Adhesions

Virtually all the failures of tendon grafting are due to this cause. Tissue links between the surrounding tissue and the tendon and graft junctions are a normal part of the healing process and resolve to permit movement to occur. The operative intervention adds to these natural adhesions and it is only by the most careful technique that these are kept to the minimum.

4. Hyperextension of the Proximal Interphalangeal Joint

One would expect this deformity to occur fairly frequently owing to the absence of sublimis action. It is not commonly seen, no doubt because many fingers

TABLE 7.6.1

TENDON   GRAFTS   1942 – 1970
Total   527

DELAY OVER 2 YEARS	77	
GRADES 1 and 2 – Hunter – 70		
RECORDS INADEQUATE	12	
NET TOTAL FOR ANALYSIS	58	
FLEXOR PROFUNDUS		5
FLEXOR PROFUNDUS & SUBLIMIS		42
FLEXOR POLLICIS LONGUS		11

TABLE 7.6.2

FLEXOR   PROFUNDUS
5   Cases

AVERAGE   DELAY   4   YEARS   (2 —   7)

AVERAGE   AGE   (AT   OPERATION)   19   YEARS   (6 — 35)

AVERAGE   FINGER   TIP   TO   DISTAL   CREASE   0·25 IN. — 0·6 CM.

AVERAGE   T.I.P. FLEXION RANGE   60°

ONE   COMPLETE   FAILURE — FROM   ADHESIONS — ARTHRODESIS

TWO   EXTENSION   LOSS — -10°,   -20°

(**4**   INCLUDED   IN   ANALYSIS)

TABLE 7.6.3

FLEXOR   PROFUNDUS   &   SUBLIMIS
42   Cases

AVERAGE   DELAY   5   YEARS   (2 —   24)

AVERAGE   AGE   (AT   OPERATION)   14   YEARS   (3 —   44)

AVERAGE   FINGER   TIP   TO   DISTAL   CREASE   0·7 IN. — 1·7 CM.

TWO   COMPLETE   FAILURES   1. FROM   ADHESIONS — AMPUTATION
                             2. FROM   RUPTURE   — ?

EIGHT   EXTENSION   LOSS   P.I.P.   JOINT — -20°,   -30°,   -30°
                          T.I.P.   JOINT — -20°,   -30°,   -30°,   -30°,   -40°

(**40**   INCLUDED   IN   ANALYSIS)

TABLE 7.6.4

FLEXOR   POLLICIS   LONGUS
11   Cases

AVERAGE   DELAY   5   YEARS   (2   — 16)

AVERAGE   AGE   (AT   OPERATION)   18   YEARS   (4   — 56)

AVERAGE   I.P.   JOINT   RANGE   61°

(ALL   INCLUDED   IN   ANALYSIS)

after tendon grafting have a slight, usually unnoticeable, flexion contracture. There is a greater risk of its occurrence in the naturally hypermobile hand. Should the volar plate of the proximal interphalangeal joint have been damaged, and preoperative hyperextension present, it is advisable to use a slip of the sublimis tendon as a restraining ligament.

5. The Lumbrical Syndrome

White[22] drew attention to this complication which he termed "extensor habitus." Littler[12] suggests that in some cases it may be due to scarring between the profundus tendon and the lumbrical muscle, causing the tendon to drag unnaturally on the lumbrical and thus extend the proximal interphalangeal joints, before acting as a flexor of the finger. Bunnell[7] spoke of this danger and advised that if the lumbrical is contracted it should not be used to cover the tendon graft anastomosis. Parkes[15] has recently reminded us of this complication and of the paradoxical extension of the proximal interphalangeal joint which it causes. The condition may be relieved by division of the lumbrical tendon.

RESULTS

It is important when comparing the results obtained under different circumstances and by different techniques that there should be a uniform method of assessment (Boyes[1]). Active flexion is recorded by measuring the distance by which the finger tip fails to reach the distal palmar crease. In cases of grafting for isolated profundus loss, the range of flexion of the distal interphalangeal joint is also included. In the thumb, the range of active flexion of the inter-

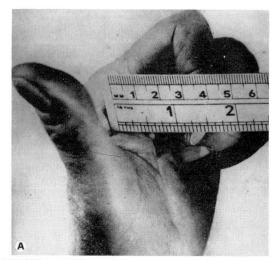

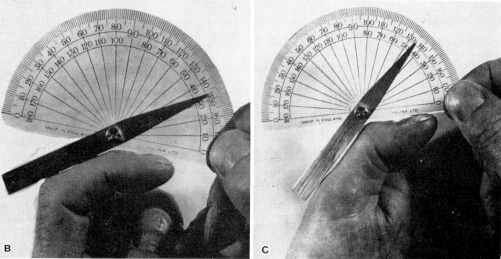

Figure 7.6.14. A. Measurement of finger flexion. The distance from the finger tip to the distal palmar crease is here one inch. *B.* Measurement of the distal interphalangeal joint range with the finger in semiflexion. *C.* Measurement of the interphalangeal joint of the thumb. (Reproduced by courtesy of the British Journal of Bone and Joint Surgery.)

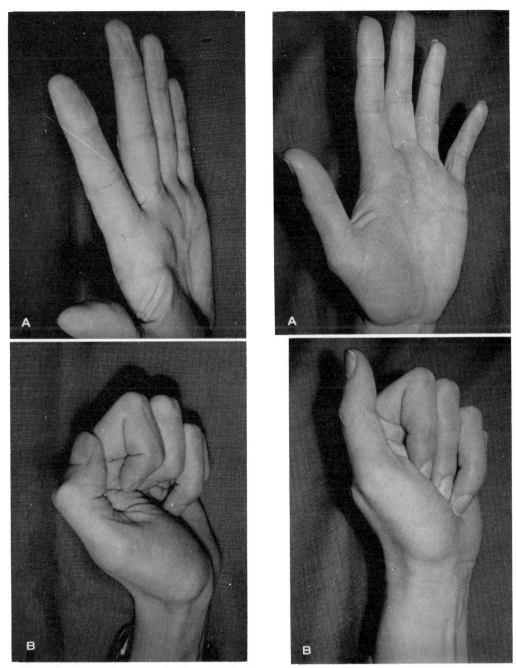

Figure 7.6.15. Result obtained by a plantaris graft to replace the profundus tendon of the ring finger. The profundus tendon was torn from its insertion and retracted into the palm. The sublimis tendon was uninjured.

Figure 7.6.16. Result obtained by a plantaris graft to replace the profundus and sublimis tendons of the ring and little fingers.

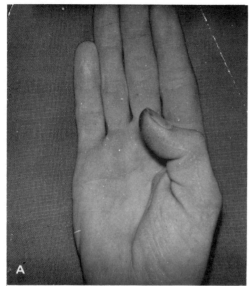

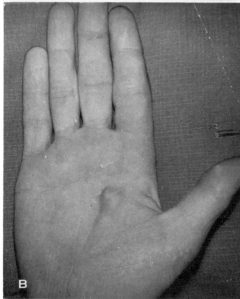

Figure 7.6.17. Result obtained by a palmaris graft to replace the flexor pollicis longus tendon.

phalangeal joint is recorded (Fig. 7.6.14). Extension in each instance is taken as complete unless otherwise stated.

In the first edition (Flynn)[10] the results obtained over a period of 13 years were stated. Since then the standard achieved has not materially altered and it appears that total success is still unattainable. The advice given to patients is that in suitable digits there is approximately 80 per cent expectation of success for profundus replacement, 70 per cent for profundus and sublimis and 90 per cent for flexor pollicis longus (Figs. 7.6.15, 7.6.16, and 7.6.17).

REFERENCES

1. Boyes, J. H. Flexor tendon grafts in the fingers and thumb. J. Bone Joint Surg., *32A:* 489, 1950.
2. Boyes, J. H., and Stark, H. H. Flexor-tendon grafts in the fingers and thumb. J. Bone Joint Surg., *53A:* 1332, 1971
3. Biesalski, K., and Mayer, L. *Die physiologiesche Schnenuerplfanzuñg.* Berlin, Springer, 1916.
4. Brand, P. W. Tendon grafting. J. Bone Joint Surg., *43B:* 444, 1961.
5. Bunnell, S. Repair of tendons in the fingers and description of two new instruments. Surg. Gynecol. Obstet., *26:* 103, 1918.
6. Bunnell, S. Repair of tendons in the fingers. Surg. Gynecol. Obstet., *35:* 88, 1922.
7. Bunnell, S. *Surgery of the Hand,* Ed. 3. Philadelphia, Lippincott, 1956, p. 450.
8. Carroll, R. E., and Bassett, C. A. L. Formation of tendon sheath by silicone-rod implants. Proc. Am. Soc. Surg. Hand. In J. Bone Joint Surg., *45A:* 884, 1963.
9. Fetrow, K. O. Tenolysis in the hand and wrist. J. Bone Joint Surg., *49A:* 667, 1967.
10. Flynn, J. E. *Hand Surgery.* Baltimore, Williams & Wilkins, 1966, p. 311.
11. Hunter, J. M., and Salisbury, R. E. Flexor-tendon reconstruction in severely damaged hands. J. Bone Joint Surg., *53A:* 829, 1971.
12. Littler, J. W. Extensor habitus. J. Bone Joint Surg., *42 A:* 913, 1960.
13. Mayer, L., and Ransohoff, N. Reconstruction of the digital sheath. J. Bone Joint Surg., *28:* 607, 1936.
14. Milgram, J. E. Transplantation of tendons through preformed gliding channels. Bull. Hosp. Joint Dis., *21:* 250, 1960.
15. Parkes, A. The "lumbricalis plus" finger. J. Bone Joint Surg., *53 B:* 236, 1971.
16. Potenza, A. H. The healing of autogenous tendon grafts within the flexor digital sheath in dogs. J. Bone Joint Surg., *46 A:* 1462, 1964.
17. Pulvertaft, R. G. Tendon grafts for flexor tendon injuries in the fingers and thumb. J. Bone Joint Surg., *38 B:* 175, 1956.
18. Pulvertaft, R. G. *The Hand.* Philadelphia, Saunders (in preparation).
19. Pulvertaft, R. G. The treatment of profundus division by free tendon graft. J. Bone Joint. Surg., *42 A:* 1363, 1960.
20. Robson, A. W. M. A case of tendon grafting. Tr. Clin. Soc. London, *22:* 289, 1889.
21. Verdan. C. E. Half a century of flexor-tendon surgery. J. Bone Joint Surg., *54 A:* 472, 1972.
22. White, W. L. Extensor habitus. J. Bone Joint Surg., *42A:* 913, 1960
23. Wood-Jones, F. *The Principles of Anatomy as Seen in the hand.* London, Churchill, 1920, pp. 131 and 190.

G.

Tendon Transfers
In the Forearm

Paul W. Brand, M.D., F.R.C.S.

GENERAL PRINCIPLES

There are three types of problem that must be solved in every operation for transfer of tendons. The first is the problem of local tissue adjustment. new blood supply may be needed for the tendon, a new gliding pathway must be opened, and adhesions must be prevented or overcome. The second problem is that of the mechanical control of the joints affected by the transfer. A few muscles have to do the work usually done by many. Finally, there is a problem in the brain; the motor units controlling the trasferred muscles must be brought under conscious control, be reeducated, and then drop back into the subconscious in a new pattern of coordination.

The Tissue Problem

Every operation involves a wound, which heals by scar tissue. The scar tends to link together every structure in the wound, both those that are static and those that should move. The following practical rules will be found useful. *The total mass of scar must be kept small.* Scar is a part of healing, therefore, there should be as little wounding as possible so that not much healing is required. Since scar fills the spaces in a wound and replaces collections of blood clot, hemostasis should be meticulous at the time of wound closure, and then, if wide dissection has been necessary, either positive pressure should be maintained externally or negative pressure continued inside the wound through fine Polythene tubes to prevent postoperative hematoma. Scar is particularly crippling and extensive when it results from infection, so the most rigid aseptic techniques must be used in tendon surgery, and great care taken to close all wounds with viable skin in hairline approximation without tension. An atraumatic technique must be practiced with an affectionate regard for every living cell. One member of the surgical team must keep constantly alert to prevent the drying of exposed tendons, automatically dribbling saline over tendons every five minutes, no matter what delicate maneuver may be in progress.

The probable orientation and attachments of scar must be predicted and planned. Some scar is necessary and inevitable, but it should not unite the tendon to an immovable structure proximal to its intended insertion. It is enough that we recognize that the consistency and alignment of a scar are influenced profoundly by the tissues with which it is in contact and

by the forces to which it is subjected. The same process that produces sound tendon union after suture may cause anchoring adhesions if a portion of the cut end of a tendon is left out of the suture line and free to organize local scar into a secondary tendon. This is the "unsatisfied end" of Bunnell.[5]

It is important, therefore, not to allow any part of any tendon end to be exposed in a wound. Tendon ends should either be fixed firmly to the insertion or to the graft to which they are supposed to attach, or they should be surrounded with tissue which will move freely with them without forming an anchor.

If the tendon cannot glide in its new pathway, the pathway must glide with the tendon. In spite of every care to prevent excessive scar, a tendon will often develop attachments to any or all of the tissues that surround it. This is especially true of a free tendon graft which, in order to survive, has to develop a new blood supply along all of its length. Thus, the cells closest to the tendon form a sort of visceral layer of paratenon. When movement is first allowed, the normal tissues that lie around this layer will begin to stretch and modify themselves to allow gliding far more easily than the scar-infiltrated layer next to the tendon. Finally, in some cases, a synovial space opens up around the tendon and true gliding is established between a visceral and parietal layer of tissue, both derived from the tissues that were there before the graft was placed. More often the so-called "gliding" is entirely due to the flexibility and stretch of connective tissue that has loosened up enough to allow unhindered movement within a certain range.

Knowing that a tendon graft may get stuck, the wise surgeon will arrange that it sticks only to mobile tissues. It is not possible to follow this advice every time but if we keep this as an ideal it will often be found possible to achieve it by placing small wounds proximally and distally, and tunnelling bluntly between them to carry tendons and grafts.

This tunnelling is by far the best way to place a graft. The surgeon probes with his blunt-nosed instrument (Fig. 7.7.1) until he finds a path along which it passes easily. The quality of tissue that allows the tunneller to pass easily is the same as that which will allow a tendon to move, or will move with a tendon which becomes adherent to it.[4]

The time factor in the mobilization of tendon transfers. If we assume that a tendon transfer or graft has been well placed, and that no gross adhesions are to be anticipated, there will nearly always be some points at which adhesions have occurred between the tendon and some fibrous septum or sling, and these adhesions have to be stretched if the tendon is to move. After any tendon operation there is an optimal time when tendon junctions are just strong enough to take a strain, and adhesions just weak enough to be stretched. It is at this time that well judged effort and exercise will be rewarded by obvious improvement in range of movement.

Many poor results in hand surgery result because

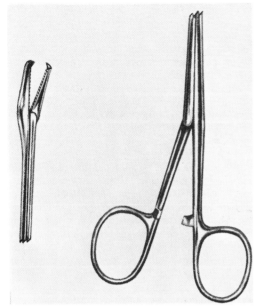

Figure 7.7.1. Tendon tunnelling forceps (Andersen). When the jaws are closed the nose is smooth rounded. The viper-shaped head places the thickest part of the tunnelling forceps just behind the nose.

the optimal time is missed. It may be that the wound is infected and must be rested, that an ambitious skin graft has had an incomplete take, or—most disgraceful of all—the surgeon has neglected to make sure that full passive mobility has been achieved before operation so that now, with the tendon transferred and ready to move, the joint is stiff. By the time the joint stiffness is overcome or the wound finally healed, the tendon adhesions have toughened and shortened so that exercises seem to produce no improvement of range, and the patient may give up his effort for lack of early response.

The Mechanical Problem

Tendon operations are usually needed for cases of paralysis, destruction, or hopeless fixation of muscles affecting the hand. The following mechanical rules and principles serve as a guide.

A muscle acts on a joint according to fixed mechanical laws. It exercises a "moment" or turning force on the joint which is directly proportional to the power of the muscle, and to the perpendicular distance between the fulcrum of the joint and the tendon as it crosses the joint.

If a tendon, on its way to move a distal joint, bowstrings across a proximal joint, its mechanical advantage at the proximal joint will be so great that it may force that joint into unwanted movement and also may use up all its amplitude so that it cannot move the distal joint. For example, in cases of severe paralysis of forearm muscles, surgeons have tried using the biceps

for flexion of the fingers. This has often failed because the tendon bowstrings across the elbow and therefore can flex the fingers only when the elbow is extended.

When most of the muscles of a hand have been paralyzed, there is a great temptation to make a remaining muscle perform multiple tasks, either by acting upon each of several joints crossed by the tendon, or by splitting the tendon so that each slip does a different job. This is sometimes useful but the following limitations must be borne in mind.

1. A muscle can have a "selective" action on two joints that it crosses only if it is opposed by a different muscle at each joint.

Consider a thumb (Fig. 7.7.2) which has lost all of its short muscles and has only the long flexor to flex both its joints, and the long extensor to extend them. When it is faced with an opposing thrust as from an index finger in the action of "pinch," it opposes this thrust by contracting the flexor pollicis longus (*M*). This tendon will have equal tension along its length, and will have a flexion turning moment on each of the two joints in proportion to its distance from the joint fulcrum at the point of crossing. The backward thrust from the index finger has a greater mechanical advantage against the proximal joint (×5 cm) than against the distal joint (×2 cm) so if the flexor exerts enough tension only to flex the distal joint, the proximal joint will retreat into extension (Fig. 7.7.3). Further effort will now only increase the deformity.

To prevent this situation the surgeon must *either* add a separate flexor, just for the proximal joint, *or* he must arthrodese one of the joints so that he may obtain full control of the other with existing muscles.

2. If a tendon is split and inserted so that each half affects a different joint then both joints must always move together. One action cannot be opposed and stopped without stopping the other.

Before splitting any tendon, therefore, the surgeon

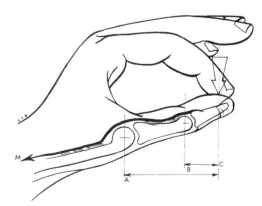

Figure 7.7.2. Diagram of a tendon that crosses more than one joint. The external force of pinch, represented by the arrow at *C* has a tendency to force joints *A* and *B* into extension. The turning moment at *A* is proportion to *A-C* while that at *B* is proportional to *B-C*.

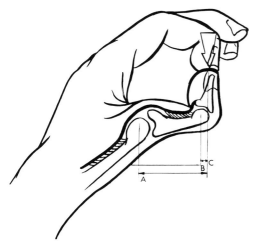

Figure 7.7.3. The deformity that results from having only one flexor tendon crossing two joints. See text for explanation.

must make sure that each of the actions he wants to achieve needs equal amplitude and that they are always needed simultaneously.

The Problem in the Brain

Even when tendon transfers are well designed mechanically and lie in good gliding pathways, their usefulness depends on the ability of the brain to direct them. Most surgeons do not place enough emphasis on reeducation. The surgeon should work closely with the therapist and should discuss the case with him or her before deciding on the final plan of surgery. This is only possible if the therapist can be part of the team, and not changed on some system of rotation.

The surgeon must decide whether the patient is mentally capable of learning the new pattern of muscular control. For example, if a wrist-moving muscle is needed to flex a finger, it is better to use a wrist extensor than a wrist flexor because the wrist is usually extended as the fingers flex.

Tendon Tension

At operation, the tension of a tendon transfer is best judged while the hand is placed in the position it will assume when the new tendon contracts. In that position, the tendon is sutured without tension and without loose redundancy. In any case where reeducation is likely to be a problem it is better to attach transferred tendons at a rather higher tension than usual. This brings the new muscle more readily into consciousness as stretch reflexes are set up when opposing muscles restore the neutral position of the limb.

Summary of General Principles

These are the rules of tendon transfer as laid down by our great teachers from Leo Meyer[11] to Bunnell.[6] Before transferring a tendon be sure: (1) that it can be

spared from its original place; (2) that it is strong enough for its new task; (3) that it has amplitude enough for its new movement; (4) that it is under conscious voluntary control; (5) that its old action is synergistic with its new, or at least retrainable to it; (6) that it can reach its new insertion without a sharp change of direction; (7) that it can get there without going through dense scar, tough fascia, or across bare bone; (8) that the movement it is expected to produce is already freely possible by passive movement; (9) that there is no avoidable hazard of infection; and (10) that the patient understands what is to be done, and is ready to accept the postoperative discipline of exercises and training.

USEFUL TENDON TRANSFERS

There are certain patterns of paralysis that occur fairly frequently and it is worth recording a few patterns of transfer which have proved useful for these cases.

Ulnar Paralysis

The ulnar nerve is particularly liable to injury and degeneration at the level of the elbow, and it is at this level that most leprosy cases suffer complete ulnar paralysis. The loss of flexor carpi ulnaris and of the ulnar half of flexor profundus is not usually serious, and does not call for tendon transfers unless there is some accompanying median or radial nerve loss. If the patient notices the weakness in flexion of his ring and little fingers then it is worth attaching the flexor profundus tendons of the ring and little fingers to the flexor profundus of the middle finger in the forearm. The adjacent surfaces of the tendons to the little finger, ring finger, and middle finger are scarified and stitched side to side. The index finger profundus should be left free.

The chief defect in ulnar palsy is the loss of the intrinsic muscles of the hand. This usually causes clawing of the ring and little fingers, and quite frequently perceptible clawing of the index and long fingers as well. In addition to the clawing of the fingers there is a weakness in the thumb which can also be described as "clawing." On attempting to pinch, the terminal joint of the thumb flexes sharply and the metacarpophalangeal joint tends to hyperextend. This is due to the paralysis of the adductor pollicis and part of the flexor pollicis brevis, both of which act as flexors of the metacarpophalangeal joint.

Claw Hand

The paralyzed intrinsics are concerned with the flexion of the metacarpophalangeal joints and the extension of the interphalangeal joint as well as with abduction and adduction movements of the fingers. Since it is not possible to find enough muscles to restore all of these actions independently it is usual to concentrate on providing a prime flexor for the metacarpophalangeal joints. The same tendon can also assist in the extension of the interphalangeal joint but this is not essential, providing that the long extensor muscles are working normally.

The surgeon should hold the patient's hand with the metacarpophalangeal joints supported in flexion, and then ask the patient to straighten his interphalangeal joints. If he can do this easily, then an immediate tendon transfer is indicated. If he fails to do it because of interphalangeal joint stiffness then a course of preliminary exercises and splintage is necessary. If he fails in spite of mobile joints it must be due to weakness of his extensor digitorum or to some failure in the dorsal extensor tendon apparatus. The whole hand needs to be reassessed and other tendon transfers advised along with that for intrinsic paralysis.

In a recent case of ulnar paralysis the clawing may not be very marked; in fact, the hand may seem to function almost normally. This is because the anterior capsule of the metacarpophalangeal joint prevents hyperextension and therefore allows the long extensor muscles to extend all the joints of the finger. As time passes, however, the capsule of the metacarpophalangeal joint becomes stretched, the joint hyperextends, and the full picture of the claw hand develops. Because a tight metacarpophalangeal joint capsule seems to control claw hand, various operations have been described to limit extension of the metacarpophalangeal joint passively and thus avoid the need for tendon transfers. These operations are successful in allowing interphalangeal extension, and thus correct "claw hand." However, the most serious defect in intrinsic paralysis is the failure in active flexion of the metacarpophalangeal joints. When an object is grasped in an intrinsic paralyzed hand, the whole force of grasp comes through the tips of the fingers rather than through the whole volar surface. This is particularly harmful in insensitive fingers where bruising and ulceration of finger tips is often followed by progressive absorption. Zancolli[19] has described a technique for capsuloplasty combined with pulley advancement at the MP joint. This is designed to give the long flexors a better mechanical advantage at the MP joints. Riordan[13] has described a tenodesis in which tendon strips cross the wrist joint on the dorsal side and the metacarpophalangeal joints on the volar side. This operation gives active intrinsic action when the wrist flexes and puts the tenodesis on the stretch. Both these operations are suitable for use when there is a shortage of muscles available for transfer.

Operations for Instrinsic Replacement for Fingers

Stiles[16] and Bunnell[6] described operations in which tendons of the flexor sublimis digitorum were used as motors for intrinsic replacement. It has been found satisfactory to use a single motor for all four fingers. The flexor sublimis tendon from the ring or middle fingers may be used. The tendon is divided at its insertion, pulled out in midpalm and split longitudinally into four strands. Each strand is passed along the line of a lumbrical tendon into a finger and attached to the dorsal expansion just proximal to the interphalangeal joint. This operation is satisfactory in most cases but has the disadvantage that a sublimis has to be removed from a finger, and that the same muscle which previously was a flexor of an interphalangeal joint becomes an extensor of the same joint. This sometimes results in hyperextension of the joint that was previously flexed ("intrinsic plus"). This is avoided if a wrist-moving muscle is used rather than a finger flexor. In this case the tendon must be extended by free grafts. Techniques have been described by Littler[9] and Brand.[4]

The best motor to use is the extensor carpi radialis longus. The tendon is divided through a short transverse incision at the end of the radius. It is identified halfway up the forearm and pulled out through another short transverse incision. The tendon is then tunnelled through an incision 2½ inches proximal to the wrist crease on the front of the forearm, and is there anastomosed to a free graft (Fig. 7.7.4). A plantaris tendon is long enough to be folded to make two grafts, so the anastomosis is made to the center of the plantaris, and then the ends are each split so that four "tails" arise from one motor tendon. In the absence of a plantaris, a strip of fascia lata half an inch wide may be used and split into four in its distal half.

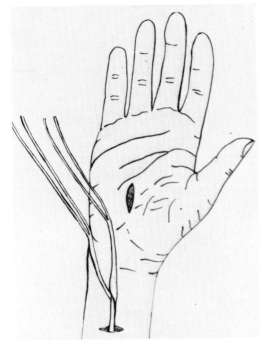

Figure 7.7.4. The many-tailed graft, for ulnar paralysis. The tendon of extensor carpi radialis longus has been tunnelled from the dorsum of the midforearm to an incision proximal to the front of the wrist. Here it is attached to a four-tailed graft.

The tendon tunneller is then inserted through a small longitudinal incision in the proximal part of the palm. It is advanced proximally along the dorsal part of the carpal tunnel and then the wrist is extended to bring the nose of the forceps into the forearm wound where the four ends of the graft are grasped and withdrawn into the palm.

From the palmar incision each tendon slip is passed separately along the line of a lumbrical tendon to the side of the dorsal expansion (Fig. 7.7.5). The attachment in each finger is made on the radial side of the dorsal expansion except that in the index finger it is placed on the ulnar side, otherwise the fingers tend to spread apart. If abduction of the index finger seems important, this may be added separately by a rerouting of the tendon of extensor indicis proprius to the radial border of the index finger.

While suturing the tendons to their insertions one should keep the wrist 40° flexed and the metacarpophalangeal joints 80° flexed, and the interphalangeal joints straight. With the hand in this position the tendon grafts should be slightly pulled and then allowed to relax and stitched under neutral tension in the position of relaxation (Fig. 7.7.6).

Another operation for this condition is Fowler's[7] procedure in which the extensor digiti minimi tendon and the extensor indicis proprius tendon are each divided, leaving the extensor digitorium tendons to extend the fingers. The divided tendons are each used for the intrinsic action of two adjacent fingers. They are passed through the interosseous spaces between the metacarpals and passed anterior to the deep transverse metacarpal ligament and then on to the lateral border of the dorsal expansion on each finger. If this operation is to be a success a high tension must be used. In some cases a slip of the extensor digitorum from the ring finger will need to be used to extend the little finger because often the extensor digiti minimi is the only effective extensor of the little finger.

Recovery of intrinsic function after high laceration of the ulnar nerve is so uncommon that it is wise to carry out a muscle-balance operation soon after nerve suture. By acting early, joint stiffness will be avoided and the volar capsule of the metacarpal joint will never become stretched.

Ulnar Weakness in the Thumb

Sometimes the clawing of the thumb proves to be quite a disablement, particularly in the right hand. In

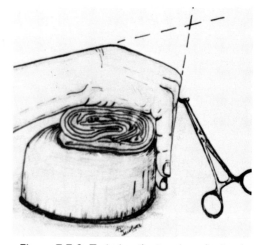

Figure 7.7.6. To judge the tension of a tendon graft, it has to be relaxed at each joint that it crosses.

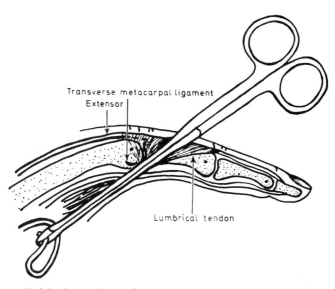

Figure 7.7.5. One tail of the four-tailed graft is picked up in midpalm by a tunneller that will bring it out beside the lumbrical tendon where it is to be attached.

such cases the acute flexion of the terminal joint of the thumb is best corrected by providing a prime flexor for the metacarpophalangeal joint of the thumb to replace the paralyzed adductor pollicis and flexor pollicis brevis. For this purpose a tendon should be directed to the proximal phalanx of the thumb from about the middle of the palm. The extensor indicis proprius has been used successfully for this but if the strength of the pinch is really important it is worth expending a sublimis from the ring finger which is brought out in mid-palm and then tunnelled from that point, superficial to the palmar fascia, and inserted into the edge of the dorsal expansion on the back of the proximal phalanx, 1.5 cm distal to the metacarpophalangeal joint. The real adductor pollicis is inserted on the ulnar side of the thumb, but in ulnar-median palsy it is better to reinforce the opposition of the thumb by inserting the new adductor on the radial side. This should also be done in ulnar palsy from leprosy because the median nerve may be paralyzed later (Fig. 7.7.7).

Median Nerve Paralysis and Ulnar-Median Paralysis at the Wrist

When the median nerve is injured at the wrist there are often tendon injuries at the same time to complicate the picture. In leprosy the median nerve is frequently destroyed at the level of the wrist and may be perfectly normal proximal to this. In these cases the

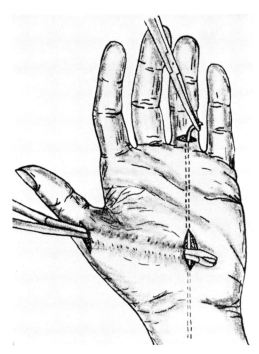

Figure 7.7.7. For ulnar palsy, a flexor sublimis tendon is rerouted to the proximal phalanx of the thumb using the palmar fascia as a sling. In this diagram both the palmar incision and the thumb incision should be a little more distal. See text.

ulnar nerve is usually paralyzed at the same time. In any median nerve lesion the sensory loss is extremely grave because it affects the important sensitive areas of the pulps of the thumb and index finger. If islands of sensitive skin are to be transferred this should be planned in advance, before any widespread tendon surgery, otherwise scarring may make the mobilization of the neurovascular bundles more difficult.

In a pure median palsy the abductor pollicis brevis and opponens of the thumb are paralyzed but the adductor muscles are normal. A new tendon will be needed which abducts and pronates the thumb. Probably the best is a flexor sublimis tendon because this is long enough to reach its new insertion without a graft and the heel of the palm is a particularly difficult area for a tendon graft because of the number of fibrous septa to which it can become adherent.

The problem becomes much more difficult when ulnar palsy is combined with median palsy because in this case all the intrinsic muscles of the thumb are lost and therefore one should provide both an abductor and adductor for the carpometacarpal joint and also an abductor, adductor, and short flexor for the metacarpophalangeal joint. Since it is quite unreasonable to spare this number of muscles for transfer, one has to try to achieve all these actions with one, or at the most two, transferred muscles.

The thumb should be held by the surgeon and twisted into full opposition and then pulled forward in this position, away from the palm to test the width of th web. It will often be found that the dorsal skin is tight. No tendon surgery should be attempted until this tight skin has been divided along the whole length of the second metacarpal. The fascia underlying it should also be divided until the thumb can lie in a good position of abduction and opposition. The defect on the back of the hand should then be filled with a free skin graft. Only occasionally will the thumb web be found to be so narrow that a Z-plasty will be needed for the free margin of the web in addition to the skin graft on the dorsum.

If only one tendon is to be transferred for low ulnar-median paralysis of the thumb, that tendon should be the flexor sublimis from the ring or middle finger. It should approach the thumb either from the direction of the pisiform bone (Bunnell)[6] or across the palm from a point just distal to the carpal tunnel (Thompson[17]). The former gives wider abduction, the latter gives a stronger pinch (Fig. 7.7.8A and *B*). In either case the tendon should approach the thumb through a subcutaneous tunnel directed towards the metacarpophalangeal joint. It should be brough out through a short incision about an inch proximal to the joint and split into two strands; one strand should pass on the radial side of the metacarpophalangeal joint ventral to the fulcrum of the joint. The other strand should cross the neck of the metacarpal, dorsal to the metacarpophalangeal joint, and should cross the joint itself on the ulnar side. The first slip may be attached to the dorsal expansion or extensor tendon between the metacarpophalangeal joint and the interphalangeal

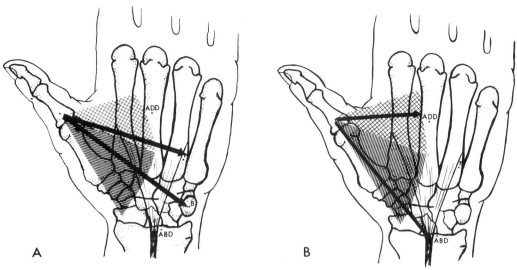

Figure 7.7.8. Diagrams indicating the way in which the intrinsic muscles fan out to give stability to the thumb. The cross-hatched area of the fan represents the ulnar-supplied muscles and the parallel shading the median supplied muscles. *A.* When one tendon only is used for intrinsic paralysis, the *lower arrow* shows direction recommended by Bunnell, the *upper arrow* shows direction recommended by Thompson. *B.* When two tendons are used, the *upper arrow* indicates the direction of the adductor replacement, the *lower arrow* the abductor replacement. Both tendons pronate.

joint and the second slip may be attached to the tendon of the adductor pollicis just distal to the metacarpophalangeal joint. Thus, the two halves of this tendon will have exactly opposing actions on the metacarpophalangeal joint, and as such will serve to stabilize the joint without moving it. It has been made clear in the early part of the chapter why one cannot expect one muscle to act separately and independently on the different joints which it crosses. Thus, it is impossible to control each joint of the thumb separately if only one tendon is transferred in cases of complete intrinsic paralysis. I suggest, therefore, that no attempt be made to control the movement of the metacarpophalangeal joint. The carpometacarpal joint should be under control and so should the interphalangeal joint. The dorsal slip should be attached first with about 1 cm of tension with the thumb in full abduction and opposition. The other slip should be attached afterwards and with at least 0.5 cm more tension than the first so that it will hold the metacarpophalangeal joint slightly abducted and slightly flexed, and will have a tendency also to hold the interphalangeal joint extended. The main effect of this whole tendon, however, will be the abduction and opposition of the thumb as a whole at the carpometacarpal joint. The tensions may be adjusted at the time of operation after testing the action of the transfer by dorsiflexing the wrist (Fig. 7.7.9).

If this operation is carried out carefully with regard to the position of each joint at the time of suture, and the over-all tension as well as the relative tension of the two halves of the tendon it should be possible to obtain an effective abduction and opposition of the

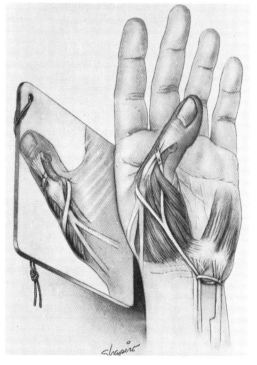

Figure 7.7.9. Low ulnar and median palsy. If only one tendon is to be transplanted, it should be a flexor sublimis with a double insertion. (White,, W. L.: Surg. Clin. North Am. *40:* 427, 1960, which was used in Campbell's Operative Orthopaedics)

thumb but it will rarely result in a really strong pinch because of the lack of an adductor and short flexor.

For this reason we prefer to transfer two tendons in most cases of low ulnar-median palsy. The extensor indicis proprius may be used for abduction and a flexor sublimis for adduction and for flexion of the metacarpophalangeal joint, both of these tendons will also pronate the thumb (Fig. 7.7.10*A* and *B*).

The extensor indicis proprius is divided at the metacarpophalangeal joint of the index finger and is withdrawn about 6 cm proximal to the wrist joint. A tendon tunnelling forceps is passed through a transverse incision at the proximal volar wrist crease, on the ulnar side of the palmaris tendon. It is passed obliquely, proximally and dorsally, passing to the ulnar side of the flexor tendons, and through a weak part of the interosseus membrane between radius and ulna. The tendon of extensor indicis proprius is gasped and withdrawn to the front of the wrist (Fig. 7.7.11). Note that the muscle rather than the tendon lies in the interosseus space. The tendon is now tunnelled subcutaneously to the dorsum of the thumb and is attached to the insertion of adductor pollicis (Fig. 7.7.12).

The flexor sublimis of the ring or middle finger is divided in the proximal segment and is withdrawn through a short longitudinal incision just to the radial side of the midpalm. From here it is tunnelled subcutaneously to the radial side of the middle of the proximal phalanx of the thumb and is attached to the extensor pollicis longus (Fig. 7.7.7).

In reeducation the extensor indicis acts in the open-hand phase, while the sublimis acts in the closing and pinching phase. Both are truly synergistic and they combine to produce a well balanced thumb (Fig. 7.7.13).

If the pinch proves to be unstable or weak after either operation the fault will usually be due to imperfect stabilization of the metacarpophalangeal joint. The best corrective operation for these conditions is an arthrodesis of the metacarpophalangeal joint in about 15° of flexion, about 5° of abduction, and some rotation in the direction of pronation so that the pulp of the thumb squarely faces the pulp of the index finger.

High Median Palsy

This is a very disabling condition because of the almost complete loss of grasp except in the ring and little fingers. If the ulnar-supplied half of the profundus is strong and active, it is best to connect the profundus tendons of the index and long fingers to the tendons of the ring and little finger in the forearm, proximal to the wrist, thus allowing the ulnar-supplied profundus to flex all four fingers. The flexor carpi ulnaris tendon can be split and attached half to the flexor carpi radialis and half to its own flexor carpi ulnaris insertion. The extensor carpi radialis longus can be detached at its insertion, pulled out half way up the forearm, and tunnelled anteriorly to be anastomosed to the flexor pollicis longus. The extensor carpi ulnaris can be brought around the ulnar side of the forearm and extended by means of a free graft to produce abduction

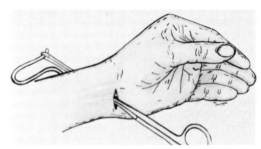

Figure 7.7.11. For median palsy, the extensor indicis proprius is rerouted from the dorsal aspect of the forearm, between the radius and ulna to appear on the ulnar side of palmaris longus.

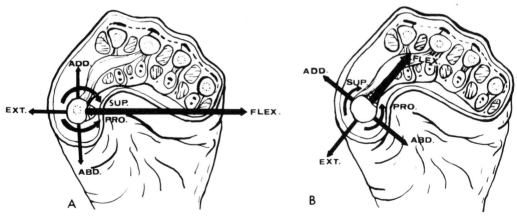

Figure 7.7.10. The strong muscle of the thumb is the long flexor. Its strength is wasted by being directed across the palm (*A*) unless the pronators of the thumb turn it around to face the fingers (*B*). Therefore, most tendon transfers for the thumb should be attached on the radial side to reinforce pronation.

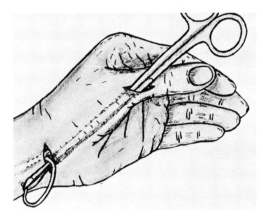

Figure 7.7.12. For median palsy, the tendon of extensor indicis proprius tunnelled subcutaneously to the dorsum of the thumb.

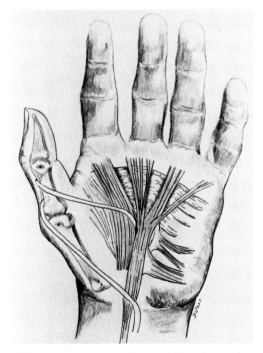

Figure 7.7.13. Low ulnar and median palsy. When two tendons are to be transferred a tendon of flexor sublimis becomes adductor and pronator and the tendon of extensor indicis proprius becomes abductor and pronator.

of the thumb. This also has the effect of tending to pronate the forearm and compensate for the loss of the median-supplied pronators (Fig. 7.7.14).

Radial Nerve Palsy

Following high radial nerve paralysis, the wrist needs an extensor, the fingers and thumb need exten-

sors, and the carpometacarpal joint of the thumb needs an extensor to replace the abductor pollicis longus. If there is no defect in the other nerves or muscles, it is reasonable to transfer three or perhaps four muscles to cover these needs.

The most basic need is for a wrist extensor. Robert Jones[8] recognized that the pronator teres makes an ideal transfer for this purpose.

When the pronator has been freed, the brachioradialis and extensor carpi radialis longus are allowed to fall back and cover the raw area of bone, while the pronator crosses these and comes to lie over the musculotendinous junction of extensor carpi radialis brevis. The pronator tendon is sutured, raw surface down, to the surface of the extensor brevis, and then the edges of the extensor are picked up and sutured together over the pronator to cover tag ends and minimize adhesions. This operation is so simple and effective that it is justifiable to do it at the same time as nerve suture in cases of high radial nerve laceration, even when there is a fair prognosis for ultimate recovery. It gives the patient many months of activity without the need for a cock-up splint. His fingers and thumb retain enough extensor power through their intrinsic musculature to make the hand useful during the period of recovery.

To provide extension for the fingers, it is best to use a wrist flexor since this is synergistic with finger extension. At one time it was common to transfer all wrist flexors in cases of radial palsy, but Zachary[18] pointed out the need to keep stability on the flexor side too. Boyes[1] has also emphasized the importance of keeping the flexor ulnaris in its position to give the important movement of ulnar deviation. This leaves us with flexor carpi radialis and palmaris available for transfer. The flexor carpi radialis has enough power to extend all four fingers. It should be divided at its insertion; pulled out through a small transverse incision half way up the forearm, and then tunnelled around the radial border of the forearm to appear in a dorsal incision which exposes the lower three inches of the back of the forearm and extends over the wrist. It is possible to tap the tendon into each of the digital extensors, while keeping them in continuity, but it is worth spending the extra time to divide the extensor tendons at their musculotendinous junctions, and do a formal anastomosis with proper change of direction of each tendon. This leaves a lot of potentially exposed tendon ends, and therefore a lot of adhesions. These can be avoided by burying each cut tendon end. The digital extensors are often multiple and have cross connections. After careful testing, four good tendons are chosen and divided at their musculotendinous junctions. They are then withdrawn distally without incising the extensor retinaculum. They are now redirected towards a point over the distal end of the radius, overlying the intact retinaculum, where they meet the flexor carpi radialis. They are retested for effective action in case the change of direction has placed some cross-connection under tension.

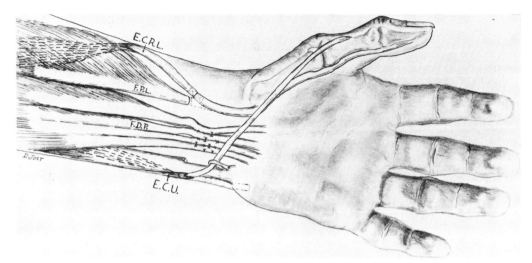

Figure 7.7.14. High median palsy. Extensor carpi radialis longus transferred to flexor pollicis longus. Extensor carpi ulnaris transferred with a free graft to abduct and pronate the thumb. The ulnar supplied part of the flexor profundus attached side by side to move the median supplied part as well.

The two best tendons are left long to join the motor tendon, while the other two are joined to their neighbors more distally. Each tendon junction is made by passing the lesser tendon through a slit in the greater, and then burying its end in a second slit. Each suture should include a small bite of each edge of the slit and of the tendon passing through. Each tendon is first fixed with a single stitch and left long until the relative tensions of all tendons can be tested. Passive flexion of each finger in turn will demonstrate whether its extensor tendon has a fair share of the tension. When all are equal the anastomosis is completed by adding more stitches to each tendon junction and then turning each cut end inwards to be buried in a tendon slit. The cut end of the motor tendon is finally buried by surrounding it with the two tendons which are attached to it (Fig. 7.7.15).

The value of the palmaris longus in radial palsy was first emphasized by Starr[15] as a result of experience in the first world war. If palmaris longus is present, it should be used for thumb extension. The extensor pollicis longus is divided at its musculotendinous junction, and the tendon is withdrawn just proximal to the metacarpophalangeal joint. It is then tunnelled subcutaneously to an incision just anterior to the tendon of abductor pollicis longus at level of the wrist. The palmaris longus is divided as far distally as possible and withdrawn half way up the forearm. From there it is tunnelled subcutaneously to the incision where it is to be anastomosed, end to end, to the extensor pollicis longus tendon. In the absence of a palmaris, the thumb extensor may join the finger extensors to be powered by the flexor carpi radialis.

Boyes[1][2] likes to use two flexor sublimis tendons as extensor of the fingers. He divides them in the distal palm and withdraws them in the forearm. He takes them through the interosseous membrane, one on each side of the flexor profundus muscle mass. One sublimis is used for extension of the thumb and index finger and the other for the remaining fingers. This leaves the flexor carpi radialis free to be used for the abductor longus and the extensor brevis of the thumb. Although it is synergistically improper to use a finger flexor as a finger extensor, this operation seems to give good results if reeducation is undertaken with care.

High Median, High Ulnar Paralysis

With only radial nerve muscles remaining the extensor carpi radialis brevis must be left in position as wrist extensor, while the extensor carpi radialis longus is brough around the forearm to flex the fingers via the flexor profundus tendons. The extensor indices proprius and the extensor digiti minimi become metacarpophalangeal flexors using Fowler's[7] technique and the extensor carpi ulnaris comes around the ulnar side of the forearm to activate the flexor pollicis longus. The metacarpophalangeal joint of the thumb is arthrodesed, and abduction of the thumb is achieved by rerouting the extensor pollicis brevis so that it approaches the thumb from the middle of the front of the wrist (the tendon of palmaris forms a nice sling if it is cut an inch or so back and stitched to the pisiform bone). The brachioradialis may be held in reserve to compensate for whatever weakness is found to be disabling after the first operation.

High Median, and High Radial Paralysis

With only ulnar-supplied muscles remaining, the profundus tendons must all be stitched side-to-side. The abductor digiti minimi may be used to abduct the thumb, using the technique of Littler[10], and the insertion of adductor pollicis transferred to the radial side

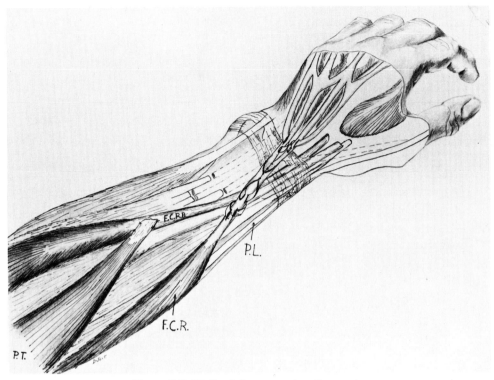

Figure 7.7.15. Radial nerve palsy. See text.

of the thumb to assist pronation. The metacarpophalangeal joint of the thumb should be fused. The wrist may be fused or the biceps may be used for dorsiflexion of the wrist. At this stage the patient should be encouraged to use the hand, to see which of the residual weaknesses bothers him most. The flexor carpi ulnaris may then be transferred either to become an extensor of the fingers or a flexor of the thumb, or if the biceps has been used as wrist extensor, it may be better to leave the flexor carpi ulnaris as a wrist flexor, split between the insertions of flexor carpi radialis and ulnaris.

Multiple Paralysis

A hand is sometimes left with very few muscles indeed, sometimes only one or two below the elbow. In such cases it is particularly important for the surgeon to consult with the patient, with his social worker, and with his vocational advisor to be sure to provide the kind of movement most needed by the patient in his future work. The patient must clearly understand that very few movements will be possible. He may choose a form of pinch or of grasp. In a sensitive right hand a pulp-to-pulp pinch between the thumb and index and long fingers will usually be the choice. In an insensitive hand, or in a sensitive left hand where there is a good right hand, some patients will choose a grasp, planned for the handle of a tool, say 1½ inches in diameter. In other cases a pinch may be preferred between the pulp of the thumb and the side of the index finger—the "key" pinch.

In either of these cases a number of joints will have to be arthrodesed and others controlled by tenodesis. The following examples may serve as a guide.

When only one muscle remains in the forearm, unless that muscle is a finger flexor, it should be made into a wrist extensor to act on the insertion of the extensor carpi radialis brevis. All the interphalangeal joints of the hand and the metacarpophalangeal joint of the thumb should be arthrodesed and a bone block should be used to fix the thumb opposed to the index and long fingers. The arthrodeses should be in such positions that the pulps of the thumb, index, and long fingers meet as a tripod pinch. Subsequently the flexor profundus tendons of the index and long fingers should be embedded in the radius in the forearm, producing a tenodesis in such a position that dorsiflexion of the wrist brings the fingers firmly down on to the thumb. This is the "flexor hinge hand" of Nickel,[12] developed for the quadriplegic who is sometimes left with only wrist extensors. A preliminary period of training in the "flexor hinge" splint is a real advantage to these patients, or they may prefer to use the flexor hinge splint permanently to avoid the multiple arthrodesis.

If the only remaining muscle in the forearm is a finger or thumb flexor, then this should not be disturbed. It may be transferred to a more important finger by adjustments in the forearm or sutured side-to-side to include other fingers. In such cases, the wrist must be provided with a dorsiflexor or else stabilized. A biceps transfer should be considered.

If two muscles remain in the forearm, one should be made into a wrist dorsiflexor and the other into a finger flexor. If there are three muscles, the third can be used as a finger extensor; if there are four muscles available, it may be possible to do without the bone block at the carpometacarpal joint of the thumb and provide instead an abductor opponens motor. Alternatively, the thumb may be left fixed and the interphalangeal arthrodesis of the fingers may be avoided by providing a lumbrical replacement with the extra motor unit. This will allow th patient to use his fingers either against his thumb in a pinch or to surround an object in a grasp.

NOTE: Diagrams 1, 4, 5, 6, 7, 11 and 12 were used in my chapter "Paralysis of Intrinsic Muscles of the Hand" in Volume Eleven, Operative Surgery, Second Edition, edited by Rob and Smith and published by Butterworths.

Diagrams 8-A, 8-B, 10-A and 10-B were used in my manuscript "Tendon Transfers for Median and Ulnar Nerve Paralysis" published by Orthopedic Clinics of North America, Vol. 1, No. 2, November 1970.

REFERENCES

1. Boyes, J. H. Tendon transfers for radial palsy. Bull. Hosp. Joint Dis.; *21:* 97, 1960.
2. Boyes, J.H. Selection of a donor muscle for tendon transfers. Bull. Hosp. Joint Dis., *23:* 1, 1962.
3. Brand, P. W. Paralytic claw hand with special reference to paralysis in leprosy and treatment by the sublimis transfer of Stile and Bunnell. J. Bone Joint Surg., *40B:* 618, 1958.
4. Brand, P.W. Tendon grafting. Illustrated by a new operation for intrinsic paralysis of the fingers. J. Bone Joint Surg., *43B:* 444, 1961.
5. Bunnell, S. Contractures of the hand from infections and injuries. J. Bone Joint Surg., *14:* 27, 1932.
6. Bunnell, S. Tendon transfers in the hand and forearm. American Academy of Orthopedic Surgeons Instructional Course Lectures, Vol. 6. Ann Arbor, J. W. Edwards, 1949.
7. Fowler, B. Quoted by Riordan.[13]
8. Jones, R. Tendon transplantation in cases of musculo-spiral injuries not amenable to suture. Am. J. Surg., *35:* 333, 1921.
9. Littler, J. W. Tendon transfers and arthrodeses in combined median and ulnar nerve paralysis. J. Bone Joint Surg., *36A:* 10, 1949.
10. Littler, J. W., and Cooley, S. G. E. Opposition of the thumb and its restoration by abductor digiti quinti transfer. J. Bone Joint Surg., *45A:* 1389, 1963.
11. Mayer L. The physiological method of tendon transplantation. Surg. Gynecol. Obstet., *22:* 182, 1916.
12. Nickel, V. L., Perry, J., and Garrett, A. L. Development of useful function in the severely paralyzed hand. J. Bone Joint Surg., *45A:* 933, 1963.
13. Riordan, D. C. Tendon transplantations in median-nerve and ulnar-nerve paralysis. J. Bone Joint Surg., *35A:* 312; 1953.
14. Riordan, D. C. Surgery of the paralytic hand. American Academy of Orthopedic Surgeons Instructional Course Lectures, Vol. 16 St. Louis, Mosby, 1959.
15. Star, C. Army experiences with tendon transference. J. Bone Joint Surg., *4:* 3, 1922.
16. Stiles, H. J., and Forrester-Brown, M. F. *Treatment of Injuries of Peripheral Spinal Nerves,* London, Henry Frowde and Hodder and Stoughton, p. 180.
17. Thompson, T. C. A modified operation for opponens paralysis. J. Bone Joint Surg., *24:* 632, 1942.
18. Zachary, R. B. Tendon transplantation for radial palsy. Br. J. Surg., *23:* 358.
19. Zancolli, E. A. Claw hand caused by paralysis of the intrinsic muscles. A simple surgical procedure for its correction. J. Bone Joint Surg., *39A:* 1076, 1957.

H.

Salvage of Scarred Tendon Systems Using Tendon Prosthesis

James M. Hunter, M.D.

BACKGROUND AND DEVELOPMENT

This chapter deals with the problem of tendon salvage in the hand and forearm. During recent years, hand surgery techniques and knowledge have advanced so that today the severely damaged hand is challenged and no longer considered hopeless. The last link in the chain of functional restoration is the tendon motor unit. Surgery after injury, infection, and disease may render the tendon and its gliding bed a wasteland of firm, fibrous scar tissue. Loss of gliding tendon function is usually accompanied by stiffness of the joints and atrophy of muscles. Attempts to recover motion by conventional tendon reconstruction procedures are usually met with limited success. More often, the surgeon finds scar has trapped his tendon graft or transfer, resulting in little, if any, functional improvement. This is particularly the case on the flexor side of the hand and forearm where the functional anatomy is more complex. The development of a tendon prosthesis and its suggested clinical applications have evolved from a need to study a different approach for the management of tendon salvage problems.

Since Lange's classic silk tendon study in 1910,[33] many investigators have searched for new techniques to overcome the "stuck tendon" problem and the research has fallen into essentially three groups: (1) blocking devices; (2) pseudosheaths; and (3) artificial tendons.

The first group[3,4,19,20,21,24,25,32,39,49] interposed a foreign substance between two tissue planes called the "blocking device." This concept attempted actually to fence out new scar tissue by an impermeable or semipermeable membrane.

The second group of investigators[1,5,13,14,18,23,26,37,38,39,46] took a compromise approach by attempting to make scar tissue work for the surgeon by using foreign material implants to build "pseudosheaths." This method takes advantage of the tendency for scar to layer and form a "mesothelial-like" membrane as it matures around an inert surface concealed within the body. Dr. Leo Mayer's[37] classic investigation in 1936 brought forth the true understanding of the pseudosheath concept. He boldly approached scarring of the flexor tendon gliding system by pointing directly to the problem with a practical solution (Fig. 7.8.1). Unable at that time to find a flexible, inert material, he abandoned this method and his brilliant concept remained dormant for many years. Carroll,[14] in 1959, using flexible silicone rods, added passive motion of the hand and advanced Mayer's concepts.

The third group of investigators[2,17,22,24,31,33,44,45] also attempted to bridge a gap of scar tissue by interposing a foreign material. They varied their approach, however, by attempting to achieve active motion with their materials. Lange[33] in 1900, worked with a silk tendon concept. There followed a lag of many years until new materials, such as braided tantalum wire, was introduced. A dual material concept, using Nylon fish line running through two polyethylene tubes was introduced in 1956 and, since then, other materials have been used with limited success. Best known were wire or silk covered with polyethylene tubes, Teflon rods, Nylon and Tetron, arterial tissue and Nylon thread.

Many materials utilized in these experiments were not inert and foreign reaction occurred. Other materials were stiff, precluding their use in the hand. Passive motion was not permitted and stiffness of the fingers developed. In addition to these factors, the feature of mechanical inefficiency is brought out in the tube cord idea. Tubes offer a continual threat of dead space for collection of fluid, blood, and bacteria. They are subjected to excessive frictional wear and tend to kink on extremes of flexion.

One is forced to conclude from these reviews that a single material was not available to reproduce the needs of a complete tendon replacement and that known dual material concepts had failed on a mechanical basis. It also seemed apparent that the important significance of Leo Mayer's celloidin tube new sheath investigation had not been correlated with artificial tendon concepts.

In 1960 a case of extensor tendon reconstruction

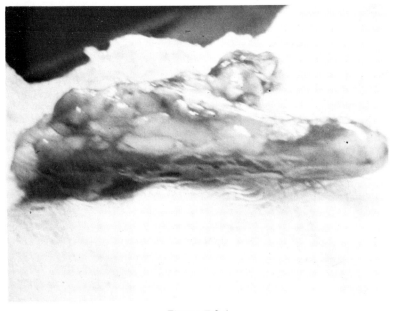

Figure 7.8.1.

being carried out in our Hand Clinic presented a missing clue to the problem. A simple unreinforced Silastic rod was introduced into the index finger of a 22-year-old female to replace an extensor mechanism which had completely sloughed due to prior infection. The area of slough extended over the dorsum of the proximal phalanx. The skin covering was tenuous, but acceptable, and proximal interphalangeal joint motion was adequate. Otherwise, the patient presented a good picture for reconstruction. At surgery, a flexible silicone rod was introduced to build a new functioning sheath. The rod was interwoven through the remaining tendon and No. 5-0 wire sutures were utilized in such a way as to eliminate a cutting effect on the silicone rubber. The patient was examined five months later. It was apparent at that time that the proximal and distal anastomosis of the silicone rod to the tendon remnant had held and passive dynamic motion was occurring. Active flexor tendon motion brought the proximal interphalangeal joint to 90° and, upon relaxation, the elastic recoil of the silicone rubber rod carried the middle phalanx to about 20° of extension. This patient had, in effect, an "intrinsic rubber band" or a passive dynamic prosthesis that actually satisfied her daily needs. The patient was very happy with the result and if a small wire had not presented itself at the proximal anastomosis, the patient would not have permitted exploration. Approximately five months from the time of implantation, the dorsal surface of this finger was again explored and a shiny mesothelial-lined membrane was noted. The silicone rod was removed and a tendon graft was placed in the new sheath. Acceptable function followed a conventional period of immobilization and rehabilitation. A fortunate accident had dramatically emphasized some of the unique properties of silicone rubbed. The simple silicone rubber rod possessed an inert surface for implantation. It could be molded to the appropriate size and shape of a tendon. Furthermore, it seemed to possess a physiologic bounce that complemented soft tissue during motion.

Silicone, however, lacked strength and tear resistance, and, also, as nothing would adhere to it, a method of anastomosis. We concluded, however, that a Silastic rod could be reinforced with a strong, nonreactive material in such a way that the unique properties were retained, a "single unit tendon prosthesis" could be developed. Currently used passive gliding designs will be discussed later. Readers interested in the quest for a complete tendon replacement should read the author's 1965 article where the problem of active tendon prosthesis is further discussed and 29 clinical cases are reviewed.[26]

Many questions, particularly in the area of new sheath formation, remain unanswered and offer new challenges for the future. After basic studies in dogs in our laboratories, the following conclusions were reached.[28]

Mesothelial cells were found aligned on the surface of the implant as early as five days and by three weeks, a well developed bursa had formed (Fig. 7.8.1). The type of implant (stiff, rigid, or flexible) did not affect pseudosheath formation provided no joint motion was involved. Studies with several types of Dacron-reinforced silicone gliding tendon prostheses in dogs and humans (Fig. 7.8.2A and B) showed a more advanced sheath formed when there was gliding and fluid resembling synovial fluid was found to be lubricating the prosthesis. When the prosthesis was removed and replaced by a tendon graft, the sheath seemed to afford nourishment and a gliding surface for the central one-third of the graft. On all occasions, the tendons remained viable both grossly and histologically. Since the presentation of these laboratory findings, our progressively improving clinical results in the salvage of fingers with severe tendon injuries has led us to believe that a reliable tendon prosthesis inserted as one stage in tendon reconstruction is the additional step needed to improve the results of flexor-tendon reconstructive surgery.

The method has been applied in more than 200 tendon reconstructions of various types. It is the purpose of this chapter to describe the presently used two-stage technique for flexor-tendon reconstruction in hands in which the conditions are less than optimum based on results in 74 of 86 consecutive cases in which this method has been employed.[30]

THE PROSTHESIS

The prothesis is constructed of a woven Dacron core (Fig. 7.8.3) (proximal end of prosthesis) which is molded into radiopaque silicone rubber. The surface finish is smooth and the cross sectional design is ovoid to aid optimal tendon sheath development. The prosthesis has the necessary combination of firmness and flexibility, as well as the smooth glistening surface required to ensure ease of insertion and free passive gliding throughout the finger, palm, and forearm.

The prosthesis is currently available through the manufacturer* in four sizes: 3mm x 23 cm, 4 mm x 23 cm, 5 mm x 25 cm, and 6 mm x 25 cm. At the time of insertion, the prosthesis may be trimmed at the distal end for proper length with a scalpel.

Currently, yarns and cables, made of stainless steel, Titanium, tantalum, and new synthetic fibers, are being tested in the hope that, with improved designs and fabrication of the yarn and the addition of end devices, an active tendon prosthesis can be developed which may be used for extended periods before a second-stage procedure for tendon grafting is required.

INDICATIONS

There is sufficient evidence to suggest that the surgeon trained in hand surgery should consider using a tendon prosthesis in selected primary injuries where the tendon gliding bed has been severely damaged.[41, 47, 48] The results also indicate that a failed primary suture in "no-man's-land" need not compromise the

*Extracorporeal Medical Specialties, Inc., Royal and Ross Rds., King of Prussia, Pa. 19406.

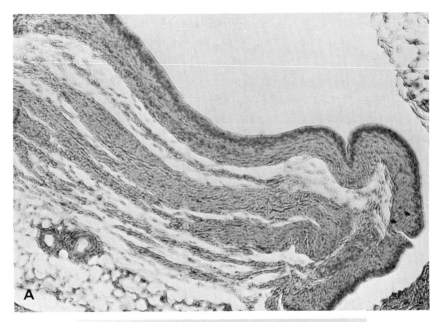

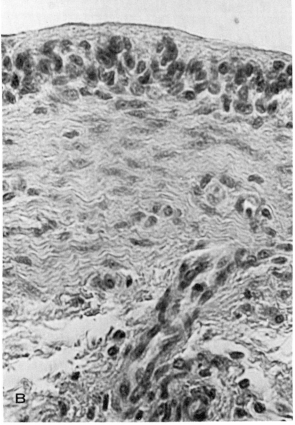

Figure 7.8.2.

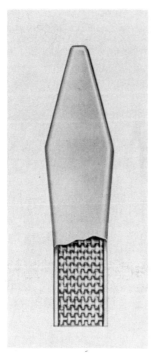

Figure 7.8.3.

secondary flexor tendon graft if this two-stage technique is used.[30]

Staged tendon reconstruction, using the tendon prosthesis prior to tendon grafting is indicated in most instances where the tendon gliding bed has been damaged. In fact, all patients in need of tendon grafts are potential candidates for this procedure since only at surgery can the true extent of damage to the tendon bed be determined.

For the purposes of evaluation, the patients' status at their initial examination and prior to Stage II was graded according to the following classification, modified from the one proposed by Boyes.[8,9]

Grade 1 (good): Good soft tissues, supple joints, and no significant scarring. (No Grade 1 patients were included in this series, since, in all of these, conventional tendon grafts can be used.)

Grade 2 (scar): Deep cicatrix, resulting from injury or previous surgery, as well as mild soft-tissue contractures which, in a few instances, were severe enough to require preliminary plastic procedures.

Grade 3 (joint): Limitation of passive joint motion, usually in the proximal interphalangeal joint, sufficient to require mobilization by traction and dynamic splinting. Grade 3 patients may show scarring of the tendon bed. (Those with significant scarring should be classed Grade 5.)

Grade 4 (nerve): Nerve damage with associated trophic changes in addition to scarring of the tendon bed and joint stiffness.

Grade 5 (multiple): Soft tissue scarring or joint changes in more than one digit, or a combination of injuries in a single digit of such character that Grades 2, 3, and 4 did not apply, and in addition, involvement of the palm in many cases.

Grade 6 (salvage): Joint stiffness, borderline circulation, nerve deficits. Finger, however, can be useful to the hand if reconstructed. Certain fingers may require amputation rather than reconstruction.

The results in each patient should be correlated with the preoperative grade.

TECHNIQUE

Patients selected for the two-stage tendon reconstruction should have a preoperative hand therapy program, designed to mobilize stiff joints[15,16] and to improve the condition of the soft tissues as much as possible before the first stage.

Stage I

The damaged flexor tendons and their scarred sheaths are exposed. In the finger, this is done through a zig-zag incision (Fig. 7.8.5) as popularized by Bruner.[11] In the palm, exposure is accomplished through a transverse incision or through a proximal continuation of Bruner's zig-zag incision.[11] In the forearm, an ulnarly curved volar incision (Fig. 7.8.5) is made to expose the proximal portions of the flexor tendons and their musculotendinous junctions. A stump of the profundus tendon (Fig. 7.8.5), 1 cm in length, is left attached to the distal phalanx. Scarred tendons, sheath, and retinaculum are then excised. If the excision is stopped in the palm at the lumbrical level, the contracted and scarred lumbrical muscle is excised.[40] Contracted or scarred lumbricals should always be excised. This is done to prevent the paradoxical motion of the lumbrical which is seen after some tendon grafts. This motion causes the finger to extend at the P.I.P. joint rather than flex as the patient attempts to flex the finger completely.

Undamaged portions of the flexor fibro-osseous retinaculum (pulley system) which are not contracted are retained. Any portion of the retinaculum that can be dilated instrumentally with a hemostat is also preserved. The rest is excised. The retinacular pulley system should be preserved or reconstructed proximal to the axis of motion of each joint or, otherwise, normal gliding of the tendon will not be restored. Four pulleys are preferred: one proximal to each of the three finger joints and one at the base of the proximal phalanx.

New pulleys may be fashioned from available tendon material to be discarded. The tendon graft should be fixed securely to the fibro-osseous remnant of the old pulley on the lateral borders of the metacarpal, proximal, or middle phalanx. The pulley diameter should be of ample size to permit easy gliding of the prosthesis.

Meticulous care of the prosthesis is most important. The prosthesis* is normally supplied sterile; if, however, it should become contaminated the manufactur-

---

*Extracorporeal Medical Specialties, Inc., Royal and Ross Rds., King of Prussia. Pa. 19406.

er's instructions regarding cleaning and sterilizing should be kept in a lint free receptacle.[5] When handled at operation, gloves should be freshly moistened with sterile saline or Ringer's solution before contact with the implant, or sponges wet with sterile saline or Ringer's solution should be used to hold the device. A large tendon prosthesis (5 mm) is preferred. It is first placed on sponges moistened with sterile saline or Ringer's solution on the volar aspect of the forearm, and then a tendon passer, with a diameter slightly larger than that of the prosthesis, is passed proximally from the palm through the carpal tunnel into the forearm. The distal end of the prosthesis is secured to this and pulled into the palm, whence it can be pushed through the retinaculum and pulleys to the distal end of the finger, a process facilitated by moistening the prosthesis with sterile saline or Ringer's solution. An alternate method is to inset the prosthesis in a proximal direction by seeking a free plane in the carpal canal by blunt instrumentation. The superficialis and profundus tendons may be transected either proximal or distal to the carpal canal. If proximal, the tendon is sutured to the fascia beneath the flexion crease of the wrist. The purpose of this suture is (1) to prevent the muscle (a potential motor for the free tendon graft to be inserted during Stage II) from shortening, (2) to provide for some isometric function of the muscle during the interval between Stage I and II, and (3) to facilitate identification of the muscle during Stage II and hence to reduce the amount of dissection required.

The distal end of the prosthesis is sutured beneath the stump of the profundus tendon after resecting all but the most distally attached fibers of the tendon (Fig. 7.8.4). A figure-of-eight suture of No. 32 or 34 monofilament stainless steel wire on an atraumatic taper-cut needle is used. In addition, medial and lateral wire sutures of No. 35 multifilament wire should be passed through the tendon, the prosthesis, and the fibroperiosteum for further fixation. Any excess of profundus tendon is resected distally. Traction is then applied on the proximal end of the prosthesis in the forearm, to be sure that the attachment of the prosthesis is distal to the distal interphalangeal joint and its volar plate and that there is no binding of the tendon during flexion and extension. The prosthesis is also observed during passive flexion and extension of the finger (Fig. 7.8.5), to make sure that it glides freely with no binding or buckling distal to some part of the pulley system which is too tight. If any portion of the system is tight, it must be removed and replaced with a new pulley constructed from a free tendon graft.

The proximal end of the prosthesis should also be observed during passive flexion and extension to make sure that it glides properly. Preferably, this end of the prosthesis should be in the forearm so that the newly formed sheath will extend to the region of the musculotendinous junction of the motor muscle. The prosthesis may be placed superficial or deep to the antebrachial fascia or deep in one of the intermuscular planes. The bed for the prosthesis can be fashioned by separating tendon mesenteries with the moistened

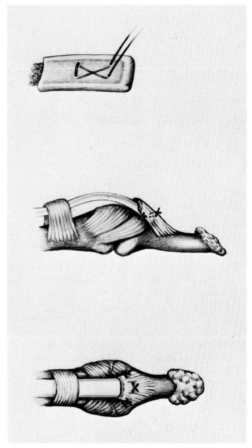

Figure 7.8.4.

gloved finger. If such a bed cannot be established by spreading and adjustment of the tissues, the prosthesis should be shortened so that, when the finger is fully extended, the proximal end of the prosthesis lies just proximal to the flexion crease at the wrist.

When multiple prostheses are threaded through the carpal canal, the superficialis tendons are generally removed from the canal. To date, carpal tunnel syndrome has not been observed with one or more prostheses traversing the canal.

Finally, before the wound is closed, traction should again be applied to the prosthesis and the amount of active finger motion determined and recorded. If this maneuver does not produce full flexion or a weak pulley ruptures, it may be necessary to modify the pulley system. This is a most important point and is a unique feature of the two-stage technique.

Postoperative Technique

Following skin closure, a standard postoperative hand dressing is applied, with the wrist and metacarpophalangeal joints in moderate flexion (40° to 50°) and the interphalangeal joints in slight flexion (20° to 30°). Where there were joint contractures prior to insertion of the prosthesis, intermittent stretching splints

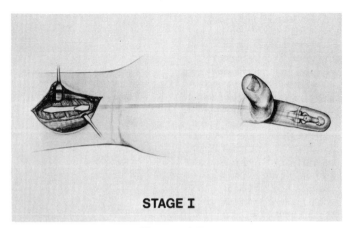

STAGE I

Figure 7.8.5.

may be required to prevent recurrence of the contracture. Intermittent elastic finger traction may be started during the first postoperative week. Gentle passive motion of all joints is started gradually during the second to the fourth week. Regular passive stretching, under the supervision of a hand therapist, is begun in the fifth week and the patient is taught at this time to flex the finger whenever possible, using an adjacent finger hooked over the damaged one. Usually, by the sixth week, there is a functional range of passive motion. During this time the hand should be examined regularly for evidence of synovitis in the new sheath. If this has not developed within the first six weeks, it is not likely to occur and the patient may resume normal activities, including going back to work, until he is ready for the second stage.

A small amount of barium sulfate is impregnated in the prosthesis so that its function can be checked roentgenographically at six weeks and again just before insertion of the tendon graft (Fig. 7.8.6). Anteroposterior and lateral roentgenograms of the hand and distal one-half of the forearm are made with the fingers and wrist in full extension and full flexion. These roentgenograms will demonstrate how much the proximal end of the prosthesis moves with respect to the distal end of the radius. If there is a full range of motion of the wrist and all fingerjoints, an excursion of 5 to 7 cm is not unusual. These roentgenograms will also show any evidence of buckling. Slight or intermittent buckling may cause no difficulty. However, if there is appreciable buckling, synovitis is likely to occur and the patient should be followed carefully. If synovitis develops, as evidenced by swelling, the finger and wrist should be immobilized promptly and, if the synovitis persists, the distended joints should be carefully mobilized daily and the sheath may decompress to the surface. The second-stage procedure should be done early before chronic fibrosis develops. A clean draining synovitis, managed by good surgical principles, is not a contraindication to Stage II tendon grafting.

The interval between Stage I and Stage II should be two to six months, or long enough to permit maturation of the tendon bed to the point where it can nourish and lubricate the gliding tendon graft. In fingers in which fixed flexion contractures of many months' duration are mobilized for the first time at the Stage I procedure, Stage II should be delayed until maximum softening of the tissues and mobilization of the stiff joints have been achieved. Each case must be individualized and the decision to do second-stage procedure must be made by the surgeon on the basis of the findings in the hand.

Stage II

When Stage II is begun, the limits of extension and flexion of the finger must first be accurately measured and recorded. The distal end of the zig-zag incision is opened to locate the distal end of the prosthesis where it is attached to the distal phalanx (Fig. 7.8.7). This attachment is left intact and the ulnarly curved volar incision is made in the forearm through the original Stage I incision to expose the proximal end of the prosthesis and the musculotendinous junction of the superficialis or profundus tendon, whichever is to be used as a motor for the tendon graft.

While the prosthesis is still in place, the excursion of the proximal end of the prosthesis should also be measured as an additional check on the amount of excursion that the motor muscle must have to provide full finger motion.

A long tendon graft is then obtained from one leg, the plantaris preferably, but, if this is missing, a long toe extensor tendon may be used. If a toe extensor tendon must be employed, the graft is obtained using a modified Brand tendon stripper[10] through two or more incisions, so that the portion of the tendon proximal to the ankle retinaculum is obtained. Any attached fat or muscle is removed and one end of the graft is sutured

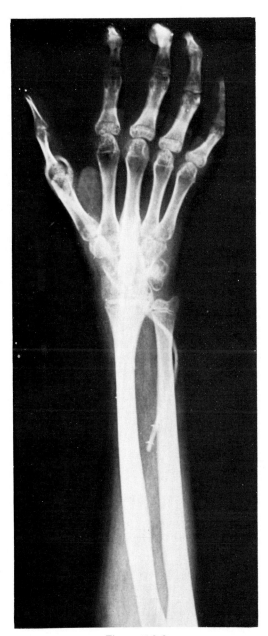

Figure 7.8.6.

the button on the fingernail. Medial and lateral reinforcing sutures through the profundus tendon stump are placed. Traction is now applied to the proximal end of the graft and the predicted range of active flexion, measured as the distance of the finger pulp from the distal palmar crease, is determined. After this maneuver, the attachment of the graft to the distal phalanx is inspected, to check on the security of the fixation.

The condition of the tissues at the site of the proximal anastomosis is critical. Atraumatic technique should be used during the dissection. Scar tissue and thickened antebrachial fascia are excised to minimize motion-restricting adhesions. When the firm fascia is carefully dissected away from the newly formed tendon sheath, the sheath is found to be soft, with loose mesentery-like attachments to the surrounding tissues (Fig. 7.8.7 and Fig 7.8.24 and B). If the sheath is thickened or scarred as the result of synovitis, it is resected far enough distally so that there will be no scar in the region of the tendon suture. If the anastomosis is small in diameter, the sheath may be placed around it. This is not always possible, however, due to the bulk of the graft-tendon junction. In this event, the sheath is either dissected away completely so that there is no contact between the anastomosis and the sheath, or the sheath may be left open so that one side of the anastomosis glides on the sheath.

In most patients in the series reported here, the proximal anastomosis was in the forearm. For the index finger, when either the superficialis or the profundus muscle was available as a motor, the graft was anastomosed to the proximal segment of the motor tendon according to the method of Pulvertaft.[43] For the long, ring, and little fingers, on the other hand, the graft was woven through oblique stab incisions in the common profundus tendon securing the different tendons together as one-tendon unit, following Pulvertaft techniques as closely as possible. In a few instances in which the palm was not involved, a palmaris longus graft was used and the proximal end of the graft was sutured to the profundus tendon at the origin of the lumbrical muscle. If the proximal anastomosis is done in the palm, the superficialis or profundus of the injured finger or the superficialis of an adjacent finger may be used as the motor. If the forearm is the site of the anastomosis, the same three options are available.

It is essential to adjust the length of the graft accurately. The excursion of the tendon graft should now be checked by pulling on the graft, starting with the finger in full extension (Fig. 7.8.8). Having determined the excursion necessary to produce a full range of flexion, the excursions of the available motors are then determined and the one is selected which is the requisite excursion. Obviously, if the motor lacks sufficient excursion, active motion will not be complete, even if the anastomosis is exact and the tendon graft glides perfectly.

The tension of the graft is adjusted so that, with the wrist in neutral, the involved finger rests in slightly

to the proximal end of the prosthesis with a catgut or polyester suture (Fig. 7.8.7). Leaving the distal end of the prosthesis attached to the distal phalanx, the rest of the prosthesis, with the attached tendon graft, is pulled distally, thereby threading the graft through the new sheath. The prosthesis is then removed and discarded. Free motion of the graft in the sheath can now be confirmed by grasping each end of the graft with a hemostat and pulling it proximally and distally.

The tendon graft is secured to the distal phalanx using a Bunnell button-pull-out wire suture,[12] with

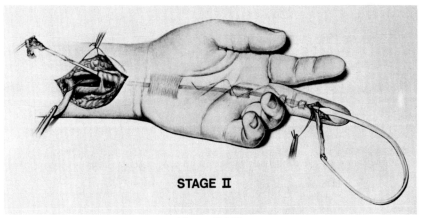

STAGE II

Figure 7.8.7.

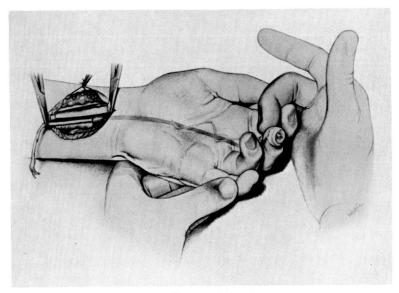

Figure 7.8.8.

more flexion than that of the adjacent fingers. When the anastomosis has been completed, the tension is checked with the wrist in both flexion and extension to assess the tenodesis effect and to make sure that the tension of the graft is correct. Uncomplicated Stage II procedures may be done under local anesthesia, supplemented with a sedative analgesic drug (Innovar). A pneumatic arm tourniquet is used intermittently during the procedure. After the distal anastomosis is completed and the distal wound is closed, the graft is sutured tentatively to the motor tendon and, after the tourniquet has been deflated for 10 to 15 minutes, the patient is asked to flex and extend the finger. If the predicted amount of active flexion is not achieved, the tension of the graft is readjusted or a motor tendon with a better excursion is selected. When the patient can accomplish the predicted

amount of flexion, the anastomosis is completed and the wound is closed and dressed.

This procedure eliminates the guess work in establishing optimum tension in the graft and the results to date have been very encouraging. Removal of the tendon graft from the leg under this type of anesthesia has not caused difficulty. If a tendon stripper is used, the patient may have some, but not excessive discomfort, although no patient has complained that the procedure was unduly uncomfortable. Some patients are better adapted to a choice of general anesthesia.

When the proximal anastomosis is completed, the peritenon may be pulled distally and sutured to the proximal end of the newly formed sheath or to the surrounding tissues as far distally as possible. The wound is irrigated with sterile saline solution and then closed, and the final dressing is applied, with a plaster splint to maintain the wrist and metacarpophalangeal joints in moderate flexion and the interphalangeal joints in slight flexion.

Postoperative Technique

Early protected active flexion of the grafted finger is encouraged, while a padded dorsal splint prevents sudden forceful extension. Each patient is instructed at the first postoperative dressing, usually after five to seven days, to splint the metacarpophalangeal joints while the proximal and distal interphalangeal joints are actively flexed and extended. Intermittent splinting may be continued during the fourth week while the pull-out suture and button are still in place. In the fifth week, the pull-out wire is removed and light passive stretching exercises may be started if necessary. Some vigorous patients with full excursion of the graft may require intermittent splinting during the fourth week to protect the proximal anastomosis from excessive stress. If stubborn contractures were present prior to tendon grafting, a supervised program of passive stretching and splinting may be required after the fifth week. Patients must be carefully instructed how to slide the tendon graft through the new sheath by holding the M.P. joints against the table in extension during flexion of the distal joints. This basic technique is also applied when squeezing the Bunnell wood block and small aspirin bottles. These training techniques may be required for several months. Therefore, constant supervision and prodding by the surgeon or a hand therapist is essential. Most patients should achieve their predicted range of active motion by the fourth or fifth month.

COMPLICATIONS

The complications related to the Stage I and Stage II operations were analyzed separately.

Stage I

The complication of synovitis is characterized by the following (singly or in combination): pain in the fingertip, swelling along the volar surface of the finger, and swelling and erythema at the site of the incision in the forearm. In some of the earlier cases, this complication was caused by soiling of the prosthesis. After the technique was perfected, synovitis occurred only occasionally, caused by excessive motion of the prosthesis too soon after surgery or when there was mechanical obstruction (tight pulleys) to the gliding of the prosthesis, producing buckling. If the synovitis does not respond to five to seven days of immobilization followed by gradual resumption of activity, the Stage II procedure should be performed earlier and the thickened synovium excised in the region of the proximal anastomosis.

Stage II

There are two complications after Stage II tendon grafting that deserve discussion: (1) adhesions along the tendon graft or at the proximal anastomosis, and (2) repture of the anastomosis of the tendon graft.

Restrictive adhesions may occur along the tendon graft, particularly at sites of dense scar and tight pulleys where sheath nutrition is poor if good freely lubricated movement of the graft is not established early after surgery.

Restrictive adhesions may form around the proximal anastomosis particularly when there has been previous trauma to this area with subsequent scarring. The functional significance of adhesions about the proximal end of the tendon graft cannot be overemphasized. These adhesions, of course, are part of the normal healing reaction but, at times, they may be the only adhesions preventing good function. Under these circumstances, the adhesions can best be released under direct vision.

If tenolysis is necessary, it is performed three to six months after Stage II using local anesthesia, Innovar analgesia, and a tourniquet. Since tourniquet ischemia rather consistently produces paralysis of the extrinsic muscles after 25 minutes and of the intrinsic muscles after 30 minutes, the tourniquet should be released at 25-minute intervals. By this means, it is possible to visualize the problem while the patient actively flexes and extends his fingers. The region of the proximal anastomosis should be explored first, with attention directed initially to the junction of the new tendon sheath and the tendon graft; next, to the proximal anastomosis; and, lastly, to the tendon graft within the new sheath. Only adhesions which actually restrict motion should be lysed.

After surgery, immediate active motion of the lysed tendon graft is necessary to preserve the increased ranges of motion.

RESULTS

The results in two series are compared in Table 7.8.1, eliminating Boyes' cases which were classified good. The incidence of fingers which postoperatively could flex sufficiently to bring the pulp to within 2.5 cm or less of the distal palmar crease is strikingly higher in our series. Although our series is considerably smaller, the comparison, nonetheless, strongly suggests that the procedure described here can produce results better than those attained by the conventional method in less than optimum cases.

White[50] classified his cases as good and less than good preoperatively, and reported that, of the 48 patients with less-than-good fingers, 35 per cent could flex the pulp of the involved finger postoperatively to within 2.5 cm of the distal palmar crease. Of our 69 patients, all with a less-than-good rating preoperatively, 80 per cent could flex their finger to within 2.5 cm or less of the distal palmar crease at follow-up. These results represent a considerable improvement over those reported by White.

Pulvertaft[43] grouped all of his tendon grafts together

TABLE 7.8.1

Comparison of results with Boyes'[8],[9] in hands graded 2, 3, and 5:* Preoperative grade vs. distance of fingertip pulp from distal palmar crease

Stage	Grades	0	1.3	2.5	3.8	No. of Cases
I						
Hunter and	2 Scar	16†	57	85	85	12
Salisbury,	3 Joint	31	62	85	85	13
1970	5 Multiple	25	45	79	79	44
	Total cases					69
II						
Boyes, 1955	2 Scar	8	24	49	82	79
	3 Joint	12	30	64	82	33
	5 Multiple	2	6	45		64
	Total cases					176

*No Grade 1 fingers included in this series.
†Figures are in percentages which are cumulative.

and reported that 70 per cent of his 90 patients achieved pulp-to-crease flexion of 2.5 cm or less. Again, our results compare very favorably.

Finally, it is worth noting that, in their good cases, 2.5 cm pulp-to-crease flexion was achieved in 84 per cent by Boyes (Grade 1) and in 79 per cent by White. The percentages in these good cases are essentially the same as the percentages in our cases, all of which were less than good.

CASE REPORT

M. D., a left-handed female cafeteria worker, had sustained a severe laceration of the left palm on a broken bottle. Primary skin closure was performed, followed one month later by tenorrhaphies in the palm. Six months later, the patient was referred for treatment of her persistent numbness and lack of flexion of the left long, ring, and little fingers.

Four neurorrhaphies were performed and the scarred superficialis tendons of the long and ring fingers were excised. Five months later, after the patient had received intensive physical therapy and had acceptable sensation and active flexion of the long and ring fingers but not in the little finger, a Stage I procedure was performed on the little finger. This included excision of dense scar which extended from the base of the finger proximally for the full extent of the tendon bed in the palm. The tissues in the finger were atrophic, an appearance consistent with what would be expected after absence of function for one year. A medium prosthesis was inserted from the distal phalanx to the forearm and the finger pulleys were preserved or reconstructed. The potential range of motion was then from full extension to full flexion and the finger was assigned Grade 2, since the defect was primarily scarring of the bed.

The postoperative course was uneventful and, five months later, a Stage II procedure was performed. A long toe-extensor tendon was used as the graft. In the forearm, the common tendon of the profundus muscle of the ring and little finger was used as the motor.

Two months later, the pulp of the little finger could be actively flexed to within 0.6 cm of the palmar crease, and one month later, flexion was complete (Fig. 7.8.9*A* and *B*).

The good result in this patient is believed to be significant because this finger was of the type in which a conventional graft is often attempted with a poor result. Typically, the tissues are soft and the joints are mobile but there is extensive scarring of the tendon bed in the finger and in the palm.

The excellent result obtained in this little finger

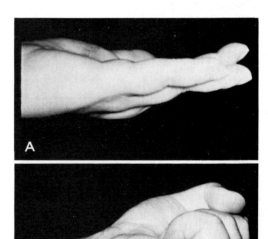

Figure 7.8.9.

suggests that this procedure has a place in the treatment of borderline injuries which do not belong in the salvage category, yet often do not do well after conventional tendon graft.

SUMMARY

The two-stage procedure for tendon reconstruction using a gliding silicone Dacron-reinforced prosthesis has important advantages. A new tendon bed and anatomic pulley system, with gliding surfaces, is established prior to insertion of the graft. At the first stage, it is possible to do multiple procedures, such as digital neurorrhaphy, osteotomy, and capsulotomy, in addition to resection of scar, construction of the pulley system, and insertion of the prosthesis. By careful preoperative planning, it is therefore possible to reduce the number of operations necessary to reconstruct a severely damaged hand. It should be emphasized, however, that fingers which are stiff, as the result of severe injury or repeated unsuccessful operations, cannot be benefited by this procedure. Restoration of a tendon sheath and a gliding tendon will not mobilize a stiff finger.

When there has been extensive damage to the palm, the two-stage procedure, with a long graft and the proximal anastomosis in the forearm, has great advantages and is the procedure of choice. When this is done, the proximal anastomosis may be placed beneath the profundus peritenon, within the superficialis peritenon, or within the newly formed sheath, thereby reducing the formation of restrictive adhesions.

The evidence from our clinical experience suggests that the sheath which forms about the gliding tendon prosthesis after Stage I procedure can provide the nutritional requirements of a free tendon graft with minimum or no adhesions. When the gliding prosthesis is removed, the sheath which has formed around it apparently has both the physiologic and the anatomic characteristics necessary to nourish a tendon graft.

Results in the salvage of fingers with severe tendon injuries has led us to believe that a reliable tendon prosthesis inserted as one stage in tendon reconstruction is the additional step needed to improve the results of flexor tendon reconstructive surgery.

Although the results with the passive prosthesis have been distinctly encouraging, it would seem that a reliable active prosthesis would have advantages under certain circumstances. From our earlier experience, it would appear that an active tendon prosthesis results in better organization of the tissues in the region of the proximal anastomosis so that at the Stage II procedure there is a good connective tissue mesentery which can be preserved when the graft is inserted. As a result there is an earlier return of function after grafting. In addition, with an active prosthesis, the muscle which is to be the motor for the graft continues to function, fewer adhesions form, and functional training after grafting is simplified.

Continuing research with porous synthetic and metal fabrics, metal end devices, indicates the basic direction for further research in the development of active artificial tendons in the future.

The prosthesis, as it is now produced should be used primarily as a passive gliding device with no proximal attachment. However, in carefully selected and closely supervised patients, the prosthesis may be made active by suturing its proximal end to the proximal tendon stump or musculotendinous junction of the motor muscles in the palm or forearm.

REFERENCES

1. Anzel, S. H., Lipscomb, P. R., and Grindlay, J. H. Construction of artificial tendon sheaths in dogs. Am. J. Surg., *101:* 355-356, 1961.
2. Arkin, A. N., and Siffert, R. S. The use of wire in tenoplasty and tenorrhaphy. Am. J. Surg., *85:* 795-797, 1953.
3. Ashley, F. L., Polak, T., Stone, R. S., and Marmor, L. Healing of tendons in silicone rubber sheaths. Bull. Dow-Corning, *4:* 3, 1962.
4. Ashley, R. L., Stone, R. S., Alonso-Artieda, M., Syverud, J. M., Edwards, J. W., and Mooney, S. A. Experimental and clinical studies on the application of monomolecular cellulose filter tubes to create artificial tendon sheaths in digits. Plast. Reconstr. Surg., *23:* 526-534, 1959.
5. Bassett, C. A., and Campbell, J. B. Keeping silastic sterile. Bull. Dow-Corning, *2:* 1, 1960.
6. Biesalski, K. Ueber Sehnenscheidenauswechslung Dtsch. Med. Wochnschr., *36:* 1615-1618, 1910.
7. Biesalski, K., and Mayer, L. *Die physiologische Sehnenverpflanzung.* Berlin, Springer, 1916.
8. Boyes, J. H. Flexor tendon grafts in the fingers and thumb. An evaluation of end results. J. Bone Joint Surg., *32A:* 489-499, 1950.
9. Boyes, J. H. Evaluation of results of digital flexor tendon grafts. Am J. Surg., *89:* 1116-1119, 1955.
10. Brand, P. Principles of free tendon grafting, including a new method of tendon suture. J. Bone Joint Surg., *41B:* 208, 1959.
11. Bruner, J. M. The zig-zag volar-digital incision for flexor-tendon surgery. Plast. Reconstr. Surg., *40:* 571-574, 1967.
12. Bunnell, S. *Bunnell's Surgery of the Hand,* Ed. 4, revised by J. H. Boyes. Philadelphia, Lippincott, 1964.
13. Bunnell, S. [Editor]. *Hand Surgery in World War II.* Medical Department of the United States Army. Washington, Office of the Surgeon General, Department of the Army, 1955, p. 49.
14. Carroll, R. E., and Bassett, A. L. Formation of tendon sheath by silicone-rod implants. Proceedings— American Society for Surgery of the Hand. J. Bone Joint Surg., *45A:* 884-885, 1963.
15. Curtis, R. M. Joints of the hand. In *Hand Surgery,* edited by J. E. Flynn. Baltimore, Williams and Wilkins, 1966, pp. 350-375.
16. Curtis, R. M. Capsulectomy of the interphalangeal joints of the fingers. J. Bone Joint Surg., *36A:* 1219-1232, 1954.
17. Cushman, P. Personal communication.
18. Davis, L., and Aries, L. J. An experimental study upon the prevention of adhesions about repaired nerves and

tendons. Surgery, 2: 877-888, 1937.

19. Goenicdtian, S. A. A new method of canalization tendon sutures with vein grafts. Arch. Surg., 26: 181, 1949.

20. Gonzalez, R. I. Experimental tendon repair within the flexor tunnels: Use of polyethylene tubes for improvement of functional results in the dog. Surgery, 26: 181-198, 1949.

21. Gonzalez, R. E. Experimental use of Teflon in tendon surgery. Plast. Reconstr. Surg., 23: 535-539, 1958.

22. Grau, H. R. The artificial tendon: An experimental study. Plast. Reconstr. Surg., 22: 562-566, 1958.

23. Hanisch, C. M., and Kleiger, B. Experimental production of tendon sheaths. A preliminary report on the implantation of a flexible plastic in the tissues of rabbits and guinea pigs. Bull. Hosp. Joint Dis., 9: 22-31, 1948

24. Henze, C. W., and Mayer, L. An experimental study of silk-tendon plastics with particular reference to the prevention of postoperative adhesions. Surg. Gynecol. Obstet., 19: 10-24, 1914.

25. Hochstrasser, A. E., Broadbent, T. R., and Woolf, R. Sheath replacement in tendon repair. Experimental study with Ivalon. Rocky Mt. Med. J., 57: 30-33, July 1960.

26. Hunter, J. M. Artificial tendons. Early development and application. Am. J. Surg., 109: 325-338, 1965.

27. Hunter, J. M. Artificial tendons—their early development and application. In Proceedings of the American Society for Surgery of the Hand. J. Bone Joint Surg., 47A: 631-632, 1965.

28. Hunter, J. M., Salem, A. W., Steindel, C. R., and Salisbury, R. E. The use of gliding artificial tendon implants to form new tendon beds. In Proceedings of the American Society for Surgery of the Hand. J. Bone Joint Surg., 51A: 790, 1969.

29. Hunter, J. M., and Salisbury, R. E. Use of gliding artificial implants to produce tendon sheaths. Techniques and results in children. Plast. Reconstr. Surg., 45: 564-572, 1970.

30. Hunter, J. M., and Salisbury, R. E. Flexor tendon reconstruction in severely damaged hands. J. Bone Joint Surg., 53A: 829-858, 1971.

31. Iwauchi, S., Shoji, N., and Abe, I. Experience with artificial tendon-grafting in the hand. In Proceedings of the Fourth Annual Meeting of the Japanese Society for Surgery of the Hand. J. Bone Joint Surg., 43A: 152, Jan. 1961.

32. Koth, D. R., and Sewell, W. H. Freeze-dried arteries used as tendon sheaths. Surg. Gynecol. Obstet., 101: 615-620, 1955.

33. Lange, F. Ueber periostale Sehnenverpflanzungen bei Lähmungen. Münch. Med. Wochnschr., 47: 486-490, 1900.

34. Littler, J. W. Free tendon grafts in secondary flexor tendon repair. Am. J. Surg., 74: 315-321, 1947.

35. Littler, J. W. Principles of reconstructive surgery of the hand. In Reconstructive Plastic Surgery, edited by J. M. Converse. Vol. 4. Philadelphia, Saunders, 1964, pp. 1612-1674.

36. Mayer, L. The physiological method of tendon transplantation. Surg. Gynecol. Obstet., 22: 182-197, 1916.

37. Mayer, L., and Ransohoff, N. Reconstruction of the digital tendon sheath. A contribution to the physiological method of repair of damaged finger tendons. J. Bone Joint Surg., 18: 607-616, 1936.

38. Milgram, J. E. Transplantation of tendons through preformed gliding channels. Bull. Hosp. Joint Dis., 21: 250-295, 1960.

39. Nichols, H. M. Discussion of tendon repair with clinical and experimental data on the use of gelatin sponge. Ann. Surg., 129: 223-234, 1949.

40. Parks, A. The "lumbrical plus" finger. J. Bone Joint Surg., 53B: 236-239, 1971.

41. Potenza, A. D. Tendon healing within the flexor digital sheath in the dog. An experimental study. J. Bone Joint Surg., 44A: 49-64, 1962.

42. Pulvertaft, R. G. Experiences in flexor tendon grafting in the hand. J. Bone Joint Surg., 41B: 629-630, 1959.

43. Pulvertaft, R. G. Tendon grafts for flexor tendon injuries in the fingers and thumb. A study of technique and results. J. Bone Joint Surg., 38B: 175-194, 1956.

44. Sakata, Y. Experimental study on the combined use of arterial tissues with Nylon thread in artifical tendon formation. J. Jap. Orthop. Assoc., 36: 1021, 1962.

45. Sarkin, T. L. The plastic replacement of severed flexor tendons of the fingers. Br. J. Surg., 44: 232-240, 1956.

46. Thatcher, H. vH. Use of stainless steel rods to canalize flexor tendon sheaths. South. Med. J., 32: 31-18, 1939.

47. Tubiana, R. Greffes des tendons fléchisseurs des doigts et du pouce. Technique et résultats. Rev. Chir. Orthop., 46: 191-214, 1960.

48. Verdan, C. E. Primary and secondary repair of flexor and extensor tendon injuries. In Hand Surgery, edited by J. E. Flynn. Baltimore, Williams and Wilkins, 1966, pp. 220-275.

49. Wheeldon, T. The use of cellophane as a permanent tendon sheath. J. Bone Joint Surg., 21: 393-396, 1939.

50. White, W. L. Secondary restoration of finger flexion by digital tendon grafts. An evaluation of seventy-six cases. Am. J. Surg., 91: 662-668, 1956.

chapter eight

Injuries to Joints

A.

Fractures and Dislocations of the Carpal Bones

John C. Molloy, M.D.

Fractures and dislocations of the carpal bones, although quite common, cause great difficulty in diagnosis and confusion in treatment. Accurate diagnosis is essential to development of a rational plan of treatment of these injuries.

Seven small bones comprise the carpal mechanism. The two rows of the carpus are stabilized by the scaphoid which spans both rows. Many ligaments connect the bones and these permit only small degrees of motion between the individual bones, but considerable motion at the radiocarpal and midcarpal joints (Fig. 8.1.1).

As McLaughlin illustrates so well,[9] the radiocarpal joint accounts for the major portion of motion of the wrist, except rotation (Fig. 8.1.2).

The proximal row consists of the scaphoid, lunate, and triquetrum, the distal row the trapezium, trapezoid, capitate, and hamate. The pisiform does not really participate in the mechanics of the carpus.

Carpal fractures and dislocations are caused primarily by forced extension of the wrist (Fig. 8.1.3). In all dislocations there is disruption of the relationship between the capitate and lunate. As the force continues and as the relationship between the two rows becomes more disrupted, the scaphoid must either fracture or dislocate.

Most reported series of carpal dislocations find dislocations of the lunate to be the most common, followed by transscaphoperilunar dislocation and perilunar dislocation.[1,6,12]

The key to diagnosis of the injury of the wrist is the lateral x-ray. The axes of the radius, the lunate, the capitate, and the third metacarpal should fall on a straight line with the wrist in neutral position. The outline of the lunate is usually readily apparent, and it is sometimes helpful to outline the lunate, capitate, and scaphoid with a wax pencil to clarify their relationships. The PA film should be observed for any alteration in the relationships of the capitate, lunate, and scaphoid to each other, for any increase in the width of the joint space between these bones, which should be symmetrical, and for any alteration in the relationship between the scaphoid and lunate and their articular notches on the radius (Fig. 8.1.4).

DISLOCATION OF THE LUNATE

Dislocation of the lunate may occur as a primary injury, by a fall on the extended hand forcing the capitate and the radius together, causing displacement of the lunate volarward (Fig. 8.1.5) or it may occur as the final stage of a perilunar dislocation in which continued force has displaced the lunate forward and allowed realignment of the capitate with the radius.[1]

The dislocated lunate (Fig. 8.1.6) may cause compression of the median nerve and the flexor tendons within the tight carpal tunnel. The disability of the hand is often the symptom which causes the patient to seek treatment for his injury.

Treatment

When seen early, closed reduction is usually successful, but with delay open reduction becomes necessary. General anesthesia is helpful in providing adequate relaxation for reduction and traction on the wrist combined with extension and direct pressure over the dislocated lunate are the most useful maneuvers in securing reduction. The wrist should be immobilized in moderate flexion for three to four weeks following reduction.

When closed reduction fails, operation should be carried out. In view of the poor results following excision of the lunate, this should not be done as a primary procedure. Avascular necrosis of the lunate is rare, even though the approach is made through a volar incision.[1]

The dorsal incision is preferable, however, for several reason: the approach is simpler and more direct; the relationship between the navicular and lunate may have to be restored, and exposure for this is more readily attained thru a dorsal incision; there is no disturbance of the volar blood supply to the lunate which may be its only remaining blood supply.

Reduction of the lunate followed by excision of the proximal row of the carpus if symptoms persist is preferable to primary excision of the lunate.

PERILUNATE DISLOCATION

Perilunate dislocation indicates a more extensive injury to the intercarpal ligaments, with only the lu-

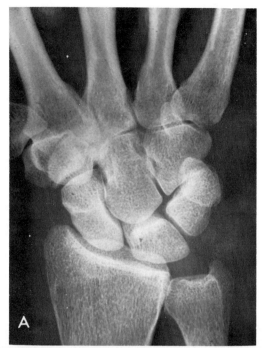

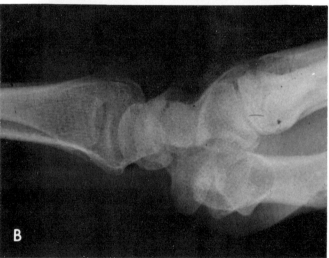

Figure 8.1.1. Normal wrist. *A.* PA x-ray of the wrist shows the equal spacing between the small bones, the articular notches on the radius for articulation with the scaphoid and lunate, the quadrilateral shape of the lunate, and the profile of the scaphoid spanning the proximal and distal rows of the carpus. *B.* Lateral x-ray of the wrist, the key to diagnosis of dislocations of the wrist. With the wrist in neutral position a straight line drawn through the central axis of the radius should pass through the central axis of the lunate and capitate. This wrist is in slight dorsiflexion, but the relationship between the radius, lunate, and capitate are all shown. A line drawn through the central axis of the scaphoid should intersect the line drawn through the radius at an angle of 40 to 50°.

nate maintaining its normal relationship with the radius (Fig. 8.1.7). The extensive ligament disruption makes the reduction of this dislocation easier than the reduction of a lunate dislocation, but it also makes the maintenance of the exact anatomic relationship more difficult. When perilunate dislocation occurs, the scaphoid must either fracture or dislocate; therefore, when the dislocation is reduced, the relationship between the scaphoid and the lunate tends to remain disrupted and a rotary dislocation of the scaphoid may occur.[14]

Maintenance of the relationships between the carpal bones may be impossible by closed means, and if the relationships cannot be restored and held anatomically closed, open reduction and fixation by Kirschner wires is indicated.

It is difficult to obtain a good result after perilunate dislocation, but it is nearly impossible if precise restoration of the anatomy is not obtained (Fig. 8.1.8).

TRANSSCAPHOPERILUNATE DISLOCATION

Since the scaphoid bridges both rows of the carpus, as a force is applied which causes a perilunate dislocation, the scaphoid must either dislocate from its proximal attachments or fracture. In the latter instance its proximal pole remains attached to the lunate (Fig. 8.1.9).

Reduction of the dislocation is carried out by traction and flexion of the distal portion with direct pressure over the displaced segments. The reduction tends to be unstable due to the extensive ligament damage,

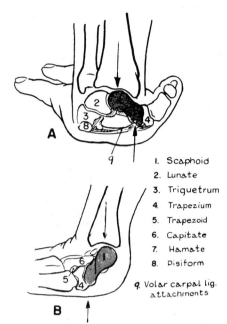

1. Scaphoid
2. Lunate
3. Triquetrum
4. Trapezium
5. Trapezoid
6. Capitate
7. Hamate
8. Pisiform
9. Volar carpal lig. attachments

Figure 8.1.3. Mechanism of wrist injury. A. The volar carpal ligament and canal in cross section. When a person falls on the fully extended hand, the force of the impact *(arrows)* is primarily accepted by the waist of the scaphoid. B. Lateral view of the carpal bones. A fall on the fully extended hand also centers the force of the impact *(arrows)* at the narrow midportion of the scaphoid. Since this bone cannot adjust itself simultaneously to the plane of both the common cause of fracture of the scaphoid. (From McLaunghlin, H. L.: Saunders., p. 143).

and it may be impossible to obtain and maintain accurate reduction of the scaphoid fragments short of open reduction and internal fixation. Imperfect reduction may result in delayed union or nonunion of the scaphoid fracture. The scaphoid fracture, if not well approximated following reduction of the dislocation, should be fixed by a screw or Kirschner wire as a primary procedure.

Early internal fixation of the scaphoid fracture provides the additional benefit of stabilizing the dislocation since the scaphoid is the connection between the two rows of the carpus.

The reduction should be checked frequently during the course of treatment to assure maintenance of the reduction of the scaphoid. If reduction is not maintained, the chances of nonunion and avascular necrosis are grately increased.

DISLOCATION OF THE SCAPHOID

Dislocation of the scaphoid may occur as a primary injury to the wrist, or it may occur following reduction

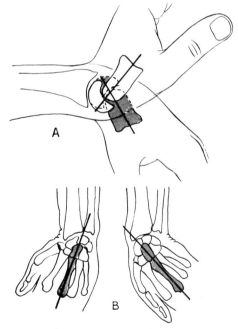

Figure 8.1.2. Motions of the wrist joint. A. Flexion and extension are mainly products of radiocarpal motion. The axis of the capitate bone changes much more in relation to the radius than to the lunate. B. Abduction and adduction are mainly products of radiocarpal motion. There is little motion between the carpal bones. (From McLaughlin, H. L.: *Trauma*. Saunders Co., p. 142).

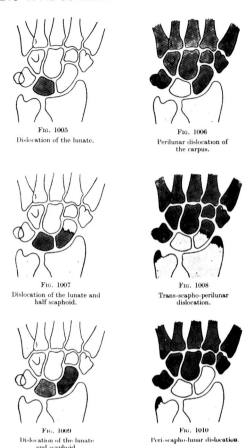

FIG. 1005
Dislocation of the lunate.

FIG. 1006
Perilunar dislocation of the carpus.

FIG. 1007
Dislocation of the lunate and half scaphoid.

FIG. 1008
Trans-scapho-perilunar dislocation.

FIG. 1009
Dislocation of the lunate and scaphoid.

FIG. 1010
Peri-scapho-lunar dislocation.

Figure 8.1.4. Classification of dislocations of the carpus. The dislocated bones are shown in dark shading and the undisplaced bones in pale shading. Note that in each pair, the dislocation on the left is the counterpart of that on the right. (From Watson-Jones, *Fractures and Joint Injuries,* Ed. 4, Edinburgh and London, Livingston, 1956, p. 623).

of a perilunate dislocation (Fig. 8.1.7*B*). The dislocation is rotary, with the distal pole rotating volarward. This gives the x-ray signs, as seen in Figure 8.1.7*C*, (1) increased distance between the scaphoid and the lunate, (2) medial shift of the lunate, (3) loss of height of the scaphoid on the posterior-anterior projection, and (4) on the lateral view displacement of the long axis of the scaphoid so that its axis approaches nearly a right angle with the long axis of the radius.

Dislocation of the scaphoid is easily overlooked. The widening of the space between the lunate and the scaphoid is the clue which should lead one to the diagnosis.

Reduction is difficult to maintain in the early case and may be impossible in the late case. Early reposition and fixation with Kirschner wires is the treatment of choice.

Good results have been reported following open

reduction six weeks or more after injury, [12,14] but in our experience the results after late open reduction have been poor in two cases and both have required further surgery.

FRACTURES OF THE CAPITATE AND LUNATE AND DISLOCATIONS OF THE CAPITATE

These injuries are rare and are usually seen only in very severe injuries of the wrist. The essential injury is a form of perilunate dislocation. The dislocation should be reduced, and any small displaced fragments should be removed. Any large displaced fragments should be replaced and fixed. The wrist should be immobilized in moderate flexion to permit soft tissue healing.

More definitive procedures, *i.e.,* excision of the proximal row or arthrodesis, should be delayed until an evaluation of the degree of residual disability can be satisfactorily carried out.

FRACTURES OF THE SCAPHOID

Fracture of the scaphoid is a common injury; it may cause significant disability to the patient, and it may be a cause of great consternation to the surgeon. A proper plan for treatment of these injuries must be developed. The following is a plan which has been helpful to me and which is based, I hope, on some sensible principles. The difficulty with laying down rigid principles for treating wrist injuries is that every time a principle suggests itself, several reasons for not following it emerge as well.

For instance, the adage that every wrist sprain must be treated as a fracture of the scaphoid until proven otherwise seems somewhat excessive. Many untreated scaphoid fractures probably go on to uneventful union; many certainly go on to strong, painless fibrous union which remains undetected until a subsequent injury results in an x-ray being taken, which shows a long standing pseudarthrosis. These are obviously stable fractures, ones in which the articular cartilage is intact, and which are difficult to locate at time of operation if bone grafting is attempted. These fractures must be clearly differentialed from unstable fractures which eventually result in painful arthritis of the wrist joint if left untreated.

The proximal one-half of the scaphoid is intraarticular and has no soft tissue attachments. It, therefore, is subject to the same problems in healing that apply to the femoral neck and the body of the talus, *i.e.,* nonunion and aseptic necrosis.

The distal one-third of the scaphoid is completely covered by soft part attachments, has an excellent blood supply, is extraarticular, and heals promptly almost regardless of what type of treatment is applied.

Fractures through the waist of the scaphoid may be intra- or extra-articular and thus are on the borderline between those which heal promptly and those which may not heal at all.

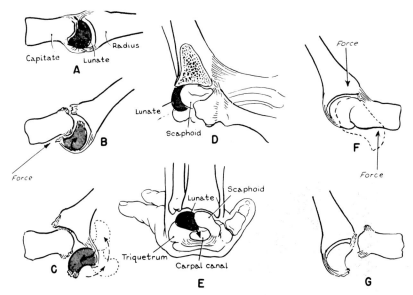

Figure 8.1.5. Dislocations of and on the lunate. *A.* Normal relations, lateral view. *Arrows* indicate vascular supply to the lunate. *B.* An appropriate force, with the wrist moderately extended, may extrude the lunate from between the radius and the capitate bone. *C.* The displaced lunate rotates around the soft part hinge, which is its only remaining source of blood supply. The capitate bone is forced against the radius. *D.* and *E.* The extruded lunate encroaches upon the flexor tendons and the median nerve in the volar carpal canal. *F.* and *G.* An appropriate force to the hyperextended carpus tends to displace the other carpals on the lunate. Impact of the proximal end of the scaphoid against the radius may fracture this bone so that only the distal fragment accompanies the capitate bone into a dislocated position. (From McLaughlin, H. L.: *Trauma.* Saunders, 1959, p. 160).

On the PA view of the wrist (Fig. 8.1.10) it may be seen that the radial styloid lines up directly with the waist of the scaphoid. This accounts for the prevalence of fractures in this region as well as the beneficial effect of radial styloidectomy on fractures of the navicular.

Otto Russe[11] states that 10 per cent of scaphoid fractures occur in the distal third, 70 per cent in the middle third and 20 per cent in the proximal third.

Stable fractures through the waist or midportion of the scaphoid are held securely by soft tissue attachments or intact articular cartilage (Fig. 8.1.10). In these cases very little motion occurs at the fracture even on motion of the wrist. Healing can be expected within four to eight weeks with immobilization in a snug-fitting plaster cast. The cast should be applied with the thumb metacarpal in abduction and opposition to the index finger and need extend only to the metacarpophalangeal joint.

Unstable, or displaced fractures of the scaphoid (Fig. 8.1.11) may as Campbell[2] contends often or always be the result of a transscaphoperilunar dislocation which is incompletely reduced. This represents a more severe and extensive injury to the wrist than a simple scaphoid fracture, and the best chance of a successful result will follow open reduction and internal fixation with a screw or Kirschner wires.

Mandsley[8] reports a series of 62 patients treated by screw fixation for fracture of the carpal scaphoid by McLaughlin's technique combined with radial styloidectomy. Of 20 patients treated for recent fracture (within three months of operation) all 20 were satisfied with their result and 19 had united. Of 15 treated by this method for delayed union (failure to unite within a year of injury), all 15 were satisfied and had returned to normal work, eight fractures united and seven did not, with some discomfort and restriction of full use in five. Of 19 patients treated for nonunion (when a clear gap was present at the fracture line after more than a year) 17 were satisfied with the result and resumed normal work. Only two of the fractures united, however, and one required an arthrodesis.

These patients were not immobilized in plaster following operation. Mandsley feels that by stabilizing the wrist, by restoring the scaphoid bridge between the carpal rows, the integrity of the wrist is restored and symptoms are relieved or prevented, whether the fracture unites or not.

He advocates screw fixation in (1) displaced recent fractures, (2) perilunartransscaphoid dislocations as the method of choice, (3) cases of delayed union where conventional management with splints or casts prevents work, (4) cases of nonunion without secondary arthrosis when symptoms persist after an adequate period of immobilization.

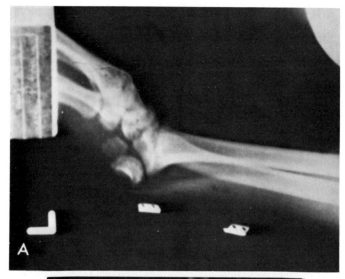

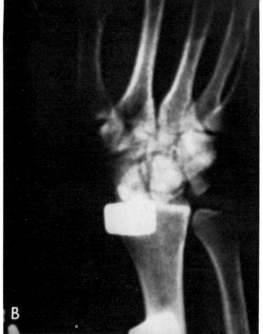

Figure 8.1.6. Dislocation of the lunate. *A.* Lateral view shows the lunate displaced from its normal relation to the radius, and rotated ninety degrees. The space between the capitate and radius is decreased. *B.* PA view reveals that the anatomy of the wrist is disrupted but it is not clear from this view what the pathology is, although it is well seen on the lateral view.

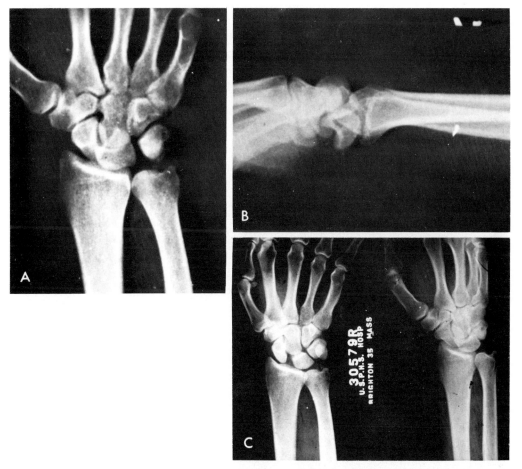

Figure 8.1.7. Perilunate dislocation. *A.* and *B.* AP and lateral view shows the relationship between the lunate and radius maintained, with the remainder of the carpus dislocated dorsally. Again, the lateral view is the key to the diagnosis. *C.* This man was treated by closed reduction, placed in a cast, and when initially seen by us was found to have a rotary dislocation of the scaphoid. The key to this diagnosis is the gap between the scaphoid and lunate, the change in the profile of the scaphoid and the shift ‘ulnaward of the lunate on the PA x-ray. Open reduction and internal fixation was necessary to realign the scaphoid.

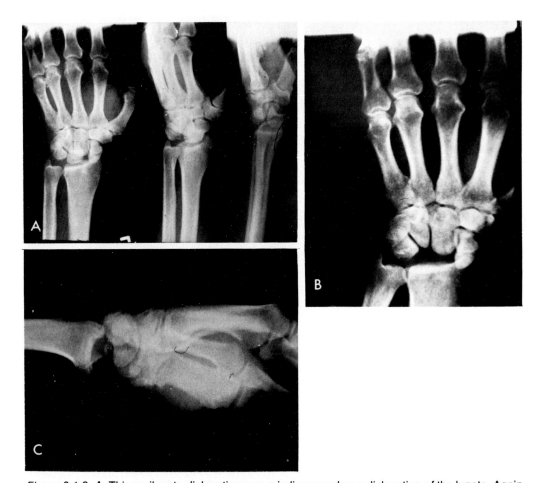

Figure 8.1.8. A. This perilunate dislocation was misdiagnosed as a dislocation of the lunate. Again, the diagnosis is obvious on the lateral film, the lunate maintaining its relationship with the radius. The error in diagnosis was followed up by an erroneous treatment, and the lunate was excised (*B.* and *C.*)

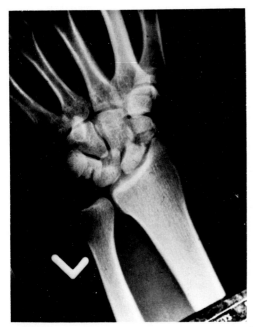

Figure 8.1.9. PA x-ray of the left wrist of a man who jumped from a second story window, sustaining severe injuries to both wrists and a dislocation of the left elbow. The left wrist shows a transscaphoperilunar dislocation with a fracture of the proximal pole of the capitate and a small fracture of the lunate. Open reduction and stabilization of the scaphoid was necessary together with excision of the small fragments of the capitate and lunate. The prospects for a good result in cases such as this are dim.

Fresh fractures should be immobilized in a lightly padded plaster cast. The healing should be evaluated at monthly intervals with discontinuance of the casts as soon as evidence of bony trabeculae crossing the fracture line appear. If after three months of immobilization there is still no evidence of healing a reevaluation of the course of treatment should be made. The alternatives should be carefully explained to the patient. The cast should be discontinued at this point and a trial of exercise should be instituted. The patient may have a stable fibrous union which requires no further treatment. For younger patients and for patients in whom symptoms occur with use of the wrist, bone grafting is indicated.

We have found the technique of bone peg grafting to be unsuccessful, and recently have been using the technique of Otto Russe[11] for treatment of symptomatic, ununited fractures of the scaphoid. The approach is through a longitudinal incision on the volar aspect of the wrist, just radial to the flexor carpi radialis tendon. The fracture site is visualized, it being usually in line with the tip of the radial styloid. The bone ends are freshened and a cavity is formed, extending well into

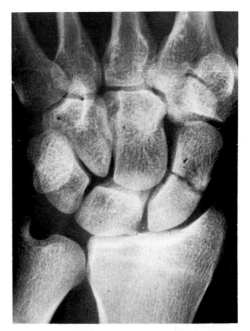

Figure 8.1.10. Stable fracture through the waist of the scaphoid. Prompt healing or at least a stable fibrous union can be expected in fractures of this type.

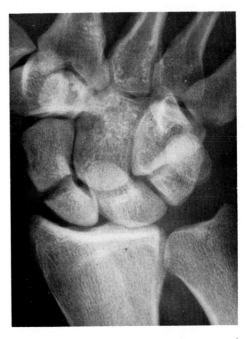

Figure 8.1.11. Fracture of the scaphoid with displacement. This indicates a more severe injury to the wrist, and warrants a more aggressive approach to treatment than a simple undisplaced fracture.

the adjacent fragments. An oblong piece of cancellous bone is taken from the iliac crest and packed into the cavity. Small chips are used to fill the remainder of the cavity. If good stability is not attained by packing the cavity, Kirschner wire fixation may be added. A plaster cast is worn for 12 to 16 weeks until union occurs. Russe reports a success rate of 80 to 90 per cent using this method in 120 cases. In his own series of 22 cases, there had been a delay of more than one year between accident and operation in 15 of them, and, of the 22 cases, 20 (90 per cent) united.

Small fragments of the proximal third of the scaphoid are best treated by excision and any operative intervention on the scaphoid for fixation or bone grafting should be accompanied by radial styloidectomy.

SALVAGE PROCEDURE

Any discussion of carpal injuries would be incomplete without some comment about the wrist injury so severe or of such prolonged duration that repair or realignment is impossible. Multiple fractures and dislocations of the carpal bones, perilunar dislocations in which treatment has been unsuccessful, avascular necrosis of the scaphoid or lunate bone, painful ununited fractures of the scaphoid and certain other conditions fall into this catagory.

For these cases removal of the proximal carpal row holds the greatest promise of success. Many authors who have reviewed excision of the three proximal carpal bones — the scaphoid, lunate, and triquetrum — have been enthusiastic about the results.[1-4,7,10,12,13]

Th proximal carpal row is excised without difficulty through a dorsal incision. The arm should be immobilized in a below elbow cast for four to six weeks.

Jorgensen[4] reports that his best results occurred in those patients who were operated on soon after injury. All of his 20 patients reported a subjective feeling of weakness in the involved wrist as compared to the normal wrist. Only one of his patients showed degenerative changes by x-ray at the time of follow-up.

A painless, mobile wrist can be anticipated following this procedure, although there is usually some weakness as compared to a normal wrist. The radial and ulnar ligaments shorten and provide a satisfactory degree of stability. If the procedure fails, a radiocapitate or radiometacarpal fusion can be performed subsequently.

Resection of the proximal carpal row is contraindicated in those wrists which are already severely involved by arthritis, particularly of the radial articular surface. Arthrodesis of the wrist is more apt to achieve a satisfactory result in these cases.

REFERENCES

1. Campbell, R. D., Jr., Lance, E. M., and Yeoh, C. B. Lunate and peri-lunar dislocations. J. Bone Joint Surg., *46B:* 55-72, 1964.
2. Campbell, R. D., Jr., Thompson, T. C., Lance, E. M., and Adler, J. E. Indications for open reduction of lunate and peri-lunate dislocations of the carpal bones. J. Bone Joint Surg., *47A:* 915-937, 1965.
3. Crabbe, W. D. Excision of the proximal row of the carpus. J. Bone Joint Surg., *46B:* 708-711, 1964.
4. Jorgensen, E. C. Proximal row carpectomy. An end result study of twenty-two cases. J. Bone Joint Surg., *51A:* 1104-1111, 1969.
5. Linschied, R. L., Dobyns, J. H., Beabout, J. W., and Bryan, R. S. Traumatic instability of the wrist. J. Bone Joint Surg., *54A:* 1612-1632, 1972.
6. MacAusland, W. R. Perilunar dislocations of the carpal bones and dislocations of the lunate bone. Surg. Gynecol. Obstet., *79:* 256-266, 1944.
7. Marek, F. M. Avascular Necrosis of the Carpal Lunate. Clin. Orthop. *10:* 96, 1957.
8. Mandsley, R. H., and Chen, S. C. Screw fixation in the management of the fractured carpal scaphoid. J. Bone Joint Surg., *54B:* 432-441, 1972.
9. McLaunghlin, H. L. *Trauma.* Philadelphia and London, Saunders, 1959, pp. 140-178.
10. McLaughlin, H. L., and Baab, O. D. Symposium on orthopedic surgery carpectomy. Surg. Clin. North Am., *31:* 451-461, 1951.
11. Russe, O. Fracture of the carpal navicular. J. Bone Joint Surg., *42A:* 759-768, 1960.
12. Russell, T. B. Intercarpal dislocations and fracture dislocations. A review of fifty-nine cases. J. Bone Joint Surg., *31B:* 524-531, 1949.
13. Stark, J. K. End results of excision of carpal bones. Arch. Surg., *57:* 245-252, 1938.
14. Thompson, T. C., Campbell, R. D., Jr., and Arnold, W. D. Primary and secondary dislocation of the scaphoid bone. J. Bone Joint Surg., *46B:* 73-82, 1964.
15. Watson-Jones, *Fractures and Joint Injuries,* Ed. 4. Edinburgh and London, Livingstone, 1956, pp. 606-628.

B.

Joints of the Hand

Raymond M. Curtis, M.D.

The joints of the hand are the means by which the power of the muscles moving the bones of the hand bring about useful function. When these joints are stiffened by fibrosis, destroyed by disease, or deformed by dislocation or fracture, the function of the hand is impaired or even destroyed.

DISCUSSION: CAUSES OF JOINT STIFFENING IN THE HAND

The primary factors behind stiffening of the joints of the hand are: (1) lack of motion in the joints; (2) swelling of the hand. To decrease the edema and swell-

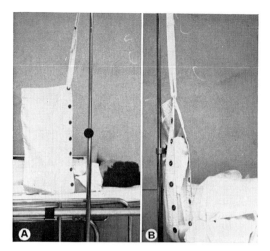

Figure 8.2.1. Canvas sling with zipper to use for elevation of injured or postoperative hand and forearm to minimize swelling.

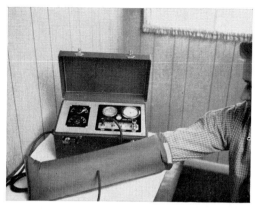

Figure 8.2.2. Intermittent compression unit which aids in mobilizing stiffened joints and reduces swelling.

ing in the injured hand or in a postoperative hand, we find the following is necessary: (1) elevation of the parts; (2) mechanics' waste as a dressing for mild pressure; (3) elimination of pain, which causes disuse, edema, and stiffening of the joints.

Bunnell[6] has stated that all uninjured parts should be kept unrestrained and free to move. This is the functional treatment of fractures as described by Böhler[4] and Watson-Jones.[55] Moberg[38] has emphasized that contraction of the muscles pumps the tissue fluids through the limb, preventing edema and stasis, and keeping the tissues nourished.

CONSERVATIVE METHODS OF TREATING STIFFENED JOINTS

Elevation

Elevation of the injured part as shown in Figure 8.2.1 is important in that it minimizes the degree of swelling. This should be used immediately after all surgery on the hand and one should be sure that the patient, when ambulatory, keeps the hand elevated as well.

Elastic Splints and Elastic Traction

These should be used early and continuously. The amount of tension used should not produce swelling.

Intermittent Compression Unit* (Fig. 8.2.2)

This therapy has been very helpful in reducing the swelling in the post-traumatic and postoperative hand, and in mobilizing the stiff interphalangeal joints. The hand is placed in the sleeve with the fingers in extension for 5 min, under pressure, and then in flexion for 5 min. One uses the amount of pressure that can be

---

*Jobst Intermittent Compression Unit.

easily tolerated by the patient, increasing the time in the pneumatic sleeve gradually from 30 min to one hour, one or more times a day, and gradually increasing the millimeters of mercury pressure in the sleeve.

Local Heat Therapy

Physiotherapy in the form of warm water soaks or whirlpool is helpful, as is hot wax therapy.

Stellate Ganglion Blocks

The local nerve blocks, or blocks with local anesthesia of the painful trigger areas, are very helpful. When indicated in the sympathetic dystrophy, the stellate ganglion block or sympathectomy can be an aid in relieving pain and decreasing edema.

Active Exercise

One cannot overemphasize the need for active use of the hand in mobilizing stiff joints.

DISLOCATION OF THE METACARPALS ON THE CARPUS

This is a very disabling injury. When the injury is seen while new, attempts should be made at closed reduction. If closed reduction is not successful, immediate open reduction should be carried out with fixation of the metacarpals in their proper position with Kirschner wires. This will be almost impossible to achieve three to four months after injury. This dislocation of the metacarpals on the carpus upsets the muscle balance in the hand, as shown in Figure 8.2.3. (Hsu and Curtis[27]).

The chronic dislocation that one sees with this deformity can be corrected only with open surgery. One may not be able to free the bases of the metacarpals and lever them back into a normal relationship with the carpus. If not, a repositioning of the metacarpals

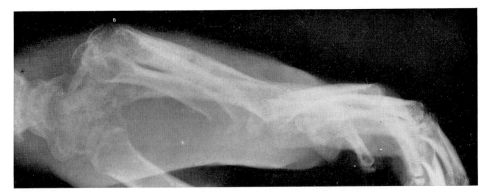

Figure 8.2.3. Old carpometacarpal dislocation. X-ray shows bases of middle, ring, and little finger metacarpals dislocated on carpus. Muscle imbalance characterized by hyperextension of proximal phalanx on metacarpal head and flexion at proximal interphalangeal joints.

is best achieved by resection of the bases that overlap the carpus, freeing the soft tissues about the distal end of the carpus so that the metacarpals can be pushed down into their normal relationship.

THE THUMB

Carpometacarpal Joint

Dislocation

This occurs as a result of a rupture of the volar accessory ligament and may be associated with a fracture of the base of the thumb metacarpal. If it is associated with a small chip fracture and proper alignment of this fracture is not achieved by closed reduction, then an open reduction should be carried out. An incision is made along the radial border of the thumb metacarpal and curved across the flexion crease of the wrist at the base of the thumb. The thenar muscles are stripped partly away from the thumb metacarpal. The incision is deepened to expose the long abductor tendon at its point of insertion into the base of the metacarpal. This tendon is retracted and the dorsal portion of the articular capsule opened. This allows one to reposition the fracture fragment using a Kirschner wire to anchor it in position.

The chronic subluxation at this joint brings considerable weakness in grip between the thumb and the object which the patient is gripping. This can best be corrected, if one desires to maintain motion in the carpometacarpal joint, by the method of Littler[35] using a portion of the flexor radialis tendon.

Chronic Arthritis

Clinically it manifests itself by pain in the region of the carpometacarpal joint with some radiation of this pain up towards the metacarpophalangeal joint. Palpation may elicit roughness and crepitus in this joint.

If there is a marked degenerative change throughout the joint, this may be corrected by excision of the grea-

ter multangulum, as reported by Gervis.[18] A fusion of the carpometacarpal joint may also be done.

With arthrodesis of this joint in a position of function, *i.e.,* opposition, there will be very little loss of motion in the thumb, as a result of the movement of the navicular, except for the position of marked abduction. Bunnell[6] feels that arthrodesis gives a more certain result.

Excision of the greater multangulum with prosthetic replacement (Swanson[51] and Niebauer[40]) may be preferred where there is marked arthritic change in the remainder of the carpus and one expects that pain will be present on motion of the greater multangulum as it moves against the adjacent carpal bones, or where total abduction of the thumb is desired.

Metacarpophalangeal Joints

Forced abduction of the thumb produces a rupture of the ulnar collateral ligament. With rupture of this ligament pain, swelling, local tenderness, abnormal mobility, and weakness on pinch appear.

Stener[50] studied the total rupture collateral ligament of the metacarpophalangeal joint at operation in 39 patients. He found that the ligament, when ruptured distally, which was most usual, often displaced so that the ulnar expansion of the dorsal aponeurosis, "adductor aponeurosis," became interposed between the ruptured end of the ligament and the site of its attachment on the phalanx (Fig. 8.2.4). Such displacement of the ligament was found in 25 of the 39 cases. In other instances the ligament was displaced without interposition of the abductor aponeurosis, with a gap between the ruptured end and the site of its attachment on the phalanx.

Since there is such a high instance of interposition of the abductor aponeurosis, the patient in whom this injury is suspected should be explored, and the ligament should be repaired by simple suture technique or pullout wire technique.

In old injuries, excision of the dorsal capsule will aid in the exposure of this ruptured ligament. Despite exposure of the ligament, one is not able to reinsert the ligament properly, and if motion at the metacarpophalangeal joint is to be preserved, reconstruction can be best accomplished by a tendon graft (Fig. 8.2.5).

Dislocation of the Metacarpophalangeal Joint of the Thumb with Hyperextension Injuries

Stener[49] points out that the degree of hyperextension determines the degree of injury to the joint ligaments. This can be associated with fracture of the

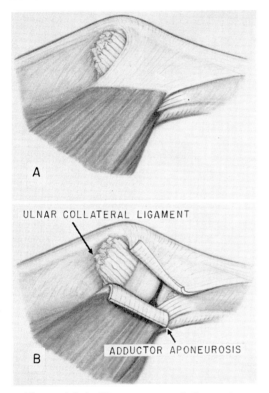

A

ULNAR COLLATERAL LIGAMENT

ADDUCTOR APONEUROSIS

B

Figure 8.2.4. Ulnar aspect of the metacarpophalangeal joint of the right thumb. *A.* After distal rupture the ulnar collateral ligament has been folded over. The torn end protrudes proximal to the adductor. *B.* Aponeurosis shown divided.[50]

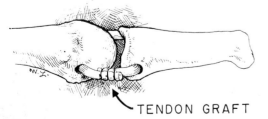

TENDON GRAFT

Figure 8.2.5. Surgical technique for repair of rupture of ulnar or radial collateral ligament of metacarpophalangeal joint of the thumb with a free tendon graft.

sesamoid bones as well as a rupture of the flexor pollicis brevis muscle near its insertion (Fig. 8.2.6).

When the proximal palmar ligament has ruptured, the proximal phalanx is displaced dorsally. However, if in this injury the phalanx itself is not forced back at a right angle to the head of the metacarpal, but rather is simple subluxated, closed reduction may be successful and a good result can be obtained by immobilization in slight flexion for four weeks. If however, the proximal phalanx is forced into extreme hyperextension and is found clinically to rest at a right angle with the head of the metacarpal, there will be a severance of the accessory collateral ligaments, and the palmar ligament and the collateral ligaments may be partially severed. In this type of injury the ruptured ligaments may become caught between the two surfaces of the joint, and a reduction will be impossible without open operation.

Stener[49] prefers a radiopalmar incision, because it provides better exposure of the injury and of the musculature. The incision runs along with the most proximal skin crease of the thumb and is extended as required in a proximal direction radial to the metacarpal bone (Fig. 8.2.6). Immobilization after repair is carried out for four to five weeks.

THE FINGERS

Metacarpophalangeal Joints
Anatomy

The metacarpophalangeal joints of the four fingers can be flexed and extended. When the hand is open in extension the fingers can also be abducted and adducted; thus they perform the four movements which comprise circumduction and are called condyloid joints.

The collateral ligament is attached to a pit in front of the eccentrically placed tubercle on the head of the metacarpal and is composed of two parts: a dorsally placed portion or "cord" ligament and a fan-shaped volar portion, the accessory collateral ligament, which extends from the metacarpal to the sides of the palmar or volar plate (Fig. 8.2.7).

For allowance of flexion and extension, the anterior and posterior parts of the capsule must be lax. Dorsally there are no ligaments to these joints. Here the extensor or dorsal expansion of the extensor tendons effectively serve the part. The synovium of the joint closes the joint dorsally.

Ankylosis

Anatomic structures that limit the metacarpophalangeal joint flexion: (1) insufficient skin coverage or scar of the skin over the dorsum of the hand, as in a burn; (2) adhesions of the extensor tendons over the dorsum of the hand or adhesions of the extensor hood mechanism over the metacarpophalangeal joints; (3) thickening of the dorsal capsule of the metacarpophalangeal joints; (4) contracture of the collateral ligament (cordlike portion); (5) adherent volar plate gives a bony block within the joint.

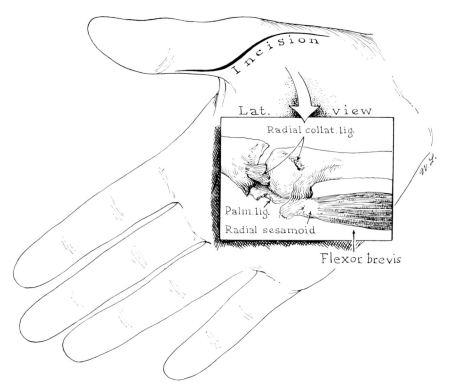

Figure 8.2.6. Incision for exposure of radial and volar aspect of metacarpophalangeal joint of thumb. Insert shows rupture of radial collateral ligament, palmar ligament, and tendon of flexor pollicis brevis (redrawn from Stener[49]).

Of primary importance is the prevention of this very disabling abnormality. It can be best prevented by: (1) early motion of the metacarpophalangeal joints; (2) elevation of the injured extremity with prevention of edema; (3) elimination of plaster casts which immobilize the metacarpophalangeal joint; (4) early elastic band traction in patients who are developing this clinical entity.

Treatment by Splinting and Physiotherapy. In patients who are seen early after injury, attempts should be made to carry out rubber band traction along with the use of a small volar plaster splint, worn 12 or 24 hours a day, or the practical Bunnell[6] knuckle bender splint, to determine what can be achieved with such conservative treatment.

This type of therapy can be coupled with various forms of physiotherapy. Alternating positive pressure, with a compression unit, can be of great help in reducing the edema of the hand and mobilizing the joints. In addition, active exercise should be carried out.

If one is making progress with this form of treatment, the operative release should be delayed. If, on the other hand, one finds after several months of this type of conservative treatment that there is no progress as far as the range of active or passive motion is concerned in the metacarpophalangeal joints, then there will be an indication for surgical release of the metacarpophalangeal joints.

Capsulectomy

If there is no flexion at the metacarpophalangeal joint, but an intrinsically good joint, then one can expect to achieve a good result from the release of the tight capsular ligaments and extensor tendon mechanism. On the other hand, as 75° of active motion is approached in the metacarpophalangeal joint, there is less indication for surgical intervention.

Do not perform capsulectomies on the metacarpophalangeal joints if the patient flexes as much as 65° in these joints. These patients should continue physiotherapy and special splinting.

The choice between arthroplasty and capsulectomy or capsulotomy in a given situation where there is an ankylosis in the metacarpophalangeal joint will depend on the appearance of the metacarpal head and the base of the phalanx in the roentgenogram. Frequently a good range of motion in the metacarpophalangeal joint can be achieved even in instances where by roentgenogram there has been considerable joint destruction.

The technique allows one to release the cordlike portion of the collateral ligament from the tubercle of the metacarpal on either side of the metacarpophalangeal joint after excision of the dorsal capsule, and as a result of the maintenance of continuity between the cordlike portion of the collateral ligament and the accessory collateral ligament, there is in essence still an attachment of the cordlike portion of the collateral ligament to the metacarpal itself. This attachment is enough to prevent ulnar deviation (Fig. 8.2.8).

Operative Technique of Capsulectomy. The exten-

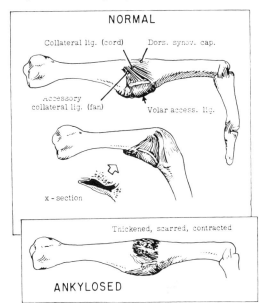

Figure 8.2.7. Top, diagram of normal anatomy of capsular ligaments of metacarpophalangeal joint. Bottom, diagram of contracture of capsular ligament, with ankylosis of metacarpophalangeal joint.

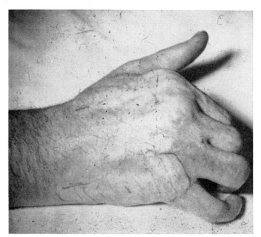

Figure 8.2.8. Ulnar drift of fingers after capsulectomy of the metacarpophalangeal joints caused by too radical resection of the radial collateral ligaments.

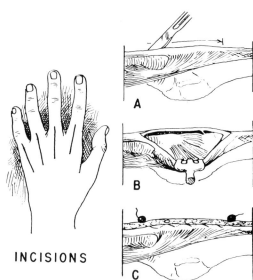

Figure 8.2.9. Technique of L.D. Howard for exposure of capsular ligaments of metacarpophalangeal joints of fingers for capsulectomy. A. Splitting extensor tendon. B. Retraction of extensor hood to expose capsular ligament. C. Closure of extensor tendon with running 4-0 stainless steel wire (redrawn from Bunnell[6]).

sor tendons are exposed by four straight longitudinal incisions over the metacarpals (Fig. 8.2.9). The extensor tendon is then split longitudinally for a distance of approximately one inch on either side of the metacarpophalangeal joint (Howard[26]). The aponeurotic hood, or extensor hood, is then retracted to either side (Fig. 8.2.9), and the attachments of the extensor tendon to the base of the proximal phalanx are severed when these are present. The synovium which forms the dorsal part of the capsule of the joint between the base of the phalanx and the head of the metacarpal is excised, for this may be greatly thickened in severe cases. This dorsal capsule is excised from one collateral ligament across to the opposite collateral ligament over the dorsum of the joint (Fig. 8.2.10).

Since it is the cordlike portion of the collateral ligament that limits flexion, it can be released from its attachment just beneath the tubercle on either side of the head of the metacarpal, leaving it attached to the accessory collateral ligament, but freeing any adhesions which may have formed between the cord portion of the collateral ligament and the head of the metacarpal. Pressure against the base of the proximal phalanx will then carry the proximal phalanx into flexion beneath the head of the metacarpal (Fig. 8.2.11).

In those patients with much thickening in the collateral ligament, a section of the cordlike portion of the ligament should be removed near the tubercle on either side of the head of the metacarpal. One must also take care not to sever the attachment of the in-

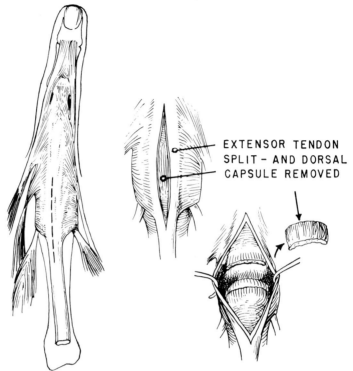

EXTENSOR TENDON
SPLIT- AND DORSAL
CAPSULE REMOVED

Figure 8.2.10. Exposure of joint by dorsal approach through extensor tendon, with excision of thickened synovium which forms dorsal part of capsule.

terosseous tendon into the base of the phalanx just distal to the attachment of the collateral ligament to the phalanx, for this may also lead to ulnar deviation of the fingers.

If the phalanx does not drop into flexion beneath the head of the metacarpal, then a curved periosteal elevator should be inserted around the head of the metacarpal to recreate the volar pouch beneath the head of the meatcarpal, for, in long standing cases, this pouch becomes obliterated when the volar plate becomes adherent to the metacarpal head.

The excursion of the extensor tendons over the dorsum of the hand should be checked. If these are not gliding freely, they should be tendolyzed over the dorsum of the hand, and if necessary over the dorsum of the wrist, and into the forearm. In addition, one may need to free the extensor hood well on to either side of the metacarpophalangeal joint.

The extensor tendon is closed with a running suture of 4-0 stainless steel wire as illustrated in Figure 8.2.9C. The hand is dressed in a pressure dressing with the metacarpophalangeal joints in moderate flexion; however, not in such a severe degree of flexion as to cause the extensor tendons to open over the metacarpophalangeal joint. This pressure dressing is left in place for 72 hours, at which time it is removed and a volar plaster splint applied so that one may begin rubber band traction by leather loops about the proximal phalanges for flexion.

The elastic splinting must be continued as long as

necessary, both day and night. After four to six weeks, a Bunnell[6] knuckle bender splint may be used. During the period of elastic splinting one allows some active extension as well. Occasionally it is necessary to alternate between splinting in flexion and in extension.

Complications. There are certain complications which may follow the operative procedure of capsulectomy.

1. Ulnar deviation of the fingers as a result of a too radical resection of the collateral ligament on the radial side, particularly in the presence of ulnar nerve palsy, and also if one inadequately releases the collateral ligament on the ulnar side of the joint.

2. Disruption of the extensor tendons over the metacarpophalangeal joint in those patients in whom one has not adequately tendolyzed the extensor tendons, also in those patients in whom there has been considerable shortening of the extensor muscles themselves.

3. Recurrence of the ankylosis may occur where one has inadequately corrected the abnormality at surgery, or where one has failed to maintain adequate rubber band traction after surgery. If one does not obtain a good result the procedure can be repeated after four to six months.

Arthroplasty

This procedure is indicated for patients who have such severe destruction of the metacarpal head and/or the base of the proximal phalanx, that release of the capsular ligament may not provide a satisfactory range of motion.

Vainio,[54] in his "Arthroplasty of the Metacarpophalangeal Joint for Rheumatoid Arthritis," excises ½ inch of the head of the metacarpal and carries a portion of the extensor tendon down between the base of the proximal phalanx and the reshaped head of the metacarpal, suturing it to the volar plate and then resuturing the divided extensor. In this instance the extensor tendon is shortened approximately ½ inch, this being made necessary by the excision of the metacarpal head. Tupper[52] prefers to bring the volar plate dorsally and attach it to the metacarpal rather than interpose the extensor tendon. A good result can be obtained by the use of joint implants or prothesis implant as suggested by Swanson[51] and Niebauer.[40]

Locking of the Fingers due to Abnormalities at the Metacarpophalangeal Joints

Recurrent locking of the metacarpophalangeal joints may occur as a result various changes in and about the joint. This must be remembered in the differential diagnosis of stenosing tenosynovitis.

Bruner[5] has reported a case in which this problem was caused by a thin crescentic membrane within the joint which caught the head of the metacarpal when the joint was in strong flexion. Flatt[16] reported a case where an abnormal relationship of the sesamoid and the metacarpal head resulted in locking, and Allbred[1] reports a case where the locking was caused by a torn collateral ligament which caught the metacarpal head and prevented extension. All these cases required operative correction.

Acute Dislocation

Reduction of the acutely dislocated metacarpophalangeal joint is usually accomplished without difficulty. In those patients in whom the reduction is not obtained after several attempts and the displacement persists, open reduction will be necessary. In the operation, one usually finds that a portion of the capsule has impinged itself between the two bones, preventing reduction. Umansky[53] has reported that in children the displacement of the proximal phalanx may be more to the ulnar than to the dorsal side and that there is frequently a shirring type of osteocartilagenous fracture of the ulnar side of the metacarpal leading to periosteal callus on the ulnar side of the metacarpal.

Chronic Dislocations

One frequently sees patients in whom dislocation has existed for several months or more. In some instances repeated reductions have been attempted without success. In these patients, reduction may still be possible by exposing the joint dorsally and opening the extensor tendon mechanism in the longitudinal technique as described for capsulectomy of the metacarpophalangeal joint.

A capsulectomy of the collateral ligaments on either side of the metacarpophalangeal joint will, as a rule,

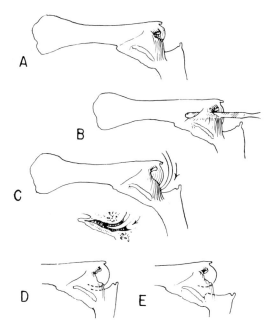

Figure 8.2.11. Technique for capsulectomy with the release of the "cord" portion of the ligament. Flexion is obtained but continuity is maintained between the distal portion of the "cord" ligament and the accessory collateral ligament to prevent ulnar deviation even when a small wedge of the "cord" portion of ligament is excised. A. Dorsal capsule excised and "cord" portion released at point of attachment to metacarpal. Accessory collateral ligament still intact. B. Elevator frees adhesions between ligament and head of metacarpal. C. Elevator releases adherent volar capsule and recreates a normal pouch beneath metacarpal head. D. Proper relation of the phalanx to the metacarpal. E. With inadequate release of the volar capsule, the phalanx does not rest beneath head of metacarpal.

be necessary to achieve a reduction. One may find, as in Figure 8.2.12, that it may be necessary to excise the excess bone to reposition the head of the metacarpal correctly.

Dislocation of the Extensor Tendon at the Metacarpophalangeal Joint

The extensor tendon may shift either to the ulnar side or the radial side of the metacarpophalangeal joint, coming to occupy a place between the two heads of the metacarpals, as a result of a laceration of the extensor expansion.[32,37,46] It may also be shifted as a result of a large exostosis that may form on one side or the other of the metacarpal head, or as a result of a thinning out and attenuation of the extensor hood, as in the rheumatoid arthritic hand.

This is best treated by a proper repair of the extensor expansion in the acute injury with a row of interrupted sutures. In the rheumatoid hand this is best repaired by

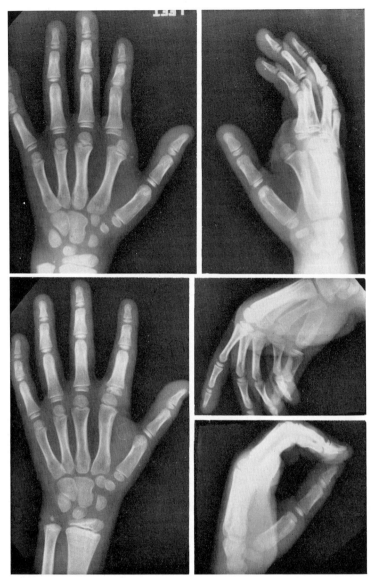

Figure 8.2.12. Case T.P., age 8. Chronic dislocation of metacarpophalangeal joint for 1½ years. X-ray views show preoperative view of dislocation (*top*) and postoperative reduction after capsulectomy and excision of ulnar border of metacarpal (*bottom*).

imbricating the attenuated extensor hood and suturing with two rows of sutures (Fig. 8.2.13).

The extensor tendon can also be held in its normal anatomic position by a free tendon graft sutured to the extensor tendon dorsally and passed around the metacarpal head to be anchored to the transverse metacarpal ligament volarly on either side of the flexor tendon (Fig. 8.2.14).

Rupture of the Collateral Ligament

The collateral ligament of the metacarpophalangeal joint of the fingers may be ruptured with acute injuries, the rupture usually occurring at the point where

the collateral ligament attaches to the tubercle of the metacarpal.

One rarely needs to perform an operative repair of an isolated ruptured ligament when it is present in the fingers, except when it occurs in the collateral ligament on the radial side of the metacarpophalangeal joint of the little finger. In this latter instance, the short abductor of the little finger may tend to pull the little finger in acute ulnar deviation.

Proximal Interphalangeal Joint

Dr. Sterling Bunnell[6] has pointed out that it is the narrow joint space present in the interphalangeal joints which produces limitation of motion when there is even the slightest shortening of the capsular ligaments as might be produced by non-use or edema of the ligaments and subsequent fibrosis.

Anatomy

The proximal interphalangeal joint is constructed on essentially the same plan as the metacarpophalangeal joint. It possesses collateral ligaments, a palmar fibrocartilage, and a loose dorsal capsule of synovial tissue guarded by an extensor expansion. This is considered a hinge joint since movements are restricted to flexion and extension by the anteroposterior flattening of the ends of the bones.

An important fascial structure covers the collateral ligaments on either side of the joint. This has been described in detail by Landsmeer[33] as being composed of a transverse portion extending from the extensor tendon dorsally to the lateral border of the volar plate. The oblique portion of the ligament passes from the proximal phalanx to the extensor tendon over the middle phalanx. Stack[48] feels that this ligament is really a portion of the extensor tendon mechanism. Kaplan[29] has described this as a deep fascial cuff.

Dislocation of Middle Phalanx of Proximal Interphalangeal Joint

If this occurs acutely it will, as a rule, rupture the volar capsular ligament from its attachment to the proximal phalanx. If the force has been great enough to force the middle phalanx back at a right angle to the proximal phalanx, then in addition, a portion of the lateral capsular ligament will be torn (Fig. 8.2.15). Spinner[47] reports tear of the central tendon in certain closed dislocations.

For the acute injury, immediate reduction, with splinting in a position of flexion of approximately 20° at the proximal interphalangeal joint, will frequently be followed by a satisfactory result.

This injury is frequently followed by limitation of

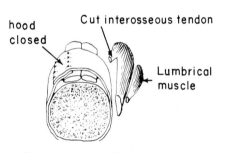

Schema of relationships

Figure 8.2.13. Cross section of metacarpal showing method of imbricating attenuated extensor expansion at metacarpophalangeal joint in the rheumatoid arthritic hand to reposition extensor tendon.

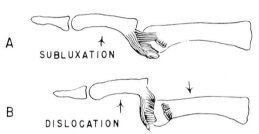

Figure 8.2.15. Capsular ligament injury in dislocation of proximal interphalangeal joint. *A.* Subluxation of middle phalanx due to rupture of volar ligament and accessory collateral ligaments. *B.* Dislocation of middle phalanx on proximal phalanx due to rupture of volar ligament and total severance of collateral ligaments.

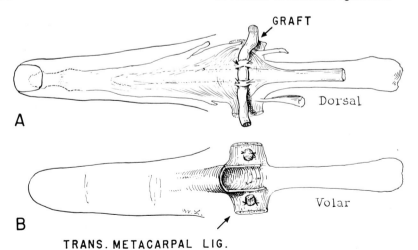

TRANS. METACARPAL LIG.

Figure 8.2.14. Technique of holding extensor tendon in normal anatomical position over metacarpophalangeal joint by tendon graft sutured volarly to transverse metacarpal ligament. *A.* Dorsal view. *B.* Volar view.

flexion and extension in the proximal interphalangeal joint. It may take months in some patients with the use of the Bunnell[6] finger splint of the knuckle bender type, and the Bunnell safety pin splint to gain full flexion and extension.

If there is evidence of tear of the central tendon from the middle phalanx, immediate surgical repair is indicated (Spinner[47]). In the chronic dislocation of the proximal interphalangeal joint (Fig. 8.2.16A), reduction usually can be accomplished by an excision of the scar-bridged collateral ligaments on either side of the joint and a tendolysis of the extensor tendon. Once reduction is obtained, a Kirschner wire holding the middle phalanx in flexion on the head of the proximal phalanx, is left in place for 10 days, and active motion started, preventing full extension of the joint, for a total of three weeks.

Occasionally, for correction of the severe contracture in the extensor tendon mechanism, an osteotomy of the proximal phalanx, with resection of ¼ inch of bone, may be necessary (Fig. 8.2.16B).

A useful range of motion may be obtained in these dislocated joints as long as six months after injury.

Chronic Subluxation with Rupture of the Volar Capsular Ligament

The proximal interphalangeal joint hyperextends (Fig. 8.2.17), and in the hyperextended position the extensor tendon mechanism, at the proximal interphalangeal joint, rides up into a more central position directly over the center of the joint, dorsally; when the patient attempts to flex the finger, there is a snapping sensation as the patient forces the lateral part of the extensor hood down over the lateral aspect of the joint.

The treatment of this abnormality is best accomplished by use of one-half of the flexor sublimus tendon, as illustrated in Figure 8.2.18, the tendon being left attached distally at its point of insertion but being inserted into the proximal phalanx through a drill hole by the use of a pullout wire. This free tendon

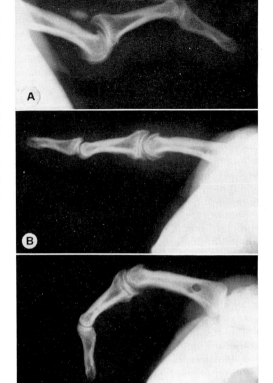

Figure 8.2.17. Case R.M. *A.* Rupture of volar capsular ligament of proximal interphalangeal joint, with dorsal subluxation of the middle phalanx. Repair of volar capsule with tendon graft as shown in Fig. 8.2.18. *B.* Postoperative result for extension in proximal interphalangeal joint. *C.* Postoperative result for flexion in proximal interphalangeal joint.

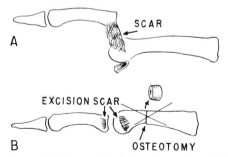

Figure 8.2.16. Old dislocation of middle phalanx on proximal phalanx, with operative reduction. *A.* Scar bridging the torn lateral capsular ligaments. *B.* Reduction after excision of scarred lateral capsular ligaments on either side of joint. Resection of a portion of the proximal phalanx may be necessary to give length to the contracted extensor mechanism to obtain reduction.

graft across the proximal interphalangeal joint prevents hyperextension.

Another surgical approcah is to reattach the volar capsular ligament to the distal end of the proximal phalanx (Howard[24]). Technically, however, it is as a rule better to repair this abnormality by the former technique.

Subluxation with Fracture of the Base of the Middle Phalanx

In the acute cases, this is best treated by the technique described by McElfresh *et al.*[36] where closed reduction is achieved and the middle phalanx held in moderate flexion to approximate it to the fracture fragment attached to the volar plate, using a curved aluminum splint dorsally to maintain the correction allowing early flexion but limiting early extension.

If the dislocation is associated with a badly comminuted fracture of the base of the middle phalanx the preferred treatment is that described by Robertson, Cawley, and Faris[45] (see Fig. 8.2.20). On the other hand, if the fragment is a single one, open reduction may be indicated, with Kirschner wire fixation. The operative approach is by a lateral incision with exposure of the proximal interphalangeal joint by section of the transverse retinacular ligament. The repositioning of the fracture fragment is done under direct vision with Kirschner wire fixation, so that the proper alignment of the joint surface can be achieved. The retinacular ligament is resutured (Fig. 8.2.19).

Chronic Dislocation with Fracture at the Base of the Middle Phalanx

When patients are seen late with this clinical abnormality, operative intervention is the only solution, for a closed reduction of this abnormality once it has existed for more than a few days is usually not possible.

At the time of operation in this chronic problem, as a rule, one will not be able to reduce the dislocated middle phalanx under the head of the proximal phalanx until a capsulectomy of the lateral capsular ligaments has been performed.

A dorsal incision allows excision of the lateral capsular ligaments and scar. The incised transverse retinacular ligament exposes the joint. The fracture fragment which is displaced along the shaft of the middle phalanx can be elevated with a small osteotome repositioned to form the correct contour of the base of the middle phalanx, and then a Kirschner wire

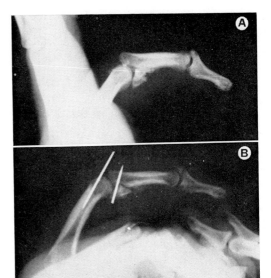

Figure 8.2.19. A. Fracture-dislocation of proximal interphalangeal joint. The preferred treatment is traction as in Figure 8.2.20, or (B) open reduction and Kirschner wire fixation of fracture with temporary Kirschner wire to prevent recurrence of subluxation.

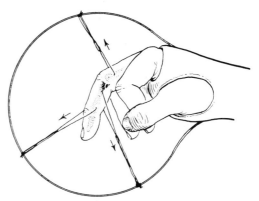

Figure 8.2.20. Method of treatment for acute fracture-dislocation of the proximal interphalangeal joint, with Kirschner wire in proximal and middle phalanges (from Robertson, Cawley, and Faris[45]).

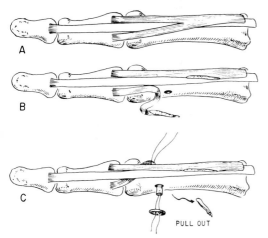

Figure 8.2.18. Technique of repairing rupture of volar capsular ligament of the proximal interphalangeal joint by tendon graft from one-half of the flexor sublimis tendon. A. Diagramatic view of flexor sublimis tendon at proximal interphalangeal joint. B. Splitting off one-half of flexor sublimis tendon at point of division. C. Tendon passed through drill hole and held with proper tension by pullout wire through finger.

is inserted to anchor the fracture fragment. A second Kirschner wire is used across the proximal interphalangeal joint to hold the finger in a moderately flexed position at this joint (Fig. 8.2.19).

The wire across the proximal interphalangeal joint should be removed in two weeks. A dorsal aluminum splint is used on the finger to prevent hyperextension at the proximal interphalangeal joint, but active motion for flexion is begun at the end of two weeks (Fig. 8.2.21).

If the middle phalanx cannot be reduced on the head

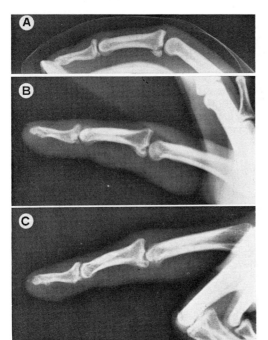

Figure 8.2.21. A. Fracture at the base of the middle phalanx with subluxation with inadequate reduction. *B.* Operative reduction failed to correct the subluxation completely. *C.* Traumatic arthritis has developed due to articulation of proximal phalanx with poorly aligned joint surface.

of the proximal phalanx, then an osteotomy with excision of approximately ¼ inch of the proximal phalanx will allow one to achieve reduction of this chronic dislocation (Fig. 8.2.15).

Sprains

This type of injury may occur with varying amounts of injury to the capsular ligaments about the joint from minute tears of the ligament to more extensive damage.

These injuries should receive careful attention, in the acute stage, being splinted in slight flexion for two to three weeks. If possible, the splint should be removed periodically with careful flexion and extension guarding against forced flexion and extension.

Local injection of the joint with Xylocaine and triamcinolone acetonide (Kenalog, E.R. Squibb & Sons, Inc.) may be helpful in relieving pain in the chronic case. The solution is prepared by mixing .5 cc Xylocaine and 4 mg triamcinolone acetonide (Kenalog). Of this mixture, 0.2 cc is used for the proximal interphalangeal joint and 0.5 cc for the metacarpophalangeal joint.

Total or Partial Finger Joint Transfer

This is a useful procedure for those patients who have had a completely destroyed metacarpophalangeal or interphalangeal joint where a joint

prosthesis would be contraindicated. This destruction may follow trauma, rheumatoid arthritic disease, or tumor.

The distal end of the fifth metatarsal may be used to replace the metacarpal head. A portion of phalanx of a toe may be used to replace that portion of a phalanx of a finger which has been destroyed.

Hendrick Wolff is reported by Bunnell[6] to have recorded the first case of grafting of a half of a joint in 1910. Other early reports on joint transplantation were presented by Judet[28] and Lexer.[34] Later interest in his subject has been demonstrated by Graham and Riordan,[20] Herndon and Chase,[23] Entin,[13] Erdelyi,[14] and Graham.[19]

A useful range of motion can be obtained after the transplant. In several cases reported by Graham,[19] 70° of motion were present in the metacarpophalangeal joint after the transplanataion of a metatarsal head and its capsular ligaments. Graham[19] and Stephenson obtained 70° of motion in a child with complete transplantation of the metatarsophalangeal joint to the thumb.

Ankylosis of the Proximal Interphalangeal Joint in Extension

The surgeon about to correct a limitation of flexion of the proximal interphalangeal joint must have in mind the various anatomic structures in the finger that may limit this motion. These structures are: (1) scar contracture of the skin over the dorsum of the finger; (2) contracted long extensor muscle or adherent extensor tendon; (3) contracted interosseus muscle or adherent interosseus tendon; (4) retinacular ligament adherent to capsular ligament; (5) contracted capsular ligament, particularly the collateral ligament; (6) boneblock or exostosis; (7) volar capsular ligament adherent to the proximal phalanx; (8) flexor tendons adherent within the flexor sheath.

Bunnell, Doherty, and Curtis[7] have described various test positions of the hand and fingers to determine which structures are to blame.

Operative Technique and Postoperative Treatment. The interphalangeal joint is approached by a dorsal curvilinear incision (Fig. 8.2.22). (It may also be approached by a lateral incision on both its sides.) This incision is deepened through the skin and subcutaneous tissue to expose the extensor tendon over the dorsum of the finger. The skin flaps are reflected laterally to allow exposure of the retinacular ligaments on either side of the joint. The retinacular ligament is preserved so that joint stability may be maintained after the collateral ligaments have been excised. The collateral ligament of the proximal interphalangeal joint is best demonstrated by approaching the joint from the base of the middle phalanx after elevating the retinacular ligament and retracting it proximally. As much of the collateral ligament as possible should be excised from its attachments to the base of the middle phalanx and to the distal end of the proximal phalanx on both sides of the joint. A small portion of the distal edge of

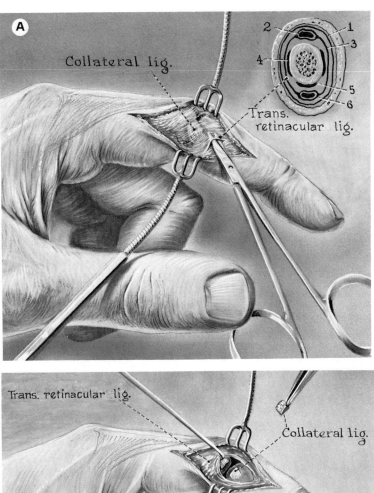

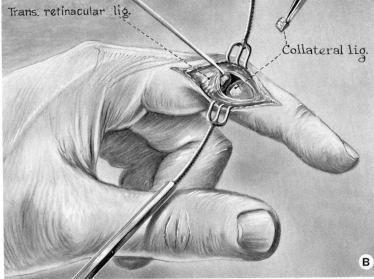

Figure 8.2.22. A. Capsulectomy of proximal interphalangeal joint. Diagram shows operative approach for capsulectomy of proximal interphalangeal joint. Skin incision is developed down to deep fascial cuff, which is lifted with point of scissors to show approach to collateral ligament. *Inset.* Cross section of finger at level of base of middle phalanx with deep fascial cuff extending from extensor to flexor. *1.* Superficial fascia. *2.* Extensor tendon. *3.* Transverse retinacular ligament. *4.* Collateral ligament of joint capsule. *5.* Volar plate of capsule. *6.* Flexor tendon. *B.* Capsulectomy of proximal interphalangeal joint. The transverse retinacular ligament has been retracted, and a block of collateral ligament has been excised (from Curtis[11]).

the retinacular ligaments can be excised, if necessary, in order to expose either collateral ligament. In some longstanding cases, the volar synovial pouch becomes obliterated and must be re-formed with a small curved elevator or by forcing the base of the middle phalanx into flexion.

In some instances, it may be necessary to incise the retinacular ligament in a prolonged extension contracture. It can be removed from the distal end of the proximal phalanx to achieve complete flexion. When this is required the ligament should be resutured at the end of the operation to preserve joint stability.

Once the collateral ligament has been excised, the finger should be tested to determine whether some other structure within the finger is still limiting flexion. Where there is an associated contracture of the interosseous muscle, it is lengthened by tenotomy at the junction of the longitudinal fibres with the middle slip of the extensor tendon and allowed to slide proximally where it is sutured to the extensor aponeurosis. Excising a triangular portion from the lateral band on both sides of the finger at the level of the proximal phalanx, as suggested by Littler and Howorth,[35] is also effective. Such a tenotomy or excision relieves the mild contracture, but in more severe cases, tenotomy of the tendon must be carried out just proximal to the metacarpophalangeal joint in order to gain an adequate release.

When the extensor tendon is adherent dorsally, it can be freed where necessary. In some instances there is a thickening dorsally of the synovium of the proximal interphalangeal joint and it may be necessary to incise it with the use of a small curved osteotome in order to achieve flexion.

At the end of the operation it should be easy to flex the joint passively. If the obstructing structures all have been released to the point where the finger can be flexed with the same ease as the normal adjacent finger, then a good result can be anticipated.

Once the finger has been stiff in extension, the flexor tendons frequently become adherent in their bed. The operator should routinely check function of these tendons by identifying them through a small incision in the palm of the hand and by placing traction on them in order to be certain that, with the joint freed surgically, they will completely flex the finger. It is sometimes necessary to free them not only through the palmar incision but also by exposing them in the finger by reflecting the original skin flaps laterally over the proximal phalanx (Fig. 8.2.23).

The injection of 2 mg of triamcinolone acetonide into the interphalangeal joint before wound closure sometimes seems to be of value.

Following wound closure, the hand is placed in a compression dressing, with the fingers in moderate flexion, for the first 72 hours to prevent excessive swelling and to achieve perfect wound healing. Seventy-two hours postoperatively, rubber bands are attached to the fingertips with adhesive tape and trac-

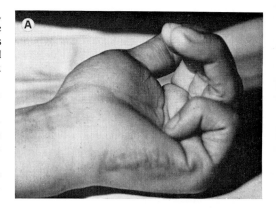

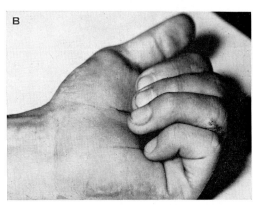

Figure 8.2.23. A. Limitation of flexion caused by tight collateral ligaments, contracture of interossei, and adherent flexor tendons, after fractures of proximal phalanges of index, middle, ring, and little fingers. B. Degree of improvement after capsulectomy of collateral ligaments, tenotomy of the interossei, and tendolysis of the finger flexors (from Curtis[11]).

tion started slowly to pull the fingers into the completely flexed position.

Splinting is continued until the patient can maintain, by active and passive exercise, the range of motion achieved at surgery. In some instances, this has necessitated part-time splinting for as long as three or four months. Physical therapy, with active motion and careful passive motion, is also commenced as soon as wound healing will permit. Of particular value in the late postoperative care is intermittent compression therapy using the Jobst unit, in which the hand, with fingers flexed, is slipped into a bag which is alternately inflated and deflated by a small compressor.

Analysis of the results indicates that when the proximal interphalangeal joint may be actively flexed to 75° or more, it is better judgment to rely on conservative measures of further physiotherapy and special splinting to achieve further flexion.

If the only limiting factor for flexion in the interphalangeal joint is a capsular ligament, then capsulectomy of the collateral ligaments gives a good result both for flexion and extension. On the other hand, if it is necessary to free the extensor tendon over the proximal phalanx, to perform a tenotomy of the interosseus tendons and a capsulectomy of the collateral ligaments to obtain flexion of the proximal interphalangeal joint, then the end result achieved by surgery will not be as successful. This is particularly true of the finger bound by cicatrix.

Carroll[9] approaches this problem of ankylosis of the proximal interphalangeal joint by resection of the distal end of the proximal phalanx. Backdahl[2] also has resected the distal end of the proximal phalanx to correct some rheumatoid deformities of this joint. This may produce a joint which has lost some of its lateral stability when in extension, however.

A joint prosthesis may be the procedure of choice where there is gross abnormality in the joint surfaces.[40][51]

Ankylosis of the Proximal Interphalangeal Joint in Flexion

The anatomic structures that limit extension of a finger at the proximal interphalangeal joint may be: (1) scar of the skin over the volar surface of the finger; (2) contraction of the superficial fascia in the finger, as in Dupuytren's contracture; (3) contracture of the flexor tendon sheath within the finger; (4) contracted flexor muscle or adherent flexor tendon; (5) adherence of the oblique fascia of Landsmeer to the collateral ligament; (6) contraction of the volar plate of the capsular ligament; (7) adherence or contracture of the accessory volar ligaments; (8) bony block or exostosis. Frequently, more than one structure is involved in this flexion contracture.

In congenital flexion contracture of the finger, all tissues from skin to bone may be involved, for the skin may be too short, the flexor sublimus tendon contracted, and the volar capsule and the collateral ligaments may limit extension.

Similarly in the patient with Dupuytren's contracture that has existed for a long period of time and where there is marked flexion contracture of the proximal interphalangeal joints, the skin will be short, there will be a thick strand of contracted superficial fascia, the flexor sublimus tendon may be contracted, and the volar capsule and the collateral ligaments will adhere in such a way as to prevent extension.

Operative Technique. Operative release of the finger in an acutely flexed position is usually carried out through a midlateral incision which is deepened to expose the flexor tendon sheath and the joint itself. A Z-plasty on the flexor surface of the finger may be preferable in Dupuytren's and congenital flexion contracture. A good approach is to excise a portion of the flexor tendon sheath over the flexor tendon and see whether or not this simple excision will allow any extension. In some instances, it may be the only structure which is contracted.

This is then followed by a checking of the flexor tendons to see whether they are adherent over the proximal phalanx o. whether they are contracted. If they are severely contracted, it may be necessary to tenotomize and lengthen the flexor tendons in the forearm.

The oblique retinacular ligament is freed from the lateral capsular ligament, and the volar capsule is then excised from the proximal interphalangeal joint. When necessary (Fig. 8.2.24), the accessory collateral ligament is incised on either side of the proximal interphalangeal joint through separate incisions. Subluxation of the middle phalanx may occur if the cord portion of the lateral ligament is completely severed. In some instances, it will be necessary to divide the transverse and oblique retinacular ligaments. A surgical release of the contracted structures will then allow one to extend the proximal interphalangeal joint. The joint is fixed in moderate extension by a Kirschner wire across the proximal interphalangeal joint, the Kirschner wire being removed in one week and active motion for flexion and extension begun with rubber band traction to improve the degree of extension and maintain the gain that was achieved operatively.

Arthrodesis of Finger Joints

Arthrodesis of the proximal interphalangeal joint is indicated when there is no way to restore function and the joint is not aligned for proper use. It may also be indicated for persistent pain in a joint and in some arthritic deformities. This procedure is most useful where there is a good motion in the metacarpophalangeal joint. The angle of fusion to achieve best function should be ascertained preoperatively for each patient, for it varies with the range of motion of the other joints and the needs of the patient.

The metacarpalphalangeal and interphalangeal

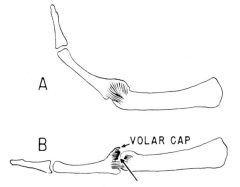

Figure 8.2.24. Capsulectomy for release of flexion contracture of finger. *A.* Fixed flexion contracture. *B.* Excision of portion of volar capsule and release of accessory collateral ligament, leaving cord portion to maintain stability of joint.

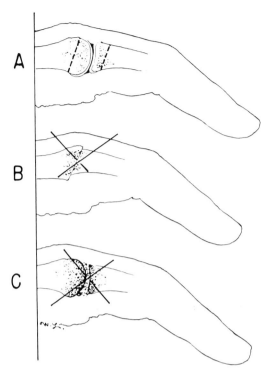

Figure 8.2.25. Alternate techniques for arthrodesis of proximal interphalangeal joints of the fingers. *A.* Resection of articular margin, proximal and middle phalanges. *B.* Kirschner wire fixation. *C.* Articular cartilage removed, proximal and middle phalanges, joint packed with cancellous bone. Kirschner wire fixation.

joints are approached through a dorsal incision. Several techniques for fusion are described. When the joint is already fused, then resection type of fusion is preferred as in Figure 8.2.25. If there is a movable joint the joint can be opened and the cartilage curreted away. The joint is then packed with cancellous bone and positioned in that degree of flexion felt to be most useful for the patient. The joint is immobilized in this position by Kirschner wire fixation across the joint. An alternate technique (Carroll[10]) shapes the proximal phalanx and inserts it into middle phalanx.

REFERENCES

1. Allbred, A. A locked index finger. J. Bone Joint Surg., *36B:* 102-103, 1954.
2. Backdahl, M. Lesions of the extensor aponeurosis in the rheumatoid hand. Presented at the meeting of the Second Hand Club of Great Britain. May, 1963.
3. Bate, J. T. An operation of the correction of locking of the proximal interphalangeal joint of finger in hyperextension. J. Bone Joint Surg., *27:* 142-144, 1945.
4. Böhler, L. *The Treatment of Fractures.* Baltimore, William Wood, 1932.
5. Bruner, J.M. Recurrent locking of an index finger due to internal derangement of the metacarpophalangeal joint. J. Bone Joint Surg., *43A:* 450-452, 1961.
6. Bunnell, S. *Surgery of the Hand,* Ed. 4. Philadelphia, Lippincott, 1964.
7. Bunnell, S., Doherty, E. W., and Curtis, R. M. Ischemic contracture, local, in the hand. Plast. Reconstr. Surg., *3:* 424-433, 1948.
8. Campbell, W.C. *Operative Orthopedics.* St. Louis, Mosby, 1939.
9. Carroll, R.E. Digital arthroplasty of the proximal interphalangeal joint. J. Bone Joint Surg., *36A:* 912-920, 1954.
10. Carroll, R.E., and Hill, N.A. Small joint arthrodesis in hand reconstruction. J. Bone Joint Surg., *51A:* 1219-1221, 1969.
11. Curtis, R.M. Capsulectomy of the interphalangeal joints of the fingers. J. Bone Joint Surg., *36A:* 1219-1232, 1954.
12. Drury, B.J. Para-articular fusion of the proximal interphalangeal joint of the hand. Calif., Med., *90 (1):* 37-38, 1959.
13. Entin, M.A., Alger, J.R., and Baird, R.M. Experimental and clinical transplantation of autogenous whole joints. J. Bone Joint Surg., *44A:* 1518-1536, 1962.
14. Erdelyi, R. Reconstruction of ankylosed, finger joints by means of transplanation of joints from the foot. *31:* 140-150, 1963.
15. Flatt, A.E. *The Care of Minor Hand Injuries,* Ed. 2. St. Louis, Mosby, 1963.
16. Flatt, A.E. Recurrent locking of an index finger. J. Bone Joint Surg., *40A:* 1128-1130, 1958.
17. Fowler, S.B. Mobilization of metacarpophalangeal joint, arthroplasty and capsulotomy. J. Bone Joint Surg., *29:* 193-202, 1947.
18. Gervis, W.H. Excision of the trapezium for osteoarthritis of the trapeziometacarpal joint. J. Bone Joint Surg., *31B:* 537-542, 1949.
19. Graham, W.C. Transplantation of joints to replace diseased or damaged articulations in the hands. Am. J. Surg., *88:* 136-144, 1954.
20. Graham, W.C., and Riordan, D.C. Reconstruction of a metacarpophalangeal joint with a metatarsal transplant. J. Bone Joint Surg., *30A:* 848-853, 1948.
21. Grant, J. C. B. *A Method of Anatomy,* Ed. 4. Baltimore, Williams & Wilkins, 1948.
22. Harris, C., Jr., and Riordan, D.C. Intrinsic contracture in the hand and its surgical treatment. J. Bone Joint Surg., *36A:* 10, 1954.
23. Herndon, C.H., and Chase, S.W. Experimental studies in the transplantation of whole joints. J. Bone Joint Surg., *34:* 564, 1952.
24. Howard, L.D., Jr. Treatment of postraumatic recurvatum deformity of the proximal interphalangeal joint with occasional locking but with otherwise free joint mobility. In *Symposium on the Hand,* Vol. III, p. 33. St. Louis, Mosby, 1971.
25. Howard, L.D., Jr., Pratt, D.R., and Bunnell, S. The use of Compound F (hydrocortisone) in operative and non-operative conditions of the hand. J. Bone Joint Surg., *35-38:* 994-1002, 1953.
26. Howard, L.D. Cited by S. Bunnell in *Surgery of the Hand,* Ed. 2. Philadelphia, Lippincott, 1948, p. 301.
27. Hsu, J.D., and Curtis, R.M. Carpometacarpal dislocations on the ulnar side of the hand. J. Bone Joint Surg., *52A:* 927-930, 1970.

28. Judet, H. Essai sur la gresse ces tissues articulaires. C.R. Acad. Sci., *146:* 193, 1908.

29. Kaplan, E.B. *Functional and Surgical Anatomy of the Hand.* Philadelphia, Lippincott, 1953.

30. Kaplan, E.B. Dorsal dislocation of the metacarpophalangeal joint of the index finger. J. Bone Joint Surg., *41A:* 1081, 1959.

31. Kessler, I., and Heller, J. Complete avulsion of the ligamentous apparatus of the metacarpalphalangeal joint of the thumb. Surg. Gynecol. Obstet., *116:* 95-98, 1963.

32. Kettlekamp, D.B., Flatt, A.E., and Molds, R. Traumatic dislocation of the long finger extensor tendon. Proceedings American Society for Surgery of the Hand. J. Bone Joint Surg., *53A:* 815, 1971.

33. Landsmeer, J.M.F. The anatomy of the dorsal aponeurosis of the human finger and its functional significance. Anat. Rec., *104:* 31, 1949.

34. Lexer, E. *Die Freien Transplantationen.* Stuttgart, F. Enke, 1924.

35. Littler, J.W., and Howorth, M.B. *A Textbook of Orthopedics.* Philadelphia, Saunders, 1952, p. 251.

36. McElfresh, E. C., Dobyns, J. H., and O'Brien, E. T. The conservative and functional management of the common fracture-dislocation of the proximal interphalangeal joint. Proceedings American Society for Surgery of the Hand. J. Bone Joint Surg., *54A:* 907-908, 1972.

37. Michon, J. and Vichard, P. Lateral luxations of the extensor tendons with regard to the metacarpophalangeal articulation. Rev. Med. Nancy, *86:* 595-601, 1961.

38. Moberg, E. and Stener, B. Injuries to the ligaments of the thumb and fingers. Diagnosis, treatment, and prognosis. Acta Chir. Scand. *106:* 166-186, 1953.

39. Muller, G.M.: Arthrodesis of the trapeziometacarpal joint for osteoarthritis. J. Bone Joint Surg., *31B:* 540-542, 1949.

40. Niebauer, J.J. Dacron-silicone prosthesis for the metacarpophalangeal and interphalangeal joints. In *Symposium on the Hand,* Vol. III, p. 96. St. Louis, Mosby, 1971.

41. Nydahl, M.J. Fractures and dislocations of the hand and fingers. Minn. Med., *40:* 849-852, 1957.

42. Peacock, E.E., Jr. Reconstructive surgery of the hands with injured central metacarpophalangeal joints. J. Bone Joint Surg., *38A:* 291-302, 1956.

43. Peacock, E.E., Jr. Preservation of interphalangeal joint function: a basis for the early care of injured hands. South. Med. J., *56:* 56-63, 1962.

44. Pratt, D.R. Joints of the hand and fingers — their stiffness, splinting and surgery. Calif. Med., *66:* 22-24, 1947.

45. Robertson, R.C., Cawley, J.J., Jr., and Faris, A.M. Treatment of fracture, dislocation of the interphalangeal joints of the hand. J. Bone Joint Surg., *28:* 68-70, 1946.

46. Roca, C.A., Santoro, J.C., and Ramos, V.J. Habitual luxation of the extensor tendons of the hand. Semana Méd., *122:* 97-103, 1963.

47. Spinner, M., and Choi, B.Y. Anterior dislocation of the proximal interphalangeal joint. J. Bone Joint Surg., *52A:* 1329-1336, 1970.

48. Stack, H.G. Muscle function in the fingers. J. Bone Joint Surg., *44B:* 899-909, 1962.

49. Stener, B. Hyperextension injuries to the metacarpophalangeal joint of the thumb, rupture of ligaments, fracture of sesamoid bones, rupture of flexor pollicis brevis. An anatomical and clinical study. Acta Chir. Scand., *125:* 279-293, 1963.

50. Stener, B. Displacement of the ruptured ulnar collateral ligament of the metacarpophalangeal joint of the thumb. A clinical and anatomical study. J. Bone Joint Surg., *44B:* 869-879, 1962.

51. Swanson, A.B. Flexible implant arthroplasty for arthritic finger joints. Rational technique and results of treatment. J. Bone Joint Surg., *54A:* 435-455, 1972.

52. Tupper, J. Volar plate-plasty. American Society for Surgery of the Hand letters, April, 1969.

53. Umansky, A.L. The dislocated index metacarpalphalangeal joint. J. Bone Joint Surg., *45A:* 216, 1963.

54. Vainio, K., and Pulkki, T. Surgical treatment of arthritis mutilans. Ann. Chir. Gynaecal., Fenn., *48:* 361-367, 1959.

55. Watson-Jones, R. *Fractures and Other Bone and Joint Injuries.* Baltimore, Williams & Wilkins, 1940.

C.

Surgery of the Rheumatoid Hand

Paul R. Lipscomb, M.D.

Before World War II, surgical measures for correction of deformities of the hand and wrist caused by rheumatoid arthritis were almost unheard of. Among the pioneers in this field of surgery were Steindler, Kestler, Kellgren and Ball, and Bunnell. The principles of surgery resulting from the treatment of rheumatoid knees, hips, feet, and elbows also have been of inestimable value. Riordan and Fowler of the United States, Vainio and colleagues of Finland, and Vaughan-Jackson of England were among the first to make new contributions to the surgical treatment of the rheumatoid hand. As our medical colleagues, especially the rheumatologists, became aware of the benefits available to their rheumatoid patients through surgery, the horizons have been extended by the joint effort of those charged with the care of such patients.

ETIOLOGIC FACTORS

The cause of rheumatoid arthritis is unknown. Many patients with the disease apparently have an hereditary tendency for its development. Although various infectious agents were indicated in the past and the disease was once called "chronic infectious arthritis," it is now believed that auto immune mechanisms may be the underlying cause. Females are affected twice as often as males, even in juvenile arthritis. The small joints of the hands and feet are often the first joints to be affected; larger joints become involved later.

PATHOGENESIS

The tendon sheath (tenosynovium), as well as the synovial lining of the joint, frequently is involved by rheumatoid arthritis. A proliferation of subsynovial fibrous tissue and of the synovial membrane results in a villosynovitis. A thick mucinous fluid distends the joint capsule and tendon sheath together with the thickened synovial membrane. The hyaline cartilage and the subchondral bone of the joint are destroyed by the pressure produced in a confined space as well as by the enzymatic action of the fluid and by granulation-like tissue. Likewise, the ligaments and capsule of the joint become stretched, attenuated, and in some instances actually destroyed, resulting in secondary deformities (Fig. 8.3.1). In a similar manner, when rheumatoid tenosynovitis is present, the tendons may be invaded and destroyed by the thickened synovium and fluid. Rice bodies formed by the deposition of fibrin may be present. It is likely that interference with blood supply from pressure in a confined space has a part in the destructive process.

Microscopically, rheumatoid synovium or tenosynovium is characterized by a perivascular infiltration of plasma cells and lymphocytes. The synovial lining of joints and tendon sheaths are not the only tissues involved by this pathologic process (Fig. 8.3.2).

Striated muscle, cardiac muscle, supporting ligaments, tendons, and even bone also are involved.

Muscles that surround joints, which include the intrinsic muscles of the hand, may be involved primarily or secondarily. Steindler first proposed that the joint deformities in rheumatoid arthritis of the hand were produced by the imbalance of muscular stresses acting across inflamed and weakened articular surfaces. The inflamed joints are pulled into the position affected by the predominant antagonists that cross them; the capsule is stretched on the side of the weaker antagonists, and permanent contracture results as the involved structures undergo fibrosis. To Steindler's concept probably should be added the effects of destruction of tendon attachments and those of tendon rupture, blockage of tendon excursion, and the pull of gravity.

Thus a fixed flexion contracture of the proximal interphalangeal joint of a finger may occur in rheumatoid arthritis after the destruction of the central slip of the extensor mechanism. Similarly a drop of the distal phalanx, a mallet deformity, may be produced.

Destruction of the radial collateral ligament and the attachment of most of the fibers of the first dorsal interosseous tendon together with the pull of the long extensors and flexor tendons, of the first volar interosseus muscle, and of gravity itself may be instrumental in producing ulnar drift or deviation of the index finger on the second metacarpal head.

In the normal finger ulnar excursion at the metacarpophalangeal joint is greater than radial excursion. The hypothenar muscles and particularly the abductor digiti minimi, which is a comparatively large intrinsic muscle, may have a considerable role in causing ulnar

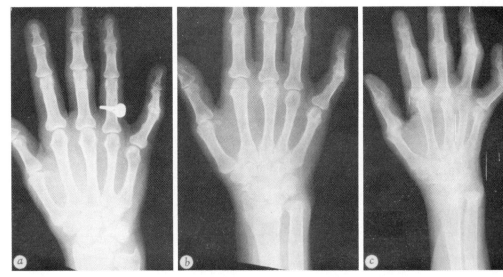

Figure 8.3.1. Right hand and wrist with rheumatoid arthritis. *a.* Soft tissue swelling and destruction of joints is minimal. *b.* Destruction of carpal and radioulnar joints particularly has advanced (approximately two years after *a*). *c.* Destruction of metacarpophalangeal, interphalangeal, carpal, and radioulnar joints is far advanced, and secondary deformities have occurred (approximately five years after *b*).

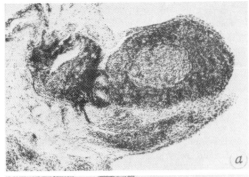

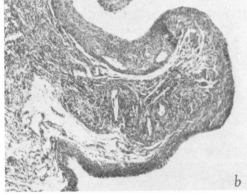

Figure 8.3.2. a. Synovium from rheumatoid joint. Note perivascular collection of small round cells and large collection of these cells, giving appearance of a granoloma (Hematoxylin and eosin; × 41). *b.* Villus from the tenosynovium in the carpal tunnel in probable rheumatoid arthritis. Note proliferation of synovial cells, increased vascularity, and small round cell infiltration (hematoxylin and eosin; × 78).

dislocation or drift of the little finger; gravity probably has its role. The long and ring fingers are deformed in similar manners. A finger which has drifted in an ulnar direction may cause, by pressure, an ulnar dislocation of the adjoining finger.

A fixed deformity at one joint is usually accompanied by the reverse deformity at the next joint. For example, the so-called "intrinsic-plus" contracture described by Bunnell in which the metacarpophalangeal joint is flexed and the proximal interphalangeal joint is hyperextended is accompanied by a flexion contracture of the distal joint. Also, the flexion deformity of the proximal interphalangeal joint, caused by rupture of the central slip of the extensor hood, is accompanied by hyperextension of the distal joint.

The metacarpophalangeal joint of the thumb usually becomes unstable and flexed when involved by rheumatoid arthritis. The interphalangeal joint goes into the reverse deformity of hyperextension and also becomes unstable.

In most patients with rheumatoid arthritis, the wrist assumes a position of slight radial deviation and flexion. Early in the involvement of the wrist, the distal radioulnar joint is affected; the attaching ligaments and triangular cartilage are likely to be destroyed, and the head of the ulna dislocates dorsally. The ulna is lengthened, comparatively, by the narrowing not only of the radiocarpal joints but also of the intercarpal joints. The dislocated head of the ulna then tends to hold or push the wrist into a position of flexion and slight radial deviation.

Carpal Tunnel Syndrome

When proliferation of the tenosynovium (tenosynovitis) occurs in the carpal canal, the boundaries of which are rigidly fixed, secondary compression of the median nerve is likely to be produced; this results in pain, paresthesia and, as a late sequel, weakness and atrophy of the thenar muscles.

Trigger Finger

Tenosynovitis at the level of the proximal pulleys of the digital synovial sheaths in the palm produces an adherent thickening and enlargement of the flexor tendons, a stenosis of the pulley, or both. This in turn causes a catching, snapping, or locking as the tendon passes through the pulley, resulting in the so-called trigger finger. The ring and long fingers are involved more often than are the little and index fingers and the thumb.

Rupture of Tendons

The proliferation of the tenosynovium may be so marked that the relatively avascular tendons are completely deprived of their blood supply and may become necrotic and may rupture spontaneously. Compression of blood vessels likely has a part in diminution of the vascularity.

The most common site of the rupture of tendons is the dorsum of the wrist where the extensor tendons of the fingers pass beneath the dorsal carpal ligament and are surrounded by tenosynovium. In many instances the tendons are actually sawed in two as a result of their passing back and forth over a sharp spicule of bone. Such a spicule may be produced when the distal part of the radioulnar joint is destroyed and the head of the ulna is dislocated dorsally. The extensor tendons to the little finger usually rupture first and may be followed successively by rupture of the tendons of the ring, long, and index fingers.

The extensor pollicis longus tendon is located in a separate compartment and ruptures at the level of Lister's tubercle. Occasionally one or more of the flexor tendons will rupture in the carpal canal or in the digit itself.

DIAGNOSIS

Involvement of the hand by rheumatoid arthritis is usually evident, but, early in the course of the disease, the cause of localized tenosynovitis, synovitis, intrinsic muscle contracture, carpal tunnel syndrome, or tendon rupture may be difficult to establish at times.

When the diagnosis is not evident, a history of polyarticular involvement, rheumatoid arthritis in other members of the family, and absence of trauma should be suggestive of rheumatoid arthritis as a likely cause of disability of the hand. The presence of rheumatoid nodules may be helpful in the diagnosis of rheumatoid arthritis of the hand. An elevated sedimentation rate of the erythrocytes, a positive agglutination test for rheumatoid factor, biopsy of inflamed synovium or tenosynovium, and analysis of joint fluid also may be helpful in establishment of the diagnosis.

CONSERVATIVE TREATMENT

The keystones of conservative treatment at the present time include adequate rest, the use of aspirin in large doses, and the application of general measures that will help the patient resist the onslaught of the disease.

Since rheumatoid arthritis is a systemic disease, it is unusual for the hands to present the only problem. Thus, the conservative treatment of active inflammation in the hand is largely the treatment of the disease itself.

Heat applied locally in the form of paraffin baths at 100 to 110° F, warm soaks, and infrared irradiation helps to allay local inflammation and make the patient's hands and wrists more comfortable.

Elevation and gentle massage of the hands and controlled active exercises help prevent undue edema and the concomitant stiffness.

Gentle, active exercises help to overcome stiffness and to prevent contractures. These active exercises and occupational therapy also will help prevent undue weakness of the intrinsic muscles. Passive exercises are to be condemned since they cause more inflammation, pain, stiffness, and deformity.

Mild deformities due to spasm or to early contracture of the intrinsic muscles should be helped, at least theoretically, by the patient's extending the metacarpophalangeal joint fully while flexing the proximal and distal interphalangeal joints completely. Dynamic splints, as described by Bunnell, may be of value in the prevention and correction of mild contractures and deformities.

Contractures that are not fixed can be overcome, at times, by the use of series of plaster casts. These seem to be most efficacious when applied by the technique of Brand. The affected part, usually a finger, is well greased with petroleum jelly and covered with two or three circular layers of plaster. Gentle corrective force is applied as the plaster sets. After 24 or 48 hours, the plaster is soaked in water and removed by the patient by peeling the bandage away. The finger or hand is heated and exercised by the patient for at least two hours, after which time the process is repeated.

Injections of hydrocortisone into the joints or the tendon sheaths may be of value for the treatment of mild synovitis or tenosynovitis; they may be especially valuable in cases of trigger finger or de Quervain's syndrome.

The paresthesia associated with a carpal tunnel syndrome may, in early stages of the disease, be relieved by decreased use of the hand during the day, by injection of hydrocortisone into the carpal canal, and by splintage of the wrist in the extended position with a cock-up splint at night.

Labor-saving devices and self-help appliances are of great aid to the paitent with rheumatoid arthritis.

SURGICAL TREATMENT (MEASURES)

Surgical treatment of the rheumatoid hand is concerned not only with the prevention of specific deformities and syndromes but also with their correction.

Rheumatoid arthritis is a systemic disease and usually involves joints in addition to those in the hand. In the acute stages of the disease, the patient is likely to be debilitated and anemic. The erythrocyte sedimentation rate is usually elevated, and the patient may have marked deformity and atrophy of the musculoskeletal system, both from disease and from disuse. After prolonged administration of steroids the patient often demonstrates hypercortisonism. These effects resemble Cushing's syndrome and include, besides amenorrhea, the characteristic facies and buffalo bump, thin parchment-like atrophic skin, and fragility of blood vessel walls accompanied by a tendency to bleeding.

Formerly it was recommended that elective surgical procedures should not be carried out during the active stage of rheumatoid arthritis, but now it is realized that such delay is unnecessary provided that the disease is not in the florid stage. Even when active, the disease usually can be reduced to a less active stage by the administration of aspirin, phenylbutazone (Butazolidine), indomethacin, gold, or steroids. Likewise when a flare of the disease occurs after an operation, it usually can be controlled by modern therapy.

Often surgical procedures on the hands can be combined with procedures that are required for other joints, such as the hip, knee, or foot, thereby effecting a substantial saving to the patient in time and money.

One of the most distrubing complications is profound surgical shock, which may occur after relatively minor surgical procedures in those patients whose adrenals are atrophic because of the steroids they have received. When the patient has had significant steroid therapy six months before a contemplated surgical procedure, a 200-mg dose of hydrocortisone should be given intramuscularly 48 hours before the operation. Injections should be repeated 24 hours before and on the morning of the operation to prevent profound surgical shock and possible death. The injection 48 hours before the operation may be omitted if preparation is made to administer hydrocortisone intravenously during or after the surgical procedure. The patient must be monitored carefully during and after the operation to detect the first signs of shock. If there is doubt about the need for steroids immediately before, during, or soon after the operation, it is advisable to administer some hydrocortisone parenterally. The patient who receives steroids should not be given morphine because of the tendency toward respiratory depression.

Anesthesia

For anesthesia, axillary block of the lowermost portion of the brachial plexus by injection of a 2 per cent solution of lidocaine (Xylocaine) containing epinephrine is efficacious for most surgical procedures of the rheumatoid hand and wrist. With adequate preoperative sedation, the upper arm tourniquet, which is used routinely, is tolerated for as long as two hours without complaint by the average patient.

When operation is to be confined to one or two digits, digital blocks with local anesthesia are preferable to axillary block.

When the surgical procedure is to be performed only for a carpal tunnel syndrome or for trigger finger, local infiltration of 1 per cent lidocaine solution is often sufficient.

Excision of Rheumatoid Nodules

Rheumatoid nodules that are seen in some patients are usually infiltrative and may develop on the sides of joints, on phalanges, on pressure points, in the tendon sheaths, and on tendons (Fig. 8.3.3). The nodules should be excised when their location or their size interferes with function of the digit.

Treatment for Carpal Tunnel Syndrome (Figs. 8.3.4 A and 8.3.5)

The incision is made in line with the thenar crease and is curved toward the base of the hypothenar eminence where it crosses the wrist creases at angles of at least 45° (Fig. 8.3.4 A). If a tenosynovectomy is indicated, the incision is extended proximally in a curvilinear manner. The palmaris longus tendon, if present, is identified, and the distal 1 inch of the tendon is resected. The proximal end of the transverse carpal ligament, which begins just distal to the distal wrist crease, is incised in a longitudinal direction and on the ulnar side of the median nerve. Care is taken to section the entire thickness and breadth of the transverse carpal ligament; this ligament is more distal than is often realized. A ¼-inch segment of the transverse carpal ligament is usually excised. Next, the volar carpal ligament is incised; this ligament, although continuous with the transverse carpal ligament, is proximalward and much thinner. The median nerve is carefully dissected from the thickened rheumatoid tenosynovium; the motor branch is identified as it pierces the distal end of the transverse carpal ligament and is carefully preserved. When the tenosynovium is greatly thick-

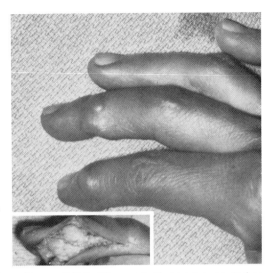

Figure 8.3.3. Rheumatoid nodules on index and long fingers. *Inset.* Rheumatoid nodule of index finger at excision.

ened, the nerve should be retracted radialward and the tenosynovium should be excised from about the digital flexor tendons that occupy the carpal canal. If there is gross evidence that the nerve has been constricted markedly, an external or an internal saline neurolysis, or both, may be performed. At this time, the pneumatic tourniquet is released and hemostasis is accomplished. A solution containing 25 mg of hydrocortisone is placed about the tendons. The tourniquet may be reinflated while only the skin is sutured (Fig. 8.3.5).

After the operation, a modified, bulky hand dressing that leaves the fingers and thumb partly free is applied and a cock-up splint is incorporated in the dressing. The bulky dressing and the splint are removed four or five days after the operation, and normal motion of the digits and wrist is encouraged.

Release of Trigger Finger

The incision is made parallel to the distal palmar crease, and the proximal pulley overlying the beginning of the digital synovial sheath is partially excised (Fig. 8.3.4A). A local tenosynovectomy is performed, and especially tissue that is densely adherent to the tendons is excised. Since the operation is usually performed with the use of local anesthesia, the patient can flex and extend the finger on request and thereby can demonstrate whether the locking or catching has been relieved. The pneumatic tourniquet is released, and hemostasis is accomplished. A few drops of hydrocortisone solution is placed about the tendons, and only the skin is sutured.

When extensive tenosynovitis is present in a finger, it may be advisable to make a midlateral incision on the finger and to perform a tenosynovectomy throughout the length of the finger (Fig. 8.3.6a). Fibrous pul-

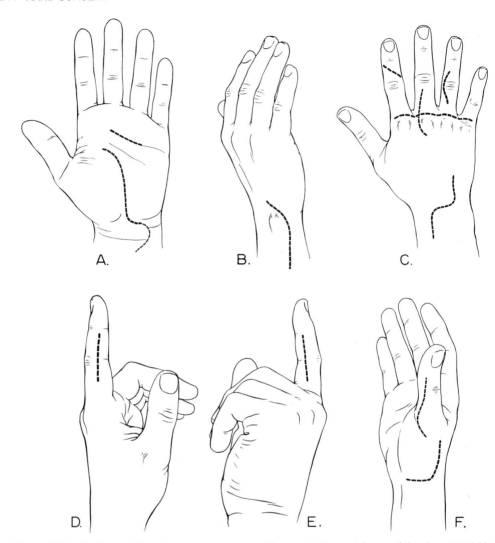

Figure 8.3.4. Outlines of incisions commonly used for surgical procedures of the rheumatoid hand. *A.* For relief of carpal tunnel syndrome and release of trigger finger. Incision only along the *heavy dotted lines* is necessary when tenosynovectomy is not to be performed. The incision may be extended as indicated in the *lighter dotted line* when tenosynovectomy is necessary in carpal tunnel syndromes. *B.* For tenosynovectomy of extensor carpi ulnaris tendon, for resection of distal end of ulna, and for subtotal synovectomy of the wrist. This incision may be used for arthrodeses of the wrist. *C.* For repair of ruptured extensor tendons on the dorsum of the wrist. This incision also can be used for arthrodeses of the wrist. For operation at the level of the metacarpophalangeal joints, the curved longitudinal incision is used when the procedure is a localized one and the transverse incision is used when all of the metacarpophalangeal joints or their contiguous structures are to be exposed. For arthrodeses of an interphalangeal joint, the curved incision across is utilized. For section of the lateral bands in boutonniere deformities, the oblique incision on the dorsum of the middle phalanx is useful. *D.* On radial (lateral) aspect of finger *E.* On ulnar (medial) aspect of finger. *F.* For exposure of thumb at levels of metacarpocarpal, metacarpophalangeal, and interphalangeal joints.

leys, approximately ¼ inch wide, are preserved over the middle part of the proximal and middle phalanges (Fig. 8.3.6*b*).

When only the proximal fibrous pulley has been sectioned and a limited tenosynovectomy performed, a small protective dressing is applied to the wound and early motion of the digit is encouraged. When the dissection is fairly extensive, a large, bulky hand dressing is applied and is left in position; the acute postoperative pain and edema subside usually in four or

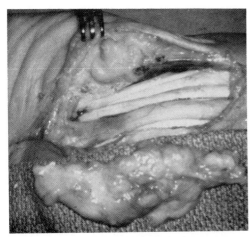

Figure 8.3.5. Inflamed synovium removed from about flexor tendons of left hand of patient with carpal tunnel syndrom. Note bruising of median nerve at level of transverse carpal ligament, which has been excised partially.

five days. At the end of this time, complete active excursion of the tendons is encouraged.

Excision of Distal Ulna and Partial Synovectomy of the Wrist (Figs. 8.3.4 *B*, 8.3.7, 8.3.8 *A*, 8.3.9, and 8.3.10)

A 3-inch curved incision with the base dorsalward is made on the ulnar side of the wrist, and the skin flap is elevated. The dorsal branch of the ulnar nerve sometimes comes off the ulnar nerve at the level of the neck of the ulna and must be protected; if present at this level, it is retracted volarward. The thickened and hypertrophied tenosynovium is excised from the extensor carpi ulnaris tendon, which may be displaced volarward. The distal ¾ inch of the dislocated, abnormally mobile ulna is resected. The ulna is severed obliquely at the level of its neck. The fragment to be removed is grasped with a Lewin clamp, bone-holding forceps, or a towel clip, and is resected subperiosteally. No more than 1 inch of the ulna should be excised lest the insertion of the pronator quadratus muscle becomes distrubed unduly, thereby interfering with pronation and producing more instability of the ulna. The ulnar side of the radiocarpal joint is exposed widely on removal of the distal part of the ulna. A large amount of synovial tissue can then be excised easily from the ulnar side and the dorsal and volar aspects of the wrist joint. If there is any evidence of instability, the carpus is pinned to the distal end of the radius with Kirschner wires; these are removed after six to eight weeks. After resection of the distal part of the ulna, the motion at the wrist usually is freer. The hand can be placed in dorsal extension, and ulnar deviation at the wrist is possible whereas such may have been impossible previously. The pneumatic tourniquet is released, and hemostasis is accomplished. Bäckdahl advocated re-

placement of the extensor carpi ulnaris tendon to its normal position on the dorsum of the ulna and fixation with a loop of the palmaris longus tendon. It is usually sufficient to use a band either of fascia or of the dorsal carpal ligament, which is left attached dorsally, to form the loop that holds the extensor carpi ulnaris tendon in its proper position (Fig. 8.3.7). The wound is sutured.

After the operation, a bulky, mildly compressive hand dressing, with a plaster of Paris splint to hold the wrist in extension and in slight ulnar deviation, is applied.

Arthrodesis of the Wrist

Occasionally when there is severe deformity, instability, or pain as a result of destructive changes, arthrodesis of the wrist is indicated. The technique described by Bunnell is used in most instances. Resection of the distal end of the ulna usually is advised at the time the radiocarpal joints are arthrodesed. Although fusion of one wrist may be of great help to the patient, fusion of both wrists should not be performed because acts connected with bathing and toilet cannot be performed satisfactorily when both wrists are in a fixed position.

Osteotomy of Distal Radius

Occasionally when there is a fixed flexion deformity of the wrist but little pain and instability, a cuneiform osteotomy of the radius through the distal metaphysis allows correction of the deformity and

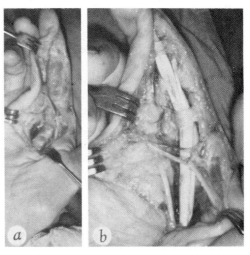

Figure 8.3.6. Rheumatoid tenosynovitis of flexor sheath of right index finger. *a.* Thickened and swollen tendon sheath has been exposed. *b.* Sheath has been excised, but narrow pulleys preserved. Both neurovascular bundles can be visualized. Note erosion of profundus tendon as it lies between the slips of the sublimus tendon at the level of their insertion.

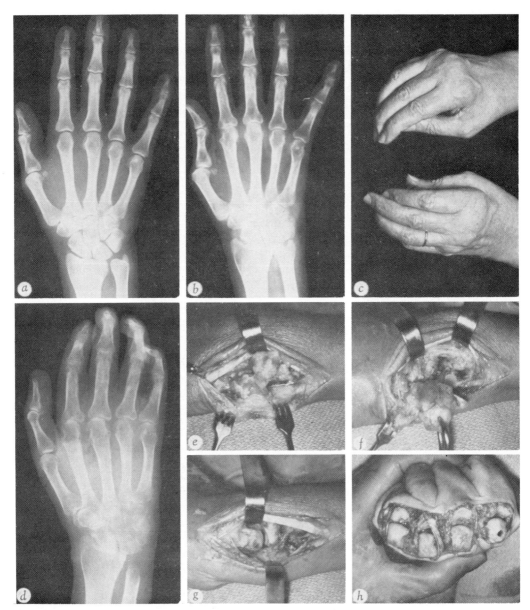

Figure 8.3.7. Serial rocentgenograms of the right hand, preoperative appearance of both hands, and surgical findings in left hand of patient with rheumatoid arthritis. *a.* Right hand is almost normal. *b.* Right hand has moderate synovitis, osteoporosis, and destruction of small joints (seven years after *a*). *c.* Preoperative appearance of both hands. *d.* Right hand immediately after excision of distal part of ulna and synovectomy of wrist and metacarpophalangeal joints. *e.* Exposure of extensor carpi ulnaris tendon and distal part of ulna. Note marked synovial reaction. *f.* Head of ulna has been severed from shaft and is held by Lewin clamp as it is being excised. *g.* Head of ulna has been removed, and synovectomy of wrist has been performed. *h.* Metacarpophalangeal joints of left hand. Note eyst in head of second metacarpal.

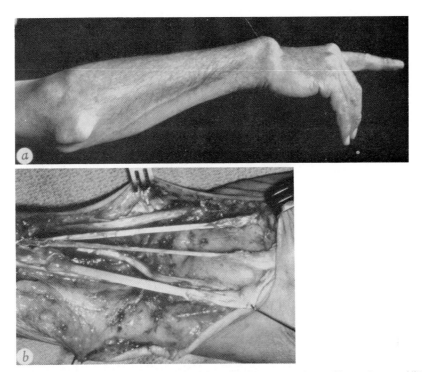

Figure 8.3.8. a. Dorsal dislocation of ulna with rupture extensor tendons of long, ring, and little fingers of right hand. Note large rheumatoid nodule at elbow. *b.* Repair of ruptured extensor tendons with long plantaris graft to reestablish continuity for tendons of long and ring fingers and palmaris longus graft for extensor digiti minimi tendon.

maintenance of the range of motion present at the wrist. Resection of the distal end of the ulna usually is advised at the same time.

Repair of Ruptured Tendons (Figs. 8.3.4 C, 8.3.8, 8.3.11, and 8.3.12)

The most common site of tendon rupture is the dorsum of the wrist. Rupture of the long extensor tendons of the fingers is evidenced by inability of the patient to extend the metacarpophalangeal joints actively. An S-shaped incision, approximately 4 inches long, is made on the dorsum of the hand, wrist, and distal part of the forearm. The ulnar end of the dorsal carpal ligament is incised longitudinally and reflected radialward; the radial end is left attached. The tenosynovium and scar are excised, and a search is made for sharp spicules of bone that may have eroded the tendons; if found, the spicules are removed. Usually, the distal end of the ulna, which is dislocated dorsalward, is excised. A gap of 2 to 4 inches usually is present between the ends of healthy tendon when the fibrillated, thinned, and degenerated portions of the tendon are excised. At this time, the pneumatic tourniquet is released and hemostasis is accomplished. The tendons may be repaired by free tendon grafts, by suture of the distal tendon ends to adjacent healthy tendons, or by transfer of the extensor indicus proprius

tendon or of the extensor carpi ulnaris tendon to the distal ends of the finger extensor tendons. The source of the tendon grafts can be the palmaris longus, the plantaris, or both. The tendon sutures are accomplished while the wrist and fingers are held in moderate extension. The dorsal carpal ligament, which was reflected on the intact attachment, is placed anterior to the reconstituted tendons and held with two or three sutures, as advocated by Riordan and Clayton. A smooth gliding surface is thereby provided by the ligament beneath the tendon grafts. The wound is sutured (Fig. 8.3.8).

Essentially the same technique is used for repair of a ruptured extensor pollicis longus tendon as for repair of ruptured long extensor tendons of the fingers; the former tendon is not placed around Lister's tubercle but rather it is displaced to the radial side of the wrist (Fig. 8.3.11).

When a flexor tendon ruptures, the repair follows the same principles as those used for the much more common rupture of the extensor tendons. In such an instance, repair is accomplished while the wrist and digits are in a slightly flexed position (Fig. 8.3.12).

After the operation, a bulky, lightly compressive hand dressing is applied and a plaster of Paris splint is incorporated to maintain the wrist and digits in the position that will relax tension on the repaired ten-

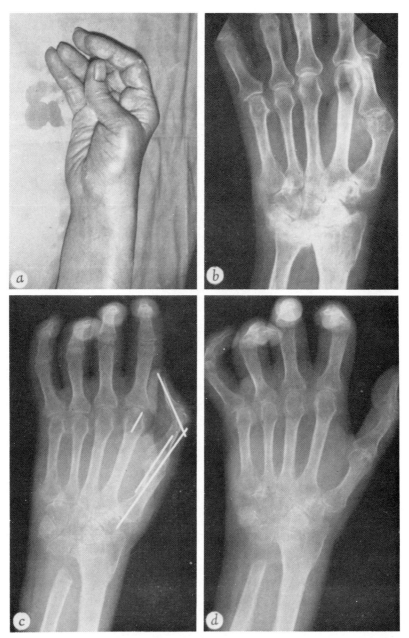

Figure 8.3.9. Deformity of a right thumb in rheumatoid arthritis. *a.* Flexion contracture of metacarpophalangeal joint and extension deformity of interphalangeal joint. *b.* Preoperative view demonstrates deformity of thumb and of distal part of radioulnar and carpal joints. *c.* Postoperative view demonstrates Kirschner wire fixation of metacarpophalangeal joint after surgical arthrodesis, interphalangeal joint after surgical arthrodesis, interphalangeal joint after advancement of volar plate, and temporary fixation of extensor tendons of index fingers over center of second metacarpophalangeal joint. Note that distal end of ulna has been excised. *d.* Position of thumb after removal of Kirschner wires. Metacarpophalangeal joint is fused, and interphalangeal joint no longer hyperextends. Distal end of ulna has been resected.

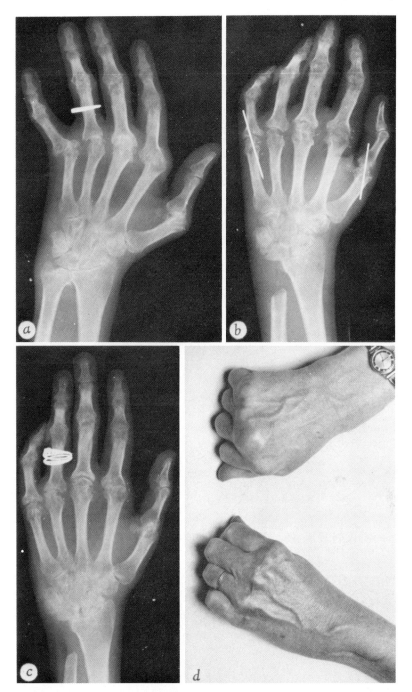

Figure 8.3.10. a. Left hand shows flexion deformity and dislocation of metacarpophalangeal joint of thumb, ulnar drift of fingers at metacarpophalangeal joints, and destruction of distal part of radioulnar joint. *b.* Left hand after arthrodesis of metacarpophalangeal joint of thumb, Littler releases of extensor hoods, synovectomy of metacarpophalangeal and wrist joints, reduction of dislocated metacarpophalangeal joints with temporary internal fixation of the thumb and little finger, and relocation of extensor tendons. *c.* Left hand six months after surgical correction of deformities. *d.* Both hands six months after surgical correction of multiple deformities of left hand. Before operation, deformity and synovitis of left hand and wrist was about the same as that seen in right hand.

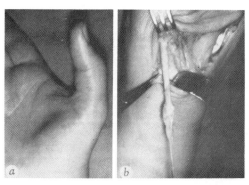

Figure 8.3.11. Rupture of extensor pollicis longus tendon. *a*. Distal phalanx of right thumb is unable to be fully extended. *b*. Frayed appearance of extensor pollicis longus tendon.

taken to preserve the dorsal intermetacarpal veins. Because of the associated tendency for ulnar drift of the finger, the extensor hood and underlying joint capsule are divided in a longitudinal direction just medial to the extensor tendon. The underlying joint is thereby exposed throughout its length and breadth as the extensor tendon is retracted radialward. As much as possible of the thickened synovia is excised from in and about the joint. It may be advisable at times to section the collateral ligament on one side of the joint, thereby allowing complete access to all surfaces of the joint, as it is dislocated on the intact collateral ligament; thus, a more complete synovectomy is accomplished. Small rongeurs and curettes are helpful in picking away the snyovial lining in the recesses of the joints. Usually the dorsal capsule is so thin and attenuated that it is impossible to perform a thorough synovectomy and still maintain the capsule. I have observed no particular

dons. The dressing and splint usually are not removed for three to four weeks. In extensor tendon repair, the wrist is supported with a cock-up splint for an additional two weeks while active extension and flexion of the digits is encouraged.

Synovectomy of metacarpophalangeal and interphalangeal joints (Figs. 8.3.4*C*, 8.3.7, 8.3.10, 8.3.13, and 8.3.14). Continued and prolonged synovitis destroys the hyaline cartilage and subchondral bone of joints and also stretches ligaments and capsules. Synovectomy should be performed when possible before these undesirable secondary effects occur. At present, the trend is to perform synovectomy of the finger joints early in the course of the rheumatoid disease (Fig. 8.3.10).

Synovectomy of two or more of the metacarpophalangeal joints of the fingers usually is performed through a transverse incision over the distal end of the metacarpal heads. Synovectomy of a single metacarpophalangeal joint is performed through a 1½-inch, curved incision on the side of the joint. With either transverse or curved incision, great care should be

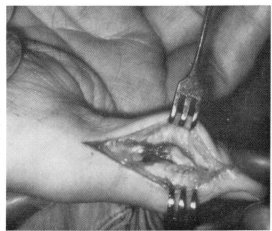

Figure 8.3.12. Acute rupture of flexor pollicis longus tendon, proximal to level of interphalangeal joint in extensive rheumatoid tenosynovitis.

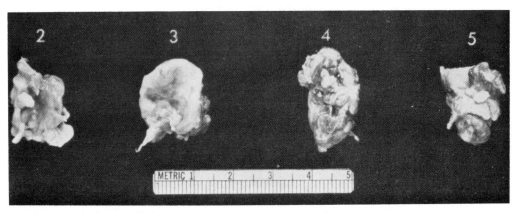

Figure 8.3.13. Synovium excised from the second, third, fourth, and fifth metacarpophalangeal joints a typical rheumatoid hand.

harm to the joint from partial removal of the dorsal joint capsule. The procedure is repeated on each of the metacarpophalangeal joints that needs synovectomy.

At this time in the operation, the pneumatic tourniquet is released and hemostasis is accomplished (Fig. 8.3.13). Usually, it is advisable to fix temporarily the proximal phalanx to the metacarpal in the desired position with a Kirschner wire across the joint.

The Kirschner wire is cut at the level of the skin so that it can be removed easily. The extensor tendon is carefully repositioned over the center of the joint, and either it is held with a loop formed from the wing tendons of the extensor hood on the radial side of the joint or it is tacked in position with one or two fine absorbable sutures. The skin wound is then closed.

When there is a tendency for volar subluxation of the base of the proximal phalanx on the metacarpal head, the extensor tendon may be tenodesed to the base of the proximal phalanx as advocated by Fowler.

After the operation, a bulky, mildly compressive hand dressing with a plaster of Paris splint incorporated is applied. When there is no tendency to contracture of the intrinsic muscles, the fingers are placed in the position of function. When an intrinsic contracture is present, the metacarpophalangeal joints are immobilized in extension and the interphalangeal joints are immobilized in flexion (Fig. 8.3.14).

When only a synovectomy has been performed, the dressing is removed in 10 or 12 days and active motion of the fingers is commenced. However, longer immobilization is usually indicated since it often has been necessary to section a collateral ligament, to reposition the extensor mechanism, to tenodese the extensor tendon, and to transfix the joints with Kirschner wires or hypodermic needles. In most instances, therefore, the dressing and sutures are first removed at the end of three weeks. The Kirschner wires, the ends of which lie just under the skin, are removed at this time or a few days later.

Mobilization is by active exercise. At first a dynamic reverse knuckle bender splint may be indicated, and later a knuckle bender splint may serve the purpose best.

Release of Intrinsic Contractures (Figs. 8.3.1, 8.3.4 C, 8.3.7, 8.3.9, 8.3.10, and 8.3.14)

This procedure is performed frequently in association with synovectomy of the metacarpophalangeal joints. In rheumatoid disease the Littler release should be only one step in surgery at the level of the metacarpophalangeal joints; almost always the surgeon should combine the releases with synovectomies or arthroplasties. An intrinsic contracture is characterized by a flexion deformity of the metacarpophalangeal joint and by hyperextension of the proximal interphalangeal joint. Frequently, an ulnar drift of the finger also is present. The oblique fibers of the extensor hood on the ulnar sides of the proximal phalanges should be released when an intrinsic contracture is present. Often it is necessary to also release the oblique fibers on the radial sides to afford a more complete correction and to prevent recurrence of the deformity. However, the fibers of the first dorsal interosseous tendon, which insert into the proximal phalanx of the index finger, are not sectioned. On resection of the oblique fibers of the extensor hood, the metacarpophalangeal joints can be extended while the interphalangeal joints are flexed and the fingers straightened on the metacarpal in the horizontal plane. The fingers are splinted in this position after the operation. The pneumatic tourniquet is released, hemostasis is established, and the wound is sutured (Fig. 8.3.14).

The postoperative care is the same as that for synovectomy.

Correction of Ulnar Drift (Figs. 8.3.9, 8.3.10, and 8.3.14)

The procedures are the same as for synovectomy and release of intrinsic contracture. After release of contractures and the performance of synovectomies as indicated, the capsule and fibrous tissues on the radial sides of the metacarpophalangeal joints are reefed to hold the finger in the corrected position. Almost always the fingers should be fixed temporarily in the corrected position by placing Kirschner wires across the joints. The extensor tendon is relocated carefully across the center of the joint and may be either tenodesed to the proximal phalanx, or tacked with two or three sutures to the surrounding soft tissues. A crossed finger intrinsic transfer may be added. After the operation, immobilization is continued for three to four weeks.

Arthroplasty of Metacarpophalangeal Joints (Figs. 8.3.4 C, 8.3.14, and 8.3.15)

When severe destruction of the metacarpophalangeal joints has occurred and is accompanied by dislocation of the proximal phalanx, not only is synovectomy performed but also it is usually necessary to do a modified arthroplasty to place the fingers in correct and stable position on the end of the metacarpals. The same approach as that described for synovectomies is used. The metacarpal head is resected, and the neck that remains is fashioned into the shape of a transverse wedge. Enough bone is resected so that a space of 1 cm is present between the end of the refashioned metacarpal and the base of the proximal phalanx. The neck of the metacarpal not only is cut into the shape of a wedge but also is angulated slightly so that there is no longer an inclination for the proximal phalanx to slip ulnarward. No bone is removed from the proximal phalanx. The pneumatic tourniquet is deflated, and hemostasis is accomplished. As a rule no interposition membrane is placed between the proximal phalanx and the metacarpal although a loop of the extensor tendon that is divided at the base of the proximal phalanx may be

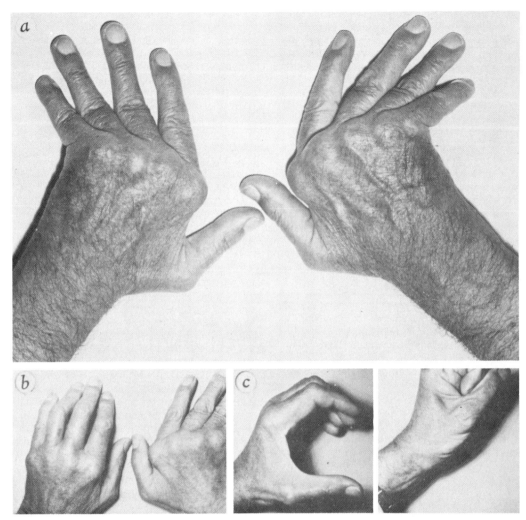

Figure 8.3.14. a. Rheumatoid deformity of hands prior to surgical treatment. *b.* Correction of deformity and improvement in function six months after operation on left hand. *c.* Ability of patient to open hand and grasp four years after Littler releases, synovectomies, and arthroplasties of metacarpophalangeal joints together with relocation of extensor tendons of left hand. Note: Surgical correction of right hand was never undertaken because of patient's age (73 years) and of severe bleeding from a gastric ulcer after operation on left hand. (Reproduced from Linscheid and Lipscomb[33] by permission of Bruce Publishing Company.)

interposed. When this is done, the cut end of the distal tendon is sutured to the proximal end of the tendon just proximal to the interposed loop. Temporary fixation of the proximal phalanx to the metacarpal with the use of Kirschner wires or hypodermic needles as described previously is next accomplished. If the interposition of the extensor tendon has not been done, the extensor tendon should be fixed to the proximal phalanx by the technique (described under heading "Synovectomy of Metacarpophalangeal Joints").

Another technique is to tack the tendon to the periosteum and the remains of the capsular attachment to the base of the phalanx. Next the skin is sutured.

The postoperative care is the same as for synovectomy. Immobilization of the metacarpophalangeal joints is maintained with internal fixation wires or needles for three to four weeks. The interphalangeal joints may be freed, and active motion is begun in these joints at the end of two weeks. It is unusual for the patient to have more than 45 to 60° of motion at the metacarpophalangeal joints after arthroplasty. In fact, stability in the horizontal plane, which usually is ob-

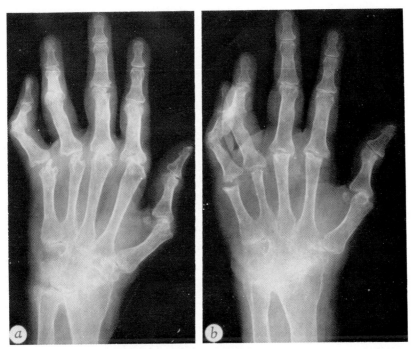

Figure 8.3.15. Left hand of a patient with rheumatoid arthritis. *a*. Before arthroplasties on metacarpophalangeal joints. *b*. Eight months after arthroplasties.

tained by a partial fibrous ankylosis of the joint after arthroplasty, is preferable to a full range of flexion and extension and to lateral instability (Fig. 8.3.15).

Synovectomy of Interphalangeal Joints (Fig. 8.3.4 *D* and *E*)

Through side incisions, between the dorsal and volar creases, 1 inch long on each side of the proximal interphalangeal joint, both dorsal and volar synovectomy can be performed without disturbing the collateral ligaments. By an incision on the ulnar side of the joint and division of the collateral ligament on this side the joint then can be dislocated with the intact ligament used as a hinge, and a complete synovectomy can be performed with ease. After reduction, if there is undue instability with the joint in 30° of flexion, a pin or needle for temporary fixation is placed obliquely across the joint.

After the operation, active motion is encouraged four to 10 days later. The time depends on the degree of joint destruction and instability found at the time of surgery.

Correction of Flexion Deformity of Interphalangeal Joints

A fixed flexion or boutonniere deformity of an interphalangeal joint usually is due to detachment of the central slip of the extensor tendon from the middle phalanx. If the deformity is severe (more than 60°) and

long standing, the articular cartilages are likely to be degenerated to such an extent that no procedure short of arthrodesis of the joint will be satisfactory. However, if the deformity is of recent onset and passive correction can be demonstrated, a more conservative surgical procedure may be tried. The simplest and most rewarding conservative operation is that described by Fowler. Through a small oblique incision on the dorsum of the middle phalanx, the underlying extensor tendon, which at this level consists of the two lateral bands, is severed obliquely (Fig. 8.3.4*C*). Severing allows the distal phalanx, which has been hyperextended, to flex and allows the entire extensor hood proximal to the cut to shift proximally. Thus the central slip, which has been reattached to the base of the middle phalanx by attenuated scar tissue, again becomes functional; the lateral bands assume more dorsal positions rather than lateral positions across the proximal interphalangeal joint as this joint extends.

Arthrodesis of Small Finger Joints (Figs. 8.3.4 *C* and 8.3.16)

When severe, long standing flexion deformity or marked instability of an interphalangeal joint is present, no procedure short of arthrodesis is likely to furnish a satisfactory permanent result. The interphalangeal joint to be fused is approached through a slightly curved incision on its dorsolateral aspect, and the extensor mechanism is divided in a longitudinal direction.

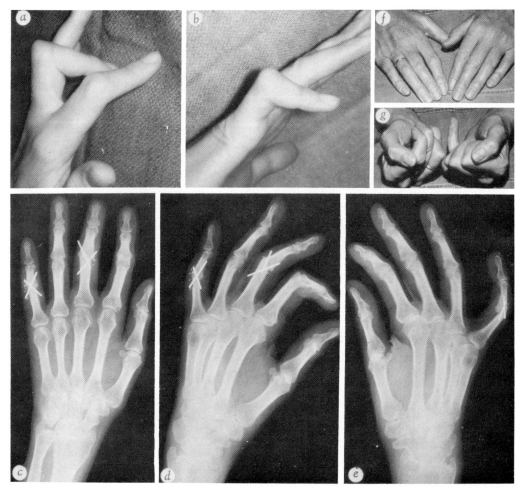

Figure 8.3.16. Severe flexion or boutonniere deformities of long fingers of left hand and little finger only of right hand in a patient with rheumatoid arthritis. *a.* Long finger of left hand. *b.* Little finger of right hand. *c.* Anteroposterior view of left hand five weeks after arthrodesis. *d.* Oblique view of left hand five weeks after arthrodeses. *e.* Anteroposterior view of right hand five weeks after arthrodeses. *f.* Appearance of hands four years after operation. *g.* Function, four years after operation. Patient had no pain, could again wear gloves, and was pleased with results.

The cartilage and subchondral cortical bone is excised as is any thick redundant snynovial membrane. In cases of severe flexion contracture, it is necessary to remove a comparatively large amount of bone to correct the deformity. The remaining cancellous surfaces are approximated carefully and held in 30 to 40° of flexion with two Kirschner wires or with hypodermic needles that are drilled across the joint to be fused. Care is exercised that the finger is not rotated and that, when it is flexed at the metacarpophalangeal joint, the touch pad of the distal phalanx is in line with the tubercle of the navicular bone. It is helpful to countersink a small bone graft in a groove that is made longitudinally across the dorsal aspect of the joint. This is particularly necessary if the joint is fused because of instability. If the distal end of the ulna has been excised during the same operative procedure, the graft is fashioned from this part; otherwise the graft is removed from the crest of the upper part of the ulna through a short incision. The wounds are closed.

If extensive surgical procedures have been carried out elsewhere in the hand and wrist, a large, mildly compressive, fluffy dressing is applied; if not, only the operated digit requires dressing.

After the operation, the internal fixation wires or needles are left in position until roentgenograms demonstrate solid fusion. From eight to 12 weeks, or even longer, frequently is required for such fusion to occur (Fig. 8.3.16).

Endoprosthesis

Prosthetic replacement of the interphalangeal and metacarpophalangeal joints in selected patients was advocated by Flatt who used metal. More recently Swanson has advocated their replacement by silicone rubber implants, Niebauer *et al.* by silicone dacron hinge prosthesis and Reis and Calnan with a polypropylene hinge joint. Savill, Vaughn-Jackson and Vainio favored excisional arthroplasty at a workshop on Artificial Finger Joints, attended by the principal proponents of prosthetic replacement. It seems fair to state that prosthetic replacement of finger joints is still in the experimental stage.

Surgery for the Rheumatoid Thumb (Figs. 8.3.4F, 8.3.9, and 8.3.10)

The most common deformity of the thumb is that of flexion of the metacarpophalangeal joint and hyperextension of the interphalangeal joint. If the joint surfaces are preserved, synovectomy of these joints, combined with prolonged (six to eight weeks) internal fixation in the position of function, usually results in marked improvement of stability and function with preservation of some motion in these joints.

When there is marked destruction and instability of the interphalangeal joint but stability of the metacarpophalangeal joint is still present, arthrodesis of the interphalangeal joint and synovectomy of the metacarpophalangeal joint is the procedure of choice.

When both the interphalangeal and metacarpophalangeal joints are destroyed and unstable, arthrodesis of both joints may be necessary. In such instances, it is desirable that good position and motion be present in the first metacarpotrapezial joint, but unfortunately this joint may also be severely destroyed.

When the first metacarpotrapezial joint is destroyed and unstable, the surgeon has the choice of performing a modified arthroplasty by excising the trapezium piecemeal through an L-shaped incision as was described by Goldner and Clippinger or by performing an arthrodesis. The modified arthroplasty procedure is usually applicable and advisable for deformity that results from rheumatoid arthritis. Excision of the trapezium allows the surgeon to reposition the thumb, thereby overcoming mild adduction contractures and, at the same time, preserve some motion at the base of the thumb. This preservation of motion is particularly desirable when it is necessary to arthrodese the interphalangeal and metacarpophalangeal joints of the thumb. After the trapezium is excised, the base of the first metacarpal is pinned to the distal articular surface of the navicular bone by means of Kirschner wires for three or four weeks. The degree of motion, freedom from pain, and stability are usually gratifying.

Occasionally a severe adduction contracture of the thumb is present, and excision of the trapezium alone will not allow the surgeon to reposition the thumb so that its touch pad will oppose those of the index and long fingers. In such instances the contracted thumb web may have to be released by a Z-plasty of the skin and by severance of the insertion of the adductor tendon; in addition, the trapezium is excised.

COMMENTS

The problems presented by the patient with rheumatoid arthritis must be considered individually before surgical procedures are performed on the hands. It is seldom that only the hands need correction of deformity by surgical means. Often surgical procedures on the hands can be combined with correction of deformities of the feet, knees, and hips during the same hospital stay, thereby materially decreasing the total time necessary for rehabilitation of the patient. Use of the hands for cane and crutch walking because of involvement of the lower extremities by rheumatoid arthritis is often necessary. It is important that surgical procedures on the hands be timed correctly and that the surgeon consider this timing in the over-all care of the patient. If this is not done, the patient may be rendered almost completely helpless while even one hand is healing. Likewise a potentially good result that follows surgical correction of deformities of the hand may be negated by the necessity for early use of crutches or canes during the convalescent period.

When operation is warranted for involvement of the hands by rheumatoid arthritis, usually a combination of surgical procedures is indicated. Not only careful techniques but also meticulous planning are essential to obtain the best possible results from the surgery on the hands.

REFERENCES

1. Addison, N. V. Spontaneous ruptures of extensor tendons at the wrist-joint. B. J. Surg., *41:* 511, 1954.
2. American Rheumatism Association Committee: Nineteenth rheumatism review. Arthritis Rheum., *13:* 457-711, 1970.
3. Bäckdahl, M. The caput ulnae syndrome in rheumatoid arthritis: A study of the morphology, abnormal anatomy and clinical picture. Acta Rheum. Scand, Suppl. 5, 1963, 75 pp.
4. Bäckdahl, M., and Myrin, S. O. Ulnar deviation of the fingers in rheumatoid arthritis and its surgical correction: A new operative method. Acta chir. scand., *122:* 158, 1961.
5. Boyes, J. H. Personal communication to the author.
6. Brand, P. W. Fundamental principles involved in tendon transfers. Read at the Symposium on the Neuromuscular Tendinous Disorders of the Upper Extremity, University of Pittsburgh Medical Center, September 21, 1960.
7. Brewerton, D. A. Hand deformities in rheumatoid disease. Ann. Rheum. Dis., *16:* 183, 1957.
8. Brower, T. D. Rheumatoid arthritis of the hands. Surg. Clin. North Am., *40:* 541, 1960.
9. Bunnell, S. Splinting the hand. In *The American Academy of Orthopaedic Surgeons: Instructional Course Lectures,* Vol. 9. Ann Arbor, Mich., Edwards, 1952, p. 233.
10. Bunnell, S. Ischaemic contracture, local, in the hand. J. Bone Joint Surg., *85A:* 88, 1953.
11. Bunnell, S. Surgery of the rheumatic hand. J. Bone Joint Surg., *37A:* 759, 1955.
12. Bunnell, S. *Surgery of the Hand,* Ed. 5, edited by J. H. Boyes, Philadelphia, Lippincott, 1970.

13. Clayton, M. L. Surgery of the thumb in rheumatoid arthritis. J. Bone Joint Surg., 44A: 1376, 1962.
14. Cregan, J. C. F. Indications for surgical intervention in rheumatoid arthritis of the wrist and hand. Ann. Rheum. Dis., 18: 29, 1959.
15. Díaz, C. J., García, E. L., Merchante, A., and Perianes, J. Treatment of rheumatoid arthritis with nitrogen mustard: Preliminary report. J.A.M.A., 147: 1418, 1951.
16. Ehrlich, G. E., Peterson, L. T., Sokoloff, B., and Bunim, J. J. Pathogenesis of rupture of extensor tendons at the wrist in rheumatoid arthritis. Arthritis Rheum., 2: 332, 1959.
17. Fearnley, G.R. Ulnar deviation of the fingers. Ann. Rheum. Dis., 10: 126, 1951.
18. Flatt, A. E. The Care of the Rheumatoid Hand, Ed. 2. St. Louis, Mosby, 1968.
19. Flatt, A. E. Prosthetic replacement of joints in rheumatoid arthritis. Read at the Continuation Course in Orthopedic Surgery, University of Minnesota, November 23, 1963.
20. Fowler, S. B. Surgery of the arthritic hand. Read at the meeting of the Clinical Orthopaedic Society, Hermitage Hotel, Nashville, Tennessee, October 18, 1963.
21. Fowler, S. B. Operative treatment of the rheumatoid hand. Read at the meeting of the Continuation Course in Rheumatoid Arthritis, University of Minnesota, November 22, 1963.
22. Goldner, J. L., and Clippinger, F. W., Excision of the greater multangular bone as an adjunct to mobilization of the thumb. J. Bone Joint Surg., 41A: 609, 1959.
23. Hench, P. S., Kendall, E. C., Slocumb, C. H., and Polley, H. F. The effort of a hormone of the adrenal cortex (17-hydroxy-11-dehydrocorticosterone: compound E) and of pituitary adrenocorticotropic hormone on rheumatoid arthritis: Preliminary report. Proc. Mayo Clin., 24: 181, 1949.
24. Henderson, E. D., and Lipscomb, P. R. Rehabilitation of the rheumatoid hand by surgical means. Arch. Phys. Med., 42: 58, 1961.
25. Henderson, E. D., and Lipscomb, P. R. Surgical treatment of rheumatoid hand. J.A.M.A., 175: 431, 1961.
26. Hindenach, J. C. R. Wrist joint surgery in the rheumatoid arthritis. Rheumatism, 19: 24, 1963.
27. Howard, L. A., Jr. Surgical treatment of rheumatic tenosynovitis. Am. J. Surg., 89: 1163, 1955.
28. Kellgren, J. H., and Ball, J. Tendon Lesions in rheumatoid arthritis: A clinico-pathological study. Ann. Rheum. Dis., &: 48, 1950.
29. Kestler, O. C. A surgical procedure for the painful arthritic hand. Bull. Hosp. Joint Dis., 7: 114, 1946.
30. Kuhns, J. G. The preservation and recovery of hand function in rheumatoid arthritis. Bull. Rheum. Dis., 10: 199, 1959.
31. Laine, V. A. I., Sairanen, E., and Vainio, K. Finger deformities caused by rheumatoid arthritis. J. Bone Joint Surg., 39A: 527, 1957.
32. Laine, V. A. I., and Vainio, K. J. Spontaneous ruptures of tendons in rheumatoid arthritis. Acta orthop. scand., 24: 250, 1954-55.
33. Linschoid, R. L., and Lipscomb, P. R. Advances in surgical treatment of the rheumatoid hand. Minn. Med., 45: 273, 1962.
34. Lipscomb, P. R. Recent advances in surgical treatment

35. Lipscomb, P. R. Tenosynovitis of the hand and the wrist: Carpal tunnel syndrome, de Quervain's disease, trigger digit. Clin. Orthop., 13: 164, 1959.
36. Lipscomb, P. R. Surgery of the hand, (Bunnell Memorial Lecture). Mayo Clinic Proc., 40: 132, 1965.
37. Littler, J. W. Quoted by C. Harris, Jr. and D. C. Riordan. Intrinsic contracture in the hand and its surgical treatment. J. Bone Joint Surg., 36A: 10, 1954.
38. Marmor, L. The role of hand surgery in rheumatoid arthritis. Surg. Gynecol. Obstet., 116: 335, 1963.
39. Niebauer, J. J., Shaw J. L., and Doren, W. W., Silicone-dacron hinge prosthesis: Design, evaluation, and application. Ann. Rheum. Dis., 28: Supp. 56-1969.
40. Paul, W. D., Hodges, R. E., Bean, W. B., Routh, J. I., and Daum, K. Effects of nitrogen mustard therapy in patients with rheumatoid arthritis. Arch. Phys. Med., 35: 371, 1954.
41. Phalen, G. S., and Kendrick, J. I. Compression neuropathy of the median nerve in the carpal canal. J.A.M.A., 164: 524, 1957.
42. Pratt, D. R. Exposing fractures of the proximal phalanx of the finger longitudinally through the dorsal extensor apparatus. Clin. Orthop., 15: 22, 1959.
43. Pulkki, T. Rheumatoid deformities of the hand. Acta rheum. scand., 7: 85, 1961.
44. Reis, N. D., and Calnan, J. S. Integral hinge joint, Ann. Rheum. Dis., 28: Suppl. 59-62, 1969. (This is a polypropylene hinge joint.)
45. Riordan, D.C. Personal communication to the author.
46. Riordan, D. C., and Fowler, S. B. Surgical treatment of rheumatoid deformities of the hand. J. Bone oint Surg., 40A: 1431, 1958.
47. Scherbel, A. L. Schuchter, S. L., and Weyman, S. J. II. Intraarticular administration of nitrogen mustard alone and combined v 'h a corticosteroid for rheumatoid arthritis. Cleveland Clin. Quart., 24: 78, 1957.
48. Stecher, R. M. Ankylosis of the finger joints in rheumatoid arthritis. Ann. Rheum. Dis., 17: 365, 1958. Gynecol. Obstet., 45: 476, 1927.
49. Steindler, A. Orthopedic reconstruction work on hand and forearm: Report on early and late results. Surg. Gynecal. Obstet., 45: 476, 1927.
50. Steindler, A. Arthritic deformities of the wrist and fingers. J. Bone Joint Surg., 88A: 849, 1951.
51. Straub, L. R. The rheumatoid hand. Clin. Orthop., 15: 127, 1959.
52. Straub, L. R. Analysis and correction of deformity of the finger. Read at the Clinical Congress of the American College of Surgeons, San Francisco, California, November 1, 1963.
53. Straub, L. R., and Wilson, E. H., Jr. Spontaneous rupture of extensor tendons in the hand associated with rheumatoid arthritis. J. Bone Joint Surg., 38A: 1208, 1956.
54. Swanson, A. B. The need for early treatment of the rheumatoid hand. J. Mich. Med. Soc., 60: 348, 1961.
55. Swanson, A. B. Finger joint replacement by silicone rubber implants and the concept of implant fixation by encapsulation. Ann. Rheum. Dis., 28: Suppl. 47-55, 1969.

of rheumatoid arthritis of the hand. Read at the meeting of the American Rheumatism Association, San Francisco, June 20 to 21, 1958.

56. Vainio, K., and Julkuncn, H. Intra-articular nitrogen mustard treatment of rheumatoid arthritis. Acta rheum. scand., *6:* 25, 1960.
57. Vainio, K. Quoted by Flatt, A. E.[18]
58. Vainio, K. and Oka, M. Ulnar deviation of the fingers. Ann. Rheum. Dis., *12:* 122, 1953.
59. Vaughan-Jackson, O. J. Rheumatoid hand deformities considered in the light of tendon imbalance. J. Bone Joint Surg., *44B:* 764, 1962.
60. Workshop on Artificial Finger Joints, Supplement to Ann. Rheum. Dis., *28:* 10, 1969.

D.

The Upper Extremity in Gout

Robert A. Chase, M.D.
Donald A. Nagel, M.D.

The antiquity of gout as a malady is well documented.[2][5] The disease was described by ancient writers such as Hippocrates and Heron of Syracuse (5th century). A classic description of the disease was given by Guillaume de Baillou in 1642. Unequivocal prima facie evidence of the existence of gout historically was noted by Smith and Jones.[13] They found a large tophi in the great toe and other joints in the skeleton of an elderly man exhumed from a first century cemetery in Nubia in upper Egypt. Chemical analysis of the tophi showed urates. The 17th century scholar and physician, Thomas Sydenham, wrote a classic description of the disease in 1683.[2] Sydenham himself suffered the misery of acute gout attacks. Similarly, Sydney Smith, in a letter to Lady Carlisle, September 5, 1840, described gout with colorful accuracy: "What a singular disease gout is; it seems as if the stomach fell down to the foot. The smallest deviation from the right diet is immediately punished by limping and lameness and the innocent ankle and blameless instep are tortured for the vices of the nobler organs. A plum, a glass of champagne, excess in joy, excess in grief, any crisis however small is sufficient for redness, swelling and large shoes. Gout is the only enemy that I do not wish to have in my feet."[14]

Gout has historically been known as a disease of the higher social strata since it has been known to occur after dietary and alcholic indiscretions as well as during periods of emotional turmoil. Today the disease might be considered a status symbol if it were to fall to Vance Packard's classification. Recently the origin of the word "gout" has been reviewed by Hartung.[5] It is interesting that for 2000 years it was called arthritis and podagra, the latter literally meaning a trap for the feet. Chiragra was the term used by Aretaeus to refer

to the arthritic symptoms in the hands. Since various humors were thought by medical leaders of antiquity to be fundamental in understanding disease, arthritis was considered a flowing of humors or fluid from one part of the body to another. Thus the word rheumatism is derived from the root rheuma which literally means flowing. Gout comes from the Latin gutta, literally meaning a drop, referring to the humoral concept of the disease. Tophus is from the Greek tofus, meaning rough, crumbling rock.

Clinically, the disease is divided into primary and secondary gout. Primary gout is undoubtedly an inherited metabolic trait.[15] Secondary gout occurs secondary to other diseases, largely those of the myelopathic group such as a polycythemia vera, hemolytic anemia, lymphomas, leukema, and pernicious anemia with liver therapy.[19] The disease is relatively common, occurring in approximately 1 per cent of the population. It is generally a long-term, progressive malady with intermittency of symptoms a classic feature. It is painful and disabling and results in multiple complications if untreated. These fall into the categories of renal calculi, tophaccous deposits in bones, joints, bursa, tendons, blood vessels, the mitral valve and cardiac muscle, nephrosclerosis with deposits in the renal parenchyma hypertension, and atherosclerosis.

Mustard *et al.*[10] have shown clotting mechanisms to be more active than normal in gout.

PATHOGENESIS

There is a positive family history in approximately 15 per cent of patients with primary gout.[11] Talbott[20] has noted that approximately 20 per cent of next of kin of gouty patients have an increase in uric acid in the serum without other evidence of gout. It seems that the human organism is capable of synthesis of uric acid from carbon dioxide glycine and ammonia and that dietary purines contribute only small amounts of uric acid to the "miscible pool" of uric acid within the body.[11]

There has been controversy on the part of the educated theorists concerning the mechanism for hyperuricemia. There is general increasing support for the overproduction theory against the renal reabsorption theory for the hyperuricemia in gout.[17] Weingaarden[22] in his study of the intermediary purine metabolism, feels that the overproduction of urates in primary gout is entirely tenable on the basis of biochemical analyses. Kelly and his associates[6] have reported that some patients with gout have deficiencies of the enzyme hypoxanthine-guanine phosphoribosyltransferase and the overproduction of uric acid.

There is increasing evidence that acute symptoms of gouty arthritis are due to crystal inflammation, that is, crystals of uric acid free within the joints causing chemotaxis, phagocytosis by polymorphonuclear-leukocytes, and then liberation of lysosomal enzymes which cause the inflammation.[3] Still the exact interaction of all the various factors has not been worked out.

CLINICAL PICTURE IN GOUT

The classic clinical picture of acute gouty arthritis is such that if one's index of suspicion is attuned he would be unlikely to miss the diagnosis of gout. The sudden onset of severe pain in an otherwise healthy man after some characteristic provocation with complete subsidence in several days without residual symptoms is standard. A dramatic response to colchicine and an elevated serum uric acid are substantiating factors in the diagnosis. The characteristic history of sudden onset coupled with extremely severe pain, with the duration of the first attack being five to 10 days, should prompt the physician to search for the other important diagnostic features. Nearly 50 per cent begin with podagra (great toe involvement). The characteristic purple-red color resembles cellulitis.[11] There is extension into neighboring soft tissues around the primary involved joint with marked tenderness, swelling, and redness. After six or seven days desquamation over the site of inflammation is characteristic. Acute gouty arthritis may affect any joint or bursa, and occasionally the patient may present with an acute tenosynovitis of the upper extremity. The disease may initially occur at any age but generally the younger the patient the more likely he is to have a polyarticular onset. It is classically a disease of men, although it is said to occur in women 5 per cent of the time.[11][15] The precipitating factors in initiating the first attack may be surgery, emotional or physical stress, injections of liver or thiamine, diuretic drug use, recent excess of food or alcohol, transfusion, penicillin, or chlorothiazide (for hypertension). Dietary contents which are high in purines may initiate the first attack. These food substances are liver, kidney, sweetbreads, anchovies, and rich gravies. High intake of fats and alcohol also are known to provoke gouty arthritis. In an acute attack of gouty arthritis, there may be leukocytosis, elevation of sedimentation rate, mild albuminuria, and frequently, although not reliably, an elevation of serum uric acid. The serum uric acid is elevated in 75 per cent of cases at some time in the disease.[11] The finding of uric acid elevation is helpful in making the diagnosis but it cannot be relied on to rule out gout as the diagnosis. Certain drugs are uricosuric and may create a false-positive uric acid elevation. Such drugs are the salicylates, steroids, phenylbutazone or its analogs, probenecid, ethyl biscoumacetate (Tromexan), and bishydroxycoumarin (Dicumerol). Certain diseases also may create a false positive elevation in uric acid. Such diseases as urticaria, chronic eczema, and psoriasis are examples of this. The 24-hour urinary excretion of uric acid is usually elevated in patients with gout, but this test is rarely positive without elevation of the serum uric acid. More recently snyovial fluid has been studied for crystals with positive findings in gout.[7]

Graham[4] has pointed out that gout frequently goes unrecongized because it is not considered by the examining physician. The reasons given for this are that it is thought by many to be a European disease, although in fact it is more common in North America than it is in Europe at present. The classic, obese, red-faced "Colonel Blimp" is not the usual picture. Dependence on uric acid elevation with dismissal of gout when the level is normal results not infrequently in diagnostic failure. The dependence on absence of tophi with the finding of podagra and reliance on x-ray which is negative in early gout are other factors mitigating against one's suspicious of gout. The periodicity of attack of acute gouty arthritis at 6-, 12-, to 18-month intervals is frequently diagnostic. In uric acid analyses the upper limit of normal is 5 mg per 100 cc in men with a lower range for gouty men at 6 mg per 100 cc. Both of these figures are slightly lower in women as a general rule.

CHRONIC GOUTY ARTHRITIS

Repeated intermittent attacks of acute gouty arthritis may lead imperceptibly into the chronic articular changes typical of chronic gout. With the passage of time urate crystals are deposited radially in superficial portions of articular cartilages, in synovial and capsular tissues, in periarticular tissues, tendons, and subchondral bone marrow (Figs. 8.4.1, 8.4.2, 8.4.3, and 8.4.4). These geographic locations suggest that

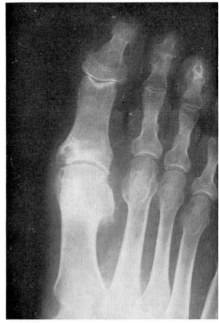

Figure 8.4.1. Classic roentgenographic changes in the great toe in chronic gouty arthritis. Urate deposition has resulted in radiolucent month-eaten appearance adjacent to the metatarsophalangeal joint.

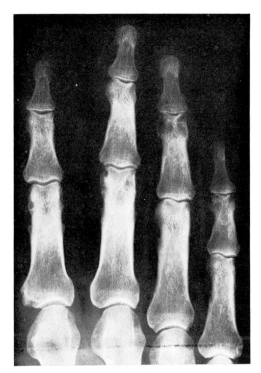

Figure 8.4.2. Involvement of hand phalanges with typical periarticular decalcification and destruction in chronic gout. Punched-out areas represent interosseous tophi.

the urates enter from the synovial fluid. The affected portions of cartilage undergo nonspecific degenerative changes with disintegration which leads to a picture not unlike osteoarthritis. Massive obliteration of joint structures occurs and chronic topaceous synovitis appears. The punched-out lesions of bone that occur in the epiphyseal areas of bone represent marrow tophus deposits replacing calcium salts. With the deposition of uric acid salts in bone and articular areas during the chronic stage of gout, deposits also occur elsewhere forming typical tophi. Commonly these occur in the ear, over the olecranon bursa, and in the Achilles area. Tophi may be studied for diagnostic confirmation by polarized light microscopy for crystals. Uric acid crystals dissolve in formalin; therefore, materials must be fixed in absolute alcohol for pathologic study. Whether the deposit of urates is metastatic that is a result of excessive quantity of uric acid in blood presented to tissues from exogenous or endogenous sources, or whether the deposits are dystrophic occurring as a result of urate deposition in tissue because the latter have undergone some primary pathologic alteration is as yet unclear. The tophus is a multicentric deposit of urate crystals with intercrystalline matrix. A typical foreign body granuloma is evoked by the presence of crystalline uric acid in tissues. In the chronic stage of gout the differential diagnosis may present some difficulty. By x-ray, chronic

gout shows characteristic cystic changes in the epiphyseal portion of bone as well as cartilage and synovial destruction[8] (Figs. 8.4.5, 8.5.6, and 8.4.7). Differentiation from acute rheumatic fever, rheumatoid arthritis, and osteoarthritis must be made. Helpful facts in making the differential diagnosis are the following: statistically women are more likely to be suffering from rheumatoid arthritis than gout; the duration of the acute attack is longer in rheumatoid arthritis than the short, totally reversible period of five to 10 days in acute gouty arthritis; in rheumatoid arthritis the cystic areas in bone by x-ray are located peripherally in the

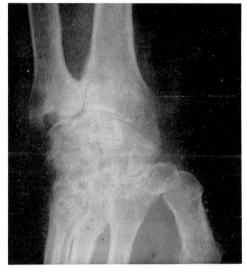

Figure 8.4.3. Chronic gout with involvement of the radius, ulna, and carpals. Perisynovial location suggests deposition from joint fluid or concentration in the synovia.

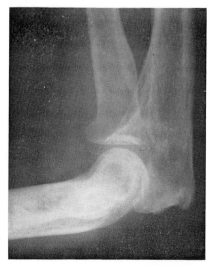

Figure 8.4.4. Tophaceous deposits present in olecranon bursa. Note changes in the olecranon.

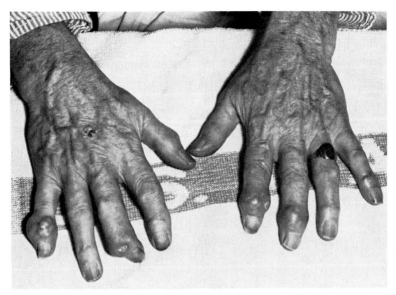

Figure 8.4.5. Urate deposits forming soft tissue tophi adjacent to phalangeal joints. The chemical foreign bodies in this case set the stage for infection which finally resulted in the fifth digit amputation for sepsis.

heads of the phalanges. The hands are more suscep-tible than the feet in rheumatoid arthritis, and the hands show characteristic coolness and hyperhydrosis in rheumatoid disease which does not appear in gout. Excessive synovial fluid in the proximal interpha-langeal joints with involvement of the metacarpo-phalangeal joints is characteristic in rheumatoid ar-thritis. C-reactive protein and sheep cell agglutina-tions are positive only in rheumatic disease, not in gout. The differential diagnosis may rest on cell counts and differential, Ropes test, or polarized light microscopy of synovial fluid or may rest on chemical or histologic examination of biopsy of a nodule, syno-vial tissue, or a section of bone. At least 10 per cent of patients with well developed rheumatoid arthritis will have a uric acid concentration greater than 6 mg per 100 cc which makes it an invalid single factor on which the differentiation can be made.[8] In osteoar-thritis, acute articular episodes are unusual and al-though Heberden's nodes may suggest small urate de-posits, the x-ray changes in hypertrophic osteoarthritis are so classically different from those in gout that the differential diagnosis should not be difficult with the usual laboratory studies. In the x-ray study of patients with gout the recent introduction of a magnification procedure has permitted a more precise evaluation of the changes. Talbott *et al.,*[18] in discussing the x-ray findings, point out that early decalcifications progress-ing to complete loss of calcium in the cystic areas are easier to identify with the magnification technique. Subchondral bone is the usual site of early changes in gout as noted by x-ray. Subcutaneous tophi may be identified by x-ray as soft tissue swelling but the tophi are usually radiolucent, although occasionally they are calcified and more radiopaque.

TREATMENT OF GOUT

In discussing treatment, one must summarize the above discussion by stating that gout appears to be a disease of stages and each stage will require different treatment.[11] [20] [21]

Stage 1: Asymptomatic hyperuricemia. Because few patients with hyperuricemia develop gouty ar-thritis there is serious question of whether any medical treatment is indicated. If, on the other hand there is hyperuricosuria not controlled by diet and increased fluid intake, treatment is indicated to prevent renal stones. Diet, with omission of high purine foods and a single uricosuric agent, such as high dosage of salicy-lates (greater than 3 gm/day), or probenecid (Benemid 1.5 to 2.5 gm/day) and a large fluid intake are adequate to control the disease, prevent renal stone formation, and avoid overt attacks of acute gouty ar-thritis.

Stage 2: Acute gouty arthritis with complete remis-sion between attacks. The first acute arthritic attack of gout is best treated with colchicine as response to this drug is helpful in the diagnosis of gout. Prescribe 0.65 mg colchicine with one glass of hot water hourly for six to eight doses depending on the development of gastrointestinal symptoms, nausea, or diarrhea. Gen-erally the colchicine dosage must be pushed to near gastrointestinal toxicity to become effective in abating the acute attack. Response to treatment is rapid and gratifying. A repeat course is given in 48 hours, if there is still troublesome joint pain. Colchicine's ef-fect in acute gout appears to be the inhibition of chemotaxis, thereby stopping inflammation.[9]

For subsequent attacks, after the diagnosis is thoroughly established, the drug of choice appears to

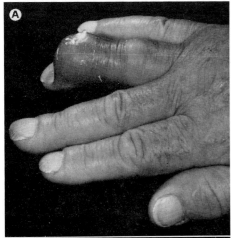

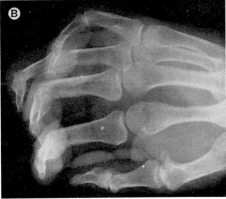

Figure 8.4.6. A. Sinus tract from a digital urate deposit in gout. Here a portal of entry and urate foreign body have set the stage for sepsis. *B.* Note bone and interphalangeal joint changes as well as soft tissue deposition of urates.

be phenylbutazone or oxyphenylbutazone (generally 200 mg three times a day for three to five days),[8] because these drugs are usually not associated with the gastrointestinal morbidity seen with colchicine. These drugs do, however, produce rare, but serious, side affects on occasion. For such short duration therapy, this would most usually be activation of a gastric or duodenal ulcer. Such an ulcer would be an absolute contraindication. If the gouty arthritis attack occurs postoperatively and the patient is not able to take drugs by mouth, a single dose of 3 mg of colchicine has been found to be helpful and by giving the drug intravenously, gastrointestinal symptoms are bypassed.

Stage 3: Chronic gouty arthritis with or without tophus formation. The institution of diet, uricosuric drug, colchicine, and physical therapy has been recommended for this stage. Surgical excision of tophi is recommended especially if ulceration is iminent. A large fluid intake is helpful in avoiding progressive tophus formation.

In chronic gout which has gone untreated, large

tophi and cystic changes in bone will have already occurred. It is gratifying to know that some of these changes are reversible.[1] Tophi may decrease in size and the cystic areas in bone may recalcify on proper treatment. Improved renal function may also be achieved by appropriate treatment. The best treatment is to avoid late problems by institution of proper therapy early in the disease after its recognition. Bartels[1] has shown dramatic evidence of reversal of destructive changes in bone.

Renal changes occur in gout and there has been controversial discussion as to the possible renal origin of the disease.[16] [17] [22] Renal insufficiency is frequent in chronic gout. Gout patients are repeatedly prone to the development of hypertensive and arteriosclerotic vascular diseases which may have their basis in renal changes. There are specific anatomic lesions in the kidney with microtophaceous rate deposits in the renal pyramids giving rise to gout nephrosis. The severity of renal changes is not always in proportion to the skeletal changes and the name primary renal gout has been given to gout nephrosis with apparent articular disease.

If the kidneys are functioning properly Probenecid appears to be the drug of choice in chronic gout. The dose of the drug must be titrated for the patient with frequent checks of the serum uric acid level.

If the patient has renal disease, Allopurinol may be used with caution. This drug is an inhibitor of xanthine oxidase which is important in the production of uric acid. Oxipurinol is another xanthine oxidase inhibitor and both drugs in addition to this function, have been shown to inhibit early steps of purine synthesis. Again, these drugs must be used in varying doses (200 to 800 mg/day) to titrate the level of blood uric acid desired. The prescribing physician must be aware of the many complications from the use of this drug before it is prescribed. Such information may be found in the literature accompanying the drug or in recent articles such as The Drug Letter written by Stanley L. Wallace.[21] If the drug is used, small doses of colchicine

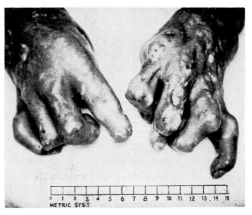

Figure 8.4.7. Far advanced destructive gouty arthritis in a patient who had suffered from chronic gout for several decades.

may be given along with these xanthine oxidase inhibitors to prevent the acute gouty attacks that occasionally occur with mobilization of uric acid from the joints.

SURGERY IN GOUT

Surgical intervention is reserved for complications of gout where medical therapy cannot reverse the physical changes.

Surgery has no role in the management of acute gout. Acute synovial and articular disease is completely reversible by proper medical management.

Chronic gout not infrequently results in deformity which can be diminished by surgical intervention. Symptomatic and unsightly tophi can be excised but the patient must know that recurrence is likely unless diligent medical management is adhered to. Breakdown of soft tissue with sinus tract formation should be treated by tophus excision wherever anatomically possible. This may avoid secondary bacterial infection. Established progressive infection requires vigorous surgical therapy.

A constant high index of suspicion of gout in any patient with severe, sudden joint discomfort should be the watchword of surgeons who examine hands frequently. One of the historical figures in hand anatomy, Wood Jones, had the disease and is said to have stated during an acute attack that if he sees a fly on the ceiling of his bedroom he is filled with consternation, lest the fly lose its hold and drop on his foot.[4] Such descriptions of the acute pain and tenderness in joints involved with articular gout should be constantly borne in mind as we deal with our daily patient examinations.

REFERENCES

1. Bartels, E. Treatment of gout. In *Symposium on Gout*. Metabolism, *6:* 297-307, 1957.
2. Graham, W., and Graham, K.M. Martyrs to the gout. In *Symposium on Gout*. Metabolism, *6:* 209, 1957.
3. Gout and Uric Acid Metabolism. Nineteenth Rheumatism Review, Arthritis Rheum., *13:* 557, 1970.
4. Graham, W. Gout and gouty arthritis. Postgrad. Med., *30:* 555, 1961.
5. Hartung, E. Historical considerations. In *Symposium on Gout*. Metabolism, *6:* 196, 1957.
6. Kelley, W.N., Rosenbloom, F.M., Henderson, J.F., *et al.* A specific enzyme defect in gout associated with overproduction of uric acid. Proc. Natl. Acad. Sci., *57:* 1735, 1967.
7. Kohn, N.N., Hughes, R.E., McCarty, D.J., Jr., and Faires, J.S. The significance of calcium phosphate crystals in the synovial fluid of arthritic patients: The "pseudogout syndrome," II. Identification of crystals. Ann. Intern. Med., *56:* 738, 1962.
8. Lockie, L.M. Diagnosis. In *Symposium on Gout*. Metabolism, *6:* 269, 1957.
9. Malawista, S.E., and Seegmiller, J.E. The effect of pretreatment with cholchicine on the inflammatory response to microcrystalline urate. Ann. Intern. Med., *62:* 648, 1965.
10. Mustard, J.F., Digby, J.W., Montgomery, D.B., and Ogryzlo, M.A. Blood coagulation in gout and its relation to atherosclerosis. Second American Congress on Rheumatic Diseases, 1959.
11. Rottenberg, E.N. Diagnosis and treatment of gout. J. Mich. State Med. Soc., *60:* 1304, 1961.
12. Seegmiller, J.E., Howell, R.R., and Malawista, S.E. The imflammatory reaction to sodium urate, its possible relationship to the genesis to acute gouty arthritis. J.A.M.A., *180:* 469, 1962.
13. Smith, G.E., and Jones, F.W. *The Archeological Survey of Nubia,* Report for 1907-08, Vol. 2. Cairo National Printing Department, 1910, pp. 44, 269.
14. Smith, S. *Letters of Sydney Smith.* Toronto, Oxford University Press, 1954.
15. Smyth, C. Hereditary factors in gout. In *Symposium on Gout*. Metabolism, *6:* 218, 1957.
16. Sokoloff, L. The pathology of gout. In *Symposium on Gout*. Metabolism, *6:* 230, 1957.
17. Stetten, D., Talbott, J. H., Seegmiller, J. E., Wyngaarden, J.B., and Laster, L. The pathogenesis of gout. Letter to the Editor. Metabolism, *6:* 88, 1957.
18. Talbott, J.H., Culver, G.J., Mizraji, J., and Crespo, D.I. Roentgenographic findings — description of a magnification technic. Metabolism, *6:* 277, 1957.
19. Talbott, J.H. Blood dyscrasias and gout. Medicine, *38:* 173, 1959.
20. Talbott, J.H. The diagnosis and treatment of gout. Med. Clin. North Am., *45:* 1489, 1961.
21. Wallace, L. The treatment of gout. Arthritis Rheum., *15:* 317, 1972.
22. Wyngaarden, J.B. Intermediary purine metabolism and the metabolis defects of gout. In *Symposium on Gout*. Metabolism, *6:* 244, 1957.

E.

Flexible Implant Resection Arthroplasty in the Upper Extremity

Alfred B. Swanson, M.D., F.A.C.S.
G. de Groot Swanson, M.D.

One of the most interesting challenges of reconstructive surgery is to restore function to the joints of the hand and the upper extremity.[2] Appropriate treatment includes synovectomy, release of tendons and joints, reconstruction of tendons, arthroplasty, and arthrodesis.[19, 40, 41, 43]

Attempts to replace joints with metal implants have met with mixed success and limited acceptance, for in most cases the bone has not tolerated the metal. Bone absorption and metal corrosion have negated many of the early good results obtained. However, the concept of prosthetic joint replacement is excellent since restoration of early motion with some joint stability has obvious advantages over resection arthroplasty or joint fusion. The development of synthetic materials which can be used in the human body has provided new approach to joint reconstruction by resection arthroplasty, especially in the upper extremity.[22]

PRINCIPLES OF IMPLANT RESECTION ARTHROPLASTY

The basic concepts for using flexible implants for arthroplasty surgery differ from the total joint replacement idea. These differences are important to understand for the proper application of these implants in the selection of patients, correct surgical and postoperative techniques. The ideal arthroplasty should be mobile, stable, pain-free, and durable. The flexible implant is a dynamic spacer used as an adjunct to resection arthroplasty. The use of a well designed flexible implant with appropriate operative and postoperative technique will help to: (1) obtain more predictable results immediately and later; (2) improve the range of motion; (3) provide better relief of pain; (4) achieve greater stability; (5) facilitate rehabilitation.

The perfect implant requires proper design and the development of the ideal implant material. This requires a compromised balance of: (1) Engineering principles; (2) Anatomic factors; (3) Physical characteristics of material; (4) Patient's needs.

Flexible Implant Characteristics

Since 1962 we have carried out a full time research project (John A. Hartford Foundation, Inc.) for the development of flexible implants for reconstructive surgery of the extremities. The use of silicone rubber for implants to replace diseased or destroyed joints was suggested by our previous experience in developing an intramedullary-stemmed silicone rubber implant to cushion the end of long bones in lower extremity amputations to improve their weight-bearing characteristics.[21] Since that time we have designed, developed, tested mechanically and in laboratory animals 23 different silicone rubber implants (Silastic,® Dow Corning Corporation, Midland, Michigan). The most frequently used flexible implants in humans include those to replace the metacarpophalangeal and proximal interphalangeal joints of the fingers,[23 24 27 28 34] the trapezium,[29 35] carpal scaphoid and lunate,[30] the ulnar and radial heads, the wrist, elbow, and shoulder joints,[37] the tibial plateau, the first metatarsophalangeal joint,[36] and to control the bone overgrowth problem in the juvenile amputee (Fig. 8.5.1). The implants are made in a variety of sizes and can be sterilized by autoclaving.

Flexible implants have been used in more than 10,000 patients in most countries in the world and carefully evaluated in our own clinic and in 293 participating Field Clinics. The results of our clinical,

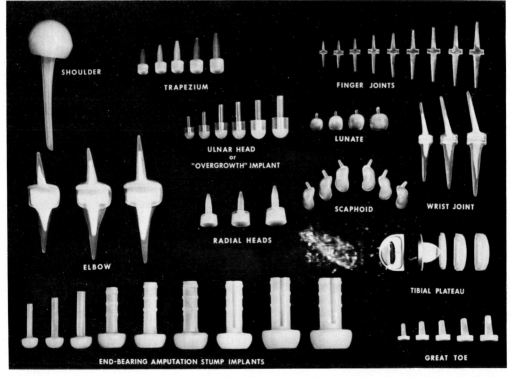

Figure 8.5.1. The 12 most frequently used flexible implants for reconstructive procedures of the extremities.

roentgenographic, and biochemical evaluation of these implants has demonstrated that silicone rubber is well tolerated by the host tissues and that it has been both physically and chemically stable. The silicone rubbers are heat-stable, do not appear to deteriorate in time,[3][18][42] they have excellent flexion characteristics and force-dampening properties but will tear if a laceration occurs in the surface. Correct design of the prosthesis can greatly improve the flexural durability of the silicone implant. Machine-testing has shown that a one piece, heat-vulcanized implant has much better wear advantages than a hand-carved or hand-molded implant or one that is reinforced with Dacron or other materials. The medical-grade silicones with which we are dealing do not produce tissue reaction when properly sterilized and should not be confused with industrial silicones that have additives which may be toxic. They are as biologically inert as any material known and, being softer than bone, they are not so likely to stimulate bone absorption as metal implants.

Development of a flexible, heat-molded silicone rubber implant for MP and PIP joint arthroplasties has proceeded through many changes in design. Eight years of testing were involved in the development of the final design. The latest model has been machine tested for more than 600 million flexions without evidence of breakdown (Fig. 8.5.2).

Concept of Fixation by Encapsulation

"Joint Resection + Implant + Capsule
= New Joint"

Simple joint resection arthroplasty works well in the hand if the joint space and alignment can be maintained. This can frequently be achieved only by prolonged postoperative fixation with pins and external support that may decrease the expected range of motion. In a considerable number of these cases, the joint space gradually narrows and stiffness and subluxation may result. Excellent results do occur, however, if an adequate supportive fibrous joint capsule develops during the period when a guarded range of progressive motion is started.

In finger arthroplasty, it is difficult to obtain the proper amount of flexion-extension, appropriate lateral movement and reduction of dorsopalmar subluxation necessary for a good result. Therefore, one of the most important functions of a flexible implant is to act as a dynamic joint spacer to provide sufficient internal stability to maintain the alignment and space between the bone ends while early motion is started. Early motion is essential to promote the development of a new functionally adapted fibrous capsule. The finger joint silicone rubber intramedullary stemmed implant is a flexible hinge that acts as an internal mold for this important phenomenon which we have named the "encapsulation concept."[26] In the early stages of healing, the orientation and the tension of the developing capsule are extremely important. In fact, the immediate

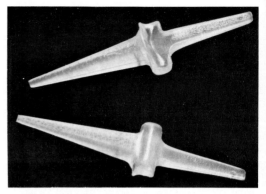

Figure 8.5.2. The flexible intramedullary stemmed silicone rubber finger joint implant acts as a dynamic spacer to maintain proper joint alignment and spacing. It serves as an internal mold to support the new capsuloligamentous system which develops around the implant. The stems of the implant are not fixed. This allows a slight gliding of the implant stems in the intramedullary canals. This implant has been used successfully in more than 10,000 patients around the world.

postoperative positioning and control of joint movement during the first six to eight weeks after reconstruction by dynamic bracing and physiotherapy are as important as surgery itself.[31]

Because the implant becomes so well stabilized by the encapsulation process, it is felt that no other fixation of the implant is required and, in fact, is contraindicated. Fixation of an implant with crossed pins, cement or a Dacron cover[12] on the intramedullary stems has led to early breakage of the implant at the junction of the stem and the central portion such as noted in our earlier cases and mechanical testing.[15] We have demonstrated that lateral stability could not be obtained simply by fixing the stems of the flexible implant and, in fact, it becomes decreased in time because of bone absorption. We have now removed most of these implants and found that the Dacron in a synovial lined cavity causes severe inflammatory reactions which in turn enlarges the joint capsule and results in instability. An implant should cause no inflammatory reaction if it is to be long tolerated. The smooth stems of our flexible implants are included in the encapsulation process and the implant glides one or two millimeters on flexion-extension movements. A slight amount of piston movement of the stems increases the life of the implant because forces that are developed around the implant on flexion and extension movements are not concentrated in one particular area but rather spread over a broader section. The surrounding bone is also protected from excessive stress. Gliding of the implant also allows a greater range of motion to occur and permits the flexible implant to find the best position with respect to the axis of rotation of the joint. A rigid implant or one fixed tightly would not have this advantage. The gliding, flexible implant, therefore, is subjected to less strain and in turn causes less stress on the surrounding bone.

Preparation of the Implant

Medical-grade silicone elastomers are extremely inert but, if contaminated by lint, fingerprints, and other foreign materials, they can cause a foreign body reaction. Every effort should be made to eliminate the chance of contamination throughout the entire procedure. The implants should be handled with instruments rather than gloves. The following cleaning and sterilization procedure is recommended if the implants become contaminated and are not sterilized before packaging:

1. Boil the implants in distilled water and a nonoily soap for 20 minutes.
2. Rinse thoroughly in distilled water.
3. Wrap in lint-free cloth or place in a clean open tray and autoclave by one of the following methods: (a) High speed instrument sterilizer, 3 min at 270° F; (b) Standard gravity sterilizer, 30 min at 250° F; (c) Prevacuum high-temperature sterilizer, normal cycle at 250° F.

SURGICAL TECHNIQUE

Arthroplasty and reconstructive surgery of the upper limb requires consideration of the following factors: (1) good general condition of the patient; (2) good neurovascular status; (3) adequate skin cover; (4) sufficient bone stock; (5) possibility of a functional musculotendinous system; (6) availability of good postoperative therapy; (7) a cooperative patient. Specific indications for each procedure are listed separately.

THE METACARPOPHALANGEAL JOINT

Indications

Indications for flexible implant arthroplasty of this joint are a fixed or stiff joint, roentgenographic evidence of joint destruction or subluxation, ulnar drift not correctable by surgery of the soft tissues alone, contracted intrinsic and extrinsic muscles, and associated stiff interphalangeal joints.[33] Excessive manual labor and awkward hand weight bearing such as occasionally occurs in some crutch walkers should be avoided after surgery.

Surgical Technique

The technique described below is for a rheumatoid hand (Fig. 8.5.3). A transverse skin incision is made on the dorsum of the hand over the necks of the metacarpals. The dorsal veins which lie between the metacarpal heads are carefully released longitudinally and retracted laterally. The radial portion of the extensor hood is usually stretched out and the extensor tendon displaced ulnarward. A longitudinal incision is made over the ulnar aspect of the extensor hood paral-

lel to the extensor tendon. The hood and capsule are carefully dissected from the underlying synovium, preserved and retracted to the radial side to expose the metacarpal head.

The neck of the metacarpal is transected with an air drill, motor saw, or cutting forceps leaving part of the flair of the metaphysis. The head of the metacarpal is then grasped, the collateral ligament and capsular attachments are incised and the head with the attached synovial tissue are removed "en masse." A pituitary rongeur is then used to complete the synovectomy of the joint cavity.

A comprehensive soft tissue release is essential so that the base of the proximal phalanx can be displaced dorsal to the metacarpal. This may require division of the palmar plate and the collateral ligaments at their attachments to the proximal phalanx. The insertion of the ulnar intrinsic tendon is identified and pulled up into the wound with a blunt hook and, if it is tight, it is sectioned at the myotendinous junction. The tendons of the abductor digiti minimi and flexor digiti minimi are identified on the ulnar aspect of the fifth metacarpophalangeal joint and sectioned, taking care to preserve the ulnar digital nerve.

The intramedullary canal of the metacarpal is prepared with a curette, broach, or air drill with a special smooth leader point (Hall International, Inc., Santa Barbara, California) that prevents from cutting through the cortex of the metacarpal. No bone resection is performed at the base of the proximal phalanx except for trimming of marginal osteophytes. Too much reaming of the canals should be avoided especially in patients with thin bones. Test implants are used to select the proper size. The stem of the implant should fit well down into the canal so that the transverse midsection of the implant abuts against the bone end. The largest possible implant should be used (usually sizes 4 through 8). Reshaping of the implant should be avoided because modification might create mechanical weakness. Shortening of the end of the stem is permissible.

A rectangular hole is made in the joint surface of the proximal phalanx with an osteotome, knife, broach, or air drill and the intramedullary canal is reamed in the same fashion as for the metacarpal. The end of the bones should be free of any sharp points that might damage the implant surface.

The wound is thoroughly irrigated with saline to remove all debris. The implants are inserted with blunt instruments using a no-touch technique. The proximal stem of the implant is first inserted into the metacarpal intramedullary canal. The distal stem is then flexed and guided into the proximal phalanx with the joint flexed and distracted. With the joint in extension there should be no impingement of the bone ends on the implant. If so, either the soft tissue release or bone resection has been inadequate.

The radial portion of the sagittal fibers of each extensor hood is reefed in an overlapping fashion to bring the extensor tendon slightly to the radial side of

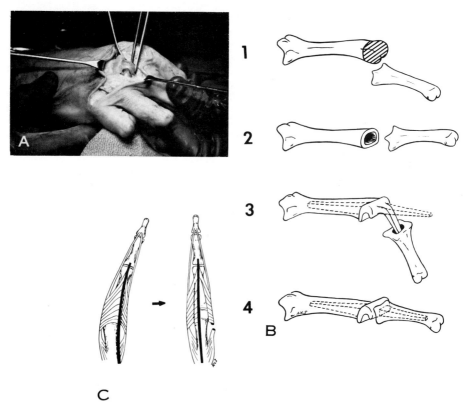

Figure 8.5.3. Operative technique for the MP joint. *A.* Through a transverse skin incision, the metacarpal heads are exposed taking care to preserve the longitudinal views. *B.* The metacarpal heads are removed leaving part of the flair of the metaphysis. A synovectomy of the joint is performed. It is essential to reduce completely the joint by resection of bone and release of all soft tissue contractures. On passive extension of the joint, there should be no impingement of the midsection of the implant by the bone edges. *C.* The ulnar aspect of the extensor hood is incised longitudinally parallel to the extensor tendon. The ulnar intrinsics, if tight, are sectioned at the myotendinous junction. The extensor tendon is brought slightly to the radial side of the center of the joint by reefing the radial side of the extensor hood.

the center of the joint. From three to five 4-0 Dacron sutures are used with a buried-knot technique.

Occasionally in patients who have an inadequate first dorsal interosseous muscle or a tendency for pronation deformity of the index finger, a reconstruction of the radial collateral ligament of the metacarpophalangeal joint is indicated. A distally based flap is made from the radial half of the palmar plate and related capsular structures which are separated from the underlying intrinsic muscles and flexor tendons. This flap which would be 1½ to 2 cm in length and 5 to 8 mm wide, is attached around the radial aspect of the neck of the metacarpal to a hole in the dorsal-radial cortex of the neck of the bone (Fig. 8.5.4).

The skin incision is closed with 5-0 nylon sutures and two small drains made of strips of silicone sheeting are inserted under the skin. A voluminous conforming hand dressing is applied with a narrow plaster splint fitted to the palmar aspect (Fig. 8.5.5). During the postoperative period, elevation of the hand and forearm is maintained with a special sling attached to a intravenous stand.

The wound is inspected on the second day and the drains are removed. On the third or fifth postoperative day, a light dressing is applied to the hand and forearm and the dynamic brace (Pope Brace Co., Kankakee, Illinois) is fitted to allow the patient to start finger movement through a protected arc of 0° to 90° of flexion[31] (Fig. 8.5.6). The joints have a tendency to tighten up during the second week after surgery. Therefore, early flexion-extension movements in a slightly radially deviated position are encouraged within the limits of the patient's pain and fatigue. Gonimeter readings of joint flexion should be recorded. If the patient does not reach or maintain 70° of flexion, the flexion cuff should be used one to two hours three to four times a day to encourage flexion passively. The extension part of the brace is usually worn night and day for three weeks except by the patients who may require intermittent flexion assistance.

The brace is then worn at night for approximately three more weeks and sometimes longer by patients who have a tendency for extensor tendon lag or recurrent deformity. Bracing should be continued until the patient has a suitable range of motion. A carefully controlled follow-up and rehabilitation program should be provided including passive and active movements for at least three months postoperatively.

Surgery on a rheumatoid extremity should not last more than one and a half to two hours. The steps of the surgical technique must be carefully followed. The longitudinal arch of the hand must be rebalanced including the wrist joint or collapse deformity of the digits using temporary Kirschner wire fixation of the proximal interphalangeal joints as necessary. Other associated reconstructions of the thumb, proximal distal interphalangeal joints, the wrist and elbow may be performed at the same sitting depending on the time involved. Frequently other affected joints of the lower extremity, such as the knee or foot, can be operated simultaneously by another surgical team.

PROXIMAL INTERPHALANGEAL JOINT

The proximal interphalangeal joint can be disabled by rheumatoid, degenerative, and traumatic arthritis. The deformities presented are usually a swan-neck deformity, a boutonniere deformity, or a fixed flexion or extension deformity.[33] Treatment of the deformities of

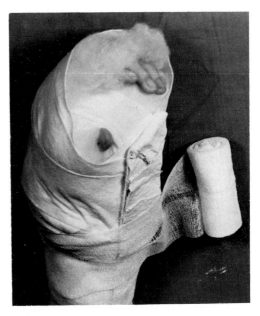

Figure 8.5.5. Gauze fluffs are placed loosely between the fingers. A roll of Dacron batting is placed across the palm and on the dorsal and palmar aspects of the hand and forearm. A short palmar plaster splint is applied and a nonelastic type bandage such as Kling is used to secure the dressing. The completed dressing which should support the wrist and fingers in a functional position is worn for three to five days.

the interphalangeal joints is challenging, not only because of the destruction of the joints, but also because of the often associated muscle imbalances.[13][20] Restoration of a stable, mobile, pain-free proximal interphalangeal joint is an important consideration to restore reasonable hand function.[4][7][11] The distal interphalangeal joint should also be placed in the position for best function.

Indications

Implant resection arthroplasty of the proximal interphalangeal joint is indicated for destroyed or subluxated joints, stiffened joints when simple soft tissue release would be inadequate.

Resection arthroplasty for severe disability of the proximal interphalangeal joint using an intramedullary stemmed flexible implant has been successful if enough bone stock is present and if an adequate tendon mechanism can be reconstructed.[10][32] An arthrodesis of the index proximal interphalangeal joint in 40° of flexion and implant resection arthroplasty of the other fingers would be preferable for a man doing heavy work. The more stable index finger can be used for pinch activities and the flexion obtained from arthroplasty of the other digits should facilitate grasping.

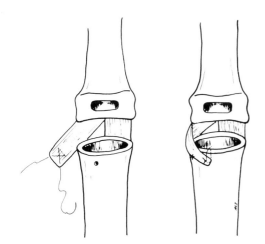

Figure 8.5.4. Reconstruction of the radial collateral ligament of the MP joint: The palmar plate and its attachments are incised longitudinally through the middle. The sesamoid bone, if present, is resected. A distally based flap of 1½ to 2 cm is made of the radial portion of the palmar plate and collateral ligament which are separated from the underlying intrinsic muscle and tendon. This flap is attached around the radial aspect of the neck of the metacarpal to a hole in the dorsal radial portion of the bone with non-absorbable suture material.

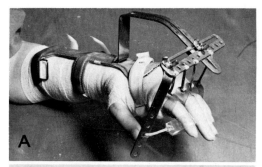

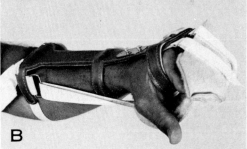

Figure 8.5.6. A. The adjustable dynamic brace is placed over a slightly padded dressing after the third to fifth day. Early flexion-extension movements are encouraged in a slightly radially deviated position. *B.* A flexion cuff may be used intermittently to assist flexion movements. Proper use of bracing is essential to ensure an adequate range of motion.

Surgical Technique

A longitudinal S-shaped incision is made over the dorsum of the joint, taking care to protect the dorsal veins. If surgery of the flexor-tendon mechanism is also indicated, a midlateral incision is used. The extensor mechanism is exposed by blunt dissection. The central tendon is incised longitudinally from its insertion on the base of the middle phalanx proximally along the distal two-thirds of the proximal phalanx. Each half of the extensor mechanism is gently dislocated palmarward as the joint is flexed. The collateral ligaments are released from their attachment to the proximal phalanx, but the distal insertion of the central tendon must be left intact. If the extensor mechanism cannot be dislocated, the head of the proximal phalanx is sectioned transversely through the neck with an air drill and then removed piecemeal. The collateral and accessory collateral ligaments are completely released from the proximal phalanx. Adequate release of the joint is essential for a good result. If there is a flexion contracture, this may require excision of the collateral and accessory collateral ligaments and the palmar plate.

The intramedullary canal of the proximal phalanx is carefully reamed and shaped with the smooth leader tip burr to accept the rectangular stem of the implant. The intramedullary canal of the middle phalanx is pre-

pared in a similar fashion. The base of the middle phalanx is not resected but osteophytes, if present, are trimmed.

Implant sizes 0 through 3 are most frequently used. The largest implant size that will fit properly is selected. The implant is inserted in the same fashion as for the metacarpophalangeal joints. There should be no impingement of the implant by the bone ends during passive extension of the joint. The extensor mechanism is brought together and sutured with 4-0 or 5-0 Dacron or other nonabsorbable suture using an inverted-knot technique. If the central slip has been cut, it should be reattached to the base of the middle phalanx with a suture passed through a small drill hole. A small drain is inserted in the wound and a voluminous conforming hand dressing is applied.

The wound is inspected on the third postoperative day and the drain removed. An active exercise program is started supporting the proximal phalanges with a brace, cast or other exercise device. Flexion and extension movements are encouraged as fully as possible without causing pain or swelling. Small aluminum splints are taped on the fingers to hold them in extension at night for three to six weeks after surgery. Occasionally passive flexion exercises with a flexion cuff or dorsal strap may be necessary to increase flexion starting three weeks after surgery.

Reconstruction of a swan-neck deformity

The reconstructive procedure for a fixed swan-neck deformity varies slightly from that for a nondeformed stiff proximal interphalangeal joint. The central tendon is separated from the dorsally displaced lateral tendons which are allowed to relocate volarward (Fig. 8.5.7). It is then divided in a step-cut fashion and released from the proximal phalanx. After insertion of the implant, the cut ends of the central tendon are reapproximated with interrupted sutures with a buried-knot technique thereby lengthening it. If the distal joint is severely flexed, it is fixed in extension by an intramedullary Kirschner wire to increase the flexion force on the proximal phalanx during the early postoperative period.

Postoperatively, the proximal interphalangeal joint is held in 20° of flexion with a small taped-on aluminum splint for approximately 10 days. Active flexion and extension exercises are then started with the proximal phalanx supported. Hyperextension of the reconstructed joint must be avoided for the first three to six weeks to obtain a slight flexion contracture and maintain the correction of the hyperextension deformity.

Reconstruction of a Boutonniere Deformity

In a boutonniere deformity, implant arthroplasty must be accompanied by reconstruction of the extensor mechanism.[9] [14] [38] In a rheumatoid deformity, the central tendon is usually lengthened and the lateral tendons are displaced volarly. The connecting fibers are stretched out. Two methods of reconstruction have

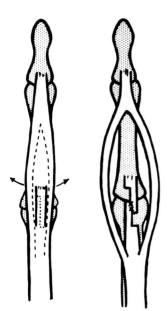

Figure 8.5.7. Extensor mechanism reconstruction in a swan-neck deformity: The central tendon is incised in a step-cut fashion. The lateral bands are released and allowed to relocate palmarward. After insertion of the implant, the central tendon is sutured in a lengthened fashion with nonabsorbable sutures.

been used (Fig. 8.5.8). In one, the attachment of the central tendon to the base of the middle phalanx is repaired by suturing the stretched-out central tendon to the base of the middle phalanx through a small drill hole. In the other method, a lateral tendon, usually the radial one, is attached to the insertion of the central tendon to reinforce it.[17] If passive flexion of the distal interphalangeal joint cannot be accomplished, the lateral tendons may be released proximal to the insertion of Landsmeer's ligament to correct the hyperextension deformity of the distal joint.

After approximately 10 days of immobilization of the finger with a taped-on aluminum splint, guarded flexion movements are allowed (Fig. 8.5.9). The proximal interphalangeal joint is held in extension part time for three to six weeks according to the degree of extension lag (Figs. 8.5.10 and 8.5.11).

THE BASAL JOINTS OF THE THUMB

Arthritic changes at the base of the thumb can seriously interfere with normal function of the hand.[39] The disability may result most frequently from osteoarthritis or rheumatoid arthritis and also from traumatic arthritis.[1 5 6] Pain and swelling at the base of the thumb are the most common complaints. As the disease progresses, instability, crepitation, deformity, and loss of motion and strength are also noted. Adduction contracture of the first metacarpal and swan-neck deformity of the thumb may also be seen.

A study of the roentgenograms of patients selected

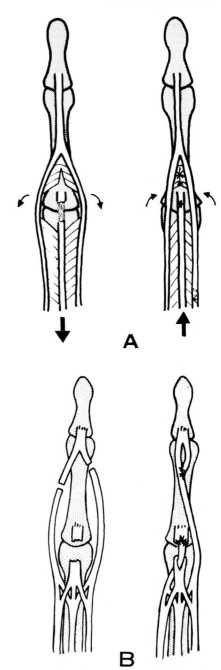

Figure 8.5.8. Repair of the extensor mechanism in a boutonniere deformity. *A.* Preferred method of repair: The lengthened central tendon is advanced and sutured to a small drill hole in the base of the middle phalanx. The lateral tendons are released and relocated dorsally by suturing their connecting fibers. *B.* Matev's method of repair: The lateral tendon (usually on the radial side) is used to reconstruct the central tendon. The remaining lateral tendon is reattached in a relatively lengthened position distally.

for reconstructive surgery of the thumb demonstrated that the arthritic changes most frequently occur at the trapeziometacarpal joint but that the trapezio-scaphoid, trapeziotrapezoid, and trapezio-second-metacarpal joints are also involved in a significant number of cases.[35] The trapezium was the center of the arthritic process in all cases of osteoarthritis and of traumatic arthritis. Rheumatoid patients may have a similar localized involvement of the basal thumb joints. They may also have severe absorptive changes of the trapezium and base of the metacarpal which produces a result not unlike a resection arthroplasty. If the joint is reasonably stable, mobile, and pain-free, no surgery is indicated.

We have designed an intramedullary stemmed silicone implant to preserve the anatomic relationship after excision arthroplasty of the trapezium by acting as a space filler. The stem of the implant is fitted in the intramedullary canal of the first metacarpal and its concave base seats over the scaphoid bone. The implant is available in five anatomic sizes and has been mechanically tested to 150 million compression and sheer stress movements without failure.

Indications

Trapezium implant resection arthroplasty is indicated in presence of the following conditions whether the disability is due to degenerative, posttraumatic, or rheumatoid arthritis:

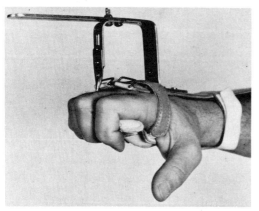

Figure 8.5.9. The dynamic brace can be adjusted to support the proximal phalanx as the patient performs flexion and extension exercises of the PIP joint.

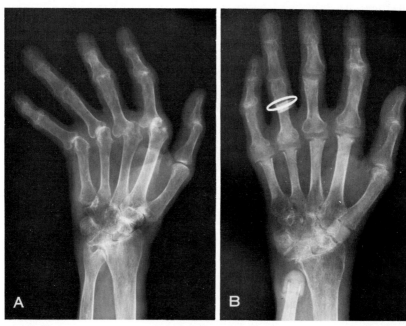

Figure 8.5.10. Case illustrating the use of flexible implants for reconstruction of finger joints, the base of the thumb and the ulnar head. *A.* Preoperative roentgenogram of a 65-year-old woman with rheumatoid arthritis of 15 years duration. Note the destruction of the MP joints of the fingers with severe ulnar drift and the arthritic changes of the proximal interphalangeal joint of the index, middle, and little fingers, at the basal joints of the thumb, the wrist, and the distal radioulnar joint. *B.* Two years after surgery the roentgenogram demonstrates the correction of the deformities and the good tolerance of the implants by the bone and the soft tissues. Implant arthroplasties of the PIP joint of the middle finger, the base of the thumb and the ulnar head were carried out at the same time as the reconstructions of the MP joints of the index, middle, ring and little fingers. The patient was relieved of pain and had an excellent cosmetic and functional improvement.

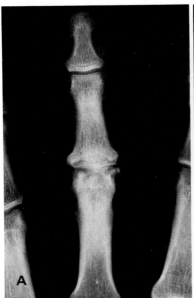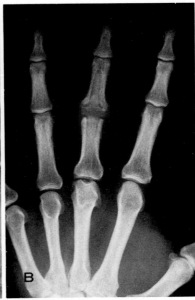

Figure 8.5.11. A. Preoperative roentgenogram demonstrating severe post-traumatic arthritis in an active 29-year-old football coach following a fracture-dislocation injury. *B.* The postoperative roentgenogram taken six years after surgery demonstrates the excellent tolerance of the implant. The patient has a strong, stable, pain-free finger with an excellent cosmetic and functional result. He has a range of motion from full extension to 90° of flexion.

1. Localized pain and palpable crepitation during circumduction movements with axial compression of the thumb.
2. Loss of motion with decrease of normal pinch and grip strength.
3. Radiologic evidence of arthritic changes of the trapeziometacarpal, trapezioscaphoid, trapeziotrapezoid, and trapezio-second-metacarpal joints, singly or in combination.
4. Unstable, stiff or painful distal joints of the thumb or swan-neck collapse deformity.

Surgical Procedure

A 5- to 7-cm curved radiopalmar incision or preferably a longitudinal radial incision centered over the trapezium parallel to the extensor pollicis brevis tendon is used. The branches of the superficial radial nerve are identified and carefully retracted (Fig. 8.5.12). The joint capsule is incised longitudinally and reflected by sharp dissection from the base of the metacarpal. It is very important to preserve the capsule for its later reclosure. The dissection is carried close to the bone to avoid injury to the branches of the radial artery, overlying tendons, and the capsuloligamentous structures both palmarly and dorsally.

The trapezium is then removed either piece-meal or en bloc including its medial portion. Any osteophytes or irregularities on the distal end of the scaphoid are trimmed to eliminate any block to proper seating of the implant. The base of the metacarpal is squared off with a rongeur leaving most of the cortical and subchondral bone intact. The intramedullary canal of the first metacarpal is prepared to receive the stem of the implant. The canal should not be opened more than necessary to fit the stem easily. This must be done carefully to avoid perforation of the lateral walls of the bone. A size implant that will comfortable fit into the space left by the resection of the trapezium and allow full stable thumb circumduction is selected from one of the five available sizes. The stem of the implant should fit snugly. The base of the implant should seat properly on the scaphoid bone. Infrequently shortening of the proximal end of the first metacarpal is required to further decompress the joint space.

The stem of the implant is inserted into the intramedullary canal using a no-touch technique. It is important that the collar of the implant be in intimate contact with the base of the metacarpal to avoid wobbling. The thumb is held in abduction to place the implant well into the recess left by the trapezium removal.

It is essential that the implant be thoroughly secured by the capsuloligamentous structures at the end of the surgical procedure. These structures should be carefully preserved during dissection. Before inserting the implant, the anterior capsule and ligaments should be inspected in the depths of the wound for inadvertent tears; these must be sutured securely to provide a firm supporting capsule on the volar surface of the implant. If there are only mild or moderate destructive changes around the trapezium, the normal capsuloligamentous structures will suffice to maintain the implant in position. The dorsal radial capsular structures are brought together tightly over the implant and are carefully sutured with 3-0 Dacron or other nonabsorbable suture material using multiple interrupted sutures and an inverted knot technique. The proximal reflection of the capsule on the scaphoid should be incorporated in this repair. Adequate exposure of the capsule for suture placement is obtained by proximal retraction of the radial artery. If the capsule is loose, it should be imbricated. If it is thinned out, it should be reinforced using a portion of the abductor pollicis longus tendon (Fig. 8.5.13A). This tendon is split in half 5 cm proximally from its insertion to the base of the first metacarpal. A tendinous slip 5 cm in length composed of one half of the split tendon (left attached at its distal end) is placed dorsally directly over the implant and under the weakened area of the capsule which is plicated or overlapped and sutured over the tendon slip. The remaining portion of the tendon is then pulled back over the capsule and sutured in place with 3-0 Dacron.

A slip of the flexor carpi radialis tendon may be used to reconstruct an ulnar oblique ligament between the first and second metacarpals. This is especially important in patients who have had subluxation of the metacarpal off the trapezium with stretching out of this ligament and in patients who will be expected to do heavy work. Strong pinch forces require stability of the base of the metacarpal to prevent subluxation and a simple capsular repair may not be adequate. The flexor carpi radialis is exposed either by extending the initial longitudinal incision in a palmar proximal direction or through a separate incision. A slip 5 to 7 cm long and 8 to 12 mm wide formed of the radial portion

of the flexor carpi radialis is prepared leaving its distal insertion at the base of the second metacarpal intact. The slip is dissected proximally and passed through the carpal tunnel of the flexor carpi radialis to be withdrawn into the area left by the resected trapezium. It is then further dissected longitudinally from the main flexor carpi radialis tendon. With a small hemostat a tunnel is developed under the capsule and the tendon slip is brought around the base of the metacarpal between the capsule and the bone and pulled tight to provide a check ligament between the base of the second and first metacarpals. The slip is then sutured to the capsule, passed underneath the insertion of the abductor pollicis longus tendon and sutured across the dorsal capsule. (Fig. 8.5.13B).

The insertion of the abductor pollicis longus tendon is advanced distally on the metacarpal as the closure is completed. The first dorsal compartment is routinely released longitudinally to improve the moment force of the abductor pollicis longus and the extensor pollicis brevis as well as to relieve the frequently associated tendinitis in this area.

If there is an adduction contracture and the angle between the first and second metacarpals does not reach 45° or more, proximal release of the origin of adductor pollicis muscle from the third metacarpal can be done through a separate palmar incision.[25] Sufficient abduction is essential to assure proper seating of the implant. If the metacarpophalangeal joint hyperextends from 10° to 20°, a Kirschner wire is placed obliquely across the joint in 10° of flexion. The wire is extracted when the case is removed four to six weeks after surgery. If hyperextension of the metacarpophalangeal joint is greater than 20°, stabilization is

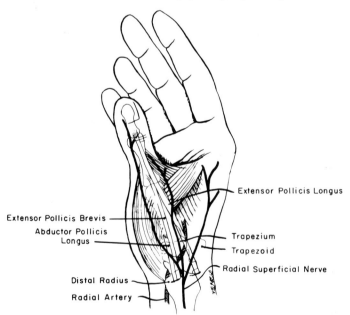

Extensor Pollicis Longus

Extensor Pollicis Brevis

Abductor Pollicis Longus

Trapezium

Trapezoid

Radial Superficial Nerve

Distal Radius

Radial Artery

Figure 8.5.12. Anatomic relationship of the abductor pollicis longus, extensor pollicis brevis and longus tendon, superficial radial nerve, radial vein, and artery at the base of the thumb.

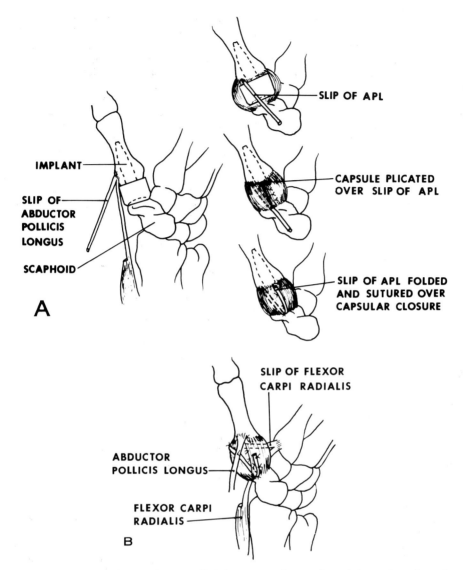

Figure 8.5.13. A. A slip of the abductor pollicis longus can be used to reinforce a weakened capsule. Note the proper seating of the implant over the scaphoid bone. *B.* An ulnar-check ligament can be reconstructed using a slip of the flexor carpi radialis in patients who had longstanding dislocations of the trapeziometacarpal joints. This is also important in patients who are expected to do heavy work.

an absolute necessity either by palmar capsulorrhaphy or by fusion.

Postoperative Care

The patient's hand and forearm are placed in a voluminous conforming dressing with a roll of cotton or Dacron batting between the first and second metacarpals to maintain 40° to 60° of palmar abduction. A plaster splint is applied over this dressing. A scaphoid type forearm cast is applied after three to four days and worn for four to six weeks. When the cast is removed, aduction and opposition movements of the thumb are encouraged. If there is a tendency for adduction contracture, a roll of soft material or a 1½-to 2-inch cylinder of wood or plastic is given to the patient to hold across the palm of the hand and the thumb web space. As far as the arthroplasty is concerned, full unguarded movements are usually possible in six to ten weeks.

THE CARPAL SCAPHOID AND LUNATE BONE

Flexible implant resection arthoplasty for diseases of the carpal scaphoid and lunate bones has been successful in our clinic for the last five years. If intercarpal stability and a good capsuloligamentous system is present, long-term good results can be obtained.[30] These implants act as a spacer to maintain the relationship of the adjacent carpal bones but, because ligaments cannot attach to the implants, they must be supported on all sides by bone or a firm capsuloligamentous system.

The scaphoid and lunate implants have a stabilizing stem that fits into an adjacent carpal bone. The stem of the scaphoid implant is inserted into the trapezium and the stem of the lunate implant into the triquetrum bone. The trapezium and the triquetrum bones were selected for fixation points because there is the least intercarpal motion between these bones and the replaced one. The main function of the stem is to help provide stability during the early postoperative period. Adequate capsuloligamentous support around these implants is essential for early and late stability and must be obtained at surgery. if there is a collapse deformity of the wrist as may be seen following severe hyperextension injuries of this joint with associated damage to the carpal ligaments, the scaphoid and lunate bones, instability will continue unless the ligamentous structures are repaired. After soft tissue healing and completion of the encapsulation process, the tendency for rotation or dislocation of these implants decreases.

THE SCAPHOID IMPLANT

Indications

Scaphoid implant resection arthroplasty is indicated in the following conditions:
1. Acute fractures
   A. Comminuted
   B. Grossly displaced
2. Pseudoarthroses, especially with small proximal fragment
3. Preisser's disease
4. Avascular necrosis of a fragment
5. Failures due to previous surgery

The procedure should not be used, of course, in cases where arthritic involvement is not localized to the scaphoid articulations if complete relief of symptoms is to be expected. Any situation where loss of support for the implant or instability of the carpus would be present is a contraindication for the use of the implant. In cases where there is severe diminution of the size of the scaphoid through longstanding disease, there may be inadequate room for placing the implant.

Surgical Procedure

A 5- to 7-cm volar or as preferred dorsolateral incision is made. The superficial sensory branches of the radial nerve and the radial artery must be meticulously preserved. The joint is approached between the tendons of the extensor pollicis longus and extensor carpi radialis longus. The capsule must be carefully preserved. Positive identification of the scaphoid bone must be made using roentgenograms if necessary. The scaphoid bone is completely removed en bloc or

piece-meal. Any bony fragments left behind may compromise the result. A hole is fashioned into the trapezium with a drill or a curette to accept the stem of the implant which should be directed at an angle so that it will be anatomically oriented. A size implant that will comfortably fit into the space left by the excision of the scaphoid is selected from one of the five graduated sizes available for each the right and left carpus (Fig. 8.5.14).

Before inserting the implant, the anterior capsule must be checked for inadvertent tears. These must be repaired. After insertion of the implant, the dorsal capsule is securely repaired with 4-0 Dacron using an inverted knot technique. A firm capsuloligamentous support around the implant is essential to obtain good results in scaphoid replacement implant arthroplasty. A small drill hole may be placed in the distal radius to help secure the capsular closure.

THE LUNATE IMPLANT

Indications

Lunate implant resection arthroplasty is indicated for: (1) avascular necrosis, Kienböck's disease; (2) longstanding dislocations.

The procedure should not be used in cases where arthritic involvement is not localized to the lunate articulations if complete relief of pain is to be expected. In cases of longstanding dislocations or old cases of Kienböck's disease, the space for the lunate may be markedly diminished and proper fitting of the implant may be difficult. Loss of integrity of the capsular structures may be a contraindication to the implant procedure unless the relationship of the carpal bones can be reestablished and the ligaments repaired.

Surgical Procedure

A 5- to 7-cm dorsal longitudinal incision is used for surgery in Kienböck's disease. When the lunate bone is dislocated, a volar approach is suggested. Care should be taken to avoid the superficial sensory branches of either the radial or ulnar nerve. The wrist capsule is transversely incised between the third and fourth dorsal compartments and carefully preserved. Exposure is made between the extensor pollicis longus and the extensor digitorum communis tendons.

The lunate is removed en bloc or piece-meal with great care to avoid injury to the palmar radiocarpal and ulnocarpal ligaments. Positive identification of the lunate bone must be made using roentgenograms if necessary. A hole is made in the triquetrum bone to accept the stem of the implant. A size implant that will comfortably fit in the space left by the resection of the lunate is selected from one of the four available sizes (Fig. 8.5.15).

Before inserting the implant, integrity of the anterior capsuloligamentous structures must be verified, tears or weaknesses must be repaired. The posterior capsule which is preserved during dissection is tightly sutured with nonabsorbable sutures using an inverted

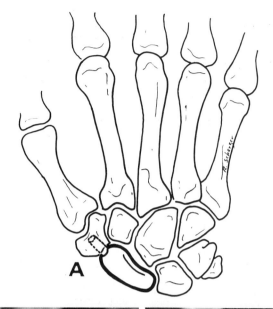

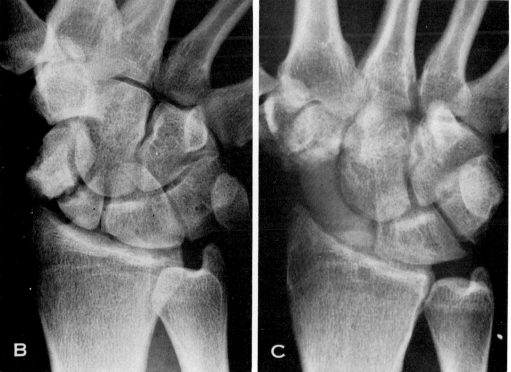

Figure 8.5.14. A. The stabilizing stem of the scaphoid implant should be anatomically oriented to fit in the trapezium bone. *B.* Preoperative roentgenogram showing the nonunion of the scaphoid of three years duration in a 21-year-old active college student. He complained of pain and weakness of the wrist and inability to carry on competitive sports. *C.* Roentgenogram three years after implant replacement arthroplasty of the scaphoid. This patient has a pain-free, strong, stable wrist, is active in skiing and football, and works as a logger during the summer.

knot technique. If necessary, two small drill holes may be placed in the distal radius to help secure the capsular closure.

Postoperative Care of Scaphoid and Lunate Implant Arthroplasty

A voluminous conforming dressing including a posterior molded splint is worn for the first week. A short-arm scaphoid type cast is then applied and worn for four to six weeks. Full wrist activity is resumed at 12 weeks.

ULNAR HEAD IMPLANT REPLACEMENT ARTHROPLASTY

Resection of the distal end of the ulna and replacement with an intramedullary-stemmed silicone rubber implant has definite advantages over simple resection methods.[8][16] Less bone is removed and the physiologic length of the ulna is maintained to help prevent ulnar carpal shift and provide greater wrist stability. A smooth articular surface for the radius and carpus is provided to allow freer movements of the distal radioulnar and carpoulnar joints. The overlying extensor tendons glide over a smooth surface. The incidence of bone overgrowth is decreased. Reconstruction of the ligaments is possible including the rerouting of the important extensor carpi ulnaris tendon over the dorsum of the ulna. The cosmetic appearance of the wrist is improved.

Indications

The ulnar head implant replacement arthroplasty may be considered for disabilities of the distal radioulnar joint in rheumatoid, degenerative or post-traumatic dysfunctions of this joint. Specific indications include pain and weakness of the wrist joint not improved by conservative treatment, instability of ulnar head, and roentgenographic evidence of dorsal subluxation and erosion of the ulnar head.

Surgical Technique

A 6- to 8- cm longitudinal incision centered over the ulnar head is made taking care to preserve the dorsal cutaneous branch of the ulnar nerve. The extensor retinaculum of the sixth dorsal compartment is incised in such a fashion as to preserve a narrow radially based distal flap and a broad ulnarly based proximal flap (Fig. 8.5.16). If a synovectomy of the dorsal compartments is indicated, it must be carried out at the same time. The extensor carpi ulnaris which is usually subluxated ulnarward off the ulnar head is retracted. The ulna is exposed subperiosteally at the neck, retractors are placed to protect the underlying structures, and the ulna is sectioned at the neck with an air drill. The periosteum is not stripped off the distal ulna but muscular attachments on the anterior surface of the ulna are released over the distal 2 cm. A synovectomy is performed. The cut edge of the distal ulna is

trimmed with a rongeur. Bone irregularities that may be present, especially at the undersurface of the ulna, are smoothened. The intramedullary canal of the ulna is prepared to receive the stem of the implant which is available in six sizes. The stem of the implant must fit snugly in the intramedullary canal and the cuff must fit loosely over the bone. Manipulation and insertion of the implant must be carried out using a no-touch technique. A nonabsorbable suture passed through the cap of the implant and through a drill hole in the distal ulna holds the implant in place. Sutures should not ordinarily be passed through silicone rubber implants because of potential tear propagation. However, in our experience, this capping ulnar head implant does not undergo much flex, compression, shear or rotatory torque loads and, therefore, the advantages of the suture outweigh the disadvantages. The retinaculum of the sixth dorsal compartment can be used as a check ligament to hold the dorsally displaced ulna in a reduced position. The ulnar portion of the cut retinaculum is sutured over the ulna into the soft tissues of the radius and the retinaculum of the fifth dorsal compartment. A small strip of retinaculum can be used to secure the extensor carpi ulnaris in a dorsal position over the ulna. Digital extensors which may occasionally be ruptured as a result of the ulnar head syndrome should be repaired.

On the third postoperative day, the volar splint is changed to a short-arm cast with the hand in slight dorsiflexion and radial deviation for three to four weeks.

RADIAL HEAD IMPLANT REPLACEMENT ARTHROPLASTY

Resection of the radial head is indicated for certain types of fractures and for disabilities secondary to rheumatoid or degenerative arthritis. A significant number of these cases develop dysfunctions of the distal radioulnar joint secondary to the shortening of the proximal radius. A limited resection of the radial head at the proximal metaphysis and replacement with a radial head implant has decided advantages: (1) It prevents bone formation at the proximal end of the radius; (2) it maintains the physiologic length of the radius to prevent proximal displacement of the radial shaft while providing a smooth articulating mechanism for the radiohumeral and proximal radioulnar joints; (3) it provides an improved stability, joint space relationship, and range of motion; (4) it facilitates postoperative rehabilitation. Excessive postoperative immobilization which could compromise the range of useful motion is not required.

Indications

The radial head implant arthroplasty is indicated in dysfunctions of the radiohumeral joint in the following clinical conditions:

1. Pain and limitation of movement secondary to incongruity of the joint surfaces.

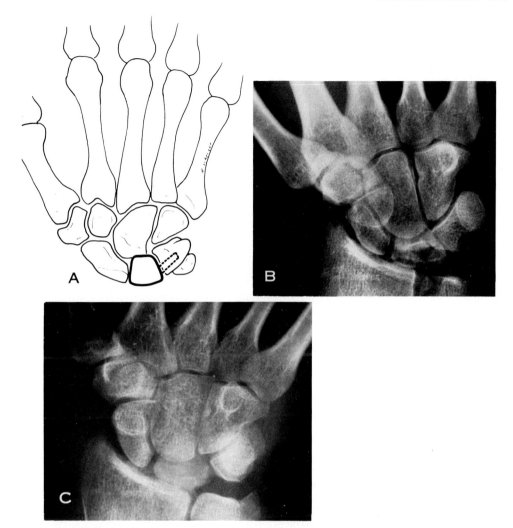

Figure 8.5.15. A. The stabilizing stem of the lunate implant should be anatomically oriented to fit in the triquetrum bone. *B.* Preoperative roentgenogram showing a Kienböck's disease in a 20-year-old student. He complained of weakness of the wrist with pain and restriction of motion. *C.* The roentgenogram shows the lunate implant in place. Three years after surgery the patient maintains a pain-free wrist with good strength and motion.

2. Roentgenographic evidence of joint destruction or subluxation.
3. Replacement following previous resection of the radial head for rheumatoid, degenerative or post-traumatic arthritic conditions.
4. Primary replacement following radial head resection for fracture.

The radial head implant arthroplasty is contraindicated in growing children with opened epiphyses, in dislocations of the radius on the ulna that would not allow a radiohumeral articulation, and in the presence of inadequate bone stock.

Surgical Procedure

The radiohumeral joint is entered through a dorsolateral approach between the anconeus and the ex-

tensor carpi ulnaris muscles taking care to preserve the motor branch of the radial nerve which passes at the radial neck. The radial head is resected at the epiphyseal metaphyseal junction, under the protection of retractors, preserving the annular and quadrate ligaments. A synovectomy of the elbow joint may be performed at the same time. The intramedullary canal of the radius is prepared to receive the stem of the implant. The implant cuff should overlap the radius and the stem fit snugly in the canal (Fig. 8.5.17). A choice from the three available sizes should provide proper fit of the implant. The implant is inserted using a no-touch technique and blunt instruments to avoid contamination with foreign materials or injury to the implant. The prosthetic head should articulate snugly but smoothly with the capitellum on flexion, extension,

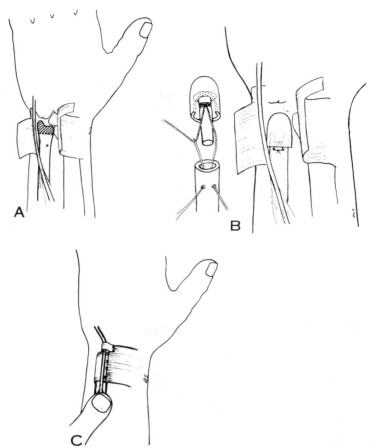

Figure 8.5.16. Ulnar head implant resection arthroplasty. *A.* The extensor retinaculum of the sixth dorsal compartment is incised preserving a narrow radially based distal flap and a broad ulnarly based proximal flap. The ulnar head is resected leaving part of the flair of the metaphysis. The periosteum is not stripped. *B.* The implant must be secured to the end of the ulna by a suture technique. We now prefer to secure the implant by tying a strong non absorbable 2-0 Dacron suture around the base of the stem such as shown in figure 16-B. The ends of the suture are passed through two small drill holes made in the distal ulna and securely tied together once the implant is well seated over the bone end.

and rotation movements of the joint as noted during passive movements of the forearm. The capsule, anconeus, and extensor carpi ulnaris muscles are sutured using nonabsorbable sutures and a buried-knot technique. A drain is inserted in the wound. A conforming dressing including a posterior plaster splint is applied.

Postoperative Care

On the third postoperative day, the plaster splint is removed and guarded progressive movements are allowed. Full activity is resumed at six weeks. The early postoperative movement facilitates rehabilitation and increases the range of motion.

WRIST IMPLANT RESECTION ARTHROPLASTY

A flexible intramedullary-stemmed implant has been successfully used in our clinic as an adjunct to re-

section arthroplasty of the radiocarpal joint of the wrist. This procedure has allowed us to avoid wrist fusion in patients with an unstable and subluxating wrist joint secondary to rheumatoid arthritis.

Indications

The wrist implant arthroplasty is indicated in cases of (1) instability of the wrist due to subluxation or dislocation; (2) severe deviation of the wrist causing muscle tendon imbalance of the digits; (3) stiffness of the wrist in nonfunctional position; and (4) stiffness of a wrist where movement is a requirement for hand function.

Surgical Technique

Through a gently curved or straight dorsal longitudinal incision, the extensor retinaculum is opened in the fashion illustrated in Figure 8.5.16*A.* Part of the proximal carpal row is usually absorbed and displaced palmarward of the radius. The remaining portion of the scaphoid and lunate bones are resected taking care to avoid injury to the underlying tendons and neurovascular structures. The distal end of the radius is squared off so that it will fit against the distal carpal row (Fig. 8.5.18). A portion of the base of the capitate and the triquetrum are removed. The radiocarpal subluxation should be completely reduced. Because the distal carpal row is important to maintain the stability of the metacarpal bases, it is preferable to shorten the distal radius rather than remove more carpal bones to reduce completely the radiocarpal subluxation. The intramedullary canal of the radius is prepared to receive the proximal stem of the implant. The distal stem fits through the capitate bone into the intramedullary canal of the third metacarpal. The distal ulna is trimmed back to about one centimeter from the distal end of the radius and an ulnar head implant is used to cap this bone. The proximal stem of the wrist implant is introduced first. Once the implant is in place, extension of the wrist on passive manipulation should be possible. Usually a space of 1 to 1½ cm of separation between the bone ends is adequate. The capsuloligamentous structures are sutured over the im-

plant passing the sutures through small drill holes in the dorsal cortex of the radius to assure good capsular fixation. This should allow 45° of flexion and extension and 10° of ulnar and radial deviation on passive manipulation. The extensor retinacular flaps are closed as shown in Figure 8.5.16C. The pull of the wrist extensor tendons should be evaluated and rebalanced by either shortening or transfer as necessary to obtain wrist extension without lateral deviation. Ruptured digital extensor tendons are repaired if indicated.

The wound is closed in layers and a small drain is inserted subcutaneously. A voluminous conforming dressing including a plaster splint is applied. After three to five days, a short arm cast is applied with the wrist in neutral position and left in place for approximately four to six weeks. The patient is then started on an exercise program to obtain an active range of motion.

SUMMARY

Since 1962 we designed, developed, and tested 23 flexible implants to be used in reconstructive surgery of

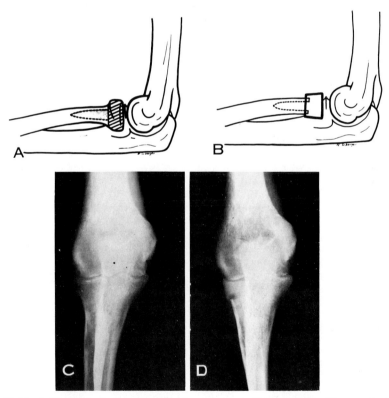

Figure 8.5.17. Radial head implant resection arthroplasty. *A.* The radial head is resected at neck and the intramedullary canal is prepared taking care to preserve the annular and quadrate ligaments. *B.* The correct size implant articulates smoothly with the capitellum on passive flexion, extension, and rotation of the elbow and forearm. *C.* Preoperative roentgenogram showing narrowing of the radiohumeral joint and erosion of the capitellum in a 41-year-old patient with rheumatoid arthritis. *D.* Roentgenogram two years after surgery showing the radial head implant in position.

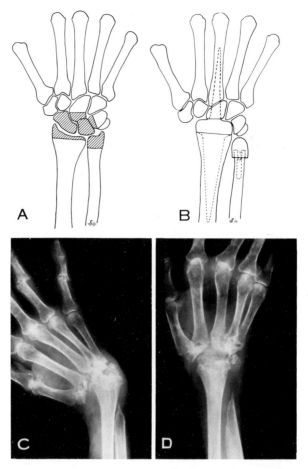

Figure 8.5.18. Wrist implant resection arthroplasty. *A.* Amount of bone usually resected from the distal radius, ulna and carpal bones in preparation for the wrist implant insertion. *B.* The stem of the implant should fit snugly in the intramedullary canal and the cuff should fit loosely over the resected bone-end. The implant is maintained in position with a strong non absorbable (2-0 Dacron) suture tied around the base of the stem. The ends of the suture are passed through two small drill holes made in the distal ulna, and securely tied together once the implant is in good position over the bone end.

the extremities. The concepts and principles of flexible implant arthroplasty are discussed. The surgical indications, technique, postoperative care, and points of special surgical attention are briefly discussed for each of the following implant arthroplasty procedures: the metacarpophalangeal and proximal interphalangeal joints, the trapezium, the scaphoid and lunate bones, the ulnar and radial heads, and the wrist joint.

REFERENCES

1. Aune, S. Osteo-arthritis in first carpo-metacarpal joint. An investigation of 22 cases. Acta Chir. Scand., *109:* 449-456, 1955.
2. Barron, J. N. Assessment of suitability for surgery in general: Timing of operation. International Workshop on Artificial Finger Joints. Ann. Rheum. Dis. (Suppl.), *28:* 74-76, 1969.
3. Braley, S. The silicones as tools in biological engineering. Med. Electron, Biol. Eng., *3:* 127-136, 1965.
4. Carroll, R. E., and Taber, T. H. Digital arthroplasty of the proximal interphalangeal joint. J. Bone Joint Surg., *36 A:* 912-920, 1954.
5. Carstam, N., Eiken, O., and André, N. Osteoarthritis in the Trapezio-scaphoid joint. Acta Orthop. Scand., *39:* 354-358, 1968.
6. Clayton, M. L. Surgery of the thumb in rheumatoid arthritis. J. Bone Joint Surg., *44 A:* 1376-1386, 1962.
7. Curtis, R. M. Capsulectomy of the interphalangeal joints of the fingers. J. Bone Joint Surg., *36 A:* 1219-1232, 1954.
8. Darrach, W. Anterior dislocation of the head of the ulna. Ann. Surg., *56:* 802-803, 1912.
9. Dolphin, J. A. Extensor tenotomy for chronic boutonnierè deformity of the finger. J. Bone Joint Surg., *47A:* 161-164, 1965.
10. Elliot, R. A. Injuries to extensor mechanism of the hand. Orthop. Clin. North Am., *1:* 335-354, 1970.
11. Granowitz, S., and Vainio, K. Proximal interphalangeal joint arthrodesis in rheumatoid arthritis. Acta Or-

thop. Scand., *37:* 301-310, 1966.

12. Kessler, I., Niebauer, J. J., and Howard, L. D., Jr. Studies on the response of the medullary canal of long bones toward Dacron D-119. Plast. Reconstr. Surg., *39:* 307-310, 1967.

13. Landsmeer, J. M. F. A report on the coordination of the interphalangeal joints of the human finger and its disturbances. Acta Morphal. Neerl.-Scand., *2:* 59-84, 1959.

14. Littler, J. W., and Eaton, R. G. Redistribution of forces in the correction of the boutonnière deformity. J. Bone Joint Surg., *49 A:* 1267-1274, 1969.

15. Liotta, D. Personnal communication (Houston, Texas).

16. Lugnegard, H. Resection of the head of the ulna in posttraumatic dysfunction of the distal radio-ulnar joint. Scand. J. Plast. Reconstr. Surg., *3:* 65-69, 1969.

17. Matev, I. B. Transposition of the lateral slips of the aponeurosis in treatment of long-standing boutonnière deformity of the fingers. Bri. J. Plast. Surg., *17:* 281-286, 1964.

18. Roberts, A. C. Silicones and their applications as implant materials. Bio-Med. Eng., *2:* 156-160, 1967.

19. Swanson, A. B. The need for early treatment of the rheumatoid hand. J. Mich. State Med. Soc., *60:* 348-351, 1961.

20. Swanson, A. B. Pathomechanics of the swan-neck deformity. J. Bone Joint Surg., *47 A:* 636, 1965.

21. Swanson, A. B. Improving the end-bearing characteristics of lower extremity amputation stumps. New York University, Inter-Clin. Inform. Bull., *5:* 1-7, 1966.

22. Swanson, A. B. A flexible implant for replacement of arthritic or destroyed joints in the hand. New York University, Inter-Clin. Inform. Bull., *6:* 16-19, 1966.

23. Swanson, A. B., and Yamauchi, Y. Silicone rubber implants for replacement of arthritic or destroyed joints. In *Proceedings of The American Academy of Orthopaedic Surgeons, Scientific Exhibits.* J. Bone Joint Surg., *50 A:* 1272, 1968.

24. Swanson, A. B. Silicone rubber implants for replacement of arthritic or destroyed joints in the hand. Surg. Clin. North Am., *48:* 1113-1127, 1968.

25. Swanson, A. B. Surgery of the hand in cerebral palsy and muscle origin release procedures. Surg. Clin. North Am., *48:* 1129-1138, 1968.

26. Swanson, A. B. Finger joint replacement by silicone rubber implants and the concept of implant fixation by encapsulation. In *International Workshop on Artificial Finger Joints.* Ann. Rheum. Dis. (Suppl.), *28:* 47-55, 1969.

27. Swanson, A. B. Silicone rubber implants for replacement of arthritic or destroyed joints in the hand. In *The Rheumatoid Hand.* Groupe d'Etude de la Main. Monograph No. 3, edited by Raoul Tubiana. Paris,

L'Expansion, 1969, pp. 176-189.

28. Swanson, A. B., and Matev, I. B. The proximal interphalangeal joint in arthritic disabilities and experiences in the use of silicone rubber implant arthroplasty in the upper extremity. In *Proceedings of The American Academy of Orthopaedic Surgeons, Scientific Exhibits.* J. Bone Joint Surg., *52A:* 1265, 1970.

29. Swanson, A. B. Arthroplasty in traumatic arthritic joints in the hand. Orthop. Clin. North Am., *1:* 285-298, 1970.

30. Swanson, A. B. Silicone rubber implants for the replacement of the carpal scaphoid and lunate bones. Orthop. Clin. North Am., *1:* 299-309, 1970.

31. Swanson. A. B. A dynamic brace for finger joint reconstruction in arthritis. In *Surgery of Rheumatoid Arthritis,* edited by R. L. Cruess and N. Mitchell. Philadelphia, Lippincott, 1971, pp. 199-203.

32. Swanson, A. B. Surgery of established rheumatoid deformity in the hand. In *Surgery of Rheumatoid Arthritis,* edited by R. L. Cruess and N. Mitchell. Philadelphia, Lippincott, 1971, pp. 177-198.

33. Swanson, A. B., deGroot, G. A., Hehl, R. W., Waller, T. J., and Boeve, N. R. Pathogenesis of rheumatoid deformities in the hand. In *Surgery of Rheumatoid Arthritis,* edited by R. L. Cruess and N. Mitchell. Philadelphia, Lippincott, 1971, pp. 143-158.

34. Swanson, A. B. Flexible implant arthroplasty for arthritic finger joints — rational, technique and results of treatment. J. Bone Joint Surg., *54 A:* 435-455, 1972.

35. Swanson, A. B. Disabling arthritis at the base of the thumb — treatment by resection of the trapezium and flexible (Silicone) implant arthroplasty. J. Bone Joint Surg., *54 A:* 456-471, 1972.

36. Swanson, A. B. Implant arthroplasty for the great toe. Clin. Orthop., *85:* 75-81, 1972.

37. Swanson, A. B. *Flexible Implant Arthroplasty in the Hand and Extremities.* St. Louis, Mosby, 1973 (in publication).

38. Tubiana, R. Surgical repair of the extensor apparatus of the fingers. Surg. Clin. North Am., *48:* 1015-1031, 1968.

39. Tubiana, R., and Valentin, P. Opposition of the thumb. Surg. Clin. North Am., *48:* 967-977, 1968.

40. Vainio, K., Reiman, I., and Pulkki, T. Results of arthroplasty of the metacarpophalangeal joints in rheumatoid arthritis. Reconstr. Surg. Traumat., *9:* 1-7, 1967.

41. Vaughan-Jackson, O. J. Rheumatoid hand deformities as considered in the light of tendon imbalances. J. Bone Joint Surg., *44 B:* 764-775, 1962.

42. Wesolowski, S. A., Martinez, A., and McMahon, J. D. Use of artificial materials in surgery. In *Current Problems in Surgery.* Chicago, Year Book, 1966.

43. Zancolli, E. *Structural and Dynamic Bases of Hand Surgery.* Philadelphia, Lippincott, 1968.

chapter nine

Injuries to Nerves

A.

Peripheral Nerve Injuries in the Hand: General Considerations

William F. Flynn, M.D.

INTRODUCTION

In this century, the management of peripheral nerve injuries in the hand has evolved from an ill defined, empirical approach to a plan of precise evaluation of the elements of injury, repair, and technique. New understanding of the response to injury of the mesenchymal environment of the intraneural fibrils, as well as the whole wound, permits better decisions concerning extent of primary debridement of the wound, and provides a clearer understanding of a rational selection of cases for delayed as opposed to primary repair. Progress in technique, which extends to all phases of surgery, is producing further refinement in surgical performance, with improved visualization of the finer structures to be repaired.

HISTORY

The earliest available record of nerve repair relates to Baudens (1836) who performed repair of median and ulnar nerves, approximated stumps by suture of adjoining tissues, and avoided contact of the nerve itself by the materials used. The first organized investigation of nerve injuries was undertaken during the American Civil War, at the instigation of W. A. Hammond, Surgeon General of the Federal Armies. Work began in May 1863 at an army hospital in Turner's Lane, Philadelphia, with Silas Weir Mitchell[24] in charge. After fifteen months he and his co-workers published a little book which is the foundation of our knowledge of nerve injuries. A more complete work was published in 1872.[25] In 1864 Nelaton and also Houel performed primary sutures of nerve injuries.

Claims were made for sensory and motor recovery in a few days.[46] In 1893 Howell and Huber collected 84 cases of primary nerve sutures and concluded that function is likely to return, partially or completely.

In 1908 Sherren reported 50 cases and analyzed the various types of return of function. He reported that pain sensibility occurred in from five to 25 weeks, that touch sensibility returned in 19 to 46 weeks, and that tactile sensibility was near complete in two years. Motor return occurred after one year for lacerations at the wrist and two years at the elbow level. Platt and Bristow in 1923 reported on nerve injuries in World War I and offered the opinion that "extreme perfection" was possible after primary suture and incomplete recovery occurred after most secondary sutures. In 1928 Gonzalez and Aquilar advocated suture as soon as possible after myelin remains had been removed from the distal stump and at a time of maximal Schwann cell activity, about 30 days after division of the nerve. In 1937 Herbig reported four primary and 13 secondary sutures, the latter performed from two to 12 months after injury. He observed that primary repairs gave better results than secondary sutures. In 1937 Platt and Bristow studied primary and secondary nerve sutures and advocated primary repair for small clean wounds, failure being likely on bruised or infected wounds. In 1942 Tolley reported on his experience in the Spanish Civil War. A number of primary nerve sutures was done, but this method was abandoned later on the advice of Diaz, who felt that secondary suture was superior. Infection was a great hazard in these cases. Pollock and Davis[30] offered the opinion which is controverted by few, namely that primary suture in a clean wound, healing by primary intention, offers the advantage of the best possible conditions under which end-to-end suture may be performed.

In animal experimentation, under aseptic conditions, primary repairs give optimal functional result. Comparable situations occur after accidental or planned nerve division occurring in the course of an operation.

And finally in 1942 there was inaugurated what Woodhall[46] has referred to as the beginning of modern history of nerve surgery when an organized and objective study was begun on an ultimate 15,000 cases of nerve injury.

PATHOLOGY

Etiology

Most peripheral nerve injuries seen in civilian practice are nonoccupational, and are caused by kitchen accidents or personal trauma. Knife cuts and broken glass are most common causes, and the porcelain faucet is now seldom involved. Sharp nerve cuts are frequent, and these are often clean wounds. Avulsed or tearing injuries are often slight and usually caused by falls on broken glass. Rarely seen are the violent injuries common in wartime, crushes, bullet wounds, contusions and hematomas, and extensive soft part and bone damage.

Nerve injuries occurring early after a fracture may be caused by traction, and in these recovery is often slow and paralysis may be permanent.[4] Early evidence of nerve injury from compression may, however, also follow fractures, and these are amenable to local excision of the lesion.[38] It may be impossible to decide on clinical grounds whether traction or compression or a combination of both is the cause, and exploration of the injured nerve may be necessary to determine whether effective treatment may be performed.

Repair

When nerve fibrils are divided there is a local swelling and proximally there is a degeneration of myelin sheath and axone fibrils to the nearest node of Ranvier. Regeneration of both sheath and fibrils occurs and in a few days, if nerve ends are in apposition, down-growing axones "cross the gap." If there is no repair and local escape of axone fibrils with other cellular elements occurs, a local mass, a neuroma, forms.

In the distal nerve stump, the products of Wallerian degeneration are removed by phagocytes and it may be many months or as long as two years before the distal endoneurial sheaths are cleared of degenerating myelin. The distal sheaths become narrowed by fibrous proliferation if penetration by new down-growing axone fibrils does not occur. Within the distal sheaths, the Schwann cells increase soon after injury, and at the point of nerve transection these cells grow out to form the distal "glioma," which grows toward the proximal stump.[18] If junction occurs between outgrowths from both stumps, channels are formed through which regenerating axones are guided into the distal endoneurial tubes. Perineurial fibroblasts aid the formation of satisfactory junctions by growing out with the Schwann cells, from which in humans they can be distinguished only with difficulty, to secure the longitudinal orientation of the tissue connecting the stumps.[9] If junction fails, new axones will grow in many directions in the scar between the two stumps, forming a "neuroma."

After successful junction, fibrils grow down endoneurial tubes filled by Schwann cells and ultimately reach an end organ, grow larger and are covered by new myelin sheaths growing down from the proximal stump. Axones entering the end organ survive; others atrophy.

Neuromas in continuity occur when nerve fascicles are divided within an intact epineurial sheath producing a fusiform swelling. Although linear integrity is apparently preserved, the nerve may be functionally severed. Kline and Nulsen[19] report their experience with 66 peripheral nerve neuromas in continuity. Management is difficult because it is impossible to predict the outcome if the lesion is left alone. Knowledgement of the milestones of regeneration for each nerve, an appreciation for signs which can be misleading, the judicious use of electric stimulation and electromyography will help to decide whether regeneration is proceding satisfactorily and whether continued conservative management or operation is necessary. Of utmost importance in the evaluation of nerve trauma is the state of the wound in which nerve trauma occurs. A clean incised wound with an incised nerve should be repaired primarily. A wound with minimal soft tissue crush or avulsion and minimal crush or avulsion of the nerve may, with proper debridement, be repaired primarily. A wound with extensive crush or avulsion of soft tissues and nerves requires a delayed reconstruction of the nerves.

CLASSIFICATION

The traditional classification of injuries of peripheral nerves under headings of contusion and severance, partial and complete, has the advantage of simplicity and applicability to most injuries seen in civilian practice. Seddon[37] has proposed a classification that moves toward closer correlation of the nerve disorder with certain causative mechanisms, and at the same time introduces the concept of histologic change along with that of functional impairment. He distinguishes three types of injury: that associated with complete transsection of the nerve, neurotmesis; that of nerve fiber degeneration without disruption of nerve stroma, axonotmesis; that resulting in brief paralysis, whether partial or complete, neurapraxia.

Neurotmesis

Neurotmesis indicates complete separation by division of fibers of proximal and distal segments of the nerve. This includes complete separation by division of injury, or functional separation by fibrous change with some preserved anatomical continuity. In this category fall nerve injuries caused by gunshot, traction, injection of medications, such as sulfonamides, and ischemic changes, such as those resulting from Volkmann's contracture, as well as the common types of complete division.

Axonotmesis

Axonotmesis refers to structural division of nerve fibers without division of the total nerve structure. The damage to the nerve fiber is sufficient to result in axonal interruption and peripheral degeneration while the stroma of the nerve remains in continuity. The endoneurial tubes remain intact, and regeneration of high grade quality is achieved as recovering axons make their way through intact channels to their peripheral connections. This lesion can be produced experimentally by focal crushing, but does not occur often in civil or wartime trauma, except in fractures involving peripheral nerves in which this disturbance follows with considerable regularity. Initially there is no way of differentiating neurotmesis and axonotmesis; in both there is total loss of function distal to the lesion, the clinical picture of complete functional interruption.

Neurapraxia

This is a benign disturbance of short duration. Seddon states that the paralysis is predominantly motor, with little muscle atrophy and no change in electric excitability. Subjective sensory disorders are common, *e.g.*, tingling, burning, and numbness. Objective evidence of cutaneous sensory loss is less pronounced than motor disturbance and may be absent. The lesion is predominantly one of myelin sheaths, possibly explaining why motor and proprioceptive fibers, the largest myelinated peripheral nerve fibers, are chiefly affected. The axones remain in continuity and recovery usually occurs in a few days, or at the most, several weeks. This is the usual lesion resulting from tourniquet injury.

Shutta and Bogdanoff[36] have recently described pointers in the clinical diagnosis of acute peripheral nerve injuries. Pain, paresthesias, or intense burning in the sensory distribution of a nerve suggest injury to the nerve. Loss of sensation and muscle function may also reveal nerve injury. When assessing sensory loss, it is important to remember that there is considerable overlap between adjacent nerve supply territories. Motor function is often difficult to assess because the patient is reluctant or unable to cooperate because of pain.

VASOMOTOR AND NUTRITIONAL DISTURBANCES

Injuries to peripheral nerves lead to changes in the vasomotor and nutritional state of the area innervated. Nutritional changes previously h   been referred to as "trophic changes" the development of which has not been well understood. Vasomotor and nutritional changes occur inconstantly after nerve injuries, and appear to be more commonly associated with injuries of major sensory nerves (*e.g.*, median) rather than motor (*e.g.*, radial) in the upper extremity, and are more pronounced after partial than complete nerve divisions.[32]

In his discussion of vasomotor and trophic disorders, Richards[33] concludes that vasoconstrictor paralysis explains the warm phase immediately following nerve division, and that the later cold phase, although not completely understood, coincides with possible sensitization to epinephrine and the loss of local vasodilator response to trauma. Atrophy of skin and nail changes are explained by disuse and a persistently reduced circulation. Nerve irritation is seldom if ever a factor in vasomotor and nutritional disturbance, and if it occurs the mechanism is probably that of interaction of nerve fibers at the site of injury, a cross-channelling through artificial synapses.

ELECTRIC REACTIONS

There are three methods available for electric diagnosis of nerve injures: (1) the use of an electric shock to produce excitation of nerve or contraction of muscles; (2) the detection of minute and transient electric changes arising in active nerve and muscle tissues; and (3) the use of electric techniques to measure changes indirectly concerned with nerve function, such as skin resistance and skin temperature.[35]

Electrodiagnosis by stimulation is used to assess two properties of excitable tissue. The first property is the normal polarization of healthy nerve and muscle cell boundaries which can be altered by the application of an external electromotive force, *e.g.*, the galvanic-faradic test and intensity-duration curves. The second is the accommodative property of the cell membrane whereby a constant stimulus tends to become ineffective with the passage of time.

Seddon[40] uses five types of investigation: (1) strength-duration curve; (2) nerve stimulation; (3) electromyography; (4) motor nerve conduction; and (5) nerve action-potential recording.

Depolarization Tests

The galvanic-faradic test is a depolarization test utilizing shocks of widely different durations to identify normal and denervated muscle.[34] Normal muscle can readily be made to contract by the application of the output from a faradic coil. Denervated muscle will not respond to faradic current of moderate intensity, but will contract under stimulation from a galvanic current, as from a battery source. Normal muscle, which is responsive to brief faradic shocks, is in fact excited through its nerve content. Denervated muscle is excited directly and requires a longer lasting stimulus.

The measurement of intensity-duration curves in testing for nerve injury has become practicable with the development of modern electronic apparatus especially devised for this purpose.[1] With the use of "square shocks," pulses for which rise and fall are very short compared with their persistence it is possible to make these determinations with greater efficiency than with previous methods.

Measurement of Accommodation

If a stimulus of gradually increasing intensity is

applied to excitable tissue, a high value may be reached before reaction occurs.[31] Living tissue has the power of adapting its polarized state to a gradual stimulus in such a way that a shock sufficient to cause excitation when suddenly applied may not produce excitation if the peak of the stimulus is reached over a period of time. The threshold value for excitation by a gradually increasing stimulus may be many times that for sudden stimulation. The ratio of the two values is the measure of accommodation of a tissue. The accommodative powers of nerve are much greater than those of muscle alone, and this provides a means of distinguishing innervated from denervated muscle. Three tests that are dependent on assessment of accommodation are: (1) the galvanic-tetanus ratio; (2) progressive current testing; and (3) alternating current intensity-frequency curves.

The galvanic-tetanus ratio requires a determination of the rheobase and the application of a galvanic current up to a point of continuous contraction. The ratio of current required for this tetanus to rheobase is about five for normal muscle and less than two for denervated muscle. This test is reported to be simple and rapid, but may produce skin burns because of high and prolonged currents needed to produce contractions.

Progressive current testing requires an increasing shock with a period of rise and peak value that can be recorded. The ratio of the threshold for progressive current to threshold for sudden shock stimulation expresses the relative elevation of the gradual stimulus to the instantaneous impulse, and is a true measure of accommodation.[31]

The determination of alternating current intensity-frequency curves involves the application of variable frequency AC to muscle or nerve and the measurement of the intensity required at each frequency; this reveals a frequency-intensity relationship which shows a definite optimal frequency. The diagnostic possibilities of the method rest in the fact that the optimal frequency for minimal intensity stimulation is 60 cycles per second for normal, and two cycles per second for denervated human muscle.

An extended discussion of variables attending identification of neuromuscular complexes and the validity of assessments in various tests is given by Ritchie.[35] In summary it is suggested that electrodiagnosis is worth doing if done thoroughly. An examination consisting of an ID curve based on eight to 10 readings with an accommodation measurement by galvanictetanus ratio should give as much information about a muscle as can be gained from artificial stimulation. With electromyography as an adjunct, these methods should provide recognition of regeneration several weeks before clinical recovery in the majority of cases.

While testing motor response to nerve stimulation, in evaluating nerve recovery after injury or after surgical repair, our chief experience has been with bipolar neural stimulation, through two hypodermic needles,

1 cm apart, inserted in close proximity to the nerve. A current is applied to secure a confined bipolar stimulation of the nerve trunk. It is not necessary that the needles be in contact with the nerve trunk, but if they do it is not harmful. The intensity of stimulus required for maximal stimulation of the nerve trunk is very small, and the make-and-break shock delivered by two 1½-volt flashlight batteries toned down by a simple rheostat is adequate. Stimulation through the intact skin is easier, but may yield negative results when positive results are obtained with bipolar needle electrodes. Deep nerves, such as the radial, are tested with the latter method, which is much more reliable in beginning recovery.[45] If Tinel's sign is positive at the level of nerve that is stimulated, similar paresthesias should be referred to the sensory area of supply with each electric stimulus, indicating an adequate stimulation of the nerve and serving as a control of the adequacy of the current intensity in the event of failure of motor response. First motor response by this nerve stimulation test will precede voluntary motor response by several weeks. Care must be exercised in adjusting the rheostat as considerable discomfort is complained of by some people during this test.

DIAGNOSIS

In all wounds involving the upper extremity, damage to nerves must be considered and motor and sensory tests done. Simple methods are used for the examination of all forms of sensibility. The inaccuracy of using cotton wool with varying pressure in estimating touch sensibility has led to the use of von Frey hairs, calibrated by pressure against a known weight in a balance.[39] Pain is most easily tested by pinprick, although this method is subject to the same inaccuracy of varying pressure as cotton wool. Postural sensibility is determined by moving the part through flexion and extension, with the patient indicating position in the opposite normal hand. Thermal sensibility is not universally recommended because it offers no helpful additional information.

The area of sensory supply of the median nerve is usually the volar surface of the thumb, index, and long fingers, lateral half of the ring finger, and the palm lateral to the fourth metacarpal bone extending proximally to the base of the thenar eminence. It also includes the dorsal aspect of the distal ends of these fingers.[27] The ulnar nerve supplies the rest of the palmar surface of the hand, and through its dorsal branch arising above the wrist, the skin of the medial half of the dorsum of the hand with the exception of the area at the distal ends of the fingers. These are supplied by the volar branches.

The radial nerve commonly supplies the dorsum of the lateral aspect of the hand over the first two metacarpals, and the dorsum of the thumb and index finger over two phalanges. Its supply to the long finger is usually limited to the area over the proximal phalanx. Much variation is described with either the radial or ulnar supplying the entire surface, and overlap or replacement by the cutaneous nerves of the forearm.

Anomolous innervation should be suspected if the area of sensory deficit varies from the usual zone of cutaneous sensory supply.[39] Seddon has found that the autonomous zone of the median nerve may be smaller than expected, and limited to the tips of the thumb, index, and long fingers. Similarly, the autonomous zone of the ulnar nerve may be limited to the short finger and the ulnar border of the hand. The autonomous zone of the radial nerve may be completely lacking.

Tinel's sign has been established as a valuable diagnostic aid in nerve recovery by Henderson,[16] who in studying a series of patients who were not surgically explored, found that with a strong Tinel's sign at the level of injury and persistent absence distally, regeneration did not occur. A strong sign at level of the lesion with the development of a weak sign distally indicated poor regeneration. However, a strong Tinel's sign at the point of injury that gradually diminished as sensitivity of the distal part increased, progressed peripherally and faded centrally, was a definite indication that satisfactory recovery was in progress.

Tinel's sign is determined by percussing the nerve trunk distal to the lesion in such a way that the nerve junction is not distrubed. Pressure applied to skin between the point of suture and the distal point tested prevents stimulation by tapping from that source. When paresthesias occur and are referred to the area of sensory supply of the nerve trunk, positive proof exists of continuity of sensory axons from the point percussed to the central nervous system.[45] Tinel's sign is believed to indicate the presence of poorly myelinated axons in the area percussed.

When the Tinel's sign progresses distally at a fairly rapid rate of 3 to 4 mm a day, as it commonly does, this is clear evidence that some regeneration is going on, but not proof that satisfactory regeneration will occur. More than three-quarters of the nerve lesions which required resection and suture later had been associated with a properly advanced Tinel sign.[45]

Motor Examination

Median Nerve

The median nerve arises in the brachial plexus by two heads from the anterior divisions of motor roots from C5 to T1, descends with blood vessels (Fig. 9.1.3) and enters the forearm between the two heads of the pronator teres.[8] It descends in the forearm between the sublimis and profundus muscles, upon the tendon of the flexor profundus to the index finger until at the wrist joint it is lateral to the sublimis and directly under the palmaris longus tendon (Fig. 9.1.1). Beneath the lower edge of the transverse carpal ligament, it gives off the thenar motor branch, and divides into digital branches in a plane superficial to the tendons and deep to the superficial arterial palmar arch. Proper

digital branches to both sides of the thumb and the lateral side of the index finger arise distal to the origin of the thenar motor nerve and two common volar digital nerves continue into the palm where they divide into proper digital nerves supplying the adjoining sides of the second and third digital clefts. Here they have reversed their proximal relations and the proper volar digital nerves lie superficial to the accompanying arteries.

Motor branches of the median nerve above the elbow supply the humeral head of the pronator teres muscle. Motor branches from in front of the elbow supply the remainder of the pronator teres and also the flexor carpi radialis, the palmaris longus, and the flexor digitorum superficialis. The anterior interosseus nerve arises at the upper border of the pronator teres (Fig. 9.1.2) and supplies the deep flexors of the fingers on the radial side, the flexor pollicis longus and the pronator quadratus. At the lower border of the transverse carpal ligament, the thenar motor branch supplies the opponens muscle of the thumb, the abductor pollicis brevis, one-half of the flexor brevis muscle to the thumb, and the two lateral lumbrical muscles.

Division of the median nerve at the level of the elbow causes loss of flexion of thumb, index, and long fingers at the proximal and distal interphalangeal joints through loss of function of the superficial and deep flexors. Flexion of the wrist is weak with ulnar deviation from loss of flexor carpi radialis. Both pronators are denervated, as is the palmaris longus. There is loss of function of the "median intrinsics" in the hand.

Median nerve injury at the wrist results in "opponens paralysis" of the hand caused by paralysis of the short abductor and opponens muscles to the thumb. Abductor loss results in inability to open the hand for grasping large objects, and abductor-opponens loss results in inability to oppose the thumb to the ring finger, that is to approximate it in flat, pad-to-pad contact. "Opponens paralysis" is absent at times in median nerve transections because of anomalous innervation into the whole thenar eminence by the ulnar nerve. Loss of function in the two lateral lumbrical muscles is not clinically apparent as a rule.

Ulnar Nerve

The ulnar nerve arises in the branchial plexus from the inner cord which derives from C8 to T1 roots, and descends in the arm at the inner side of the brachial artery (Fig. 9.1.3), leaving this vessel in the lower third of the arm along the inner head of the triceps muscle, to pass through the angle formed by the medial epicondyle and olecranon under the dense bridging fascia. It passes between the ulnar and humeral heads of the flexor carpi ulnaris muscle, descends between this muscle and the ulnar half of the flexor digitorum profundus, giving several branches to both muscles (Fig. 9.1.2). It is accompanied by the ulnar artery on its side. Above the wrist, the dorsal sensory

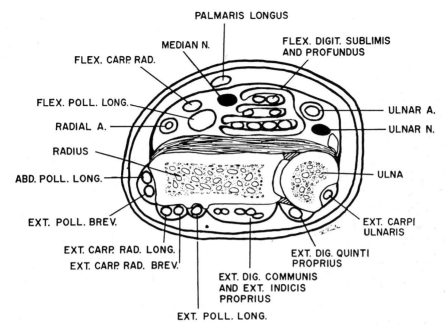

Figure 9.1.1. Cross section through the forearm above the wrist showing relation of median and ulnar nerves to the tendons and blood vessels at this level.

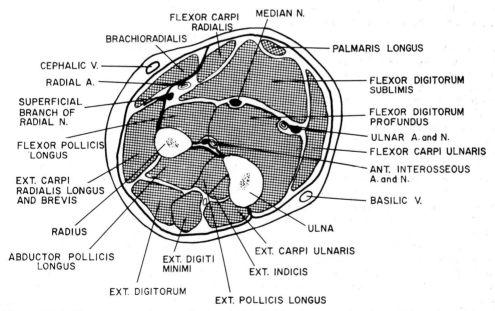

Figure 9.1.2. Cross section through the upper third of the forearm showing relation of median and ulnar nerves to muscles and blood vessels at this level.

branch winds around the lower end of the ulna to supply the dorsum of the ulnar part of the hand (Fig. 9.1.1).

At the wrist, the ulnar nerve passes through an opening in the transverse carpal ligament, and its sensory branch sends a medial proper digital branch to the little finger and a common volar branch from which arise proper digital nerves to the adjoining sides of the ring and little fingers at the fourth cleft. Motor branches of the ulnar nerve to the flexor carpi ulnaris muscle and ulnar portion of the flexor profundus digitorum to the ring and little fingers arise at the elbow

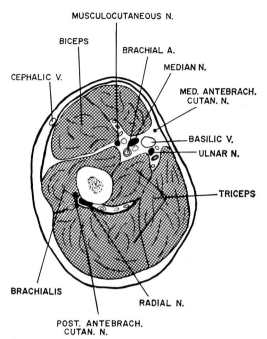

MUSCULOCUTANEOUS N.

BICEPS

BRACHIAL A.

MEDIAN N.

CEPHALIC V.

MED. ANTEBRACH.
CUTAN. N.

BASILIC V.

ULNAR N.

TRICEPS

BRACHIALIS

RADIAL N.

POST. ANTEBRACH.
CUTAN. N.

Figure 9.1.3. Cross section through the middle third of the humerus showing relation of radial nerve to bone and muscle, and other anatomical relations of median and ulnar nerve at this level.

level, and at a lower level another branch to the flexor carpi ulnaris also arises. The deep palmar motor branch of the ulnar nerve descends between the abductor and flexor muscles of the little finger, winds around the hook of the hamate on its ulnar side, and travels across the palm with the deep volar arterial arch, supplying successively the palmaris brevis, the hypothenar muscles, the two medial lumbricals, all the interossei, one-half the flexor pollicis brevis, and the adductors of the thumb.

Injuries to the ulnar nerve occur chiefly with lacerations at or above the wrist, or with penetrating wounds in the palm or fingers. Less commonly it is involved at the elbow joint in fracture or dislocation, or later involvement in callus.[8]

Severance of the ulnar nerve at the wrist results in loss of function of the ulnar intrinsic muscles enumerated above, with loss of lateral motions of the fingers, and inability to flex the proximal and to extend the two distal finger joints in the little and at times the ring finger. Function in the long flexors of one or both of these fingers leads to ''claw deformity,'' hyperextension at the metacarpophalangeal joint with flexion at the proximal and distal interphalangeal joints of the fingers involved. Muscular atrophy leads to flattening of the hypothenar bulge of the hand, and interosseous atrophy leads to conspicuous grooving in the interosseous spaces noted on the dorsum of the hand. Also loss of the stabilizing function of the adductor muscle

of the thumb and the first dorsal interosseus leads to instability in pinching the thumb against the index finger, and this ''loss of pinch'' results in inability to hold firmly a perfect circle with the thumb and index finger.

Radial Nerve

The radial nerve arises from the posterior cord of the brachial plexus and provides extension to the elbow, wrist, and digits, aided in the distal two finger joints by the intrinsic muscles of the hand. The radial nerve descends in the arm close to the humerus, curves around it in its musculospiral groove (Fig. 9.1.3), pierces the intermuscular septum and continuing under the brachioradialis muscle, divides below the elbow into its sensory and motor branches, the superficial radial and posterior interosseus nerves. The superficial radial branch continues under the brachioradialis muscle and enters the dorsum of the forearm in the subcutaneous tissue, continuing to supply sensory fibers to the radial aspect of the dorsum of the hand and fingers. The posterior interosseus nerve penetrates the supinator brevis muscle, and supplies this muscle with the extensors of the wrist, fingers, and thumb, and the long abductor of the thumb.

Severance of the radial nerve in the elbow region or above results in a sensory deficit of a part of the dorsum of the arm and forearm, and in a triangular area on the radial aspect of the dorsum of the hand of variable size. This area is unimportant for tactile sensation. Injury to the sensory branch at the wrist or below may escape attention because of the small size of the fibrils involved but may lead to formation of a painful neuroma.

Radial nerve paralysis occurs with injuries in the axilla by prolonged pressure, as in an alcoholic stupor, in the arm by injury in fracture of the humerus or later involvement in its callus, and below the elbow by penetrating wounds or surgical trauma, as in operations on the head of the radius. The characteristic motor deficit of radial paralysis, wrist drop, consists in loss of extension of the wrist, fingers, and thumb, with adduction of thumb which may interfere with flexion of the fingers. Pronation of the arm is present if the injury is above the innervation of the supinator, and triceps paralysis with inability to extend the elbow may accompany trauma at the level of the axilla.

Combined median and ulnar nerve injuries, resulting from injuries at the wrist or forearm, are very disabling. Anesthesia extends through the whole palm, volar surface of fingers and thumb, and most of the dorsal segments of the fingers. The hand is flat with loss of muscle tone in thenar and hypothenar eminences, and the thumb cannot be moved actively away from the index ray. The metacarpophalangeal joints fall into extension unless their volar capsules are tight, and marked clawing of the fingers results from flexion of the distal joints if the nerves are divided below the muscle branches to the long flexors of the fingers.

Clawing is less in injuries above the motor branches. Contractures occur and may be slowly responsive to treatment. Proper splinting, physical therapy, and close observation are essential, and early reexploration of the nerves should be performed if any doubt exists as to the quality of the initial repair or if electrodiagnostic evidences of regeneration are unsatisfactory.

TREATMENT

The correct treatment of peripheral nerve injuries begins in the accident admitting room where the wound is assessed as to location, causative agent, direction of causative force, contaminating environment, elapsed time, and presence of bleeding. Wound bleeding is controlled with sterile compression, sensory and motor tests performed, tendon deficits noted, and the need for x-rays determined. Immediate exploration is indicated by the syndrome of nerve division, or a wound in or near the line of a nerve, and especially so in those unable to cooperate with testing, such as adult alcoholics and excited children. General anesthesia or axillary nerve blocking is usually selected and a tourniquet is applied to the extremity which has been rendered bloodless by an Esmarch elastic bandage. Local anesthesia is advised for certain secondary explorations which require nerve stimulation in a conscious patient to determine conduction through a damaged nerve segment.

Wound Diagnosis and Preparation

Preparation of the extremity includes suitable cleansing with agents such as Phisoderm and Zephiran, the wound being protected with sterile gauze, and then a thorough irrigation of the wound with sterile saline or Ringer's solution. At this time a careful wound survey is made which is further refined into precise wound diagnosis during the wound exploration and debridement which follows final cleansing of the skin. In a clean incised wound, or a minimally contused or contaminated wound confidently converted to a clean state, a decision to perform primary repair is made. The decision for a delayed repair, usually in a crushed, avulsed or contaminated wound confidently converted to a clean state, a decision to perform primary repair is made. The decision for a delayed repair, usually in a crushed, avulsed or contaminated wound, rests on five factors: (1) the possibility of the wound being made bacteriologically clean by irrigation and wound excision; (2) the assurance of obtaining uncomplicated primary healing of the wound by complete debridement of severely traumatized and devitalized soft tissue; (3) the ability to detect the true extent of damaged nerve and to debride that amount of injured nerve necessary for healing and a good nerve junction; (4) the availability of adequate facilities for a good repair; and (5) the absence of associated damage of high priority. If any of these conditions is not favorable, the nerve is approximated by a visible black silk suture, the wound is closed, and definitive repair postponed to a later date. Debridement should include the search for and the surgical removal of the diffuse hematoma which suffuses through areolar planes along tendons and nerves as these are not always apparent nor removed by even prolonged wound irrigation. These provide a chemical stimulus for the development of dense mature collagen, and if allowed to remain in the wound, these hematomas may be followed by persistent induration and edema,[28] which occasionally occur in wounds otherwise cleanly debrided. The aim is to secure in the healed wound the best possible environment for the function of a nerve junction. Too much emphasis cannot be placed on the necessity for painstaking preparation of the wound, always including prolonged irrigation and careful scrutiny of the wound in evaluating the total effect of the causative trauma. A correct wound diagnosis leads to a correct decision as to the proper type of treatment, either primary repair, or wound closure and delayed repair. The following indications for delayed repair are offered by Larsen and Posch[20] (1) severe crush or tearing type of trauma; (2) marked wound contamination; (3) associated injury of high priority; (4) inadequate facilities for operation.

Exposure of Nerves

The exposure of nerves after injury requires incisions which should be so placed as to avoid scar contractures. Flexion creases should be avoided, but when necessary incisions across flexion creases are made in a sinuous pattern, or in a linear manner with a transverse step in the flexion crease, a bayonet type or a "Z" incision.[27]

Digital nerves in the fingers are exposed by a midlateral incision, and in the palm by an incision in the line of a flexion crease, extending the existing laceration if possible. In the fingers, it is at times necessary to produce a T-shaped incision, since the laceration producing digital nerve injury is often a transverse cut.

In the proximal palm, the median nerve is exposed by an incision parallel to the proximal palmar crease extending to the wrist, and crossing the flexion crease in a sinuous pattern or transverse "step" when it is necessary to view the nerve in the forearm. To the motor branch of the ulnar nerve in the palm, a useful approach is through an incision in the middle palmar crease carried proximally along the medial aspect of the hypothenar eminence to the flexion crease of the wrist, avoiding the bulge of the pisiform bone. This is carried laterally in the flexion crease before curving upward along the line of the flexor ulnaris tendon for forearm exploration.

Above the wrist, the ulnar nerve is exposed by a linear incision along the edge of the flexor carpi ulnaris, and at the elbow by a lateral incision posterior to the medial epicondyle. The median nerve in the forearm may be approached by a short linear anterolateral incision which may be extended in a sinuous pattern across the antecubital space on the ulnar aspect of the arm. A linear extension into the arm may be made for higher exploration.[27]

The radial nerve in the arm is approached by a medial incision between the triceps posteriorly and the biceps and other muscles anteriorly. Laterally, an approach is made along the long head of the triceps down to the medial edge of the brachioradialis at the elbow. The deep branch of the radial nerve is exposed by an incision which divides the fascial plane between the brachioradialis muscle and biceps over the distal humerus, descends laterally to the antecubital fossa, and posteriorly over the upper portion of the forearm between the brachioradialis and extensor carpi radialis. It is advisable to locate the nerve in a normal state at or just above the elbow joint and to follow it distally to the point of injury, preserving all motor branches to the larger muscles arising at this level.[22]

Seletz[41] has recently described anatomic surgical approaches to peripheral nerves. New incisions and surgical approaches were developed in order to provide more direct surgical approach to peripheral nerves with adequate exposure, avoidance of injury to other structures bridging extensive gaps, and prevention of scar contracture. Surgical anatomy and incisions used in repair of specific nerves are illustrated.

Technique of Repair

An adequate incision having been made, lengthening when necessary the initial laceration and avoiding linear incisions across flexion creases, and a wound diagnosis having established that primary repair is to be done, wound debridement is performed and nerve ends drawn into the field. The nerve ends are "squared" with a new knife blade or razor against a firm surface, such as a small board, never with scissors which always cut with a slight contusing force. Alignment is aided by the somewhat oval shape of larger nerves; the vascular marking is a definite landmark. The use of a magnifying lens is helpful and Bruner[6] strongly recommends the inexpensive low power loupe, with two power magnification, in the repair of digital nerves and the identification of small nerves during palmar fasciectomy. The operating microscope offers further advantages. Current investigations have led to enthusiastic preliminary reports of improved nerve junctions and earlier return, both motor and sensory, of a better quality. Dilute methylene blue, applied to nerve ends, stains fibrous tissue and nerve fibrils differentially and aids in determining the extent of the necessary dissection, and the placement of sutures without injury to neurofibrils, when instruments of higher magnification are used.[42] Final decision of the value of the operating microscope in nerve suture awaits reports of long term studies of a well controlled large series.

Fine sutures of silk (7-0) or tantalum (No. 40) are first placed in opposite corners, including epineurium only, and in number sufficient to produce a water-tight closure, and to prevent escape of regenerating axons. Otherwise a lateral neuroma may result. Evidence is offered that fine (6-0) stainless steel wire is superior to other materials of similar size, such as silk, chromic catgut, and Mersilene. In histologic examination 42 days after nerve sutures performed in rabbits, the inflammatory reaction was gone from nerves sutured with wire, but was present in all others (Granberry and Wilson[12]). In discussion of this work, Hardy[15] emphasized the basic principles of nerve suture; (1) small caliber suture material with atraumatic needles should be used; (2) there should be minimal trauma incident to insertion of sutures; (3) suture material that sets up minimal fibroblastic reaction should be used; (4) the surface area of suture in contact with neural tissue should be reduced to a minimum; (5) sutures should be placed in the epineurium since more reaction results if the perineurium is pierced; (6) the nerve ends should be approximated without torsion or tension; and (7) there should be good hemostasis so that the repair can be done in a dry operative field.

Nerve repair should be done after any necessary deep tendon repair. It is of primary importance to release the tourniquet before nerve suture is done to prevent formation of a trapped hematoma within the repaired junction, one which in fibrous resolution will produce some disorganization of the junction area and may ruin an otherwise excellent nerve junction. The injection of saline into small nerves in the hand to produce a larger structure by temporary edema makes nerve repair easier technically. The injection of larger amounts of saline 1.0 cm proximal to a completed sutured line to demonstrate adequacy of "water-tight closure" and scar-free stroma, and to align nerve fibrils by flowing into the distal segment, may offer further advantage in nerve suture. Woodhall advises the placing of opaque wire markers 1 cm from the suture line on each side of the nerve so that a postoperative anteroposterior x-ray picture may reveal separation in the event of suture line disruption, and a second exploration be done without delay. The use of insulating materials, such as tantalum foil, vein segments, or various membranes around a nerve junction, is generally condemned. These provide a barrier to the invasion of local blood supply which is necessary for healing and for the preservation of nutrition in nerve segments, which may have been mobilized by dissection through a distance.

After repair of nerves, the extremity is flexed into a position that provides suitable relaxation for nerve healing, and the wound is closed, isolating the deep repair from the skin closure by a loose interposition of superficial fascia or subcutaneous fat. The skin is closed by vertical mattress sutures of fine nylon, which are well tolerated for long intervals. Subcuticular sutures of fine material may be placed and the skin closed with simple or mattress sutures; these tension-free incisions tend to heal well with thin scars. Suitable flexion of wrist and elbow is maintained for three weeks with anterior and posterior molded plaster splints. Elbow flexion is released at three weeks, and neutral positioning of the wrist established at four weeks. Support is provided with a removable molded anterior plaster splint. Passive motions are begun at three to four weeks, and active motion at about four weeks. Plaster splint protection is continued for four to five weeks after injury. Brown[5] has reported on factors influencing the success of the surgical repair of peripheral nerves. He suggests that the generally poor results in the surgical repair of injured peripheral nerves suggests the need for greater understanding of the physiology and pathology of neural tissue and for more sophistication in the surgical handling of this tissue. The success ratio in the managing of these injuries is influenced by the understanding of seven factors: (1) type of injury, mixed or unmixed nerves; (2) age of patient; results are usually better in younger patients; (3) level of the injury; peripheral lesions present a better regenerative potential of the distal neuron than a more proximal injury; (4) length of defect; (5) associated injuries; (6) surgical technique; (7) time factor; the sooner nerve repair is done, the better are the chances of success.

Special Considerations

Certain special considerations in the treatment of nerve injuries are worthy of emphasis. The repair of digital nerves in the palm and fingers, as far distally as they can be seen and sutured, is advisable.

When a partial laceration of a major nerve is found it is recommended that primary repair is of special importance.[20] At this time the injury is clearly seen and accurate suture is easily performed. Delayed repair of partial lacerations after a long interval is difficult, as the scar at and around the point of injury obscures intact fibers and makes their identification most difficult. If primary repair is not done for any reason, secondary repair should be done as soon as possible, ideally at three to four weeks, or as soon thereafter as the condition of the wound permits.

The recovery of function of intrinsic muscles after median nerve injury is by no means as great a problem as after ulnar nerve injury. There is evidence that repair of pure nerves, as in the motor branch of either median or ulnar nerve, has a better prognosis for intrinsic muscle return than in repairs done in the mixed motor-sensory nerves at the wrist. It is occasionally possible to recognize a small bundle on the anterolateral edge of the median nerve at the wrist (Fig. 9.1.4) which represents the aggregate of motor fibrils of the thenar motor nerve above the point of branching. In local nerve suture this is to be selectively approximated to its distal counterpart, so that the mixed nerve repair becomes in effect a repair of two pure nerves. This method of selective bundle repair may be also performed in the ulnar nerve, in which the deep motor bundle, a larger aggregate of fibrils than the thenar motor bundle, may at times be clearly seen above its branching take-off.

Better intrinsic muscle reinnervation, with restora-

tion of quick and skillful hand movements, occurs after early repair of the motor branch of the ulnar nerve, which may be performed at various points between the hypothenar muscles and the adductor pollicis muscle.[3] Regeneration is evidenced by voluntary activity of the first dorsal interosseous muscle, and is present in from three to 14 months after repair. Gaps which occur after ulnar motor injuries in which there is loss of substance, as in gunshot wounds, are overcome by rerouting the proximal nerve through the carpal tunnel after dividing the palmaris brevis laterally and the hypothenar muscle origins to preserve intact their nerve supply. The motor component may be split off the main ulnar nerve well up into the forearm, if length is needed for a good nerve junction.

Gaps in nerves in the forearm may also be reduced by the method described by Larsen and Posch[20] in which a 4-inch (10-cm) gap in the median nerve at mid forearm level was closed by successive mobilization and advancement, and bulb suture and posturing in each of several successive reconstructive operations. First evidence of sensory return was present at six months, and at two years sensation was found to be almost normal. At this time there was electromyo-

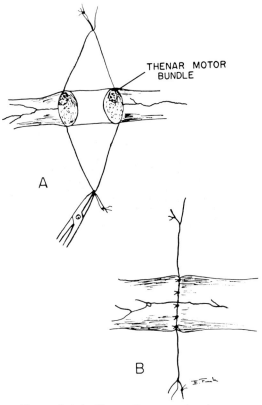

Figure 9.1.4. Shows the occasional appearance of the thenar motor bundle in the median nerve at the wrist, and the placement of sutures and use of vascular markings in aligning nerve for repair.

graphic evidence of reinnervation of thenar muscles, but clinically the degree of functional return was not impressive.

It is established that injuries to the posterior interosseous branch of the radial nerve are amenable to surgical repair. The reluctance to attempt repair, which existed formerly, was based on the belief that gaps could not be overcome because of the straight course of the nerve, and that widespread arborization prevented end-to-end suture. Mayer and Mayfield[22] have shown that arborization often occurs one or more inches below the supinator muscle. The nerve is exposed by a lateral incision extended downward below the elbow on the posterolateral aspect of the forearm between the brachioradialis and the extensor carpi radialis. The radial nerve is identified between the brachioradialis and the biceps tendon and is dissected downward to the site of the injury below the supinator, thus separating the extensor carpi radialis and extensor digitorum communis muscles. Gaps up to 5.0 cm are readily overcome by freeing the nerve and flexing the elbow to 90°. More than 70 per cent of cases repaired by end-to-end suture gained a high degree of recovery.

Buncke[7] reports that digital nerve injuries, which are very common, are best treated by careful debridement and microsurgical repair with fine suture material. Protective sensation can uniformly be restored and a two-point discrimination of under 6 mm can be expected in 60 per cent of patients.

Late Repair of Nerves

When clinical and physiologic testing at six months after injury have yielded no evidence of nerve regneration, Woodhall[46] recommends exploration under local anesthesia followed by general anesthesia after distal sensory testing. The extremity is draped so that all passive joint movements may be carried out and the results of nerve testing readily seen. The use of a tourniquet is warranted because of the great value of a bloodless field, which must be balanced against occasional "unpredictable involvement" of normal nerve structures by tourniquet injury. The nerve is exposed proximally and distal to the point of trauma, and testing compared with preoperative tests.[46]

The evaluation of the neuroma presents certain difficulties.[46] A stony, hard lesion probably signifies a major local disruption of fibrils, but a small firm lesion gives no assurance that regeneration will occur. Inability to inject saline through a point of injury does not rule out the possibility of regeneration, but a gross solid scar, revealed by a longitudinal incision through the neuroma, justifies resection. The levels of neuroma resection are established by trial razor cuts revealing scar-free nerve ends with distinct and unfixed fibrils proximally. Free bleeding must cease before nerve suture. Smaller distal nerve ends are distended with saline, and end suture is performed with fine arterial silk or tantalum with sufficient sutures so that the junction is water-tight to subsequent local instillation. Opaque wire marker sutures are placed to mark a point 1.0 cm on either side of the junction, and an x-ray is made at three to four weeks to check on possible separation of the suture line. In positioning the part, extreme flexion is avoided, and immobilization is secured by a plaster half-shell. This is continued for three weeks, and gradual extension, up to the point of paresthesia, is performed until neutral position is attained. Rigid circular casts are not used as they may favor development of unrecognized venous and lymphatic stasis which may impede neuroregeneration, and favor atrophy of intrinsic hand muscles.

In the postoperative period, muscle training is provided by passive, active-assisted, and active exercises. Tension splints are provided if hand contractures exist. For wrist drop, a cock-up splint is provided, with thumb and fingers free. Extension of metacarpophalangeal joints is avoided, lest the well recognized shortening of collateral ligaments which is apt to occur in splinted extension should prevent later full flexion. If there is a tendency to clawing, a simple removable "knuckle duster" plaster cast, fitted snugly from proximal end of metacarpals to proximal interphalangeal joint, maintains the metacarpophalangeal joint in 25° to 30° of flexion until tone returns in the medial lumbricals. Postoperative median nerve repairs may be fitted with plastic splints to maintain relaxation of the opponens-abductor group of muscles. If these are not available, a simple opponens sling of elastoplast or 1-inch adhesive looped around the thumb and attached medially above the ulnar styloid, is quite adequate.

Delayed exploration of nerves previously repaired will usually be indicated by evidence available four to six months after injury. In instances of further delay, some return of motor function may be obtained two years after injury, and some sensory return is stated to be obtainable up to six years.

RESULTS

Best results in treatment of nerve injuries are obtained when early axonal downgrowth is established through a well constructed nerve junction. Factors working against this are several. Delay in repair favors narrowing of distal tubules and increase of fibrous interstitial elements in the distal nerve segment. These factors are operative in some degree, possibly in combination with other influences not now well understood, when the distal nerve segment is a long one, as in transections high in the arm. Technical errors are of various types. (1) Faulty alignment leads to haphazard channeling in mixed nerves, with lowered quality of the sensory and motor return. (2) Loose suturing of the nerve junction favors focal escape of downgrowing axones and the development of lateral neuromas. (3) Deep placement of sutures or the use of large suture material leads to fibrosis of the suture line with internal disorganization of varying degree. (4) Suture line separation that follows suturing under too much tension or too rapid extension of the flexed extremity before the time of firm healing produces fibrosis of the junction area with total block of axonal regeneration. Even with preservation of good apposition of repaired nerve ends, and effective protection through the period of healing, a mesenchymal reaction of unexpected degree may lead to failure of regeneration. At times "the more primitive healing process predominates over a superlative effort at neural regeneration" for reasons not well understood nor amenable to control.

After nerve repair, sensation returns before motion, with sensation progressing downward to the tip of the extremity, coarse touch and pinprick response preceding light touch, and deep sensibility preceding stereognostic return.[8] Paresthesias in response to various stimuli are present in diminishing degree for one to three years, at which time sensation approaches but does not attain the "normal state."

Rates of advance of axone tips have been investigated clinically in limbs requiring amputation[47] for nonmalignant conditions, and determinations of a rate of 4.4 mm per day determined for a digital nerve. From examination of muscle biopsies there was evidence[2] that outgrowth of new axones was not less than 3 mm per day after nerve crush. These are in general agreement with studies based on Tinel's sign.

The nature of the lesion in the nerve trunk influences the rate of outgrowth of axone tips[49] and the rate of advance of recovery of function. These rates are more rapid after a simple crush injury than after nerve suture or an extensive lesion in continuity. There is an initial delay before the axone tips reach the distal stump of the nerve, and there is a longer delay before there is clinical evidence of recovery. The initial delay and the delay before clinical recovery are shorter after a simple crush injury than after a suture. In man there appears to be a progressive decline in the rate of outgrowth of axone tips as measured by Tinel's sign, and also in the rate of recovery of function. This seems to vary in individual cases, and there is evidence to suggest that the level of the lesion plays a significant part in that the higher the lesion the more rapid appears to be the initial progress of recovery.[39] Therefore the average rates of recovery quoted from various sources can only be used with reserve as rough approximations.

The value of reports of end results of nerve suture depends on: (1) strict adherence to accurate criteria for each important phase of recovery; (2) adequate and comparable periods of postoperative observation for all cases; and (3) a simple and clear method of analysis.[49] A method that records the numbers of patients who reach particular grades of recovery when a given time has elapsed after suture is a useful index of the chance of final success. The method avoids the vagueness of general descriptive terms, such as "good," "poor," without further definition, and also avoids reference to functional recovery in terms of occupation or employment, as in return to a certain type of job. The method does address itself to neurologic recovery, which will usually correlate with better function and greater occupational skill.

Zachary[49] has pointed out that repair of a divided nerve gives an even chance of useful recovery, and a return of sufficient function to make suture worthwhile. The results vary from nerve to nerve, and are influenced by such factors as condition of wound, level of suture, delay before suture, and gap after resection of the damaged portion. Results will probably be considerably better in cases resulting from peacetime accidents, as compared with results of war injuries. Perfect recovery possibly never occurs, but there is an approach to perfection in a few radial nerve repairs and in some sutures of the median nerve in children. In almost one-third of radial nerve sutures, even under good conditions, there is still defective independent movement of the fingers, and after median nerve repair two-point discrimination was regained in only 10 per cent of cases. Ulnar nerve repairs had a bad reputation because the familiar test of lateral movement of fingers was passed only by patients with the highest grade of recovery. Useful return of intrinsic power occurred, however, in 70 per cent of low sutures.

Results with war injuries have been reported by Zachary[49] in the Medical Research Council Report (M.R.C.R.) 1954, and those presented by Woodhall et al.[45] 1956 in the American Veterans' monograph entitled "Peripheral Nerve Regeneration." Rank and Wakefield[32] report good results with primary repair under ideal circumstances.

Such, then, is the record of results obtained in nerve suture. For the future, it seems that improvement will be obtained with attention to all phases of wound evaluation and management, especially of the nerve wound and its environment, so that primary suture of nerves will be limited to clean wounds, sharply incised, and avulsed or contused wounds held over for delayed repair. Favoring better results, too, will be constant attention to technical details of operating, directed toward producing a clean environment for a nerve junction which has been made with an absolute minimum of disturbance to the conducting tissues. Added improvement may come from the use of magnifying aids in nerve suture, more intelligent supervision of the postoperative period, and the use of muscle stimulation during the convalescent period, if early reports of more favorable results are sustained in long term studies.

REFERENCES

1. Bauwens, P. Electrodiagnosis and electrotherapy in peripheral nerve lesions. Proc. Roy. Soc. Med., *34:* 459, 1941.
2. Bowden, R.E.M., and Gutmann, E. Clinical value of muscle biopsies. Lancet, *2:* 768, 1945.
3. Boyes, J. Repair of ulnar motor branch in palm. J. Bone Joint Surg., *37A:* 920, 1955.
4. Brooks, D. M. Nerve injuries and fractures. In *Peripheral Nerve Injuries.* H.J. Seddon (Editor). Her

Majesty's Stationery Office, London, 2954, p. 83-105.

5. Brown, P.W. Factors influencing the success of the surgical repair of nerves. Surg. Clin. North Am., 52, 5: 1137-1156, 1972.

6. Bruner, J.M. Use of low power magnifying loupe for routine surgery of hand. Meeting of American Society for Surgery of the Hand, Chicago, Jan. 17, 1964.

7. Buncke, H.J., Jr. Digital nerve repairs. Surg. Clin. North Am., 52, 5: 1267-1286, 1972.

8. Bunnell, S. Surgery of the Hand, Ed. 3. Philadelphia, Lippincott, 1944, (a) p. 382-384; (b) p. 391.

9. Denny-Brown, D.B. Importance of neural fibroblasts in regeneration of nerve. Arch. Neurol. Psychiat., 55: 171, 1946.

10. Doupe, J.J. Studies in denervation: observations concerning adrenaline. J. Neurol. Psychiat., 6: 121, 1943.

11. Flynn, J.E., and Flynn, W.F. Median and ulnar nerve injuries. Ann. Surg., 156: 1002, 1962.

12. Granberry, W.M., and Wilson, J.N. Experimental comparison of suture materials in repair of small nerves. J. Bone. Joint Surg., 45A: 884, 1963.

13. Gutmann, E. Reinnervation of muscle by sensory nerve fibres. J. Anat., 79: 1, 1945.

14. Gutmann, E., and Young, J.Z. The reinnervation of muscle after varying periods of atrophy. J. Anat., 78: 15, 1944.

15. Hardy, S. B. (Discussion of Granberry, W. M., and Wilson, J.N.). J. Bone Joint Surg., 45A: 884, 1963.

16. Henderson, W.R. Clinical assessment of peripheral nerve injuries. Tinel's test. Lancet, 2: 801, 1948.

17. Highet, W.B. Quoted by Zachary, R.B. Results of nerve suture. In Peripheral Nerve Injuries, edited by H.J. Seddon. London, Her Majesty's Stationery Office, 1954, p. 355.

18. Holmes, W., and Young, J.Z. Nerve regeneration after immediate and delayed suture. J. Anat., 77: 63, 1942.

19. Kline, D. G., and Nulsen, F. E. The neuroma in continuity: Its preoperative and operative management. Sur. Clin. North Am., 52, 5: 1189-1210, 1970.

20. Larsen, R.D., and Posch, J.L. Nerve injuries in upper extremity. Arch. Surg., 77: 474, 1958.

21. Lewis, T., and Pickering, G.W. Circulatory changes in fingers in some diseases of the nervous system, with special reference to digital atrophy of peripheral nerve lesions. Clin. Sci., 2: 149, 1936.

22. Mayer, J.H., and Mayfield, F.H. Surgery of posterior interosseous branch of radial nerve. Surg. Gynecal. Obstet., 84: 979, 1947.

23. Meagher, S.W. Personal communication.

24. Mitchell, S.W., Morehouse, G.R., and Keen, W.W. Gunshot Wounds and Other Injuries of Nerves. Philadelphia, Lippincott, 1864.

25. Mitchell, S. W. Injuries of Nerves and their Consequences. Philadelphia, Lippincott, 1872.

26. Moberg, E. Criticism and study of methods for examining sensibility in the hand. Neurology, 12: 8, 1962.

27. Nichols, M. Hand Injuries, Ed. 2. Year Book, Chicago, 1960, (a) pp. 196-197; (b) pp. 233-235.

28. Peacock, E. Tendon repairs; some aspects of wound healing affecting restoration of gliding function.

Meeting of the American Society for Surgery of the Hand, Chicago, Jan. 17, 1964.

29. Phalen, G.S., and Kendrick, J.I. Compression neuropathy of the median nerve in the carpal tunnel. J.A.M.A., 164: 524, 1957.

30. Pollock, L.J., and Davis, L. Peripheral Nerve Injuries. New York, Hoeber, 1923.

31. Pollock, L.J., Golseth, J.G., Arieff, A.J., and Mayfield, F. Electrodiagnosis by means of electric currents of long duration. Surg. Gynecol. Obset., 81: 192, 1945.

32. Rank, B.K., Wakefield, A.R., and Heuston, J.T. Surgery of Repair as Applied to Hand Injuries, Ed. 3. Edinburgh, Livingstone.

33. Richards, R.L. Vasomotor disturbances in hand after injuries to peripheral nerves. Edinburgh M.J., 50: 449, 1943.

34. Ritchie, A.E. The electrodiagnosis of peripheral nerve injury. Brain, 67: 314, 1944.

35. Ritchie, A.E. The electrical diagnosis of peripheral nerve injury. In Peripheral Nerve Injuries, edited by H.J. Seddon. London, Her Majesty's Stationery Office, 1954, pp. 246-262.

36. Schutta, H.S., and Bogdanoff, B.M. Pointers in the clinical diagnosis of acute peripheral nerve injuries. Surg. Clin. North Am., 52, 5: 1123-1136, 1972.

37. Seddon, H.J. Three types of nerve injury. Brain, 66: 237, 1943.

38. Seddon, H.J. Nerve injuries complicating certain bone injuries. J.A.M.A., 135: 691, 1947.

39. Seddon, H.J. Methods of investigating nerve injuries. In Peripheral Nerve Injuries, edited by H.J. Seddon. London, Her Majesty's Stationery Office, 1954, (a) pp. 6-8; (b) p. 19, (c) p. 24.

40. Seddon, H. Electrical Phenomena in Surgical Disorders of Peripheral Nerves. Baltimore, Williams and Wilkins, 1972, pp. 57-67.

41. Seletz, E. Anatomic surgical approaches to peripheral nerves. Surg. Clin. North Am., 52, 5: 1211-1234, 1972.

42. Smith, J.W. Discussion of Bruner, J.M. Use of low power magnifying loupe for routine surgery of hand. Meeting of the American Society for Surgery of the Hand, Jan. 17, 1964.

43. Tanzer, R. The carpal tunnel syndrome. J. Bone Joint Surg., 41A: 626, 1959.

44. Tolnick, B., and Beck, W.C. Histamine flare in evaluation of peripheral nerve injuries. War Med. Chicago, 8: 386, 1945.

45. Woodhall, B., Nulsen, F.E., White, J.C., and Davis, L. In Peripheral Nerve Regeneration, Chap. VII. United States Government Printing Office, 1956, pp. 581-583.

46. Woodhall, B. Peripheral nerve injury. Surg. Clin. North Am., (a) 1147, (b) 1162, (c) 1165, 1954.

47. Young, J.Z. Advances in Surgery, Vol. 1. New York, Interscience, 1949, p. 215.

48. Zachary, R.B., and Holmes, W. Primary suture of peripheral nerves. Sur. Gynecol. Obstet., 82: 632, 1942.

49. Zachary, R.B. Results of nerve suture. In Peripheral Nerve Injuries, edited by H.J. Seddon. London, Her Majesty's Stationery Office, 1954, p. 354.

B.

Methods for Examining Sensibility of the Hand

Erik Moberg, M.D.

In a review in 1946 on neural mechanism of cutaneous sense, Bishop wrote that "the selection of four fundamental modalities for the classification of cutaneous sensations is...a compromise between simplicity and confusion...." In summarizing, he stated that "the concept of sensory modality has become a strait-jacket from which the study of sensation may profitably be released, to the extent of relegating this vestment to the status of a loose-fitting generalization." Recently, Noordenbos[36] clearly pointed out the extent to which a cutaneous stimulation was described as touch or as pain according to the instrument applied. If a pin was used, the sensation was named pain, if cotton wool, touch. "It would appear that the concept of the four sensory modalities...is the results of incorrect verbalization of our clinical findings." Until recently, however, almost every neurologic examination in practical clinical work was based on the theory, that the four modalities, the appreciations of touch, pain, warmth, and cold, taken together, should represent the sensibility of a given point, and that the routine standard tests for the modalities therefore should give all the information necessary.

Rarely did earlier publications on surgical hand problems discuss sensibility. A splendid description of the functional loss following impaired sensibility was given by Bell[3] as early as 1833 in his monograph on the hand. The first clear account of the role of sensory function is to be found in Bunnell's *Surgery of the Hand.*[9] Independent of this work, Hilgenfeldt[17] in Germany stressed how neglected but important the sensory function was, when reconstructive hand surgery was discussed. Both these authors obviously felt that the sensory function had to be graded and that a high quality was necessary for good hand function. Bunnell stresses "stereognosis," Hilgenfeldt Fingerspitzengefühl.

To Seddon and his coworkers[43] [44] we owe the important distinction between "academic" recovery, judged by the response to the conventional tests for touch and pain, and "functional" recovery.

The examination of sensibility performed by the neurologists usually has as its main purpose to diagnose or locate a central or generalized lesion to the nervous system. The conventional tests for the four modalities were invented during the second half of the 19th century by physiologists to distinguish between the different modalities (Blix,[5] von Frey[14]). This is a different purpose than that for which neurology now uses them. The examination performed by the hand surgeons often has an entirely different aim, *i.e.*, to find out the functional value of the sensibility in the periphery. His questions usually are: (1) How many tasks for which a hand is needed can it perform with the sensibility present? (2) Is improvement possible? The hand surgeon will soon realize that this usual approach for examination of the modalities is quite different from the method always accepted when dealing with other nerve functions, *e.g.*, when sight or hearing is tested. For sight it is always felt necessary to examine function, to find out what the eye can see and not only a physiologic detail, as for example that appreciation of light is possible quite apart from stereoscopy, capacity of distinguishing colors, or acuity of vision. Why should not the same approach be the rule when testing sensibility of the hand? Why not examine what the hand in question can do with sensibility present? (Fig. 9.2.1).

We have found how little the results of those tests corresponded with the amount the patient was actually able to use his hands. In a thorough examination of the functional value of the cutaneous sensibility of the hand with various lesions and stages of recovery after them it was found (Moberg) that the two-point discrimination test, variously assessed by different workers (Head *et al.*,[16] Pollack and Davies,[38] Hutchinson *et al.*,[18] Onne[37]), was the only one of the known tests that was useful for examining the functional value of hand sensibility.

It was found necessary to devise tests that could better distinguish between different qualities of sensory function and could give, if not an entirely true, at least a useful picture of the functional value of hand sensibility. To the two-point discrimination test were added two new tests, the "picking up" test and the "ninhydrin fingerprinting" test. *The tests for touch and pain were given up entirely.*

The grasping functions of a hand are, besides the necessary amount of mobility, strength, and stability, dependent on the ability of the digits to feel what they are holding, and to appreciate how and with what strength they are holding it. In addition, the functions are dependent on an alarm system, which gives notice of any mechanical or thermal factor that may cause in-

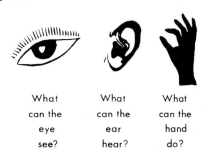

| What can the eye see? | What can the ear hear? | What can the hand do? |

Figure 9.2.1. Function must also be tested when hand sensibility has to be evaluated.

jury to the hand. Finally, more or less included in the requirements mentioned above is proprioception.

The degrees of cutaneous sensibility now possible to distinguish in practice are:

1. Tactile gnosis. This is the quality of sensation that makes a precision sensory grip possible, such as that necessary to screw a nut on a bolt, wind a wrist watch, sew with a needle, knot a string, lift a teacup with the thumb and index, and button and unbutton (usually median nerve area) without the help of the sight. A hand with impaired sensibility in the gripping area cannot perform these actions rapidly and skillfully, even if the motor function is normal.

The term tactile gnosis now seems to be widely accepted in this field where terminology has previously been lacking or ambiguous. The concept here is also wider, including all factors in the complex sensibility, which gives a grip "sight" (Fig. 9.2.2).

2. Sensibility good enough for gross grips as for work with a heavy handle, a spade, for holding a bottle, or carrying a basket. However, without tactile gnosis even these grips cannot be performed with normal speed and skill.

3. Cutaneous protective function, which can be present or absent. Whenever the precision sensory grip with tactile gnosis is possible, protective function is always present. On the other hand, it is possible to have enough sensibility for gross grips without protective sensibility. Also an abnormal reaction for stimuli, not to be confused with sensibility, may give enough

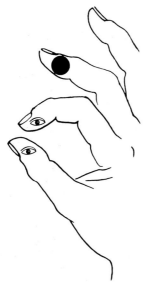

Figure 9.2.2. Fingers with normal sensibility, *i.e.,* where tactile gnosis is present, are able to "see," what they are doing without the help of the sight. If tactile gnosis is lost, the finger is blind and the function greatly impaired, even if the four sensory modalities seem to be present, according to routine methods for examining them.

protection when sensibility is not good enough for gross grip. Here one must discuss a very important distinction, unfortunately not often observed, between useful sensibility and the abnormal nerve reactions of stimuli variously referred to as "wicked" pain (Boring[6]), hyperpathia (Noordenbos[36]), hyperalgesia, or paresthesia. Sensibility is from a functional point of view a plus factor, the other a minus factor. When returning "sensation" after a nerve suture is examined, it is possible to obtain normal figures from these tests or even figures "better" than normal from areas, which from a functional point of view are useless for work due to lack of sensibility.

The division of skin sensibility into protopathic and epicritic components, as Head *et al.*[16] suggested, is often mentioned. What Head called protopathic sensibility has little to do with the gripping functions of the hand. In fact, this form of "sensibility" is not always enough for protection, since the threshold for stimuli may be high and the response often comes too late. His epicritic sensibility would be equivalent to the sensibility needed for tactile gnosis.

TESTS FOR TACTILE GNOSIS

Three valuable tests, the picking-up test, the ninhydrin finger printing test, and the two-point discrimination test, will now be described and technical details given. Their practical value in different situations and their limitations will be discussed.

The Picking-up Test

The subject is asked to pick up a number of small objects on a table and to put them as quickly as he can into a small box, first with one hand and then with the other. After he has done this a few times he is asked to do the same thing blindfolded. It is then studied how rapidly and efficiently he picks up the objects; comparison is made between his right and left hands, and likewise between his performance when he is blindfolded and when he is not. The test with blindfolding can be made harder by asking him to identify the objects as he picks them up. If his hand possesses normal sensibility, it can "see" even when the subject is not helped by his eyes. If sensibility in the median nerve regions is impaired, the subject grasps the objects in a grip with the thumb against the ring and little fingers (Fig. 9.2.3) instead of with thumb and forefinger as he normally would.

It is also observed if the grip is performed in an unusual way, *i.e.,* if the grip moves from areas with impaired sensibility to others with a normal one, but perhaps less good or less comfortable motor function. This often takes place when smaller objects are picked up. If the thumb has lost median nerve sensibility, the patient may often be observed searching for objects and even picking them up with the sides of the distal phalanx of the thumb, innervated from the dorsal side by the radial nerve, avoiding the use of the central pulp

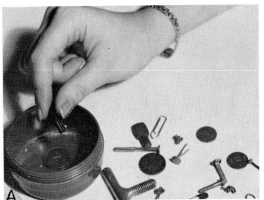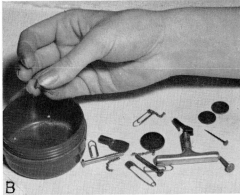

Figure 9.2.3. A. The "picking-up" test. B. If tactile gnosis in the median nerve area is lost, the grip will move to fingers where tactile gnosis is present, often even without the patient being aware of it. (Reprinted with permission of *Journal of Bone and Joint Surgery.*)

area on the tip. When examining children, a small trick is very useful. Let them play with small pieces of colored writing chalk. It makes it very easy to see their finger pulps where useful sensory function is present and where it is absent.

The Ninhydrin Printing Test

The secretion of sweat is regulated by the sympathetic nervous system. The fibers of this system enter the brachial plexus in the cervical region in the form of postganglionic fibers. They then follow the sensory pathways to the periphery, branching in the same way as the bundles carrying tactile gnosis. When a peripheral nerve is severed, the sweat glands in the skin of the region supplied by this nerve lose their innervation. The same area will become dry and sensibility will be lost. All the technique and conclusions now to be described, therefore, apply to injuries to the peripheral sensory nerves distal to the point where sympathetic nerves enter the brachial plexus. The overwhelming majority of nerve lesions of interest to a hand surgeon are located in the arm distally to this level. Amino acids and lower peptides are present in the sweat in small quantities, about 0.4 mg per cc, and ninhydrin is very sensitive to these substances. Fingerprints will show in which area of the pulps innervation of the sweat glands is present or absent. As the site of the nerve lesion is usually known or indicated by the presence of a scar or a neuroma, the cutaneous sensibility of the skin between the pulp and the nerve lesion can be estimated from the prints (Fig. 9.2.4).

Technique

It must be emphasized that exact and clean work is necessary for reliable prints. These prints differ from those used for criminal identification purposes. The aim is to show the orifices of the functioning sweat glands only as dots on a strip of paper (Fig. 9.2.5). From a blurred print like the one in the same picture it

is impossible to tell if sensory function is present or whether the surface examined has been contaminated by moisture from other areas, *e.g.*, from fingers close to a denervated area of the hand. Hypersecretion is often present around a denervated area and the moisture from this may easily be the cause of blurred prints, even from the denervated area, and so lead to misinterpretation. Thus only good punctiform prints give reliable results. The prints are obtained by pressing the pulps of the fingers one at a time steadily against a strip of paper about 3 by 15 cm in size. The outline of the fingertip is traced on the paper with a lead pencil that contains no soluble dye. Sometimes it is useful to roll the tip of the finger slowly and steadily over the paper from one side to the other, to get its lateral surfaces on the print, especially for the thumb, where the border zones of the radial nerve are of great practical importance (Fig. 9.2.6). The same is very often the case also with the doubly innervated pulp of the ring finger.

For comparison, prints are always made from both hands. If the fingers are too moist, they can be cleaned with alcohol or ether. If they are too dry the secretion can be stimulated by exercise. For example, the patient may run up and down a staircase. Better prints can also be obtained by pressing the finger more firmly against the paper and keeping it in place longer. To induce some form of mental stress in the patient may be helpful, for example in the form of an arithmetic problem. To apply a blood pressure cuff at 300 mm Hg was found useful by Onne.[37] As a rule, however, good prints are obtained at ordinary room temperature in Sweden (about 18°C or 64°F) without any previous preparation of the patient. The quality of the paper used is very important, but good glossy writing paper is usually sufficient. (Paper strips made for this purpose as well as the Nin Spray can be obtained from AB Spray Master, Nyodlingsvägen 4R, 19102 Sollentuna 2, Sweden.) The prints are developed in a 1 per cent ninhydrin solution in acetone, mixed with a few

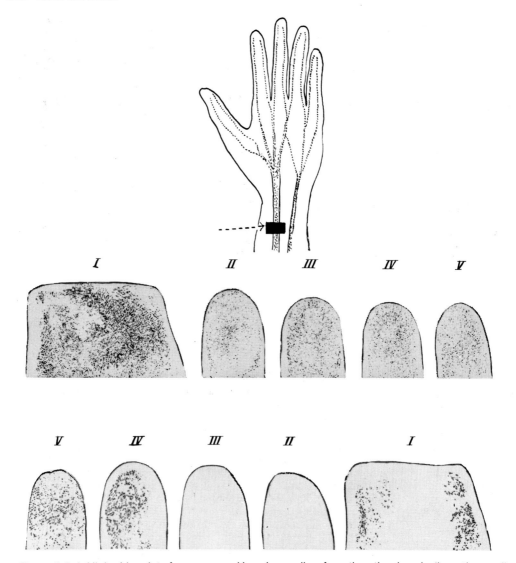

Figure 9.2.4. Ninhydrin prints from a normal hand as well as from the other hand, where the median nerve was severed one inch above wrist level. The prints have mapped out very accurate the areas, where tactile gnosis is present. The thumbs have been rolled over the paper from side to side to show, in addition, the lateral parts innervated from the dorsal side by the radial nerve. Here these branches are supplying a greater area than usual, and therefore the thumb has retained a better functional value.

drops of glacial acid or in ready-made stable Nin Spray solution. After drying and air-warming at 100 to 120°C for five to 10 minutes, the dots become visible. Permanent copies are easily made in the form of Xerox prints.

The Two-Point Discrimination Test

This test is described in every textbook of neurology. A few additional points are given here. The patient should be comfortably seated with the hand outstretched, relaxed, and in a position of rest, and must be unable to watch the test. It is important that the sub-

ject does not try to move the fingertips against the points. Therefore I usually keep the patient's distal phalanx fixed against the table with one of my hands and have the points in my other hand, which is also rested against the table to give satisfactory support (Fig. 9.2.7). The test has been converted from a time-consuming, moderately difficult test to a very handy one by a small variation of the test instrument. Instead of the compass, the writer now is using the instrument show in Figure 9.2.7 made from a small paper clip. The ends are blunt and the weight is inconsequential. It is better to start with the points fairly wide apart and then shorten the distance. The points must be applied simultaneously. Usually 7 correct answers out of 10 tests are felt to be a standard that could be accepted in practical work. A good description on how to perform the test is given by Önne,[37] who also discusses its threshold values. A normal finger pulp can usually discriminate between points 2 to 4 mm apart or, if the skin is used in hard work and is tough, between 4 and 6 mm apart. At the base of the fingers the discrimination is 1 to 2 mm less than at the tip. On the dorsum of the hand values of about 8 to 10 mm are normal. When two-point discrimination is worse than 12 to 15 mm, tactile gnosis is not present. Good tactile gnosis is hardly present if values are higher than 8 mm.

VALUE OF TESTS

The value of these three tests in different situations can be summarized in the following way.

The Picking-Up Test

1. It is function which is tested.
2. Cheating is very difficult or almost impossible.
3. The test is very simple.

Limitations

Active mobility is necessary, but impaired motor function only occasionally affects tests results. Only

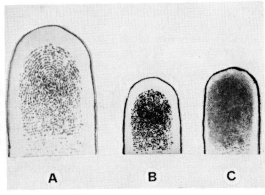

Figure 9.2.5. A. A good print, showing the gland openings as dots. B and C are too blurred and will not permit exact evaluation; prints of this quality should not be used.

gripping surfaces can be tested. If sensation in only one of the two arms of the pincer grip is impaired, some picking-up function may still be present. Such a "one-shank" sensory grip, while undoubtedly inferior to a normal grip, is still not useless (Fig. 9.2.8).

The Ninhydrin Fingerprinting Test

1. The method is objective. Cooperation is not required (children, intoxicated people, malingerers).
2. The test maps out loss of tactile gnosis with greater accuracy than other methods. The broder lines exactly given. Therefore, this test is the best base for planning reconstructive surgery in this field. The prints can be used in a similar way as x-ray pictures are used in bone surgery.

It is astonishing to see how small are the tactile areas when a tool is used in a normal hand, *e.g.*, when a hammer or a pair of pliers is used (Fig. 9.2.9). The exactitude in which the printing test can map out areas with tactile gnosis can hardly be demonstrated better than in such cases where sensibility has been brought to a denervated part of a hand with the help of a neurovascular flap (Fig. 9.2.10).

3. Remaining function in a sensory nerve after a crush has been demonstrated and prognosis was therefore determined early in cases where no other method was of use (Fig. 9.2.11).

4. In high lesions of the brachial plexus, it is sometimes possible to get normal prints, where all sensibility (and motor function) is lost. The lesion must in such cases be proximal to the entrance of the sympathetic fibers in the plexus. A lesion at this level means that no recovery of value is to be expected. As in Paragraph 3 also here the test is helpful in making a correct prognosis early.

Limitations

1. Technical accuracy is necessary.
2. After nerve suture the test is useful only when prints are absent. If prints are positive, the picking-up test and the two-point discrimmination test must be added.

After a nerve suture, it is often something like a year before some sudomotor function is established. Many cases will never have it, but it has been shown by Moberg, Stromberg *et al.*,[46] and also by Önne,[37] that

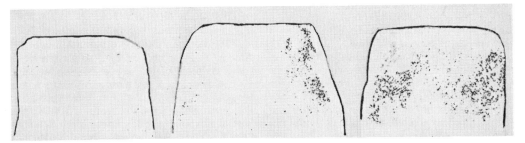

Figure 9.2.6. Loss of median nerve sensibility in the thumb in three different hands. Lateral parts are innervated by dorsal branches from the radial nerve. Great anatomical variations occur.

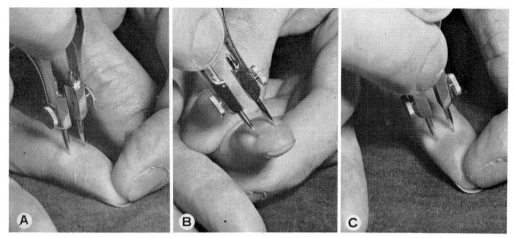

Figure 9.2.7. Correct (*A*) and unreliable (*B* and *C*) ways to perform the two-point discrimination test.

nerve suture under ideal conditions and also a number of such sutures under less favorable conditions, will make it possible for small diameter nerve fibers to grow through the suture line carrying sudomotor function and what has been described under the name paresthesia or wicked pain in advance of the thicker fibers carrying tactile gnosis. Therefore, after a nerve suture, if the printing test shows no dots or just a few, tactile gnosis is absent. In this respect the test is entirely reliable. In other cases, however, when normal or almost normal prints are obtained this does not mean that tactile gnosis has also returned. This degree of sensibility must be checked with the other tests described.

3. Limitations in injuries to brachial plexus and for grafts and flaps.

The Two-Point Discrimination Test

This test is sensitive to defects in sensory quality too small to be demonstrated by other methods. It is reliable also after a nerve suture and for grafts and flaps.

Many papers are published on the possibility that grafts and flaps may gain sensibility. So far, few investigations seem to have taken into account that the result obtained always will be the sum of the function of uninjured receptors beneath and around the transplant in the receptor area, the (dys-)function of unavoidable microneuromas around borders of the transplant, and the function of wild growing axons passing the borders. The graft itself will probably be responsible for a very small part of the total reaction. As shown by Moberg and Mannerfelt,[23] skin transplants will never get a higher quality of sensory function and therefore it is not too often necessary to examine their sensory function. If necessary, however, the two-point discrimination test will usually be the only test of use.

Limitations

Cooperation is necessary. Very narrow areas, as, *e.g.,* the lateral borders of the thumb, innervated by the radial nerve, cannot be tested.

Evaluation of Lower Qualities of Sensory Function

If tactile gnosis is absent, a lower degree of sensibility of some use for gross grips may be present. It is not rare to get this degree of sensibility back as a result of a nerve suture in adults, where recovery of true tactile gnosis is very rare. Values obtained by the two-point discrimination test, values worse than 12 to 15 mm but better than 30 to 40 mm, as well as testing practical function in every-day grips, will reveal the presence of this limited sensory function.

Protective Sensibility

This may be evaluated according to the history the patient gives. If he states that blisters, small cuts, and other cutaneous lesions repeatedly occur without any pain being felt, one must conclude that protective sensibility is absent. Where these lesions or scarring from them are observed, it is of course an objective sign, indicating this lack of protective sensibility.

PROPRIOCEPTION

It has been the custom to distinguish between exteroception and proprioception, the latter being the *conscious* perception of motion, position, and force applied. The idea was that those qualities had their distal receptor system located in the joint structures, a theory accepted as a fact since the days of the German physiologist, Goldscheider, about 1890. On the other hand the *cutaneous end organs* were believed to register only impulses belonging to the exteroception sys-

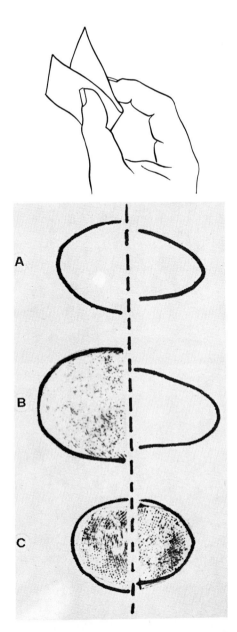

Figure 9.2.8. The ninhydrin test used for planning reconstructive surgery. Should restoration of lost opposition of the thumb be undertaken or not? *A.* Median nerve severed at the wrist level. None of the two pincers in a grip have tactile gnosis. The patient will never use the grip if another is available and therefore a tendon transfer for opposition is not worthwhile. *B.* Volar nerves to the thumb severed. The index has tactile gnosis. A one-shank sensory grip is possible. Normal pinch cannot be obtained, but one of some limited value can probably be developed. *C.* Polio. Normal tactile gnosis in both pincers pres-

tem. My own studies, however (Moberg), have clearly shown that the skin, without any joint structures or receptors involved, is able to register in a normal way all the three factors mentioned.

Usuaully it can be stated that if exteroception is normal, proprioception also will be normal. When exteroception is absent, proprioception also is absent.

OTHER WAYS TO JUDGE HAND SENSIBILITY

Practically, a most important way to evaluate the sensibility in the hand has so far not been mentioned, the direct observation of the hand surface. This is, with training, of great use. A hand that has lost tactile gnosis in its best gripping area will immediately move the grip to another part of the hand, where this sensibility is present, even if the new grip has much less strength or is not neary as handy. When the grip alters in this way, the skin surface of the original grip area will lose its staining, the scratches, callosities, and other signs of normal use. With the three tests already described it is then easy to check the deficit, but before this is performed a trained examiner can confirm his result by palpation. Bunnell[9] as early as 1944 wrote, ''The skin in an anesthetic area is so characteristic, that one can by feeling with the finger determine the area almost as accurately as by testing with an applicator. The finger glides over it smoothly with a satiny feel: it does not jump along as it does on normal skin, in which the sweat glands are working. Atrophic skin appears smooth.''

Other ways occasionally used for examination of sensory functions are as follows: (1) to test the ability to say from where the sensation comes; (2) to test capacity to differentiate between sharp and blunt with a point and head of pin; (3) digit writing; (4) vibration test.

A thorough examination of these four tests (Moberg) showed that none of them can be relied on as a help in hand surgery or give information not obtained by the methods described before.

When discussing functional capacity after hand lesions the ability of the human hand to compensate for loss must always be remembered.

In leprosy, where no doubt total anesthesia often is present in both hands, sight is the leading sense. In darkness those patients are almost entirely helpless. Their hands are acting as two pairs of forceps, but not as hands. Similarly, the surgeon is able to perform with forceps quite a few grips with precision, but is lost when there is trouble with the lamp. The difference between normal function and, as in leprosy, an ability to perform slowly a few simple tasks must be understood, and the great importance these factors

ent. The value of the pinch will be determined only according to how much motor function can be obtained. Usually it is possible to get a valuable pinch.

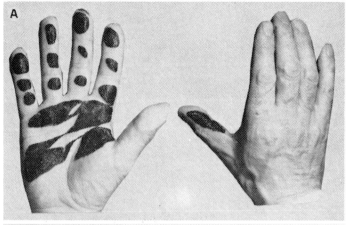

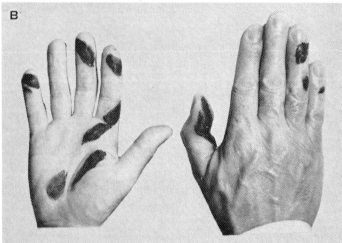

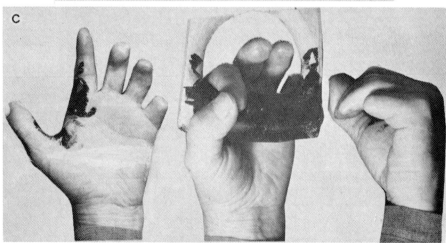

Figure 9.2.9. Only limited areas of the hand take part in a grip. The handles were stained and the gripping areas are therefore black. The grips shown are from *A,* a hammer; *B,* a pair of pliers; *C,* a spade gripped by a hand with loss of volar sensibility in the ulnar three fingers. Motor function and mobility enough for a grip were left. Still these fingers were not used for the hold.

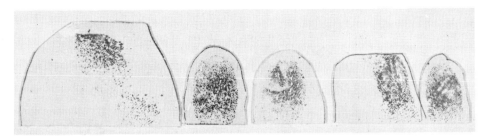

Figure 9.2.10. Prints from a hand in which a neurovascular flap tactile gnosis has been transferred to a denervated thumb. The prints permit mapping out the areas of normal sensibility with an accuracy not obtainable with other tests.

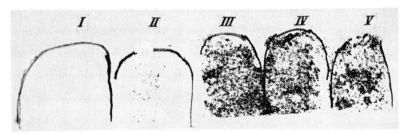

Fibure 9.2.11. Crush injury to the arm above the elbow. No clinical signs of median nerve function present. The prints show some small dots in median nerve distribution to index and thumb indicating that a few axons are still functioning. Accordingly a favorable prognosis could be determined early. (Reprinted with permission of Jounral of Bone and Joint Surgery.)

have for making a living today. For anyone in doubt there is a simple and harmless test, which can be recommended. I have performed it on myself. It is to block one's own median nerve at wrist level with 2 cc of Xylocaine or another anesthetic and then try to use the hand. The motor loss is usually not important. The personal experience of what a loss of sensibility means is most helpful.

Due to the unsatisfactory tests usually relied on, great confusion exists today about the results of nerve surgery. It seems necessary that in the future much more rigid requirements should be applied for such studies.

Work is going on in several centers aiming at better understanding and better tests for the different aspects of sensory function. The author has tried to visit such places and to find out what is coming in this field. So far, however, in spite of interesting trials, real additions of practical value for the surgery can hardly be said yet to exist. It is of paramount interest to get ahead in this field.

This could not be demonstrated better than in the extensive monograph "Surgical Disorders of the Peripheral Nerves" (1972) by Sir Herbert Seddon.[44] He, who has during a long and active life done more than anyone else for the development of this field, says in the perface to this book: "What is so astonishing is that in spite of the devoted efforts of many workers the riddle of sensibility is still not yet solved." In the special parts of this book in which our present methods of testing sensibility are described, no basically new or improved method appears.

The only trials recently to get ahead, worthwhile to mention here, are (1) on the line of the vibration tests (Talbot et al.,[47] McQuillan,[25]); or (2) variations of the two-point discrimination test. So far none of the variations of the vibration tests have reached a development which could make them helpful to the hand surgeons. The variations of the two-point discrimination test consists of letting the finger pulp identify steel type letters 1.0 by 0.3 cm in size (Porter[39]) or small triangles cut in plastic blocks (Edshage[12]). I have myself in special cases several times used plastic letters of different size. They can also be used in the mouth and the result compared with the tactile gnosis of the finger pulps.

A negative contribution is given by Almquist and Eeg-Olofsson[2] who could clearly demonstrate that the conductive speed in sensory nerves could not be used to determine the functional value of a nerve suture. Quite useful function could go together with low speed and also bad functional results with fair recovery of conductive speed.

Nothing could, however, better than all these trials elucidate the need for better methods in this very difficult field. It is to be hoped that the necessary further development will come from the hand surgeons who have need for those tests. As already said, neurology has other problems and only a limited interest in the functional value of the periphery.

REFERENCES

1. Afanassieff, A. La valeur pratique du test a la ninhydrin dans les lésions des nerfs de la main. Thèse pour le doctorat en médicine. Paris, 1962.
2. Almquist, E., and Eeg-Olofsson, O. Sensory nerve conduction velocity and two-point discrimination in sutured nerves. J. Bone Joint Surg., 52A: 4, 1970.
3. Bell, C. The Hand. London, William Pickering, 1833.
4. Bishop, G. H. The relation of nerve fiber size to modality of sensation. In Cutaneous Innervation, edited by W. Montagna. London, Pergamon, 1960, p. 88.
5. Blix, M. Experimentelle Beiträge zur Lösung der Frage über die specifische Energie der Hautnerven. Z. Biol., 20: 141, 1884; 21: 145, 1885.
6. Boring, E.G. Cutaneous sensation after nerve division. Q. J. Exp. Physiol., 10: 1-95, 1916.
7. Bowden, R.E.M. Factors influencing recovery. In Peripheral Nerve Injuries, edited by H.J. Seddon, London, Her Majesty's Stationery Office, 1954, pp. 298-353.
8. Bowden, R.E.M., and Napier, J.R. The assessment of hand function after peripheral nerve injuries. J. Bone Joint Surg., 43: 3, 1961.
9. Bunnel, S. Surgery of the Hand. Philadelphia, Lippincott, 1944.
10. Clarkson, P., and Pelly, A. The General and Plastic Surgery of the Hand. Oxford, Blackwell, 1962.
11. Dhuner, K. G., Edshage, S., and Wilhelm, A. Ninhydrin test — an objective method for testing local anesthetic drugs. Acta anaesthesiol. scand., 4: 189-198, 1960.
12. Edshage, S. Cutaneous sensibility in the hand. Presented at Annual Meeting of American Society for Surgery of the Hand, 1971, to be published.
13. Flynn, J.E., and Flynn, W.F. Median and ulnar nerve injuries. A long range study with evaluation of the ninhydrin test, sensory and motor returns. Ann. Surg., 156: 6, 1962.
14. Frey, M. von. Untersuchungen über die Sinnesfunktionen der menschlichen Haut. Ber. d. Verhandl. d. K. Sachs. Gesellsch. d. Wissensch. z. Leipzig. Math.-Phys. Classe, 47: 166-184, 1895.
15. Head, H. Studies in Neurology. London, Oxford, 1920.
16. Head, H., Rivers, W.H.R., and Sherren, J. The afferent nervous system from a new aspect. Brain, 28: 99-155, 1905.
17. Hilgenfeldt, O. Operative Daumenersatz. Stuttgart, Ferdinand Enke Verlag, 1950.
18. Hutchinson, J., Tough, J.S., and Wyburn, G.M. Comparison of the cutaneous sensory pattern of different regions of the body. Br. J. Plast. Surg., 1: 131, 1948.
19. Ingvar, D., and Moberg, E. To be published.
20. Iselin, M., Manetta, F., and Afanassieff, A. Le syndrome d'interruption partielle du nerf médian. Mem. Acad. chir., 88: 20-21, 1962.
21. Littler, J.W. Neurovascular pedicle transfer of tissue in reconstructive surgery of the hand. J. Bone Joint Surg., 38: 4, 1956.
22. Mackenzie, I.G., and Woods, C.G. Causes of failure after repair of the median nerve. J. Bone Joint Surg., 43: 3, 1961.
23. Mannerfelt, L. Evaluation of functional sensation of skin grafts in the hand area. Br. J. Plast. Surg., 15: 136, 1962.
24. Marks, J.H. Peripheral nerve injuries. Proc. Mine Med. Off. Assoc., 41: 380, 1962.
25. McQuillan, W. Sensory recovery after nerve repair. Hand, 2: 1, 1970.
26. Moberg, E. Discussion. American Orthopedic Association Meeting, 1954. J. Bone Joint Surg., 37: 2, 1955.
27. Moberg, E. Objective methods for determining functional value of sensibility in the hand. J. Bone Joint Surg., 40: 3, 1958.
28. Moberg, E. Examination of sensory loss by the ninhydrin printing test in Volkmann's contracture. Bull. Hosp. Joint. Dis., 21: 296, 1960.
29. Moberg, E. Evaluation of sensibility in the hand. S. Clin. North Am., 40: 357, 1960.
30. Moberg, E. Grip reconstruction of the hand with transfer of small neurovascular island flaps. Acta orthop. scand., 31: 3, 1961.
31. Moberg, E. Peripheral nerve and hand function. J. Bone Joint Surg., 43: 3, 1961.
32. Moberg, E. Criticism and study of methods for examining sensibility in the hand. Neurology, 12: 1, 1962.
33. Moberg, E. Aspects of sensation in reconstructive surgery of the upper extremity. First Sterling Bunnell Memorial Lecture. J. Bone Joint Surg., 46A: 4, 1964.
34. Napier, J.R. The return of pain sensibility in full thickness skin graft. Brain, 75: 147, 1952.
35. Neilson, J.M.M., Bordman, A.K., McQuillan, W.M., Smith, D.N., Hay, R.L., and Anthony, J.K.F. Measurement of vibro-tactile threshold in peripheral nerve injury. Lancet, Sept. 27, 669, 1969.
36. Noordenbos, W. Pain. Amsterdam, Elsevier, 1959.
37. Önne, L. Recovery of sensibility and sudomotor activity in the hand after nerve suture. Acta chir. scand. (Suppl.), 300, 1962.
38. Pollock, L.J., and Davies, L. Peripheral nerve injuries. Am. J. Surg., 15: 411, 571, 1932.
39. Porter, R.W. New test for fingertip sensation. Br. Med. J., 2: 927, 1967.
40. Rivers, W.H. Instinct and the Unconscious. Cambridge, 1920.
41. Robins, R.H.C. Injuries and Infections of the Hand. London, Arnold, 1961.
42. Schink, W. Handchirurgischer Ratgeber. Berlin-Göttingen-Heidelberg, Springer Verlag, 1960.
43. Seddon, H.J. Peripheral Nerve Injuries. London, Her Majesty's Stationery Office, 1954.
44. Seddon, H.J. Surgical Disorders of the Peripheral Nerves. Edinburgh-London, Churchill-Livingstone, 1972.
45. Souquet, R., and Chancholle, A.R. Plaies de la Main. Paris, G. Doin, 1959.
46. Strömberg, W.B., Jr., McFarlane, R.M., Bell, J.L., Koch, S.L., and Mason, M.L. Injury of the median and ulnar nerves. One hundred and fifty cases with an evaluation of Moberg's ninhydrin test. J. Bone Joint Surg., 43: 5, 1961.
47. Talbot, W. T., Smith, D., Kornhuber, H. H., and Mountcastle, V. B. The significance of flutter-vibration: Comparison of the human capacity with response patterns of mechanoreceptive afferents from the monkey hand. J. Neurophysiol., 31: 301, 1968.
48. Tubiana, R., and Dupare, J. Restoration of sensibility in the hand by neurovascular skin island transfer. J. Bone Joint Surg., 43: 3, 1961.
49. Zachary, R.B. Results of nerve suture. In Peripheral Nerve Injuries, edited by H.J. Seddon. Medical Research Council Special Rep. Ser. No. 282. London, Her Majesty's Stationery Office, 1954, p. 354.

C.

Management of Peripheral Nerve Injury Producing Hand Dysfunction

Frank E. Nulsen, M.D., F.A.C.S., and David G. Kline, M.D., F.A.C.S.

No individual requires a more intimate knowledge of the anatomy and physiology of the upper extremity than does the surgeon who must manage peripheral nerve injuries producing hand dysfunction. Central to developing logical guidelines for the management of such injuries is a firm understanding of not only the importance of the mechanisms of injury but also the time table required for recovery for each nerve and the limitations of clinical and electrophysiologic testing to predict the need for exploration and neurolysis or neuroma resection and anastomosis. In addition, the surgeon must develop a practical understanding of the limitations of motor and sensory recovery for each nerve even when the repair is timed correctly, performed accurately, and associated injuries are minimal.

MECHANISM OF INJURY

Knives, glass, or jagged metal may lacerate soft tissues such as muscles, tendons, and vessels, but also frequently produce either partial or total injury to nerve.[40][45][52] This type of injury results in *neurotemesis* which consists of disruption of the perineurium and endoneurium of the nerve as well as of the axons and their covering of myelin.[47] When deficit distal to such an injury is complete, the need for repair is fairly obvious. Civilian experience, as well as some experimental studies, suggest that such sharply created injuries, particularly when they involve the distal portion of an upper extremity nerve such as the median or ulnar nerve at the wrist, can be repaired primarily along with associated muscle, tendon, and vascular injuries.[16] Prior to exploration, the surgeon must perform an accurate and extensive examination of hand sensory and muscle function in order to establish a baseline against which to project future recovery or lack thereof.

Thus, if the deficit secondary to a lacerating injury is complete, then primary repair of the nerve injury may be indicated. On the other hand, if the nerve defi-

cit distal to the injury is partial those fibers already lacerated may be only a small fraction of the total. Thirty per cent retained function can increase to 70 per cent in a few weeks as axons recover from *neuropraxia;* and to 90 per cent after several months as axons suffering from *axonotemesis* regenerate spontaneously.

Blunt injuries are usually due to shell fragments, vehicular accidents, often associated with fractures. Such injuries will sometimes have an element of *neuropraxia* consisting of both large fiber-motor and sensory loss which may be reversible within several days to three weeks. More likely, *axonotemesis* which consists of axon loss with preservation of the connective tissue framework of the nerve as well as neurotemesis will be present particularly if there is an element of stretch injury. For example, a gunshot wound to the upper extremity can have completely transected the nerve but more frequently contuses and stretches the nerve, leaving a lengthy segment of neurotemesis and axonotemesis with perhaps a small element of neuropraxia. Blunt injuries are less likely to transect the nerve completely than sharp injuries but are, on the other hand, more likely to produce a mixture of different types and grades of injury to the nerve. The decision whether or not to explore such an injury is most difficult, and, indeed, when operation is decided upon, the surgeon may be confronted with a lesion in continuity and does not know whether to resect or to leave the lesion alone.[27][56] For this reason, exploration of upper extremity peripheral nerve injuries due to blunt trauma should be delayed for three to eight weeks after injury even though the nerve may be fully transected. Ability to resect adequately damaged nerve ends is a major factor in producing results with delayed repair which surpass, on the average, those achieved with primary repair.[13][56][58] Technically excellent nerve anastomoses are constantly encountered with failure to regenerate because the approximated nerve ends had shared in the damage and gone on to fibrosis.

Compressive injuries with secondary ischemic nerve damage such as that produced by pressure from a hematoma or edema in a closed fascial compartment, by a cast applied too tightly over a nerve trunk, or by unfelt compression of a nerve in deep sleep or intoxicated states, may produce total but potentially reversible paralysis. Less frequently, extraneural soft tissue tumors in juxtaposition to a nerve can cause partial paralysis. Decompressive surgery or excision of the offending mass may sometimes be beneficial, particularly if compression has occurred in an area where the nerve is likely to be entrapped, such as the ulnar nerve at the level of the olecranon notch or the median nerve at the elbow level as it runs beneath the lacertus fibrosis or at the wrist as it runs beneath the transverse carpal ligament. A patient with a bullet or stab wound near the axilla complaining of a progressive numbness or weakness of the hand may lose function due to expansion of a false aneurysm from a lacerated axillary or brachial artery. An aneurysm of this type may compress the median and/or ulnar nerve and, in addition to progression of deficit, can be suspected if pain and/or a bruit develops. Another example of a progressive lesion is Volkmann's contracture due to hemorrhage and edema occurring about a fractured elbow. Here, the median nerve sustains progressive ischemic damage because it is entrapped beneath the unyielding lacertus fibrosis which spans the antecubital space of the elbow. If there is a large element of neuropraxia with this type of injury, then some degree of recovery should occur spontaneously by three weeks.

Another but, fortunately, infrequent mechanism of injury is the passage of electric current through the nerve which produces severe intraneural changes as well as damage to skin, vessels, and bone. Associated necrosis of muscle is particularly severe and often limits the degree of functional return to the hand despite satisfactory recovery of the peripheral nerves. Here, nerve surgery offers nothing. Drug injections into or close to a nerve cause major injuries in continuity and are frequently seen in relation to the radial nerve where injections meant for the deltoid region are given at the level of the lateral midhumerus. The deficit is usually due to intraneural neuritis and scar tissue rather than extraneural scarring.[9] [24]

It should be stressed that if there is positive evidence favoring substantial retention of neural function distal to a lesion, this suggests but does not guarantee an eventual favorable result, particularly with partial lacerations where the loss may never improve significantly. If there is some distal functional sparing in a nerve with diffuse damage, then all of the spared motor and sensory axons are scattered throughout the cross section of involvement. When a significant proportion of these axons has escaped initial dysfunction none have suffered the totally disruptive injury of neurotemesis, but instead will have suffered only from axonotemesis. Regeneration with this type of injury far exceeds whatever the surgeon can achieve by suture.

TIME TABLE FOR RECOVERY

Once a thorough baseline evaluation of function of the hand is made and primary exploration and repair are delayed in the absence of visualizing transected nerve the surgeon must re-evaluate the extremity periodically, looking for evidence of autonomic, sensory, and motor return. In order to define regeneration adequately, one must know when return of sensory perception is proof positive of reinnervation as opposed to changing sensory patterns secondary to overlap innervation.[33] [37] One must also know when visible muscle contractions are supplied solely by the nerve in question. The examiner cannot afford to be fooled either by compensatory movements or by the all too common anomalies of nerve supply to the hand which falsely suggest peripheral nerve recovery.[38]

Fine fiber autonomic recovery as manifested by ability to sweat may occur during the early months following peripheral nerve injury or repair. Evidence of sweating can be found by examining the distal digits, particularly in the autonomous zones, with the aid of the plus 20 lens of an ophthalmoscope or by using a Ninhydrin sweat test. If sensory return to gross touch and painful stimuli occurs in an autonomous zone, this is more encouraging and usually but not always predicts useful motor return.

By comparison, recovery in motor function which is not due to trick or substitutive movements, provides definite evidence for useful functional reinnervation. The step-ladder or domino arrangement of muscles innervated by a given nerve must be known by the physician caring for upper extremity nerve injuries.[20'] [52] If he has some idea of the distance between the injury and the muscle immediately distal and closest to the injury or repair, he can predict when initial recovery should occur. New axons must not only penetrate the area of injury but must first replace proximal stump Wallerian degenerative changes which occur retrograde to most injuries.[18] The axons must then penetrate the connective tissue disarray of the injury site itself and this requires a few weeks. Upon reaching the distal stump, the motor axons then regenerate at a rate of 1 mm a day or 1 inch a month.[51] This rate can be faster for lesions involving the proximal upper extremity where the regenerating axon is closer to the mother neuron in the spinal cord and also in children who tend to regenerate more rapidly. Axonal regrowth will be slower, on the other hand, for injuries involving the distal portion of the nerve in adults. Once axons reach their muscle destinations, two to four weeks are required for functional regeneration of the motor-end plates. These specifics are important, but it is sufficient for the clinician to calculate dead-lines at one inch per month. Thus, with radial nerve injury at the mid-humeral level, brachioradialis function should occur by three to four months, if all is going well. With wrist-level median nerve injury, four to five months may be required for abductor pollicis brevis function to return. Since there is such a delay between the time when satisfactory axonal regeneration begins and the beginning evidence of such regeneration that can be gained by clinical examination, special clinical and electrical tests may help one decide whether to explore the injury before the calculated deadline for muscle return is met.[26]

Clinical and Electrical Tests for Regeneration or for Partial Injury

During the early weeks after injury or repair, fine sensory axons will, if regeneration is processing satisfactory, penetrate into the distal segment. If one taps over such a distal nerve site, paresthesias will be produced in the distribution of the tested nerve, and this is called a *Tinel's sign*.[21] Similar sensations can be elicited by tapping over the injury or repair site in most patients and are useful to define the most proximal point of injury after extensive wounding. When the Tinel's sign progresses down the distal stump of the nerve, advance of fine fiber regeneration is suggested. Unfortunately, the Tinel's sign can progress favorably with *any* degree of regeneration — hence its presence in no way portends *adequate* regeneration. But it is a valuable sign from a negative standpoint — its failure to develop by six weeks is conclusive evidence for gross discontinuity of injured nerve, or regeneration failure after suture.

Stimulation of the nerve trunk by means of surface electrodes or bipolar needle electrodes inserted to reach a deep-lying nerve can sometimes elicit muscle function distal to an injury which cannot be obtained when the patient is asked to try to contract the muscle voluntarily. Such early evidence of motor return may antedate voluntary function by two to four weeks.[43] If the time interval is correct, a positive stimulation test provides definite evidence of satisfactory regeneration, whereas, if it does not produce muscle function by the appropriate deadline following injury, the test provides conclusive evidence against useful regeneration. If an injury is explored under local anesthesia, one can also stimulate distal to the injury to see if the patient reports sensation and/or paresthesias in the distribution of the tested nerve, for this will suggest some regeneration to the distal stump when time has been insufficient to permit motor response.

The *electromyograph* (EMG) can provide qualitative but, unfortunately, not quantitative evidence of denervation and/or reinnervation. Within three weeks of a serious injury, muscle recording will show fibrillations and denervation potentials in muscles whose nerve has undergone some degree of Wallerian degeneration. If neuropraxia is present, distal musculature will not contract voluntarily but fibrillations and deinnervation potentials, although present, will be minimal in number. Furthermore, stimulation of the nerve distal to the injury site will produce muscle contractions. With a nonneuropraxic injury which is regenerating, the number of fibrillations and deinnervation potentials will decrease and nascent potentials may be recorded. These findings may occasionally prevent an unnecessary operation but may also offer false encouragement unless the clinician realizes that the EMG documents qualitative and not necessarily adequate functional reinnervation.[17][29]

More recent development of noninvasive methods of recording *evoked potentials* directly from nerve offer promise, for one can evaluate axonal conduction through the injury in a serial fashion without exploring the nerve and recording directly from it.[11][14] In our laboratory, the use of preamplifiers, amplifiers, oscilloscope, and a small computer permits the recording of a number of single evoked responses from the skin level which can then be summated, to provide semiquantitative information about the axon population at the recording site. Such a potential may be due to preservation of a portion of the axonal population by the original injury, recovery of neuropraxically injured axons, or regeneration into the distal stump which has not yet reinnervated muscle.

During the early weeks after injury, stimulation of a neuroma in continuity can document partial injury and, if three to six months have elapsed, early return of muscle function can also be demonstrated by this technique.

SPECIFIC NERVE INJURIES

Median Nerve

Wrist is a frequent site for median nerve injury particularly due to accidental or purposeful laceration. At this level the median nerve lies between the tendons of the flexor carpi radialis and the palmaris longus and these structures frequently suffer from associated injury as does the nearby radial artery.[46] The median nerve lies somewhat volar to the flexor pollicis longus and flexor digitorum profundus and then enters the carpal tunnel beneath the carpal ligament where it begins to branch to supply the median innervated hand intrinsic muscles, particularly the abductor pollicis brevis. Care must be taken not to interrupt this branch when the nerve is being mobilized. The most essential function of the median nerve is to supply sensation to the median distribution of the hand which includes the radial half of the palm, the palmar surface of the thumb, index and long fingers, and sometimes the radial half of the ring finger, and a variable portion of the dorsal surface of these fingers. This sensory supply is absolutely necessary for man's grasping function, for digital dexterity, and for identification of small objects. It is surprising but well recognized how small the actual sensory deficit is with a complete median nerve lesion because of overlap innervation from both the ulnar and the radial nerves. The autonomous zone for median nerve innervation includes only the volar surface of the terminal two phalanges of the index finger and the very tip of the thumb (but this is crucial for hand function). Loss in this area means median denervation while return in this same area provides very definite evidence favoring regeneration of the median nerve and not overlap innervation from either ulnar or radial nerves.[33] Autonomic fiber loss provides absence of sweating especially in the autonomous zone. Loss of sensation in the median distribution of the hand is the major reason for repairing the median nerve at any level and this is particularly true at the level of the wrist where the more proximal flexor muscles of the fingers are spared and where the patient learns very often to substitute for median innervated intrinsic hand muscle loss.

The major intrinsic muscle loss is difficulty in abducting and opposing the thumb due to abductor pollicis brevis and opponens pollicis loss. Flexion of the proximal phalanx of the thumb is preserved since flexor pollicis brevis retains, in most cases, innervation from the ulnar nerve. Flexion of the distal phalanx will be spared since the flexor pollicis longus obtains its innervation from the median nerve in the forearm. Median nerve lesions at the wrist level give loss of lumbricales function to the index and long fingers although that to the latter digit may be only partial due to dual innervation from the ulnar as well as the median nerve. Lumbricales function is tested for by holding the metacarpalphalangeal joint in extension and then asking the patient to extend the second phalange of the finger against resistance. The most reliable test is that for abductor pollicis brevis function and this is done by asking the patient to abduct the thumb at right angles to the palm of the hand. One can palpate the thenar emminence and feel the muscle contract. Atrophy in the hand due to a wrist-level median nerve lesion is most evident in the region of the abductor pollicis brevis along the thenar emminence.

After neurorrhaphy at the wrist level, the earliest sensory return in autonomous zones may require four months. By five months one should also see some return of abductor pollicis brevis and/or opponens pollicis function. Despite this relatively early return, the ability to use the thumb and fingers for coordinated, highly skilled tasks involves retraining and re-education to overcome poor localization of sensory input despite the fact that the latter appears good quantitatively. Total median sensory loss is much more disabling than most people realize and, as a result, it would be a great disservice to a patient to resect a lesion in continuity which had the potential for establishing better sensory localization than could be possible with the best of nerve sutures. In this regard the use of stimulation which may show motor return as early as three months and the use of evoked potential recording which may indicate good regeneration as early as eight to 10 weeks become very important in the management of wrist-level median nerve lesions in continuity.

Injury to the median nerve in and around the elbow results in forearm muscle paralysis in addition to the above described intrinsic muscle loss. Pronation is usually spared unless the lesion is somewhat proximal to the elbow since branches for the pronator teres usually originate above the elbow. Flexor pollicis longus denervation causes inability to flex the tip or distal phalanx of the thumb. As the patient makes a fist, his third, fourth, and fifth fingers usually behave normally despite some loss in strength from flexor sublimis paralysis. But the index finger does not flex at its distal phalanx and flexion is reduced or absent at the middle phalanx. In testing these muscles, one must be careful to hold the other fingers in extension so that one is dealing with only a single flexor tendon.

The median nerve may be located in the bicipital groove between the biceps and the triceps along the medial surface of the upper arm where it runs in close relationship to the brachial artery and vein. In the midupper arm the nerve also travels along with the ulnar nerve which eventually deviates to run towards the olecranon groove. When the median nerve reaches the flexor crease of the elbow, it runs beneath the lacertus fibrosis and through the antecubital fossa of the forearm. At this point, the nerve dives deep into the superficial muscles of the forearm making mobilization distal to this point very difficult due to tethering by muscle branches running to the flexor carpi radials, palmaris longus, and the flexor superficialis and profundus muscles. Length can be best gained by mobilizing the nerve towards the axilla, sacrificing some of the pronator teres muscle branches, and by flexing the elbow. When dealing with median nerve injury in the midforearm, one does best to expose the nerve at the elbow level or above, and then to expose the nerve at the wrist level. Then tracing both ends towards the deeply situated forearm permits dissection through muscle planes with minimal sacrifice of muscle substance. Although flexion of the forearm on the upper arm will gain length, transposition of the nerve does not. Repair of the median nerve about the elbow will, if successful, usually result in return of flexor carpi radialis and palmaris longus function by two or three months. A little longer period is required for flexion of the fingers and up to six months may be necessary for return of flexor pollicis longus function. Reinnervation of the abductor pollicis brevis and opponens pollicis will require 10 to 12 months, and functional recovery may be inadequate after this delay. A tendon transfers or fusions may be necessary to provide some degree of thumb to finger opposition. In spite of intervals to 12 months required for sensory regeneration, a helpful return of median innervated sensation will follow satisfactory recovery of proximal median muscles.

Axillary and upperarm level lesions to the median nerve will give pronator teres loss as well as the deficits described for an elbow-level median nerve lesion. It is important to recognize that the median nerve takes its origin from both the medial and lateral cords of the brachial plexus and, thus, total injury to one of these cords suggests a partial median nerve deficit. Lateral cord damage, for example, results in a typical median distribution sensory loss and forearm flexor weakness, but with retention of median hand muscle function. At the same time, the musculocutaneous nerve's supply to biceps will be affected. Medial cord injury, on the other hand, will affect only the small hand muscles in the median nerve's domain, while all ulnar nerve motor and sensory functions are involved. When only one nerve is injured, a stimulator will identify the nerves that are functioning.

Repair of the median nerve at the axillary or upper arm level is worthwhile, for what little critical median sensation can result, provided a plan can be visualized to provide useful mechanical function. This will have to be managed with realization that useful reinnervation of the median intrinsic hand muscles will not occur and that forearm flexor function may be poor. Nine months may be necessary for flexor superficialis and/or profundus function to recur and another two months for flexor pollicis longus function to come about. This possible return of flexion to the fingers and the thumb adds an extra benefit to repair of the lesion at this level. There is a need to explore injuries at a high level a little earlier than elsewhere because a delay will add a further period of denervation at a time when clinical signs may not.

There is no question that functional results following suture of the median nerve can be related to the level of the repair. World War II experience indicated that useful abductor pollicis brevis function ocurred in only 32 per cent of patients with repair of the median nerve at the wrist level but this figure was even lower with patients with repair at the axillary level (19 per cent).[48] [58] Sensory return can be expected in a little over half the patients. Certainly the use of electrical techniques preoperatively and at the operating table are of great importance with axillary and upper arm level median nerve injuries. If stimulation produces distal muscle contraction with a neuroma in continuity, then it should be left alone because the result in terms of hand sensation will be so much better than whatever one could achieve by suture. In a similar fashion, if stimulation produces no function and the time after injury is relatively short, then the use of evoked potential recording becomes very important. A good potential evoked through such a lesion indicates either sparing of a proportion of the large and medium-sized fibers or adequate regeneration of these fibers. Such regeneration or sparing will produce an end result much better than could be hoped for by suture repair at this level.

Ulnar Nerve

Wrist-level injuries to the ulnar nerve result in sensory loss in the ulnar distribution of the hand which includes both the volar and the dorsal surfaces of the little finger and either all or half of the ring finger. The autonomous zone for the ulnar nerve is on the volar surface of the distal phalanx of the little finger. At the wrist, the ulnar nerve lies on the radial side of the flexor carpi ulnaris and as it enters the hand, it divides into superficial and deep branches at the level of and on the radial side of the pisiform bone. The superficial branch innervates the motor muscles of the hypothe-nar emminence and provides sensation to the ulnar half of the hand whereas the deep palmar branch runs beneath the flexor tendons to reach the palmar interosseus muscles, the first dorsal interosseus muscle, and the adductor pollicis. There is considerable overlap and anomalous innervation shared with the median nerve, making the picture of motor loss in the hand somewhat variable. One can count, however, on weakness of the hypothenar emminence muscles and this includes loss of abductor digiti quinti minimi and opponens digiti quinti function. The interossei will be weak or paralyzed, particularly the first dorsal interosseus muscle which abducts the forefinger away from the middle finger. In addition, the loss of adductor pollicis function is compensated by action of the flexor pollicis muscles innervated by the median nerve to move the thumb towards the palm. The resultant flexion of the distal phalanx of the thumb against forefinger is called a Froment's sign. The most readily discernible deficit with wrist-level ulnar lesions is inability to extend the middle phalanges of the ring and little fingers due to lumbricales loss. This leads to a flexion or claw deformity of these fingers. Inability to extend the fingers with ulnar nerve injury appears to be paradoxical until one analyzes what the lumbricales muscles do. These muscles serve to stabilize the metacarpal phalangeal joint. With loss of this stabilization, the intact radial innervated extensor muscles tend to pull the MP joints into extension, thereby wasting their action to extend the more distal phalanges of the digits. Both the flexor superficialis and the flexor profundus to the ring and little fingers are no longer balanced by a competent extensor system and these muscles tend to abet clawing of the fourth and fifth fingers by pulling the phalanges into flexion.

Presence of minimal function through an ulnar lesion at the wrist is evidenced by preservation of sensation in the ulnar autonomous zone on the volar aspect of the fifth finger and by visible contraction in the bellies of the abductor digiti quinti, opponens digiti quinti, or first dorsal interosseus muscles. If there is any question of partial motor function, stimulation of the ulnar nerve at the level of the wrist will resolve whether the ulnar nerve is actually supplying muscles clinically suggesting ulnar function.

Surgical exposure is readily accomplished at the wrist level, where the nerve runs between the flexor carpi ulnaris and the flexor superficialis tendons and passes superficial to the transverse carpal ligament. Due to its juxtaposition, the ulnar artery is frequently injured along with the ulnar nerve. If nerve length is needed, it may be gained by mobilizing proximally, for distal mobilization is of little benefit since the nerve quickly splits at the level of the pisiform bone into the superficial and deep branches. Some length may be gained by mobilizing the nerve into the forearm where it runs between the two heads of the flexor carpi ulnaris. Length can also be gained by flexing the wrist on the forearm but gaps of over 5 cm require mobilization of the proximal nerve to well above the elbow. When this is done, the nerve should be transposed volar to the elbow and buried in the pronator teres so as to gain length with elbow flexion. In this fashion, gaps of nearly 10 cm in the ulnar nerve can be overcome by combining mobilization and transposition with flexion of both the wrist and the elbow.

Suture of the ulnar nerve at the wrist gives variable results although, in general, averaged return in terms of normal function from World War II American and British statistics was about 73 per cent.[48 58] However, if attention was paid to independent and coordinated finger function, then only 16 per cent of the patients regained useful function. Unfortunately, the muscles which are most difficult to regain are the lumbricales which permit proper extension of the little and ring fingers so as to overcome disabling clawing and the interossei which permit the typist, pianist, and the mechanic to work swiftly and deftly. Lack of lumbricales function can and should be substituted for very early by a tendon transfer such as the technique described by Brand where either a portion of the median innervated flexor superficialis, plantaris tendon, or fascia lata is attached to extensor carpi radialis and inserted into the dorsal expansions of the first phalanges of the ring and little fingers so as to permit stabilization of the MP joint and prevent claw deformity.[4]

After ulnar suture at the wrist, sensation to the hypothenar emminence and little finger region usually return in three to five months as does hypothenar emminence muscle function. Six to eight months may be required for first dorsal interosseus function to occur. Beginning recovery in adductor pollicis is hard to recognize. When an ideal repair of the ulnar nerve is achieved because of proper timing and good surgical technique, good return of strength to each individual ulnar innervated muscle results as confirmed by nerve stimulation, but coordinated and synchronized movement of these muscles may not result. Eight months or more may be required to define which tendon transfers are required, if any, to improve the result.

A frequent higher site for injury to the ulnar nerve is at the level of the elbow where the nerve is relatively superficial, lying on top of the bone of the olecranon notch behind the medial epicondyle. Injury at this level is enchanced by the relatively small space available to the nerve as it travels through the notch. Many patients with elbow-level ulnar nerve lesions have sparing of flexor carpi ulnaris function because major branches to this muscle may leave the nerve above the elbow level to run into the proximal belly of the muscle. Flexion of the fingers is the primary function of the median nerve but complete injury to the ulnar nerve at the elbow level will result in paralysis of the flexor profundi muscles to the ring and little finger. In addition to a possible loss of flexor carpi ulnaris function and definite loss of ulnar innervated flexor profundus function, the patient with a complete, elbow-level lesion will show all of the deficits described with wrist-level lesions, but the clawing may be less marked.

Upon exploration, the nerve can be readily located as it passes through the olecranon notch and then traced into the proximal upper arm as well as into the distal forearm. Irrespective of whether a neuroma in continuity is found and stimulation and/or evoked potential recording shows either that the lesion should be left alone or be resected and sutured, the nerve should be transposed volar to the elbow and buried in the pronator teres musculature. This maneuver tends to reduce later trauma to the injury site. When resection and suture are necessary it will aid in making up lost length. More frequently, however, one must prepare a bed for the nerve within the pronator teres by sectioning through fascia and the upper layers of the muscle and then loosely closing some of the muscle over the repair or injury site taking care not to strangulate the nerve. With transposition, the surgeon must also split the intermusclar septum of the upper arm as well as the connective tissue raphe of the proximal forearm so that the nerve will not buckle around these structures. This important point is frequently overlooked and upper arm and/or forearm entrapment is substituted for olecranon notch entrapment.

Results with elbow-level repair are somewhat worse than those with wrist-level repair, for the distance that axons must regenerate is greater. Once again, though muscle function will return, it seldom does so in a synergistic fashion. Tendon transfers will almost always be needed to supply extension of the fourth and fifth fingers although clawing, with elbow-level lesions, is not as severe as with wrist-level lesions. Repair of axillary-level ulnar nerve lesions can be frustrating since return of hand intrinsic muscle function is so poor, and low-grade sensory recovery to the fifth finger is a limited goal, as compared to the functional value of median nerve sensation. One can early utilize tendon transfers for prevention of "claw hand" by stabilization of fourth and fifth MP joints. Since the ulnar nerve travels with the median nerve in the axilla and midupper arm, it is in juxtaposition to the brachial artery and radial nerve and, as such, is frequently involved in combined vascular and nerve injuries. In this setting where the median nerve should be repaired in the hopes of at least providing some sensation to the hand, one might as well repair the ulnar nerve lesion. The entire ulnar nerve originates from the medial cord of the brachial plexus as does that portion of the median nerve supplying hand intrinsic muscle function.

REFERENCES

1. Barber, K. W. Benign extraneural soft tissue tumors of the extremities causing compression of nerves. J.

Bone Joint Surg., *44A:* 98, 1962.

2. Barnes, R. Traction injuries of the brachial plexus in adults. J. Bone Joint Surg., *31B:* 10-16, 1949.

3. Bonney, G. The value of axon responses in determining the site of lesion in traction injuries of the brachial plexus. Brain, *77:* 588-609, 1954.

4. Brand, P. Tendon grafting. J. Bone Joint Surg., *43B:* 444-453, 1961.

5. Brown, H. A. The value of early neurolysis in contused injuries of peripheral nerves. West. J. Surg., *61:* 535-537, 1953.

6. Brown, B. A. Internal neurolysis in treatment of traumatic peripheral nerve lesions. California Med., *110:* 460-462, 1969.

7. Campbell, J. B. Peripheral nerve repair. In *Clinical Neurosurgery,* Vol. 17. Baltimore, Williams & Wilkins, 1970, pp. 77-98.

8. Campbell, J. B., and Lusskin, R. Upper extremity paralysis consequent to brachial plexus injury. Surg. Clin. North Am., *52:* 1235-1245, 1972.

9. Clark, K., Williams, P., Willis, W., and McGavran, W. L. Injection injuries of sciatic nerve. In *Clinical Neurosurgery,* Ch. VIII. Baltimore, Williams & Wilkins, 1970.

10. Davis, L., Perret, G., and Carroll, W. Surgical principles underlying the use of grafts in the repair of peripheral nerve injuries. Ann. Surg., *121:* 686-699, 1945.

11. Dawson, G. D. Nerve conduction velocity in man. J. Physiol., *31:* 436-451, 1956.

12. Ducker, T. B., and Hayes, G. J. Experimental improvements in use of silastic cuff for peripheral nerve repair. J. Neurosurg., *24:* 582-587, 1968.

13. Ducker, T. B., Kempe, L., and Hayes, G. The metabolic background for peripheral nerve surgery. J. Neurosurg., 1969, *30:* 270-280, 1969.

14. Gilliat, R. W., and Sears, T. A. Sensory nerve action potentials in patients with peripheral nerve lesions, J. Neurol. Neurosurg. Psychiat., *21:* 109-118, 1958.

15. Goldner, J. L. *Function of the Hand Following Peripheral Nerve Injuries.* American Academy of Orthopedic Surgeons, Instruction Course, Lectures 10. Ann Arbor, Edmonds, 1953, p. 268.

16. Grabb, W. G. Median and ulnar nerve suture: An experimental study comparing primary and secondary repair in monkeys. J. Bone Joint Surg., *50A:* 964, 1968.

17. Grundfest, H., Oester, Y. T., and Beebe, G. W. Electrical evidence of regeneration. In *Peripheral Nerve Regeneration,* VA Monograph. Washington, U.S. Gov't Printing Office, 1957, pp. 203-240.

18. Guth, L. Regeneration in the mamalian peripheral nervous system, Physiol. Rev., *36:* 441-478, 1956.

19. Guttmann, E., and Young, J. Z. Reinnervation of muscle after various periods of atrophy. J. Anat., *78:* 15-43, 1944.

20. Haymaker, W., and Woodhall, B. *Peripheral Nerve Injuries: Principles of Diagnosis.* Philadelphia, Saunders, 1953.

21. Henderson, W. R. Clinical assessment of peripheral nerve injuries. Tinels test. Lancet, *2:* 801-805, 1948.

22. Kettlekamp, D. B., and Alexander, H. Clinical review of radial nerve injury. J. Trauma, *7:* 424-432, 1967.

23. Kempe, L. *Operative Neurosurgery,* Vol. 2. New York, Springer-Verlag, 1970, pp. 158-170.

24. Kline, D. G., and DeJonge, B. R. Evoked potentials to evaluate peripheral nerve injuries. Surg. Gynecol. Obstet., *127:* 1239-1248, 1968.

25. Kline, D. G., Hackett, E. R., Davis, G. D., and Myers, M. B. Effect of mobilization on the blood supply and regeneration of injured nerves, J. Surg. Res., *12:* 254-266, 1972.

26. Kline, D. G., Hackett, E. R., and May, P. R. Evaluation of nerve injuries by evoked potentials and electromyography. J. Neurosurg., *31:* 128-136, 1969.

27. Kline, D. G., and Nulsen, F. E. The neuroma in continuity: its pre-operative and operative management. Surg. Clin. North Am., *52:* 1189-1209, 1972.

28. Lehman, R., and Hayes, G. Degeneration and regeneration in peripheral nerve. Brain, *90:* 285-296, 1967.

29. Licht, S. *Electrodiangosis and Electromyography,* New Haven, E. Licht Publisher, 1961.

30. Liu, C. T., Benda, C. E., and Lewey, F. H. Tensile strength of human nerves. Arch. Neurol. Psychiat., *59:* 322-336, 1948.

31. Liu, C. T., and Lewey, F. H. The effect of surging current of low frequency in man on atrophy of denervated muscles. J. Nerv. Ment. Dis., *105:* 571-581, 1947.

32. Littler, J. W. Tendon transfers and arthrodesis in combined median and ulnar nerve paralysis. J. Bone Joint Surg., *31A:* 225-234, 1949.

33. Livingston, W. K., Evidence of active invasion of denervated areas by sensory fibers from neighboring nerves in man. J. Neurosurg., 1947, *4:* 140-145, 1947.

34. Marmor, L. Nerve grafting in peripheral nerve repair. Surg. Clin. North Am., *52:* 1177-1187, 1972.

35. Mayfield, F. H., *Causalgia.* American Lecture Series. Springfield, Charles C. Thomas, 1951.

36. Melzack, R., and Wall, P. Pain mechanisms: a new theory. Science, *150:* 970-979, 1965.

37. Moberg, E. Criticism and study of methods for examining sensibility in the hand, Neurology, *12:* 8-19, 1962.

38. Murphey, F., Kirklin, J. W., and Finlayson, A. I. Anomalous innervation of the intrinsic muscles of the hand. Surg. Gynecol. Obstet., *83:* 15-23, 1946.

39. Murphey, F., Hortung, W., and Kirklin, J. W. Myelographic demonstration of avulsing injury of the brachial plexus. Am. J. Roentgenol., *58:* 102-105, 1947.

40. Nickolson, O. R., and Seddon, H. J. Nerve repair in civil practice. Br. Med. J., *2:* 1065-1071, 1957.

41. Nulsen, F. E., Lewey, F. H., and Van Wageman, W. D. Peripheral nerve grafts. In *Peripheral Nerve Regeneration,* edited by B. Woodhall and G. W. Beebe, Ch. 9. VA Monograph. Washington, 1957.

42. Nulsen, F. E., and Slade, H. W. Recovery following injury to the brachial plexus. In *Peripheral Nerve Regeneration,* edited by B. Woodhall, and G.W. Beebe, Ch. 9. VA Monograph, Washington, 1957.

43. Nulsen, F. E., Lewey, F. H. Intraneural bipolar stimulation: A new aid in the assessment of nerve injuries. Science, *106:* 301, 1947.

44. Riordan, D. C. Tendon transplantations in median nerve and ulnar nerve paralysis, J. Bone Joint Surg., *35A:* 312-320, 1953.

45. Robles, J. Brachial plexus avulsion. A review of diagnostic procedures and report of six cases, J. Neurosurg., *28:* 434-438, 1968.

46. Sakellorides, H. Follow-up of 172 peripheral nerve in-

juries in upper extremity in civilians. J. Bone Joint Surg., *44A:* 140-148, 1962.

47. Seddon, H. J. Three types of nerve injury. Brain, *66:* 238-288, 1943.

48. Seddon, H. J. *Peripheral Nerve Injuries,* Med. Res. Council Special Report Series No. 282. London, Her Majesty's Stationary Office, 1954.

49. Spurling, R. G., and Woodhall, B. *Surgery in World War II.* Neurosurgery, Vol. II. Washington, Office of the Surgeon General, Department of Army, U.S. Gov't Printing Office.

50. Sunderland, S. Funicular suture and funicular exclusion in the repair of severed nerves. Br. J. Surg., *40:* 580-587, 1953.

51. Sunderland, S. Rate of regeneration in human peripheral nerves. Arch. Neurol. Psychiat.,*58:* 251-295, 1947.

52. Sunderland, S. *Nerve and Nerve Injuries.* Baltimore, Williams & Wilkins, 1968.

53. Tarlov, I. M. How long should an extremity be immobilized after nerve suture? Ann. Surg., *126:* 336-376, 1947.

54. Weiss, P. Technology of nerve regeneration: A review.

J. Neurosurg., *1:* 400-450, 1944.

55. Whitcomb, B. B. Techniques of peripheral nerve repair. In *Medical Department United States Army, Surgery in World War II: Neurosurgery,* Vol. 2, Part II-Peripheral Nerve Injuries, edited by R. G. Spurling and B. Woodhall. Washington, U.S. Gov't Printing Office, 1959.

56. White, J. C. Timing of nerve suture after gunshot wound. Surgery, *48:* 946-951, 1968.

57. White, W. L. Restoration of function and balance of the wrist and hand by tendon transfers. Surg. Clin. North Am., *40:* 427-459, 1960.

58. Woodhall, B., Nulsen, F. E., White, J. C., and Davis, L. Neurosurgical implications. In *Peripheral Nerve Regeneration.* VA Monograph. Washington, 1957, pp. 569-638.

59. Yeoman, D. M., and Seddon, H. J. Brachial plexus injuries: Treatment of the flail arm, J. Bone Joint Surg., *43B:* 493-500, 1961.

60. Zachary, R. B., and Holmes, W. Primary suture of nerves. Surg. Gynecol. Obstet., *82:* 632-651, 1946.

D.

Median and Ulnar Nerve Injuries at the Wrist: A Long Range Study with Evaluation of Sensory and Motor Return

J. Edward Flynn, M.D., and William F. Flynn, M.D.

Evaluation of sensory regeneration after nerve repair may be on the basis of (1) return of pain sensibility which occurs usually before tactile sensibility; (2) Tactile sensibility; Moberg has done more than anyone to emphasize the functional importance of restoration of tactile gnosis, on the basis of the two-point discrimination test of Weber,[11] the picking-up test of Moberg,[4] and the coin test of Riddock.[7]

The autonomic nerves which supply the skin have much the same distribution as the sensory fibers. Guttmann[2] has been chiefly responsible for arousing interest in this subject: (1) the starch and iodine method elaborated by Önne;[6] (2) the quinizarin method of Guttmann;[2] (3) the Moberg[4] ninhydrin test; (4) the Sakuurai and Montagna[8] test.

Electro-diagnosis[10] is developing on the basis of (1) strength-duration curve; (2) nerve stimulation; (3) electromyography; (4) motor nerve conduction; (5) nerve action-potential recording.

In our study we selected the two-point test of Weber, the ninhydrin test, the Riddock coin test, and the Moberg picking-up test,[4] to determine sensory regeneration, and Highet's criteria[12] for motor recovery. Sensory function in the hand cannot be determined accurately by the cotton wool test for touch, pinprick for pain, and ordinary methods of testing sensations of warmth and cold.

In 1966, we reported on results of repair of transected median and ulnar nerves one to 12 years after operation in 80 cases. In all cases the nerves were transected at the wrist level and primary repair was performed. A continuing study reveals the same results.

CUTANEOUS SENSIBILITY IN THE HAND

We agree with Moberg[4] that there are three grades of cutaneous sensibility in a hand: precision sensory grip, gross grip, and protective sensibility. A hand

TABLE 9.4.1
Low medium and ulnar nerve injuries

Years between Repair and Evaluation	Low Median 40 Cases	Ulnar 40 Cases
2	1	
3		1
5	2	7
6	6	7
7	10	4
8	4	3
9	5	2
10	3	9
11	7	4
12	2	3

that lacks tactile perception is blind. It cannot be used without the aid of the eyes, and one does not know whether or how the hand holds an object, or what the object is.

Grade I. Precision Sensory Grip

This is required for buttoning a shirt, turning a bolt, tying a bundle, sewing, and winding a watch. Loss of this sensation can be determined objectively by the ninhydrin test. Subjective tests of value are the Weber two-point discrimination test, Seddon's coin test, and Moberg's picking-up test.

Grade II. Gross Grip

This may be evaluated objectively by examining for the presence of calluses, or by testing ability in lifting a shovel, hammer, bottle, or basket.

Grade III. Protective Sensibility

This may be judged from the history. Lesions such

AGE	TIME SINCE INJURY	PROTECTIVE SENSIBILITY	PRECISION SENSORY GRIP	GROSS GRIP	TWO POINT		
3 YRS.	7 YRS.	++	++	++	3 mm.		
16 YRS.	8 YRS.	++	++	++	3 mm.		
10 YRS	2 YRS.	++	++	++	6 mm.		
23 YRS.	8 YRS.	++	++	++	12 mm.		

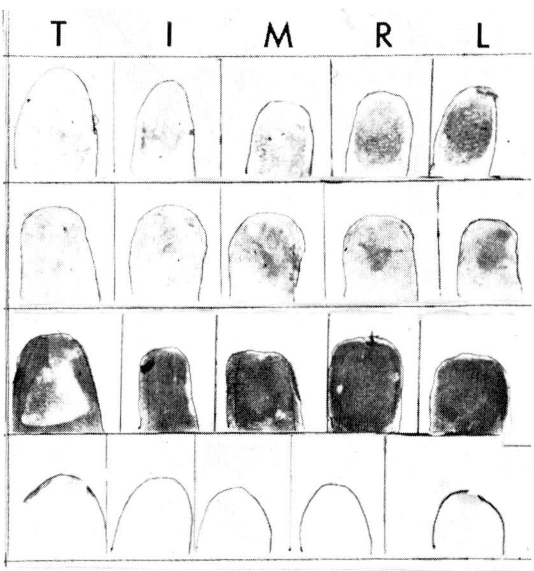

AGE	TIME SINCE INJURY	PROTECTIVE SENSIBILITY	PRECISION SENSORY GRIP	GROSS GRIP	TWO POINT		
7 YRS.	7 YRS.	++	++	++	12 mm.		
24 YRS.	6 YRS.	+	+	+	12 mm.		
16 YRS.	2 YRS.	+	+	+	>26 mm.		
52 YRS.	11 YRS.	+	+	+	>40 mm.		

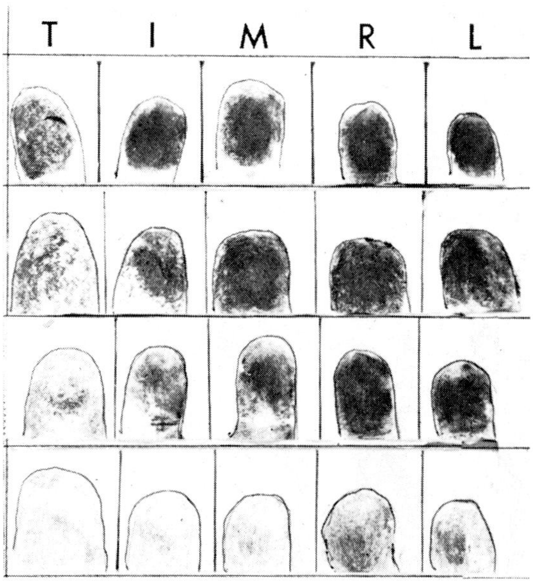

Figure 9.4.1. Median nerve loss.

as burns and infected wounds may provide further evidence. It is interesting how rarely precision sensory grip is restored after transection and repair of median and ulnar nerves in the wrist.

COMPARISON BETWEEN TACTILE SENSIBILITY AND SUDOMOTOR FUNCTION

There were 40 cases of median nerve and 40 cases of ulnar nerves transected and repaired primarily at the wrist level examined from 1 to 12 years after operation (Table 9.4.1).

The results of the ninhydrin test were compared with the results of the two-point discrimination test, the Seddon coin test, and the Moberg picking-up test.

Normal sudomotor function is indicated by 3, moderately reduced by 2, greatly reduced by 1, and absent by 0. Normal precision sensory grip, gross grip and protective sensibility are indicated by +++, moderately reduced by ++, greatly reduced by +, and absent by 0.

In eight cases of median nerve repair it is interesting that return of sudomotor function as evidenced by the ninhydrin test is comparable to return of two-point discrimination. With return of two-point discrimination of 12 mm, a ninhydrin test of 2 is noted. With two-point discrimination of greater than 26, a ninhydrin test of one is noted (Fig. 9.4.1).

More detailed study of sensory return with median nerve repair shows that sudomotor function is comparable to two-point discrimination test and to other

TABLE 9.4.2
Median and ulnar nerve sensory restoration

Age Injury (Yr)	Time Intervals		Grip Function				Two-Point Discrimination in Pulp (mm)					Sudomotor Function				
	Injury to Repair (Hr.)	Repair to follow up (Months)					Median			Ulnar		Median			Ulnar	
3	10	84	++	++	++	++	3	3	4			2	2	2		
10	2	24	++	++	++	++	6	8	8			2	2	2		
23	4	96	+	+	+	+	12	14	16			2	2	1		
26	2	84	+	+	+	+	14	12	14			1	2	1		
24	4	72	+	+	+	+	12	12	12			2	1	2		
16	8	96	+	−	−	−	26	26	26			1	1	1		
52	10	132	+	+	−	−	40	40	40			1	1	1		
16	2	24	+	+	−	−	26	26	22			1	2	1		
43	3	132	+	+	−	−				11	7				2	2
27	2	24	+	+	−	−				7	15				2	2
18	5	36	+	+	−	−				12	12				2	2

Sudomotor function: normal, 3; absent, 0.   Grip function: normal, +++; absent, 0.

AGE	TIME SINCE INJURY	PROTECTIVE SENSIBILITY	PRECISION SENSORY GRIP	GROSS GRIP	TWO POINT	T	I	M	R	L
43 YRS.	11 YRS.	+	+	+	9 mm.					
27 YRS.	2 YRS.	+	+	+	11 mm.					
18 YRS.	3 YRS.	+	+	+	12 mm.					

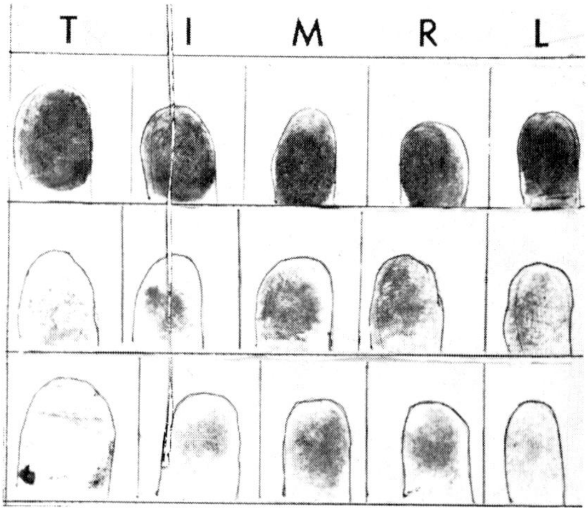

Figure 9.4.2. Ulnar nerve loss.

subjective tests. With sudomotor function of two and two-point discrimination of 12 mm or less, there is usually some return of precision grip (and a positive picking-up test). With a ninhydrin test of one and a two-point discrimination of 26 mm or more, usually there is loss of precision sensory grip, negative picking-up test, and often a negative gross grip (Table 9.4.2).

In three cases of ulnar nerve repair, it is also noted that return of sudomotor function is comparable to the return of two-point discrimination. With two-point discrimination of from 9.0 mm to 12 mm, a ninhydrin test of two is noted (Fig. 9.4.2).

The more detailed study of ulnar nerve repair shows that precision sensory grip and the picking-up test are frequently negative, even when the two-point discrimination is 12 mm or more and the ninhydrin test is two (Table 9.4.2).

An analysis of the results of median and ulnar nerves sutured at the wrist was made. Sensory and motor recovery were studied and were compared with the results reported by others. Sensory and motor recovery were assessed separately and recognized grades of restoration from total paralysis to complete recovery were recorded.

Sensory recovery is graded from SO failure to S4 excellent. The criteria for different grades are noted in Table 9.4.3.

These criteria were compared to criteria suggested by Highet in a memorandum addressed to the British Nerve Injuries Committee.[12] Highet's criteria for sensory recovery are:

Stage 0. Absence of sensibility in the autonomous zone of the nerve.

Stage 1. Recovery of deep cutaneous pain sensibility within the autonomous zone.

Stage 2. Return of some degree of superficial pain and tactile sensibility within the autonomous zone.

Stage 3. Return of superficial pain and tactile sensibility throughout the autonomous zone with the disappearance of over-response.

Stage 4. Return of sensibility as in Stage 3 with the addition that there is recovery of two-point discrimination within the autonomous zone.

Study of return of sensory functions with median and ulnar nerve suture reveals that the greatest percentage of results is in S1, poor, to S2, fair (Table 9.4.3). These compare with results reported by Zachary[12] (Table 9.4.4).

Motor recovery with median nerve suture is graded from M0, failure, to M5, excellent. These criteria are

Stage 1. Return of perceptible contraction in proximal muscles.

Stage 2. Return of perceptible contraction in both proximal and distal muscles.

Stage 3. Return of function in both proximal and distal muscles to such an extent that all important muscles are of sufficient power to act against resistance.

Stage 4. Return of function as in Stage 3 with the addition that all synergic and isolated movements are possible.

Stage 5. Complete recovery.

Our study of return of motor function with median nerve suture shows that more than half the cases are graded from M2, poor, to M3, fair. These results compare with those of Zachary (Table 9.4.5).

TABLE 9.4.3
Percentage sensory recovery, 40 median, 40 ulnar nerve repairs

	Two-Point Discrimination	Grip	Protective Grip	Sudomotor Function	Sensibility
S0 failure	0	0	0	0	0
Median	3	3	3	3	3
Ulnar	0	0	0	0	0
S1 poor	0	0	0	+	½
Median	27	27	27	27	27
Ulnar	30	30	30	30	30
S2 fair	>20	0	+	++	1
Median	50	50	50	50	50
Ulnar	50	50	50	50	50
S3 good	12-20 mm	+ or −	++	++	2
Median	17	17	17	17	17
Ulnar	20	20	20	20	20
S4 excellent	<12 mm	+++	+++	+++	3
Median	3	3	3	3	3
Ulnar	0	0	0	0	0

Normal grip function, +++; normal sudomotor function, 3.

TABLE 9.4.4
Sensory recovery of median and ulnar nerve repairs

	Median		Ulnar	
	Our %	Zachary 5 yrs. %	Our %	Zachary 5 yrs. %
S4 excellent	3	9	0	S3 + 3
S3 good	17	29	20	S3 28
S2 fair	50	15	50	15
S1 poor	27	47	30	54
S0 failure	3	0	0	0
Totals	40	278	40	390

Motor recovery with ulnar nerve suture is graded from M0, failure, to M5, excellent. Criteria are based on the angles of deformity in the three joints with clawing, strength of thumb-index pinch, and active flexion of distal phalanges of the ring and little fingers (Table 9.4.6). Our findings with return of motor function with ulnar nerve suture show that the greatest percentage is in M1, poor, to M2, fair and comparable with those of Zachary (Table 9.4.6).

SUMMARY

The ninhydrin test is a valuable adjunct in determining sensory return after suture of median and ulnar nerves at the wrist. This test is comparable to the Weber two-point discrimination test and other subjec-

tive tests. The two-point discrimination test is better to show normal differences in the pulp of finger and volar aspect of base of proximal phalanx, and between volar aspect of proximal phalanx and palm. The main value of the ninhydrin test is that it is objective and records are permanent. This printing test is valuable in demonstrating small degrees of sensory function in a damaged nerve and in showing regions with and without sensation.

Repair of divided median and ulnar nerves at the wrist gives a fair chance of useful recovery. Perfect recovery is rare and possibly never occurs, but was closely approached in one repair in a child. Forty per cent of median nerve repairs were motor failures or poor. Tendon transplants were not performed in all of this group. Absence of abduction and opposition may be so well compensated for by the flexor pollicis longus, extensor pollicis longus, and the adductor pollicis that there is good grasp. Our indication for tendon transfer in median nerve palsy is when the thumb cannot be abducted sufficiently to grasp an object such as a drinking glass.

Seventy per cent of ulnar nerve repairs were either motor failures or poor. Tendon transfer, to stabilize the second metacarpophalangeal joint and provide for firm pinch between the thumb and index finger, was performed in most cases after transection of the ulnar nerve at the wrist. Proper splinting of the metacarpophalangeal joints in 30° of flexion with a plaster cuff allows the extensor digitoriam communis to extend the middle and distal phalanges and control clawing. Tendon transfer to correct clawing is performed when this disability is so pronounced that an apple or orange cannot be grasped. Tendon transfers for clawing were performed in about 30 per cent of cases of ulnar nerves transected at the wrist.

TABLE 9.4.5
Median nerve, motor recovery

| | Classification | | Results | |
	Flexion of interphalangeal joints	Abduction of thumb	Our %	Zachary 5 yrs. %
M5 excellent	90° each	60-90°	7	6
M4 good	50-90°	45-60°	15	13
M3 fair	30-50°	20-45°	38	41
M2 poor	10-30°	0-20°	25	28 M1 +
M1-M0 failure	0-10°	0	15	12 M1
Totals			40	290

TABLE 9.4.6
Ulnar nerve motor recovery

	Classification							
		Clawing					Motor recovery	
Hyperextension	Hyperextension, M. P. joints	Flexion deformity I. P. joints	Digital abduction and adduction	Thumb index pinch	Flexion distal joint ring and little	Our %	Zachary 5 yrs. %
M5 excellent	0	0	Normal	Normal	50-90°	0	0
M4 good	5°	10-20°	½ Normal	½ Normal	30-40°	8	5
M3 fair	5-10°	20-40°	Poor	¼ Normal	20-30°	15	14
							M2+27
MS poor	10-20°	40-80°	0	Weak	10-20°	57	M2 49
M1-M0 failure	10-20°	40-80°	0	Weak	M1 0-10°	20	5
					M0 0°		
Totals						40	384

Long range examination of 40 median and 40 ulnar nerves transected at the wrist and repaired primarily reveals good sensory return in about 20 per cent with each nerve. Good motor recovery was noted in about 22 per cent of median nerves and 8.0 per cent of ulnar nerves. However, little practical disability occurred as most patients returned to their regular occupations.

REFERENCES

1. Flynn, J. E., and Flynn, W. F. Median and ulnar nerve injuries at the wrist: A long range study with evaluation of sensory and motor return. In *Hand Surgery*, edited by J. E. Flynn. Baltimore, Williams & Wilkins, 1966, pp. 482-487.
2. Guttmann, L. Topographical studies of disturbances of sweat secretion after complete lesions of peripheral nerves. J. Neurol. Psychiatr., *3:* 197, 1940.
3. Hier, S. W., Cornbleet, T., and Bergeim, O. The amino acids of human sweat. J. Biol. Chem., *166:* 327, 1946.
4. Moberg, E. Objective methods for determining the functional value of sensibility in the hand. J. Bone Joint Surg., *40B:* 454, 1948.
5. Oden, S., and Hofsten, B. Detection of fingerprints by ninhydrin reaction. Nature, *174:* 449, 1954.
6. Önne, L. Recovery of sensibility and submotor activity in the hand after nerve suture. Acta chir. Scand., Suppl. 30, 1962.
7. Riddock, G. Phantom limbs and body shape. Brain, *64:* 197, 1941.
8. Sakurai, M., and Montagna, W. The skin of the primates. J. Invest. Dermatol., *42:* 411, 1964.
9. Seddon, H. J. Methods of investigating nerve injuries. In *Peripheral Nerve Injuries*, edited by H. J. Seddon. Medical Research Council Special Report Series No. 282. London, Her Majesty's Stationery Office, 1954, p. 1.
10. Seddon, H. J. Electrical phenomena. In *Surgical Disorders of the Peripheral Nerves*. Baltimore, Williams & Wilkins, 1972, pp. 57-67.
11. Weber, E. H. Cutaneous sensation. In *Textbook of Physiology*, edited by E. A. Schafer. New York, MacMillan, 1900, p. 928.
12. Zachary, R. B. Results of nerve suture. In *Peripheral Nerve Injuries*, edited by H. J. Seddon. Medical Research Council Special Report Series No. 282. London, Her Majesty's Stationery Office, 1954, p. 354.

E.

Compression Neuropathies

Radford C. Tanzer, M.D.

CARPAL TUNNEL SYNDROME

History

The carpal tunnel syndrome, also termed acroparesthesia, median compressive neuropathy, median neuritis, and tardy median palsy, is a chronic, disabling condition characterized by nocturnal hand discomfort, numbness of fingers in median nerve distribution, and thenar muscle atrophy. Sir James Paget[51] quoted two cases of median neuritis of traumatic origin, both of whom developed trophic ulceration. Woltman[77] described typical symptoms occurring in 10 patients with acromegaly; he also referred to the first instance of treatment of carpal tunnel syndrome by division of the flexor retinaculum, a case treated with dramatic relief by Sir James Learmonth. The first comprehensive report, a study of 38 cases by Cannon and Love,[9] demonstrated the advantage of the longitudinal incision.

Anatomy

A glance at a cross section of the carpal tunnel reveals the vulnerability of the median nerve to compression (Fig. 9.5.1). The carpal bones are tightly bound together to form a trough which conducts the long flexor tendons and median nerve into the hand. The trough is transformed into a canal by the flexor retinaculum, or transverse carpal ligament, a dense, nonresilient roof attached on the medial side to the pisiform and hook of the hamate, and on the radial side to the tubercle of the navicular and crest of the greater multangular. The proximal third of the flexor retinaculum, which averages 2.5 mm in thickness, changes abruptly to a thickness of approximately 3.6 mm in its middle and distal thirds (Tanzer[67]).

The flexor synovialis, which invests the flexor tendons, normally contains no appreciable fluid between its visceral and parietal layers, although thickening, fibrosis, and loss of luster of the superficial portion of the flexor synovitis has been consistently noted in adult wrists studied at autopsy or after amputation (Tanzer,[67] Yamaguchi, Lipscomb, and Soule[78]). The median nerve courses through the canal within a thin perineural sheath which merges imperceptibly with the flexor synovialis. The motor branch occasionally appears within the canal, but usually branches at, or distal to, the distal edge of the retinaculum. Abbott and Saunders[1] have pointed out that the median nerve transmits most of the sympathetic nerve supply to the hand, explaining the aching and trophic changes associated with this disease.

McCormack[41] has drawn attention to the fact that incomplete sectioning of the transverse carpal ligament is the most common cause for unsatisfactory results by stating, "the inexperienced operator is frequently surprised at how far out the distal edge of the volar carpal ligament really is located." A detailed anatomic study by Robbins[58] showed that a distance of

3 to 4 cm beyond the distal volar crease of the wrist one encounters a thinned-out distal margin of the transverse carpal ligament which may be mistaken for the mid-palmar fascia. Johnson *et al.*[30] showed that at this level the motor branch of the median nerve occasionally separates itself from the sensory trunk to enter the thenar muscles, thus providing another reason for hesitation in transecting that part of the ligament.

Pathology

In its earliest manifestation compression produces merely a segmental area of hyperemia of the nerve, usually near the junction of the proximal and middle thirds of the flexor retinaculum. In the more advanced form an actual constriction of the nerve takes place at this level, and in the most compressed state a deep indentation and flattening of the nerve is flanked by atrophic degeneration distal to the point of constriction and a pseudo-neuromatous swelling proximal thereto (Fig. 9.5.2).

Etiology

The syndrome can probably be produced by several mechanisms, involving either an increase in the vol-

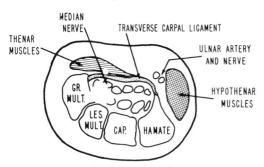

Figure 9.5.1. Cross section of the wrist at level of distal carpal row.

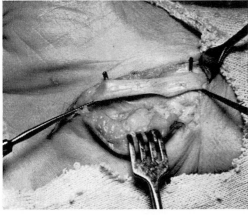

Figure 9.5.2. Carpal tunnel opened, showing compression of median nerve distally and pseudoneuroma proximally.

ume of tunnel contents, in the presence of an unyielding wall, or a decrease in tunnel diameter. Acute conditions, such as severe burn, acute hemorrhage within the tunnel, or violent hand exercise, may be accompanied by a sudden onset of symptoms (Adamson *et al.*[2]).

Thickness of the retinaculum in cases of carpal tunnel syndrome, compared to that in a control series studied at autopsy, has shown no significant difference (Tanzer[67]). The point of the retinaculum at which the thickness abruptly changes, nevertheless, is the site at which nerve compression is usually more prominent.

Symptoms may stem from the presence of space-filling lesions, such as osteophytes, sclerosed hemangiomata, synovial cysts, and anomalous lumbrical or flexor digitorum sublimis muscles within the carpal tunnel (Entin[17]). Cannon and Love[9] described compressive symptoms in several cases of fracture about the base of the radius and of the carpus. Lynch and Lipscomb[39] found that patients with Colles' fracture treated by immobilization in full flexion are more vulnerable to the development of carpal tunnel syndrome. Stein[64] has also described a more subtle effect of wrist fracture — Sudeck's atrophy without the usual sensory deficit and delay in conduction time, responding dramatically to division of the retinaculum.

The prevalence of the syndrome at or near the menopause affords one example of the association of carpal tunnel syndrome with physiologic and pathologic endocrine disturbances. Wallace and Cook[76] and Layton[37] have noted the syndrome during pregnancy and have ameliorated symptoms by the use of estrogens. Sabour and Fadel[59] have found a direct correlation between the carpal tunnel syndrome and the taking of oral contraceptives. Acromegaly and myxedema may both produce compressive symptoms (Woltman,[77] Schiller and Kolb[60]).

Tenosynovitis of a nonspecific variety has been a common concomitant in the cases reported by Phalen[53] and Yamaguchi, Lipscomb, and Soule.[78] These authors, as well as Michaelis,[45] Vicale and Scarff,[75] Grokoest and DeMartini[24] and Crow[11] have established a linkage with the rheumatoid state, manifested as a specific rheumatoid tenosynovitis of the flexor synovialis.

Oppenheim[49] noted that certain occupations (stokers, blacksmiths, laundry women, milkmaids, and ironers) were peculiarly vulnerable to median nerve paresthesia. Tanzer[67] noted that half of his patients with symptoms of median nerve compression had been engaged, for varying periods of time prior to the onset of symptoms, in prolonged activity involving forceful flexion of the fingers, with the wrist flexed.

Experiments on dynamic pressures within the carpal tunnel need clarification. Brain[6] found that pressure readings, taken with tambours in the carpal canal, were three times as high with the wrist in extension, as in flexion, a finding that was substantiated by Kendall.[33] On the other hand, Abbott[1] and Meadoff[43] demonstrated that solutions injected through the carpal canal along the nerve sheath flowed with ease when the wrist was extended, but with difficulty when the wrist was flexed. Tanzer[67] demonstrated increased pressure within the proximal half of the carpal canal when the wrist was flexed or extended. This observation, which has been confirmed by Hunt et al.,[27] lends itself to graphic explanation in a longitudinal cross-section of the wrist (Fig. 9.5.3). Contraction of finger flexors while the wrist is flexed squeezes the nerve between the flexor tendon mass and the unyielding flexor retinaculum.

A residual group of patients, whose symptoms defy explanation, is usually referred to as the "spontaneous" variety. There is some slight evidence to indicate a familial tendency. Zabriskie,[79] Stephens and Welch,[65] and Tanzer[67] have all had instances of multiple occurrence within families. The latter also noted an increased incidence of congenital anomalies about the wrist and carpal canal.

Diagnosis

Carpal tunnel syndrome, occurring twice as frequently in females as in males, is a disease predominantly of middle age, although it occurs rarely in children (Tanzer[67]). It is much more frequent in the right hand than the left; both are involved in about one-half of the cases. The appearance of symptoms in the second hand, when the affected dominant hand is put at rest, is common.

Numbness and tingling in the tip of the middle finger is an early manifestation; later the tips of the two adjacent fingers and thumb may become involved. Sparing of the little finger is often not noted until the patient's attention is directed thereto. Numbness in the little finger, however, does not rule out carpal tunnel syndrome. As might be expected from the large sympathetic element in the median nerve, coldness and sweating are common.

The prominent feature of well established cases is a poorly described, burning, aching discomfort, often accompanied by a feeling of swelling or tenseness, which not only involves the affected hand, but which may also extend proximally into the wrist and forearm, usually on the volar and ulnar side, occasionally running even into the upper arm. This discomfort comes on characteristically two or three hours after retiring, responds somewhat to shaking or rubbing the hand, or hanging over the bedside, but recurs repeatedly until return to morning activity. Relief may persist as the day progresses, but active use of the hand, driving for example, may exacerbate symptoms.

When irreparable damage to the median nerve occurs, the patient may reach a point at which hand discomfort disappears. This loss of protective sensation occasionally results in trophic ulceration of the affected finger tips, a feature noted in Sir James Paget's original description of the disease.

Objective Findings

Isolated thenar muscle atrophy is a most important sign. Selective paresis of the abductor pollicis brevis and, to a lesser extent, of the flexor pollicis brevis, gives a characteristic shelf atrophy which precedes the more complete flattening of the thenar pad (Fig. 9.5.4). Tenderness to pressure over the course of the median nerve at the wrist, fluctuant swelling representing an associated tenosynovitis, and a pseudoneuromatous mass just proximal to the edge of the flexor retinaculum should be sought for. A palpable abnormality in bony contour about the wrist may implicate an old fracture; in fact, roentgenograms should be an integral part of the study.

Tinel's sign, a tingling in one of more digits elicited by tapping the nerve at the wrist, is usually present in well established cases. Acute flexion of the wrist, maintained for one minute, will usually reproduce the characteristic numbness and tingling. A sensory deficit usually appears first on the pulp of the middle finger tip, later on the ring and index fingers and thumb. Moberg's[46] ninhydrin test of sweating gives a graphic representation of the degree of sensory nerve impairment in more advanced cases.

The tourniquet test of Gilliatt and Wilson[22] has been

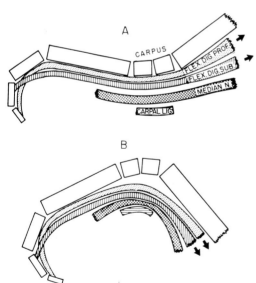

Figure 9.5.3. Schematic representation of longitudinal section of hand, wrist and lower forearm. A. With wrist extended and fingers forcefully flexed, the median nerve within the carpal canal is free of compression. B. With wrist flexed and long digital flexors under tension, the median nerve is compressed against the transverse carpal ligament. (Reprinted from The Carpal-tunnel Syndrome, by R. C. Tanzer, J. Bone Joint Surg., 41A: 626-634, 1959, by permission of the editor.)

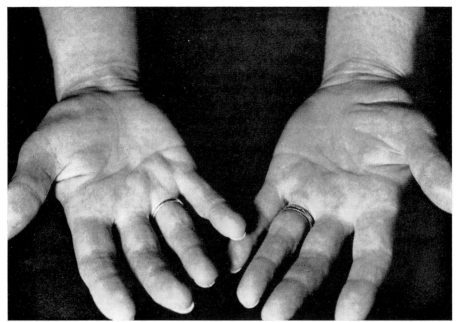

Figure 9.5.4. Advanced bilateral thenar muscle atrophy associated with median nerve compression.

used extensively as a diagnostic aid, although it is less helpful in the borderline cases than in more obvious types. In the presence of median nerve compression, shutting off of the circulation proximal to the wrist often reproduces characteristic aching and burning in the hand, sometimes spreading to the wrist and lasting seven to eight minutes after release of the tourniquet.

Measurement of nerve conduction time, although requiring proficiency in testing, has become one of our most valuable aids in diagnosing equivocal cases of carpal tunnel syndrome. Simpson,[63] using an electrical stimulus to the median nerve at the wrist, and pick-up electrodes in the abductor pollicis brevis and opponens muscles, demonstrated a slowing of conduction time in the presence of median nerve compression, followed by a return to normal when compression was relieved. His findings have been confirmed by others (Carpendale,[10] Thomas *et al.*,[71] Goodman and Gilliatt,[23] Johnson and Melvin[31]). A simpler test using surface electrodes over the thenar musculature has proved quite adequate. Determination of the conduction time of sensory, rather than motor, nerves between the digits and the wrist requires more precise technique because of the small electrical potentials involved, but does afford another quantitative test to measure nerve compression (Dawson and Scott,[13] Gilliatt and Sears,[20] Campbell,[8] Thomas *et al.*[71]).

Normal motor conduction delay or latency, is less than 5 msec, but in patients with carpal-tunnel syndrome, the delay may be as long as 20 msec.

Prolonged sensory latency or failure to evoke an action potential on stimulation of the afferent fibers of the median nerve occurs frequently with carpal-tunnel syndrome.[31] [55] Increased sensory latency more than 3.7 msec is usually present before any motor latency.

Electrodiagnostic studies are especially valuable in patients in whom objective signs of carpal-tunnel syndrome are absent, although subjective complaints suggest the diagnosis. Such studies are helpful in the differential diagnosis of cervical root compression and median nerve entrapment in the forearm (anterior-interosseous-nerve syndrome). Electrodiagnostic studies are of value in providing good objective signs of clinical improvement postoperatively.[44]

Differential Diagnosis

Cervical disc disease, hypertrophic cervical arthritis, and cervical spondylosis cause neuritic symptoms in the hand, but associated symptoms such as neck and shoulder pain, aggravation by coughing and straining, and diminished tendon reflexes usually identify the source of the compression. The carpal tunnel syndrome occasionally occurs coincidentally with cervical root compression. Diabetic neuritis involving the hand is particularly difficult to differentiate, although involvement of the median nerve alone is unusual. Conduction velocity studies are particularly helpful in evaluating the role of nerve compression in these equivocal cases.

Localized compression of the median nerve in other areas, including the palm, forearm, and upper arm, must be considered in the differential diagnosis. Seyfarth,[62] Bell and Goldner,[5] and Kopell and Thompson[35] have described the so-called "pronator syndrome'' due to compression or kinking of the nerve as it passes between the two heads of the pronator teres and under the arch of the flexor digitorum sublimis. Symptoms resemble those of carpal tunnel syndrome; however, aching in the wrist and forearm, sharply localized spot tenderness on the thenar eminence, palpable increase in firmness of the pronator teres, and a positive Tinel's sign aid in the identification of compression at this level.

Treatment

Not all patients with carpal-tunnel syndrome need surgical treatment. In some mild cases no specific treatment is needed. Splinting for a few weeks aids those whose wrist is being subjected to much stress. Injections should be given no more frequently than once every two weeks. No more than three injections are given before insisting upon surgery. The drugs of choice are 1 ml (10 mg) of triamcinolone acetonide or methylprednisolone acetate.[55]

Division of the flexor retinaculum furnishes immediate, dramatic relief of symptoms. When nerve constriction has been severe, some numbness may persist, although the aching and burning disappear. Improvement in muscle wasting may be anticipated in half of the cases, but full return of function is unusual. Under local or block anesthesia, and using a pneumatic tourniquet, a curved incision around the base of the hypothenar eminence is extended between, and parallel to, the wrist creases for about 1 cm ulnarward (Fig. 9.5.5). The palmar cutaneous nerves, if identified, should be preserved, but these have usually branched sufficiently to make their isolation difficult. The palmaris longus tendon if present may be either divided or retracted. The flexor retinaculum, after exposing its entire length, is carefully divided and the contents of the canal are inspected. Should markedly edematous tendons bulge from the canal, they may be restrained by the use of a pull-out suture technique described elsewhere (Tanzer[69]).

Single-layer closure of the wound is followed by a

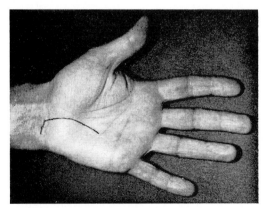

Figure 9.5.5. Incision for exploration of carpal tunnel.

week of wrist immobilization in dorsiflexion by means of a padded volar plaster splint. Gentle finger motion can be started on the day after operation.

Prompt and dramatic relief of discomfort is the almost invariable result, although numbness may persist in some degree. A significant disability due to loss of opposition should lead to consideration of an opponens transfer either at the time of the initial operation, or as a later procedure.

RECURRENCE OF CARPAL-TUNNEL SYNDROME

Surgical release of the transverse carpal ligament for the relief of symptoms resulting from median nerve compression results in a high incidence of success.[12] [54] [57] [78]

Langloh and Linscheid[36] report of re-exploration of 34 wrists in the decade prior to 1969. During that period a total of 2,053 median nerve decompressions were performed. Three conditions seemed to account for recurrent or unrelieved median neuritis. These existed as single entities or in various combinations with each other: (1) incomplete sectioning of the transverse carpal ligament; (2) tenosynovitis of the flexor synovialis; (3) fibrous proliferation within the carpal canal: incomplete sectioning is the most common cause.

ULNAR PALSY AT THE ELBOW

History

Speaking before the Académie de Médicine in Paris in 1887, Panas[52] described four cases of slowly progressive ulnar nerve paresis associated with bony abnormalities of the elbow. In 1916, the name "tardy or late paralysis of the ulnar nerve" was coined by Hunt[29] to describe a late complication of fracture dislocation of the elbow joint in children. Hunt recognized the important role that cubitus valgus and deformity of the ulnar groove play in the production of symptoms, appreciated the existence of other inciting factors such as chronic hypertrophic arthritis, cysts, and tumors, and suggested transposition of the ulnar nerve anteriorly as a means of relieving tension on the nerve.

Pathogenesis

The ulnar nerve pierces the medial intermuscular septum in the midarm and, approaching the elbow in the posterior compartment, traverses the ulnar groove, posterior to the medial epicondyle, before dipping between the two heads of the flexor carpi ulnaris onto the surface of the flexor digitorum profundus. Although lying in a loose fascial compartment in the groove itself, the nerve dips, at the distal limit of the groove, into a more constricted area bounded superficially by an aponeurotic arch joining the olecrenon with the medial epidondyle and deeply by the ulnar collateral ligament of the elbow joint. As the elbow is flexed the nerve becomes angulated and, if associated with a shallow ulnar groove, may actually dislocate anteriorly. When local trauma has been the precipitating agent, one often finds fibrosis about the nerve sheath, fixation of the nerve in a deformed ulnar groove, and a pseudoneuromatous, fusiform swelling of the nerve which may extend throughout the ulnar groove (Fig. 9.5.6).

Etiology

Platt[56] has called attention to the occurrence of fracture of the external or internal condyle of the humerus, complicated by an ulnar neuritis which persists long after the fracture has healed and which is relieved by transplanting the nerve from its bed into a more anterior position. Most cases of ulnar neuritis lack this close association with injury. Denny-Brown and Doherty[14] have demonstrated the production by nerve stretching of pseudoneuromata which persist for months. Hunt and others have felt that the valgus deformity of the elbow incident to fracture of the external condyle, or to osteoarthritis about the elbow, produces tension on the ulnar nerve, which is exacerbated by flexion of the elbow and relieved by transposition of the nerve.

Others have postulated a friction neuritis, due to the repeated sliding back and forth of a hypermobile nerve across the medial epicondyle or across some post-traumatic or osteoarthritic irregularity. McGowan[42] has listed a number of cases with a history of repeated minor occupational trauma. Bed-ridden patients may develop paresis from sustained pressure on the ulnar nerve (Mumenthaler[47]). Occasionally one finds an actual impingement upon the nerve by an expanding lesion such as a synovial cyst.

There remains a group of slowly progressive ulnar palsies in which no obvious cause is apparent. Osborne[50] operated upon some of these cases and found a band of fibrous tissue bridging the heads of the flexor carpi ulnaris, fixed at the medial epicondyle but movable at the olecrenon. He postulated a mechanism analogous to the compression of the median nerve in carpal tunnel syndrome. Feindel and Stratford[18] pursued this thesis and demonstrated significant local constriction of the nerve as it passes through the so-called "cubital tunnel" just distal to the ulnar groove. The nerve proximal to the point of constriction forms a fusiform pseudoneuroma, creating a picture identical to the median nerve configuration as it is compressed in a tight carpal canal.

Diagnosis

A slow, insidious onset, sometimes extending over a period of years, is characteristic. Paresthesias are frequent and may be associated with a positive Tinel's sign, but actual diminution in sensation is a late symptom, often absent. The symptom which usually stirs the patient to seek advice is progressive generalized weakness of the hand, with diminished grip and difficulty in executing finer movements. Pain is unusual but vasomotor symptoms, particularly coldness of the hand, may be present.

Objectively atrophy of the small muscles of the

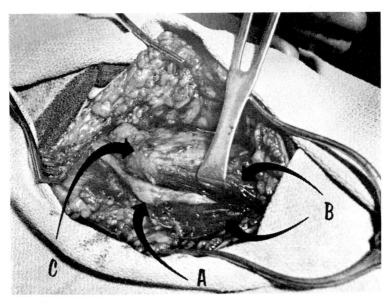

Figure 9.5.6. Fusiform neuroma of ulnar nerve (A) in the ulnar groove, and narrowing of the nerve distally, associated with fall on elbow one year previously. Divided heads of flexor carpi ulnaris (B) will permit shifting of nerve anterior to medial epicondyle (C). (Courtesy of Dr. Robert Fisher.)

hand supplied by the ulnar nerve is a consistent finding. In well developed cases actual clawing of the ring and little fingers may result. Weakness of flexion of the tips of the ring and little fingers, when demonstrable, connotes a lesion proximal to the hand itself. Sparing of the flexor carpi ulnaris muscle places the site of nerve damage distal to the ulnar groove.

A careful search, including roentgenograms of the elbow, should be made for evidence of old condylar fracture, or fibrosis about the ulnar groove, or of arthritic irregularities or other masses which might produce compression. Careful palpation of the nerve in the ulnar groove shows varying degrees of nontender fusiform swelling in about half of the cases.

In the event of an uncertain diagnosis, electrical studies of the conduction velocity of the ulnar nerve and electromyography are most helpful in localizing the level at which compression is producing slowing of electrical impulses within the nerve itself (Simpson,[63] Dawson and Scott,[13] Gilliatt and Sears,[20] Thomas et al.,[72] Gilliatt and Thomas[21]).

Treatment

Osborne,[50] Feindel and Stratford,[18] and Vanderpool et al.[74] have shown that, when an exploration of the nerve reveals definite evidence of constriction within the "cubital tunnel," and particularly when this is associated with a pseudoneuroma in the ulnar groove, a simple release of the nerve in the ulnar groove by splitting the aponeurosis between the two attachments of the flexor carpi ulnaris is usually sufficient to relieve symptoms. In the event that this relatively minor procedure is ineffective, or in cases in which the presence of gross scarring or of distortion of structures in the region of the ulnar groove, the anterior subcutaneous transplantation of the nerve, as suggested by Hunt,[28] Murphy,[48] and McGowan[42] is indicated.

The anterior transplantation requires a longitudinal incision along the middle of the medial aspect of the elbow, posterior to the medial epicondyle, and extended proximally and distally several centimeters along the course of the ulnar nerve. A flap is reflected anteriorly off the deep fascia, preserving if possible both branches of the medial antibrachial cutaneous nerve. If necessary, one or both branches may be divided and anastomosed at the end of the operation. The fascia overlying the ulnar groove is opened and the ulnar nerve dissected proximally to the intermuscular septum which is resected at that point to allow the nerve to swing forward freely. The aponeurotic arch between the olecrenon and the medial epicondyle is divided and the two heads of the flexor carpi ulnaris muscle are separated in order to free the intervening nerve. The articular branch to the elbow is usually sacrificed but the nerve branches to the two heads of the flexor carpi ulnaris muscle can usually be mobilized by cutting the nerve sheath and separating these motor bundles from the main trunk (Learmonth[38]). The nerve can then be transplanted anterior to the medial epicondyle where it is retained by suturing the superficial fascia of the anterior flap to the deep fascia, forming a tunnel to contain the nerve.

If a subcutaneous transplant causes the nerve still to lie in a kinked position, or in a bed which is scarred or deficient in adequate fatty cover, the embedment of the nerve beneath the flexor-pronator muscle mass, as suggested by Adson,[3] Learmonth,[38] and Platt[56] may be necessary.

McGowan[42] and Brooks[7] have emphasized the importance of early operation.

ULNAR PALSY AT THE CARPUS

Historical

Ulnar palsy in the hand is a sharply localized lesion which is almost invariably due to a mechanical compression of the ulnar nerve at the carpal level. Gessler,[19] in a study of a progressive muscular wasting in gold polishers, described the disease accurately, but mistakenly he attributed it to a degeneration of motor nerve endings. Hunt[29] provided a classic description to which little has been added, directing attention to compression as the etiologic agent. The term "ulnar tunnel syndrome" has been applied to the condition more recently (Dupont et al.,[15] Kleinert and Hayes[34]).

Anatomy

As the ulnar nerve, in close association with the radially placed ulnar artery, reaches the wrist, it enters a compartment, the tunnel of Guyon, bounded ulnarward by the pisiform and pisohamate ligament, radialward by the flexor retinaculum and the hook of the hamate, and roofed by a sheet-like expansion from the flexor carpi ulnaris tendon and the antibrachial fascia. Within this canal the ulnar nerve splits into its superficial and deep branches.

Etiology

It is now recognized that most cases of ulnar paralysis of the hand have an occupational basis. Magee,[40] granting that single episodes of trauma may produce symptoms, calls attention to the factor of repeated minor trauma which may often be overlooked. The disease has been noted in gold and brass polishers, jewelers, cobblers, machinists, and motorcyclists. The most common actue injuries, aside from actual laceration of the nerve, causing an ulnar nerve deficit include fractures of the pisiform, hamate, and bases of the fourth and fifth metacarpal bones (Howard[26]).

Kleinert and Hayes[34] have noted thickening of the palmaris brevis muscle and thrombosis of the ulnar artery in several cases. Phalen[53] described calcification adjacent to the pisiform as an etiologic factor which can be recognized by appropriate roentgenograms. Seddon[61] drew attention to the frequency of carpal ganglion as a cause of ulnar neuritis of the hand and noted that the superficial hypothenar muscles are usually not affected in these cases.

A rare and unusual cause for compression of ulnar nerve is by an anomalous muscle in the canal of Guyon.[25] Thomas[70] described a single case. Swanson et al.[66] described three cases. The anomalous muscle is described as originating in the forearm and coursing through Guyon's canal to insert with the flexon digiti quinti brevis. The nerve and blood supply comes from the ulnar nerve and artery.

Diagnosis

Ulnar nerve lesions of the hand can be divided into three groups (Ebeling et al.[16]). The largest is characterized by weakness of all hand muscles supplied by the ulnar nerve, excepting the hypothenar group, and by the absence of sensory loss, indicating compression of the deep palmar branch after the nerves to the hypothenar muscles have been given off. A second group presents all of the symptoms of the first, and in addition paralysis of the hypothenar muscles, indicating a lesion in a narrow segment just before the nerve dips into the hypothenar musculature. The third group, which involves a sensory deficit in addition to full motor loss, indicates a lesion at the nerve trunk or immediately after its division.

The sharply localized nature of the symptoms usually makes the diagnosis evident. Ulnar palsy from a lesion at the elbow may simulate the condition, particularly when the flexor carpi ulnaris muscle is spared. In the presence of atrophy of the small muscles of the hand, without sensory disturbance, the possibility of a neuritis of the deep palmar branch, early amyotrophic lateral sclerosis or myelopathic muscular atrophy (Aran-Duchenne disease) should be considered (Bakke and Wolfe[4]). When the diagnosis is in doubt, studies of electrical conduction times may prove of particular value in determining the presence or absence of nerve compression (Simpson,[63] Thomas, Sears, and Gilliatt[72] Thomas et al.,[71] Ebeling et al.[16]).

Treatment

If the history of occupational trauma can be elicited, improvement may be anticipated when the source of trauma is eliminated. In the event of paralysis following fractures about the carpus, the status of ulnar nerve function should be followed carefully; failure to improve over a period of eight weeks calls for an exploration of the nerve (Howard[26]). A persistent paralysis unassociated with a history of occupational trauma or isolated injury suggests compression by a space-filling lesion, the most common of which, according to Seddon,[61] is carpal ganglion.

The canal of Guyon is most easily approached by an incision similar to that used in exploring the carpal tunnel (Fig. 9.5.5). The incision curves longitudinally to the radial side of the hypothenar eminence and then swings transversely along the distal wrist crease towards the ulnar side of the wrist. Extensions distally or proximally may be used as needed. In addition to unroofing the canal, any entrapment of the nerve at its entrance to the hypothenar musculature should be sought for and released (Thompson and Kopell[73]), and a search for carpal ganglion should be made particularly in the region of the hamate hook where a protrusion into the floor of the canal is most likely to appear.

REFERENCES

1. Abbott, L. C., and Saunders, J. B. deC. Injuries to the median nerve in fractures of the lower end of the radius. Surg. Gynecol Obstet., 57: 507, 1933.
2. Adamson, J. E., Srouji, S. J., Horton, C. E., and Mladick, R. A. The acute carpal tunnel syndrome. Plast. Reconstr. Surg., 47: 332, 1971.
3. Adson, A. W. The surgical treatment of progressive ulnar paralysis. Minnesota Med., 1: 455, 1918.
4. Bakke, J. L., and Wolfe, H. G. Occupational pressure neuritis of the deep palmar branch of the ulnar nerve. Arch. Neurol. Psychiatr., 60: 549, 1948.
5. Bell, G. E., Jr., and Goldner, J. L. Compression neuropathy of the median nerve. South. Med. J., 49: 966, 1956.
6. Brain, W. R., Wright, A. D., and Wilkerson, M. Spontaneous compression of both median nerves in the carpal tunnel: Six cases treated surgically. Lancet, 1: 277, 1947.
7. Brooks, D. M. Nerve compression by simple ganglia. A review of thirteen collected cases. J. Bone Joint Surg., 34B: 391, 1952.
8. Campbell, E. D. R. The carpal tunnel syndrome: investigation and assessment of treatment. Proc. R. Soc. Med., 55: 401, 1962.
9. Cannon, B. W., and Love, J. G. Tardy median palsy; median neuritis; median thenar neuritis amenable to surgery. Surgery, 20: 210, 1946.
10. Carpendale, M. T. F. Conduction time in the terminal portion of the motor fibers of the ulnar, median and peroneal nerves in healthy subjects and in patients with neuropathy. M.S thesis (Phys. Med.), University of Minnesota, 1956.
11. Crow, R. S. Treatment of the carpal-tunnel syndrome. Br. Med. J., 5186: 1611, 1960.
12. Czeuz, K. A., Thomas, J. E., Lambert, E. H., Love, J. G., and Lipscomb, P. R. Long-term results of operation for carpal-tunnel syndrome. Mayo Clin. Proc., 41: 232, 1966.
13. Dawson, G. D., and Scott, J. W. Recording of nerve action potentials through skin in man. J. Neurol. Neurosurg. Psychiatr., 12: 259, 1949.
14. Denny-Brown, D., and Doherty, M. M. Effects of transient stretching of peripheral nerve. Arch. Neurol. Psychiatr., 54: 116, 1945.
15. Dupont, C., Cloutier, G. E., Prévost, Y., and Dion, M. A. Ulnar-tunnel syndrome at the wrist. J. Bone Joint Surg., 47A: 757, 1965.
16. Ebeling, P., Gilliatt, R. W., and Thomas, P. K. A clinical and electrical study of ulnar nerve lesions in the hand. J. Neurol. Neurosurg. Psychiatr., 23: 1, 1960.
17. Entin, M. A. Carpal tunnel syndrome and its variants. Surg. Clin. North Am., 48: 1097, 1968.
18. Feindel, W., and Stratford, J. The role of the cubital tunnel in tardy ulnar palsy. Can. J. Surg., 1: 287, 1958.

19. Gessler, H. Eine eigenartige form van progressiver muskelatrophie bei goldpolirerinnen. Med. Cor. Bl. w¨urrtemb. ¨artzl ver., 66: 281, 1896.

20. Gilliatt, R. W., and Sears, T. A. Sensory nerve action potentials in patients with peripheral nerve lesions. J. Neurol. Neurosurg. Psychiatr., 21: 109, 1958.

21. Gilliatt, R. W., and Thomas, P. K. Changes in nerve conduction with ulnar lesions at the elbow. J. Neurol. Neurosurg. Psychiatr., 23: 312, 1960.

22. Gilliatt, R. W., and Wilson, R. G. A pneumatic tourniquet test in the carpal-tunnel syndrome. Lancet, 2: 595, 1953.

23. Goodman, H. V., and Gilliatt, R. W. The effect of treatment on median nerve conduction in patients with the carpal tunnel syndrome. Ann. Phys. Med., 6: 137, 1961.

24. Grokoest, A. W., and DeMartini, F. E. Systemic disease and the carpal tunnel syndrome. J.A.M.A., 155: 635, 1954.

25. Guyon, F. Note sur une disposition anatomique propre á la face anteriéure de la région du poignet et non encore décrite par le docteur. Bull. Soc. Soc. Anat. Paris, 2nd series, 6: 184, 1861.

26. Howard, F. M. Ulnar-nerve palsy in wrist fractures. J. Bone Joint Surg., 43A: 1197, 1961.

27. Hunt, G. M., Abbott, K. H., and Roberts, W. H. The median nerve and carpal tunnel syndrome: historical features, anatomical basis and clinical experiences. Bull. Los Angeles Neurol. Soc., 25: 211, 1960.

28. Hunt, J. R. Occupational neuritis of the deep palmar branch of the ulnar nerve: a well defined clinical type of professional palsy of the hand. J. Nerv. Ment. Dis., 35: 673, 1908.

29. Hunt, J. R. Tardy or late paralysis of the ulnar nerve. A form of chronic progressive neuritis developing many years after fracture dislocation of the elbow. J.A.M.A., 66: 10, 1916.

30. Johnson, E. W., Wells, R. M., and Duran, R. J. Diagnosis of carpal tunnel syndrome. Arch. Phys. Med., 43: 414, 1962.

31. Johnson, E. W., and Melvin, J. L. Sensory conduction studies of median and ulnar nerves. Arch. Phys. Med., 48: 25, 1967.

32. Johnson, R. K., and Shrewsbury, M. M. Anatomical course of the thenar branch of the median nerve, usually in a separate tunnel through the transverse carpal ligament. J. Bone Joint Surg., 53A: 269, 1970.

33. Kendall, D. Non-penetrating injuries of the median nerve at the wrist. Brain, 73: 84, 1950.

34. Kleinert, H. E., and Hayes, J. E. The ulnar tunnel syndrome. Plastic Reconstr. Surg., 47: 21, 1971.

35. Kopell, H. P., and Thompson, W. A. L. Pronator syndrome: confirmed case and its diagnosis. N. Engl. J. Med., 259: 713, 1958.

36. Langloh, N. D., and Linscheid, R. L. Recurrent and unrelieved carpal-tunnel syndrome. Clin. Orthop., 83: 41, 1972.

37. Layton, K. B. Acroparesthesia in pregnancy and the carpal tunnel syndrome. J. Obstet. Gynecol., 65: 823, 1958.

38. Learmonth, J. R. A technique for transplanting the ulnar nerve. Surg. Gynecol. Obstet., 75: 792, 1942.

39. Lynch, H. C., and Lipscomb, P. R. The carpal tunnel syndrome and Colles' fractures. J.A.M.A., 185: 363,1963.

40. Magee, K. R. Neuritis of deep palmar branch of ulnar nerve. Arch. Neurol. Psychiatr., 73: 200, 1955.

41. McCormack, R. M. Carpal-tunnel syndrome. Surg. Clin. North Am., 40: 517, 1960.

42. McGowan, A. J. The results of transposition of the ulnar nerve for traumatic ulnar neuritis. J. Bone Joint Surg., 32B: 293, 1950.

43. Meadoff, N. Median nerve injuries in fractures in the region of the wrist. Calif. Med., 70: 252, 1949.

44. Melvin, J. L., Johnson, E. W., and Duran, R. Electrodiagnosis after surgery for carpal-tunnel syndrome. Arch. Phys. Med., 49: 502, 1968.

45. Michaelis, L. S. Stenosis of carpal tunnel, compression of median nerve and flexor tendon sheaths, combined with rheumatoid arthritis. Proc. R. Soc. Med., 43: 414, 1950.

46. Moberg, E. Evaluation of sensibility in the hand. Surg. Clin. North Am., 40: 357, 1960.

47. Mumenthaler, M. Die ulnaris lähmungen über 314 (nicht-traumatische) eigene Beobachtungen. Schweiz. Med. Wochenschr., 90: 815, 1960.

48. Murphy, J. B. Cicatricial fixation of ulnar nerve from ancient cubitus valgus-release and transference to new site. Clin. John B. Murphy, 5: 661, 1916.

49. Oppenheim, H. Die lähmung des n. medianus. Lehrb. Nervenkrankh., 1: 589, 1913.

50. Osborne, G. V. The surgical treatment of tardy ulnar neuritis. J. Bone Joint Surg., 39B: 782, 1957.

51. Paget, J. Lectures on Surgical Pathology, Ed. 1. Lindsay, Philadelphia, Blakiston, 1854, p. 40.

52. Panas, P. Sur une cause peu connue de paralysie du nerf cubital. Arch. G´en. M´ed., 2: 5, 1878.

53. Phalen, G. S. Calcification adjacent to the pisiform bone. J. Bone Joint Surg., 34A: 579, 1952.

54. Phalen, G. S. The carpal-tunnel syndrome. Seventeen years' experience in diagnosis and treatment of 654 hands. J. Bone Joint Surg., 48A: 211, 1966.

55. Phalen, G. S. The carpal-tunnel syndrome. Clin. Orthop., 83: 29, 1972.

56. Platt, H. The pathogenesis and treatment of traumatic neuritis of the ulnar nerve in the post-condylar groove. Br. J. Surg., 13: 409, 1926.

57. Rietz, K. A., and Onne, L. Analysis of 65 operated cases of carpal-tunnel syndrome. Acta Chir. Scand., 133: 443, 1967.

58. Robbins, H. Anatomical study of the median nerve in the carpal-tunnel syndrome. J. Bone Joint Surg., 45A: 953, 1963.

59. Sabour, M. S., and Fadel, H. The carpal tunnel syndrome, a new complication. Am. J. Obstet. Gynecol., 107: 1265, 1970.

60. Schiller, F., and Kolb, F. O. Carpal tunnel syndrome in acromegaly. Neurology, 4: 271, 1954.

61. Seddon, H. J. Carpal ganglion as a cause of paralysis of the deep branch of the ulnar nerve. J. Bone Joint Surg., 34B: 386, 1952.

62. Seyffarth, H. Primary myoses in the m. pronator teres as cause of lesion of the n. medianus (the pronator syndrome). Acta Psychiatr. Neurol. Scand. Suppl. 74, 251, 1951.

63. Simpson, J. A. Electrical signs in the diagnosis of carpal tunnel and related syndromes. J. Neurol. Neurosurg. Psychiatr., 19: 275, 1956.

64. Stein, A. H. The relation of median nerve compression to Sudeck's syndrome. Surg. Gynecol. Obstet., 115: 713, 1962.

65. Stephens, J., and Welch, K. Acroparesthesia: a symptom of median nerve compression at the wrist.

Arch. Surg., *73:* 849, 1956.

66. Swanson, A. B., Biddulph, S. L., Baughman, F. A., Jr., and deGrout, G. Ulnar nerve compression due to an anomalous muscle in the canal of Guyon. Clin. Orthop., *83:* 64, 1972.

67. Tanzer, R. C. The carpal-tunnel syndrome: a clinical and anatomical study. J. Bone Joint Surg., *41A:* 626, 1959.

68. Tanzer, R. C. *The Carpal Tunnel Syndrome.* Clinical Orthopaedics No. 15. Philadelphia, Lippincott, p. 171, 1959.

69. Tanzer, R. C. The carpal tunnel syndrome. In *Reconstructive Plastic Surgery,* edited by J. M. Converse. Philadelphia, Saunders, 1964.

70. Thomas, C. G. Clinical manifestations of an accessory palmar muscle. J. Bone Joint Surg., *40A:* 929, 1958.

71. Thomas, J. E., Lambert, E. H., and Cseuz, K. A. Electrodiagnostic aspects of the carpal tunnel syndrome. Arch. Neurol, *16:* 635, 1967.

72. Thomas, P. K., Sears, T. A., and Gilliatt, R. W. The range of conduction velocity in normal motor nerve fibres to the small muscles of the hand and foot. J. Neurol. Neurosurg. Psychiatr., *22:* 175, 1959.

73. Thompson, W. A. L., and Kopell, H. P. Peripheral entrapment neuropathies of the upper extremity. N. Engl., J. Med., *260:* 1261, 1959.

74. Vanderpool, D. W., Chalmers, J., Lamb, D. W., and Whiston, T. B. Peripheral compression lesions of the ulnar nerve. J. Bone Joint Surg., *50B:* 792, 1968.

75. Vicale, C. T., and Scarff, J. E. Median neuritis owing to compression in the carpal tunnel in the absence of osseous disease of the wrist. Trans. Am. Neurol. Assoc., 187, 1951.

76. Wallace, J. T., and Cook, A. W. Carpal tunnel syndrome in pregnancy: a report of two cases. Am. J. Obstet. Gynecol., *73:* 1335, 1957.

77. Woltman, H. W. Neuritis associated with acromegaly. Arch. Neurol. Psychiatr., *45:* 680, 1941.

78. Yamaguchi, D. M., Lipscomb, P. R., and Soule, E. H. Carpal tunnel syndrome: a clinicopathologic study to determine the pathogenesis. Read at the meeting of the American Society for Surgery of the Hand, Jan. 25-26, 1963. Minn. Med., *48:* 22, 1965.

79. Zabriskie, E. G., Hare, C. C., and Masselink, R. J. Hypertrophic arthritis of cervical vertebrae with thenar muscular atrophy occurring in three sisters. Bull. Neurol. Inst. N. Y., *4:* 207, 1935.

F.

Surgery of the Hand in Cerebral Palsy

Alfred B. Swanson, M.D., F.A.C.S.

Cerebral palsy is a "condition characterized by paralysis, weakness, incoordination, or any aberration of motor control centers of the brain" (Perl-stein,[21]). It is a challenging problem for those who would treat it.

Some form of brain damage manifested by cerebral palsy occurs in one to five newborns per every 1,000 births in the United States.[6][11] The improvement of prenatal care and obstetrical methods are the main factors contributing to the decreased incidence of this disorder. There are an estimated 600,000 cases of cerebral palsied newborns in the United States: one of every seven cases dies, two of every seven cases will require custodial care for severe mental handicaps, one of every seven cases will require custodial care for severe physical handicaps, two of every seven cases will require some moderate treatment and one will require some mild treatment.

The classification of cerebral palsy has been the subject of many debates. The most logical classification seems to be made in reference to the type of manifestation of the central motor disorder and the distribution of the peripheral involvement.

Classification of types of cerebral palsy:

Type	*Incidence*
Spastic	70 per cent
Athetoid	20 per cent
Ataxia	
Tremor	10 per cent
Rigidity	
Others	

Few patients have a single diagnostic involvement. Most have a mixed involvement with one type predominating. Approximately 25 per cent of these patients have a severe loss of sensibility that will prevent usage of their hands even though their motor ability is adequate.[33]

Classification of peripheral involvement in cerebral palsy:

Involvement	*Incidence*
Quadriplegia	50 per cent
Hemiplegia	40 per cent
Para-, mono-, triplegia	10 per cent

A comparison of the intelligence quotient between the general population and the cerebral palsied patients shows the following values:

I.Q. in "Normal"	*I.Q. in C.P.*
z 90 = 75 per cent	z 90 = 25 per cent
x 70 = 3 per cent	x 70 = 50 per cent

The complications presented by the cerebral palsied patient further handicap this unfortunate child and increase the difficulties of the rehabilitation program. Speech defects are present in 75 per cent of these patients, visual defects in 50 per cent, hearing defects in 10 per cent, some convulsive disorders in 30 per cent, and laterality in 40 per cent. A certain number of these patients also have nutritional problems, marked distractibility, incontinence, and drooling. Their psychological development and adjustment can be poor and is further complicated by parental attitudes of guilt, intolerance, or rejection.

DISTURBED MUSCLE PHYSIOLOGY AND PRINCIPLES OF TREATMENT

Separate muscle units can be affected differently in cerebral palsy. They may be spastic, flaccid, normal, weak, or contracted. Long-standing flexion deformities commonly result in myostatic contractures. This is often coupled with disturbances in the stretch reflex mechanism. There is a direct relationship between the length to which a muscle is stretched and the amount of tension developed. As the tension increases, the stretch reflex or contractile response of the muscle increases.[1] This reflex is present in all normal skeletal muscles but is overactive in the spastic muscle (Fig. 9.6.1).

Spasticity of muscles, especially of the flexors of the wrist and fingers, is common in the upper extremity of a patient with cerebral palsy. Myostatic contractures can be prevented to some degree by physical methods of stretching with casts or braces. Hyperactive stretch reflexes can be abolished by destroying any portion of their arc. Selective neurectomy has been used in the past but has become contraindicated because it resulted in excessive muscle weakness.

Temporary abatement of the spasticity may be produced by injecting the muscle or the peripheral nerves with 1 per cent procaine. This apparently reduces the activity of the gamma system without completely decreasing the motor control. It has been pointed out that hyperactivity of the gamma motor neurons to the muscle spindle is the main cause of spasticity.[23] Recent work has suggested that dilute chemolytic agents injected directly into a peripheral nerve may selectively destroy the gamma motor fibers to decrease spasticity without seriously affecting the larger motor or sensory pathways.[2 19] Two to 5 per cent phenol has been used for direct injection into the motor branches of the ulnar and median nerves in the forearm after surgical exposure. It should not be injected in sensory nerves and therefore should not be injected into mixed nerves. Most cases demonstrate only a short-term effectiveness. A long-term appraisal of these agents will be necessary before they are included in the treatment of cerebral palsied extremities.

Overactive reflexes and spasticity can be relieved in part by judicious shortening of the muscle to prevent its over-stretching. This can be achieved by either lengthening the tendon distally or releasing the origin of the muscle and sliding it proximally as will be discussed below.

The ideal treatment for relieving spasticity, when it is finally discovered, will be a pharmacologic agent or surgical procedure that will differentially decrease

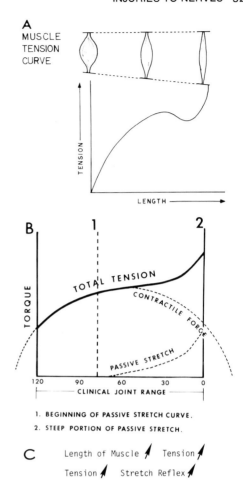

1. BEGINNING OF PASSIVE STRETCH CURVE.
2. STEEP PORTION OF PASSIVE STRETCH.

C   Length of Muscle ↑ Tension ↑

        Tension ↑   Stretch Reflex ↑

Concept of Muscle Release Procedures in C. P.

        Short Muscle = Less Tension

        ∴ Less Stretch Reflex

Figure 9.6.1 A. This curve demonstrates the direct relationship between the length of the muscle as it is stretched and the tension developed: the longer the stretch, the greater the tension and the greater the stretch reflex.

Figure 9.6.1 B. The total tension curve developed in voluntary muscles is in relationship to the torque and the motion of the related joints. As the passive stretch increases, the contractile force decreases and the total tension increases steeply as manifested by an increased stretch reflex. The graph denotes flexion and extension of the proximal interphalangeal joint.

Figure 9.6.1 C. This summarizes the concept of muscle release procedure in cerebral palsy.

spasticity at the motor end-plate without affecting voluntary movements.

Any physician responsible for the rehabilitation program of a cerebral palsied individual must be aware of the problems briefly summarized above to evaluate properly the potential of each patient, adequately select the candidates for surgical improvement, and apply the proper treatment.

PREOPERATIVE EVALUATION

Definite plans for rehabilitation of a cerebral palsy case cannot be formulated after a single consultation. The patient must be carefully evaluated several times by the physician and members of the team, including the physical and occupational therapists, before the treatment patterns can be established.

The functional part of the evluation is done by questioning the parents, the patient, when possible, and observing his patterns of hand activities with handling test objects. This functional evaluation must include the observation of speed, coordination, and strength in the use of the hand, skill and coordination, hand adaptation patterns, hand-eye coordination, reach, hand placement, handedness, bilaterality, and the ability to handle test objects. The questions and observations must also be directed towards defining the patient's intelligence and his capacity to perform activities of daily living.

The physical examination must include observation of the patient's voluntary control, his grasp and release patterns. A grasp and release pattern must be present in a cerebral palsied patient if improvement is to be expected from a surgical procedure. Spasm, accessory movements, and muscle imbalances must be noted. The muscle tone may be flaccid, normal, or spastic in various muscle groups of the same extremity. The presence and degree of joint instability and its repercussions on hand function should be recorded. The presence of resistant deformities and the sensory status must be determined. The functional value of sensibility must also be determined. A simple sensory test may be the the the blind differentiation between a marble and a cube.

The results of tenodesis operative procedures can be evaluated in advance by taping small aluminum splints on the digits to simulate the postoperative condition. Although rarely indicated, should a wrist arthrodesis be considered, the application of a plaster cast or a brace can demonstrate the postoperative functional possibilities of the patients or the best fusion position of the wrist. Because the spastic patients are especially dependent on the reciprocal flexion of the wrist to obtain finger extension, a wrist fusion can be disastrous.

DEFORMITIES AND IMPAIRMENTS

Common deformities in the cerebral palsied upper extremity include internal rotation of the arm, flexion of the elbow, pronation of the forearm, flexion of the wrist and digits, extension of the digits with swan-neck deformities, thumb-in-palm deformity, unstable joints, motor deficiencies, and sensibility defects.

Pronation deformity is common in cerebral palsy. The pronation position is functional for many hand activities and therefore no surgical treatment may be indicated. This deformity cannot be well treated by conservative method of stretching or exercises. Tendon releases of the insertion of the pronator teres and/or pronator quadratus may be of some benefit in certain cases. Release of the pronator teres origin as performed in the flexor-pronator origin release procedure can also improve the problem. The Green procedure can also be of benefit. Occasionally this deformity may be associated with posterior dislocation of the head of the radius or altered relationship of the shaft of the radius to the ulna. A long oblique osteotomy of the shaft of the radius may be necessary to bring the hand to the neutral position. In general, if supination to $0°$ is possible, no other treatment should be indicated. Specific surgical treatment for this deformity alone is uncommon and the results frequently unrewarding.

The major handicap of the hand in cerebral palsy is the patient's inability to open the hand for grasp. Often the hand has good strength for closing but does not have efficient extension or the necessary speed of extension which is so important for normal function. Another common handicap of the hand in cerebral palsy is instability of the finger joints. This is especially true in hyperextension deformities of the fingers so common in this condition. These deformities preclude a strong pinch and grasp pattern. The collapse of the normal flexion arc of the digit, associated with hyperextension of the proximal interphalangeal joint and flexion of the distal interphalangeal joint, known as the swan-neck deformity, is functionally disabling and also cosmetically unattractive. These deformities are particularly severe in individuals with inherently lax ligamentous structures. The loss of the normal flexion arc of the interphalangeal joints also contributes to the inability to extend the metacarpophalangeal joint properly. Extension of the metacarpophalangeal joint is facilitated by proximal interphalangeal joint flexion.[34]

The normal function of the contiguous articulations in the fingers and hand are interdependent. Any disturbance in one joint will affect other related joints. In cerebral palsy these interrelated functions are profoundly affected and it may be difficult to determine if a deformity is primary or secondary to other imbalances.

INDICATIONS FOR SURGERY

Most patients with cerebral palsy involvement of the upper extremity are not candidates for surgical reconstructive procedures. In 10 to 20 per cent of the cases, certain selective operative procedures may assist in the patient's rehabilitation.[8][15][22][25][27][28] We have developed a group of operations over a period of years in our clinic that appear to be useful. It is our impression that this type of surgery can best be carried out in a clinic situation where many patients are seen and a team approach to their rehabilitation is available. The need for careful preoperative evaluation of the patient's functional potential is obvious.

The indications for surgery in the cerebral palsied hand include a rehabilitation potential for disabilities that are correctable by surgery in presence of a good potential for functional and cosmetic improvement. Approximately 50 per cent of these cerebral palsy patients are seeking cosmetic improvement. Patients with severe athetoid manifestations usually present incoordinations that will probably not benefit from any surgical procedure.

The ideal surgical candidate is one with sufficient intelligence, emotional stability, and a cooperative disposition. He is usually a spastic hemiplegic patient with good voluntary grasp and release patterns and adequate sensation in the hand. He must have a good functional and cosmetic potential. He is handicapped usually by defects such as pronation deformity of the forearm, flexor muscle overactivity with contracture, and spasm of the wrist and finger muscles, thumb-in-palm attitude, and hyperextension or swan-neck deformities of the proximal interphalangeal joints. Surgical procedures are designed, therefore, to improve the following: (1) the inability to open the hand, (2) the thumb-in-palm deformity, and (3) the swan-neck deformities.

SURGICAL TREATMENT

Flexion Deformity of the Wrist

Treatment of this deformity includes the following methods:
1. Conservative stretching by means of bracing or a cast.
2. Selective lengthening of flexor tendons.
3. Transfer of the flexor carpi ulnaris.
4. Flexor muscle origin release procedure.
5. Combination of the above.
6. Postoperative bracing.
7. Wrist arthrodesis.

Conservative attempts to correct the wrist flexion deformity by means of bracing or casts should precede any surgical procedure. The flexor carpi ulnaris transfer, as described by Green and Banks,[10] is our procedure of choice for patients who present a flexion-pronation deformity of the wrist with weakness of the wrist extensors. This procedure is occasionally done in association with a flexor muscle origin release procedure for finger-flexion deformity. In this situation the proximal origin of the flexor carpi ulnaris is left intact. Bracing must always be applied postoperatively and usually for a prolonged period of time.

Arthrodesis of the wrist is most infrequently per-

formed in our clinic because of the particular dependency of the cerebral palsied patient on wrist flexion to achieve finger extension. It is most important to evaluate preoperatively the potential for finger extension as the wrist is maintained in the desired position of fusion with a plaster cast or brace. This procedure has been occasionally done in an attempt to obtain cosmetic improvement in athetoid patients.

Flexor Carpi Ulnaris Transfer

Careful assessment of the degree of deformity present before surgery and measure of the tendon balance at the wrist are important to anticipate the muscle power balance after the flexor carpi ulnaris tendon transfer. It is also critical to determine whether an increase in the extensor power or merely a decrease in flexor power should be obtained in order to adjust correctly the tightness of the tendon transfer. The degree of wrist flexion needed to enable the patient to extend the fingers is noted. Increased extension of the wrist is provided at surgery when good finger extension is available preoperatively. If reasonable finger extension is not present, the tendon transfer should not be pulled so tight as to prevent some wrist flexion. The power of the wrist extensor muscles can be evaluated more accurately by temporarily blocking the flexors with a local anesthetic.[28]

The basic steps of the Green procedure are the following (Fig. 9.6.2). A longitudinal incision is carried out from the area of insertion of the flexor carpi ulnaris distally, along the ulna over the muscle belly proximally. The flexor carpi ulnaris tendon is identified and sectioned far enough distally to obtain sufficient length. The muscle is then carefully dissected from the ulna proximally to its origin taking care to preserve its neurovascular supply. An oblique subcutaneous tunnel is made from the origin of the muscle, along the forearm and around the dorsum of the wrist to the level of the extensor carpi radialis brevis tendon distally. This tendon is the favored recipient for the transfer because it is a neutral extensor of the wrist. The flexor carpi ulnaris tendon is then rerouted through this tunnel and securely woven through the extensor carpi radialis brevis tendon about 2 to 4 cm proximal to the wrist. The tension of the transfer is carefully adjusted and the tendon is firmly fixed with multiple interrupted nonabsorbable sutures. The extremity is immobilized in a long arm cast with the wrist in moderate dorsiflexion and the forearm in supination. The cast is worn for approximately six weeks.

Flexion Deformity of the Fingers

Flexion deformity of the fingers is the result of the severe spasticity and myostatic contracture of the flexor muscles and is usually associated with flexion and pronation of the wrist. Treatment of this deformity include the following methods:
1. Attempts at conservative stretching of the muscle contracture with bracing should always pre-

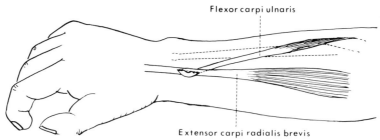

Flexor carpi ulnaris

Extensor carpi radialis brevis

Figure 9.6.2. The Green produce for transfer of the flexor carpi ulnaris subcutaneously to the extensor carpi radialis brevis is the preferred method of treatment of flexion deformity of the wrist in cerebral palsy.

cede any surgical procedure.

2. Release of the flexor muscles origin.
3. Lengthening of individual tendons participating in the deformity.
4. Lengthening of multiple tendons.
5. Continued bracing after the surgical procedure.

Flexor Muscle Origin Release

Release of the origin of the flexor muscles, which we first performed in cerebral palsied patients in 1963, has been a most useful and successful operation in our hands. It allows the flexor muscles to reattach distally without interrupting their main neurovascular supply. The purpose of releasing the origins of the flexor muscles is to obtain a new shorter resting or postural length, thereby decreasing the tension developed and the stretch reflex as explained previously. This decreases the strength as well as the spasticity and contracture. The flexor origin release procedure is most useful to rebalance the extensor-flexor forces and to improve the function of the hand.[5 9 12 20 24 29 32 35]

The flexor origin procedure is specifically indicated for patients who have a voluntary grasp and release pattern but are handicapped by flexor muscle contractures forcing them to flex the wrist to obtain finger extension. When it is noted that the patient is unable to extend the fingers completely with the wrist in more than 30° of flexion or when there is obvious contracture on passive extension of the fingers with the wrist from 30° to 70° of flexion, a proximal flexor release procedure is indicated. Injection of a dilute solution of procaine into the flexor mass can also help determine the degree of spasticity and myostatic contracture. Additional release of the pronator teres in this operation also improves the frequently associated pronation deformity. Occasionally, the lacertus fibrosus may be incised, especially if a flexion contracture of the elbow is present.

The flexor release procedure is carried out through an incision starting approximately 3 cm proximal to the medial epicondyle and carried down over the ulnar proximal two-thirds of the forearm (Fig. 9.6.3). The pronator-flexor mass is sectioned from the capsular structures over the medial epicondyle and advanced distally. The median nerve is identified and avoided. The dissection is carried along the ulna, avoiding the proximal motor branches of the ulnar nerve and sectioning all the musclar attachments from the proximal ulna and interosseous membrane distally. If the flexor pollicis longus is to be recessed, an additional incision over the radial aspect of the forearm is made to expose the radius. Most frequently, this is not done. The released pronator-flexor muscle mass can then be demonstrated to move 3 to 5 cm distally by hyperextending the fingers and wrist. The pronator teres, flexor digitorum sublimis and profundus, flexor carpi radialis, flexor carpi ulnaris, and palmaris longus have now been moved to a new resting length position. The muscle mass, especially the pronator teres, may be sutured to the underlying structures at the desired level for reattachment. If the motor branches of the ulnar nerve appear to be under tension, the ulnar nerve can be transposed out of its groove and rerouted anteriorly. Multiple drains are placed in the wound or a negative pressure drainage apparatus is used for two days to prevent a postoperative hematoma. The fingers and wrist are held in hyperextension to maintain the distal positioning of the muscle origins in the operative dressing. The proximal interphalangeal joints are flexed to 30°. A voluminous conforming dressing and a plaster cast are applied with the elbow at 90° of flexion, the wrist and metacarpophalangeal joints in 0° of extension, and the forearm in supination. This cast is worn for approximately three weeks. A physical and occupational therapy program is then started. The patient is instructed to wear a modified pancake brace between treatments for a period of three to six weeks. The brace is worn at night for an additional three months or longer as necessary.

The flexor carpi ulnaris origin has been left intact proximally and the tendon used for a Green transfer in patients who presented excessively weak wrist extensors preoperatively or in some patients who desired, for cosmetic reasons, the assurance that their wrist would no longer present a flexion deformity. White[35] has performed a wrist arthrodesis in association with the flexor origin release procedure; however, we do not believe that this is necessary.

Individual Tendon Lengthening

In patients presenting contracture of selective flexor tendons of the wrist or digits, Z step-cut lengthening

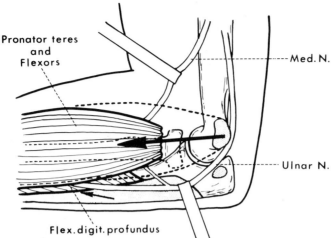

Figure 9.6.3. Release of the flexor-pronator muscles origins in the forearm. The proximal attachments are released and allowed to move 3 to 5 cm distally. The neurovascular supply is left intact. The muscle mass, especially the pronator teres, may be sutured to the underlying structures at the desired level. The length of the muscles being decreased, the stretch reflex is decreased and consequently the flexion deformity of the fingers and wrist are relieved.

of individual tendons at the musculotendinous junction in the forearm can provide adequate release. This may be especially important in the flexor pollicis longus or the flexor sublimis tendons.

Multiple Tendon Lengthening

Patients presenting severe clasping of the fingers into the palm with inability to extend the fingers until wrist flexion is greater than 70° can be candidates for multiple tendon releases in the forearm. These patients usually have poor functional potential, inadequate sensibility, and do not demonstrate voluntary grasp and release patterns. This type of release is appropriate for severe cases of flexion contracture of the digits and wrist to allow the patient to get the fingers permanently out of the palm for cosmetic and hygienic reasons. The surgery consists of step-cut lengthening of the tendons or, as we prefer now, a transfer of the cut ends of the sublimis to the profundus tendons.[4]

The surgical procedure is carried out at the distal forearm; the sublimis tendons are cut distally and the profundus tendons proximally. The proximal ends of the sectioned sublimis tendons are approximated to the distal ends of the sectioned profundi tendons at the correct tension as the fingers and wrist are in the neutral position. The fingers and wrist are immobilized in extension in a long arm cast for approximately six weeks.

The rehabilitation program should include physical and occupational therapy in an attempt to obtain useful functional adaptations to use the hand as an assistive hand. Night-time splinting to maintain extension should be continued for many months until the balance of extensors and flexors are stabilized.

Intrinsic muscle tightness may become more obvi-

ous when the long finger flexors are released. Swanneck deformities may become severe. We have done the sublimis tenodesis procedure at the proximal interphalangeal joint to correct this problem. Intrinsic muscle release procedures could be appropriate if a severe intrinsic plus deformity occurs. This has not been necessary in our cases. Selective preoperative local anesthetic blocks of the ulnar nerve at the wrist can assist in predicting the postoperative condition and should be used.

Thumb-in-Palm Deformity

The thumb-in-palm deformity in cerebral palsy can be most disabling by further interfering with already handicapped pinch and grasp patterns of the hand. This deformity has several components and the treatment must consider each factor contributing to the disability. As the patient flexes his fingers, the thumb may be drawn across the palm in the adducted position, or the metacarpal may be adducted and contracted with a tendency for hyperextension deformity of the metacarpophalangeal joint. The goal of the treatment is to achieve an adequate active abduction of the thumb. Pulp pinch can seldom be obtained in the reconstruction of these thumbs; however, lateral or key pinch can be adequately restored and is probably more useful to these patients.

The first step in the treatment of this deformity as of any other cerebral deformity should be the application of conservative methods and bracing. When the patient presents a contracture or moderate spasticity of the intrinsic muscles, the origin of the adductor pollicis and the flexor pollicis brevis are released from the third metacarpal.[13] [17] [29] If active abduction of the thumb is weak, it can be reinforced with a tendon transfer, using the brachioradialis or the flexor carpi radialis. If there is an extension deformity or instability of the metacarpophalangeal joint of the thumb, a capsulorrhaphy of this joint is done in children or an arthrodesis in later age groups. A flexion deformity of the distal phalanx of the thumb can be corrected by lengthening the flexor pollicis longus at its myotendinous junction or by reinforcing the extensor pollicis brevis. The intermetacarpal bone-block procedure has been avoided for the treatment of the thumb-in-palm deformity in our clinic because the fixed post cannot provide accurate pinch to the fingers of an uncoordinated cerebral palsy hand. Among other drawbacks, it also is a problem for the hand of a patient who requires crutches for walking.

Thumb Intrinsic Muscles Origin Release

Release of the intrinsic muscle origin is performed through a palmar incision paralleling the thenar crease (Fig. 9.6.4). The arteries and nerves in the area are identified and carefully retracted. The transverse and oblique heads of the adductor pollicis are identified and their origin released. Blunt dissection by pulling the muscle fibers from the bone with forceps works well. The deep ulnar motor branch to the interosseous muscles is preserved. The motor branch of the median nerve to the thenar muscles is identified and carefully avoided. Both heads of the flexor pollicis brevis, opponens pollicis, and the distal two-thirds of the abductor pollicis brevis muscles may also be sectioned at their origins to the volar carpal ligament and recessed distally. This is usually not necessary. The attachment of the first dorsal interosseous to the first metacarpal may also be released in the depths of the wound after adequate retraction of the released muscles; however, this has usually not been found necessary. Care is taken to avoid the perforating branch of the radial artery. The wound is closed and subcutaneous drains are inserted. A bulky conforming dressing and a plaster cast are applied with the first metacarpal widely abducted. It is important to make sure that the metacarpal and not the phalanges of the thumb are abducted. A Kirschner wire can be passed between the first and second metacarpals for temporary fixation in severe cases.

Capsulorrhaphy of the Metacarpophalangeal Joint

Capsulorrhaphy of the metacarpophalangeal joint of the thumb can be done successfully in children who have hyperextension deformity of this joint. The palmar aspect of the joint is approached through a lateral incision. The proximal membranous insertions of the palmar plate are incised. The sesamoid bones and their tendinous attachments are left intact. The periosteum is stripped from the volar aspect of the neck of the metacarpal and two small drill holes made through the bone in a vertical direction are connected with a curette to form a cavity on the volar side. The dorsal aspect of the palmar plate is roughened and fixed into the bony depression with a pull-out wire suture exiting dorsally over a button. The suture is placed through the palmar plate flap as to obtain 10° to 15° of flexion

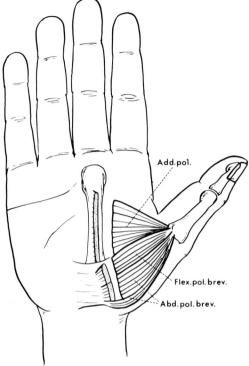

Figure 9.6.4. Release of the origin of the intrinsic muscles of the thumb for thumb-in-palm deformities involving spastic adduction of the metacarpal. The transverse head and a portion of the oblique head of the adductor pollicis are released at their origin. The flexor pollicis brevis and two-thirds of the abductor pollicis brevis may occasionally be released from the transverse carpal ligament. The attachment of the first dorsal interosseous to the first metacarpal may also be released if necessary. The motor branches of the ulnar and median nerve may be preserved.

of the metacarpophalangeal joint and a Kirschner wire is placed obliquely across the joint to hold the desired degree of flexion. The pull-out suture is removed in three weeks and the Kirschner wire in six weeks. This procedure has worked very well as a correction for hyperextension deformity if attention is paid to obtain bony union of the palmar plate to the metacarpal.

Fusion of the Metacarpophalangeal Joint

The metacarpophalangeal joint is fused in 10° of flexion, 10° of abduction, and slight pronation. A longitudinal wire is placed in a retrograde fashion across both the interphalangeal and the metacarpophalangeal joints and is left extruding 5 to 10 mm from the tip of the thumb. A second wire is inserted obliquely across the metacarpophalangeal joint to maintain the position desired. The fusion area is firmly compressed to assure good contact of the raw bone surfaces. The longitudinal wire is removed in six weeks, the oblique wire may be left in place.

Tendon Transfers for the Thumb

In patients presenting weak abduction and extension of the thumb, the abductor power can be reinforced with a tendon transfer. The common tendon transfers used for the thumb in cerebral palsy include the transfer of the flexor carpi radialis or the brachioradialis to the abductor pollicis longus, the extensor pollicis brevis or the extensor pollicis longus. We prefer using the brachioradialis for this transfer because it has good strength and, if well dissected proximally, it offers adequate amplitude of 3 to 4 cm.

Transfer of the brachioradialis muscle is performed using a dorsoradial incision starting at the elbow and exposing the full length of the musculotendinous unit (Fig. 9.6.5). The brachioradialis tendon is cut distally and the dissection is carried proximally to the origin of the muscle. Care must be taken to preserve the radial neurovascular unit and its branches to the brachioradialis muscle. A good release will allow a greater contractural excursion of the short belly muscle. The appropriate extensor compartment is incised longitudinally to allow either the extensor pollicis longus or brevis or the abductor pollicis to reroute in the line of pull of the abductors. The tendon of the brachioradialis is interwoven through the selected recipient tendon for the transfer. After carefully adjusting the tension, the transfer is firmly secured with multiple nonabsorbable sutures. We usually prefer the transfer to the extensor pollicis longus. The metacarpophalangeal joint must be stabilized by either fusion or capsulorrhaphy to prevent hyperextension tendencies. The wound is closed in layers and drains are placed subcutaneously. A voluminous conforming dressing and a full arm plaster cast are applied with the elbow at 90° of flexion, the wrist in neutral position, and the thumb widely abducted. After six weeks of immobilization, active use of the hand is resumed with special attention to abduction exercises.

Swan-neck Deformity of the Fingers

The swan-neck deformity in the cerebral palsied hand is common and has been studied using local anesthetic nerve blocks to determine the muscle group primarily causing the deformity. It has been stated in the literature that the swan-neck deformity is due to overactive intrinsics. In some cases it was noted that, when the intrinsics were paralyzed through a distal medial and ulnar block, the deformity disappeared. In other cases, anesthetizing the interosseous branch of the radial nerve was necessary to block the long extensor muscle action before the swan-neck deformity disappeared. It was felt that both extrinsic and intrinsic muscles contributed to the deformity. However, it appears that the main cause of the swan-neck deformity in the cerebral palsied hand is the result of a muscle imbalance caused by a chronic flexion of the wrist and the metacarpophalangeal joint and secondary ligamentous and capsular relaxation at the proximal interphalangeal joints.[14 16 26 27 29 30 31 34] The deformity is produced, basically, by the relative shortness of the middle extensor band, as compared with the lateral band. It is due to chronic tension from the long extensor muscle and the intrinsic muscles to the middle band. Stretching of the volar capsule and ligaments allows hyperextension of the proximal interphalangeal joint to occur. The distal interphalangeal and metacarpophalangeal joints go into flexion. The fingers frequently lock in extension, and the force of pinch and grasp is lost. Extension of the metacarpophalangeal joint is affected because of the loss of proximal interphalangeal joint flexion, and the patients are frequently concerned about the appearance of the affected hand. Once the digit goes into this swan-neck collapse deformity, surgical treatment is indicated.[27 29 32]

If the deformity is not too severe, the surgical treatment can be directed toward relief of the overloading forces on the extension side of the proximal interphalangeal joint by either lengthening the extensor communis tendon or by blocking its extension by

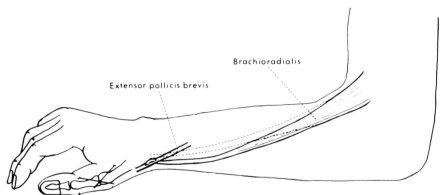

Brachioradialis

Extensor pollicis brevis

Figure 9.6.5. Transfer of the brachioradialis to the extensor pollicis brevis or longus or the abductor pollicis longus. Stabilization of the metacarpophalangeal joint of the thumb by either fusion or capsulorrhaphy is necessary to prevent hyperextension tendencies.

tenodesis at the proximal phalanx. Relocating the dorsally displaced lateral tendons palmarward toward the center of axis of rotation of the joint will improve the balance of the retinacular ligament system and to maintain the lateral tendons in this position may be important. Resection of the spiral or the oblique fibers of the extensor expansion from the intrinsics to the middle band may relieve some of the overloading of the medial band attachment. If the hyperextensibility of the proximal interphalangeal joint is too great, the deformity will recur. In these cases it is necessary to prevent hyperextension if the normal flexion arc of the finger is to be restored. The simplest and most effective procedure, in the flexible swan-neck deformity is to place the proximal interphalangeal joint in some initial flexion by palmar capsulorrhaphy of the proximal interphalangeal joint or preferably by the sublimis tenodesis procedure. The flexor sublimis tenodesis procedure, such as we have originally described, is a most useful technique to correct satisfactorily the swan-neck deformity of cerebral palsied hands.

Flexor Sublimis Tenodesis

Tenodesis of the sublimis tendon to the neck of the proximal phalanx creates a check-rein to hyperextension. Placing the proximal interphalangeal joint in 20° to 40° of flexion, depending upon the extent necessary to establish a functional flexor arch, re-establishes the position of the lateral tendons and the retinacular ligament and also allows the flexors to produce proximal interphalangeal joint flexion without further locking the joint in hyperextension. Correction of the hyperextension of the proximal interphalangeal joint also improves initial extension at the metacarpophalangeal joint. This procedure such as used in our clinic has successfully corrected the deformity and markedly improved the function of these hands for the past 18 years.

Through a midlateral incision, the flexor sheath is exposed at the proximal interphalangeal joint and incised longitudinally to expose the flexor tendons (Fig. 9.6.6). The palmar plate is partially resected at its

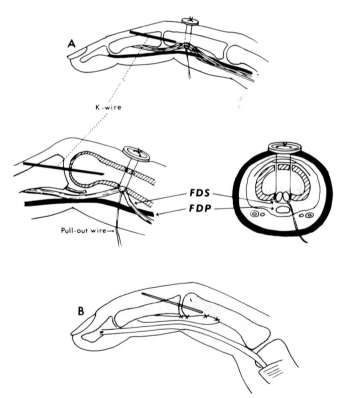

Figure 9.6.6 A. Sublimis tenodesis procedure to correct swan-neck deformities of the fingers. After placing two small drill holes through the neck of the proximal phalanx, a bed of raw-bone is prepared for firm attachment of the tendon. The sublimis is pulled up well into the bone with a pull-out type suture left in place for four to five weeks. The proximal interphalangeal joint is immobilized in 20° to 40° of flexion with a Kirschner wire for a period of six to eight weeks or longer if necessary.

Figure 9.6.6 B. Alternative method of tenodesis of the sublimis tendon stump which can be done when the sublimis tendon is used for tendon transfers in the cerebral palsy hand.

proximal portion so that it will not interfere with the tenodesis. It should be noted that tenodesis of the flexor digitorum sublimis at this level will not interfere with the action of the flexor digitorum profundus. In this procedure, it is important to obtain good healing between the tendon and the bone to avoid recurrences of the deformity. Two small drill holes are placed approximately one quarter of an inch apart through the palmar aspect of the neck of the proximal phalanx and connected with a curette. This will prepare a broad, bony bed for the attachment of the sublimis tendon. The end of the sublimis tendon is well scarified and drawn up into the bone with a Bunnell type pull-out suture.[3] The tension of the tenodesis should be adjusted as to allow 20° to 40° of extension lag at the proximal interphalangeal joint. A small Kirschner wire is inserted across the proximal interphalangeal joint to maintain the desired degree of flexion throughout the healing period. The end of the wire is cut immediately under the skin.

The deep structures including the retinacular ligament are resutured with absorbable material. The skin is sutured and a small drain is inserted subcutaneously. A voluminous conforming dressing is applied. If a plaster cast is used, it should include the elbow to prevent its proximal migration that could produce a straightening effect at the proximal interphalangeal joints.

The pull-out wire is removed in four to five weeks and the Kirschner wire in six to eight weeks. Small aluminum splints may be taped on the fingers to hold the proximal interphalangeal joint in flexion if the Kirschner wire needs to be removed prematurely or if further immobilization is desired. It should be explained to the patient that the goal of the procedure is to obtain some degree of flexion contracture; otherwise the patient might misunderstand and make efforts to mobilize his fingers in extension. This procedure can be performed in conjunction with other reconstructive procedures in the cerebral palsied hand.

The sublimis tenodesis procedure has been performed on the hands of 70 patients in our clinic for the past 18 years. It has been used to control disabling hyperextension deformities of the proximal interphalangeal joint from residuals of cerebral palsy, poliomyelitis, and rheumatoid arthritis. A postoperative recurrence of the deformity was noted in four index fingers. These failures were due to inadequate fixation of the tendon to the bone and inadequate postoperative fixation of the joint. Proper application of the sublimis tenodesis procedure as described above should obviate these problems.

The flexor sublimis tenodesis procedure can restore the flexor arc of the digit by restricting extension to less than neutral position, preferably to 20° to 40° of flexion. Full flexion of the joint is possible from this position and therefore the procedure has definite advantages over arthrodesis of the joint. Restoration of flexion of the proximal interphalangeal joint also secondarily improves extension at the distal and metacarpophalangeal joints.

BRACING OF THE SPASTIC HAND

Flexor muscles should not be stretched by extending the finger joints, as this may be a major cause of hyperextension deformities of the proximal interphalangeal joints. The normal arches of the palm and fingers should be respected and maintained.

Myostatic contractures of the finger and wrist flexor muscles are best stretched by extending the wrist, not the fingers. The muscles should never be stretched at the expense of the joints.

A recommended night splint for a spastic hand is a modified pancake splint shaped of aluminum and covered with leather (Fig. 9.6.7).[29][32] It is built up under the palmar arch and the proximal interphalangeal joints. The thumb is held abducted and extended to stretch the intrinsic muscles and the long thumb flexor. Finger and wrist flexors are then stretched by dorsiflexing the wrist portion of the splint.

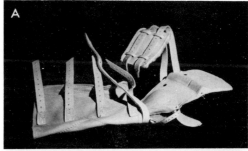

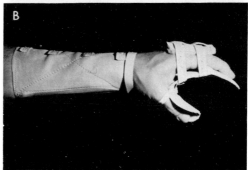

Figure 9.6.7. The pancake shaped night splint for stretching of flexion contractures in spastic hands. *A.* The splint is made of shaped aluminum and covered with leather. It allows stretching of the contracted wrist and fingers flexors at the same time, stabilizing and protecting the integrity of the finger joints and maintaining the arches of the palm and digits. Thumb is held in extension and abduction to stretch the intrinsic muscles and flexor pollicis longus. *B.* The brace can be bent at the wrist. Myostatic contractures of finger and wrist flexor muscles are best stretched by extending the wrist and not the fingers. Muscles should never be stretched at the expense of finger joints.

CONCLUSIONS

The results of operative procedures for cerebral palsy in the upper extremity are difficult to predict and reproduce. Careful preoperative and postoperative evaluations are especially important in these patients. A useful classification of results for the hand can be denoted by the following characteristics:

Excellent
Integrated digit function
Good grasp and release
Tip, lateral, pulp pinch
Good hand placement
Good control
Extension of fingers with
    wrist to $+30°$
Supination $\rangle45°$
Stable joints
Good sensibility
Good activities of daily
    living

Good
Good grasp and release
Lateral and pulp pinch
Good hand placement
Good control
Extension of fingers with
    wrist $0°$ to $+30°$
Supination $0°$ to $45°$
Stable joints
Good sensibility
Fair activities of daily
    living

Fair
Fair grasp and release
Lateral pinch
Fair hand placement
Fair control
Extension of fingers with
    wrist $-30°$ to $0°$
Supination to $0°$
Unstable joints
Helping hand
Fair sensibility
Poor activities of daily
    living

Poor
Hand, passive
Poor pinch, grasp, re-
    lease
Poor control
Poor hand placement
Extension of fingers with
    wrist $-30°$
No active supination
Unstable joints
Poor sensibility
No activities of daily liv-
    ing

Selected deformities in the upper extremity related to muscle imbalance, spasticity, contracture, and joint instability associated with cerebral palsy may be helped by certain surgical procedures here described. In the planning of the rehabilitation program it is most important to repeat carefully the preoperative evaluation record, the functional and anatomic disabilities, and define the functional and cosmetic potential, considering first the patient, then the extremity, and then the hand in that order. Existing functional adaptations must never be sacrificed. A continued rehabilitation program must be planned. The postoperative progress and results must be objectively evaluated. In spite of all these considerations, one cannot expect to gain a normal hand.

REFERENCES

1. Bechtol, C. O. Muscle physiology. In *Instructional Course Lectures,* The American Academy of Orthopaedic Surgeons, 1948, Vol 5. Ann Arbor, Edwards, 1948, pp. 181-189.

2. Boyd, I. A., Eyzaguirre, C., Matthews, P. B. C., and Rushworth, G. *The Role of the Gamma System in Movement and Posture.* Association for the Aid of Crippled Children, 1964, Library of Congress 64-15244.

3. Boyes, J. H. *Bunnell's Surgery of the Hand,* Ed. 4. Philadelphia, Lippincott, 1964.

4. Braun, R. M.: Personal communication.

5. Braun, R. M., Mooney, V., and Nickel, V. L. Flexor-origin release for pronation-flexion deformity of the forearm and hand in stroke patients. An evaluation of the early results in eighteen patients. J. Bone Joint Surg., *52A:* 907-920, 1970.

6. Denhoff, E., and Robinault, I. P. *Cerebral Palsy and Related Disorders: A Developmental Approach to Dysfunction.* New York, McGraw-Hill, 1960.

7. DeVries, J. S. *Encephalopathia Infantilis. A Study Based on Patients and Orthopaedic Procedures.* Asten, N. Br., Schrik's Durkkerij n.v., 1967.

8. Goldner, J. L. Reconstructive surgery of the hand in cerebral palsy and spastic paralysis resulting from injury to the spinal cord. J. Bone Joint Surg., *37A:* 1141-1154, 1955.

9. Gorynski, T., and Jedrzejewska, H. Chirurgiczne leczenie znieksztalcen i zaburzen czynnosciowych nadgarstka i palcow w porazeniah mozgowych. Chir. Narzad. Ruchu Ortop. Polska, *25:* 621-628, 1960.

10. Green, W. T., and Banks, H. H. Flexor carpi ulnaris transplant and its use in cerebral palsy. J. Bone Joint Surg., *44A:* 1343-1352, 1962.

11. Illingworth, R. S. *Recent Advances in Cerebral Palsy.* Boston, Little, Brown, 1958.

12. Inglis, A. E., and Cooper, W. Release of the flexor-pronator origin. J. Bone Joint Surg., *48A:* 847-857, 1966.

13. Inglis, A. E., Cooper, W., and Bruton, W. Surgical correction of thumb deformities in spastic paralysis. J. Bone Joint Surg., *52A:* 253-268, 1970.

14. Kaplan, E. B. *Functional and Surgical Anatomy of the Hand,* Ed. 2. Philadelphia, Lippincott, 1965.

15. Keats, S. *Operative Orthopaedics in Cerebral Palsy.* Springfield, C. C. Thomas, 1970.

16. Landsmeer, J. M. F. The anatomy of the dorsal aponeurosis of the human finger and its functional significance. Anat. Rec., *104:* 31-44, 1949.

17. Matev, I. Surgical treatment of spastic "thumb-in-palm" deformity. J. Bone Joint Surg., *45B:* 703-708, 1963.

18. Moberg, E. Objective methods for determining the functional value of sensibility in the hand. J. Bone Joint Surg., *40B:* 454-476, 1958.

19. Mooney, V., Frykham, G., and McLamb, J. Current status of intraneural phenol injections. Clin. Orthop., *63:* 122-131, 1969.

20. Page, C. M. An operation for the relief of flexion-contracture in the forearm. J. Bone Joint Surg., *5:* 233-234, 1923.

21. Perlstein, M. A. Infantile cerebral palsy. Classification and clinical correlations. J.A.M.A., *149:* 30-34, 1952.

22. Phelps, W. M. Long-term results of orthopaedic surgery in cerebral palsy. J. Bone Joint Surg., *39A:* 53-59, 1957.

23. Samilson, R. L., and Morris, J. M. Surgical improvement of the cerebral-palsied upper limb. J. Bone Joint Surg., *46A:* 1203, 1964.

24. Scaglietti, O. Sindromi Cliniche Immediate E Tardive Da Lesioni Vascolari Nelle Frature Degli Arti, Ar-

chivio "Putti," Di Chirurgia Degli Organi Di Movimento, Vol. VIII, 1957.

25. Steindler, A. Pathokinetics of cerebral palsy. In *Instructional Course Lectures*. The American Academy of Orthopaedic Surgeons, 1952, Vol. 9. Ann Arbor, Edwards, 1952, pp. 118-129.

26. Sunderland, S. The actions of the extensor digitorum communis, interosseous and lumbrical muscles. Am. J. Anat., *77:* 189-217, 1945.

27. Swanson, A. B. Surgery of the hand in cerebral palsy and the swan-neck deformity. J. Bone Joint Surg., *42A:* 951-964, 1960.

28. Swanson, A. B. Considerations for Surgery of the Hand in cerebral palsy. Acad. Med., N. J. Bull., *10:* 170-174, 1964.

29. Swanson, A. B. Surgery of the hand in cerebral palsy. Surg. Clin. North Am., *44:* 1061-1070, 1964.

30. Swanson, A. B. Pathomechanics of the swan-neck de-formity. In *Proceedings of the American Society for Surgery of the Hand*. J. Bone Joint Surg., *47A:* 636, 1965.

31. Swanson, A. B. Treatment of the swan-neck deformity in the cerebral palsied hand. Clin. Orthop., *48:* 167-171, 1966.

32. Swanson, A. B. Surgery of the hand in cerebral palsy and muscle release procedures Surg. Clin. North Am., *48:* 1129-1138, 1968.

33. Tachdjian, M. O., and Minear, W. L. Sensory disturbances in the hands of children with cerebral palsy. J. Bone Joint Surg., *40A:* 85-90, 1958.

34. Tubiana, R., and Valentin, P. The physiology of the extension of the fingers. Surg. Clin. North A., *44:* 907, 1964.

35. White, W. F. Flexor-muscle slide in the spastic hand. J. Bone Joint Surg., *54B:* 453-459, 1972.

chapter ten

Stenosing Tenosynovitis: Trigger Fingers and Trigger Thumb, DeQuervain's Disease, Acute Calcification in Wrist and Hand

George S. Phalen, M.D.

STENOSING TENOSYNOVITIS

The movement of a tendon within its sheath may become restricted by an enlargement of the tendon itself, by a swelling and thickening of the normally thin synovial covering of the tendon, or by a thickening of the fibrous sheath through which the tendon glides. Although stenosing tenosynovitis may develop in any location where a tendon passes through a sheath or an osteoligamentous tunnel, this condition is found almost exclusively in the hand and wrist.

Anatomic Features

The tendon sheath, with its synovial lining, reduces friction, the annular ligaments, formed from reinforcement of the deep fascia, provode retinacula or pulleys to hold tendon close to the bones over which they pass.

Because there is a wide range of motion in both flexion and extension of the wrist, retinacula are present on both the volar and dorsal aspects of this joint.

At the level of the first metacarpophalangeal joint, the tendon of the flexor pollicis longus passes through a channel formed by a groove in the palmar surface of the first metacarpal neck and the transverse fibers of the strong proximal annular ligament. There are usually two sesamoid bones in the capsule of the first metacarpophalangeal joint; into these sesamoids are inserted the tendon of the medial and lateral head of the flexor pollicis brevis. The flexor sheath is narrowest at the level of the sesamoids, and this is the place where the flexor tendon usually is constricted.

The anatomy of the fingers is much the same as that of the thumb, except for the variable appearance of the sesamoids. The tendons of the flexor profundus and flexor sublimus pass together through a narrow osteofibrous tunnel formed by a shallow groove in the palmar surface of the metacarpal neck covered by the thick transverse fibers of the annular ligament. This is where the finger flexors are usually constricted.

Etiology

Repetitive occupational trauma must certainly play some role in the production of stenosing tenosynovitis. When the annular ligament is pressed firmly for long periods by the handle of a pair of scissors, a screwdriver, or some other tool, the tendon gliding beneath the ligament may become irritated. This irritation produces exudation, with eventual thickening of the snovial covering of the tendons, thickening of the tendons themselves, or thickening of the flexor tendon sheath, and interference with the free gliding movement of the tendons.

The most common cause of stenosing tenosynovitis is a chronic inflammation of the synovial sheath about the tendon; this inflammation is of a rheumatoid nature. Patients with true rheumatoid arthritis frquent ly have trigger fingers, too.

In reports of large series of cases of trigger fingers, the right hand is more often involved than the left, and this would give support to the theory that trauma is the primary etiologic factor in the production of trigger fingers. The increased incidence in women, however, cannot be explained on a traumatic basis. The frequent prompt therapeutic response to the local injection of steroid preparations also lends credence to the rheumatic origin of stenosing tenosynovitis. Weilby[12] has recently reviewed trigger fingers in children and adults and presents the possibility of predisposition in certain age groups.

Stenosing tenosynovitis of the flexor pollicis longus may be present at birth or may develop in early infancy. In infancy, however, a trigger thumb may bear some relation to the congenital clasped thumb.

Pathology

In stenosing tenosynovitis the inflammation occurs principally in the synovial covering of the tendon. The tendon sheath itself is often thickened to several times its normal size. When the condition has existed for some time, the tendon itself may become constricted, or a bulbous swelling may develop in the tendon both distal and proximal to the stenosis. A serious effusion may often be present. Instead of its usual smooth, white, glistening appearance, the tendon may be a dull gray.

Diagnosis

With the onset of inflammatory changes about the flexor tendon and its sheath, pain develops along the course of the tendon, and this pain may be present with the finger at rest or in motion. The point of maximal tenderness is usually over the annular band at the base of the finger overlying the neck of the metacarpal, although there may be some tenderness all along the course of the tendon in the distal palm and finger.

As the inflammatory process progresses and the tendon becomes more constricted within the tendon sheath, pain increases and active motion in the digit decreases. The bulbous enlargement on the flexor tendons usually occurs distal to the annular band with the digit in complete extension. With forceful active flexor of the finger or thumb, this bulbous enlargement is dragged through the tendon sheath and then lies proximal to the annular band in the palm (Fig. 10.1). This motion is often accompanied by a painful snap, and the digit is then locked in flexion. The flexor tendons are much stronger than the extensor tendons, so the patient is often unable to extend the digit actively and must grasp the locked digit with his opposite hand and passively straighten the finger or thumb to the accompaniment of another painful snap as the bulbous enlargement on the tendon is drawn back through the stenotic tendon sheath.

Although the local tenderness is along the midline on the palmar aspect of the metacarpophalangeal

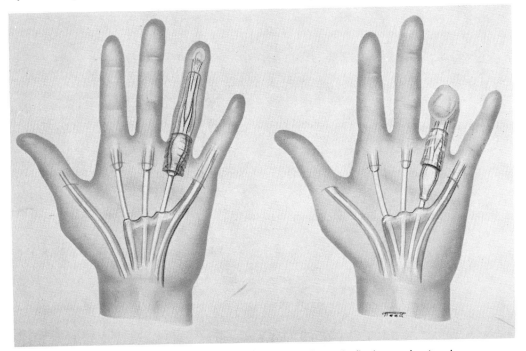

Figure 10.1. Diagram of palm, showing trigger finger in flexion and extension

joint, the snapping motion in the digit is at the proximal interphalangeal joint and often the pain is referred to this joint.

Rarely the finger or thumb may be locked in extension. This locking either is caused by so great an enlargement on the tendon that it cannot be forced through the tendon sheath, or the sheath itself may be so stenotic that the normal tendon can no longer pass through it.

When the trigger finger is locked in flexion, the patient frequently will not want to extend the finger again because of the pain that will surely occur when the finger snaps back into extension. Often the examiner or the patient may avoid this painful snap by carefully extending only the distal phalanx of the finger before extending the proximal interphalangeal joint. By moving the distal phalanx into extension, the flexor profundus tendon alone is moved, altering the relative position of the flexor sublimus and flexor profundus tendons. This alteration in position of the two tendons may be sufficient to reduce the size of the localized swelling of the tendons and to permit both tendons to be drawn through the flexor sheath without a painful snap.

Occasionally the trigger phenomenon may occur only in the morning and will disappear as the hand is used during the day. With inactivity, edema develops about the flexor tendon, and this edema is disseminated by activity, permitting the tendon to glide easily again through the tendon sheath. Symptoms may also become attentuated with time, especially if the snapping is caused largely by swelling of the tendon or edema of the vaginal covering of the tendon and not to excessive thickening of the annular band. Pressure of the examiner's finger over the annular band may occasionally produce a trigger phenomenon with a painful snap that is not present otherwise. Not all cases of stenosing tenosynovitis have a typical trigger phenomenon.

The trigger thumb in infancy presents a typical clinical picture. The condition is usually bilateral and often passes unnoticed for the first few months of life. Then the mother notices that the distal phalanx of the infant's thumb is kept constantly flexed, and when any attempt is made to extend the distal phalanx of the thumb the baby cries. The distal phalanx of the thumb may then remain extended for a long period, since any attempt at flexion of the interphalangeal joint will be accompanied by some pain. A bulbous enlargement on the flexor pollicis longus tendon may often be palpated in the region of the first metacarpal head.

Treatment

Conservative (nonoperative) treatment will cure at least 50 per cent of the patients with trigger fingers or tringer thumbs. Spontaneous recovery may occur in some patients without any treatment. If symptoms have been present for less than six weeks, immobilization of the finger or thumb for from seven to 10 days will often bring complete relief. The splint need be only long enough to span the proximal interphalangeal joint, since restricting the motion in this joint will prevent the trigger phenomenon. By placing the splint on the dorsal aspect of the digit, the tactile surface of the tip of the digit may be left uncovered so that pinch between the thumb and fingers may be unimpaired. The splint should be removed two or three times daily to permit the patient to move the interphalangeal joints *passively* through a full range of motion. Care must be taken not to move the digit actively, since this might cause snapping of the flexor tendon.

If symptoms have been present for more than 6 weeks, or if the symptoms are extremely acute, one is justified in injecting a few drops (about 0.5 ml) of a long acting corticosteroid preparation, such as triamcinolone directly ito the flexor tendon sheath. This is done with a short 25-gauge needle. Preliminary procaine infiltration is usually not necessary. The needle is plunged directly into the flexor tendon at the base of the digit and then is withdrawn slowly until the injection meets with little resistance, indicating that the end of the needle lies within the flexor tendon sheath. At times, the physician may actually palpate the material as it spreads along the flexor tendon. Immediately after the injection, the area is massaged to disseminate further the injected material, and the digit is passively flexed and extended. A finger splint is then applied and is worn for one week.

If symptoms persist after injection treatment, then surgical measures are indicated. The annular band at the base of the finger or thumb is exposed through a short transverse incision about 1 cm long. Care must be taken not to traumatize the proper digital nerves. The thickened annular band is incised longitudinally, and occasionally a longitudinal segment of the sheath may be removed if it appears that the flexor tendons are especially thickened. After the annular band has been exposed, it is easy to cut through the band in a longitudinal direction, carrying the incision through the entire flexor sheath proximally and extending the incision distally for a distance sufficient to permit the thickened flexor tendons to move freely back and forth without snapping. The surgical wound is closed by suturing only the skin.

It is imperative that the operation be performed under local anesthesia so that, after section of the annular band, the patient may actively move the involved tendons and prove both to himself and to the surgeon that the trigger phenomenon is no longer present. A pneumatic tourniquet may be left on for from 10 to 15 min. without undue discomfort. The surgeon must remember, however, that the forearm and hand are ischemic, and the patient will not be able to flex and to extend the involved digit more than two or three times without a resultant painful cramp in the flexor muscles. Active flexion and extension of all the fingers is encouraged after release of the tourniquet, and the patient can certainly tell at this time whether or not the triggering has been relieved. Upon complete extension of the digit, if there should still be some snapping present the flexor sheath must be opened more widely, and this usually is in a distal direction. Passing a flexible probe down the sheath alongside of the tendon may be helpful in determining whether or not the entire annular band has been severed. This is useful especially in children with trigger thumbs, since one obviously cannot employ local anesthesia in the very young child.

Kolind-Sorensen[5] has recently reviewed his results in the treatment of trigger finger with hydrocortisone, used topically and with intrathecal injections, and surgery. His results are comparable to ours.

DeQUERVAIN'S DISEASE

In 1895, the Swiss surgeon, Fritz DeQuervain,[3] described a form of tendovaginitis involving the abductor pollicis longus and the extensor pollicis brevis tendons in the region of the radial styloid. The same condition was termed ''washer-woman's sprain'' in the 13th edition of Gray's *Antomy* in 1893. Despite the fact that deQuervain was not the first to describe this particular syndrome of stenosing tenosynovitis, his name has become permanently associated with this clinical entity.

Anatomic features

On the dorsal aspect of the wrist are the tendons of nine muscles — three for the thunb, three for the fingers, and three for the wrist. Overlying these tendons is a band of thickened deep fascia, called the extensor retinculum or dorsal carpal ligament, which forms the roof of six separate compartments or tunnels through which the extensor tendons pass. The first of these compartments lies over the radial styloid and contains the tendons of the abductor pollicis longus and the extensor pollicis brevis (Fig. 10.2). There is a shallow groove over the radial styloid, which forms the floor of the unyielding osteoligamentous tunnel or first dorsal compartment of the wrist. The tough tranverse fibers of the dorsal carpal ligament are about 1 mm thick and 2 cm wide. Around the two thumb tendons

within this first dorsal compartment is a synovial sheath that extends for a short distance both proximally and distally to the dorsal carpal ligament.

The two thumb tendons are subject to direct trauma in the region of the first dorsal compartment. There is also a high degree of angulation of these tendons as they pass from the level of the radial styloid to the thumb, which is increased with abduction of the thumb and radial deviation of the hand. The degree of angulation is usually greater in women than in men, and Bunnell[1] has suggested that this may account for the preponderance of deQuervain's disease in women.

The extensor pollicis brevis is often a slender tendon, and is absent in at least 5 per cent of all persons. The abductor pollicis longus usually does not have a unified tendon; this tendon is composed of from two to six separate fasciculi, with one bundle inserting at the base of the first metacarpal and others passing to the greater multangular, the abductor pollicis brevis, the opponens pollicis, the volar carpal ligament, and the scaphoid.

The extensor pollicis brevis may have its own separate sheath, and the abductor pollicis longus may have two separate sheaths. Strandell[11] described two cases with a slender fasciculus of the abductor pollicis longus embedded in the wall of the main compartment beneath the abductor tendon.

For a powerful grasp, the first metacarpal must be strongly stabilized in abduction at the carpometacarpal joint; this is a function performed mainly by the abductor pollicis longus.

Etiology

DeQuervain's disease may be caused by any condition that produces a swelling or a thickening of the tendons themselves, or a change in the contour or a decrease in the diameter of the first dorsal compartment of the wrist. Repetitive occupational trauma seems to be the most logical and most frequent etiologic agent. The sheath itself may become irritated and thickened, thus further narrowing the diameter of

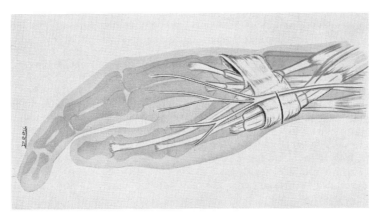

Figure 10.2. Diagram of wrist, showing first dorsal compartments, and line of recommended incision to open first compartment. This incision crosses over the radial nerve, and care must be taken to avoid injury to this structure.

the compartment through which the tendons must glide. If occupational trauma were the primary cause of deQuervain's disease, the condition would be more common in men than in women. It is widely accepted that deQuervain's disease occurs from 8 to 10 times more often in women than in men.

Occasionally deQuervain's disease may develop after a direct blow to the medial aspect of the radial styloid.

Certainly the most common cause of deQuervain's disease is a chronic inflammation of the sheath that covers the long abductor and the short extensor tendons. Such a chronic tenosynovitis is more apt to be produced by a rheumatic process than by trauma.

The majority of cases of deQuervain's disease, trigger finger, trigger thumb, and the carpal tunnel syndrome all have a similar fundamental cause — a chronic, nonspecific tenosynovitis. In one of the first published cases of carpal tunnel syndrome the patient had an associated deQuervain's disease, and in another, the patient had two trigger fingers. The coexistence of these various disorders, as well as tennis elbow, periarthritis of the shoulder, and calcific tendinitis, is all too frequent to deny that there must be some etiologic relationship. Furthermore, deQuervain's disease, trigger digit, and the carpal tunnel syndrome are almost all cured either by local injection of a steroid or by simple sectioning of the overlying fibrous retinaculum.

Diagnosis

DeQuervain's disease has often been misdiagnosed as arthritis, periostitis, neuralgia, causalgia, or a psychosomatic disorder.

Usually the patient with deQuervain's disease is a woman. Pain is the predominant symptom and may be acute or gradual in onset. In only rare instances is there a history of a single initiating traumatic episode. Pain is usually localized to the region of the radial styloid, but often radiates up the radial side of the forearm to the shoulder and down to the thumb. The pain is worse with any active use of the hand, especially any forceful grasping or pinching; wringing out a cloth or opening a jar may be impossible because of pain. Rest does not relieve the pain completely. Usually the condition is unilateral.

On examination there is often slight thickening and swelling over the radial styloid. The point of maximal tenderness is usually immediately over the radial styloid, but there may be some tenderness all along the course of the long abductor tendon and muscle. Pain is also increased by extending and abducting the thumb against resistance, with the wrist completely extended or completely flexed, or with the hand deviated ulnarward. A test, described by Finkelstein,[4] is almost always positive — a stabbing intense pain is elicited along the course of the long abductor of the thumb when the patient clasps the fingers tightly over the thumb and then flexes the wrist sharply into ulnar deviation. This maneuver, which places an unusual amount of stretch on the long abductor muscle, will produce some pain in the normal person, but in a patient with deQuervain's disease, it will produce severe pain.

Occasionally one may palpate a small ganglion lying adjacent to the edge of the first dorsal compartment.

Roentgenograms of the wrist and hand show nothing abnormal except for the rare case with evidence of some periosteal reaction at the radial styloid (Piver and Raney[9]).

Treatment

A patient with deQuervain's disease may recover spontaneously without treatment, but when the symptoms have been present for several weeks, recovery is unlikely without some local treatment. The injection of 0.5 ml of a long acting corticosteroid into the first dorsal compartment will cure at least 50 per cent of the patients. This injection is carried out as described under the treatment of trigger digits. Usually one injects 2 or 3 ml of procaine hydrochloride first to minimize the pain of injecting the steroid through the dorsal retinaculum and about the long abductor and short extensor tendons of the thumb. No more than two injections at an interval of from 7 to 10 days is advised. If two injections do not give permanent relief, then surgical treatment is indicated.

The first dorsal compartment is exposed through a 3-cm transverse incision overlying the radial styloid. Care must be taken to avoid all branches of the radial nerve. The transverse incision is recommended because it follows the skin creases and heals without an objectionable scar. A longitudinal incision is made through the entire length of the dorsal carpal ligament, exposing the tendons in the first dorsal compartment (Fig. 10.3A). These tendons may show some constriction within the compartment and some thickening proximal to the dorsal carpal ligament (Fig. 10.3B). The tendons are carefully lifted from the compartment to be sure there is not an additional tendon in a separate sheath. If the short extensor tendon of the thumb does not lie together with the long abductor tendon, a search should be made for the extra compartment or tunnel through which the extensor tendon will pass, and this compartment should also be opened. The fibrous partition between the two compartments should be excised.

Just as in the case of trigger digits, the operation is performed under local anesthesia with a pneumatic tourniquet to produce a bloodless field, and before the wound is closed, the patient is asked to move the wrist and thumb to prove that the former pain at the radial styloid is no longer present.

Postoperatively a light compression pressure dressing is applied, incorporating a splint to hold the wrist in neutral position. On the third postoperative day, this dressing is replaced by a small dry dressing, but the wrist splint is worn for one week, to promote prompt healing of the wound.

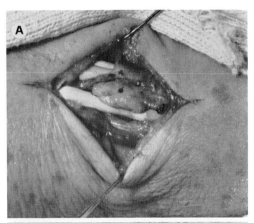

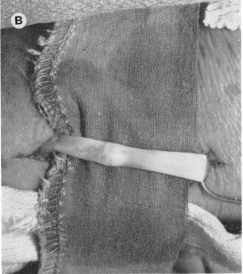

Figure 10.3 A DeQuervain's disease at operation. *B.* Long abductor tendon removed from sheath to demonstrate area of compression in the tendon.

The surgical treatment of stenosing tenosynovitis is perhaps the most simple and certainly the most gratifying surgery that the physician may perform. He may assure his patients preoperatively that they will have almost a 100 per cent chance of being relieved of their symptoms.

It has been recommended by Rais[10] of Sweden that daily intravenous injections of 150 mg of heparin be given to patients with deQuervain's disease. It is possible that such treatment might hasten the resolution of an acute tenosynovitis, but it would not enlarge the diameter of a first dorsal compartment stenosed by a greatly thickened dorsal carpal ligament.

ACUTE CALCIFICATION IN THE WRIST AND HAND

Calcific tendinitis may involve the wrist and hand, as well as the shoulder, elbow, hip, and knee. The clinical course and treatment of acute calcification in the wrist and hand is similar to an acute "calcified bursitis" of the shoulder. More than 200 cases of acute calcium deposits in the hand have now been published in the literature. That this condition is not a rarity is well attested to by Carroll's series[2] of 100 cases treated in only a few years.

Etiology

No one has as yet explained the exact pathogenesis of calcium deposition in soft tissues. Calcium salts are often deposited in diseased tissues such as tendons, bursas, lipomas, fibroids, or tuberculous glands. It is believed that there must first be an area of necrotic tissue, produced by injury or disease, into which the calcium salts may be deposited directly or through the intermediary of a soap or fatty acid. In calcific tendinitis, one may presuppose that there has been some minor trauma to the tendon, causing a tear in some of the tendon fibers and producing a zone of decreased vascularity into which the calcium salts are precipitated.

Local accumulations of calcium salts are not dependent on a generalized hypercalcemia. One may safely assume that serum calcium and serum phosphorus levels will be well within normal limits in patients with calcific tendinitis.

The simple presence of calcium within a tendon does not mean that there is pain at this site. The same cannot be said for calcific tendinitis in the hand, since the presence of a calcium deposit in the wrist, palm, or fingers is usually accompanied by considerable pain.

Calcific tendinitis in the hand is not a disease of the very young or the very old. Most of the cases reported are in the age group of from 30 to 60 years. Women have this condition a little more often than men.

No one has yet explained the mechanism of the severe inflammatory reaction accompanying an acute calcific tendinitis. The local inflammatory response associated with an acute calcific tendinitis in the hand seems out of proportion to the amount and the location of the calcium deposit.

Pathology

The calcium deposit is usually within the substance of the tendon. In cases of acute calcific tendinitis, the calcium is under tension and the local tissues are inflamed and edematous. Because few cases of calcific tendinitis in the hand require surgical treatment, little pathologic material has been available for study. In a single case of so-called "calcified pisiform bursitis"[8] (a deposit of calcium within the flexor carpi ulnaris tendon near its insertion into the pisiform bone) (Fig. 10.4), the microscopic examination of tissue removed at the time of surgery revealed focal areas of degeneration in fibrous tissue with irregular areas of amorphous calcified material. One of these foci of degeneration and calcification presented a peripheral zone of increased cellularity somewhat resembling a rheumatoid nodule, but without true palisading of the cellular elements (Fig. 10.5), and without inflammatory cells.

Diagnosis

Acute calcification in the wrist and hand always manifests itself by the sudden onset of severe pain, well localized over the tendon or ligament containing the calcium deposit. The entire hand and wrist may be

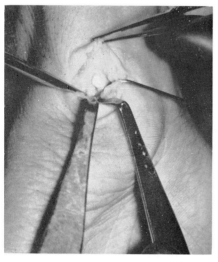

Figure 10.4. Operative appearance of calcification in flexor carpi ulnaris tendon.

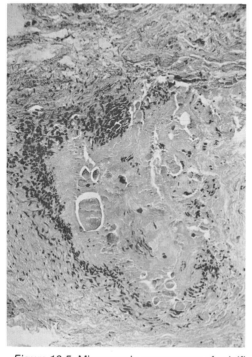

Figure 10.5. Microscopic appearance of calcification; × 70.

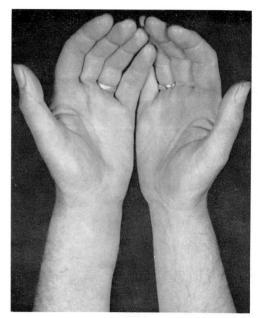

Figure 10.6. Photograph of hands and wrist of a 30-year-old woman with acute pisiform bursitis, left. There was swelling, redness, increased warmth, and marked tenderness along the ulnar side of the wrist and forearm.

swollen (Fig. 10.11), and there frequently is redness and increased warmth in the region of the calcification. The patent has no fever and no sign of toxemia, but the redness and swelling often extends proximally up the forearm with an appearance similar to an acute cellulitis and lymphangitis. There is no local lymphadenopathy (Fig. 10.6).

The disability is great: the hand is rendered practically useless by the intensity of the pain and by the aggravation of the pain with any movement. A careful, gentle examination of the hand and wrist will reveal one region of maximal tenderness that must be shown well on roentgenograms. The usual anteroposterior and lateral views may show nothing abnormal, and it is only on oblique views taken in midsupination or midpronation that evidence of the calcific deposit is demonstrated (Fig. 10.7). The intensity of the symptoms and the degree of redness and swelling seem to bear no direct relationship to the size of the calcium deposit. A small amount of calcium may be accompanied by a severe soft tissue reaction (Fig. 10.10).

In the fingers and thumb, the calcium deposits are usually found in the supporting ligaments, whereas in the palm the intrinsic musculature is involved. At the wrist, any of the flexor or extensor tendons may contain a deposit of calcium. The most common site is in the tendon of the flexor carpi ulnaris near its insertion into the pisiform bone. The deposit there is usually small and is readily overlooked in routine roentgenograms; a view of the wrist in midsupination will throw the pisiform bone into relief and readily will demonstrate even the smallest bit of calcium adjacent to this bone (Fig. 10.7).

There is usually only one site of calcification, but occasionally there may be a deposit both at the wrist or on the dorsum of the hand, as well as another deposit in the digits (Figs. 10.8 and 10.9). The calcification may spread out for some distance along the involved tendon, especially when the symptoms subside and the calcium is being absorbed.

There has been one case of compression of the median nerve produced by a massive deposit of calcium in the flexor tendons within the carpal tunnel; this was a true carpal tunnel syndrome (Fig. 10.12).

Treatment

The treatment of calcified tendinitis in the wrist and hand is essentially the same as the treatment of any calcified bursitis or tendinitis elsewhere in the body. Spontaneous recovery may occur without treatment. Splinting the wrist in neutral position may hasten recovery by reducing painful motion in the involved tendon.

Surgical treatment should be reserved for those patients who do not respond to conservative measures. Every patient deserves at least one attempt to disseminate the calcium deposit by injection of a local anesthetic. A 1 per cent solution of procaine hy-

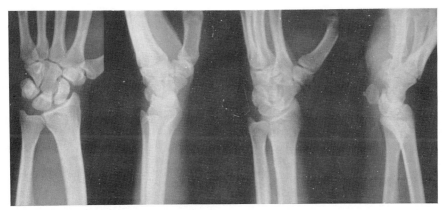

Figure 10.7. Four roentgenograms of wrist — anteroposterior view, lateral view, semipronation view, and semisupination view (*left* to *right*). A small, dense calicification adjacent to pisiform bone is visable only in the semisupination view.

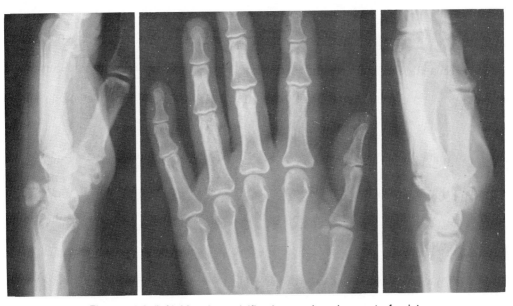

Figure 10.8 (left) Massive calcification on dorsal aspect of wrist.

Figure 10.9 (right). Appearance of wrist one month later.

drochloride, or any similar anesthetic agent, when injected into the calcium deposit, will give immediate relief from the acute pain, and all soreness will usually disappear within the next few days. If the calcium deposit is unusually large, calcific material may be aspirated, and when this occurs, the physician may feel confident that there will be prompt subsidence of symptoms. As a rule, however, the volume of the calcium deposit is small, and it is necessary to make multiple punctures with the injecting needle to be sure that the calcium deposit has been entered. In the fingers

and palm, a short 25-gauge needle and about 1 ml of local anesthetic will suffice, while in the wrist a 22-gauge needle and 2 or 3 ml of local anesthetic will be needed, especially if one anticipates the possibility of aspirating some of the calcific deposit. When injecting the flexor carpi ulnaris tendon at the wrist, care must be taken not to traumatize the ulnar nerve and vessels.

Since the advent of the corticosteroids, it has been customary to add a few drops of hydrocortisone or a similar compound to the local anesthetic that is used in the injection of a calcium deposit. It is doubtful that the addition of the hydrocortisone really increases the

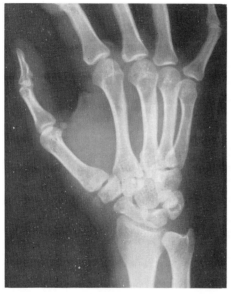

Figure 10.10. Massive calcification on dorsal aspect of wrist.

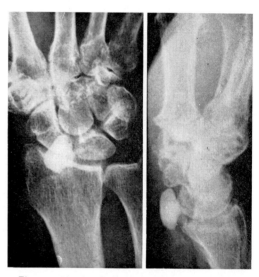

Figure 10.12. Carpal tunnel syndrome produced by large calcification in flexor tendons at wrist. (Case of J. R. Stacy, M.D.)

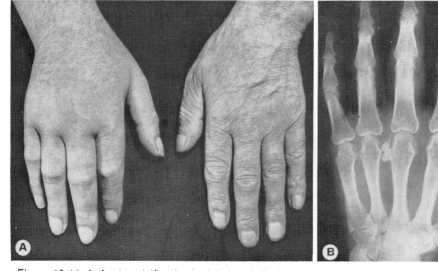

Figure 10.11. A. Acute calcification in right hand of a 60-year-old man; marked tenderness present in the third web. *B.* Roentgenogram of hand, showing calcification in third web.

efficacy of the injection. It is not advisable to use large amounts of hydrocortisone in the hand or wrist, since this material is slowly absorbed and may even act as a mechanical block to normal function. The relief of symptoms after injection of the calcium deposit is believed to be due to the release of tension within the deposit and the dissemination and absorption of the calcium salts. The addition of hydrocortisone to the injected fluid may reduce the local edema and hasten the absorption of the calcium.

Roentgentherapy is also an effective means of treating acute calcium deposits in the hand and wrist. It is entirely possible that patients who immediately respond satisfactorily to treatment by local infiltration might react equally well to roentgentherapy, although recovery probably would be more prolonged. There is no immediate relief from pain with roentgentherapy, but recovery is hastened by its use. In a series of 13 cases of calcified pisiform bursitis (calcific tendinitis of flexor carpi ulnaris), only roentgentherapy was used with an exposure of 200 r on three alternate days; all these patients had prompt relief within 24 hours.

Physical therapy, such as diathermy, whirlpool baths, paraffin baths, and warm soaks may be employed in the treatment of calcium deposits in the wrist and hand. Such treatment may be helpful in promoting a rapid absorption of the calcium.

If the symptoms of calcific tendinitis have been of long duration — one month or longer — and the calcification appears quite dense on roentgenographic examination, it is quite likely that local infiltration will not be effective in relieving the patient's symptoms. Such cases are rare, but these patients will require surgical excision of the calcium deposit.

REFERENCES

1. Bunnell, S. *Surgery of the Hand,* Ed. 3. Philadelphia, Lippincott, 1956, 1079 p.
2. Carroll, R. E., Sinton, W., and Garcia, A. Acute calcium deposits in the hand. J. A. M. A., *157:* 422-426, 1955.
3. De Quervain, F. Ueber eine Form von chronischer Tendovaginitis. Cor. -Bl. f. schweiz Aerzte, Basel, *25:* 389-394, 1895.
4. Finkelstein, H. Stenosing tenovaginitis at the radial styloid process. J. Bone Joint Surg., *12:* 509-540, 1930.
5. Kolind-Sorensen, V. Treatment of trigger fingers. Acta Orthop. Scand., *41:* 428 - 432, 1970.
6. Leonard M. H., *et al,* Electromyography in surgery of the hand. Electromyography, *10:* 239 - 52, 1970.
7. Onkelix, A. Paresthesias of fingers. J. Belge Rhumatol. Med. Phys., *25:* 53 - 58, 1970.
8. Phalen, G. S. Calcification adjacent to the pisiform bone. J. Bone Joint Surg., *34A:* 579 - 583, 1952.
9. Piver, J. D., and Raney, R. B. De Quervain's tendovaginitis. Am. J. Surg., *83:* 691 - 694, 1952.
10. Rais, O. Heparin treatment of peritenomyosis (peritendinitis) crepitans acuta. Acta Chir. Scand. Suppl., *268:* 1 - 88, 1961.
11. Strandell, G. Variations of the anatomy in stenosing tenosynovitis at radial styloid process. Acta Chir. Scand., *113:* 234 - 240, 1957.
12. Weilby, A. Trigger finger incidence in children and adults and the possibilities of a predisposition in creatain age groups. Acta. Orthop. Scand., *41:* 419 - 427, 1970.

chapter eleven

Amputations

A.

Upper Extremity Amputation

Stanley L. James, M.D.
Donald B. Slocum, M.D.

Amputations of the upper extremity, whether traumatic or elective, must be approached with a sound knowledge of upper extremity function and a program of planned reconstruction clearly in mind. The primary function of the hand is prehension, which can be conveniently categorized into digital pinch and palmar grasp. Digital pinch occurs with the thumb in opposition and opposed to one or more of the fingertips while performing one of the many variations of pinch. The most essential element for digital pinch is a mobile, normal, or reconstructed thumb capable of opposing the fingers. Palmar grasp differs in that the fingers and thumb firmly clasp an object, pressing it securely into the palm of the hand, such as when grasping a hammer. Amputation in the hand should be performed with the preservation of prehension in some form as the eventual goal. The "basic hand" to perform prehension requires durable skin coverage with sensibility, a mobile radial digit capable of contacting other elements of the hand, and at least one stable ulnar digit within reach of the radial digit.

The musculoskeletal components provide a combination of stability and mobility for upper extremity function. In the hand the skeleton forms two transverse arches and one longitudinal arch system. The proximal transverse arch is rigid and is formed by the distal carpal row. The distal, more mobile, transverse arch is formed by the metacarpal heads joined to each other by the transverse metacarpal ligament. Each finger constitutes a longitudinal arch system with a more stable proximal metacarpal segment and a mobile, articulated, phalangeal distal segment. The metacarpophalangeal joint is the keystone of the distal transverse arch system. In amputations of the hand, the function of each skeletal segment must be thoroughly considered in the terms of final function.

Preservation of sensibility, whether it be in the stump of an amputated digit or a more proximal upper extremity stump, is of utmost importance. Sensation in the hand has attained an extremely high degree of

refinement, and the hand may actually be considered a sense organ. It feeds back information from the environment to the central nervous system, relating to tactile sensation, stereognosis, and position sense, which is interpreted, and appropriate motor activity initiated. The thumb, index, and long finger are considered primary digits for exploration. Sensibility reaches its highest degree of refinement in the thumb and finger pads, and their loss through amputation seriously hampers upper extremity function.

Upper extremity prosthetic replacement is less satisfactory than in the lower extremity, and this is not a surprising fact when one considers that function in the upper extremity is a highly refined system of sensory feed-back integrated with complex motor skills. Prosthetic devices at the present state of development are unable to duplicate successfully such complex function. From a functional standpoint, the more proximal the amputation, the less satisfactory is prosthetic replacement. In bilateral amputations it is particularly beneficial to have one limb long enough to reach the buttocks and interscapular area.

Indications for amputation are trauma and its sequelae, congenital and acquired deformities, infection, tumors, and peripheral vascular disease. Amputation as a result of injury or its sequelae is the most common cause in the upper extremity. It is frequently helpful to consider the degree of involvement of the five major tissues (skin, nerves, vessels, tendons, and bone) when contemplating an amputation in the hand. If three of more of these structures have major involvement, an amputation may be indicated. Loss of blood supply is the only absolute indication for amputation regardless of other factors. Amputation may also be indicated where the final functional and cosmetic result of extensive reconstruction does not warrant the time and effort involved. For example, an unskilled laborer might prefer slight shortening of a digit, primary closure with a local flap, and early return to work. In contrast, a woman more concerned with cosmetic appearance might prefer a more lengthy reconstructive procedure.

In children, a disarticulation is preferable to amputation through the shaft of a long bone. Disarticulation saves the distal epiphysis and avoids the problem of terminal overgrowth, which frequently occurs, particularly with the humerus. Proximal phalangeal epiphyses may be retained with little worry that the terminal skin will not keep pace with growth in the remaining digit.

Open amputations in the upper extremity are not as common as the lower extremity. Closed amputations are preferable except where contraindicated by sepsis or severely contaminated wounds in which infection is imminent. Open amputations in the hand should be closed as soon as practicable because an open granulating wound leads to excessive scarring which reduces mobility so vital to hand function.

AMPUTATION THROUGH THE FINGERS AND METACARPALS

The index finger has independent activity unlike the adjacent fingers and occupies a position on the radial aspect of the hand where it is uniquely suited for function in concert with the thumb. Since length is so important to the index finger, the bone should generally not be trimmed back to achieve primary closure with local flaps. A full thickness graft, sliding flap, or pedicle flap may be used to conserve length. As the level of amputation in the index finger approaches the distal interphalangeal joint, pinch is transferred to the adjacent long finger. When the proximal interphalangeal joint is reached, the remaining stump serves only to widen the palm for stability in grasp. Frequently a stump of this nature undergoes "physiologic amputation" and assumes a hyperextended position due to inappropriate activity of the extrinsic extensors.

The long and ring fingers are not as important as the index finger; nevertheless, they do contribute significantly to hand function. The long finger contributes strength for hook type grasp, reinforces the index finger for firm lateral pinch with the thumb, and along with the ring finger is responsible for maintaining the "cup" effect of the hand. In addition, the long finger metacarpal is one element in the stable longitudinal arch of the hand and also serves as origin for the adductor pollicis muscle.

The ring finger acts in concert with the little finger and helps provide mobility to the ulnar side of the hand. It also helps fill in the span of the hand and participates in various types of pinch and grasp.

It is permissible to trim back bone in a central digit to achieve primary coverage by local flap. Retaining a proximal phalangeal stump is beneficial in that objects are not so likely to fall through the cupped hand, and the adjacent fingers will not deviate toward the gap created by complete absence of the digit. Amputation proximal to the metacarpal head removes the transverse metacarpal ligament, creating instability in the distal transverse arch of the hand and a rotary disturbance of the adjacent fingers which tend to deviate away from the lost metacarpal on flexion. This creates a narrower, three-fingered hand with improved function and appearance.

Developing a three-fingered hand from metacarpal amputation of a border finger or transfer of an adjacent finger to fill the gap created by an amputated central digit has stimulated considerable discussion. The consensus seems to be that, when soundly indicated, a symmetrical three-fingered hand is more appealing cosmetically and function is improved for most patients. Even if strength of grasp is diminished compared to the normal hand, this may be of little consequence for many people, particularly those more concerned with precision activities and desirous of improved appearance.

The little finger is considered the least important digit and its amputation is often felt to be of little consequence. However, it must be remembered that it is one of the mobile polar elements necessary for prehensile adaptability of the hand and plays an important role in adding width and stability to the palm for palmar grasp. Its loss is much more disabling to a carpenter than to an accountant. The importance of the little finger becomes more pronounced with loss of other fingers at which time the little finger may be the sole remaining pole for thumb pinch on the ulnar aspect of the hand.

TECHNIQUE OF FINGER AMPUTATION

The classic description of skin flaps in amputation of a finger is to create a long palmar and short dorsal skin flap in the ratio of two to one. The palmar flap is made tongue-shape rather than semi-circular to avoid "dog-ears" at the margins of the suture line. Unfortunately, however, when the amputation is being performed because of trauma, typical skin flaps seldom can be created. When the situation demands maintenance of length and circulation is adequate, atypical flaps and minor plastic procedures are used. Supplementary free skin grafts may be used in areas not subjected to heavy pressure and to cover the end of the stump in transverse amputation where no flaps of skin are available without re-amputation at a higher level.

To ensure adequate skin length, the dorsal flap may be cut with the finger in flexion and the palmar flap with the finger in extension. Although at the time of closure the flaps may appear to be loose, the elastic tension within the skin will draw them up snugly over the stump ends.

The bone is severed about ⅛ inch, or slightly more, proximal to the surrounding soft tissues and at a level that allows easy approximation of the skin flaps. The bone end is trimmed to a gently rounded shape and all spicules removed lest the constant irritation, which occasionally occurs, cause excessive scarring. With joint disarticulation, projecting bone from the condylar area is ronguered away to prevent a bulbous end. Articular cartilage is usually removed to promote more rapid fixation of the soft tissues to the stump end. It is usually best to lay the skin flap over the end of the stump and palpate the bone through the flap to assure the absence of projecting bone elements before closure. Where length of the middle phalanx is not a particular requirement, it is better to remove the bone to the level of the proximal interphalangeal joint.

The nerves are located anteriorly on either side of the flexor tendons and freed proximally in their beds to the point of intended section in normal, healthy, soft tissue. Usually the bed of the nerve is spread with a hemostat to the point of intended section, and the nerve is severed with a sharp knife or razor blade. There should be no injection of sclerosing substance and no use of ligatures. Care should be taken not to apply too much traction to the nerves at the time of section to avoid rupturing axons more proximally and creating painful neuromas. Blood vessels are ligated with 4−0 catgut when necessary and closure done with interrupted fine skin sutures.

The tendons are severed by simple transverse section and allowed to retract. They are never sutured over the end of the bone because of the danger of contracture and restricted motion of the amputation stump and adjacent fingers due to the interdigitation of the flexors and extensors at higher levels.

When simple closure with available skin cannot be effected and length still maintained, alternative plastic procedures may be used. Free skin grafts, either of the full thickness or split thickness type, form excellent coverage for dorsal, terminal, and lateral wounds in a freshly amputated finger. Sliding flap closure may also be of occasional use.

METACARPAL AMPUTATION

Index Metacarpal

A dorsal racket incision is used (Fig. 11.1.1). The incision starts at the level of the base of the index metacarpal and passes distalward, paralleling the ulnar border of the bone to the metacarpal head where it swings anteriorly around the finger at the level of the proximal skin crease. The extensor tendons are sectioned at the distal end of the wound and allowed to retract. The anterior soft tissues are freed by carrying the incision to the bone. This incision sections the flexor tendons which are allowed to retract proximally into the palm. The metacarpal is either sectioned at its base or disarticulated at the carpometacarpal joint. The finger is now free and is removed. The nerves are treated as in finger amputation. After hemostasis is secured, the body of the first dorsal interosseous muscle is sutured to the soft tissues about the third metacarpal to close dead space, and its tendon is attached to the base of the proximal phalanx of the long finger to reinforce lateral pinch. If it is attached to the extensor tendon or its hood, intrinisic over-pull may result.

A recently proposed alternative method to reinforce lateral pinch of the long finger is to transfer one of the flexor tendons from the amputated index ray to the long finger proximal phalanx. The tendon is placed in a small drill hole on the radial aspect at the base of the flare of the metaphysis and secured with a pull-out wire. The first dorsal interosseous is left in the web space to provide bulk. Subcutaneous tissues and skin

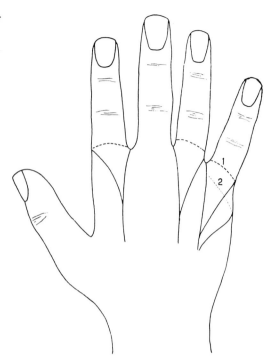

Figure 11.1.1. Incisions for metacarpal amputation. (Reproduced from *Clinical Orthopaedics* by permission of J. B. Lippincott Company.)

are approximated with interrupted sutures. The suture line is posterior, away from pressure that may occur in grasp (Fig. 11.1.2).

Long and Ring Finger Metacarpals

When the third or fourth metacarpal is amputated, a racket incision is used. A longitudinal incision is made along the dorsum of the metacarpal to the level of the metacarpal head. From this point it swings to the side of the finger at the web space and crosses the anterior aspect of the finger at the level of the proximal flexor crease, whence it follows dorsally and proximally to join the longitudinal limb of the incision. Wound closure is carried out in accordance with the standard principles so that the scar falls on the dorsal aspect of the hand. When reconstruction is practical, two procedures may be considered. The simplest method, although often not the most satisfactory, is complete excision of the involved metacarpal with collapse of the two adjacent metacarpal heads in such a manner that a scar tissue bridge will substitute for the transverse metacarpal ligaments and afford some stability. Unfortunately, this procedure provides only a fair rotary stabilization and usually some finger deviation remains; also, there is loss of width and the hand often feels tight and restricted. A second alternative is the transplant of the little finger to the position of the amputated ring finger or of the index finger to a position of the amputated long finger metacarpal (Fig. 11.1.3).

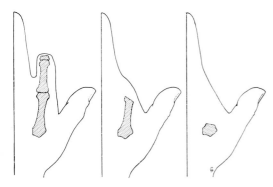

Figure 11.1.2. Amputations through the index finger. *Left.* Amputation stumps proximal to the interphalangeal joint are poor cosmetically, and they provide little function other than adding breadth to the hand. *Center.* Metacarpal shaft amputations impede the web space and provide little stability, and often they are painful in grasp. *Right.* Amputations through the base of the metacarpal or disarticulation at the carpometacarpal joint clear the web of projecting bone and add dexterity. Also, they are good cosmetically. However, they narrow the width of the palm.

When this procedure is undertaken, osteotomy should be done at the base of the metacarpal sufficiently away from the joint to insure its integrity and position secured by threaded K-wires. This yields excellent rotary stabilization and gives a good cosmetic and functional result.

Little Finger Metacarpal.

When the fifth metacarpal is to be removed, a dorsal racket incision is used. The longitudinal limb of the incision is carried along the radial side of the fifth metacarpal, and the distal end of the incision loops about the finger at the level of the proximal flexor crease. This ensures that the incision is well away from the hypothenar eminence when the wound is closed. Amputation through the distal one-half of the fifth metacarpal shaft is not a satisfactory procedure because of the mobility of the remaining bone.. When the metacarpal is amputated in its proximal one-half, the outer and dorsal aspects of the bone should be beveled to form a smooth and even contour beneath the skin. If this cannot be accomplished, the bone should be amputated at a more proximal level near the base. Either of these two bone levels gives an excellent cosmetic result (Fig. 11.1.4).

AMPUTATIONS OF THE THUMB

The thumb is the most mobile and important digit on the hand. Without the thumb to oppose the fingers, hand function is reduced largely to that of a hook type of grasp utilizing only the fingers. Maintenance of

length is of utmost importance. Amputation distal to the midportion of the proximal phalanx is performed similar to finger amputations. If primary closure without trimming back cannot be achieved, mobilization of a local flap, a cross-finger pedicle flap from the radial aspect of the index finger, or dorsum of the long finger middle phalanx, will provide good skin cover. In some instances, a full thickness skin graft is adequate. As the level of amputation approaches the metacarpophalangeal joint, consideration for deepening the web space must be made. Often this can be accomplished by a simple Z-plasty procedure, but it may also be necessary to strip the origin of the first dorsal interosseous and insertion of the adductor pollicis to acquire adequate depth, particularly in amputations at or near the metacarpal head level. Muscle stripping will provide an additional three-quarters to one inch deepening of the web space. When Z-plasty will not afford sufficient web space, a dorsal rotational flap, transpositional flap, or distance pedicle flap will be necessary. A thick, split thickness, or full thickness skin graft can be used to cover any remaining defect. If the index finger has been amputated, the thumb web space may be deepened and broadened by excision of the index metacarpal.

Thumb amputations proximal to the metacarpal head will require reconstructive procedures to restore length and thumb function.

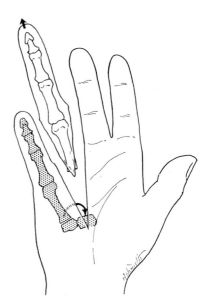

Figure 11.1.3. Amputation through the shaft of the third or the fourth metacarpal permits rotary deformities of adjacent fingers. It is corrected best by finger transplant: for the ring finger, the little finger is moved to the base of the fourth metacarpal; for the middle finger, the index finger is moved to the base of the third metacarpal.

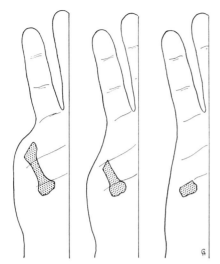

Figure 11.1.4. Amputations through the fifth metacarpal. *Left.* In disarticulation at the metacarpophalangeal joint, the metacarpal head is beveled on its lateral and dorsal aspects to create a smooth, even contour. *Center.* Amputation through the distal one-half of the metacarpal is to be avoided because of increased mobility and the prominence of the bone beneath the skin; in the proximal one-half, the side of the metacarpal is beveled to eliminate any bony projection. *Right.* Amputation through the metacarpal base results in a smooth, even contour of the hypothenar region.

MULTIPLE FINGER AMPUTATIONS

When more than one finger has been amputated, functional reconstruction must be individualized to each situation.

The general objectives are: (1) to salvage remaining digits and digital remnants; (2) to save as much length as possible in the remaining fingers; (3) to preserve the palm for stability of grasp, pushing, and holding; (4) to provide an adequate cleft between the thumb and remaining fingers; (5) to furnish two poles for pinch and grasp, consisting of a thumb or thumb substitute and finger or finger substitute; (6) to insure the approximation of these two polar elements by increasing their mobility and supplying motor elements when necessary and by changing their position through osteotomy.

A partial hand prosthesis may be helpful for some patients. Swanson points out that a partial prosthesis fills the gap between a total prosthesis and reconstruction by allowing the patient with a functioning hand remnant to have useful prehension.

The index and long finger; or index, long, and ring fingers are amputated and the thumb and the ulnar fingers are intact. No special problems are present at the finger level, provided that the stumps of the ampu-

tated fingers are sound. The little and ring fingers afford fair stability for grasp as long as the palm and remaining finger stumps are intact. An adequate cleft usually is present between the thumb and the fingers, since the palm and thumb web generally are not involved (Fig. 11.1.5). No special treatment is required.

When amputation occurs at the level of the metacarpophalangeal joints, stability is decreased and there is more likelihood of damage to the web space. Pinch may be accomplished readily by apposition of the thumb and remaining ring and little fingers. When amputation occurs at the level of the metacarpal shaft or proximalward, the problem is principally one of making a smooth, even sloping contour between the thumb and the remaining ring and little fingers. So far as the remaining ring finger is concerned, it is well to be sure that the interosseous muscle providing its radial deviation is adequate for lateral pinch and to reenforce this action by tendon transplantation as required. The third metacarpal forms the base for the attachment of the adductor tendon of the thumb as well as the pivot point about which the ring and little finger rotate in creating the palmar arch. When intact to the level of the transverse metacarpal ligaments, it should be maintained; if not, the shaft should be beveled to ensure a smooth web space.

The thumb remains intact and all fingers are amputated at the level of the metacarpophalangeal joints. The problem facing the surgeon is to provide a cleft in the web space between the thumb and the remaining fingers with sufficient depth to give greater mobility to the fifth metacarpal and still to maintain adequate palm for palmar pushing and lifting. Since the fingers are not long enough to appose the thumb with ease in pinch or to hold objects against the palm in grasp, it is desirable to increase the width and depth of the web. This is accomplished by amputation of the second metacarpal. The third metacarpal is not disturbed, because it forms the center of rotation for the palmar arch. It is well to ensure the mobility of the fourth and

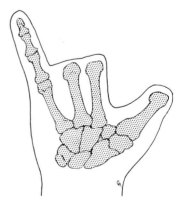

Figure 11.1.5. Where the metacarpal bone and little finger remain, a cleft may be created between the thumb and third metacarpal by removal of the index metacarpal.

fifth metacarpals by attaching the extensors and one of the long flexors to the metacarpal heads of these two bones. Mobility of the fourth and fifth rays may also be increased significantly by dividing their transverse metacarpal ligaments. If the surgeon fails to do this, the fourth and fifth metacarpals will not roll toward the thumb in pinch and grasp.

The thumb remains, the second metacarapl is amputated at midshaft, and the long, ring, and little fingers are amputated at their metacarpal heads. The problem is one of clearing the web space by resection of the second metacarpal and making sure that the metacarpals of the fourth and fifth fingers are mobilized and powered by the extensors and the long flexors. If apposition of the fifth metacarpal to the thumb cannot be accomplished well, further mobilization may be carried out by resecting the fourth metacarpal at the carpometacarpal joint and phalangization of the fifth metacarpal.

The thumb and the little finger remain intact, and all others are amputated at the metacarpal shaft or bases. The problem is one of apposing the thumb to the little finger (Fig. 11.1.6). If this cannot be done, the web space is cleared of all impediments and the thumb and the little finger are tilted toward each other by osteotomizing the metacarpals at their bases and providing motor power for opposition by an opponens transplant of the Bunnell type or the Bunnell tendon T operation.

All the fingers and the thumb are amputated at the metacarpophalangeal joint to form the so-called mitten hand (Fig. 11.1.7). The problem is to provide apposable posts for grasping and pinching objects. This is especially important in a bilateral amputee, in whom the opposite hand cannot substitute for the amputated one and bimanual activities are at their lowest ebb. There are two possibilities for reconstruction of such a hand. First, a two-digit hand may be made, the two apposing poles being represented by the thumb metacarpal and by the fourth and fifth metacarpals. To

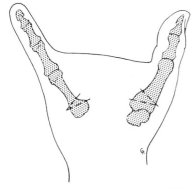

Figure 11.1.6. When the thumb and little finger remain but cannot be approximated, osteotomy will frequently be required. If motors are lacking, an opponens transplant or tendon T may be added to the operation.

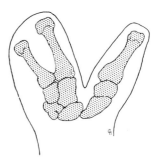

Figure 11.1.7. In a mitten hand where all fingers are amputated at the metacarpophalangeal joints, phalangization may be accomplished by removal of the second and third metacarpals together with the capitate bone.

do this, the index and the middle finger metacarpals are removed and the capitate bone is resected to increase the mobility. Motor power must be furnished to these two posts if they are to be of value. The second method of handling this situation is to form a three-digit hand by resecting the index metacarpal to deepen the thumb web and by phalangizing the fifth metacarpal by resection of the fourth at its carpometacarpal articulation. In addition to the formation of a cleft between the long and little fingers, the mobility of the fifth metacarpal is increased. Such a three-digit hand has some advantages and it has pincer action both between the thumb and the long finger and between the long and the little fingers (Figs. 11.1.7 and 11.1.8).

The thumb and the index fingers remain; and the long, ring and little fingers have been amputated at the finger level. All remaining fingers should be preserved. If the amputation is at the level of the metacarpophalangeal joints, the metacarpals should not be disturbed, for the preservation of the palm adds much to the hand.

The ring and little finger remain; and the thumb, index and long fingers have been removed at the metacarpophalangeal joints. Hook action alone remains. The thumb stump is relatively useless, but some function may be restored if a cleft is provided between it and the adjacent metacarpals. This will give some semblance of grasp and increase the mobility of the thumb metacarpal. Disarticulation of the second metacarpal with a modified Z-plasty or adjunct plastic methods will best restore the web space. Lengthening the thumb is desirable. Since finger transplant is impracticable, the only method remaining is to elongate the thumb stump itself. In principle, a transverse osteotomy is made through the distal metacarpal shaft, the distal segment and its investing soft tissues are migrated distalward, and a segment of the amputated second metacarpal bone is then interposed to fill the gap.

This distal shift is effected when the incision starts on the posterior aspect of the midmetacarpal level, swings proximally to lie near the metacarpal base at the lateral aspect of the thumb, and then passes distally

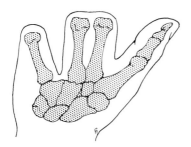

Figure 11.1.8. The ring finger metacarpal may be removed to create a three-digit hand.

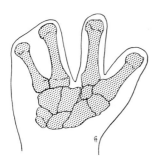

Figure 11.1.9. The third metacarpal may be removed to create a three-digit hand.

to the anterior aspect of the thumb at a level opposite the starting point. The soft tissues are mobilized and the interposing graft is placed in position at the osteotomy site, where it is fixed in position with suitable internal fixation such as an intermedullary wire. Soft tissue covering is provided about the transplanted graft and a full thickness skin graft is used to cover the skin defect left by the distal migration of the skin of the thumb.

The long and ring fingers remain, and the thumb, index, and little fingers have been amputated. The essential problem is to provide good integument and adequate grasping surface, if possible. When the thumb remains at the level of the metacarpal head, the depth of the thumb web space may be deepened by Z-plasty and disarticulation of the second metacarpal at the carpometacarpal joint. When sufficient thumb does not remain, it may be worthwhile to provide a grasping area between the fingers and the thenar eminence. One method of accomplishing this is through a posterior shift of the third and fourth metacarpals at their carpal articulations and subsequent arthrodesis. Since this posterior shift may disturb the tendon balance, tendon lengthening is carried out if necessary.

AMPUTATIONS PROXIMAL TO THE LEVEL OF THE METACARPALS

Amputations proximal to the level of the metacarpals are always carried out with a view to eventual prosthetic fitting. A comfortable and durable stump that fits well in a prosthesis may be obtained if certain general principles are followed.

1. Level of Amputation

The most distal level compatible with formation of a satisfactory stump should be selected. With modern prosthetic fittings, any level in the upper extremity may be fitted. In children the epiphyseal plate is preserved wherever possible to ensure future growth of the stump.

2. Skin

Good skin with normal sensation and mobility and an adequate amount of subcutaneous fat is an essential feature of a good stump.

3. Muscles

When transection of the limb is carried out through shafts of the forearm bones or humerus, the most important function of the muscles at the end of the stump is to provide circumferential padding.

4. Bones

Bone is divided transversely to its longitudinal axis and all bony prominences are smoothed and rounded. Periosteal stripping is minimized to prevent future new bone formation.

5. Nerves

Nerves are isolated and cleanly sectioned with a sharp knife one inch proximal to the bone end. Strong tugging and pulling is avoided. The nerve ends are allowed to retract into a soft tissue bed.

6. Blood Vessels

Hemostasis is essential to healing. Major vessels are doubly ligated with plain catgut. The smaller vessels are tied. A drain or plastic suction tube is routinely used.

AMPUTATIONS ABOUT THE WRIST

Amputations about the wrist are preferred to more proximal levels because they (Fig. 11.1.10) (1) preserve rotation of the forearm, (2) save the distal epiphysis of the radius and ulna in children, (3) are useful for pushing and holding without a prosthesis, (4) require a shorter, less cumbersome prosthesis, and (5) preserve flexion and extension of the wrist when performed at the transcarpal level. Children particularly may develop a remarkable amount of wrist motion which can be utilized with or without a prosthesis. Only about 50 per cent of available forearm rotation is transmitted to the prosthesis but this is extremely valuable.

Amputation through the Carpus

In amputation through the carpus, a long palmar

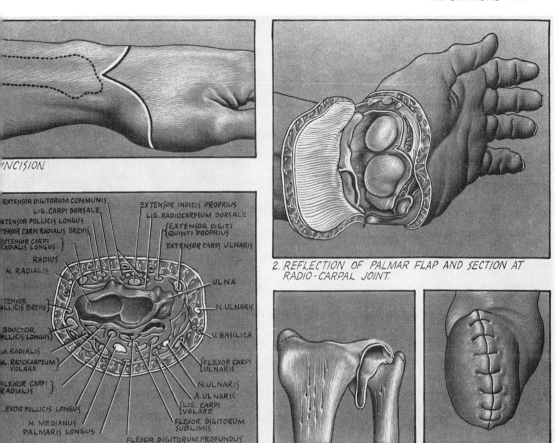

Figure 11.1.10. Wrist disarticulation. (Reproduced from *An Atlas of Amputations* by permission of C. V. Mosby.)

and short dorsal flap, in the ratio of two to one is used. The skin flap is dissected proximally to expose the soft tissues at the proper bone level. The extensors and flexors of the fingers are drawn distally and sectioned so they will retract proximally into the forearm. The flexors and extensors of the wrist are reflected proximally above the bone level and are later re-attached to the end of the bone at the most distal convenient point in line with their normal insertions. The median and ulnar nerve and the fine filaments of the radial nerve are drawn distally, sectioned, and allowed to retract proximally. The bone is then divided with a saw and fashioned to form a smooth, rounded contour with no projecting bony eminences. The skin flaps are approximated under normal tension over the bony end by interrupted sutures.

Disarticulation of the Wrist

The skin incision is stared at a level one-half inch distal to the styloid processes, and is carried over the palm and dorsum of the hand to form a long anterior flap of palmar skin and a short dorsal flap. The flaps are reflected proximally to expose the radiocarpal joint. The radial and ulnar arteries are identified, sectioned, and doubly ligated. The median, ulnar, and radial nerves are drawn down gently and sectioned so that they will retract above the level of the wrist joint. The remainder of the soft tissues are divided, starting at the radial side of the wrist and progressing toward the ulna until the wrist and hand are freed. The cartilage overlying the end of the radius and radioulnar joint is not disturbed. When the prominences of the styloid processes project unduly, they may be removed to a point where a smooth, rounded bone end is obtained. The skin flaps are approximated by interrupted sutures.

AMPUTATIONS THROUGH THE FOREARM

Amputations of the lower forearm, the so-called long, below elbow stump, may be satisfactorily fitted with the wrist disarticulation type of prosthesis when the stump is in good condition. The middle third of the forearm is the best level for amputation from the surgical viewpoint. Both stumps and prosthesis at this level are excellent. Flexion and extension are powerful. In the longer stumps within this level, careful fitting of the socket will permit pronation and supination to a certain extent.

Amputations through the upper third of the forearm correspond roughly with the short below-elbow stump of the prosthetist. The prosthetic problem is to provide adequate flexion of the elbow joint while maintaining the stump within the socket. Fitting techniques available today, along with resection of the distal one-inch of the biceps tendon, allow prosthetic fitting of stumps only one and one-half inches in length. Functionally this is preferable to an elbow disarticulation or above-elbow amputation.

With a very short, below-elbow stump, the motion multiplying variable ratio step-up hinge with split-socket may be used or a Münster-type below elbow socket may be employed. The step-up hinge is geared so that the forearm shell moves upward in a ratio of three to two in comparison with actual stump flexion, but at a scarifice in lifting strength. The Münster sock-et is set at a preflexed position of about 35° and is molded up high posteriorly around the olecranon for attachment and stability.

Techniques in the Lower Forearm

With the arm held midway between pronation and supination on an armboard at the side of the operating table, anterior and posterior flaps of equal lengths are formed with the incision starting immediately above the desired bone level. The underlying muscle and fascia are cut in a similar pattern and reflected proximally. The muscles are sectioned transversely to fall at bone level. The radial, ulnar, and median nerves are sectioned and allowed to retract proximal to the bone level. The radial and ulnar arteries are cut and doubly ligated. The tourniquet is released and hemostasis secured. The fascial flaps are approximated with plain catgut to aid in muscle grouping about the sides of the bone ends. Some surgeons do not use fascial flaps and prefer a thin layer of sublimis muscle over the bone ends. The skin flaps are approximated with interrupted sutures and a drain or plastic suction tube left in the wound (Fig. 11.1.11).

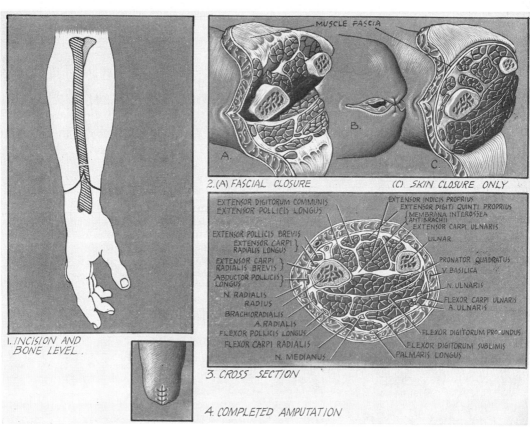

Figure 11.1.11. Amputation of the forearm. (Reproduced from *An Atlas of Amputations* by permission of C. V. Mosby.)

Technique in the Upper Third of the Forearm

Anterior and posterior flaps of equal length are preferred but from a practical point of view any available skin may be used for coverage to secure maximal stump length. Fascial flaps are used when practical. Bones are sectioned transversely and treated in the usual fashion. All excess muscle bulk is trimmed. When the biceps tendon prevents fitting of a socket in a very short below-elbow stump, it may be sectioned and allowed to retract. The brachialis muscle will provide sufficient flexion of the elbow. Skin flaps are closed in the usual fashion.

DISARTICULATION OF THE ELBOW

Amputations that lie between the supracondylar level of the humerus and the elbow joint proper utilize the elbow disarticulation-type prosthesis. This has a definite advantage over more proximal levels because the prosthetic socket fits securely about the flare of the humeral condyles and humeral rotation is transmitted to the prosthesis. In addition, the stump provides end-bearing, as in resting the elbow on a table, and in children the distal humeral epiphysis is preserved.

Technique for Elbow Disarticulation

A short anterior and long posterior skin flap are created. The medial flexor muscles attached to the medial epicondyle are divided at the joint line. The brachial artery is clamped, sectioned, and doubly ligated and the median and ulnar nerves are pulled gently downward, sectioned, and allowed to retract into a soft tissue bed. The biceps and brachialis tendons are released distally. The radial nerve is drawn down, sectioned, and allowed to retract proximally. The extensor muscles attached to the lateral epicondyle are sectioned two and one-half inches below the joint line and then the joint is disarticulated. The triceps tendon is drawn anteriorly and sutured to the brachialis and biceps tendons. The lateral extensor muscles are trimmed to form a thin muscle flap, swung medially, and attached to the medial flexor muscles to cover all exposed tendon and bony prominences. When hemostasis is achieved, the skin flaps are closed without tension and a drain or a plastic suction tube left deep to the fascia.

THE ABOVE-ELBOW OR UPPER ARM AMPUTATION

An above-elbow amputation is any level from the axillary fold proximally to the supracondylar area distally. Transcondylar amputations are managed as elbow disarticulations. The prosthesis may be fitted more satisfactorily and better control achieved with as long a stump as practicable. From a cosmetic standpoint, it is ideal to have the prosthetic elbow at the same level as the opposite elbow; and since the elbow lock mechanism extends one and one-half inches distal to the socket, the bone level should be at least one and one-half inches proximal to the joint. Externally powered prostheses are now available for the high above-elbow amputee, particularly when there is no convenient source of body power. However, they are not in general use.

Technique

Starting at the level of the intended bone length, flaps of equal length either anterior and posterior or medial and lateral are formed. Flaps may be modified in any manner necessary to preserve the stump length. The anterior muscles are sectioned to fall at bone level. Posteriorly the triceps is sectioned about one and one-half inches below the bone level to form a thin, myofascial flap. The nerves are isolated, sectioned and allowed to retract above the end of the stump. The major vessels are sectioned and doubly ligated. The skin is approximated with interrupted sutures and a drain or plastic suction tube placed in the posterior margin of the wound (Fig. 11.1.12).

AMPUTATIONS ABOUT THE SHOULDER

In amputations above the axillary fold, the stump is of little functional value. However, amputees may be successfully fitted with limbs at this level. Although the functional gains are small, the balance of the torso is maintained and prevents the development of the otherwise inevitable postural scoliosis, and the prosthesis is of value in holding functions of various types. Cosmetically, amputation through the surgical neck of the humerus is superior to shoulder disarticulation, because the head of the humerus gives the shoulder a more rounded appearance. Amputation at this level tends to produce deformity proportionate to (1) the loss of weight of the limb, (2) atrophy of disuse of the muscles, and (3) over-development of the remaining limb.

Technique

The skin incision is begun at the level of the coracoid process and continued along the anterior border of the deltoid muscle downward to its insertion, then along the posterior aspect of the deltoid to the axillary pole. The two ends of the incision are connected by a second incision passing through the axilla. The pectoralis major muscle is sectioned at its insertion and reflected medially. The interval between the pectoralis minor and the coracobrachialis muscle is developed to expose the neurovascular bundle. The axillary artery and vein are sectioned immediately below the pectoralis minor muscle. The median, ulnar, radial, and musculocutaneous nerves are isolated, drawn down, and sectioned so that they fall proximal to the pectoralis minor muscle. The deltoid muscle is then sectioned at its insertion and reflected upward together with its attached lateral skin flap; the teres major and latissimus dorsi muscles are sectioned near

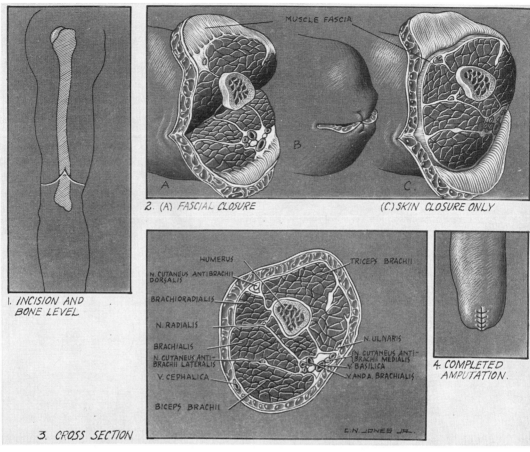

Figure 11.1.12. Amputation of the upper arm. (Reproduced from *An Atlas of Amputations* by permission of C. V. Mosby.)

their insertions at the bicipital groove and the biceps tendon, triceps, and coracobrachialis are cut at a point three-fourths of an inch distal to the bone level. The bone is transected at the level of the humeral neck. Both heads of the biceps, the long head of the triceps, and the coracobrachialis are sutured over the cut-end of the humerus, while the pectoralis major is swung laterally and sutured to the inferior pole of the bone. The skin flap with its underlying deltoid muscle is tailored for accurate approximation and sutured with interrupted skin sutures.

When the shoulder is disarticulated, the technique is essentially the same except that muscle is tucked into the glenoid cavity to give a more rounded contour to the shoulder. When the acromion is unduly prominent, its outer portion may be resected (Fig. 11.1.13).

CINEPLASTY

Cineplasty amputation is really a combination of two operations; one in which the amputation stump is created and a second procedure at a later time when a muscle motor is created to permit the harnessing and transmission of muscle power for motivation of the prosthesis. The biceps muscle with its long excursion and great strength has proved the best motor to the point where other cineplastic power sources have been abandoned. The cineplasty amputation still has a relatively limited application and should be undertaken only by a surgeon familiar with the surgical technique and postoperative rehabilitation program. It is probably most applicable for a cooperative, highly motivated forearm amputee who cannot wear a harness or whose vocation demands good manual dexterity and controlled prehension which is available with a voluntary closing terminal device on a cineplastic prosthesis.

THE KRUKENBERG AMPUTATION

The Krukenberg amputation is a very useful modification of a long forearm amputation in which the forearm bones are phalangized, forming a radial and ulnar ray pinching mechanism with tactile sensation. It is particularly adaptable for the adult and child bilateral amputee and the blind bilateral amputee. It may

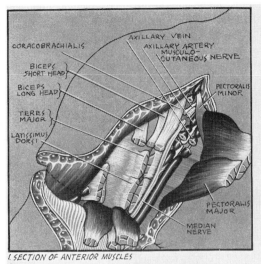

1. SECTION OF ANTERIOR MUSCLES

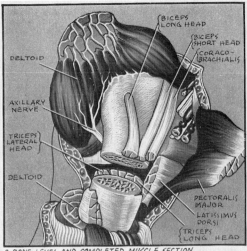

2. BONE LEVEL AND COMPLETED MUSCLE SECTION.

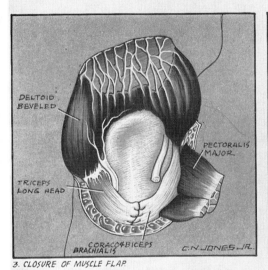

3. CLOSURE OF MUSCLE FLAP.

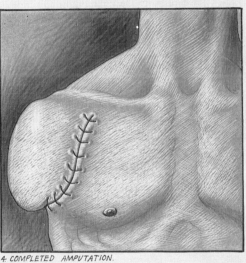

4. COMPLETED AMPUTATION.

Figure 11.1.13. Amputation of the surgical neck of the humerus. (Reproduced from *An Atlas of Amputations* by permission of C. V. Mosby.)

also be used in remote areas where prosthetic services are lacking. A prosthetic limb is used on the opposite extremity for assistance. Swanson reports that children readily adapt to the Krukenberg stump and use it as the dominant hand. Objections to the procedure have been primarily directed at its cosmetic effect, but a standard prosthesis can be used over the stump in public and removed for home activity.

REFERENCES

1. Alldredge, R. H. Surgical aspects of amputations in the upper extremity. American Academy of Orthopedic Surgeons, Instructional Course Lecture. Vol. 10, Ann Arbor, J. W. Edwards, 1953.
2. Boyes, J. W. *Bunnell's Surgery of the Hand,* Ed. 5. Philadelphia, Lippincott, 1970.
3. Capener, N. Emergency amputations, upper limb. Ann. Coll. Surg., *40:* 218, 1967.
4. Carroll, R. E. The levels of amputation in the hand. Bol. Asoc. Med. PR., *62:* 183-185, 1970.
5. Chase, R. A. Conservation of usable structures in injured hands. In *Reconstructive Plastic Surgery.* Philadelphia, Saunders, 1967.
6. Chase, R. A. Functional levels of amputation in the hand. Surg. Clin. North Am., *40:* 415, 1960.
7. Chase, R. A. The severely injured upper limb. To amputate or reconstruct — that is the question. Arch. Surg., *100:* 382-92, 1970.
8. Entin, M. A. Salvaging the basic hand. Surg. Clin. North Am., *38:* 1063-81, 1968.

9. Eversmann, W. W., Burkhalter, W. E., and Dunne, C. Transfer of the long flexor tendon of the index finger to the proximal phalanx of the long finger during index-ray amputation. J. Bone Joint Surg., *53A:* 769-73, 1971.

10. Fishman, S., and Kay, H. W: The Münster-type below elbow socket, an evaluation. Artif. Limbs, *8:* 4, 1964.

11. Flatt, A. E. *Minor Hand Injuries,* Ed. 2. St. Louis, Mosby, 1963.

12. Frantz, C. H., and Aitken, G. T.: Management of the juvenile amputee. Clin. Orthop., *14:* 40, 1959.

13. Gottlieb, O. Metacarpal amputation: The problem of the four fingered hand. Acta Chir. Scand. Suppl., *343:* 132-142, 1965.

14. Graham, W. P. Incisions, amputations, and skin grafting in the hand. Orthop. Clin. North Am. *1:* 213-218, 1970.

15. Harvis, W. R., and Houston, J. K. Partial amputation of the hand: A follow-up study. Can. Surg., *10:* 431, 1967.

16. Inglis, A. E. Traumatic digital amputations of the thumb. Bull. Hosp. Joint Dis., *32:* 4-9, 1971.

17. Joshi, B. B. One-stage repair for distal amputation of the thumb. Plast. Reconstr. Surgery, *45:* 613-5, 1970.

18. Kaplan, I. Functional levels of amputation of fingers. S. Afr. Med. J., *43:* 1113-5, 1969.

19. Karchinov, K. Phalangization of hand metacarpals. Acta Chir. Plast. (Praha), *13:* 47-52, 1971.

20. Mazet, R., Jr. Cineplasty, historical review, present status, and critical evaluation of sixty-four patients. J. Bone Joint Surg., *40A:* 1389, 1958.

21. McCash, C. R. Cosmetic aspects of hand surgery. Hand, *1:* 67, 1969.

22. Milford, L. The hand. In *Campbell's Operative Orthopaedics.* St. Louis, Mosby, 1971.

23. Napier, J. R. The prehensile movements of the human hand. J. Bone Joint Surg., *38B:* 902, 1956.

24. Peacock, E. E., Jr., Madden, J. W., and Trier, W. C. Transplantation of finger-tips. Ann. Surg., *173:* 812-26, 1971.

25. Pulvertaft, R. G. Hemiamputation of the hand. J. R. Coll. Surg. Edinb., *14:* 89-97, 1969.

26. Sharpe, C. Tissue cover for the thumb web. Arch. Surg., *104:* 21, 1971.

27. Slocum, D. B. *An Atlas of Amputations.* St. Louis, Mosby, 1949.

28. Slocum, D. B. Amputations of the fingers and hand. Clin. Orthop., *15:* 35, 1959.

29. Slocum, D. B. Amputations. In *Campbell's Operative Orthopaedics.* St. Louis, Mosby, 1963.

30. Slocum, D. B. Upper Extremity Amputation. In *Hand Surgery.* Edited by J. E. Flynn. Baltimore, Williams & Wilkins Co., 1966.

31. Simpson, D. C. External powered prosthesis. Hand, *3:* 213, 1971.

32. Simpson, D. C. Artificial hands. Hand, *2:* 211, 1971.

33. Swanson, A. B. Multiple finger amputations. J. Mich. State Med. Soc., *61:* 316, 1962.

34. Swanson, A. B. Restoration of hand function by the use of partial or total prosthetic replacement. I. The use of partial prosthesis. J. Bone Joint Surg., *45A:* 276, 1963.

35. Swanson, A. B. The Krukenberg procedure in the juvenile amputee. J. Bone Joint Surg., *46A:* 1540, 1964.

36. Swanson, A. B. Levels of amputation of fingers and hand: Consideration for treatment. Surg. Clin. North Am., *44:* 1115, 1964.

37. Tooms, R. A. Amputations. In *Campbell's Operative Orthopaedics.* St. Louis, Mosby, 1971.

38. Tubiana, R., Stack, H. G., and Hakstian, R. W. Restoration of prehension after severe mutilations of the hand. J. Bone Joint Surg., *48B:* 455, 1966.

B.

Traumatic Amputations of Phalanges and Digits

Raoul Tubiana

Traumatic amputation of phalanx and digits, excluding the thumb, show a variety of extremely different lesions, whose consequence is more or less to alter prehension.

Traumatic amputations differ from congenital ones because of the frequency of impairment of sensibility, the extensiveness of scar tissue, and further more because the injured patient will find adaptation to his amputation the more difficult the older he is.

It is well known that prehension is a complex mechanism which should not be confused with simple grip, as the hand is constantly adapting itself in terms of the sensory information it receives. Unsensitive or painful fingers are most often not used by the patient. Therefore, one must strive to give a skin coverage and a sensibility as good as possible in gripping areas.

One of the most difficult problems arising from these amputations is the organization of emergency care. Their frequency does not enable all of them to be treated by specialized hand surgeons. The aim of the early treatment should be to assess: (1) which tissues are viable and which are unlikely to survive; (2) what can be sacrificed and what must be preserved, in order to restore the most useful grips.

At the beginning of each particular case, the problem will be to judge in which cases one can shorten the bony structures to facilitate skin closure without increasing impairment, and those in which, conversely, one must try to preserve as much length of the stump as possible by making use of more sophisticated plastic procedures.

Such an evaluation is often difficult and one must take into consideration numerous factors depending on the type of amputation, the status of the patient, and the experience of the surgeon.

Before describing the different procedures necessary in these cases, we must:

1. Stress the important difference which exists between the clean laceration and the crush injury in

which, adding to the skin loss, deep lesions exist, especially of the bony structures.

2. General principles which govern the treatment of wounds also apply here: cleansing and debridement to reduce the risk of infection; stabilizing the skeleton in case of fracture; providing a skin cover as early as is safely possible; preventing stiffness by early mobilization of the finger joints.

3. Last, whatever the reconstructive stage, the treatment will take into account: (a) the general condition of the patient, his age, his occupations, his cosmetic wishes, the function of the other hand, and whether it is the dominant one or not; (b) the local condition: the amputation level and which digit is involved.

We shall describe successively: distal phalanx amputations; proximal and middle phalanx amputations; multiple amputations. Special problems such as lengthening of a digital stump, reimplantations, and prosthesis will be roughly outlined.

AMPUTATIONS AT THE LEVEL OF THE DISTAL PHALANX

In amputations of the digital extremities, one encounters contradictory problems difficult to solve. The importance of the distal phalanx is such, for sensory function and precision grip, that the treatment of finger tip amputations should be carefully selected by specialists. And yet, these lesions are so frequent that many are treated in inadequate centers by inexperienced surgeons.

We shall start by outlining a simple, safe line of treatment to be followed in emergency by the resident on duty or the isolated general surgeon. We shall then discuss the more refined procedures which should be only attempted by specialists; some of these techniques, in less competent hands, may well aggravate the initial lesions.

Common Procedures

The following can be included in this category: simple wound suture, shortening of the skeleton to allow skin covering, partial thickness grafts, and "assisted" cicatrization. These procedures all have some disadvantages which justify the use of more sophisticated techniques, but they also have the advantage of being simple.

The line of treatment is quite obvious, if sufficient skin has been preserved to allow suture without tension, or a limited bony shortening facilitates approximation of the skin edges. However, not infrequently the provision of adequate soft tissue covering is not feasible unless *the skeleton is shortened* by 1 cm or more. Bone shortening has the simultaneous advantage and disadvantage of being a "once and for all" procedure. It may be necessary in crush injuries with a comminuted fracture of the distal phalanx.

A shortened finger with a healthy stump is of much greater value than a longer digit with a painful stump. However, digital shortening of more than 5 mm to facilitate skin covering should never be performed as an emergency procedure: (1) in the thumb; (2) in the fingers, if several digits are involved; (3) in children; (4) in female patients, for cosmetic reasons. It should also be avoided as far as possible when the traumatic amputation reaches halfway down the nail as further shortening would cause the nail to tilt forward.

Partial thickness skin grafts can be used in other cases in emergency.

In some cases, a second operation will be required: at first sight, this might seem to be an obvious disadvantage, but at least future repairs are not jeopardized, the lesion is not aggravated and, not infrequently, the surface area requiring secondary repair is reduced by contraction of the tissues. The volar aspect of the forearm is usually a convenient donor area, but in female patients a less obvious skin area may be cosmetically preferable.

In the young child, *spontaneous epithelialization* with tissue retraction is so rapid that skin grafting is not required in wounds with a diameter of less than 1 cm. Spontaneous cicatrization is also worth trying for in adults for small lateral wounds by simple covering of the defect with tulle gras.

Other Procedures

Skin loss at the digital extremities can be made up for by full-thickness or partial-thickness skin grafts, composite pulpocutaneous grafts, adjacent flaps, regional flaps taken from the same hand or distant flaps. One should aim at restoring the fullest sensibility in the pulps of the thumb and index, protective sensibility for the pulps and tips of the other digits, and a cushion of subcutaneous tissue at all pressure points. But it should be remembered that the more complex the treatment, especially if several operations are required, the longer the time lost from work and the more difficult the professional readaptation, especially in the older patient.

Transverse Amputations (Fig. 11.2.1)

These are the easiest to repair.

1. If the lesion lies beyond the distal third of the phalanx, a simple Thiersch graft is usually sufficient provided the bone is not exposed.

2. If the bone is partially bared, one may use a well cushioned protective *pulpocutaneous* graft taken from a toe.

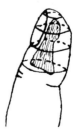

Figure 11.2.1. Transverse amputations: the different levels

This latter procedure was described by Ardao[1] and by McCash[17] who used it in more than 1,000 cases (Marchac and Rousso[16]). It consists of cutting a dome-shaped graft from the pulp of a toe, using a broad (no. 24) blade. The graft should include a few millimeters of pulpar tissue in its central part. It is gently exsanguinated and sutured to the defect. The donor area (usually the fourth toe which is the least weight bearing) can be covered with a thin graft or simply with tulle gras to promote contraction of the edges. Walking is possible at once.

3. If the bone is bared, a skin flap is usually preferable and we personally favor an *adjacent flap*. The procedure described by Kutler[15] consists of advancing two small lateral island flaps (Fig..2.2). The posterior side of the triangle should be drawn parallel to and 2 mm from the nail (Hann[9]) to preserve as many as possible of the sensory branches coming from the anterior part of the pulp. Subcutaneous fibrous adhesions which impede the free advancement of the flap should be divided especially at the level of the posterior incision.

Erler[6] and Kleinert[13] have shown that a palmar island flap, based on the V-Y principle and advanced to the defect could provide a useful sensitive covering (Fig. 11.2.3).

4. If more than half the nail bed has been lost in the injury, a decision must be taken as to whether the nail should be preserved or sacrificed. The nail requires an anterior support of at least half a centimeter distal to the lunula. If left unsupported, it tilts forward over the tip of the finger: this may be unsightly, may interfere with digital function, and may cause pain. If the stump is too short, the best solution in a manual worker, is to remove the remnant nail with its matrix. If, however, the nail is preserved for cosmetic reasons in a female patient, a regional flap may be used to pad the stump: we regard this as one of the exceptional indications for a thenar flap. It is also possible, as was suggested by Holevitch,[10] to displace the nail matrix proximally. To avoid damage to the matrix, it should be moved along with a thin layer of bone.

For proximal amputations of the distal phalanx, when the nail cannot be preserved, a dorsal flap, *e.g.*, the flag-shaped flap from the dorsal skin described by Vilain,[26] may be used (Fig. 11.2.4).

A distant flap is always necessary if we want to keep the length of an exposed bony stump.

Oblique Dorsal Amputations (Fig. 11.2.5)

1. *If the nail is only partially injured,* an attempt must be made at preserving it. The nail is an important structure cosmetically and functionally: it provides efficient support to the pulp in precision handling. One should always try to preserve it or at least to promote normal regeneration. This is possible only if the matrix is intact, if the nail bed is even and adequately depressed, and finally, as we have seen above, if the phalangeal remnant is long enough; if not, the nail will curve in and tilt forward.

If the nail has been sectioned but each fragment is still adherent to the wound, these can be approximated and sutured. If the nail is detached, the edges are trimmed and the nail replaced in its bed and, if possible, in the matrix. It is sutured to the edges of the bed and held down with a compressive dressing.

When the nail has been damaged beyond repair, Iselin[12] advocates the use of a "bank nail," to preserve the nail bed and avoid matricial synechiae which are responsible for bifid nails. A Thiersch graft may be used.

2. *If the matrix itself has been damaged beyond re-*

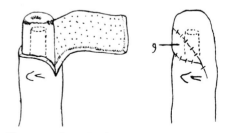

Figure 11.2.4. The Vilain procedure. *g* = skin graft

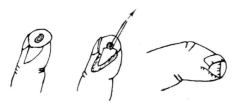

Figure 11.2.2. The Kutler procedure

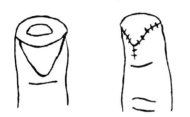

Figure 11.2.3. The Erler-Kleinert procedure

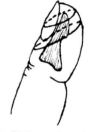

Figure 11.2.5. Oblique dorsal amputations

pair, the choice lies between a graft or a flap, again depending on the quality of the bed. But unlike lacerations of the pulp, this lesion does not require a thick or sensitive skin cover. The aim of the treatment here is to even the nail bed, reduce the hollow caused by the absence of the nail, and, if need be, prepare the area for application of an artificial nail later.

If a large surface of bone is exposed, a flap is preferable, and this, to be cosmetically satisfactory, should be very thin. This is where heterodigital flaps are useful, taken from the adjacent finger or from the dorsal skin of the proximal phalanx of the thumb (Tupper[25]

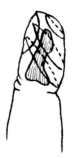

Figure 11.2.6. Oblique palmar amputations

Oblique Palmar Amputations (Fig. 11.2.6)

The problems here are more complex, as the reconstructed pulp should be sensitive and well cushioned.

1. *When the bone is not exposed,* a skin graft is possible. While thin partial-thickness grafts have the advantage of reducing the insensitive area as they retract, total or ''supratotal'' grafts provide better protection. They are usually taken from areas where the skin has similar characteristics to that of the pulp: hypothenar eminence, first commissure, or even the anterior aspect of the wrist or elbow.

2. *When bone is exposed,* a flap must be raised. Only a skin transfer with its neurovascular pedicle or a contiguous homodigital flap can preserve the normal connections between the skin and its nerve supply. The quality of sensation is extremely variable in flaps from a distance and may even be absent if the flap is thick; but it is usually sufficient for protection, although not adequate for precision handling, in heterodigital and palmar flaps. Palmar flaps leave less obtrusive scars, but the position of immobilization is less well tolerated.

These flaps may be good enough for the repair of the ulnar digits, but one should aim for a better result in the thumb, index, and even the middle finger of the dominant hand.

Three types of flaps can be used to provide pulpar sensation: an advanced or translated palmar flap, a homodigital dorsal flap, a heterodigital flap with its neurovascular pedicle.

The Advanced Palmar Flap. Dissection of the palmar digital tissues down to the fibrous flexor sheaths allows an advancement of the superficial planes of about 1 cm (Moberg[18]). The neurovascular bundles should, of course, be spared. It is also possible, as suggested by Snow,[22] to make two lateral incisions; great care must be taken to preserve the dorsal vascular branches supplying the dorsal skin of the middle phalanx, for otherwise these is a definite risk of necrosis (Nicoletis and Morel Fatio[19]). The distal obliquity of these branches makes advancement of about 1 cm possible. We have done it on several occasions without any complications. But it may be safer to follow the suggestion of Hueston,[11] who advocates the use of a single lateral incision which curves in transversely at the base of the finger (Fig. 11.2.7). This

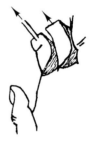

Figure 11.2.7. The advanced palmar flap (Hueston)

produces a larger rotation flap which can be advanced onto the pulp, the bare area at the base of the finger being covered over by a graft or a small dorsal transposition flap (Harrison, 1970). The advancement is facilitated if the phalanges are slightly flexed and the flexion maintained by Kirschner wires; useful extension can be recovered after a few weeks of physiotherapy.

The Translated Pulpar Flap. In cases of loss of tissue on the lateral aspect of the pulp, the teguments can be slid across to the area most useful for prehension. It may be necessary to dissect the neurovascular pedicles in the adjacent healthy zone for their own protection. Thus, if the skin loss is on the radial side of the pulp of the index, a sensitive flap is carried across from the ulnar side and the donor area is covered with a graft.

Dorsal Homodigital Flaps. Flint and Harrison[8] raise a flap centered on the dorsal neurovascular branches (in the injured finger) which arise from the palmar collateral bundles at the level of the middle and distal phalanges. This obliquely cut flap will provide cover for the pulpar defect.

Neurovascular Skin Island Transfers. Extensive pulp loss may lead to such severe functional deficit that heterodigital skin island transfers are sometimes justified. These are technically difficult and are performed at the expense of loss of sensitive skin in another digit. These island flaps are used for the thumb, sometimes for the index finger, but rarely on other digits (Tubiana and Duparc[23]).

It is now well known that these transfers, which carry a well padded, well vascularized and sensitive area of skin, are only useful if the patient can learn to re-interpret the new, displaced sensory information. Only young and active patients can be expected to adapt to this new situation. An island flap is more commonly used from the same finger to bring sensation in a useful area (Fig. 11.2.8).

AMPUTATIONS AT THE LEVEL OF MIDDLE AND PROXIMAL PHALANX

The importance of maintaining the maximum length is not as imperative in case of amputations at the level of the middle and proximal phalanx. Whereas, in distal phalanx amputations, each millimeter counts, at the level of proximal phalanges, one can often shorten the bone to ensure an easy covering of the stump.

The surgical procedure will depend of the length of the skeleton and of the importance of the digit.

Amputations of the Index Finger

In case of shortening of the index, the long finger will replace the index in terminal pinch but the patient will find writing difficult.

A long stump is useful for the key grip between the thumb and index, as well as directional grips.

When the stump is short, amputation of the finger at an elective level will be discussed. Keeping a short stump is advocated to maintain the width of the hand and as a better support for the shaft of a tool. These arguments are valid for a manual worker, but from a cosmetic consideration, amputation at the base of the second metacarpal is preferable; furthermore, it gives a better opening of the thumb web. The transfer of a muscle on the second dorsal interosseous gives a greater strength to the abduction of the long finger. It is

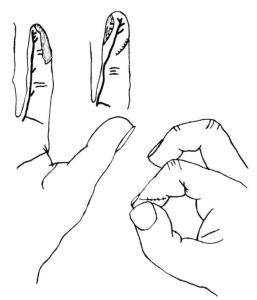

Figure 11.2.8. An island flap is brought from the ulnar side to the radial side of the index extremity.

usual to take the first dorsal interosseous as the transfer (Chase[3]), but another muscle can be used.

Amputations of the Long Finger

When the amputation is at the level of the middle phalanx, impairment is relatively moderate.

The more proximal the amputation, the more patent is the impairment. When fingers are brought together, a hollow remains through which small objects can slip. Furthermore, the key grip thumb-index loses much of its strengh because of the lack of support of the long finger. Lastly, when the stump is very short, the nonsupported index finger bends medially and its tendons deviate from their normal action. Suppression of the third metacarpal cannot alleviate this problem because the second metacarpal is fixed and the fourth has very little mobility. The best way to counteract this disturbance, when it is important, is to transfer the second ray in place of the third (Caroll,[2] Razemon[21]). An osteotomy is done at the base of the second metacarpal keeping in place the insertion of the extensor carpi brevis.

Amputations of the Ring Finger

Impairment due to the amputation of the ring finger is similar to those of the long finger but not as great. The ring finger does not, as the long finger does, take part in the terminal tripod pollici digital grip. The deficiency created by the hollow left by its amputation is partly balanced by the mobility of the fifth metacarpal which brings the little finger close to the long finger, especially if the fourth metacarpal is resected.

Transfer of the fifth ray in place of the fourth may be advocated for cosmetic consideration, but it is less justified than that of the second ray in place of the third (Duparc and Alnot[5]).

Amputations of the Little Finger

The little finger plays an important part in the palmar digital grasp. It is the key of the medial locking of the power grip. This action depends on the length of the ring finger and mobility of its joints. One must try to keep this finger as long as possible if it is mobile. If the stump is short and has only little mobility, it catches when the hand is used, and becomes troublesome. It may be better then to amputate it. The resection of the metacarpal head gives a better cosmetic result.

MULTIPLE AMPUTATIONS

Particular problems are raised by amputation of two or more fingers. One must be more conservative and try to keep the length of the remaining elements. This is to say that a wider use of skin flaps will be necessary. However, multiple injuries render the use of cross finger flaps more difficult and often one must make use of distant flaps. Several small flaps can be taken close to one another either on the opposite limb or on the thorax.

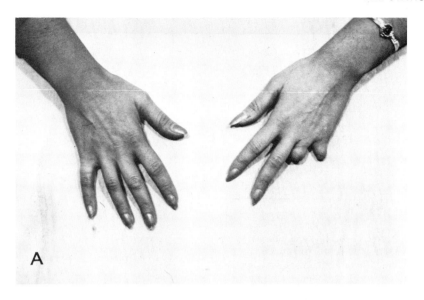

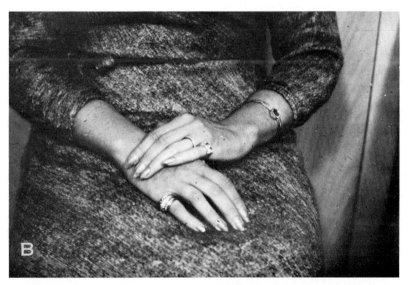

Figure 11.2.9. Cosmetic prosthesis for finger amputations (Dr. Pillet)

Even in the case of multiple amputations of the fingers, a normal thumb usually provides a useful grip against opposable stumps.

Sometimes an osteotomy to rotate a finger or a stump is indicated; it is better to do these osteotomies at the base of the metacarpal.

Phalangization of the fifth metacarpal with osteotomy in flexion and external rotation can be very useful in some cases.

Lengthening of a Digital Stump

In cases of multiple amputations, the lengthening of a digital stump can be considered. It is rarely needed for function if the thumb is intact. Conversely, it is useful if the thumb is itself stiff or shortened.

A lengthened stump is only used by the patient if the extremity is not painful and is sufficiently cushioned by sensitive teguments of good quality. These imperatives considerably reduce the possibility of lengthening by distant flaps. A toe transfer can occasionally be advocated.

The lengthening of a digital stump for purely cosmetic reasons has very rare indications. The use of a silicone finger prosthesis gives better results.

Re-implantations

Re-implantation of an amputated digital extremity has been frequently attempted but with little success. In spite of the optimistic figures of Douglas,[4] it seems unreasonable to attempt the re-implantation of a composite graft in adults without having recourse to microsurgical techniques. For one not familiar with these techniques, it is wiser to cut the skin off the amputated fragment and use it as an autograft.

In young children, however, the chances of survival are greater and immediate re-implantation by peripheral suturing is justifiable.

Cosmetic Prosthesis for Finger Amputations

The cosmetic prosthesis will be of great advantage to the finger amputee if it is capable of giving back its normal appearance to its hand (Fig. 11.2.9). For this purpose both stump and prosthesis have certain requirements.

The Stump. It must be more than 1 cm long, cylindrical, with adequate bone. If it is too thick or bulgy, remodeling will be necessary. If the stump is shorter than 1 cm, fixation will be difficult unless the stump is lengthened by a surgical procedure; but if one wishes to do lengthening and phalangization, these procedures must remain moderate as it is a purely cosmetic result that is looked for and not a functional one.

The Prosthesis. It must reproduce the shape, the skin grain, and the color of the healthy hand. The nail must be set firmly and be suitable for using the different polishes commercially available. The fabric of the prosthesis must be supple, should not harden or shrink, be easily repaired if torn and especially not get dirty or change color. In brief, it must remain stable and not be the cause of any intolerance.

These requirements were never met with polyvinyl chloride prostheses but they are today fulfilled by silicone Prostheses (Pillet[20]).

Results. If conditions for both stump and prosthesis are ideal, the cosmetic results are excellent and the amputees grateful. If conditions are not ideal, results differ, as one can see through statistical material obtained with polyvinyl chloride prostheses.

Out of 1,400 finger amputees treated by Pillet, 30 per cent were regularly followed and, from this number, 50 per cent wore their prosthesis for two years, 25 per cent from two to five years, 15 per cent from five to 10 years, and 10 per cent over 10 years.

Conclusion. Whether or not results seem good or deceiving, it is certain that a finger prosthesis gives more than cosmetic relief. It is a real treatment and as such it is given up when the patient feels "cured" that is to say adapted to his amputation. This is shown by the following case record:

Mrs. G. had an amputation at the distal phalanx of the second, third, and fourth fingers of her right hand. This amputee was so ashamed of the appearance of her hand that she refused to go out of her home. A few weeks after being equipped with her "fingers," she came back to see us very happy although the prostheses were in her bag. Questioned, Mrs. G. answered, "I am very satisfied with my prostheses. I don't use them much, but I know that I have them and can wear them if I wish to."

REFERENCES

1. Ardao. Tratamiento primario de las heridas de las manos. Thesis, Montevideo, 1959.
2. Caroll, R. E. Levels of amputation in the third finger. Am. J. Surg., *97:* 477, 1959.
3. Chase, A. The damaged index digit: A source of componets to restore the crippled hand. J. Bone Joint Surg., *50A:* 1152, 1968.
4. Douglas, B. Successful replacement of completely avulsed portions of fingers as composite grafts. Plast. Reconstr. Surg., *23:* 213, 1959.
5. Duparc, J., Alnot, J. Y., and May, P. Amputations typiques des doigts. Ann. Chir., *25:* 1363, 1970.
6. Erler, F. Zur Versorgung von Kuppensubstanzverlusten an den Fingerendgliedern. Zentralbl. Chir., *70:* 40, 1943.
7. Flint, M. H. Some observations on the vascular supply of the nail bed and terminal segments of the finger. Br. J. Plast. Surg., *8:* 186, 1955.
8. Flint, M. H., and Harrison, S. H. A local neurovascular flap to repair loss of the digital pulp. Br. J. Plast. Surg., *18:* 156, 1965.
9. Hann, J. B. The pattern of ramification of the volar digital nerve in the distal segment of the finger and the relationship of this pattern to the maintenance of sensibility following Kutler type revision of distal finger tip amputations. In *Symposium of Hand Surgery.* Göteborg, 1971.
10. Holevitch, I., and Paneva-Holevitch, E. *Chirurgie de la Main.* Sofia, 1968.
11. Hueston, J. Local flap repair of finger tip injuries. Plast. Reconst. Surg., *37:* 349, 1966.
12. Iselin, M., and Gosse, L. Le lambeau en drapeau. Son emploi systématique dans le comblement des pertes de substance limitées des doigts. Am. Chir. Plast., *7:* 1, 1962.
13. Kleinert, H. Finger tip injuries and their management. Am. Surg., *25:* 41, 1959.
14. Kuhn, H. Le traitement des amputations en coup de hache des phalanges distales. Rev. Chir. Orthopé., *53:* 469, 1967.
15. Kutler, W. A new method for finger tip amputation. J. A. M. A., *133:* 29, 1947.
16. Marchac, D., and Rousso, M. La greffe cutanéo-pulpaire aprés amputation des extrémités digitales. Ann. Chir. Plast., *16:* 51, 1971.
17. McCash, C. Toe pulp free grafts in finger tip repair. Br. J. Plast. Surg., *11:* 322, 1959.
18. Moberg, E. Aspects of sensation in reconstructive surgery of the upper extremity. J. Bone Joint Surg., *46A:* 817, 1964.
19. Nicoletis, C., Morel-Fatio, D. Etranges nécroses. Ann. Chir. Plast., *14:* 56, 1969.
20. Pillet, J. A la recherche d'une main perdue. Rev. Prat., *21:* 603, 1971.
21. Razemon, J. P. La "médialisation digitale" ou la transposition du doigt chef de file dans les séquelles d'amputation des doigts médians. Ann. Chir. Plast., *14:* 162, 1969.
22. Snow, W. The use of a volar flap for repair of finger tip. Amputations: a preliminary report. Plast. Reconstr. Surg., *40:* 163, 1967.
23. Tubiana, R., and Duparc, J. Restoration of sensibility in the hand by neurovascular skin island transfer. J. Bone Joint Surg., *43B:* 474, 1961.

24. Tubiana, R., and Malek, R. *Plaies de la Main.* Paris, Encyclopédie Médico-Chirurgicale, 1968.
25. Tupper, J. The cross-thumb pedicle flap: A study of its functional value. In *Symposium of Hand Surgery,* Göteborg, 1971.
26. Vilain, R. Les pertes de substance cutanée des doigts et leur traitement (à propos de 100 observations). Ann. Chir., *30:* 199, 1954.

C.

Reconstruction of the Thumb

John C. Kelleher, M.D.
James G. Sullivan, M.D.
George J. Baibak, M.D.
Robert K. Dean, M.D.

Absence of a thumb from an otherwise undisturbed hand leaves only a platter upon which objects may be supported or a hook on which they may be hung. Workmen's disability charts furnish numerical values for the catastrophic end product of a thumbless hand. The powerful, yet precise and diverse functioning of a normal thumb not only places a burden on one to whom it is lost, but also places before those who endeavor to replace it a very complex and delicate surgical problem.

The variety of approaches to thumb reconstruction gives evidence not only of the complexity of the problem but also to the never ending search for the near perfect solution. Virtually every procedure which is now enjoying popularity had its inception between 1870 and 1900. Phalangization of the remaining thumb metacarpal or the index metacarpal in the cases of total thumb loss was reported by Hugier in 1874 and 1875.[20] [21] Guiermonprez described techniques for migration of all digits in 1887[18] and Nicelodoni published his reports on abdominal pedicles with bone grafts in 1897,[34] and on great toe transfers in 1900.[35] All of these procedures have undergone scrutiny, revision, and refinement by inventive and arduous surgeons. Albee[1] in 1919 incorporated portions of a clavicle in a pedicle. Broadbent and Wolff incorporated the iliac bone in a one-stage approach to this technique.[3] Advances such as these in the refinement of the neurovascular island by Esser in 1917,[11] made the pedicle flap and bone graft technique a most popular one in the early half of the century as emphasized by its use in the Hand Centers of World War II.

Digit migration was revitalized in the second decade of this century by Perthes[37] and Verral[39] and nearly ten years later, in 1929, Bunnell[6] reported a neurovascular digit migration of an index stump which was the first reconstructed thumb that had both segmental movement and normal sensation including stereognosis. Subsequently (1949 thru 1950), Gossett,[16] Hilgenfeldt,[19] and Littler[29] can be credited with expanding upon and refining the migration of an intact digit as the thumb replacement. Discussion continues as to the digit most suited as a donor, when all the remaining digits are normal. The first choice as a rule is the digit which is partially injured. Reports have been submitted to support arguments in favor of each finger: Machol (1919),[30] Kleinschmidt (1931),[38] Jepson (1925),[22] and Kelleher (1958).[24] The dispute concerning the appropriate donor finger notwithstanding, digit migration has assumed a prominent position in thumb reconstruction over the past 30 years.

Toe to hand pedicle transfers have met with some success in the pre-and post-World War II era. Guelette,[17] Reid,[38] Cuthbert[8] and Clarkson[8] reported occasional good results and more recently, Freeman (1956)[12] has advocated this technique over all methods for thumb reconstruction in children where there is a congenital absence of the thumb. Advances in the use of microvascular surgical techniques by Bunke[5] and Obrien[36] have given new impetus to this approach as well as renewed interest in digit replantation.

Completeness demands recognition of two additional alternatives. It has been advised that in incomplete amputations of the thumb, additional length may be gained by the subperiosteal osteotomy stretching technique of Matev (1970).[31] Epiphyseal transplantation as a free graft (Freeman[13]) has engendered some interest in the recent past but our experience and observations have led us to believe that there is very little effective growth with this type of transplant.

In the following pages, the essentials of normal thumb function will be listed and a classification of thumb loss will be described. This classification will be related to the procedures which would be most suited to each catagory.

Essentials of Normal Thumb Function. We believe that there are four objectives which encompass the major requirements of a functioning thumb. (1) *Opposibility:* The thumb or its substitute must be capable of being placed in a position to meet the remaining fingers of the hand. (2) *Stability:* The thumb or its substitute must be free of undesirable lateral movement and hyperextension once it is brought into its working position. (3) *Length:* The value of stability and proper positioning of the thumb or its substitute may be diminished or even obviated by a lack of proper attention to length requirements. Ideally, the length should be that of the normal thumb which reaches near the middle of the proximal phalanx of the adjacent index finger with the thumb fully adducted. Lesser length can be accepted but is directly related to a reduction in the span of grasp. (4) *Sensibility:* Protective sensation in a thumb or its substitute forms a boundary, below which a less than satisfactory result is certain. Full sensibility including fine two-point discrimination and stereognosis form the ideal goal toward which all reconstructive efforts are aimed.

Restoration of as many as possible of these essentials of a normal thumb with the structures available is an easily defined goal; however, certain limitations are placed on the surgeon which may compromise these goals. It is essential for the surgeon to be aware of these limitations as ignorance of them can lead to an undesirable outcome for both the patient and the physician. A complete history and physical at the initial visit will clarify many of these areas. The patient's age and general condition mandate appropriate restrictions. As age advances, prolonged immobilization itself yeilds increasingly more disability through joint stiffness. Individual situations must be dealt with, *i.e.*, patients suffering from progressive neurologic disorders might not be candidates for digit migration or procedures requiring tendon transfers. The patient's financial resources as well as his available time must be accounted for, as procedures requiring multiple stages and lengthy rehabilitation would be inappropriate for one whose livelihood depended on a brief rehabilitation period. A patient's geographic proximity to a source of qualified care necessitates consideration in the planning of the procedure. Associated injuries or anomalies can restrict alternatives, *i.e.*, a complete amputation of the thumb and all fingers of the same hand makes a digital migration impossible and necessitates selection of other procedures. Finally, all of these factors in conjunction with the patient's activities and thumb requirements must be weighed against the individual's motivation. This factor and the skill of the attending surgeon combine to form a most reliable index of success in the reconstruction of a thumb.

CLASSIFICATION OF THUMB LOSS

This classification is intended to define the deficit present in a given injury and to aid in organizing, in light of our past experience, what we feel is the most appropriate treatment plan.   I. Traumatic
  A. Simple
    1. Soft tissue loss only with bony integrity, with or without intact tendons or capsular ligaments but necessarily with nerve loss (*i.e.*, degloving injury).
    2. Bony destruction with relatively intact skin envelope (*i.e.*, osteomyelitis, tumors, gunshot wounds etc.)
  B. Compound
    1. Group I. Amputation of a segment of the thumb distal to the MP joint but leaving an adequate functioning stump length (*i.e.*, retention of the proximal one-half of the proximal phalanx).
    2. Group II. Amputation immediately distal to or through the MP joint leaving an in-

adequate stump length (*i.e.*, proximal to the midproximal phalanx).
    3. Group III. Amputation through the metacarpal leaving adequately functioning thenar musculature.
    4. Group IV. Amputation near the carpometacarpal joint with loss of thenar muscle function but maintenance of an intact carpometacarpal joint.
    5. Group V. Amputation through or proximal to the carpometacarpal joint.
  C. Complex (any of the above with loss of other members of the same hand).
 II. Functional loss
  A. Neuromotor or proximal structural failure of the part (*i.e.*, the arm cannot be placed in the proper position to use the thumb).
  B. Loss of the opposable post for the thumb (*i.e.*, all of the fingers and metacarpals amputated but the thumb spared).
III. Congenital absence of the thumb.

PLAN OF RECONSTRUCTION

 I. Traumatic
 A. *Simple: Soft Tissue*
The choice of the word "simple" may be an unfortunate one in that it is intended to connote a loss of similar tissues in a unit fashion and, in no way, should it be interpreted as implying an easily resolved problem. Loss of the skin envelope and its closely adherent subcutaneous fat and neurovascular elements poses an immediate and serious threat to the connective tissue architecture of the thumb. Exposed bone, joint capsules, and/or tendons are subject to rapid desiccation and/or bacterial invasion and necrosis if not supplied with a suitable covering that brings in its own blood supply (Fig. 11.3.1).

The structural core of a digit lends itself poorly to the successful take of free skin graft and indeed the salvage of these parts depends upon replacement of the skin envelope with tissue of rich vascular supply. The choice is therefore limited to flap coverage of the degloved thumb.

Soft tissue loss distal to the IP joint is a somewhat less complex problem than loss proximal to this level. V-Y volar advancement flaps[2] or neurovascular island flaps[25] fill the requirements of sensibility and durability on the volar surface whereas dorsal coverage may be obtained readily by cross finger flaps (Figs. 11.3.2 and 11.3.3).

Loss of soft tissue proximal to the IP joint presents a problem of increased complexity. With no loss of skeletal length local flaps cannot be designed to encompass the thumb. Distant flaps must then be planned and applied immediately. The donor site is dependent upon the surgeon's preference. Contralateral upper extremity, thoracic, and abdominal flaps have been utilized. Our preference has been for the lower ab-

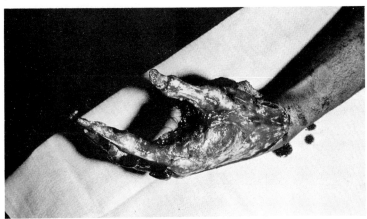

Figure 11.3.1. Twenty-four-year-old male with avulsion injury of the skin of the entire thumb and the-nar cone and entire index and distal two segments of the long finger and portion of the volar pad of the ring finger. There was a retrograde avulsion of the palmar skin.

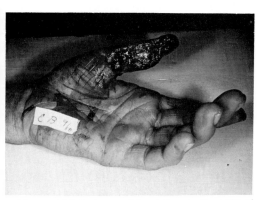

Figure 11.3.2. An avulsion injury to the skin of the volar surface of the thumb from the level of the midproximal phalanx in a 66-year-old woman.

dominal flap as described in a previous publication[25] (Figs. 11.3.4 and 11.3.5).

The donor location notwithstanding all distant flaps bear similar advantages, *i.e.,* bearing their own blood supply, and similar disadvantages, *i.e.,* somewhat bulky soft tissue coverage and poor immediate sensation.

It has been our experience that distant pedicle tissue can and often does attain high quality including stereognosis and two point discrimination (Fig. 11.3.6). This, however, requires a considerable length of time beyond that obtained by neurovascular island transfers and therefore, when feasible, the recuperative process can be hastened by procedures designed to bring neurovascular tissue to the pad of the thumb. The "binocular vision" offered by double pedicle neurovascular islands is ideal; however, single pedicle neurovascular island flaps afford the thumb substitute a sensation which is very acceptable (Fig. 11.3.7). It should be noted that improvement in island

pedicle transfer sensation continues as the neural elements from the skin surrounding the island grow into it giving some crossover in sensation.

It must be noted that the position and stability of the degloved thumb must be dealt with at the initial procedure. Fractures and/or dislocations must be reduced and immobilized. We prefer the use of intramedullary and/or transosseous K wire fixation. The thumb-index web space must be maintained. External and internal wire spreader devices are highly desirable when necessitated. by involvement of the adductor mechanism in the original injury (Fig. 11.3.8). Beyond these measures, however, structural alignment and other procedures such as tendon repair or transfers should not be attempted if it might in any way compromise circulation in an attempt to shorten the reconstructive course. Immediately following this cir-

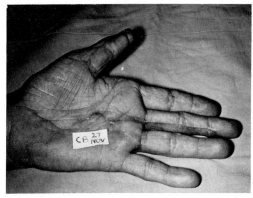

Figure 11.3.3. Final reconstruction of the patient in Figure 11.3.2. An immediate neurovascular island pedicle was constructed from the ulnar surface of the long finger and sutured in place, giving the patient good volar thumb coverage.

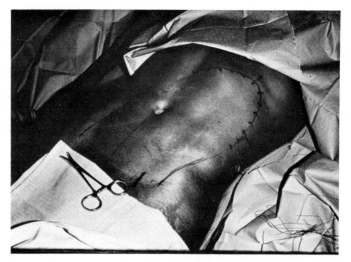

Figure 11.3.4. Exposed bony segments of the long finger were amputated and the wound closed primarily. The ring finger pad was covered with a split thickness skin graft and the palmar retrograde flap was excised and reapplied as a thick split thickness skin graft. The denuded thumb and index finger were enclosed in the pictured abdominal flap.

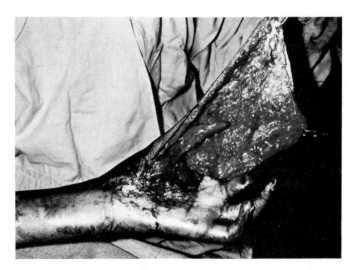

Figure 11.3.5. The detached and thinned abdominal pedicle prepared for application to the bony framework of the thumb. The long finger stump was later filleted and transferred at thumb as a double neurovascular island.

culatory assurance, joint mobility must be attended to. The physical therapist can be of great assistance in a program designed to regain joint motion through active and passive exercises of the involved parts.

B. Simple: Bone Loss

Loss of the bony elements of the thumb whether infectious, traumatic, or neoplastic in origin poses two distinctly different problems, *i.e.,* inadequate length when the phalangeal or metacarpal shaft is lost or inadequate, opposability or stability when joint surfaces or thenar muscles are destroyed. The basic principles of treatment, however, remain unchanged. Length/

and position must be maintained until bony union has occurred or until the soft tissue injuries have resolved.

We prefer to use one of two basic fixation schemes: (1) intramedullary, transarticular or transcortical K wire fixation (Fig. 11.3.9); (2) external fixation devices. The latter can be divided into two types: (a) dynamic splint, *i.e.,* the Boehler[7] splint or external K wire spreader (Figs. 11.3.10 and 11.3.11); (b) static fixation, *i.e.,* The Joe Hall Morris Appliance[33] (Fig. 11.3.12).

Although external splinting is occasionally necessary because of the nature of the soft tissue wounds,

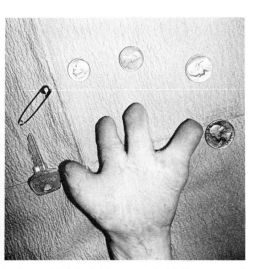

Figure 11.3.6. A 12-year-old girl, 8 years post-operative, abdominal flap coverage to all four dig-its. She is capable of identifying all of the objects pictured and has two point discrimination on the abdominal pedicle skin of 4 mm. Absence of the normal skin ligaments in abdominal pedicle coverage of hands leads to abnormal skin mobil-ity which is less than desirable.

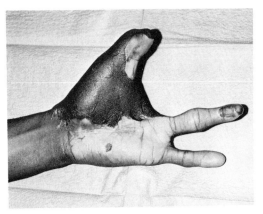

Figure 11.3.7. The final reconstruction of the patient pictured in Figure 11.3.1. This double neurovascular island flap offered the patient near normal thenar function.

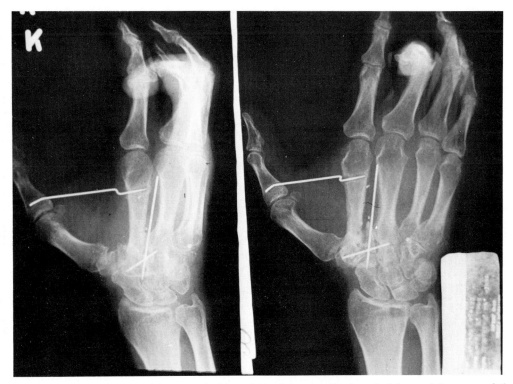

Figure 11.3.8. An internal bayonet-fashioned K wire spreader inserted for maintenance of the thumb-index web space.

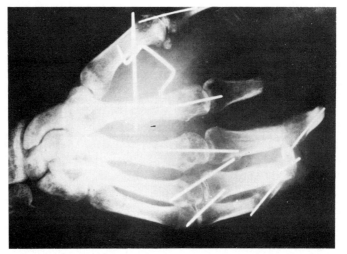

Figure 11.3.9. Examples of transarticular, intramedullary, and transcortical K wires present in this radiograph. In addition, there is an internal thumb-index K wire spreader.

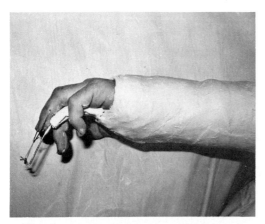

Figure 11.3.10. Boehler skeletal traction as applied to the ring finger in this photo is equally effective in maintaining length in the thumb.

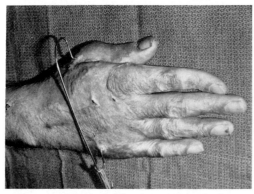

Figure 11.3.11. A Kirschner wire used as a dynamic external spreader device for the thumb-index web space.

we prefer and find most commonly that fixation can be accomplished via one of the above modalities. Interphalangeal joint destruction is best managed by joint fusion. Neither opposition, length, or stability will be significantly compromised by this procedure; however, as with fusion at any interphalangeal joint, prolonged immobilization is necessary for union to occur. The metacarpophalangeal joint likewise lends itself to fusion when the articular surface has been destroyed. Fusion at this level is accomplished more easily and yields no greater disability than fusion at the interphalangeal level. Silastic joint prostheses have been mentioned as an alternative to joint fusion at the metacarpophalangeal joint level but the need for stability of this joint because of the diversity of stresses placed upon it makes the joint prosthesis a less than satisfactory choice.

The carpometacarpal joint, however, poses a slightly different problem. Some measure of movement can be maintained by joint fusion at this level but many individuals require a greater span of movement than carpometacarpal fusion allows and therefore silastic trapezium implants or fascial arthroplasties may offer good alternatives to joint fusion at this level.

When joint surfaces are intact, the thumb length must be either maintained or regained. Proximal ulnar cortex, rib, and iliac crest have all served as donor sites for bone grafts; however, when available and of appropriate quality, other injured components of the same hand should be salvaged and used as the first choice.

We nearly always utilize a mortice and joint bone graft technique in joining the recipient phalanx or metacarpal (Fig. 11.3.13). Bone lengthening procedures as described by Matev[31] may be given consideration in certain selected cases.

B. Compound

The division between Group I and Group II thumb

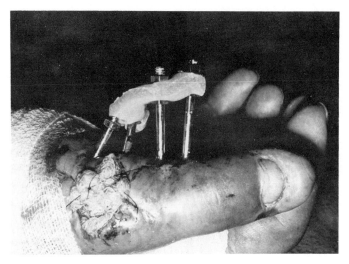

Figure 11.3.12. An external static splint to maintain the thumb length where a segment of bone has been lost.

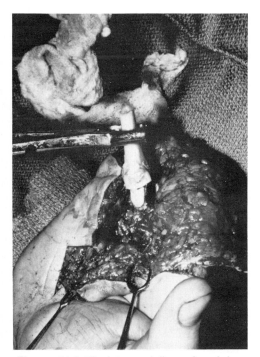

Figure 11.3.13. Intramedullary dowel bone graft.

amputations is necessarily an arbitrary one and indeed the emphasis need be placed on the retained length in the amputated thumb. The patient's requirements and motivation as well as the physician's experience may modify this division; however, it has been our experience that amputations at the metacarpophalangeal joint level will nearly always demonstrate significant disability from the standpoint of inadequate thumb length, whereas amputation at the interphalangeal joint level seldom imposes a significant length problem. We have therefore arbitrarily made the division at the midproximal phalanx recognizing and moreover encouraging the attending physician's judgement in applying this to his own experience. Accepting, therefore, this arbitrary division, Group I composite amputations leave behind one important essential of adequate thumb function, that is adequate length. The thumb index span of grasp may be slightly limited. However, this may be improved by a web-deepening procedure including a Z-plasty of the web space skin. In the use of this procedure, care must be taken to release the distal insertion of the adductor to place it more proximal on the thumb metacarpal shaft. Function in the amputation of the thumb at this level may occasionally require augmentation by deepening the thumb-index web space, however, attention must always be directed towards securing adequately padded skin with good quality sensation over the amputated end of the bone. Lateral V-Y advancement flaps or the volar advancement flap of Kleinert[2] may frequently fulfill all of these requirements; however, one must bear in mind that with the thumb shortened proximal to the level of the interphalangeal joint, pinch is accomplished on the end rather than the volar surface of the pad of the thumb (Fig. 11.3.14). Therefore, good sensory skin coverage must extend over the end of the amputated thumb and cover the surface adjacent to the index finger. In addition, thumb amputations at this level may involve disruption in the insertions of the long flexors and extensors of the thumb. Although it is recognized that this is not a common practice, we feel that reinsertion of these motors at the time of the initial procedure enhances the strength of the thumb in grasping activities.

Thumb amputations in Group II present a problem

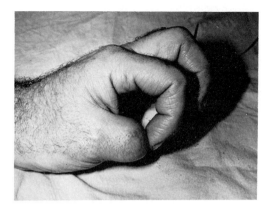

Figure 11.3.14. Pinch between the thumb and the index occurs at the end rather than at the volar pad of the shortened thumb.

of inadequate length which decidedly limits the span of grasp (Fig. 11.3.15). Adequate thenar skin, functioning thenar musculature, and a functional carpometacarpal joint are of inestimable value. The treatment plan, therefore, must be directed toward augmenting length along with good quality sensation at this level of amputation. Thumb-index web space deepening has been advocated for amputation at this level. It has been our experience, however, that only when one can afford to sacrifice the index ray can the deepening procedure produce an adequate thumb-index web space with a satisfactory functioning thumb stump. Recently, a patient was encountered eight years post Group II amputation of the thumb with no surgical intervention. Although a carpenter and claiming absolutely no disability from the injury, on close questioning, it was found that the patient's grasp occurred only between the index and long fingers. The thumb stump was not used except as a hammock to stabilize the handle of a hammer.

Gillies[14] cocked hat and Moberg's[32] technique require mention regarding amputation at this level. An additional 1.0 and 2.0 cm of length may be provided to the thumb stump by these maneuvers. Matev's[31] bone lengthening procedures can also be considered at this level of amputation. However, we have had no experience with this procedure.

The on-top plasty,[26] digit migration, abdominal pedicle, and bone graft with neurovascular island pedicle all readily fulfill the requirements for reconstruction at this level of amputation (Figs. 11.3.16 and 11.3.17).

The space alloted to us in this chapter does not permit us to present the technical details of these surgical procedures. Surgical atlases and the original publications make readily available to any surgeon these important details.

However, we do feel obliged to briefly discuss these procedures from the standpoint of the principles used in their applications. We have referred above to abdominal pedicle and neurovascular island pedicle

flaps as their use pertains to degloving injuries of the thumb. The principles are identical when dealing with the creation of additional length and good quality sensation in the thumb of inadequate length. The point in time at which a bone graft should be included in the

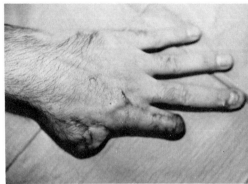

Figure 11.3.15. A Group II thumb loss with associated amputation of the index finger at the proximal interphalangeal joint level.

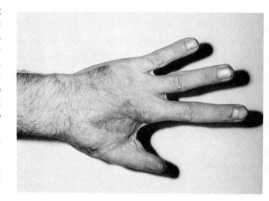

Figure 11.3.16. The span of grasp following on-top plasty transference of the index stump to the remaining thumb metacarpal.

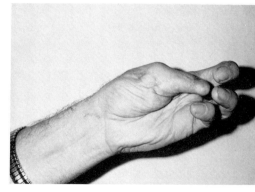

Figure 11.3.17. Flexion and opposition of the reconstructed thumb in a pinching exercise.

pedicle skin remains controversial. It has been our experience that the initial injury may be closed by an abdominal flap and, following detachment and healing, the bone graft may be inserted. If, however, the initial wound had been managed by either primary closure, skin grafting, or healing by secondary intent, the creation of a distant tube flap incorporating a bone graft within it in a single stage is justifiable. Sound arguments exist for either approach and the choice between the two is dictated not only by the experience of the surgeon but also by the severity of bacterial contamination and the presence of concomitant injuries on the initial examination.

One cannot emphasize too strongly the quantity of skin required to resurface the thenar cone in anticipation of thumb reconstruction by whatever method is chosen (Figs. 11.3.4, 11.3.5 and 11.3.20).

The presence of adequately functioning thenar musculature makes the tube pedicle-bone graft-neurovascular island flap approach to an amputation in Group II injuries a satisfactory one. It must be considered, however, that in embarking on this course, one is committed to four or five operative procedures and, therefore, a moderately lengthy reconstructive course. Digit migrations as well as the "on-top plasty" may be considered to offer significant advantages if only from the standpoint of decreasing the number of operative procedures. Immediate digit migration has been described for initial care of an injury at this level (Kaplan).[23] The advantages of this approach under appropriate circumstances are obvious. The "on-top plasty" as well as digit migration offer the advantage of the "binocular vision" of a double pedicle neurovascular island transfer. However, it must be noted that it is both safe and functionally satisfactory to transfer an injured digit on a single intact neurovascular pedicle when the skin which maintains its sensory integrity can be positioned on the opposing surface of the thumb substitute.

Two basic principles are common to "on-top plasties" and digit migrations and indeed may be of some assistance in choosing between the two procedures. We feel that it is axiomatic that where possible an injured digit should always be transferred as a partial or total thumb substitute before sacrificing any normal digit.

1. Proper digital length must be attended to. Both digital migration and the "on-top plasty" at this level should provide appropriate length for the thumb substitute. It must be born in mind, however, that creating a thumb substitute that is too long provides a disability nearly as severe as that present with a thumb of inadequate length. Indeed, when dealing with less significant discrepancies in length, errors in making the thumb substitute too short are tolerated far better than making it too long.

2. In either procedure, the composite flap is transferred on neurovascular pedicles and the success of the transfer is dependent solely on the integrity of these pedicles. We, therefore, feel strongly that the initial

dissection of the neurovascular pedicles should be begun proximally in the palm so that anomalies in the vascular origin that would preclude transfer may be detected early and preplanned alternatives chosen.[15] Should the integrity of the neurovascular pedicles be in question, however, a bridge of dorsal skin may be maintained during the tissue transfer after the method of Hilgenfeldt.

Migration of the normal digit for creation of the thumb substitute remains a controversial area in hand surgery. When dealing with thumb amputation only, the index, long, ring, and small fingers have all been recommended as donors. Critical evaluation reveals strength and weaknesses in each and although our preference remains for migration of the small finger, we feel that no dogmatic statements can be made at this time mandating the choice of one over the other three.

Thumb amputations that fall into Group III pose a transition from the preceding groups to the more complex problems in Groups IV and V. It must be emphasized that the salvage of the carpometacarpal joint and adequately functioning thenar musculature are distinct advantages. As in Group II, inadequate length of the thumb is the prime problem. However, in contrast to amputations at a more distal level in the previous groups, an amputation at this level negates the use of a web space deepening procedure or a lengthening procedure as for example Gillies' bone graft and cocked-hat procedure. In addition, amputation through the metacarpal of the thumb deprives the thenar web and eminence of so much skin that often distant pedicle tissue is necessary before an "on-top plasty," digit migration, or toe transfer could be performed to complete the reconstruction. Recent advances in microvascular surgical techniques makes replantation of a thumb an enticing concept, and where indicated, may indeed prove an invaluable tool in the armentarium of the reconstructive hand surgeon. In many injuries, the amputated segment is either crushed or mutilated beyond use and making replantation impossible.

In thumb amputation in these Groups IV and V, the problems of lack of length and thenar skin are more pronounced than those in Group III. In addition, there is a complex problem of providing a suitable replacement for the muscles of the thenar eminence (Figs. 11.3.18 and 11.3.19).

Adduction and opposition of the reconstructed thumb substitute poses a significant problem to the reconstructive surgeon. The initial management and choice of thumb substitute procedures is identical to that in Group III in that all require additional thenar skin (Fig. 11.3.20). Fusion of thumb post or thumb substitute in a position available for pinch between it and the index ray obviates the need for tendon transfers. This too readily gives up one of the valuable elements of thumb reconstruction, that is movement. Furthermore, when a thumb carpometacarpal joint has been spared as in the situation of Group IV amputations, one should make the greatest imaginative use of this residual highly desirable joint motion.

Tendon graft extension of forearm tendon transfers can reasonably substitute for the missing thumb intrinsics in the reconstructed thumb.

Other local muscles in the hand have served as functional substitutes for the thenar muscles. The location and origin of the hypothenar group of muscles provides us with a powerful bipennate muscle that exerts a great force through a short distance of movement and closely simulates the action of the opponens pollicis and extensor pollicis brevis muscles of the thenar group. The opponens digiti minimi and the other interosseous muscles are in the proper plane of action and have a strong force of movement over a short distance and can be a very suitable adductor when extended to the proper location on the thumb substitute by means of a tendon graft (Figs. 11.3.21, 11.3.22, and 11.3.23).

Amputations in Group V lack all the elements of those in Group IV, but, in addition, the carpometacarpal joint is lost along with the tendon of insertion of the abductor pollicis longus (Fig. 11.3.24).

A suitable thumb substitute can be reconstructed with a skin pedicle and bone graft into the base of the index metacarpal along with a sensory island pedicle flap, but this is devoid of the desirable qualities of movement and "binocular vision."

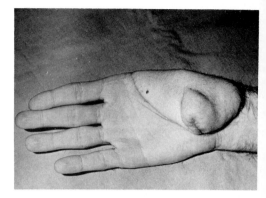

Figure 11.3.20. Patient pictured in Figure 11.3.18 following detachment of the abdominal pedicle utilized for closure of the wound.

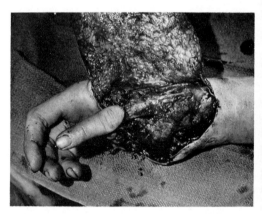

Figure 11.3.21. Small finger transposition was carried out and accomplished adequate length, sensation, and segmental movement. Transfer of the hypothenar muscles provided opposition. The remaining elements of the adductor joined to the base of the middle phalanx by a tendon graft of the flexor digitorum sublimis. The pedicle applied initially was opened, thinned, and draped to cover the new thenar cone.

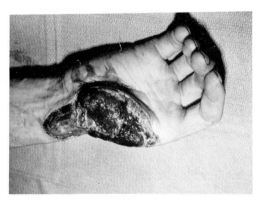

Figure 11.3.18. A Group IV amputation with carpometacarpal joint sparing (see Fig. 11.3.19). Initial coverage was obtained by immediate abdominal pedicle flap.

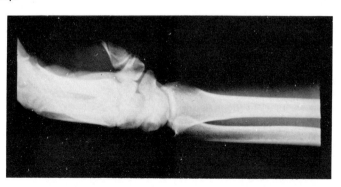

Figure 11.3.19. X-ray of Figure 11.3.18 demonstrating carpometacarpal joint sparing.

An infinitely more satisfactory thumb substitute can be had by the migration of any available digits or parts of digits along with its metacarpophalangeal joint. The neck of the transferred metacarpal is inserted into the carpus or the base of the adjacent metacarpal permitting the metacarpophalangeal joint of the transposed digit to serve as a substitute for the carpo-metacarpal joint of the thumb. Forearm tendon or intrinsic transfers can then be attached to guide the thumb substitute to its proper working position (Fig. 11.3.25). In this type of problem, it is necessary to restore strong abduction by inserting the tendon of the abductor pollicis longus into the base of the proximal phalanx of the transposed digit. Fortunately, in the case illustrated, the abductor pollicis longus was retrieved and fixed to the carpus at the original procedure thereby preserving its function. Strong adductor action is desirable as well (Fig. 11.3.26).

C. Complex

Complex injuries here are defined as those which include loss of the thumb as in any of the five previously listed groups along with one or more digits or parts of the same hand. This type of injury forms the majority of cases seen and, as mentioned in numerous occasions above, often furnishes the reconstructive surgeon with "spare parts" with which to fashion a functional thumb. Included also in this classification are the extremely destructive hand injuries as illustrated in Figure 11.3.27. Indeed it is important in these injuries to retain and salvage all possible parts for potential future use; skin, bone, joints, nerves, and tendons (Fig. 11.3.28). These little bits of tissue when added together can provide the surgeon with many

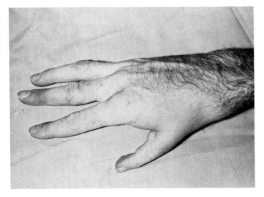

Figure 11.3.22. Extension and abduction of the reconstructed thumb.

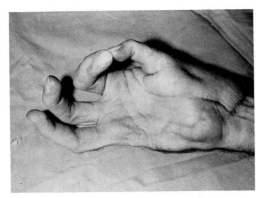

Figure 11.3.23. Pinch and opposition of the reconstructed Group IV amputation.

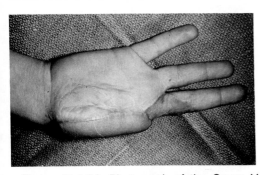

Figure 11.3.24. Photograph of the Group V amputation having been treated initially with split thickness skin graft coverage of the thenar avulsion with subsequent abdominal pedicle coverage.

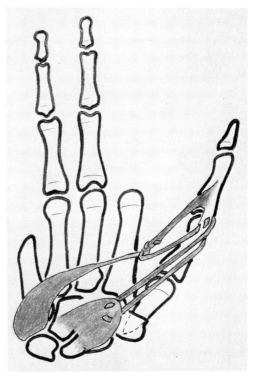

Figure 11.3.25. Thumb reconstruction by little finger transposition impaling the neck of the little finger metacarpal into the trapezium and utilization of the abductor digiti minimi as an opponens transfer and utilization of the opponens digiti minimi as an adductor.

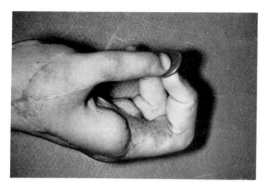

Figure 11.3.26. Function of pinch between the reconstructed thumb and the long finger with adequate strength, span of grasp, segmental movement, and sensation.

elements useful and needed in the restoration of pinch and grasp (Figs. 11.3.29, 11.3.30, and 11.3.31).

II. FUNCTIONAL LOSS

Neuromotor and/or sensory deprivation to an anatomically intact thumb rivals traumatic loss in difficulty in reconstruction. Physical therapy, appropriate joint fusions, tendon transfers, nerve anastomoses, nerve transfers, static or dynamic splinting may all be involved in the reconstruction of the functionally inactive thumb.

Detailed attention must be paid to the functional anatomic position of the thumb as importantly here as in any reconstructive effort.

Traumatic loss of the palm and all digits on a hand with an intact thumb most certainly must be regarded as functional thumb amputation (Fig. 11.3.32). A normal thumb with nothing on which to oppose is of little value. An abdominal tube pedicle with bone graft adds tissue to which the thumb may press objects in a

modified span of grasp and may, with time, develop an extreme degree of dexterity in the use of the thumb against the ulnar post (Figs. 11.3.33 and 11.3.34). Of significance in the creation of an ulnar post is the fact that in such losses no neurovascular island can be conveniently designed with which to resurface the opposing member. As noted above, despite the immediate disadvantage of a skin with poor quality sensation, this approach should not be eliminated in that, with time, the pedicle tissue will acquire a refined quality of sensation.

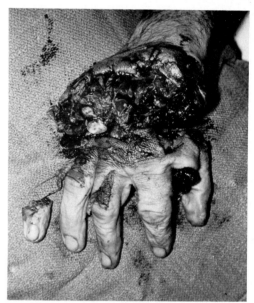

Figure 11.3.27. Complex injury with loss of the thumb equivalent to a Group IV amputation and loss of all of the fingers through the distal metacarpal level.

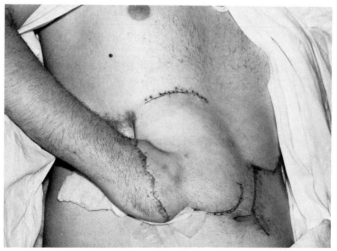

Figure 11.3.28. Immediate abdominal pedicle flap was applied to retain the exposed useful structures that remained and afforded a supple coverage for the final reconstruction.

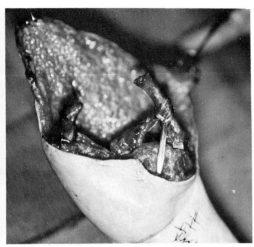

Figure 11.3.29. Remaining portion of the index, long and ring metacarpals were used to create additional length to a member in the thumb position as well as a mobile ulnar member to the two membered hand. Adduction was accomplished by crossing of the retained interossei and opposability by forearm tendon transfers.

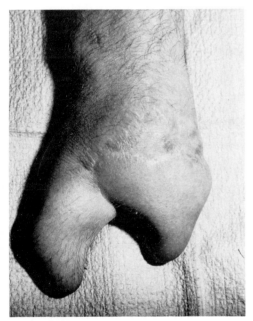

Figure 11.3.30. Three years post injury. Span of opening of the reconstructed two-membered hand accomplished by the retained abductor pollicis longus.

III. CONGENITAL ABSENCE OF THE THUMB

Edgerton, Snyder, and Weber phrased well the problem of congenital thumb reconstruction. "Con-

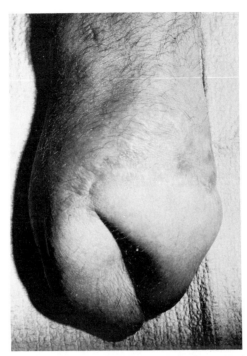

Figure 11.3.31. Firm pinch created by the interosseous adductor type transfers. The sensation in the pedicle tissues is considered quite adequate by the patient and by us.

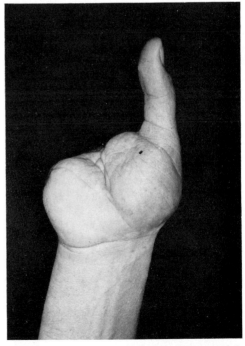

Figure 11.3.32. Loss of all of the fingers with intact thumb having normal movement and sensation.

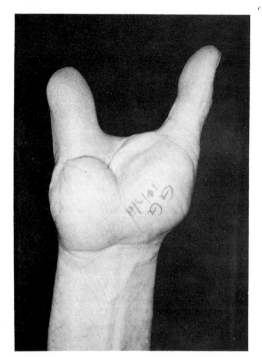

Figure 11.3.33. Demonstrates span of grasp in the final reconstruction.

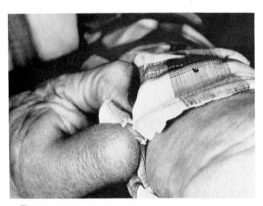

Figure 11.3.34. Demonstrates refined use of the ulnar post in an unbuttoning exercise.

genital deformities of the hand present some of the most difficult problems seen by the hand surgeon. Decisions about timing and methods of reconstruction are complicated by problems of abnormal anatomy, uncertain growth, small structures, and lack of patient motivation or cooperation.''[9] The incidence of congenital thumb absence or significant deformity is indeed difficult to determine. The above named authors determined that 16 per cent of patients with deformity limited to the upper extremity had major thumb defects, whereas upper extremity defects occur at a frequency of 1.9 to 5.4 times per 1,000 births.[10] In addition, these young patients become surprisingly facile in the use of the remaining digits on a thumbless hand.

Indeed, the acquired dexterity often found in these patients makes any surgical intervention a difficult choice. Buck-Gramcko[4] has described an index migration similar in principle to that described in compound Group V amputation. Here the intrinsic muscles of the index finger are transferred to act as adductor and opponens motors. Web space deepening, epiphyseal transplantation, bone graft techniques, digit migrations, and toe to hand transfers all contribute to thumb reconstruction in these patients and the basic principles are the same as in the traumatic thumb loss (Figs. 11.3.35, 11.3.36, and 11.3.37). Consideration need be given to operative timing. Indeed, the earlier the reconstruction is completed the less well entrenched will be the substitution movements learned by the child and more easily the adaptation to the reconstructed thumb; however, the hazzards alluded to

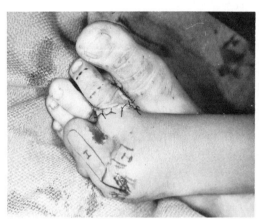

Figure 11.3.35. A pedicle transfer of the second toe to the thumb position in a hand congenitally devoid of all digits. The index metacarpal had at an earlier stage been transferred to the long finger metacarpal as diagramed on the dorsum of the hand.

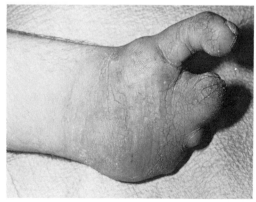

Figure 11.3.36. Span of grasp 14 years post reconstruction with evidence of callus formation over the reconstructed thumb and ulnar member indicating obvious use.

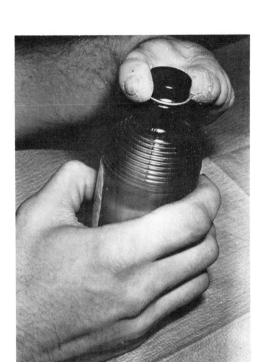

Figure 11.3.37. Demonstrates the patient using the toe-to-hand transfer in a grasping exercise.

by Edgerton, Snyder, and Weber[9] have led us to select carefully those cases amenable to early reconstruction.

SUMMARY

In summary, we would like to emphasize our approach to thumb reconstruction as it relates to our concept of the essentials of a functioning thumb.

I. Traumatic
  A. Simple: Soft tissue
    The structural core of the thumb requires skin coverage of rich vascular content and the end result is dependent to a significant degree on the final sensory function of the reconstructed thumb.
    Simple: Bone loss
    Inadequate length and/or stability as occasioned by loss of the bony shaft and/or articular surfaces must be treated by bone grafting and/or arthrodesis or arthroplasty.
  B. Compound
    Group I. Seldom requires more than adequate skin coverage with good sensation.
    Group II. Length augmentation in addition to sensory skin replacement are the requirements in this group.
    Group III. Length requirements at this level exceed those in Group II and necessitate more complex reconstructive procedures, as well as, frequent addition of distant pedicle skin prior to thumb reconstruction.
    Group IV. Additional thenar skin is nearly always necessary at this level of amputation and, in addition to the problems of the above groups, thenar muscle function must be substituted with tendon transfers.
    Group V. All of the problems listed above exist in this group of amputations. In addition, a replacement for the carpometacarpal joint must be fashioned.
  C. Complex
    These decastating hand injuries nearly always require distant pedicle coverage for "spare part" salvage. This principle forms the basic for the treatment of these hand problems.
II. Functional
  Completeness demands inclusion of this catagory and an example of an anatomically normal but functionally useless thumb is described.
III. Congenital
  Treatment plans in thumb reconstruction of congenitally absent or deformed thumbs must be coordinated with the patient's age; however, the goals of thumb reconstruction here are identical to those of the above described groups.

Acknowledgment. The authors would like to express their gratitude to Mr. Jon F. Frye, Mr. Jack Schaefer, The St. Vincent Hospital and Medical Center, and Dr. John H. Robinson for their assistance in the completion of this chapter.

REFERENCES

1. Albee, F. H. Synthetic transplantation of tissues to form new finger. Ann. Surg., *69:* 349, 1919.
2. Atasoy, E., Iokimidis, E., Kasdan, M., Kutz, J. E., and Kleinert, H. E. Reconstruction of the amputated finger tip with a triangular volar flap. J. Bone Joint Surg., *52A:* 921, 1970.
3. Broadbent, T. R., and Woolf, R. M. Thumb reconstruction with contiguous skin-bone pedicle graft. Plast. Reconstr. Surg., *26:* 494, 1960.
4. Buck-Gramcko, D. Eine ungewohnliche Behandlungsmethode eines Strocksehnenausrisses mit Knochenbeteiligung. Hand Chir., *3:* 1971.
5. Buncke, B. M., Buncke, C. M., and Schulz, W. P. Immediate Nicolodoni procedure in the rhesus monkey, or hallux-to-hand transplantation, utilising microminiature vascular anastomoses. Br. J. Plast. Surg., *19:* 332, 1966.
6. Bunnell, S. Physiological reconstruction of a thumb after total loss. Surg. Gynecol. Obstet., *52:* 245, 1931.
7. Bunnell, S. *Surgery of the Hand.* Philadelphia, Lippincott, 1956.
8. Clarkson, P. Reconstruction of hand digits by toe transfer. J. Bone Joint Surg., *37A:* 270, 1955.
9. Edgerton, M. T., Snyder G. B., and Webb, W. L. Surgical treatment of congenital thumb deformities (including psychological impact of correction). J. Bone Joint Surg., *47A:* 1453, 1965.
10. Entin, M. A. Reconstruction of congenital aplasia of phalanges in the hand. Surg. Clin. North Am., *48:* 1155, 1968.
11. Esser, J. F. S. Island flaps. N. Y. Med. J., *106:* 264, 1917.
12. Freeman, B. S. Reconstruction of thumb by toe transfer. Plast. Reconstr. Surg., *17:* 393, 1956.

13. Freeman, B. S. The results of epiphyseal transplants by flap and by free graft: A brief survey. Plast. Reconstr. Surg., *36:* 227, 1965.

14. Gillies, H., and Millard, D. R., Jr. *The Principles and Art of Plastic Surgery.* Boston, Little Brown, 1972.

15. Goldwyn, R. M. *The Unfavorable Results in Plastic Surgery: Avoidance and Treatment.* Boston, Little Brown, 1957.

16. Gosset, J. F. La pollicisation de l'index (technique chirurgicale). J. Chir., *65:* 403, 1949.

17. Guelette, R. J. Etude critique des procédés de restauration de pouce. J. Chir., *36L1,* 1930.

18. Guiermonprez. Notes sur Quelques, Resechens et Rastaurations de Pouce. Paris, P. Asselin, 1887.

19. Hilgenfeldt, O. Operativer Daumenersatz, S. 80/81. Stuttgart, Ferdinand Enke, 1950.

20. Hugier, P. C. Considerations anatomiques et physiologique pour sevir a la chirurgie du pouce et sur la chirurgie de cet organe. Arch. Gen. Med., *2:* 404, 1873.

21. Hugier, P. C. Considerations anatomiques et physiologiques pour sevir a la chirurgie du pouce. Arch. Gen. Med., *1:* 54, 1874.

22. Jepson, P. N. Transformation of middle finger into thumb. Minn. Med., *8:* 552, 1925.

23. Kaplan, I. Primary pollicization of injured index finger following crush injury. Plast. Reconstr. Surg., *37:* 531, 1966.

24. Kelleher, J. C., and Sullivan, J. G. Thumb reconstruction by fifth digit transposition. Plast. Reconstr. Surg., *21:* 470, 1958.

25. Kelleher, J. C. Plast. Reconstr. Surg., *39:* 448, 1967.

26. Kelleher, J. C., Sullivan, J. G., Baibak, G. J., and Dean, R. K. "On-top plasty" for amputated fingers. Plast. Reconstr. Surg., *42:* 242, 1968.

27. Kelleher, J. C., Sullivan, J. G., Baibak, G. J., and Dean, R. K. Use of a tailored abdominal pedicle flap for surgical reconstruction of the hand. J. Bone Joint Surg., *52A:* 1552, 1970.

28. Kleinschmidt, O. Zum Ersatz der Daumens durch die zweite Zehe. Arch. Klin. Chir., *164:* 809, 1931.

29. Littler, J. W. The neurovascular pedicle method of digital transposition for reconstruction of the thumb. Plast. Reconstr. Surg., *12:* 303. 1953.

30. Machol. Beitrag zur Daumenplastik. Beitr. Klin. Chir., *114:* 181, 1919.

31. Matev, I. B. Thumb reconstruction after amputation at the metacarpophalangeal joint by bone - lengthening. J. Bone Joint Surg., *52A:* 957, 1970.

32. Moberg, E. Aspects of sensation in reconstructive surgery of the upper extremity. J. Bone Joint Surg., *46A:* 817, 1964.

33. Morris, J. H. Biphase connector, external skeletal splint for reduction and fixation of mandibular fractures. Oral Surg., *2:* 1382, 1949.

34. Nicalodoni, C. Daumen plastik Wier. Klin. Wochnschr., *10:* 663, 1897.

35. Nicalodoni, C. Daumenplastik and organischer Ersatz der Fingerspitze (Anticheiroplastik and Daktyloplastik). Arch. Klin. Chir., *61:* 606, 1900; Weitere Erfahrungen uber Daumenplastik. Arch. Klin. Chir., *69:* 695, 1903.

36. Obrien, B. M., Crock, G. W., Bennett, R. C., Henderson, P. N., and Galbraith, J. E. K. Experimental and clinical microsurgery (abstract). Plast. Reconstr. Surg., *47:* 516, 1971.

37. Perthes, T. Uber plastichen Daumenersatz insbesodere bei verlast des ganzen Daumenstrahles. Arch. Orthop. Unfallchir., *19:* 14, 1921.

38. Reid, D. A. C. Reconstruction of the thumb. J. Bone Joint Surg., *42B:* 444, 1960.

39. Verral, P. J. Three cases of reconstruction of the thumb. Br. Med. J., *2:* 775, 1919.

chapter twelve

Burns and Frostbites

A.

Radiation Burns

Frederick C. Hansen, M.D.
Milton T. Edgerton, M.D.

INTRODUCTION

This chapter deals with injuries to the hand caused by radiant energy in its many forms. Man has always lived bathed in a low level of radiation from natural sources and this may well have played a role in the evolutionary process. As 20th century technology attempts to harness these forces, new types of injuries will now challenge the surgeon.

By the very nature of the work with these new radiation sources, a large portion of these injuries involve the hands. While the literature is filled with examples of injury from the early use of x-rays and radium, the newer more powerful radiation sources have been treated with extreme caution and only a very few injuries have been documented.

The injuries will be considered in certain broad catagories and although the degrees of injury may differ, depending on the conditions of exposure, there is a basic theme common to all radiation injuries which distinguishes their management.

HISTORICAL CONSIDERATIONS

A consideration of the historical events leading up to the first x-ray burns helps explain why they occurred in such great numbers.

On November 8, 1895, Wilhelm Konrad Roentgen first noted that a Crooke's tube caused a greenish glow near the glass jacket. In studying this he detected an emanation with the ability to penetrate dense matter and expose photographic plates. He completed his paper "On A New Kind of Ray" before the end of the year and a preliminary report was made on January 5, 1896, in the Vienna *Presse*. The news reached America the following day and on that very day Thomas A. Edison began to experiment with the new Roentgen rays.

This was the age of discovery. Many scientists had been aware of these mysterious rays and had been working with the various gas tubes and vacuum tubes capable of producing them. The truly significant aspect of Roentgen's observation was that the rays penetrated dense matter and that they were absorbed more by bone than by soft tissues so that pictures of the bones could be made through the flesh.

There was a great flurry of excitement as physicians adopted this miraculous new tool. Within a month of Roentgen's announcement, Emil H. Grubbe, a Chicago vacuum tube manufacturer and experimenter, was diagnosed as having a dermatitis induced by x-ray exposure. He went on to have 97 operations for his extensive x-ray burns. Several of Edison's laboratory assistants developed radiation dermatitis, and one of them, Clarence Dolly, went on to become the first death from x-ray-induced cancer.

Professor Elihu Thompson, of Harvard, corresponded with E. A. Codman who published the letters in the Boston *Medical and Surgical Journal*. His letter with its classical description of an acute injury is quoted: "November 21, 1896... I am just now nursing an x-ray finger which is a striking example of what x-rays may do if the exposure is long enough. Hearing of the effects of x-rays on the tissues, especially on the skin, I determined to find out what foundation the statements had by exposing a single finger to the rays. I used for this the little finger of the left hand, exposing it close up to the tube, about one and one-quarter inches from the platinum source of the rays for one-half hour. For about nine days very little effect was noticed, then the finger became hypersensitive to the touch, dark red, somewhat swollen, stiff, and soon the finger began to blister. The blistering started at the maximum point of action of the rays, spread in all directions, covering the area exposed so that now the epidermis is nearly detached from the skin underneath, and between the two there is a formation of purulent matter which escapes through a crack in the blister. It will be three weeks today since the exposure was made and the healing process seems to be as slow as the original coming on of the trouble. While the pain and sensitiveness have largely left the finger within the last day or two and the blister now covers the whole exposed back and sides of the finger, I think the finger will soon heal, but I assure you that I will make shorter exposures hereafter...."

In January of 1898, Frank Boyd, M.D., of Paducah, Kentucky, wrote to the J.A.M.A. editors to say that he had been sued for malpractice in the amount of $10,000 for producing a severe and painful x-ray dermatitis in one of his patients. He won the case on the grounds that he had exercised usual caution.

By 1949, Leddy and Rigos[23] were able to report the Mayo Clinic series of 135 cases of radiodermatitis among physicians, of which 125 cases involved the hands. The left hand was involved about seven times more often than the right hand since it was standard practice to use the left hand for a trial to determine exposure while operating the machine with the right hand.

RADIATION PHYSICS

Because the type and the course of radiation injuries may vary with the type of exposure, detailed consideration of radiation biology is necessary for rational treatment.

While it is somewhat inconsistent with the modern concepts of physics, it is both convenient and traditional to divide radiant energy into two types: electromagnetic and corpuscular.

Electromagnetic radiation is a wave type of energy which can be characterized by its wave length.

These waves may be refracted and reflected under certain conditions like ordinary light and differ from one another only in their wave length.

Corpuscular radiation consists of subatomic particles which travel with a speed which depends on their mass and energy. By subatomic particle is meant any individual part of an atom (i.e., a neutron or electron); or an atom minus one or more of its component particles (i.e., a helium nucleus or oxygen nucleus).

The naturally occurring radioactive substances such as radium, thorium, actinium, and uranium have unstable atomic nuclei and undergo a spontaneous release of energy. A portion of this may be gamma radiation but the majority will be alpha and beta particles.

Different radioactive substances will have different "half lives" and this will be an important consideration if they become implanted in tissues. (E.g., radium has a half life of 1,638 years and gives off alpha, beta, and gamma radiations which for all practical purposes will be constant throughout a lifetime. Radioactive phosphorus P^{32} has a half life of 14.3 days and emits only beta particles. After eight weeks the radiation output will be less than one-sixteenth the initial level.)

RADIATION BIOLOGY

Radiation injury results from the introduction of excessive energy into the stable chemical systems of the cells by the incident radiation. Both long wave length electromagnetic radiations and "soft" or low voltage x-rays deliver their energy chiefly by excitation. That is, the added energy causes electrons to jump from an atom's inner orbit to an outer orbit. The shorter wave length radiations of the electromagnetic spectrum and all of the corpuscular radiations deliver their energy chiefly by causing the atom to lose an electron, thus forming a positive and negative ion pair or by striking an atom and causing it to give off various type of secondary radiations.

The physiologic result of this injection of excessive energy into the cell may be alterations of membrane permeability, injury to new enzyme synthesis, or disruption of nucleic acid synthesis and cell division. The injury may be reversible or irreversible and its consequences may: temporarily alter cell function, permanently alter cell function, or destroy cell function.

It is the partially injured cells which characterize the radiation injury. The lethally radiated tissues undergo necrosis and are sloughed, leaving a wound which is based on sublethally injured tissues. The blood supply, which for the first three weeks may be increased in response to the injury, becomes greatly diminished by thrombosis and endothelial proliferation and there is a slowness or absence of fibrous tissue proliferation and capillary budding which would be seen in a normal granulating wound. If the wound re-epithelializes the tissues still remain thin and atrophic.

Low penetration radiations such as ultraviolet and soft x-rays and alpha and beta particles tend to produce maximum injury at the surface of entry and the damage falls off with depth. In contrast, the high energy radiations cause most of their damage by producing secondary radiations in the tissue so that tissues at the surface of entry, having the least other matter about it, would receive little secondary radiation and the least injury. This latter phenomenon is the so called "skin-sparing effect of high energy radiation." With structures of small volume, such as the hand, they may injure the skin at the site of exit more than at the site of entry.

The relative radio sensitivity of the tissues in the hand is important in understanding the patterns of injury. Tissues in which the cells reproduce and shed rapidly will be most susceptible to radiation injury because of its adverse effect on mitosis. A sebaceous gland, which actually secretes its cells containing oil, will be expected to have a higher cell turnover rate than a sweat gland which produces its secretion without loss of cells. The lethal dose of x-ray for a sebaceous gland is 1,200 and for a sweat gland is 2,500. The epidermis, which is constantly molting, is intermediate in sensitivity. The tissues of the hand in order of decreasing sensitivity to x-rays are: blood forming tissue of marrow, skin, endothelium of vessels, connective tissue and fat, bone, nerve muscle.

While the great bulk of experience is concerned with injuries produced by x-ray, x-ray and radioactive sources, the Department of HEW has established a

Radiation Incidents Registry which accumulates these injury reports plus any injuries related to electronic devices. This may be briefly summarized:

Microwaves

These wave lengths have produced few reports of hand injury. They cause heat in tissue by the induction of molecular motion and electric currents. Injury is most likely where circulation is poor and the heat produced is not transferred. Most reported injuries have involved the cornea and lens of the eye and the testes, but one can see the potential for injury to the cartilage of the articular surfaces.

Infra Red

These burns are superficial and ''line of sight'' in pattern. A thin layer of moisture, clothing, a ring, or bandaid may spare the area covered, whereas black garments or dirt may increase the burn to underlying skin. The thin skin of the dorsum of the hand is more susceptible to flash burns than the thick palms.

Visible Spectrum

The wide applications of laser energy has so far resulted in injuries mainly limited to the skin and eye. As the power of lasers is increased, hand injury will, undoubtedly, occur, but present indications are that they will resemble thermal injuries.

Ultra Violet

These wave lengths are stopped at the surface layers of the skin. Wave lengths from 3,200 Å to 2,900 Å cause the injury to tissues and, like x-rays, produce an injury which becomes manifest after a latent period.

Ultraviolet exposure can produce mutations in onecell organisms and in the germinal cells of insects. Normally, the injury from ultraviolet is limited to the upper, nonmitotic layers of the epidermis. However, in fair skin or thin, senile skin, the injury may reach into the germinal layers to produce premalignant changes.

TYPES OF INJURIES

The clinical picture of a radiation injury to the hand by conventional x-ray is a characteristic series of events which may be grouped according to the degree of exposure.

Moderate Acute Injury

There is no sensation or awareness of injury at the time of exposure, but a transient erythema will develop in a few hours and then fade away. After seven to 10 days of apparent normalcy, a second wave of erythema develops which, if the exposure was mild, will progress to an increase in melanin pigmentation and not much else. With greater exposure it will lead from erythema to painful blistering and superficial ulceration. Healing will be slow, taking weeks to

months for a thin, dry skin to redevelop. Telangiectasis and premalignant keratoses will develop as the years pass.

Severe Acute Injury

Again the initial course is the same except that the pain is more severe after blistering. On about the 30th day, instead of the skin healing, a painful slough begins. Usually this ulcer will not heal, but if it should, breakdown occurs in a short while (Fig. 12.1.1).

Massive Acute Injury

This type of injury is generally associated with fatal total body irradiation. Lanzl and Rosenfeld[22] report a case of 40,000 to 240,000 rads to a right hand and leg. Careful, conservative management, including percutaneous cervical electric chordotomy to control pain, was of no avail and double ampuation occurred six months after exposure. Swelling and redness comes on immediately after such massive exposure.

Chronic Injury

Repeated exposure to low levels of radiation produces insidious onset of radiation dermatitis. Characteristic changes include permature aging of the skin which becomes thin, dry, wrinkled, hyperkeratotic with loss of hair, sweat, and sebaceous glands, and atrophy of underlying fat. The nails becomes distorted, grooved, and thin. Ulceration and malignant degeneration are the ultimate result (Fig. 12.1.2).

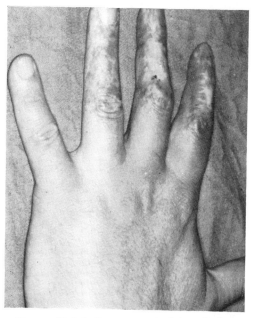

Figure 12.1.1. Severe acute injury to fingers sustained during diagnostic fluoroscopy. While this tissue healed in six months after injury, it is painful and frequently breaks down with the most minor trauma.

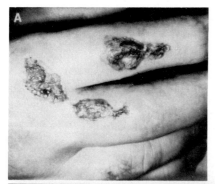

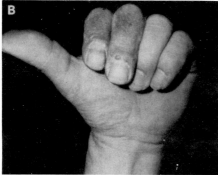

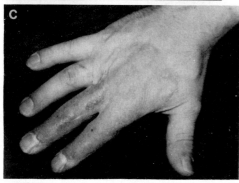

Figure 12.1.2. A. A patient of Krizek's showing ulcerations and eschar resulting three months after exposure to 19,500 rads of 110 KUP x-radiation. *B* and *C.* Result 12 months after excision and split thickness skin grafting.

There is little data on the relationship between dose and malignant degeneration but it is seen more commonly after multiple small doses for benign conditions then after large doses for malignant conditions.

TREATMENT

Treatment of the radiation injury of the hand involves all of the principles which apply generally to hand injuries but there are special additional considerations with radiated tissue.

The classical work on the treatment of the acute x-ray injury is that of Porter[31] together with Wol-

bach's[40] classical description of the pathologic histology of x-ray injuries. The basic conclusions of both of these papers remain unchallenged today, although greater efforts are made now to repair the severely damaged digit and amputation is rarely used primarily.

The victim of a heavy, acute exposure will have great anxiety. If he was aware of the exposure, he has had the 10- to 15-day asymptomastic latent period to anticipate the onset of a possibly crippling injury. At the time of the first visit to a surgeon, psychiatric consultation should be considered.

By the time most acute radiation injuries are seen by a surgeon, the latent period will be past and the most severe problem may be the management of the extreme pain. The surgeon may be implored to amputate the painful member. The patient should be reassured, if at all possible, that his hand will once again be useful. Pain should be well controlled with analgesics.

The wound should be treated conservatively with some bland dressing such as Xeroform gauze or saline dressings and gentle, active motion started.

If the wound goes on to heal in four to eight weeks, there is no need for intervention and the skin should be observed periodically, delaying any grafting until necessitated by subsequent changes. If the healed skin becomes atrophic, scarred, dry, and vulnerable to minor trauma, it is wise to recommend excision and split thickness skin grafting of the involved skin.

Excisions of localized radio dermatitis must extend beyond gross clinical changes to include a margin or normal skin. If this is not done, subsequent changes in the residual injured skin about the edges of the skin graft will likely lead to further breakdown. As in most reconstructive surgery, surface repair must coincide with or *precede* repair of deep structures. The success of repair of irradiated *hand* structures is especially dependent on the quality of repair of the integument (Fig. 12.1.3).

When the initial injury progresses to an ulceration which fails to heal, it must be excised, including any partly healed margins about the ulcer. Even though some areas may have healed in, they should be excised along with the ulcer. The entire area should be grafted immediately with split thickness skin grafts. Debridement and delayed grafting, as used sometime with thermal burns, is *not a good plan with radiation burns!* The excision may be down to tissue which appears normal but is partially injured and if covered immediately this ''marginal tissue'' will survive but, if left uncovered by skin grafts, it will result in additional tissue loss. Radiated tissue left uncovered will frequently fail to granulate but, instead, will develop a yellowish-white hyalin pseudomembrane which will not accept a graft. These ulcers are characterized by great pain and the patients may dread a change of dressing.

Should the injury uncover tendons or joint spaces, flap coverage will be required, but the tendency of

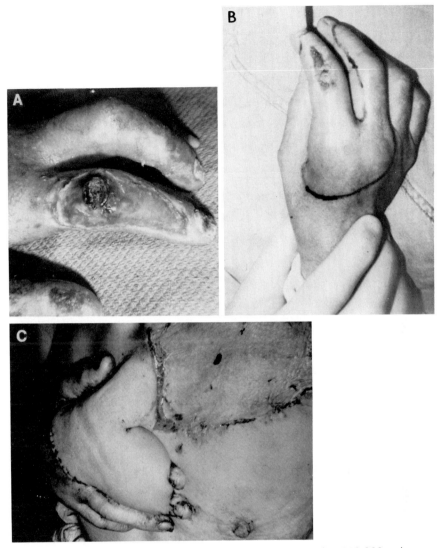

Figure 12.1.3. A and *B*. Another patient of Krizek's three months after 250,000 rad exposure from 110 KUP x-radiation. Both hands severely involded. *C*. Pectoral flap used to resurface right hand. *D, E,* and *F*. Same patient 12 months after flap coverage of excised radiation burns and ray resection of left index finger. The hands are pain free and have moderate function.

some surgeons to use a flap on *all* radiation injuries should be avoided. Think first of free grafts. Flap coverage is usually indicated when the blood supply of the base of the wound is poor or if bare tendons, joints, or bones are exposed. Again the flap edge should be carried to normal tissue. The extensor or flexor tendons may be exposed in the base of an open irradiation ulcer. If their gross structure is preserved and they are not involved by frank suppuration, they may be left under a flap after careful debridement of adjacent necrotis tissue. With very deep ulcers it may be necessary to remove not only the exposed tendons but also the cortex of exposed bone before covering with a flap (Fig. 12.1.4).

Open direct pedicle flaps are much superior to the construction and migration of tube pedicles, both from the standpoint of economy and function. Abdominal flaps tend to be excessively bulky and make management during the period of attachment somewhat difficult. In male patients or in women who will not be concerned by donor site scars, the clavicular flap offers several advantages. They are thinner, have a better blood supply, and allow a more comfortable position for the patient. Because of their thinness and excellent blood supply, more complete tailoring is possible at the time of implantation. Any flap intended for application to a radiation injury must have an excellent blood supply, for the irradiated recipient site may have

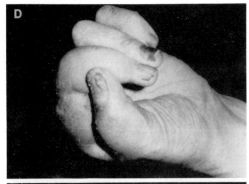

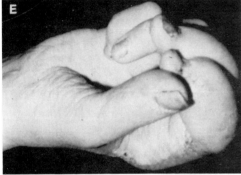

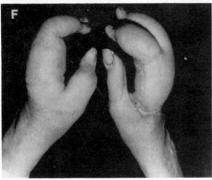

Figure 12.1.3 D — F

an injured blood supply and any flap with a poor circulation will not gain attachment. The division of the flap pedicle should be delayed for longer than usual and performed cautiously or in stages since the blood supply of the recipient base may be slow to invade the flap.

The concept of local flap rotation or advancement from the wrist to the dorsum of the hand is of particular value with irradiation ulcers. These "blood bearing" flaps give *permanent* additional circulation to the injured area. Even bone with a pathologic fracture (from irradiation) has been known to heal promptly as a result of such flap coverage.

In situations where small irradiation burns of predictable outcome are seen, the course of least debility and time loss will be to excise them and apply grafts at 12 to 24 hours after injury. At that time the first wave

of erythema demarcates the extent of the injury. Shipman,[33] cited by Brown, reports success with this treatment in small beta ray burns.

Injures to the hand have occurred with nuclear reactors or while handling radioactive substances. If these injuries are associated with sublethal total body radiation, Allen[1] has pointed out it may be prudent to do any anticipated surgery during the first two to three days after exposure so that healing will be well along before symptoms of radiation sickness develop. Conceivably ulcerations or other conditions which might result in a fatal infection during the prolonged radiation sickness may be treated and healed by taking advantage of the normal healing during the two- to three-week latent period between injury and onset.

The management of chronic exposure injuries may be divided into benign and malignant conditions but the benign conditions generally must be managed as premalignant conditions. Sailor's skin, farmer's skin, or actinodermatitis from chronic solar exposure, and the radio dermatitis from chronic x-ray exposure have more similarities than differences. The atrophic skin has mottled pigmented and depigmented areas, telangiectases, keratoses, wrinkles, crusts, fissures, and, finally, painful ulcerations. The keratoses are premalignant and they should be excised. The chronic dermatitis may become such a problem as to render the hands unfit for work. Since it is generally the dorsum of the hand which is involved, the results of excision and thick split skin grafting will be most gratifying.

Desiccation of keratoses is frequently recommended but we have preferred to excise and close or excise and graft, feeling that tissue examination for areas of malignant change is important. Any chronic ulceration or proliferative lesion must be examined for cancer. Squamous cell tumors occur most frequently but cell cancers are found and sarcomas and melanomas are reported. They tend to be low grade and a minority will show spread to regional lymph nodes.

Wide local excision is generally satisfactory for epitheliomata of the hand but an amputation of a digit, a ray, or a segment of the hand may be necessary if the cancer invades the deep investing fascia of the hand.

Scarring of the fingernails or deep grooving and distortion of them may result from radiation injury to the nail's follicle and bed. They may be bothersome by snagging on clothing and collecting debris. Excision of the complete nail follicle and bed and replacement by a nail-shaped full thickness or thick split skin graft will give improved functional and cosmetic results.

Finally consideration must be given to the hand wound contaminated with radioactive material. The physician whose responsibility it is to care for these injuries must acquaint himself beforehand with the properties of the substances he is apt to be dealing with to include the solubility, the type of emissions, and the radioactive half life. In addition, he should know how the substance is eliminated from the body and how this may be enhanced. If the radioactive material is liable

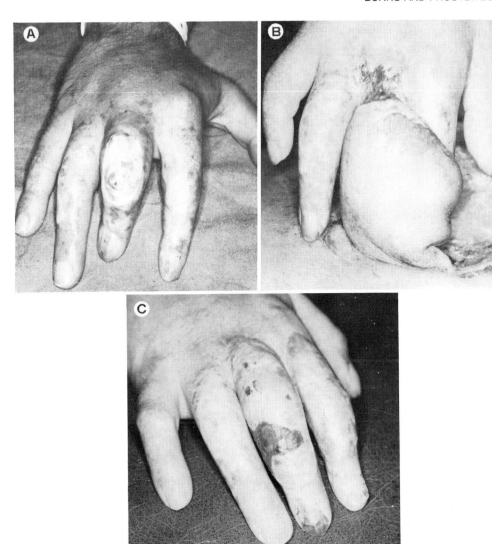

Figure 12.1.4. A. Hand of a young surgeon burned acutely during prolonged flouroscopy one year prior to photograph. Note the complete loss of skin cover and tendon with exposed joint cartilage, on middle finger. Extreme pain was the main complaint. *B.* Excision and coverage with thick flap. *C.* Early result after shaving flap off fingers leaving layer of fat and subcutaneous tissue which was covered with free full thickness grafts.

When it is important to keep the fingers slim, they may be covered with a flap to supply fat and subcutaneous tissue and a blood supply, and to clear up the infection. The finger may then be carved out of the flap so that it is normal in size and suitable for free grafting.

to be deposited in the body, the surgeon should know how this may be prevented or diminished. Proper knowledge of the factors involved will give some degree of certainty in deciding how much or how little should be done for the specific injury.

In a very real sense a radio-contaminated wound is like a snake bite and the problem is to control the material before it can enter the systemic circulation. If the wound is an open one it should be immediately washed with copious amounts of running water while brushing with a soft brush. if the water is not available, it may be wiped out with the cleanest material available and a tourniquet applied. If the tourniquet is above the arterial pressure it will prevent soluble materials from entering the circulation and, if it is between arterial and venous pressure, it will prevent venous return and produce copious bleeding so that the wound will tend to be flushed with its own blood. Whenever practical, the tissue which has been contaminated should be excised in much the same manner as a malignancy. If structures vital to the function of the portion of the hand involved have been contaminated, a more conservative excision may be done and the wound checked with the appropriate measuring device before additional tissue is taken.

Different types of radioactive materials require different detection devices (alpha counter, geiger counter, or gamma spectrometer). The use of the wrong instrument may give misleading readings.

If radioactive material is not readily removed and its presence endangers life because of spread via the blood stream, excision or amputation of important parts of the hand may be necessary. If, however, there is a higher than allowable amount of radioactive material remaining in the wound, but it is fixed in the area and does not endanger the patient, it may be left in place and observed periodically for evidence of late sequelae.

The wound caused by the accidental injection of radioactive material by a syringe, as has happened with technicians during the injection of laboratory animals, is especially difficult to treat. The wound is not open for flushing and the material is generally in solution. The only immediate first aid treatment is the application of a tourniquet above arterial pressure. Excision and flushing of the area is probably the treatment of choice. Ohlenschlaeger[28] reports a forefinger in which activity following accidental injection of Am^{241} was reduced from 244 to 0.1 by three successively larger excisions of tissue while monitoring with a counter.

The management of the patient accidentally irradiated or injected with radioactive substances will require ingenuity and resourcefulness on the part of the surgeon. Consultation with a radiophysicist may help to characterize the exposure and decide on appropriate treatment. Cystophos which can protect cells from the products of ionizing radiation may be considered, or DTPA, a chelating agent, may be used to manage contamination with transuranium elements. If the patient has received total body exposure, someone versed in transplantation biology should be consulted to consider bone marrow transplantation. Colloidal dispersion of radioactive materials may deposit in regional nodes sufficiently to warrant a node dissection. Valuable information may be obtained from HEW's Registry of Radiation Incidents which have reports on similar injuries.

While there is very little general experience available in handling these patients there is much useful, sophisticated knowledge available if one seeks it out.

REFERENCES

1. Allen, J. D. The causes of death from total body radiation. Ann. Surg., *146:* 322, 1957.
2. Blair, U. P., Brown, J. B., and Ham, W. G. The surgical treatment of post radiation verstesis. J. Radiol., *19:* 337, 1932.
3. Brown, J. B., and Fryer, M. P. Report of surgical repair in the first group of atomic radiation injuries. Surg. Gynecol. Obstet., *103:* 2, 1956.
4. Bunnell, S. *Surgery of the Hand.* Philadelphia, Lippincott, 1944, 1948.
5. Clarke, N. P., Zuidema, G. D., and Prins, J. R. Studies of the protective qualities of clothing against thermal radiation. Ann. Surg., *149:* 278, 1959.
6. Claus, W. D. *Radiation Biology and Medicine.* Reading. Mass., Addison Wesley, 1958.
7. Cole, H. N. Chronic Roentgen ray dermatosis as seen in professional men. J.A.M.A., *84:* 865, 1925.
8. Conway, H. *Tumors of the Skin.* Springfield, Charles C Thomas, 1956.
9. Cramer, L. M., Waite, J. H., Edgecoma, J. H., Powell, C. C., Touhy, J. H., VanScott, E. J., and Smith, R. R. Burn following accidental exposure to high energy radiation. Ann. Surg., *149:* 286, 1959.
10. Daland, E. M. Radiation damage to normal tissues in the diagnosis and treatment of non-malignant conditions and its surgical repair. N. Engl. J. Med., *244:* 959, 1951.
11. Davis, J. S. *Plastic Surgery.* Philadelphia, Blakiston, 1919.
12. Dunham, C. L., Cronkite, E. P., and Warren, S. Atomic bomb injury: Radiation. J.A.M.A., *147:* 50, 1951.
13. Ellinger, F. *Medical Radiation Biology.* Springfield, Charles C Thomas, 1957.
14. Frieben, E. Cancroid des rachtan Handruckens. Abst. Dtsch. Med. Wochensehr., *28:* 335, 1902.
15. Fryer, M. P., and Brown, J. D. Repair of atomic, cathode-ray, cyclotron and x-ray burns of the hand. Am. J. Surg., *103:* 688, 1962.
16. Giles, H. D., and McIndoe, A. H. The role of plastic surgery in burns due to roentgen ray and radium. Ann. Surg., *101:* 971, 1935.
17. Henriques, F. C., and Mortiz, A. R. Studies of thermal injury. Am. J. Pathol., *23:* 531, 1947.
18. Johnson, L. A. *et al.* Kinetics of lymph mode activity assumulation from sub cut PuO^2 implants. Health Physics, *18:* 416, 1972.
19. Kishn, C. L., and DesPrez, J. D. The burnt hand. Am. J. Surg., *97:* 421, 1959.
20. Knowlton, N. P. Beta ray injury of human skin. J.A.M.A., *141:* 239, 1949.
21. Krizek, T. J., and Ariyan, S. Severe acute radiation injuries of the hands. Plast. Reconstr. Surg., *51:* 14, 1973.
22. Lanzl, L. H., and Rozenfeld, M. L. Injury due to accidental high dose exposure to 10 mev. electrons. Health Physics, *13:* 241, 1967.
23. Leddy, E. T., and Rigos, F. J. Radiodermatitis among physicians. Am. J. Roentgenol., *45:* 696-700, 1949.
24. Litwin, M. S., *et al.* Burn injury after carbon dioxide laser irradiation. Arch Surg., *98:* 219, 1969.
25. Marcuse, W. Machtregz den Fall von Dermatitis and Alopacis nach Durchleuchtunge versuchen mit Roentgen strahlen. Dtsch. Med. Wochenschr., *22:* 681, 1896.
26. Mason, M. D. Irradiation dermatitis of hands. Am. Surg., *17:* 1121, 1951.
27. Michaelson, S. M. Biologic effects of micro wave exposure — Symposium Proceedings. BRH/DBE, 70-2, Sept. 1969.
28. Ohlenschlaeger, L. Report of a perforating and incised wound of the left forefinger contaminated with

strahlen therapic. Strahlentherapie, *142:* 739, 1971.

29. Padgett, E. D., and Stephenson, K. L. *Plastic and Reconstructive Surgery.* Springfield, Charles C Thomas, 1948.

30. Pearse, H. E., Payne, J. T., and Hogg, L. The experimental study of flash burns. Ann. Surg., *130:* 774, 1949.

31. Porter, C. A. The surgical treatment of x-ray carcinoma and other severe x-ray lesions (based on an anylysis of 47 cases). J. Med. Res., *21:* 357, 1909.

32. Porter, C. A. The surgical treatment of roentgen ray lesions. Am. J. Roentgenol., *13:* 31-37, 1925.

33. Shipman, T. L., cited by Brown, J. B. Personal communication. Surg., Gynecol. Obstet., *103:* 2, 1956.

34. Skeleton, H. P., Nanot, J. C., *et al.* Etude experimentals des contaminations par le curium 242 et deLeur traitement. DTPA Chelation of Certain Metals to Protect, *18:* 613, 1970.

35. Stark, R. S. *Plastic Surgery.* New York, Hoeber, 1962.

36. Sweet, R. D. The treatment of acute local radiation injuries. Clin. Radiol., *XV (1):* 55, 1964.

37. Taylor, G. W., Nathanson, I. T., and Shaw, D. T. Epidermoid cancer of extremities with reference to lymph node involvement. Ann. Surg., *113:* 268, 1941.

38. Telph, H. A., Mason, M. L., and Wheelock, M. C. Histopathologic study of radiation injury of the skin. Surg. Gynecol. Obstet., *90:* 335, 1950.

39. Vacek, A., *et al.* Protective effect of cysteamine-S-phosphate (cystaphos) on haemopoietic stem cells in irradiated mice. Folia Biol. (Praha), *17:* 340, 1971.

40. Wolbach, S. B. The pathological histology of chronic x-ray dermatitis and early x-ray carcinoma. J. Med. Res., *21:* 415, 1909.

41. Wolbach, S. B. Summary of the effects of repeated roentgen ray exposure on the human skin antecedent to formation of carcinoma. Ann. J. Roentgenol., *13:* 139, 1925.

42. Report of the U.N. Scientific Committee on the Effects of Atomic Radiation. Supplement No. 16 (A/5216), page 141.

B.

Immediate Evaluation and Treatment of the Burned Hand

Bradford Cannon, M.D.
Joseph E. Murray M.D.

Selection for local care in severe hand burns is critical. Koch noted the small amount of skin and soft tissues in relation to other parts of the body and commented that only minor debridement or wound excision in hand injury due to laceration, crush, or burn is allowable.

It is difficult immediately after a burn to determine the extent and depth of the destruction. In case of doubt, excise too little rather than too much, apply a compression dressing, and splint with the hand in the position of function, and wait for three or four days to permit more accurate analysis.

The skin and subcutaneous tissue coverings of the hand is of two types with different characteristics. Palmar skin is highly specialized, tough, resistant to withstand heavy use, flexible to permit free and and wide range of motion, firmly adherent to the palmar fascia and bony framework to minimize lateral soft tissue motion. Because of a thick surface keratin layer, it is relatively heat resistant. In contrast, dorsal skin is less in resistance in protecting it, thin with great elasticity, no deep fixation, with minimal keratin protection, and minimal subcutaneous tissue.

In thus evaluating the acute burned hand, remember that palmar skin is thick, heat resistant, and has superb healing potential from deep epithelial structures. In contrast, the burned back of the hand is often deeper than expected at first inspection. Underlying structures, the extensor tendon extending over the metacarpophalangeal and proximal interphalangeal joints, the joint capsules, and the nailbeds may be destroyed as well.

ETIOLOGY AND TYPES

There are two principal types of thermal hand burns, exposure and contact. Exposure burn, from flame or other source of intense heat, usually involves the dorsum of fingers and hand, when the patient tried to protect face or eye, to escape the heat, or to smother the fire. The hand often is flexed so palmar surface is less exposed. Commonly, both hands are burned. Often other burns occur such as the face, forearm, and other exposed parts.

Contact burns result from direct contact with hot objects. They frequently involve the palm as when a child falls against a hot stove and uses his hands to push himself away, or the worker in industry touches the hot surface of a roller or mangle. Often the burns are discrete and localized, involving only part of one hand. Other contact burns may result from spilled hot liquids, spatterings of molten metal, or by direct friction. Although these localized burns are associated only rarely with burns elsewhere, related bone fractures, tendon lacerations, and a crushed hand are not uncommon.

EVALUATION OF DEPTH AND EXTENT OF BURN

Depth and extent of burn are the two critical points in evaluation. The appearance of the area is the most accurate way to determine depth, but mode of burning provides essential correlative information. For example, brief exposure to hot liquids or momentary exposure to a flash of intense heat may produce only partial thickness damage, while prolonged exposure usually produces a full thickness burn. The significant local findings of color, moisture, and sensation are shown in Table 12.2.1.

Although other methods, such as use of radioactive tracers and intravenous dyes, have been described to estimate burn depth, they require special equipment and are not used except in some burn clinics.

Despite the efforts of many investigators, there is still no definitive test of the depth of a burn. Clinical experience and judgment are the chief bases on which the decision must be made. Allied with the evaluation of the depth of the burn is the decision about treatment. A too enthusiastic debridement is wasteful of salvageable skin which may or may not be duplicated by a skin graft. An insufficient debridement may prolong the convalescence and delay restoration of function. For these reasons most authors agree to postpone excision of damaged skin of the hand for several days or even longer.

Some surgeons divide the second-degree burn into two groups: (1) the superficial second-degree burn; and (2) the deep second-degree burn. In the former the normal abundance of epithelial tissue in the form of viable sebaceous glands and hair follicles remains in the deeper layer of the dermis, and from these healing will take place spontaneously. In the so-called deep second-degree burn, there is an *almost* complete destruction of the skin; nevertheless, islands of epithelial tissue remain, and from these some spontaneous healing could develop. However, the character of the healing from these scattered islands of tissue is of such poor quality that the burn should be considered and treated as of third degree.

It may be difficult to estimate the depth of the palmar burn because of the thickness of the skin of the palm (Fig. 12.2.1). Seldom should one consider excision of this highly specialized, irreplaceable tissue unless the damage is very obviously deep or until more accurate evaluation can be made several days later when the first dressing is removed.

Allied with the evaluation of the depth of the burn is the decision about treatment. The late Michael Mason, speaking about principles, said: "Burns are sim-

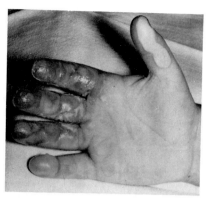

Figure 12.2.1 A contact burn in a child. Despite the obvious pallor of several areas of the volar skin suggestive of a full-thickness destruction, spontaneous healing occurred without contracture. A program of "cleanly care" initially with infrequent dressings subsequently was followed. The fingers were healed in about two weeks.

ply large open wounds and in their care these things are indicated: *first* is the protection of the open wound from further contamination and further trauma; *second,* the cleansing of the open wound and removal of dead tissue; *third,* the closing of the wound at the earliest possible moment by skin, either by spontaneous healing or by skin grafting."

PRIMARY LOCAL TREATMENT

The initial objective of local treatment should be prevention of further bacterial contamination, either from those in attendance or from debris on the skin. Thus, in the first-aid management, a clean protective covering for the hand should be applied. Gentle cleansing of the surface is desirable if the hand has been exposed to significant contamination or unnecessary handling. The attending surgeon must decide whether to apply a dressing at once or to do a preliminary washing and debridement of loose tissue. Seldom will general anesthesia be required for only primary local treatment. Rupture of blebs is undesirable, since they form an effective barrier against bacterial invasion. The bleb fluid rapidly absorbs parenterally administered antibiotics.

Identification of the necrotic tissue and its excision is the essence of the treatment of the burned hand.

The current enthusiasm for topical applications to the burned surface is not new. Each generation has its special agent — tannic acid, triple dye, magnesium sulfate jel, weak hypochlorite solution, penicillin cream, sulfamylon, silver nitrate, and many others. Improved results are reported with the use of each agent. Doubtless interest in the method increases interest in the care of the wound which of necessity influences the outcome.

Table 12.2.1
Local findings in second and third degree burns

	Partial Thickness Burn (2nd Degree)	Full Thickness Burn (3rd Degree)
Color	Red or pink but blanches with pressure	Usually blanched, pearly white or charred
Sensation	Present and usually quite painful	Anesthetic
Moisture	Blistered or weeping	Dry or charred

DRESSINGS

There is general agreement that the deeply burned hand should be splinted in the "position of function or rest." This cannot be done effectively without wrapping the hand. Most important is extension of the wrist of 40° to 45° with flexion at all metacarpophalangeal and interphalangeal joints. By splinting the wrist in extension, the powerful flexor muscles acquire an advantage which aids in flexing the metacarpophalangeal and interphalangeal joints. The thumb should be rotated toward the palm in the position of opposition. The stabilizing collateral ligaments of the finger joints are tense only in the flexed position. They are relaxed when the fingers are extended, but will tighten rapidly if the swollen fingers are left in the extended position.

"Cleanly care" must be practiced from the first examination until the hand is healed. By cleanly care is meant more than merely changing dressings at periodic intervals. Hair must be shaved, crusts must be gently lifted away, the surrounding skin must be kept free of any epithelial debris by thorough washing, and nonadherent dead tissue must be removed. By practicing the utmost gentleness in every manipulation, dressings can be changed with minimal premedication only. A single layer of fine mesh gauze, either dry or lightly impregnated with an ointment, is placed against the skin. The fine gauze can be removed with less trauma to the injured tissues and, consequently, less pain to the patient than a coarser gauze. Yet it allows unobstructed escape of exudate from the burned surface. The primary layer of gauze in turn is covered by a bulky dressing wrapped firmly in place for additional support and splinting. The term *pressure dressing* has been avoided for two reasons: (1) In the hand only minimal reduction in extravascular fluid accumulation can be anticipated by the application of pressure. The escaping plasma will merely travel proximally into undamaged tissues; (2) Even in a properly designed dressing with gauze separating each of the fingers and thumb, tight pressure creates unnecessary discomfort and may cause ischemia to the digits.

The first dressing may be left untouched for five to seven days, especially if no deep (third-degree) burn was judged present. But early removal of the outer layers of gauze may prove more comfortable and permit early passive and active motion. At five to seven days surgical debridement of the obviously deeply burned tissue will eliminate potential breeding ground for infection, and immediate or delayed (two to five days) skin-grafting will shorten the convalescence and rehabilitation. Dressings should be removed only in a fully equipped operating room with personnel and instruments for expeditious debridement and/or skin-grafting. Delay as long as 10 days before debridement and grafting is not unreasonable (Fig. 12.2.2). When faced with a clearly localized, deep burn with minimal systemic circulatory dislocation, the surgeon should consider immediate excision and skin-grafting in preference to the temporary delays proposed above.

The frequency of subsequent dressing changes is determined by the amount of drainage, twice daily if abundant, but, if dry, daily or even on alternate days may suffice.

Burns involving tendon or bone may be treated quite conservatively with a program of frequent dressings, and debridement of only that tissue which has undergone spontaneous separation. Sometimes several weeks may pass before the full extent of muscle, tendon, or bone loss can be determined. Not infrequently the outer layer of the bone or the tendon will separate, and the deeper layers will prove viable if protected from purulent exudate by covering surrounding raw surfaces with skin grafts. Enthusiastic early debridement can destroy the continuity of structure provided by these residual viable tissues. Spontaneous separation of necrotic bone or tendon progresses slowly but more tissue is saved than by arbitrary surgical excision (Fig. 12.2.3).

CHEMICAL DEBRIDEMENT

The value of topical, chemical, and enzymatic debriding agents is unconvincing. Separation of slough can be achieved just as rapidly by the meticulous care of the wound as by the agent which is used. The inefficiency of chemical or bacterial debriding agents applied topically is a compelling reason for the early surgical debridement of the burn wound when the patient's condition warrants.

ANTIBACTERIAL AGENTS

Massive antibiotic therapy is desirable in all severe burns of the hands. Cultures, both aerobic and anaerobic, from the skin at the initial examination will be helpful in deciding which agent to combine with the ubiquitous penicillin. Large systemic doses of the latter are indicated in the early care of the burn. When the patient's general condition has been stabilized, proper nutrition restored, and host resistance increased, there are valid reasons for discontinuing antibiotic therapy lest the wound organisms become resistant. Antitetanus therapy — a booster dose of tetanus toxoid or a large dose of tetanus antitoxin — is of course essential.

BURNS OF THE DORSUM OF THE HAND

Special attention must be given to the evaluation and care of burns of the dorsum of the hand. This is the part of the hand which is most frequently burned and the part in which the most disabling sequelae are encountered. The skin on the dorsum is thin with minimal subcutaneous tissue of areolar tissue and paratenon which offer little protection to the deep tendons. Even less protection is afforded the tendons where they pass over the metacarpophalangeal and interphalangeal joints.

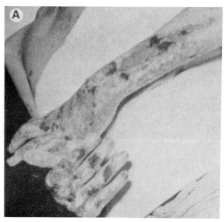
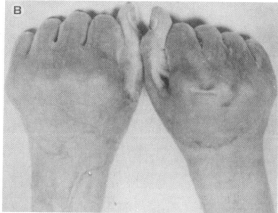
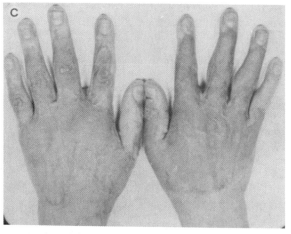

Figure 12.2.2. An excellent functional result following early grafting of a severe flame burn. This is a borderline burn between second and third degree ("deep second degree"). Excision of the partially healed scar epithelium on the dorsum and release of the developing contractures preceded the skin grafting with thick-split skin grafts. Aggressiveness in these borderline burns hastens resumption of active motion and insures a better functional result.

Obviously the best prophylaxis against infection and further destruction of tissue including tendon is prompt restoration of a healthy skin cover (Fig. 12.2.4). This goal implies removal of the damaged and dead tissue. A decision may require extraordinary judgment. The technique is challenging because of the uncertainties of determining borderline viability of important structures. When uncertainties exist, it is wiser to leave the important structure undisturbed, skin graft the adjacent healthy granulating surface, and anticipate recovery of all or part of the exposed tissue (Fig. 12.2.5).

When one carries this concept one step further it is probably prudent to forego excision if the burn is so deep that it obviously involves tendons and joints. Little functional gain is achieved by excision since spontaneous sequestration of necrotic tissue is more accurate than the surgeon's scalpel.

OPEN GRAFTING OF THE HAND

The edematous granulation tissue, which is prone to develop despite meticulous care if there are exposed tendons or open joints of the hand, is a problem of major proportions. Open skin grafting of the burned hand has proven a valuable method for early closure of the granulating surface with minimal risk of bleeding or loss of the skin graft (Fig. 12.2.6).

An unexplained but well-recognized spontaneous and firm adhesion develops between a split skin graft and a granulating surface. The temperature of the grafted skin exposed to the outside air is several degrees lower than that of grafts covered with a dressing, and the graft remains dry and thus is less likely to be destroyed by bacteria needing a warm moist environment.

Minimal handling of a freshly cut skin graft is desir-

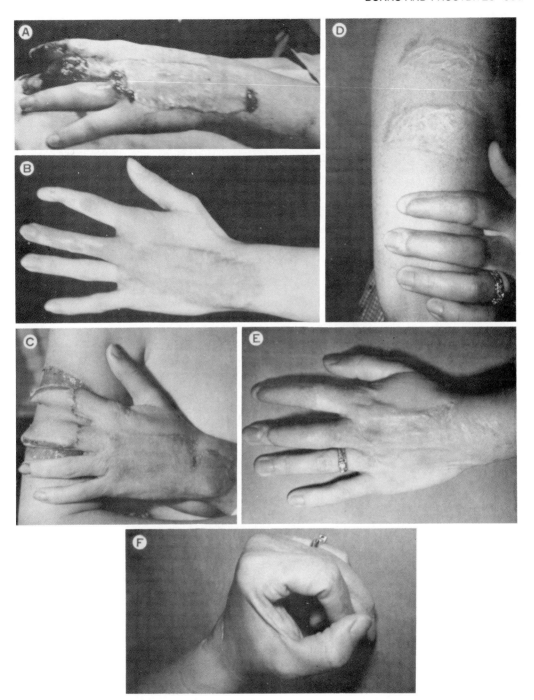

Figure 12.2.3 Mangle (contact) burn of the dorsum in a young woman. Split skin grafts used to close all granulating surfaces surrounding the extensor tendons of index and middle fingers and the open proximal interphalangeal joint of midfinger. The uncovered tendons and joint rapidly healed when no longer bathed in exudate from the marginal granulating surfaces. The thin dorsal grafts were later replaced will "cross-arm" flaps to provide a more elastic skin covering for releasing the adherent tendons and freeing the stiff joints. The flaps were separated in two stages on the 14th and 21st days. Later the two donor areas were skin grafted. A useful functional result with stable skin, good pinch, and partial restoration of motion at interphalangeal joints was secured. The middorsal contracture at the wrist was also opened and a small local flap shifted into the triangular defect.

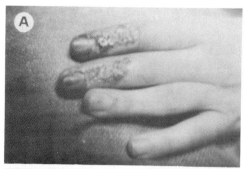

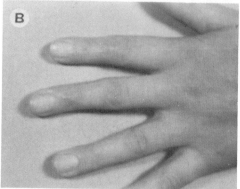

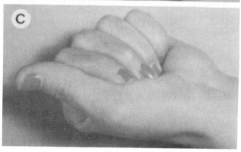

Figure 12.2.4. Small area of third-degree burn in the fingers. Limitation of function and distortion of the nails avoided by early grafting.

able. There is never any indication to ''spread it out'' on a flat surface, to wash it with saline, or to manipulate it in any other way. Likewise, the granulating surface to be grafted should have no preparation other than the meticulous care which has been practiced in doing the daily preoperative dressings. In fact, washing of the graft or the granulating surface seems to deter development of the adhesion presumably by dilution of the tissue precursors of that adhesion.

The method, of course, has limited applications. There is still no better protection for a graft than a well prepared raw surface and an accurately applied dressing. The open grafting technique offers an alternative method for securing wound closure when conditions are less than ideal. Absolute immobilization of the hand and fingers is not necessary but protection of the

grafts from mechanical dislodgement is essential.

The grafts are usually well vascularized and secure in four to five days. Daily moist dressings can then be resumed to minimize crust formation and destructive infection beneath crusts, and to insure absorption of secretions until completely healed.

The open grafting technique is stressed in this chapter because it has been found very useful in treating the deeply burned hand. These are the cases in which one failure follows another and with each failure there is irreversible deterioration of function in the hand.

RECONSTRUCTION

The most challenging of all problems is the definitive reconstruction of the healed but deformed or contracted hand. Here the surgeon must draw on a wide variety of techniques from Z-plasty to additional major skin grafting, from rotation of local flaps to multi-stage transfer of remote flaps, from tendon transplant to amputation, and from capsulotomy to arthrodesis.

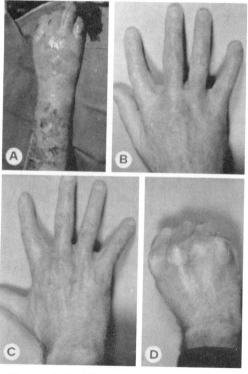

Figure 12.2.5. This is an example of a third-degree burn without tendon or joint involvement. It might have been treated by excision but the depth was uncertain and skin grafting was therefore delayed. The slough of the hand and forearm separated rapidly and early grafting (20 days) was successful. Total function was restored.

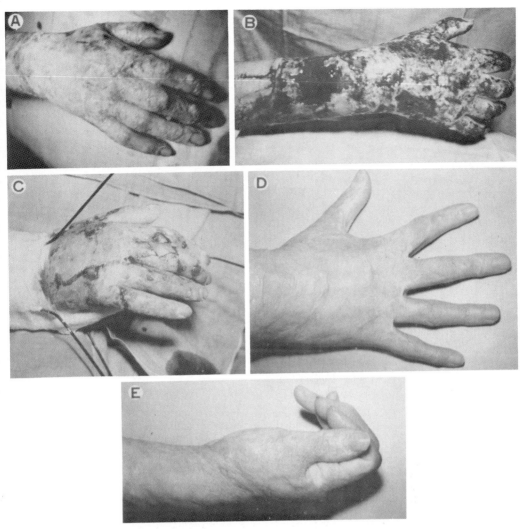

Figure 12.2.6. Typical flame burn of the hand and forearm sustained in an airliner crash. Face, neck, and opposite hand were also severely burned. Wounds bathed in purulent exudate when first seen approximately four and one-half weeks postburn. Despite daily dressings and careful mechanical debridement begun at once, the granulations remained edematous and a moderate seropurulent exudate continued. "Open grafting" technique was therefore used. Split skin grafts were laid on the granulating surfaces, leaving a narrow gap between each piece of skin for free drainage. The wrist and hand were supported by a plaster cast in which a wire protective frame was incorporated. A gauze netting was draped tightly over the frame so that no dislodgement of the grafts by outside contact was possible. All the grafts survived. Wet dressings resumed on the fifth day and the narrow gaps healed rapidly. In the final evaluation limitation of metacarpophalangeal motion was evident as was the dorsal webbing, but the skin grafts were stable and the patient was satisfied, preferring no further corrective surgery.

Opening a tight web between the first and second metacarpals (thumb-index web space) may be possible by the shifting of local flaps (Z-plasty) or may require dissection of the several muscles which occupy the space between the metacarpals and repair with a skin graft. If the former, the web is split and opposing flaps are elevated and transferred across the now relaxed gap; if the latter, the thenar and especially adductor muscle bellies are identified, displaced into a better functional positon, or occasionally detached to allow greater mobility of the thumb. The uneven surface of the several muscle bellies requires considerable care of the several contours.

The relaxing incision of the dorsal web between the

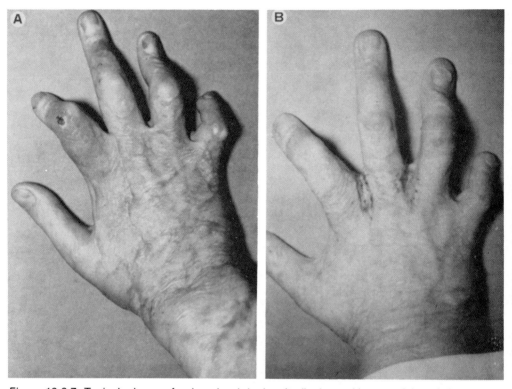

Figure 12.2.7. Typical release of a dorsal web by longitudinal cut without excision of skin. Incision does not cross the palmar web but is carried proximally beyond the heads of the metacarpals. Thick split skin graft used to close the elliptical defect. Earlier the always troublesome contraction of the fifth finger was improved by a wedge excision and fusion of the proximal interphalangeal joint and a resection of the head of the fifth metacarpal as in the arthritic hand.

fingers is made parallel to their long axis. It should extend proximally as far as the heads of the metacarpals but distally only to the edge of the normal palmar web (Fig. 12.2.7).

The Split-Thickness or Full-Thickness Graft

Since grafted skin characteristically shrinks and since the thicker the graft the less the shrinkage, selection of the appropriate free skin graft for definitive reconstruction of the burned hand depends on the capacity of the hand to minimize contraction of the graft. Thus on the dorsal surface a thick split skin graft kept stretched by action of the powerful flexor muscles contracts little, whereas this same graft on the volar surface may shrink excessively because of the relative weakness of the extensor muscles. The free full-thickness skin graft, although most inappropriate for primary closure of a granulating wound because of the uncertainties of a ''take,'' is preferable in definitive resurfacing on the volar surface because of its minimal shrinkage (Fig. 12.2.8). Almost without exception the only indication for a full-thickness skin graft in the hand is for volar surface repair; the split skin graft is indicated in all other areas.

Incisions in Definitive Procedures

Proper planning and placement of incisions for release of contractures from burns or for excision of disabling scars are essential in these as in other procedures in the hand. For example, the midline volar web which produces a contracture of the finger should seldom be excised and replaced with a skin graft. The deformity will promptly recur but now with two parallel contracting bands. Instead, the contracting web should be cut across at one or more flexion creases and individual free full-thickness skin grafts used to close each transverse defect. The intervening volar skin, hypertrophic because of tension, softens after the release and will recover much of its toughness, flexibility, and texture (Figs. 12.2.8 and 12.2.9).

Effective immobilization of the hand for any definitive procedure, especially those in which small grafts are contemplated, can be accomplished and maintained immediately after the dissection by using a one quarter inch wire mesh screen as a splint. The surgeon has free access to the dissected surface, the hand and fingers are fixed, and the assistant is free to help suture the graft in place (Fig. 12.2.10).

Hypertrophic scar tissue on the dorsal surface of the hand commonly occurs even with early skin grafting. Elimination of the inflexible scar requires either release or excision of the scar and replacement with a skin graft. All incisions should be in a transverse direction extending to the midlateral lines. If the incision must parallel the long axis of the hand, notched cuts or ''darts'' at a right angle or cuts into a web space will eliminate the foreshortening of a linear scar. Definitive resurfacing of the dissected area with thick-

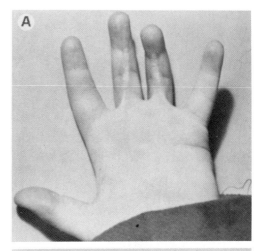

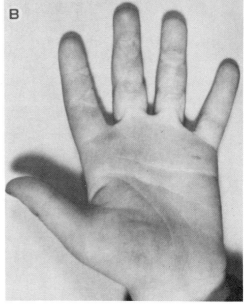

Figure 12.2.8. Volar contracture of fingers in a child. Transverse incisions at the level of the flexion creases in the second, third, and fourth digits were each carried to the midlateral line on either side. No skin or scar was excised. Free full-thickness skin grafts were used for closure of the six elliptical defects. Full functional recovery. Full-thickness skin grafts usually preferred in all definitive grafting of the volar surface of the hand or fingers because thicker grafts shrink less than the thinner ones.

split skin grafts insures a fully adequate functional covering (Fig. 12.2.11).

The Skin Flap

There are few circumstances in the burned hand where a skin flap is indicated. Only in the very deep

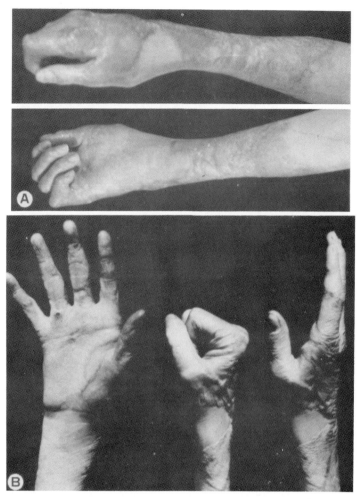

Figure 12.2.9. Example of an extreme degree of volar contracture of the fingers and thumb with extensive hypertrophic scarring of the forearm, wrist and dorsum. The flame burn was sustained many months before and no skin grafting had been attempted. Function of the hand was restored in a single operative procedure. Transverse incisions were made *across* each of the volar webs of the fingers at one or more levels, usually at the flexion creases. Each incision was extruded around the finger to the midlateral line on either side. The resulting elliptical defects totalling ten were closed with free full-thickness skin grafts from the groin. In addition a curved relaxing incision and graft at the base of the thenar eminence was necessary to release the thumb. Following release of the contractures, repair with skin grafts and the resumption of active motion, the hypertrophic scars of the hand, wrist, and forearm became softer, less red, less hypertrophic, and more comfortable. None of the volar scar of the hand was excised. This tissue recovered its flexibility and toughness and has proven stable for normal use.

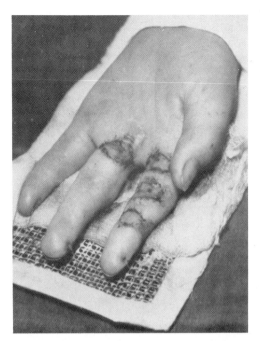

Figure 12.2.10. Effective immobilization of the hand can be secured by utilizing a one-quarter-inch wire mesh screen as a splint. The sharp edges of the wire mesh are protected with adhesive. The arm is immobilized by bandaging to the padded splint. Finally, the distal finger pads are transfixed with a wire suture and tied through the screen. The method is most useful in stabilizing the hand during and after definitive grafting of either dorsal or volar areas.

burn will the free graft or grafts fail to provide the necessary skin coverage for functional recovery. To use a remote flap before the hand is healed may be essential for the salvage of a tendon or joint but it does pose hazards of introducing infection into the remote unburned donor area. Most resurfacing with a flap is done in anticipation of definitive deep surgery on tendons, joints, or nerves after the burned hand is healed. The decision to use a remote flap implies insufficient skin and subcutaneous tissue for successful repair of the deeper structures (Fig. 12.2.12). The flap is indicated for ease of exposure, for insuring an adequare blood supply, for promise of primary wound healing, and to provide skin with a subcutaneous cushion of fat over bony prominences (Fig. 12.2.3).

Duplication of the original skin of a part is always the surgeon's goal. The skin of the hand with its thin subcutaneous tissue and its flexibility is difficult to replace. Abdominal skin, abundant and readily available, is thick, often with excessive subcutaneous fat, and ill suited for delicate hand function. The skin of the anteromedial aspect of the upper thigh is thinner with less subcutaneous fat. It is nearly as abundant as abdominal skin but the attachment of the flap is awkward and more difficult to maintain (Fig. 12.2.12). The most appropriate donor area for a flap of limited size is the opposite upper arm. The thin skin in this area resembles that of the hand in almost every respect and there is minimal subcutaneous tissue. The resulting donor site scar is seldom conspicuous. (Fig. 12.2.3).

Many details of remote skin flap transfer have been described elsewhere. The usual duration of attachment of the hand to the donor area is two and one-half to three weeks. Seldom is a shorter period desirable or necessary. Fixation can be maintained by adhesive strapping only. Frequent changes of dressing and cleanly local care to insure conditions as free of accumulated exudate as possible will hasten accommodation of the flap to its new site. If the circulation in the flap after detachment is in doubt, suturing should be delayed lest the viability of the flap be impaired by unwarranted tension.

Specialized Procedures

A number of specialized procedures useful not only after deep burns but as a sequel to many hand injuries deserve mention. These include: capsulectomy of the metacarpophalangeal joints, extensor tendon transplants especially at the metacarpophalangeal joint level in which fascia lata has proven useful in recreating the extensor hood, fusion of the interphalangeal joints in functional position by wedge excision of the joint, excision of the metacarpal head as in the arthritic hand (Fig. 12.2.7), excision of badly distorted nail beds and replacement with a skin graft, filleting of useless fingers for better covering elsewhere in the hand.

An unusual but severely disabling consequence of a burn is loss of all digits of one or both hands. Restoration of a semblance of grasp and pinch is essential for useful function. Pinch may be restored by formation of a cheft between the first and third metacarpals, sacrificing the second metacarpal unless its tip can be used to elongate a short first thumb metacarpal. If the bony stump of the thumb is shorter than that of the index finger, the head of the second metacarpal is transplanted over the end of the first metacarpal (either directly or on a vascular pedicle). The proximal shaft is then removed leaving only the base. In the formation of a cleft, a dorsal skin flap is usually transferred across its base after identification and preservation of the nerves and proximal displacement of the thenar muscles. The opposing surfaces are covered with thick split skin grafts.

Good motion of the thumb and development of considerable strength can result. The hands are converted from ineffectual stumps into useful members for pinch and for holding utensils and tools. No longer must the person be fed, dressed, and depend completely on other hands. Normal sensation in the functioning part

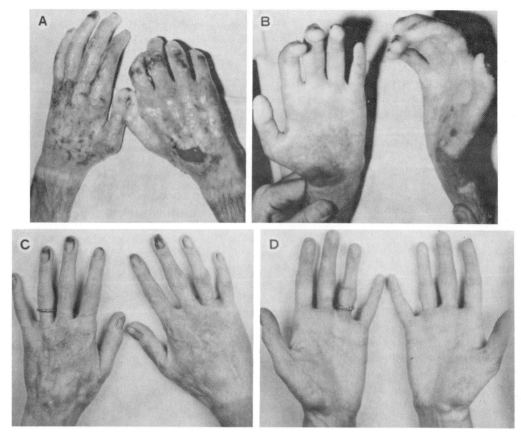

Figure 12.2.11. "Deep second" and some third-degree flame burn of the hand. Finger motion limited by shrunken skin and tight joint capsules. Treated by excision of the granulation tissue and much of the thin unstable epithelium that had spread over the dorsum of the hand and fingers. Split skin grafts used to close the surface. The skin grafts proved strong, pliable, and stable, and full functional recovery was possible.

of the hand is preserved and returns in a matter of weeks in the skin grafts (Fig. 12.2.13).

CONCLUSIONS

No definitive program of treatment of the burned hand can ever be portrayed because of variations in local circumstances. Each surgeon must consider the principles in treatment and adapt them to his particular situation.

1. Although appraisal of the severity of depth of an isolated hand burn is often perplexing, the treatment plan is dependent on it.

2. If a deep burn (third degree) can be assessed with certainty and the patient's condition warrants, prompt excision and skin grafting are indicated.

3. If the depth of the burn cannot be assessed, the hand may be wrapped, splinted, exposed, enclosed in a plastic bag or treated in any of a number of ways. Each will require different sequence in later management.

4. The first change of dressing (four to five days) should be done in the operating room with the necessary instruments ready for excision and grafting. The depth of the burn should be obvious by that time so the definitive procedure can be carried out without

Figure 12.2.12. Deep mangle burn through four extensor tendons and into the four metacarpophalangeal joints beneath. Prompt skin grafting of the raw surfaces was done. Dorsal angulation at the joints developed as the scars shortened. The graft was later removed, the scar tissue excised and a direct flap applied to the dissected surface. Dorsal webs, some fullness of the flap, and limited motion of the metacarpophalangeal joints persist. Full motion at the interphalangeal joints has proven adequate for a useful hand for the patient. Release of metacarpophalangeal joints refused.

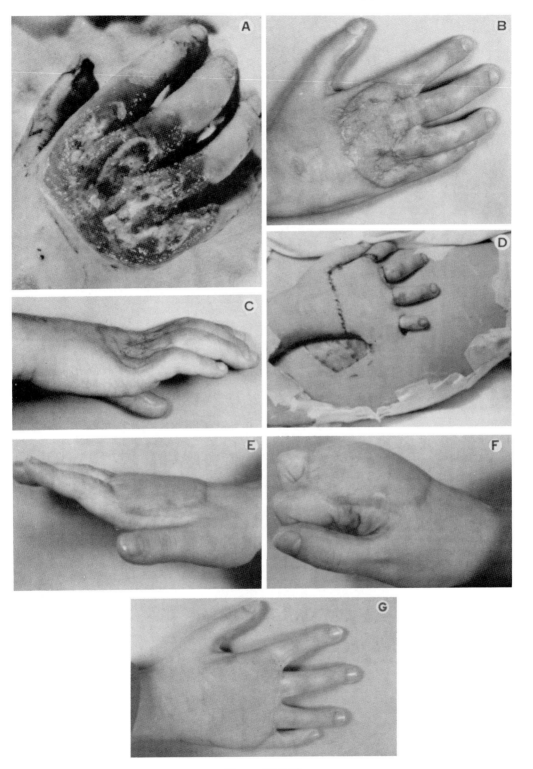

Figure 12.2.12.

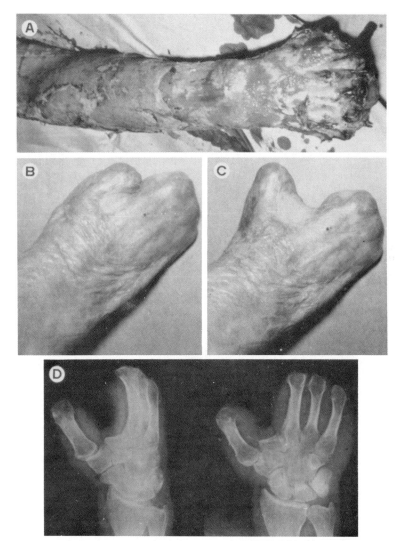

Figure 12.2.13. Destructive flame burn of the hands with loss of all ten digits. Equally severe burns of the face, scalp, skull, and legs were sustained. All areas of deep burn closed primarily with free skin grafts. Useful grasp in the crippled hands was restored by excision of the shaft and hood of the second metacarpal and lining of the cleft with thick splint skin grafts.

delay and without further manipulation or risk of contamination. If the depth is still unclear, the hand may be rewrapped, but a program of daily limited passive or active motion of the finger joints should be started.

5. When, after excision, the bleeding is excessive or difficult to control, skin grafting of the raw surface can be safely delayed for several days, but the dissected surface should not be exposed again until ready for the grafting procedure in the operating room.

6. Always to be remembered is that tough palmar skin is more resistant to heat than thin dorsal skin. The most seriously disabling burns are those of the dorsum in which tendons and joints are damaged primarily by the burn or secondarily by infection or prolonged immobilization.

7. When excising burned skin of the hand, especially the dorsum, one may wish to preseve marginally destroyed skin that has potential viability — skin which is labeled by some surgeons as deep second-degree burn. Experience has shown the fallacy of saving this skin since slow healing with hypertrophic scarring is almost inevitable, scarring which will require resurfacing at a future date.

8. A split-thickness skin graft is indicated for all primary grafting of the burned hand. It shrinks more than the thicker graft but is more certain of ''take.''

9. A full-thickness graft is indicated for definitive closure after release of volar contractures of the fingers and palm because its shrinkage is minimal and there are not powerful muscles to stretch it. By con-

trast dorsal skin is continually stretched by the power-ful flexor muscles. A split thickness graft is therefore indicated in the dorsal area.

REFERENCES

1. Allen, H. S. Treatment of the burned wound based on the experience of 1000 hospital patients. Ann. Surg., *134:* 566, 1951.
2. Artz, C. P., and Riess, E. *Treatment of Burns.* Philadelphia, Saunders, 1957.
3. Blocker, T. G., *et al.* An approach to the problem of burn sepsis with the use of open-air therapy. Ann. Surg. *134:* 574, 1951.
4. Brown, J. B., and McDowell, F. *Skin Grafting,* Ed. 3. Philadelphia, Lippincott, 1958.
5. Brown, J. B. The repair of surface defects of the hand. Ann. Surg., *107:* 952, 1938.
6. Brown, J. B., Cannon, B., Graham, W. C., Lischer, C. E., Scarborough, C. P., Davis, W. B., and Moore, A. M. Direct flap repair of defects of the arm and hand. Ann. Surg. *122:* 706, 1945.
7. Bunyan, J. Envelope method (using electrolytic sodium hypochlorite solution). Br. Med. J., *2:* 1, 1941.
8. Cannon, B. Procedures in rehabilitation of the severely burned (in the Cocoanut Grove Disaster). Ann. Surg. *117:* 903, 1943.
9. Cannon, B., Graham, W. C., and Brown, J. B. Restoration of grasping function following loss of all five digits. Surgery, *25:* 420, 1949.
10. Cannon, B. Open grafting of raw surfaces of the hand. J. Bone Joint Surg., *40A:* 79, 1958.
11. Cannon, B., and Cope, O. Rate of epithelial regeneration; effect of various agents recommended in treatment of burns. Ann. Surg., *117:* 85, 1943.
12. Cannon, B., and Zuidema, G. D. The care and the treatment of the burned hand. Clin. Ortho., *15:* 111, 1959.
13. Cave, E. F., and Rowe, C. R. Utilization of skin from useless fingers to cover hand defects. Ann. Surg. *125:* 1, 1947.
14. Cope, O., *et al.* Expeditious care of full-thickness burn wounds by surgical excision and grafting. Ann. Surg. *125:* 1, 1947.
15. Grant, A. E. Rehabilitation of the burned hand. Mod. Med., 126, 1964.
16. Greeley, P. W. Plastic repair of extensor hand contracture. Surgery, *15:* 173, 1944.
17. Koch, S. L. *Symposium on Burns.* National Academy of Sciences, National Research Council, Washington, D. C. 1951, p. 171.
18. Macomber, W. B. Relationship of superficial and deep reconstructive surgery of the hand. Plast. Reconstr. Surg. *5:* 139, 1950.
19. McCormack, R. M. Principles of treatment and reconstruction of the burned hands and fingers. In *Symposium on the Hand,* St. Louis, Mosby, 1971, pp. 66-72.
20. McDowell, F. Accelerated excision and grafting of small deep burns. Am. J. Surg., *85:* 407, 1953.
21. Moncrief, J. A. Third degree burns of the dorsum of the hand. Am. J. Surg., *96:* 535, 1958.
22. Rank, B. K., and Wakefield, A. R. *Surgery of Repair as Applied to Hand Injuries.* Edinburgh, Livingstone, 1953.
23. Ross, W. P. D. The treatment of recent burns of the hand. Br. J. Plast. Surg., *2:* 233, 1950.
24. Slater, R. M. A simplified method of treating burns of the hands. Br. J. Plast. Surg., *24:* 296, 1971.
25. Wallace, A. B. Thoughts on wound healing and wound care. Br. J. Plast. Surg., *12:* 150, 1960.
26. Whitson, T. C. Management of the burned hand. J. Trauma, *11:* 606, 1971.

C.

Frostbite

Harris B. Shumacker, Jr., M.D.

GENERAL CONSIDERATIONS

Local cold injuries are properly separated into several clinical entities: chilblains, frostbite, trenchfoot, and immersion foot and hand. Though they have exposure to cold in common as the primary inciting cause, they differ considerably with respect to the severity and duration of the exposure and to the relative importance of such contributing factors as wetness, dependency of the damaged limb, vascular stasis, and vasoconstriction. Their clinical manifestations and sequelae also have some features in common yet differ considerably from one another. Since we are here concerned solely with disorders of the hands and since trenchfoot and the immersion injuries primarily involve the lower extremities, we shall consider principally frostbite and chilblains, the former rather fully, the latter briefly.

Trenchfoot is, from all practical considerations, exclusively a military problem. It develops in personnel exposed for days or weeks to cold and wet but generally not freezing weather in situations such as to necessitate prolonged if not constant dependency of the lower extremities. After recovery from the acute episode, these patients are particularly prone to have various pains and parathesias, and especially pain in the forefoot on weight bearing, in addition to the vasospastic and cold-sensitivity sequelae common after all types of cold injury. The counterpart of trenchfoot is not observed in the hand. Immersion foot and hand develop after long continued exposure of the extremities in cold but not freezing sea water. This injury which primarily affects the lower extremities occurs mainly in times of war. A peculiar feature of its sequelae is the frequency with which major nerve paralysis is noted, a difficulty not observed following other types of cold injury.

CHILBLAINS

This condition, the mildest form of cold injury, occurs most often in individuals who are exposed repeatedly to a cold and wet environment without adequate protection of warm clothes. Its development may be dependent in part upon some intrinsic predisposition and may conceivably be related to such factors as an unusually labile vasomotor apparatus and true cold sensitivity. Often the individual is unaware of any injury during the exposure. Afterwards, he experiences intense burning and itching of the affected part, complaints which are intensified by warmth. A cyanotic rubor is likely to be present along with slight edema. A dermatitis usually develops. The skin lesions are generally bilateral and symmetrical and affect the legs, toes, and the dorsal surfaces of hands and feet. Vesicles filled with clear or bloody fluid and at times purpuric lesions may be observed. After a few days or a week or so the acute manifestations commonly disappear.

A similar recurrent skin condition characterizes chronic chilblains. It tends to be manifest in cold weather and to disappear when the weather is warm. On exposure to cold, patients with chronic chilblains complain of itching and burning. Sometimes the skin becomes erythematous and vesiculated and occasionally superficial ulcers develop. The repeated cutaneous lesions may result in scarring and atrophy of the skin and subcutaneous tissue. This chronic disorder must be distinguished from other skin diseases such as erythema induratum and bears some resemblance to the peculiar ulcerated lesions sometimes observed in association with vasoconstriction as a sequel of poliomyelitis.

Little is known about the specific management of chilblains. In treating the acute or recurrent condition one should not use excessive heat or cold applications and should make every effort to avoid secondary infections of the skin lesions. Proper warm dress in cold weather may minimize or obviate recurrences. Those who are badly affected often remain well if they can move to a warm climate. Certain observations suggest that sympathetic denervation may be indicated in the more severe cases. Chilblains does not result in lesions requiring reconstructive procedures on the hands and fingers.

FROSTBITE

This is the principal cold injury with which the hand surgeon is concerned. It results from exposure to freezing temperatures and usually to intensely cold weather. The period of exposure may be very short and the temperature very low as in high-altitude frostbite. Most ground-type injuries result from an exposure of some hours and, occasionally, days. The harmful effects of the cold can be enhanced in a number of ways. Inebriation, sleep, wounds, fear, or anything else which immobilizes the individual increases the likelihood of such injury. The same is true of anything which compromises the circulation to an extremity, such as wounds of arteries or obliterative arterial disease, constricting clothing, or cramped body positions. The possibility of sustaining frostbite is increased by wetness of the part and by inadequate clothing.

The injured limb becomes cold and numb during exposure. Muscle power becomes weak so that it may be difficult or impossible to walk or to use the extremity at all. The skin becomes pale and, if actual freezing takes place, opaque, hard, and sometimes covered with ice crystals. Afterwards the limb may remain cold, numb, and pale for a variable period but undergoes intense vasodilatation after the patient is brought into a warm environment. This period of reactive hyperemia is associated with paresthesias and burning and aching pain of variable severity and duration.

Frostbite is generally classified into four degrees according to the most severe injury present. Not infrequently the extremity exhibits more severe damage distally and progressively less damage proximally. One may, for example, have fourth degree injury of the distal phalanges, third degree damage of the proximal digits, second degree changes in the hand, and first degree alterations in the wrist.

First degree frostbite is characterized by numbness, edema, and erythema, which ordinarily last from one to three weeks. At this time superficial desquamation usually occurs. There may be also present small areas of intracutaneous hemorrhage which resolve without loss of tissue.

In second degree frostbite there occurs partial skin thickness vesiculation in addition to those findings in the milder injury. The blebs develop along with the edema and are filled with clear or bloody fluid (Fig. 12.3.1). The unruptured vesicles lose their fluid content and desquamate in from two to three weeks, leaving a thin, intact, poorly keratinized skin.

Third degree frostbite signifies full thickness involvement of the skin. Either a thick walled vesicle develops or, following the state of reactive hyperemia, an area of blue-gray edematous skin makes its appearance. Both result in a hard black eschar which, if not removed, separates in from two to eight weeks. As in the milder degrees of injury, there are usually also present erythema, edema, and partial thickness skin blebs.

The tissue necrosis is deeper than the skin in fourth degree frostbite and usually includes all soft parts down to the underlying bone. In the areas of most extensive damage vesicles are either absent or are very small, although extensive edema and vesiculation may be present proximally. The most severely injured part participates little or not at all in the phase of reactive hyperemia but tends, instead, to remain cold, cyanotic, and anesthetic. Later it becomes black, hard, and mummified if uninfected (Fig. 12.3.2), or soft, necrotic, and swollen if infection is present.

During the first days after injury there may be mild

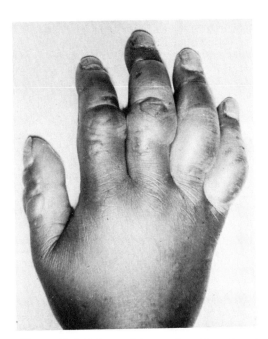

Figure 12.3.1. Second degree frostbite of hand during phase of reactive hyperemia showing edema and vesiculation.

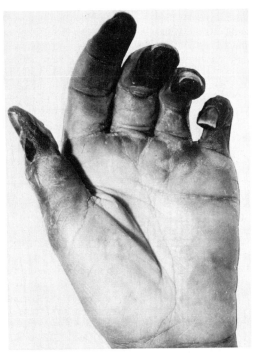

Figure 12.3.2. Fourth degree frostbite showing mummification of the digits.

or moderate stinging or burning pain, exacerbated by exposure to a warm atmosphere. Later, aching and throbbing pain may be noted and may last for several weeks. Distressing pain is not, however, a very prominent feature of frostbite. The uninfected gangrenous parts themselves are not uncomfortable. There may be small areas of hypesthesia or hypersthesia but almost never motor paralysis. Joint motion may ultimately be restricted by fibrosis.

Sympathetic overactivity is a very common sequel. Vasoconstriction tends to follow the hyperemic phase and with the onset of vasoconstriction sweat gland function returns and may become excessive. Some patients have ultimate restoration of fairly normal vasomotor and sweating activity in the injured extremity. Not infrequently, however, sympathetic overactivity and hyperhidrosis persist. This may result in troublesome maceration of the skin. The affected limb tends to be sensitive to cold and to develop numbness, aching pain, cyanosis, and pallor on exposure to cold.

Physiopathology

The body responds to exposure to cold by vasoconstriction which primarily involves the peripheral small arteries and arterioles but may, if the exposure is long enough and intense enough, affect larger arteries as well. It is known that this vasoconstrictor response represents the sum total of three different reactions. There is an intrinsic contractile response of blood vessels to cold, independent of innervation. There is also

a local vasospastic reaction of a reflex nature mediated over the regional sympathetic pathways and varying in intensity not only with the degree of cold stimulation but also with the individual's innate vasomotor tonus. In addition, there occurs a generalized reaction involving the sympathetic nerves. This is initiated by the passage of chilled blood through the vasomotor center.

Although peripheral vasoconstriction tends to conserve body heat and maintain core temperature, it jeopardizes the survival of the limb if the exposure is sufficiently long and the vasospasm sufficiently great. It results in local heat loss and in anoxia. At first the activity of the arteriovenous anastomoses in the skin provides some protection from periodic vasodilatation but they become inactive as the process goes on. Intense vasoconstriction persists with continuing exposure and the reduced blood flow brings about tissue anoxia. Stinging and burning pains develop along with loss of propioceptive reflexes and tactile sensation and decreased motor activity. This reduces further the arterial blood inflow. An additional injurious feature of the anoxic damage is the failure of normal dissociation of oxyhemoglobin at low temperatures.

Wetness of the part increases the damage by facilitating loss of heat from and transference of cold to the tissues. Wetness also tends to abolish the protective phenomenon of supercooling, or the capacity of tissues to be chilled below their actual freezing point without solidifying. In addition to the injury from anoxia, the chilled but not frozen tissue may be damaged directly by cold or, looking at it from another point of view, by loss of heat from the cells. Although the precise mechanism is not known this may result from selective inhibition of cellular anabolic processes while catabolism continues and to denaturization of cellular protein by the accumulated metabolic end products.

When actual freezing to ice takes place, as happens in some, but certainly not in all cases of frostbite, cells may be destroyed by the formation of crystals and their subsequent thawing. Cellular structure may be damaged by crystallization and thawing in a variety of ways, intra- and extracellular ionic and electrolyte imbalance, osmotic disturbances, interruption of enzymatic function, disruption of the colloidal state of protein, and mechanical rupture of cell membranes. The over-all damage is related to the makeup of the tissue and especially to its water content as well as to the intensity and rapidity of freezing and to the rapidity of thawing. It is known that tissues may be dehydrated, frozen rapidly, kept in a frozen state, thawed rapidly, and survive. Skin thus treated may be used successfully as an autograft or may serve as an allograph for a comparable length of time as does fresh skin. Cornea treated in this way serves well for transplant purposes. These conditions, of course, do not obtain in cold injuries but these considerations may explain in part the differing susceptibility of tissues to cold. Skin which has a low water content may be frozen solidly and survive. Muscle has a high water content and is especially sensitive to cold injury. These considerations also may explain in part the beneficial effect of treatment by rapidly thawing the still frozen extremity. It must be remembered, however, that actual freezing to ice does not occur in chilblains, trenchfoot, immersion foot or hand, or, as one can tell, in the majority of cases of frostbite in the temperate zone.

The intense vasoconstriction of frostbite gives way to intense reactive hyperemia after a variable period of time and usually after the patient is brought into a warm environment. It is a mistaken concept to consider the phase of hyperemia as one of full and normal circulation. The circulation to the exposed part, negligible if not absent during the exposure, is re-established through a vascular bed made hyperpermeable by the injury. Vesicles form and edema develops with fluid approximating the serum in protein content. Formed elements of the blood may also be extravasated. The damaged capillary endothelium has an increased affinity for platelets. As in other injuries, platelet adhesiveness increases and platelet aggregation takes place. Capillaries and small arterioles become filled with a red cell sludge. These changes may be reversible at first but in severe injury they tend to result in

agglutinative thrombi. True thrombus formation is observed in from 24 to 72 hours.

It seems fairly certain that tissue death in severe cold injury occurs both from direct damage to the cell and its structure and to the vasoconstriction and anoxia during exposure and the vascular reaction which follows rewarming. After the state of reactive hyperemia, the pathology gradually changes to that of tissue repair. The cutaneous epithelium proliferates from the margins of denuded areas and from islands of living cells within them. The damaged corium may become scarred and adherent to underlying structures. Small nerves and nerve endings may be caught in scar tissue. The regeneration of injured nerves is attended with the same problems as obtain in other kinds of trauma. Necrotic muscle is replaced by scar. Those structures which fail to survive develop typical ischemic necrosis and gangrene.

Epidemiologic Considerations

Previous mention has been made of the increased susceptibility to frostbite of those made inactive by such factors as inebriation and sleep. The importance of motivation to avoid cold injury cannot be overemphasized — of seeking shelter if possible, of keeping the body as warm as one can, of regular and frequent exercising of the digits and other portions of the extremities. Military experiences have confirmed on a large scale the importance of these and related factors. Frostbite increased with combat maneuvers which immobilized troops, with fatigue as estimated by days without rest from combat, by inadequacy of clothing and foot gear. Such injuries occur more commonly in those with lower army general classification test scores than those of their noninjured comrades, in those who have sustained a previous cold injury, and in Negroes as compared with whites. The marked racial difference observed was thought possibly to have been influenced by lower scores in the Negro group. Frostbite occurs more often is those reared in warm areas than in those who have grown up in cold climates. There is certainly good reason to assume that accustomization is a most important factor and very suggestive clinical and experimental data that actual acclimitazation is a protective reality.

Treatment

The effort to arrive at a valid and useful method of managing frostbite has been a painfully slow process. It has not been easy to get rid of unscientifically based concepts which have come down from the past. Accumulation of controlled clinical observations has been exceedingly difficult. Cold injury occurs primarily in times of war and especially in times of maximal combat activity, periods when it is particularly hard to make meaningful assessments. In civilian life, frostbite occurs sporadically and few individuals see and treat cases in sufficient numbers to permit adequate evaluation of measures of potential benefit. The problem is compounded by the difficulty in predicting accurately the outcome in any individual case and in matching one case of frostbite with another.

Experimental studies have contributed much to our basic understanding of the pathogenesis and management of frostbite. Laboratory studies have certain definite advantages over observations which can be made in man in that reproducible injuries can be utilized, adequate controls are possible, one can deal with statistically significant numbers in evaluating the results of any given study, and various methods which might be potentially useful can be investigated. They have, nevertheless, certain disadvantages. The readily available laboratory animals which must be utilized withstand exposure to low ambient temperatures with less hazard of local injury than man does and they have a much more stable vasomotor apparatus than man and one decidedly less reactive to cold. Although some studies have been carried out upon injuries induced by exposing small animals to a low ambient temperature, most of the investigations have been performed upon rapidly produced freezing injuries resulting from brief immersion of a limb, tail, or ear in a cool mixture. These are quite like high altitude and other quickly induced freezing injuries in man. As has been mentioned, however, most injuries are sustained after a somewhat prolonged exposure and very commonly without actual freezing of the tissues of the damaged part to ice. Although much remains to be learned, frostbite can now be treated more rationally and more effectively than in the past.

General Measures

From the first, everything possible should be done to make sure that no further damage is inflicted either from exposure to cold or from other physical factors. Body temperatures should be restored to normal without delay and further exposure to cold avoided if possible. Shelter should be obtained, wet garments removed, and the body wrapped with warm clothing or blankets. Any constricting clothing such as gloves should be removed. Attention should naturally be directed to the patient as a whole and any associated injuries such as fractures given proper attention.

Immediate thawing should not be attempted in those rare circumstances where the patient is found in an extremely cold environment with the injured hand still solidly frozen, if there is a likelihood that refreezing might take place during transporation to a suitable institution for definitive treatment. Both clinical observations and animal experimentation indicate that limbs repeatedly frozen and thawed are especially susceptible to extreme damage. More commonly the injured hand will either not be solidly frozen at the time first examined or the patient can be transported without danger of a subsequent freezing injury. The

hand should be protected by whatever measures are available against further injury during transportation, for example, by wrapping it in bulky dressings.

When the patient reaches the hospital in which definitive treatment is to be carried out he should be placed in a normally warm room. The injured hand should be protected from the pressure of bed clothing. Every effort should be made to prevent the rupture of blebs. One of the most effective ways of cleansing the damaged hand and keeping it clean is to soak it periodically in a lukewarm water bath containing some mild antiseptic and cleansing agent such as hexachlorophene, using by perference a whirlpool bath if this is available. Second and third degree vesicles which remain uninfected should be allowed to become dry and shed of their own accord. Large blebs which have been accidentally ruptured require the protection of sterile dressings. It may be necessary to place sterile gauze squares or cotton or lamb's wool between fingers if there are open lesions on adjacent digits. Obviously infected vesicles should be opened and treated with saline compresses or, if maceration is feared, with alternate compresses and dressings of a bland ointment such as bacitracin. Infected areas should be debrided of any devitalized tissue present. Cultures should be taken and appropriate antibiotic therapy instituted.

It is not clear whether antibiotics should be utilized in all cases initially nor whether antitetanus treatment should always be carried out. There would seem to be rationale for antibiotic coverage for a short period until it is evident that the injured part is not going to become grossly infected. Similarly, in the more severe injuries it would be wise to administer tetanus toxoid to those who have been immunized and tetanus antitoxin to the others. One of the cardinal principles of proper care of the cold-injured hand is to exercise conservatism with respect to debridement and amputation. Amputation should not be carried out before there is clear demarcation of the gangrenous portion so that no viable tissue will be sacrificed. Often early in frostbite one's estimate of the ultimate loss of tissue exceeds that which actually obtains. The open and denuded areas are taken care of in much the same way as are similar lesions in other injuries. Those which are best managed by application of skin grafts are so treated at the appropriate time. Since ultimate demarcation of devitalized parts and healing of blebs and ulcerated areas requires time, it is important that the hand be maintained in good position and that the patient practice active and passive exercises in order to minimize ultimate joint fibrosis and deformity.

Specific Measures

There is no question about the *initial management of the still frozen limb*. It should be thawed as rapidly as possible by immersing it in water or physiologic saline solution slightly warmer than body temperature. Numerous animal experiments have demonstrated that rapid thawing of the frozen part is by far the most effective measure for salvaging tissue which would otherwise be lost. No similar controlled observations have been made in clinical cases. Indeed, most of those especially interested in cold injuries have not had the opportunity of treating frostbite in the frozen state. Mills of Anchorage, Alaska has had, however, a very large experience and is thoroughly convinced that rapid rewarming of the still frozen limb is the single best therapeutic measure for minimizing or obviating gangrene. He recommends immediate immersion in a whirlpool bath. The water bath temperature should probably ideally be maintained at about 42°C. Animal experiments have demonstrated that rapid thawing at 38°C is not as effective and that use of temperature as high as 50°C may be actually harmful. Immersion in the water bath should be maintained only as long as is necessary to achieve actual thawing. This requires a variable time and is related to the extent and depth of the frozen tissue. On the average 15 or 20 minutes is sufficient. Judging from animal experiments, prolonged exposure to such warmth may enhance the tissue damage.

Rapid warming may be quite painful and pain-relieving medication such as morphine should be given beforehand. The addition of some mild cleansing and germicidal agent such as hexachlorophene may be very helpful. If no whirlpool bath is available one may soak the hand in an ordinary water bath. Less effective still is the use of bulky warm wet compresses.

It is not clear whether the cold but not frozen limb should be warmed rapidly in a similar fashion. Since it has not been possible to produce nonfreezing injuries in animals similar to those which occur in man, no data are available upon the value of warming quickly the extremity which has not been frozen. Studies have been carried out concerning the value of rapidly warming the cold but no longer frozen extremity of experimental animals. Although the results are far less dramatic than in the case of the still frozen limb, the data do suggest that some benefit may be derived from this method of management. Furthermore, in one clinical appraisal, benefit was noted by patients with mild frostbite who warmed their cooled extremities as compared with similarly injured patients who made an attempt to delay rewarming.

There is no place in management for delaying the natural thawing and warming process or of maintaining the damaged hand for a long period in a cool state. There is no recorded clinical experience which would indicated that the end result is improved by such measures. Experimental studies in animals with frostbite produced both by immersion of an extremity in a freezing mixture and by exposure of the body to a low ambient temperature have shown quite early that prolonged cooling not only does not prevent tissue loss which would otherwise be sustained but may indeed increase the anticipated loss.

Compression Dressings. Since some believe that edema fluid may contribute to damage in the frostbitten hand by distortion, conpression, and kinking of capillaries, one may logically wonder whether compression dressings have a place in treatment. There are no pertinent controlled clinical observations. This matter has, however, been investigated thoroughly in experimental animal frostbite utilizing both pressure dressings and plaster casts. The results have been variable and certainly not sufficiently convincing to warrant their utilization in clinical cases. Furthermore, it has been demonstrated that a comparable degree of swelling occurs during the first 24 hours in animals treated by rapid thawing and in control subjects not so treated. Despite the rapid development of equal edema, tissue loss was far less in the rapidly thawed group. The swollen hand should be kept in an elevated position but compression dressings should not be used.

Efforts to Improve the Microcirculation and Prevent Thrombosis. Since it is known that early after cold injury the microcirculation is distinctly abnormal, that platelet and endothelial adhesiveness is increased, that red cell sludging develops, that agglutinative thrombi form and that true thrombosis ultimately takes place, any effort to prevent these occurrences would appear theoretically worthwhile. One measure of potential benefit might be heparinization. It has not been possible up to the present to obtain carefully controlled observations in clinical subjects. Extensive animal experimentation has, however, been carried out. The results have been suggestive of some possible benefit, but have varied so widely as to make them of doubtful value. Furthermore, delay in heparinization for even a few hours after injury generally seemed to diminish the possible effectiveness of this agent. It is difficult to see that any harm would result from heparinization in any specific case provided no contraindication to its use existed. On the other hand, there is so little evidence, if any, of its effectiveness that its routine use can not logically be recommended.

It seems evident that the ingestion of aspirin does alter platelet adhesiveness and no harm would result from its trial in human cases. No study of this sort has been reported and no animal experiments have been described.

Experiments with low molecular dextran indicate that this may be useful in salvaging tissue which might otherwise be lost. Since this agent, which is known to have beneficial effects on the microcirculation, intravascular corpuscular clumping, erythrocyte sludging, and other factors which might lead to thrombosis, is innocuous, it might well be tried as an adjuvant in cases of frostbite. Although it has been so employed, no controlled observations have been reported.

Another agent which is thought to have similar anti-sludging properties, Pluronic F-68 (poloxalkol), has been evaluated in experimental frostbite and has been reported to reduce the incidence and extent of gangrene. It too would appear a harmless agent in man and might well be given a clinical trial.

Sympathectomy. For over 30 years patients with frostbite have been treated sporadically by temporary anesthetic blockade of the regional sympathetics or operative sympathectomy. Although some beneficial effects have been observed from the very first, only recently has immediate operative sympathectomy been established as a rational therapeutic measure for severe cases of frostbite. It was quite difficult to obtain any sort of controlled observations in man. The difficulty in predicting the outcome in any given case proved a stumbling block in arriving at clear-cut decisions. Confusion resulted from attempting to consider all together the various types of cold injuries which differ somewhat from one another. Further confusion resulted from analyzing together observations concerning operative sympathectomy, anesthetic paralysis of the regional sympathetic chain, administration of autonomic blocking agents, and the now abandoned procedure of periarterial sympathectomy. The animal experiments which have been numerous and carefully controlled have proved of little help, primarily, I believe because the animals utilized have a much more stable vasomotor tonus and a less reactive sympathetic response than man.

Gradually, however, clear-cut evidence has been forthcoming. Sympathectomy leads to earlier cessation of pain, more rapid subsidence of edema, quicker demarcation of viable and nonviable parts, earlier autoamputation, and more prompt healing of denuded areas. It is now evident that it may, in addition, also conserve tissue which might otherwise be lost. This conclusion is based upon a number of observations, for example, the better outcome in the sympathectomized extremity when this procedure is performed on one side in cases of apparently equal symmetrical involvement. It is also based upon observed preservation of tissue the loss of which was clearly to be anticipated. As an example, persistently cold, cyanotic, and anesthetic digits during the phase of reactive hyperemia have been salvaged. Sympathectomy is, therefore, recommended as an emergency measure in patients with obvious fourth degree or widespread third degree frostbite in whom the risk of operative denervation is thought to be minimal as is usually the case.

Other Methods of Treatment. A number of other measures have been studied in experimental frostbite including the use of rutin and other flavanoids and antihistaminic agents. As of the present, there would seem to be no reason for their use in man.

Management of the Sequelae of Frostbite.

Some patients recover from frostbite with no annoying sequelae. As have been mentioned previously, however, sympathetic overactivity and cold sensitivity complaints are common. Not infrequently the hand persistently exhibits a tendency towards excessive vasoconstriction and often hyperhidrosis. It is likely to be especially sensitive to cold. For more than 20 years it has been evident that sympathetic denervation has a gratifying effect upon these complaints. Most patients so treated maintain reasonably warm extremities. The hands are less sensitive to cold and not infrequently without any cold sensitivity whatsoever. Hyperhidrosis disappears. Furthermore, observations upon patients in whom sympathetic denervation has been carried out shortly after cold injury indicate that cold is readily perceived in the sympathetically denervated hand even better than in the normally innervated one and is protected from subsequent cold injury extraordinarily well. Not infrequently the patient who has had one extremity sympathetically denervated during a cold injury later requests that the same procedure be carried out upon the nonsympathectomized contralateral limb because the treated one has proved to be so much more comfortable and so free of troublesome complaints.

SUMMARY

Frostbite occurs from exposure to cold. The severity of the injury is related to the intensity and duration of exposure and to certain other contributing factors. Management of the injured hand should be characterized by conservatism with respect to debridement and amputation. Rapid thawing is of great value in the occasional patient whose treatment is begun with the hand still frozen. Immediate sympathectomy is a useful adjuvant in cases of severe frostbite. Measures which tend to improve the microcirculation, which serve as antisludging agents and which may diminish the likelihood and extent of intravascular thrombosis may deserve cautious clinical trial. Sympathetic denervation is most useful for the vasospastic, hyperhidrotic, and cold-sensitivity sequelae of frostbite.

REFERENCES

1. *Cold Injury: Transactions of the First Conference, June 4-5, 1951,* edited by M. I. Ferrer. The Josiah Macy, Jr., Foundation. Bristol, The Hildreth Press, 1952.
2. *Cold Injury: Transactions of the Second Conference, November 20-21, 1952,* edited by M. I. Ferrer. The Josiah Macy, Jr., Foundation. New York, Corbies, Macy, 1954.
3. de Jong, P., Golding, M. R., Sawyer, P. N., and Wesolowski, S. A. Role of regional sympathectomy in early management of cold injury. Surg. Gynecol. Obstet., *115:* 45, 1962.
4. Golding, M. R., de Jong, P., Sawyer, P. N., Hennigar, G. R., and Wesolowski S. A. Protection from early and late sequelae of frostbite by regional sympathectomy: Mechanism of "cold sensitivity" following

frostbite. Surgery, *53:* 303, 1963.

5. Knize, D. M. Weatherly-White, R. C. A., and Paton, B. C. Use of antisludging agents in experimental cold injuries. Surg. Gynecol. Obstet., *129:* 1019, 1969.

6. Meryman, H. T. Mechanics of freezing in living cells and tissues. Science, *124:* 515, 1956.

7. Meryman, H. T. Tissue freezing and local cold injury. Phys. Rev., *37:* 233, 1951.

8. Mills, W. J., Jr., Fish, W., and Whaley, R. Frostbite: Experience with rapid rewarming and ultrasonic therapy. Alaska Med., *2:* 1, 114, 1960.

9. Mills, W. J., Jr., Fish, W., and Whaley, R. Frostbite: Experience with rapid rewarming and ultrasonic therapy. Alaska Med., *3:* 28, 1961.

10. Minor, T. M., and Shumacker, H. B., Jr. An evaluation of tissue loss following single and repeated frostbite injuries. Surgery, *61:* 562, 1967.

11. Mundt, E. D., Long, D. M., and Brown, R. B. Treat-ment of experimental frostbite with low molecular weight dextran. J. Trauma, *4:* 246, 1964.

12. Orr, K. D., and Fainer, D. C. Cold injuries in Korea during the winter of 1950-1951. Medicine, *51:* 117, 1952.

13. Shikata, J., Shumacker, H. B., Jr., and Nash, F. D. Studies in experimental frostbite. The effect of cold acclimatization upon resistance to local cold injury. Arch. Surg., *81:* 817, 1960.

14. Shumacker, H. B., Jr. Sympathectomy in the treatment of frostbite. Surg. Gynecol. Obstet., *93:* 727, 1951.

15. Shumacker, H. B., Jr., and Kilman, J. W. Sympathectomy in the treatment of frostbite. Arch. Surg., *89:* 575, 1964.

16. Shumacker, H. B., Jr., and Kunkler, A. W. Studies in experimental frostbite. IX. Rapid thawing and prolonged cooling in the treatment of frostbite resulting from exposure to low ambient temperature. Surg. Gynecol. Obstet., *94:* 475, 1952.

chapter thirteen

Vascular Disorders

A.

Vascular Disorders of the Hand

Ralph A. Deterling, Jr., M.D.

INTRODUCTION

Significant advances in the management of vascular disorders of the hand have occurred during the past 25 years largely through applied research and increased clinical experience. With more specific understanding of the underlying pathophysiology and greatly improved methods od disgnosis, there has developed more effective coordinated medical and surgical therapy. In some instances, there has been refinement of surgical technique which has produced less risk and complications, as well as improved long-term results. During the past decade very informative and comprehensive books on peripheral vascular disease have appeared, [7] [11] [22] [40] [47] [48] [59] [67] [79] [99] [110] [118] [126] including certain ones devoted essentially to surgical technique. [49] [62] [121]

For the physician interested primarily in the hand, it would require a tedious perusal of the texts in order to delineate the specific vascular disorders which affect the hand as well as to discern the specific diagnostic procedures and methods of therapy specifically applicable to problems involving the hand. Even standard texts on hand surgery deal with the vascular disorders in rather perfunctory fashion. [15] [17] [97]

For a complete understanding, one must realize that certain apparent vascular disorders involving the hand may result from pathologic processes which are not primarily arterial or venous in origin and that those which are essentially vascular in nature may result from involvement of the intrinsic vasculature of the hand or be secondary to those located in the arm, the shoulder, or the thoracic outlet. Furthermore, some of the vascular and nonvascular lesions involving the hand may be only one area of manifestation of widespread systemic disease. It is the purpose of this chapter to describe the signs and symptoms, methods of diagnosis and treatment of those vascular conditions which affect the hand, and fingers in particular.

BASIC CONSIDERATIONS

In order to appreciate all of the causative factors in the vascular disorders of the hand one ideally should have a comprehension of the embryologic development of the arterial and venous systems, the anatomic relationships and variations encountered in the hand, and also the physiologic responses of the peripheral vessels.

Embryologically the arm bud develops during the third week of gestation through the proliferation of mesenchymal tissue and a primary axillary artery extends from a lateral aortic branch. Terminally there is a plexus of small vessels from which subsequently develop the arteries of the hand and fingers. In the next stage of development the single trunk becomes the interosseous artery. Shortly thereafter a median artery emerges from the trunk in the forearm, and connection of the interosseous artery with the digital plexus disappears. Still later the ulnar artery appears proximally and extends into the hand to form one of the palmar arches which in turn unites with that produced by the last of the major vessels, the radial artery which arises still higher from the superficial brachial artery. About this time the median artery undergoes regression and becomes the artery of the median nerve. The complete organization of the arm and hand and its component structures is complete by the end of the second month.

The development of the veins is similiar with a border vein draining a terminal plexus. From the ulnar portion of this vein develops the subclavian, axillary, and basilic veins whereas the cephalic vein arises from the radial extension of the border vein. A persistence of the primitive connections between the undifferentiated arterial and venous terminal plexes gives rise after birth to congenital arterial venous fistulae, localized for the most part in the forearm or hand. A more detailed description of normal development in the fetus may be found in medical text books, [8] [92] reports from the Carnegie Institute, and in the anatomic literature. [36] [109] [128]

The ultimate pattern of the vascular system of the hand is adequately presented in most standard text books of anatomy. The two major arteries supplying the hand are the radial and ulnar arteries. The former arises at the level of the elbow as the lesser terminal branch of the brachial artery. At the wrist it courses over the dorsal surface of the first metacarpal to pass between the heads of the first dorsal interosseous muscle and emerges on the palmar aspect of the hand to form the deep palmar (volar) arch. The ulnar artery originates in the cubital fossa as the greater terminal branch of the brachial artery. Coursing with the ulnar nerve, it soon gives rise to the common interosseous artery, an important vessel embryologically. At the wrist, the ulnar artery runs over the radial surface of the pisiform bone between the volar and transverse carpal ligaments, to form the major transverse superficial volar arch about mid palm. One must realize that considerable variation may exist in the seemingly normal hand. [36] [131] This may be appreciated only when an unexpected degree of ischemia develops in the hand and/or fingers following the interruption of one of the major arteries in the region of the wrist or palm as a result of trauma or occlusive disease.

Probably the most common and important variation is an underdeveloped or absent communication between the palmar arches (Fig. 13.1.1). This and other variations have been recognized through detailed anatomic dissection, arteriography, and mass injection of the hand (Fig. 13.1.2 A and B). [6] [18] [36] The abundant major arterial branches and communications in the hand are not present in the fingers. Although, in general, a single branch from the superficial palmar arches divides to supply the medial side of one digit and lateral aspect of the next, the artery to the index finger may supply the entire digit as well as half the middle finger. Usually the digital arteries on the medial side of the thumb, index, and fifth finger are larger than the lateral one. There are transverse anastomoses which occur regularly and interruption of one digital artery usually has little importance except in the thumb. There is an increase in the size of the contributing arterial branches to the terminal tufts as one grows beyond childhood. Of considerable importance is the distribution of the sympathetic nerves in the extremity. This has been described by Woolard[129] and others.

The physiologic function of the peripheral arteries of the hand and fingers is very important. Pulse registration and blood flow in the fingers, as demonstrated by plethysmography and other techniques, indicate rapid and often profound alternations in response to changes in posture, temperature, physical activity, internal metabolism, psychic, nervous, and hormonal state. [1] [34] [36] [42] [101] [110] [124] [126] [127] Certain drugs and chemical agents can produce intensive vasodilatation or vasoconstriction, and certain of these, if active over prolonged periods of time, may actually induce pathologic organic changes. Vasodilatation of digital arteries is greater in response to general warming of the body than from local heat, and arterial flow from vasoconstriction may be only one twentieth resting volume, but produce severe effects if prolonged. [124]

STUDY OF THE PATIENT

It may seem unnecessary to mention, but a complete history and physical examination of any patient suspected of having a vascular disorder is essential since so many conditions are not limited to the hand. Detailed and painstaking interrogation may provide sufficient information as to make exact diagnosis easily confirmed by examination and certain special studies.

Family history may reveal the presence of acquired or congenital vascular disease in several individuals. Of obvious importance is information on the use of tobacco, alcohol, and certain drugs such as ergot, lead, and arsenicals. The occupation of the patient may reveal exposure to trauma, cold, dampness, or toxic agents. Systemic review may indicate important factors such as allergies, diabetes mellitus, syphilis, rheumatic heart disease with auricular fibrillation, cerebral or cardiac arteriosclerotic disease, hypertension, hypertrophic arthritis, peripheral neuritis, or disease of the central nervous system. Recently the significance of psychiatric instability has been increasingly appreciated in relation to its effect on peripheral vasomotor tone. [29] [34] A timely addition to the medical history involves drug addiction, particularly in the youthful patient, since severe acute vasomotor and even organic effects may be observed in the hand after accidental injections of drugs into an artery of the upper extremity.

Since pain is the complaint which most frequently compels the patient with peripheral vascular disease to seek medical advice, appreciation of its exact nature is vital. One should determine the time of initial onset and whether it is persistent or intermittent. Sudden onset may suggest traumatic, embolic, or thrombotic etiology. In the drug addict, particulate matter or extremes in the pH of the injected solution may produce serious damage to the arteries of the hand and fingers, reflected initially as acute painful vasoconstriction. One must determine the factors which can produce the pain, as well as aggravate or lessen it. The severity of the pain should be evaluated in terms of the patient's general tolerance to pain. The effect on the pain by pressure, muscular activity or stress, time of day, changes in posture, heavy meals, exposure to cold, medications, and emotional disturbance should be ascertained. The association with trophic changes, dermatitis, masses, hyperhidrosis, inflammation, atrophy or enlargement of the extremity, localized swelling or generalized edema, numbness or paresthesias, color changes, alteration in cutaneous temperature, and ulceration or gangrene may provide clues to diagnosis. One should elicit an exact description of the type of pain, whether dull, aching, sharp, tearing, cramping, throbbing, "shooting", tingling, or burning. Determine if it is localized, diffuse, or radiating.

Skin sensation is at times altered in vascular conditions. Marked hyperesthesia may be observed with causalgia following trauma or in early arterial occlusion. When ischemia is advanced, a state of hypesthesia or numbness develops.

The character of color changes in an important index of vascular disease. Persistent pallor or cyanosis without edema may suggest stages of arterial occlusion, especially if accompanied by coolness. Pallor

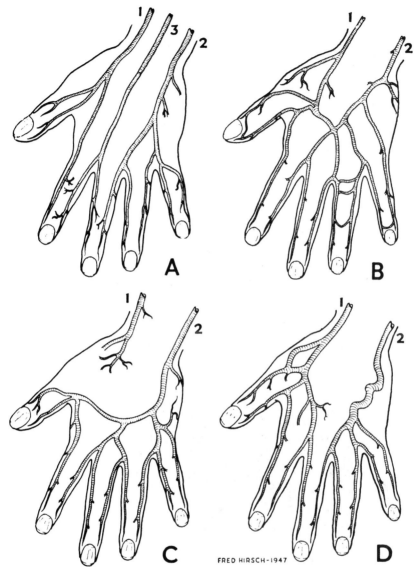

Figure 13.1.1. Important variations in the arteries of the hand as described by Jones Quain in 1847. (Reproduced from *Vascular Disease in Clinical Practice.*[131]).

with elevation of the arm indicates an arterial occlusive process. Persistent cyanosis with swelling is more suggestive of venous occlusion or acrocyanosis. Redness, heat, and swelling may indicate inflammation or a vascular condition such as hemangioma, traumatic or mycotic aneurysm, or thrombophlebitis. Parchy red to blush discoloration is observed in livedo reticularis. Intermittent color changes suggest vasospastic conditions, such as Raynaud's phenomenon or erythromelalgia. Raynaud's phenomenon consists of phasic changes in vasomotor tone due to sympathetic nervous imbalance. Characteristically, one or more fingers blanch in spotty areas or in their entirety. The palm may be involved and pain or tingling may be pres-

ent. A cyanotic phase may follow and at times an erythematous reaction. The attack may last from minutes to hours and may be elicited by exposure to cold, or emotional upset. It occurs as a part of the clinical picture of other vascular disorders, to be described in this chapter. It has also been reported with essential hypertension.[70] Warmth or sympathetic blockade are effective in reducing or abolishing the vasomotor alterations. If vasomotor changes are produced by certain positions of the arm or head, one considers mechanical interference with circulation.

The temperature of the skin is also an important index of vascular tone. The greatest variation is found in the fingers and hence the blood flow in the arm may

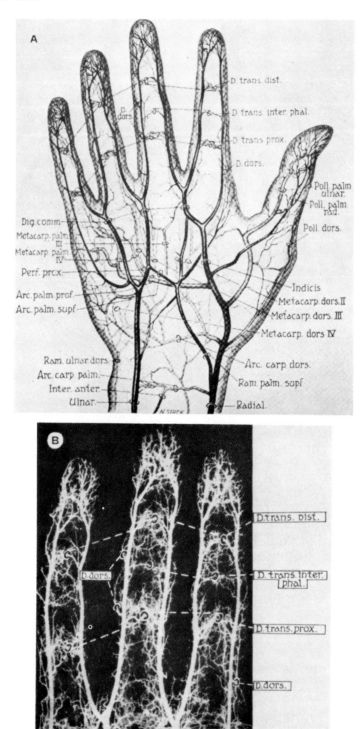

Figure 13.1.2A. A drawing of the arterial pattern of the hand from stereo-scopic study of an arteriogram of the hand from a 16-year-old boy. The superficial palmar arch is atypically proximal. There are also variations in the supply to the fingers. (Reproduced from the American Journal of Surgery.[36])

Figure 13.1.2B. Magnified view of injection arteriogram of three middle digits of the same specimen, using a mercury-barium sulfate emulsion (Reproduced from the American Journal of Surgery.[36])

not be indicated by digital cutaneous temperatures. Since the circulation provides blood to the skin, the heat measured is essentially that lost by the blood. A warm skin area may indicate increased arterial circulation, but inflammation may also elevate the temperature. A cold skin area similarly suggests arterial occlusion or vasoconstriction, although an edematous part may have decreased temperature without major deficiencies in circulation.

Ecchymosis, telangiectasis, and petechiae may suggest a process which is intrinsically a vascular condition or which may secondarily involve the vessels. Following trauma, ecchymosis is common if there has been extravasation of blood. Telangiectasis of the fingers may result from radiation burns, dermatomyositis, and lupus erythermatosis. Petechiae can occur in association with acute arterial insufficiency if pressure is applied or if anticoagulant therapy is employed. They also may indicate subacute bacterial endocarditis or polyarteritis nodosa.

In addition to discolorations, other features indicative of vascular disease should be noted by physical examination. Inspection of the skin may reveal trophic changes such as atrophy of the skin, loss of hair, and thickened nails, found with advanced arteriosclerotic disease. Pitted scars at the tips of the digits are observed in Raynaud's disease, thromboangitis obliterans, and certain other conditions. Ulcerations of the hand or fingers may result from trauma (mechanical, thermal, cold, electrical, chemical), arterial occlusive disease or embolism, Raynaud's disease, sclerodactylis, hemangioma, and congenital arteriovenous fistulae. Actual gangrene of digits may result from a variety of causes such as any type of trauma, embolism, arteriosclerotic occlusion, thromboangiitis obliterans, scalene anticus syndrome, and Raynaud's disease. Less common causes have been cryoglobulinemia, ergotism, arsenical or lead intoxication, and myocardial infarction.

Careful palpation of the arteries of the extremities, scalp and temporal region, and of the abdominal aorta will yield evidence of partial or complete occlusion, aneurysm, and arteriovenous fistula. With respect to disorders involving the hand, the equality and strength of the pulse should be determined in the subclavian, auxillary, brachial, ulnar, radial, and even digital arteries (Fig. 13.1.3). A thrill may be felt in the area or peripheral to such lesions. Ausculatation may reveal a systolic bruit produced by aneurysm or an acutely angulated or partially obstructed artery. A characteristic machinery murmur is usually heard over arteriovenous fistula. Certain venous disorders and vascular tumors may also produce a bruit.

Careful palpation will also reveal tumors which may suggest neoplasm, aneurysm, or a firm cord like structure, perhaps indicative of arterial or venous thrombosis. It should be noted that in Maffucci's syndrome, soft tissue angiomas are associated with skeletal chondromas. In one interesting case of a lady

with the hands involved primarily, there were multiple arteriovenous fistulae in the tumors involving the fingers (Fig. 13.1.4).[56] Enlargement or atrophy have been mentioned as resulting from vascular disorders. Diffuse edema may result from venous or lymphatic obstruction, if not on a systemic basis. It has even been observed in hysterical neuroses when the arm is maintained in a fixed, dependent position.[125] Prominent veins may result from hemangioma, arteriovenous fistula, axillary vein thrombosis. Atrophy and weakness may be sequelae of chronic arterial insufficiency rather than be primary neurologic effects.

Excessive sweating is produced by overactivity of sympathetic tone and is frequently seen in vasospastic conditions such as Raynaud's disease. It may also merely reflect disturbed psychosomatic balance. When severe enough, treatment by drugs such as Banthine[46] and mephobarbital[104] or even sympathetic denervation may be indicated.[123]

SPECIAL EXAMINATIONS AND TESTS

1. Maneuver to Determine Arterial Occlusion or Compression

A. Allen Test. Because of arterial occlusive disease or congenital anomaly, there may be a deficient superficial or deep palmar arch, or communication between them. In order to determine competency, a simple test may be performed to demonstrate adequacy of ulnar or radial supply to the hand.[5][7]

Both pulses are palpated at the wrist by the

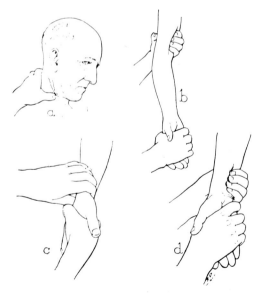

Figure 13.1.3. Method of palpating the major arteries supplying the arm and hand: A) carotid and subclavian arteries; B) brachial artery; C) radial artery; and D) ulnar artery. (Reproduced from *Peripheral Vascular Disease.*[7])

examiner facing the patient, whose palm is extended upwards. These arteries are then occluded by pressure from the thumb or the tips of the fingers of the examiner. The patient clenches his fist several times to empty blood from the hand. The patient then extends the fingers and the radial artery is released. A rapid pink flush appears in the thenar region extending into the fingers and gradually across the palm. The test is repeated, this time with release only of the ulnar artery. If there is insufficient circulation provided by the arches, the half of the hand supplied by the deficient vessel will remain pale. Obviously if one pulse cannot be felt, the occlusive test need generally be performed only on the opposite vessel.

B. Adson Test In studying patients with cervical rib or hypertrophied scalene anticus muscle, Adson noted that taking a deep breath, turning the head sharply to the suspected side, and backwards tensed the muscle, compressing the subclavian artery and obliterating the pulses at the wrist (Fig. 13.1.5). Subsequently, it has been observed that in some patients, the test is positive if the head is turned in the opposite direction. [12] It is therefore best if both maneuvers are employed in diagnosing the scalene anticus syndrome.

C. Wright Test. Recognizing that the anatomic arrangements at the shoulder could produce compression of the subclavian artery by simple hyperabduction of the arm, Wright described a suitable maneuver

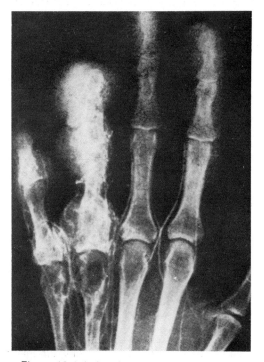

Figure 13.1.4. Arteriogram demonstrating multiple arteriovenous malformations in tumors of fingers of left hand. (Reproduced from Archives of Surgery.[56])

to test this clinically (Fig. 13.1.6A). [130]

The examiner stands behind the sitting patient while palpating the radial pulse. The arm is then hyperabducted through 180° and the quality of the pulse is noted. In a positive test, the pulse will diminish greatly or disappear. It should be performed with the patient supine, as well. [12]

D. Costoclavicular Test. Compression of the subclavian artery between the clavicle and first rib can occur in debilitated individuals or as a result of abnormal pressure on the shoulder girdle as produced by shoulder packs of soldiers. [37 76 77 103] With the examiner behind the patient and palpating the radial artery with the arms at his side, the shoulder is forced backwards and downwards. In a positive test, the pulse diminishes or disappears (Fig. 13.1.6B).

2. Angiography

During the past four decades, there has been remarkable improvement in contrast media, and roentgenographic equipment designed especially for visualization of the arteries and veins. With development of nontoxic organic iodide preparations such as Hypaque, Renografin, Conray, and others, the risk and discomfort from such a procedure is negligible. Special needles and catheters for direct and retrograde injection have been produced. Seriography is now possible for routine studies in most major hospitals dealing with the treatment of vascular disease. Sequential standard films or cinefluorography are being utilized increasingly in preference to the single film. As medical and surgical therapy have advanced, so have diagnostic methods. Since the introduction of microsurgical technique, it is possible to perform reconstructive surgery on arteries and veins less than 3 mm in diameter.[60 68] Consequently, a series of films can show the rate and degree of vascular opacification from arm to terminal digital tuft and localize single or multiple lesions amenable to surgical correction. Angiography has a role in determining the rate of progression of a disease process or improvement through development of collateral channels.

A. Arteriography. Visualization of the arteries of the extremity may be performed in a standard roentgenographic room, although a special film changer or cine-unit is desirable. Premedication reduces apprehension and pain attending the procedure. For visualization of the hand, the patient is placed supine and the antecubital space is prepared with an antiseptic solution prior to draping the area with sterile towels. One cc of 1 per cent Xylocaine is infiltrated about the brachial artery once it has been accurately located by palpation. A 19-gauge Seldinger arterial needle with guidewire or a Cournand needle are preferable to those provided for standard venipuncture. Usually operative exposure is not required. The needle is advanced through the subcutaneous tissue in a proximal direction, at a flat angle, until arterial pulsation can be felt. The needle is then advanced into the

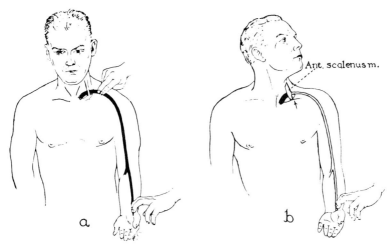

Ant. scalenus m.

Figure 13.1.5. Technique for performing the Adson test for scalene anticus syndrome. (Reproduced from Surgery, Gynecology and Obstetrics.[4])

lumen and its location inside the artery can be ascertained by briefly removing the stylet or guidewire. With this replaced, the needle is advanced 2 cm up the vessel so that with injection, particularly with automatic pressure devices, the needle will not be disengaged. It should be noted that vascular injuries have resulted from high pressure injection. [64]

Should the patient have low pain threshhold, a few cubic centimeters of 1 per cen Xylocaine (Lidocaine, (Astra Pharmaceutical Products, Worcester, Mass.) into the artery just before injecting the contrast medium may minimize pain response to the injection. Recently better visualization has been achieved by the use of reactive hyperemia or intra-arterial vasodilating drugs, prior to injection of the contrast medium. With the former technique, a blood pressure cuff is applied to the arm and inflated to just above systolic blood pressure for seven minutes. After rapid release of the cuff and the presence of arterial skin blush in the hand, the contrast material is injected for the arteriogram. A simpler and perhaps preferable approach has been to inject 20 to 25 mg of Priscoline (Tolazoline hyrochloride, Ciba Pharmaceutical Co., Summit N.J.) intravenously over a two-minute period. Thirty seconds after the injection is completed the contrast material is injected and the arteriogram obtained. Rapid injection of 10 to 15 cc of Conray and exposure of one to three films per second for approximately five seconds continuing the series with two exposures at longer intervals will allow the venous phase also to be recorded. Repeated injection may be desirable in another projection. At times a single 14 x 17 inch film may be exposed at the end of rapid injection if a more extensive area is to be examined (Fig. 13.1.7).

In order to study the subclavian, axillary, and brachial arteries, the technique used to visualize the aortic arch is now preferable to direct injection into the subclavian artery in the superclavicular space. Most commonly a Seldinger catheter is introduced percutaneously into a femoral artery and advanced up the aorta into the transverse arch orifice of the subclavian artery. Patients in whom "subclavian steal" is suspected, the caroid and vertebral arteries may also be visualized by this method (Fig. 13.1.8).

B. Venography. Following similar skin preparations, injection is made into a superficial vein distal to the area to be studied. The same equipment and dosage may be used, but since venous flow is slow, exposure of a single film after the delay of one or two seconds provides more complete visualization on a single film. Here too seriography has definite advantages in revealing the values and collateral pattern. Exact delineation of an abnormal venous lesion of the hand may be achieved by injecting a few cubic milliliters directly into the veins in the area.

3. Sympathetic Block

Infiltration of the sympathetic ganglia and chain with Xylocaine provides relaxation of sympathetic activity in the area supplied. The effects of a satisfactory block are vasodilatation and increased skin warmth, increased venous filling, and dryness, provided the vessels are responsive. Thus is afforded a means of differentiating between the degree of arterial spasm and occlusion. [122] In addition the pain in the hand of sympathetic nervous origin is relieved. Although infiltration of the upper four thoracic sympathetic ganglia from the back provides an adequate block, the simpler procedure is injection of the stellate and inferior cervical ganglia by an anterior approach.

With the patient supine, the shoulders are elevated by a small pillow to tilt the head backwards. The skin is infiltrated with 1 per cent Xylocaine at the medial edge of the sternocleidomastoid muscle immediately above the clavicle. A groove is produced by digital pressure over the wheal, and a 2-inch 22-gauge needle

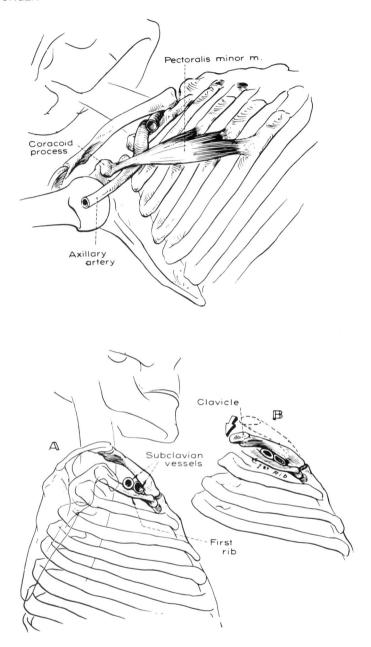

Figure 13.1.6A. Compression of the subclavian vessels by hyperabduction.

Figure 13.1.6 B. Compression of the subclavian vessels between the clavicle and first rib. (Reproduced from the journal of Thoracic and Cardiovascular Surgery.)

is advanced in a posterior, slightly lateral direction until transverse process of the sixth cervical or first thoracic vertebra is engaged. There is less chance of pneumothorax when the needle is directed toward the sixth cervical vertebra. After aspiration, 10 ml³ of 1 per cent Xylocaine is injected. With successful infiltration, the pseudovascular effects appear shortly, ac-

companied by a Horner's sign. These are not always reliable indications of vascular denervation, however. Hence, it has been wise to study the galvanic skin response in the hand or note changes in skin temperature with multiple thermal probes. If the skin temperature of the fingers rises more than 2°C, a very good response is noted.

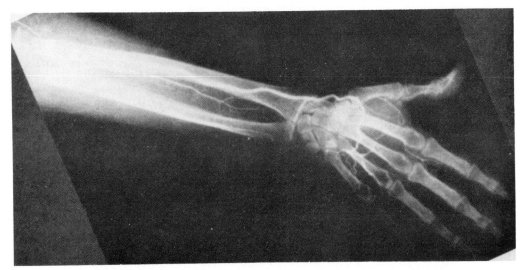

Figure 13.1.7. Arteriogram of right forearm and hand by using 10cc of Renografin 60 and a single film. The radial, interosseus, and ulnar artery are shown in the forearm, but there is occlusive disease of the ulnar artery at the wrist, as well as of certain digital vessels. (Courtesy Dr. Allen D. Callow.)

4. Diagnostic Instrumentation

A. Oscillometry. The Collens oscillometer or recording types have become available in most hospitals. Although challenged on the basis of quantitative value, oscillometric indices do provide confirmatory evidence of arterial occlusion. The cuff is wrapped about the wrist and inflated to approximately the level of systolic arterial pressure. The cuff is deflated in increments of 10 mm of mercury and the needle valve to the tambour released at each step. The deflections of the needle reflect the amplitude of the arterial pulse (Fig. 13.1.9).

B. Plethysmography. For an estimation of actual arterial blood flow in a part, the fingers are well suited to the volume displacement method. The digit is introduced through a perforated disphragm into a plastic cup-like chamber, to which the recording tube is attached. Changes in volume within the chamber are transmitted by the pneumatic system to a transducer which amplifies a signal suitable for recording. From the excursions of the pulse waves measured in the finger tip, blood flow and pulse amplitude can be estimated. Although great improvements have been made in the equipment during the past few years, this apparatus is still considered a research instrument by most clinicians. Nevertheless, increasing numbers of clinical reports include the use of calibrated plethysmography a useful diagnostic method.[42] [110] [126]

C. Skin Temperature. The patient should have fasted and be lightly clothed. The room temperature should be reasonably constant at about 70° F. There should be a period of adjustment of 30 to 60 minutes for equilebration, during which time the patient is lying down comfortably and relaxed. Cutaneous temperature is then recorded from the tips of the fingers and other specific areas of the hand and wrist, comparing the readings with those obtained from the opposite extremity.

In smokers, it is sometimes worthwhile to test tobacco sensitivity by noting response of blood pressure, pulse and cutaneous temperature after smoking two cigarettes (Fig. 13.1.10). There is a significant elevation of pressure and pulse, and fall in temperature in those patients who are particularly susceptible to tobacco.

D. Reflex Vasodilatation. With the patient essentially in a basal state as just described, a heating blanket or lighted cradle is placed over the trunk, to develop an environmental temperature of from 122° to 140° F. With patent vessels and normal vasomotor tone, there is a rapid vasodilatation of the digital arteries and corresponding rise in skin temperature at the finger tips This test has recently acquired greater clinical significance when coupled with sedation to eliminate psychomotor influence. [34]

E. Circulation Time. Obstruction to arterial or venous circulation is reflected in an increased circulation time, since blood must circulate through collateral channels. Test substances such as Evan's blue, sodium fluorescein, or radioactive sodium (Na^{24}) have been utilized to estimate location and degree of impaired circulation. If injected into the brachial artery, the build-up curve may be measured at the finger tip by photoelectric cell or scintillator, depending on the test substance. Isotopes permit counting in areas with greater mass, but results may be equivocal. Another method which has been utilized is the injection of the isotope into an involved part, and measuring the disappearance curve. These techniques are less suited to the hand and fingers than other methods already described.

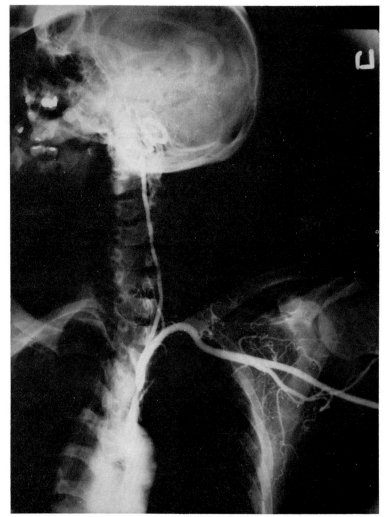

Figure 13.1.8. Occlusion of the left subclavian artery and retrograde filling via the vertebral artery is well demonstrated by a transfemoral retrograde aortic arch arteriogram. (Courtesy Dr. Allan D. Callow[19] and Dr. Paul C. Kahn.)

F. Capillary Microscopy. The superficial vasculature of the matrix and nailfold may be viewed under 50-power magnification, with proper oblique lighting. The number and character of the capillaries, as well as the speed of flow and characteristics of the red cells may be observed and photographed. This type of study has occasionally been of practical use in diagnosing unusual conditions associated with red cell agglutination, but has had greatest application as a research method.

G. Radio Isotopes. For more than two decades various isotopes have been employed sporadically to assess arterial flow and the degrees of ischemia, mostly employing sodium.

More recently there has been increasing success with the use of isotopic labeled blood products in the effort to detect intravenous thrombosis. A decade ago, Ouchi and Warren[90] reported on their use of I[131]-labeled plasma, and during the past few years Kakkar and others in Great Britain have concentrated on I[125] labeled fibrinogen for the detection of deep vein thrombosis. Virtually all of the studies have been performed in the lower extremity, although the test is applicable to patients with suspected axillary vein thrombosis. Since a high percentage of fatal pulmonary emboli originate from unsuspected deep vein thrombosis, primary interest has been directed toward the lower extremities.

H. Impedance Studies. Recently clinical studies have shown an acceptable degree of accuracy when

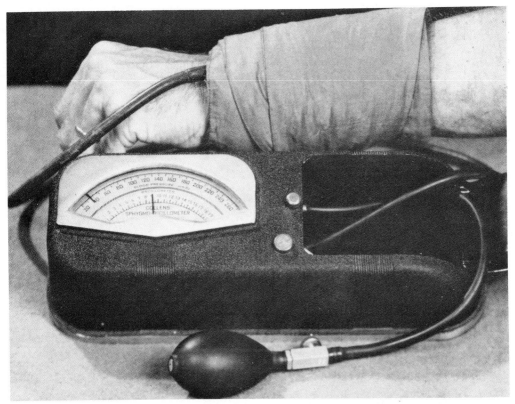

Figure 13.1.9. Sphygmo-oscillometer with partially inflated cuff on the wrist.

electrical impedance is used to estimate the local venous blood volume in an extremity.[86] Its primary use so far has been to detect deep venous thrombosis of the lower extremities and to provide a noninvasive flow meter for the clinician. Although believed to be more accurate than the ultrasonic velocity detector (Doppler), venography is still considered more accurate.

I. Ultrasound. Clinicians interested in vascular disease have been able to utilize ultrasound in two methods. The ultrasonic velocity detector (Doppler) emits a 5 to 10-million hertz beam and a receiving crystal establishes the ratio from the back scatter of high frequency sound reflected from moving red cells. The accuracy depends in a great measure on the velocity and volume of flow. An additional factor is the superficiality of the vessels under study. Simple portable battery units (Parks Electronics Laboratory, 12770 S. W. First St., Beaverton, Oregon 97005) are now available in most hospitals and the blood flow can be detected by the sound characteristics produced when the probe is placed on the skin overlying the blood vessel.[108 111]

Another somewhat similar application translates the frequency response into a graphic display (echogram). By this technique, the resistance of the beam being passed through a portion of the body is displayed on an oscilloscope either as vertical bars or in anatomic configuration of the portion of the body. It has been possible to diagnose infrarenal aortic aneurysms, and even suggest when rupture has taken place. More recently this method has been further modified to develop peripheral ultrasound arteriograms in three planes with remarkably accurate correlation with conventional arteriography.[85] With further engineering refinement, this method of diagnosis seems to hold great promise.

Recently, Yao *et al.*[132] studied 62 patients with salient features of ischemic symptoms affecting their hands and fingers by the transcutaneous Doppler ultrasound flow detection method. Subclavian or brachial arteriograms were done in 42 patients who were found to have abnormal ultrasound findings. The Doppler ultrasound flow detection method is an ideal screening procedure for uncovering arterial thrombosis in small arteries. Its use offers a new approach in the differential diagnosis of ischemia of the hands and fingers.

J. Infra-red Thermography. For several years there has been continued interest in the use of thermography for the diagnosis of neoplasms because of the increased vascularity of these lesions and the corresponding greater emanation of heat, particularly if the

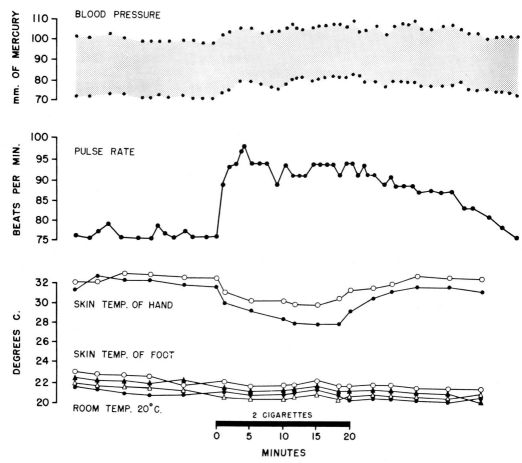

Figure 13.1.10. Moderately severe vasomotor reaction of a patient to tobacco, as reflected in the elevation of blood pressure and pulse and fall in cutaneous temperature in the hand.

tumor is close to the skin. Similarly, Winsor [126] and others have utilized thermography to diagnose vascular abnormalities of the upper and lower extremities. The method is still rather inexact and much less useful than plethysmography or ultrasonic velocity detection (Doppler). [101] Efforts are still being made to improve the instrumentation, however.

CLINICAL ENTITIES

1. Traumatic Arterial Lesions

A. Acute Arterial Spasm and Thrombosis. Being perhaps the most frequently used part of the body, the hand is injured proportionately. For the most part, daily trauma involving minor cuts, abrasions, and blunt trauma are followed by rapid resolution and no significant vascular effects. When the involvement is more serious, local vasomotor responses or vascular injury may be significant. [15 17 20 105] The most common effect is acute vasoconstriction or arterial spasm. These effects may involve the vessels in the hand even if the injury is to the larger arteries of the extremity.

The trauma is generally blunt, resulting from a blow or sustained compression. Spasm may also result from the adjacent passage of a bullet, angulation, or by bone as with fracure, dislocation, or one of the shoulder girdle syndromes. A deep wound exposing but not penetrating the vessel, and pressure from the back of a chair or from crutches all suffice to produce significant arterial spasm, which in some instances may lead to thrombosis if sifficient arterial damage occurred or if arteriosclerosis involves the artery. Repeated needling of an artery for visualization without entry into the lumen is a common cause of mild arterial spasm. In this instance, the peripheral effect is one of reflex or neural vasoconstriction and responds more readily to measures aimed at reducing sympathetic tone than is the state of spasm encountered at the site of injury where intrinsic muscular contraction also plays a role or where the stimulus is sustained. Regardless of the cause and site of major injury, profound vasoconstriction of the hand results in diffuse dull pain, pallor, coolness, and reduced arterial pulses, sufficient at time to suggest acute arterial thrombosis. It is of interest that Hunterian lectures have been devoted to acute traumatic arterial spasm[23] and Volkmann's contracture, a serious late complication.[45]

In considering the effects of local trauma to the hand, the response may be transient vasoconstriction or, if the trauma is repetitive, a chronic sensitization of the arteries to stimulus may ensue, resulting in Raynaud's phenomenon.[52][95][116]

An interesting by-product of the industrial age is the condition resulting from the use of penumatic or vibratory tools. This entity has been recognized for over a century, since pneumatic tools were introduced into French mines in 1839.[95] The relation to Raynaud's phenomenon was described by Loriga in Rome in 1911[116] and in the past two decades increasing reports have appeared in medical literature. Peters[95] has analyzed the mechanical factors involved in the production of the condition termed by some as "dead hand." The rate of vibration of heavier tools used for driving holes or breaking rock and other hard substances is generally 1,500 to 2,000 per minute. For some time, it was believed that the critical zone required for the production of vascular trauma was between 2,000 and 3,000 r.p.m. Peters studied the effects of lighter tools with frequencies of 2,000 to 2,500 r.p.m. and found the condition developing in plant workers using a tool with 2,500 r.p.m. Of 1,000 workers, 116 developed local vascular signs and symptoms. The occurrence bore a relationship to the total period of exposure. Pain of burning or throbbing nature was experienced, with a lesser incidence of numbness. Swelling was occasionally observed and the hand became stiff and weak. Raynaud's phenomeon was not encountered with high frequency tools, in contrast to the low frequency ones. Telford *et. al.*[116] found vascular disturbances in 75 or 300 workers using the low frequency tools. Raynaud's syndrome occurred frequently with attacks of blanching of the fingers, followed by cyanosis and in some by pink patchy discoloration. Ache, tingling, or loss of sensation occurred at times during the phases. The attacks lasted from minutes to hours, and rendered the patients unable to work. Attacks could be induced by exposure to cold, as in typical Raynaud's syndrome. In serious cases, sympathetic blockade and even operative denervation was necessary. Occlusion of digital arteries has also been observed, resulting in ulcers on the tips of the fingers and even gangrene.[24][95][114] In more advanced states, thrombosis of the ulnar artery has been observed.[9] In one case, thrombosis of the ulnar, radial, and brachial artery followed a crushing injury to the thumb in a machinist accustomed to using a vibratory chipping hammer.[73]

A more common type of arterial thrombosis associated with localized trauma to the hand has been observed.[14][24][68][81][91][113][120][135] This usually follows the use of the heel of the palm to hammer a wrench or similar tool. Onset of dull aching pain may be acute and be accompanied by pallor of the fingers supplied by the ulnar artery. Arteriography reveals thrombotic occlusions (Fig. 13.1.11). With intensified interest in hand surgery and traumatology during the past few years, it has become very apparent that thrombosis of the ulnar artery can occur following even minimal blunt trauma to the hand, far more commonly than has been suspected. Kleinert,[68] Zweig,[135] and others have indicated that the clinical history, examination of the hand, and the Allen test usually suffice to make the diagnosis, although brachial arteriography may be quite useful in some cases.

If collateral circulation seems adequate, conservative measures such as the use of low molecular weight dextran or anticoagulant drugs and vasodilating agents may suffice. In some patients dorsal sympathectomy has been beneficial, and is now most easily accomplished through the transaxillary approach. Although resection of the thrombosed arterial segment has been employed with benefit,[81] Kleinert has demonstrated remarkable success in restoring arterial blood flow by thrombectomy or arterial resection and reanastomosis of the ulnar artery, utilizing microsurgical techniques.[68]

Traumatic thrombosis of the arteries of the hand may follow the use of intra-arterial needles or catheters at the wrist,[132] although transient vasoplasm is more common. The author observed one such case, requiring amputation of several fingers and a portion of the hand (Fig. 13.1.12). Nach and Lohman[87] reported a drug addict developing gangrene following what appeared to be an intravenous injection of codeine at the wrist. In the past few years there has been an alarming increase in vascular damage to the hand, ranging from moderate vasomotor imbalance to gangrene of the fingers following intra-arterial injection of narcotics, hallucinogenic drugs, and barbiturates.[82] Unfortunately, the published accounts are still rare and fail to reflect what is being observed in the emergency wards of large urban city hospitals.

General sedation may be of help in managing a disturbed addict, and if vasospasm of short duration is the primary problem, injection of 5 to 10 ml of 1 per cent Xylocaine into the brachial artery may have temporary benefit. During this period it would be possible to perform a stellate block. Following this there may be a place for low molecular weight dextran or heparinazation. Gangrene of the fingers has also been reported following the accidental arterial injection of promethazine hydrochloride (Phenergan) during general anesthesia.[84]

Causalgia. The peripheral vasospastic state resulting from trauma to a major artery of the arm is usually transient unless partial injury to a major nerve has occurred. In such an instance, very painful causalgia may ensue. Mitchell described the condition in 1864 in association with military gunshot wounds, and a number of reports have appeared in the past few decades.[27][28][32][55][107][119] Usually occurring immediately after but at times even weeks after the injury, the pain is confined to the hand as a severe burning pain, at times throbbing or aching. Hyperesthesia of the skin may be so pronounced that the patient goes to ex-

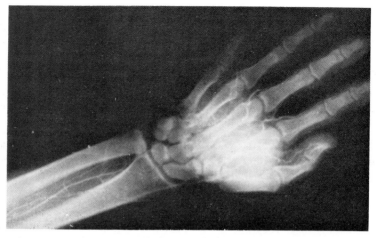

Figure 13.1.11. Arteriogram of 32-year-old mechanic who suddenly developed coolness, pallor, and pain in right hand. He had been hammering a lug wrench with the heel of his hand to loosen nuts on an automobile wheel. Seriogram reveals thrombosis of the ulnar artery and most of its branches.

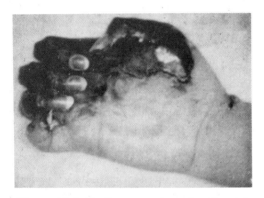

Figure 13.1.12. Gangrene involving the right hand of a 30-year-old woman in whom fine gauge catheters had been placed in the brachial artery for pressure recording and in the radial artery for intra-arterial transfusion during an operation for coarctation of the aorta.

tremes to keep the skin wet and to avoid sudden jars, or drafts. Swelling and coolness of the hand and fingers are common, and hyperhidrosis may be observed. There is some disagreement as to the dominant vasomotor state. Shumacker and Abramson[107] noted only vasoconstriction, with a decrease in skin temperature and oscillometric index, in a significant number of 142 soldiers studied. Others have observed a predominant vasodilatation in many cases, with warmth of the hand and fingers.[55, 119] All agree that the effects are those of sympathetic denervation. Other late sequelae include osteorosis and joint disorders.

Tissue injury other than the direct mechanical type produces arterial thrombosis and gangrene. Exposure to cold induces vasospasm, and if severe or prolonged produces ischemia from arteriolar constriction and capillary damage. With extremely low temperatures the tissues may actually freeze, as observed in high altitude frostbite. In serious cases most authorities agree that warming should be relatively rapid. There is immediate loss of plasma into the tissues and sludging of red cells. After two or three days, thrombi form in the vessels with gangrene developing in the involved part. Anticoagulation with heparin or low molecular weight dextran have had varying success in preventing thrombosis.[117]

Following the period of necrosis, vasospastic changes may be present, as evidenced by coldness, cyanosis, hyperhidrosis, and sensitivity on exposure to cold. Protection of the hand by gloves and use of vasodilating drugs are helpful, and sympathectomy has at times been performed. Other neurologic sequelae include sensory loss, especially involving light touch and fine temperature discrimination.

Chilblain (Pernio syndrome) results from exposure to less severe cold and dampness. It is characterized by patchy skin changes, itching or burning erythema, and swelling. Blebs may develop on the fingers. There appear to be susceptible individuals, who have always noted cold hands and feet. The acute form may last a week or more and resolve with occasional temporary brownish pigmentation. In the chronic type, the syndrome occurs in aggravated form on exposure to cold, and painful, hard, elevated red lesions appear on the fingers and extremities. After several years, progression to permanent discoloration, nodule formation, and skin ulceration occurs. Measures aimed at protection from cold and sympathetic repression form the basis of treatment. Less common vascular disorders of the fingers resulting from exposure to cold have been recognized. Cryoglobulinemia is a condition in which there is a cold precipitable protein in the serum. Patients exposed to cold have red cell agglutination resulting from the protein precipitation in the small vessels of the digits. There is coldness, blueness, and pain or burning of the fingers on exposure to cold at times with Raynaud's phenomenon.[10][58] Effects may be marked, leading to actual gangrene.[58] Prophylactic protection against cold is essential. Forbes[41] described a case of autohemoagglutination with cyanosis and numbness of the fingers developing on exposure to cold.

Injury to the vessels of the hand can result from local burns, drugs, chemicals, electricity, and radiation. There are significant skin changes and arterial thrombosis occurs in severe cases, with resulting ulceration or gangrene. Exposure to toxic drugs given systemically has produced arterial occlusion in the fingers, leading to gangrene. The more common have been ergot[66][78] and arsenic.[72]

B. Laceration or Division of Blood Vessels. In addition to contusion, partial or complete transection and laceration have been described by Luke[75] as arterial injuries requiring repair of ligation. With complete transection, normal arteries can retract and thrombus form at the contracted ends. This occurs when arterial pressure has fallen because of the shock or hemorrhage or when pressure from the hematoma slows blood loss. On the contrary with partial transection or tangential laceration, patency of the opening is maintained by the residual intact arterial wall. Significant perforations of a major artery demand urgent surgical attention, taking precedence over associated nerve or bone damage. Jagged or irregular edges must be trimmed for proper repair, at times requiring resection of a segment if too much of the circumference is involved. For simple closure, vascular clamps are placed 1 cm or more proximally and distally and a simple continuous suture employed, after removing all clot and obtaining good blood flow from proximal and distal ends. With transection, the ends are trimmed and all clot removed. This may require passage of a Fogerty catheter into the artery, as well as massage of the overlying soft tissues to extrude propagated thrombus. Once good blood flow is achieved from both ends, end-to-end anastomosis is usually possible by mobilizing several centimeters of the vessel and employing moderate traction on the vascular clamps. The least traumatic of these appear to be the fine-toothed variety. A continuous circular suture between two or three equidistant traction sutures is satisfactory. For arteries over 4 mm. in diameter, 5-0 silk or synthetic sutures are satisfactory. With vessels of smaller caliber, interrupted sutures of 6-0 down to 8-0 synthetic material are recommended. Arteries less than 2 mm. in diameter may usually be sacrificed by ligation, although satisfactory repair is possible employing micro-surgical technique, as reported by Kleinert.[68] Stapling devices produce satisfactory anastomoses but are not generally available, nor do they have any advantage over a satisfactory suture repair. Tortion and undue tension should be avoided. This at times makes the use of a graft necessary, and with open wounds or in arteries under 8 mm. in diameter,

autogenous vein grafts are preferable (Fig. 13.1.13). The techniques of repair are well described by Dye.[33]

Injection of a few cubic millimeters of 1 to 5 per cent heparin solution into the distal artery by catheter at the time of repair is optional. Some surgeons prefer general heparinazation of the patient during the period of vascular repair in order to prevent the development of sludge and thrombi in the distal circulation. This may be contra-indicated in the presence of soft tissue trauma and fractures. Hematoma, foreign bodies, and devitalized tissue must be removed from the wound. Similar repair of major veins should also be performed. Reducton of dislocations and fixation of fractures is recommended after a vascular repair in most cases to avoid angulation or compression of the vessels. Nerve repair may be deterred until later. Soft tissues should cover the vessels if the wound is to be left open. Satisfactory results may be expected if repair can be achieved within six hours of injury. Although accidents account for most vascular trauma, Hohf[53] collected a remarkable number of cases in which arterial injury occurred during the course of orthopedic operations. Arterial injury has also been reported in the course of general, gynecologic, and urologic surgery as well.

C. Aneurysm and Arteriovenous Fistula. Trauma may damage the arterial wall sufficiently so that dilatation rather than thrombotic occlusion occurs. If there is a break in the arterial wall, hematoma will form and may develop a communicating cavity. This false

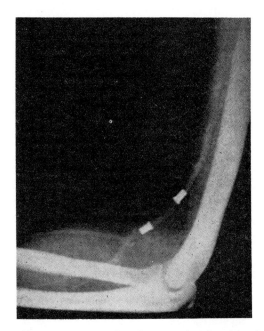

Figure 13.1.13. Arteriogram showing blood flow through one of the first vein grafts inserted with Blakemore-Lord tubes. (Courtesy Dr. Arthur H. Blakemore.)

aneurysm, or pulsating hematoma, has scar tissue for the outer wall.

If aneurysm of the major arteries of the arm fills sufficiently with clot to reduce blood flow, an ischemia of the hand will result. Resection and reconstruction of the artery will reverse the process, if performed early. With local trauma to the hand, aneurysm may occur, usually involving the superficial volar arch. Another susceptible area is the anatomic snuff box, where the radial artery is superficial (Fig. 13.1.14). Middleton[83] and others[94] [106] [134] have reported cases resulting from penetrating or blunt trauma, or resulting from reduction of a dislocation. There is usually dull pain and a palpable pulsating mass, readily visualized by arteriography. Treatment consists of ligation and excision of the involved segment. In the major vessels of the extremity, end-to-end anastomosis is usually desirable, and on rare occasions a graft may be required.[31]

Acquired arteriovenous fistula usually involves the major vessels of the arm, and results from a persistent communication between the artery and vein. The hand may be pale and cool because of diversion of arterial blood flow through the shunt. The subject has been discussed in detail by Holman in his classic monograph,[54] by Reid[98] and others. The trauma is usually penetrating as from gunshot or stab wound but may be produced by a bone spicule or needle puncture. The fistula should be closed surgically, and this may require resection of the vessels, with restoration by anastomosis or graft. On rare occasion, trauma may appear to activate congenital arteriovenous fistulae of the extremities. Greenhalgh[44] reports a man who sustained an injury to his hand at age 16 and subsequently had to have finger amputation on two occasions and finally removal of a part of the hand before cure was achieved. Despite the sequence of events which seemed to follow the traumatic episode, the arteriographic study of this hand suggested a congenital etiology.

2. Embolism

Most emboli to peripheral arteries result from cardiac disease, such as myocardial infarction, auricular fibrillation, and subacute bacterial endocarditis. Other agents are atheromatous plaques, foreign body, tumor, and fat. Emboli tend to lodge at bifurcations and involve the upper extremity less commonly than the legs. Because of the abundant collateral circulation in the scapular and pectoral region and the upper arm, embolectomy is not required often. In some instances gangrene of the fingers has resulted from ineffective treatment, however.[2]

With sudden interruption of arterial blood flow there is pain, numbness, pallor, and absence of pulses distally. The initial vasospasm can be diminished by sympathetic block and vasodilating drugs. Anticoagulation with heparin restricts propagation of clot. Experience with intra-arterial or systemic administration of fibrinolysin is too limited yet to know the exact benefits from this mode of therapy. Arteriography is helpful in determining location and extent of occlusion if operative removal is contemplated. The technique of embolectomy is well described in the operative manuals.[49] [62] [121]

Small emboli involving fingers such as produced by subacute bacterial endocarditis may cause discomfort and petechiae but require no local therapy. The author observed a case with embolization of small droplets of mercury into the brachial artery while a blood sample for gas analysis was being drawn. Following a period of marked vasoconstriction there was intense, sustained hyperemia. Pain was marked and small black spots were noticeable in the skin. With stellate blocks and supportive measures, the hand recovered completely in a few weeks. Mention has already been made of those instances in which emboli or intra-arterial thromboses follow the intra-arterial injection of drugs.

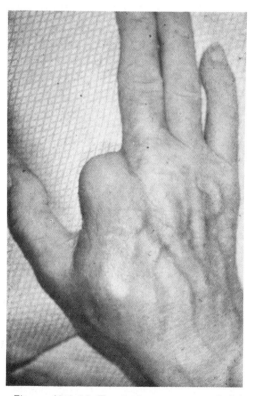

Figure 13.1.14. Traumatic aneurysm of right radial artery in a 59-year-old carpenter. The index finger had been amputated previously for trauma.

3. Arteriosclerosis Obliterans

As part of the aging process, the arteries lose elasticity and develop intimal thickening. As this progresses, thrombotic occlusion can occur suddenly with a clinical picture which mimics embolism. Involvement of the upper extremity is much less severe than that observed in the legs. Hines and Barber[50] observed Raynaud's phenomenon in 10 per cent of 280 patients but radial or ulnar occlusion in only three cases. Since the occlusion is usually gradual collateral circulation can develop and the patient remain asymptomatic. When sudden occlusion does occur, the effects are similar to those produced by embolism. Operative intervention is rarely required, however. The main danger to the patient lies in sustaining a subsequent injury to a hand which is supplied by collateral circulation. Abrasions and wounds may have marked delay in healing and ulceration or gangrene could ensue. In such a case, amputation should be withheld until demarcation and mummification, since early amputation in the presence of generalized arterial insufficiency can lead to a failure in healing of the stump of a digit.

Cerebral vascular insufficiency due to occlusion of the subclavian artery may be associated with vascular problems affecting the arm and hand. Since the description of the ''subclavian steal syndrome'' in 1961, there has been increasing awareness of the neurologic symptoms such as dizziness, positional syncope, and blurred vision with coldness and numbness of the arm and hand on exertion. The arteriosclerotic segmental occlusion occurs at the origin of the subclavian artery from the aortic arch and ends prior to the orifice of the vertebral artery. If the cross collateral circulation in the brain is competent, retrograde flow down the vertebral artery into the arm will occur when the extremity is exercised. Activity such as painting, typing, piano playing which calls for repetitive muscular contraction will soon produce an ache in the shoulder which extends down the arm and finally involves the hand. As noted, the hand may be cool, pulseless and pale. It has been estimated that 15 to 30 per cent of patients with neurologic symptoms from arteriosclerotic subclavian occlusive have symptoms involving the hand. The effects are generally minor although one patient has been reported who had gangrene of the fingers.[96]

4. Thromboangiitis Obliterans (Buerger's Disease).

Much has been written on this disease with controversy existing as to etiology, and even as to its actual existence as a separate entity. Evidence favors this being an inflammatory occlusive process, although the influence of th adrenal glands has increasingly been recognized.[43 89] Its predilection for the distal portions of the extremities, association with thrombophlebitis, occurrence in young individuals and marked predominance in males tend to differentiate it from early arteriosclerosis.[5 16 50 89] Raynaud's phenomenon may be observed in up to 30 per cent of cases. Ulceration and gangrene of the fingers is not uncommon in contrast to arteriosclerosis. Minor am-

putations are also better tolerated. Medical measures include stopping the use of tobacco, use of vasodilating drugs, and protection of the extremities. Arteriography reveals segmented occlusion of medium to small arteries, which often precludes restorative surgery although microsurgical technique may alter this attitude (Fig. 13.1.15).[60 68] Experience in vascular clinics suggests that the condition is now much less common for reasons not clearly understood.

5. Raynaud's Disease

Allen, Barker and Hines[7] have proposed criteria for differentiating primary Raynaud's disease from secondary Raynaud's phenomenon observed with many vascular disorders having a neurogenic component. Unfortunately, many reports group these conditions and it is therefore difficult to compare the course and response to therapy of the primary disease. Although typically it affects young women, males may also de-

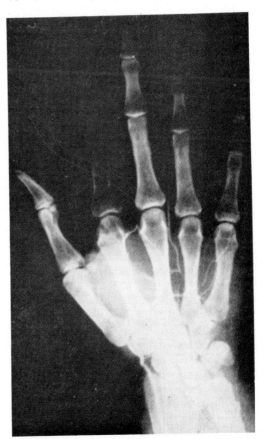

Figure 13.1.15. Arteriogram of a 32-year-old waitress believed to have thromboangiitis obliterans. There is occlusion of the ulnar artery and segmental obliteration of many of the smaller arteries of the hand and fingers. The index finger was amputated because of gangrene.

velop the condition.[51] The initial episode in most often associated with exposure to cold, but subsequently the signs and symptoms, which are those of Raynaud's phenomenon, can be produced by emotional disturbance. The neurogenic factor has been emphasized by deTakats and Fowler.[29] More recently adrenal function has been related.[25]

Comprehensive clinical descriptions have been provided by Lewis and Pickering,[71] Blain *et al.,*[13] and others. Most important of the secondary effects is the development of sclerodactyly. This is manifested by sclerosis of the digital skin and should be differentiated from diffuse scleroderma, which may have associated Raynaud's phenomenon in its early course.[17] Wright,[131] on the other hand, suggests that scleroderma is part of the Raynaud syndrome, although he admits they are not always associated. Evidence does support the view that diffuse scleroderma is primarily not a vascular condition, but a collagen disease affecting arteries by fibrous investment. Farmer *et al.*[38] in a review of 71 patients with Raynaud's disease found systemic scleroderma in only three cases.

Although early in its course, Raynaud's disease is vasomotor in nature, later there are organic changes in the digital arteries with ulcers at the finger tip and even limited gangrene in severe cases. Beyond prophylactic protective measures against cold, sedation, and psychiatric treatment have been employed. Although sympathetic block or denervation may help, there is a disappointing rate of recurrence after two years.[13] [39]

6. Miscellaneous Vasospastic Conditions

A. Acrocyanosis. The hands and feet are affected by cold by development of a persistent cyanosis, which may change to erythema on exposure to warmth. The role of emotional disturbance is contraversial. The sex ratio is about equal, in contrast to Raynaud's disease. Stiffness, edema, and hyperhidrosis have been observed. It has been considered a benign functional disorder, although Edwards[35] has described a necrotizing form. Protection against cold and sympathetic blockage or denervation are usually effective.

B. Livedo Reticularis (Cutis Marmorata). In this vasospastic disorder, the cyanosis has a mottled, blotchy pattern. Like acrocyanosis, and at times associated wth it, the color results from atomic dilatation of the capillaries and venules, producing stasis. The mild primary form appears to be common. It may be secondary to hypertension, pernio, syphilis, and nervous instability. It affects females most often, and may have arteriolar intimal proliferation and perivascular infiltration in the later stages. On occasion, ulceration may occur, usually involving the legs and toes. Sympathetic denervation may help but failures have been reported.[131]

C. Erythromelalgia. In this condition, vasomotor instability results from exposure to heat, with the appearance of burning pain-increased cutaneous temperature and marked rubor. There is evidence of in-

creased arterial circulation in the skin, and rise in capillary pressure.[1] It usually affects both sexes in middle age and may involve the palms as well as digits. Treatment is aimed at avoiding a warm environment. Various drugs have been tried without much success. Sympathectomy may aggravate the condition although there are rare reports of benefit.

7. Miscellaneous Arteritides

A. Polyarteritis Nodosa. This wide-spread arteritis involving medium sized arteries has an uncertain etiology characterized by focal inflammatory lesions. Some authors have considered it a manifestation of allergic response, and others include it among the collagen diseases. It affects males in middle age most commonly, and runs a fibrile, chronic course at times ending fatally. The perivascular infiltrations may involve the wall sufficiently to produce necrosis and aneurysm. Occasionally skin lesions are produced. Treatment has generally been ineffective.

B. Dermatomyositis. This is a rare collagen disease which may affect the arterioles secondarily, as in the case of diffuse scleroderma. Associated Raynaud's phenomenon is common. In the early course, there may be edematous, blotchy red, erythematous patches over the small joints of the hand, with telangiectasis.[1] [65] Recognition of the condition is important in the differential diagnosis of primary vascular lesions.

C. Lupus Erythematosis. In the systemic form of this collagen disease there may be widely scattered vascular lesions, with periarterial lymphocytic infiltration, endothelial proliferation, and fibrinoid deposits in the adventitia. Cutaneous lesions involve the hands and are pink, edematous, indurated plaques. Raynaud's phenomenon may be found in 20 per cent of cases, and may be a dominant clinical feature in the early course. Acute thrombosis of the larger arteries and veins may occur. The author has observed a young woman with marked Raynaud's phenomenon as well as gangrene of two fingers on each hand extending to involve one or more phalanx. Treatment has been discouraging with steroid therapy still perhaps being the most effective. Dorsal sympathectomy is disappointing, as is the use of low molecular weight dextran or anticoagulant drugs.

8. Shoulder Girdle Syndromes

A. Cervical Rib and Scalene Anticus (Naffzinger's Syndrome). Compression of the subclavian artery by the insertion of the scalene anticus muscle can produce a neurovascular involvement of the hand. The artery may develop degenerative changes at the site of compression and may thrombose.[100] In the severe form, it is characterized by paresthesias or pain, coolness, swelling cyanosis, and hyperhidrosis of the hand.[4] In certain cases, wasting may occur in the muscles of the palmar and interosseus muscles with weakening of the grip. The condition is worse in patients with cervical rib since this structure narrows the space through which the artery passes, the neck is longer because of the congenital anomaly and the insertion of the muscle is broader (Fig. 13.1.16).

In analyzing the incidence of cervical rib, Adson[4] found them in 5.6 per thousand patients at the Mayo Clinic. About 50 per cent were bilateral and there were slightly more on the left side.[4][76] At the point of compression, the artery may be thickened and even develop atheromatous plaques. Part of the symptoms are due to compression of the brachial plexus and irritation of the sympathetic components as well.[69][88][115] The neurovascular impairment may be so severe that ulceration and gangrene of the fingers develop.

In young patients or adults with mild symptoms, physiotherapy helps to strengthen and elevate the shoulder girdle. Traction to the neck may also help. Injection of 1 per cen Xylocaine into the scalenus muscle has also been beneficial.[61] Surgical treatment originally consisted of removal of the cervical rib, but in 1925 Adson and Coffey began achieving success and with less neurologic sequelae by simple division of the band of the muscle.[3] Subsequently their associates recommended resecting the anterior portion of the rib as well.[26] Relieved of pressure the subclavian artery usually is restored functionally with relief of symptoms, especially if a segment of the cervical rib is removed. Presently, most surgeons recommend the entire removal of the cervical rib for best results. Although Clagett[21] recommended the parascapular approach, Roos and Owens[102] and others[112] have demonstrated much greater simplicity, less blood loss, and better functional results with the transaxillary approach.

B. *Hyperabduction Syndrome.* Wright[130] observed that hyperabduction of the arm alone could stretch the subclavian artery sufficiently to produce occlusion in certain individuals. A clinical picture similar to the scalene anticus syndrome is produced occasionally. Raynaud's phenomenon is also present.[12] At times treatment consists of physiotherapy to improve pos-

ture and in correcting sleeping habits of those who hyperabduct the arm about a pillow. Paull[93] has reported a patient with both hyperabduction and scalene anticus syndrome.

C. *Costoclavicular Syndrome.* Neurovascular complaints may result from compression or occlusion of the subclavian artery and pressure on the brachial plexus by a narrowed space between the clavicle and the first rib.[21][37][77][100][103][112] This occurs when the shoulders are brought downward and backward. Chronic debilitation and poor posture may be responsible, as can pressure from a shoulder pack. Pain radiates from the scapular region to the neck and down the arm. The clinical involvement of the hand stimulates that of the scalenus anticus syndrome. Treatment consists of elimination of poor posture and pressure on the shoulder. Russek has obtained benefit from subscapular infiltration.[103] In severe cases, resection of the first rib may provide substantial benefit and can be achieved without too much difficulty by the transaxillary approach.

9. Congenital Anomalies

A. *Arteriovenous Fistula.* Through a persistence of fetal communications between the arterial and venous tree of the extremity functioning shunts remain after birth. The time for these to become recognizable varies, and some are not noted until about puberty. They are commonly associated with hemangiomas (Fig. 13.1.17). There may be ulceration and severe bleeding in seriously involved cases. A machinery murmur is heard only if a shunt has become sufficiently enlarged. The lesions are usually multiple and may affect circulation to the bony epiphyses so as to produce increased length and girth of the limb. There are usually few or no symptoms but medical help may be sought because of enlarged veins, hypertrophy of the limb, edema, sweating, or ulceration. The skin is warm over the area and roentgenogram of the limb may reveal vascular channels in the cortex of the bone or pheboliths. Trauma may accelerate the process.[44] Arteriography often does not reveal the actual com-

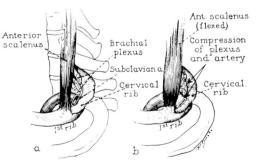

Figure 13.1.16. Anatomic relationship of the left subclavian artery and brachial plexus in sclaenus anticus syndrome associated with cervical rib. A. Head is in normal position B. With head dorsiflexed and turned to the left there is arterial compression. (Reproduced from Surgery, Gynecology and Obstetrics.[4])

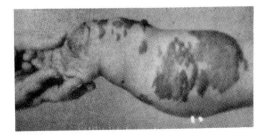

Figure 13.1.17. Arm and hand of a 3-year-old girl with multiple congenital arteriovenous fistulae associated with hemangiomata. Multiple obliterative procedures were performed because of ulceration and bleeding. Amputation was eventually necessary.

munications but suggests the diagnosis because of abundant dilated veins in the area which fill simultaneously with the artery. The oxygen content of venous blood is increased proximal to the shunts.

In mild cases, conservatism has its place since, in the attempt at excision, important muscles and nerves may be sacrificed. Also, it is not uncommon to have new channels become functional days or weeks following an apparently successful operation. In severe cases, multiple stage excisions coupled with injection of a sclerosing agent may be necessary. Skin grafts are often required if ulceration is extensive. Amputation may be required ultimately in certain patients. Similar variations of congenital arterial fistulae have been described. Arteriovenous angioma has been reported by Malan and Puglionisi.[80] In 16 patients, the lesion was extensive and active in only four; of these only one involved the hand.

B. Hemangioma. These are of several types, ranging from nevus venosus (port-wine stain), capillary hemangioma (strawberry nevus, plexiform angioma), cavernous hemangioma to massive diffuse hemagioma. The first two should be observed until after the age of six years, since some undergo spontaneous regression. Steroids may enhance the process of resolution. In some, application of Dry Ice and cosmetics may suffice.

With cavernous hemangioma, exact delineation by venography is recommended before surgical excision is undertaken. Discrete lesions may be removed, treated by injection of sclerosing drugs, or by a combination. Irradiation is frequently unsuccessful and may have serious affects on the skin and bone growth. On the other hand, if increased bone growth has occurred, as with arteriovenous fistula, epiphyseal arrest may be indicated before puberty. Surgical treatment is usually not advisable in the very extensive diffuse hemangioma which involves an entire extremity.

C. Glomus Tumor. This may arise as a benign neoplasm involving the normally present arteriovenous shunts which serve to redistribute blood in the distal part of the extremities and in visceral organs. Trauma may be an initiating cause. The tumor is usually tiny and of bluish color, often occurring under the nail. It is very sensitive, producing severe pain similar to causalgia. Reflex dilatation may produce warmth of the hand with prominent veins and increase in venous oxygen content. There may be sweating and osteoporosis. Complete removal effects a cure. Continued pain usually indicates imcomplete excision or psychiatric instability, although recurrence and multiple lesions have been reported. Sympathectomy has been performed for pain persisting after excision, but with minimal benefits.

D. Hemangiosarcoma and Hemangio-Endothelioma. These malignant lesions differ slightly in cell origin and clinical course.[7] The hemangiosarcoma has fibroblastic and vascular elements, and when near the surface is a soft, bluish red small tumor at times with satellite nodules. Thrills and bruits may be present. They may become necrotic because of rapid growth and tend to metastasize. Excisional therapy is disappointing, but some are radio sensitive.

Hemangio-endothelioma is believed to arise mainly from endothelial cells, grow slowly but may metastasize. They are soft, dark red and may have satellite nodules. Ulceration and hemorrhage may occur. Excision is reasonably successful if metastasis has not occurred. Some lesions are radio sensitive. Because of recurrence, amputation is sometimes necessary.

10. Miscellaneous Venous Disorders

A. Thrombophlebitis. The hand is rarely involved but a superficial phlebitis secondary to infection or trauma can develop. Indwelling needles or catheters in the veins of dorsum of the hand or wrist may produce a phlebitis, with thrombosis. Treatment is by resting and elevating the hand, and applying continuous warm wet compresses. Use of antibiotic and anticoagulant drugs is not usually indicated.

B. Major Venous Occlusion. Superior vena caval syndrome results from acute occlusion. It may result from trauma, malignancy, aortic aneurysm, constrictive pericarditis, stenosing mediastinitis, and tuberculous scarring. There is dusky cyanosis, swelling, and engorged veins involving the head, neck, shoulders, and upper extremities. There may be headache, vertigo, and blurred vision. In benign conditions, collateral venous channels develop rapidly and surgical relief is usually not necessary although successful correction by graft has been achieved by the author,[30] and others. Relief of obstruction caused by a malignant process is less successful, although by-pass grafts have been employed. Replacements often fail by thrombosis when employed in the venous system, whether arterial homograft, venous autograft or synthetic fabric.[30]

Axillary vein thrombosis (effort thrombosis, Paget-Schroetter's syndrome) usually results from traumatic stretching or compression. There is rapid swelling of the arm and hand, with cyanosis, coolness and sharp pain or dull ache. Muscular weakness may be noted. Venous pressure is elevated but arterial circulation is unaffected. Venography usually reveals a localized obstruction at the junction of the subclavian vein. Collateral channels develop rapidly over the chest and shoulder.

If the patient has severe clinical signs and symptoms and is seen within 12 hours, exploration and thrombectomy are usually preferred because of the persistent disability observed in many cases. Unfortunately, most patients are not seen until more than 12 hours have elapsed, and conservative therapy is usually the choice. The customary program includes elevation of the arm, anticoagulation by heparin, and trial of dorsal sympathetic block. Recently there has been success in dissolving recent clot by intravenous streptokinase or urokinase therapy. Benefits may be expected when the thrombosis is in a short segment of axillary vein and treated within two weeks.

Long term conservative therapy may include the use of prothombin depressing drugs or physiotherapy and elastic support. Activities which produce stress or hyperabduction of the arm are to be avoided for six months to a year.

SUMMARY

The various arterial and venous disorders which may involve the hand, primarily or secondarily, have been described. General guides to therapy have been suggested. The technical details of operative procedures have been omitted, because of the several choices of technique, and limitation of space. This information is supplied in several recent, well illustrated operative manuals. The surgeon engaged in surgery of the hand should be aware of the diagnostic possibilities of a vascular lesion but does well to rely on the help of a competent vascular surgeon when critical operative intervention is indicated.

REFERENCES

1. Abramson, D.I. Vascular responses in the extremities of man in health and disease. Chicago, University of Chicago Press, 1944, p. 412.
2. Abramson, P.D. Diagnosis and treatment of acral gangrene. Am. J. Surg., 57: 253, 1942.
3. Adson, A. W., and Coffey, J.R. Cervical rib; a method of anterior approach for relief of symptoms by division of the scalenus anticus. Ann. Surg., 85: 839, 1927.
4. Adson, A.W. Surgical treatment for symptoms produced by cervical ribs and the scalenus anticus muscle. Surg. Gynecol. Obstet., 85: 687, 1947.
5. Allen, E.V., and Brown, G.E. Thromboangiitis obliterans etc., Ann. Int. Med., 1: 535, 1928.
6. Allen, E. V., and Camp, J. D. A roentgenographic study of the peripheral arteries of the living subject following their injection with a radiopaque substance. J.A.M.A., 104: 618, 1935.
7. Allen, E.V., Barker, N.W., and Hines, E.A. Peripheral Vascular Disease, Ed. 4, edited by J.F. Fairbairm. Philadelphia, Saunders, 1965.
8. Arey, L.B. Developmental Anatomy, Ed.7. Philadelphia, Saunders, 1965.
9. Barker, N.W., and Hines, E.A. Arterial occlusion in the hands and fingers associated with repeated occupational trauma. Proc. Staff Meet. Mayo Clin. 19: 345, 1944.
10. Barr, D. P., Reader, G. G., and Wheeler, C. H. Cryoglobulinemia, etc. Ann. Int. Med., 32: 6, 1950.
11. Bergan, J.J. Surgery of Peripheral Vascular Diseases. Philadelphia, Lea & Febiger, 1972.
12. Beyer, J.A., and Wright, I.S. The hyperabduction syndrome with special reference to its relationship to Raynaud's syndrome. Circulation, 4: 161, 1951.
13. Blain, A., Coller, F.A., and Carver, G.B. Raynaud's Disease. Surgery, 29: 387, 1951.
14. Bugar-Miszaros. K., Okos, G., and Sas, V. Thromboangiitis obliterans on the basis of 300 cases. Acta med. Acas. sc. hung., 12: 217, 1958.
15. Bunnell, S. Surgery of the Hand, Ed. 5. Philadelphia, Lipincott, 1970.
16. Butsch, J. L. Janes injuries of the superficial palmar arch. J. Trauma, 3: 505, 1963.
17. Byrne, J. J. The Hand, Its Anatomy and Diseases. Springfield, Charles C Thomas, 1959.
18. Calenoff, L. Angiography of the hand: guidelines for interpretation. Radiology, 102: 331, 1972.
19. Callow, A.D. Surgical management of varying patterns of vertebral-artery and subclavian artery insufficiency. N. Engl. J. Med., 270: 546, 1964.
20. Cameron, J.D. Cases of severe vascular injury to the hand. Hand, 2: 74, 1970.
21. Clagett, O.T. Research and prosearch: Presidential address. J. Thoracic and Cardiovas. Surg. 44: 153, 1962.
22. Clauss, R.H., and Redisch, W. Remediable Arterial Disease. New York, Grune & Stratton, 1971.
23. Cohen, S.M. Traumatic arterial spasm: Hunterian lecture. Lancet, 246 (1): 1, 1944.
24. Conn, J., Jr., Bergan, J.J., and Bell, J.L. Hypothenar hammer syndrome: post-traumatic digital ischemia. Surgery, 68: 1122, 1970.
25. Corneleac, E. Experimental, clinical and surgical considerations on Raynaud's disease. Zentralbl. Chir., 85: 1394, 1960.
26. Craig, W. McK., and Knepper, P.A. Cervical rib and the scalenus anticus muscle. Ann. Surg., 105: 556, 1937.
27. Dale, W.A., and Lewis, M.R. Management of ischemia of the hand and fingers. Surgery, 67: 62, 1970.
28. deTakats, G. Causalgic states following injuries to extremities. Arch. Phys. Therap., 24: 647, 1943.
29. deTakats, G., and Fowler, E.F. The neurogenic factor in Raynaud's phenomenon. Surgery, 51: 9, 1962.
30. Deterling, R. A., and Bhonslay, S. B. Use of blood vessels grafts and plastic prostheses for relief of superior vena caval obstruction. Surgery, 38: 1008, 1955.
31. Deterling, R. A. Choice of arterial replacements in arterial injury. Clin. Orthop. 28: 44, 1963.
32. Doupe, J., Cullen, C. H., and Chance, G. O. Posttraumatic pain and causalgic syndrome. J. Neurol. Neurosurg. Psychiat., 7: 33, 1944.
33. Dye, W. S. Technics in arterial repair. Clin. Orthop. 28: 38, 1963.
34. Ebel, A., Rose, O. A., and Roab, K. The use of an environmental temperature vasomotor test in the evaluation of peripheral arterial disease. Angiology, 12: 310, 1961.
35. Edwards, E. A. Remittent necrotizing acrocyanosis. J.A.M.A., 161: 1530, 1956.
36. Edwards, E.A. Organization of the small arteries of the hand and digits. Am. J. Surg., 99: 837, 1960.
37. Falconer, M.A., and Weddell, G. Costoclavicular compression of the subclavian artery and vein: relation to the scalenus anticus syndrome. Lancet, 2: 539, 1943.
38. Farmer, R.G., Gifford, R.W., and Hines, E.A. Raynaud's disease with sclerodactylia. A follow-up study of seventy-one patients. Circulation, 23: 13, 1961.
39. Felder, D.A., Simeone, F.A., Linton, R.R., and

Welch, C.E. Evaluation of sympathetic neurectomy in Raynaud's disease. Surgery, *26:* 1014, 1949.

40. Foley, W.T., and Wright, I.S. Color atlas and management of vascular disease. New York, Appleton-Century, 1959.

41. Forbes, G.B. Autohaemaglutination and Raynaud's phenomenon. Br. Med. J., *1:* 598, 1947.

42. Gee, W., Masar, M.F., and Dooken, D.J. Calibrated plethysmography in arterial disease. Surg. Gynecol. Obstet., *133:* 597, 1971.

43. Gorney, D. 17-Ketosteroids and catecholamines in the urine of patients with thrombo-angiitis obliterans. Polski tygodnik lek., *15:* 1993, 1960.

44. Greenhalgh, R.M. A single congenital arteriovenous fistula of the hand. Br. J. Surg., *59:* 76, 1972.

45. Griffith, D. L. Volkmann's ischemic contracture. Br. J. Surg., *28:* 239, 1940.

46. Grimson, K. S., Lyons, C. K., Watkins, W. T., and Calloway, J. L. Successful treatment of hyperhidrosis using Banthine. J.A.M.A., *143:* 1331, 1950.

47. Haimovici, H., *et al. Surgical Management of Vascular Diseases.* Philadelphia, Lippincott, 1971.

48. Hawthorne, H. R. *Vascular Surgery,* Springfield, Charles C Thomas, 1965.

49. Hershey, F. B., and Calman, C. H. *Atlas of Vascular Surgery,* Ed. 2. St. Louis, Mosby, 1967.

50. Hines, E. A., and Barker, N. W. Arteriosclerosis obliterans: A clinical and pathological study. Am. J. Med. Sci., *200:* 717, 1940.

51. Hines, E. A., and Christensen, N. A. Raynaud's disease among men. J.A.M.A., *129:* 1, 1945.

52. Hoerner, E.F. Traumatic vasospastic disease of the hand (Raynaud's phenomenon). Indust. Med., *21:* 297, 1952.

53. Hohf, R.P. Arterial injuries occurring during orthopaedic operations. Clin. Orthop. *28:* 21, 1963.

54. Holman, E. *Arteriovenous Aneurysm.* New York, Macmillan, 1937.

55. Homans, J. Minor causalgia following injuries and wounds. Ann. Surg., *113:* 752, 1941.

56. Howard, F.M., and Lee, R.E. Jr. The hand in Maffucci syndrome. Arch. Surg., *103:* 752, 1971.

57. Hughes, E. S. R. Venous obstruction in the upper extremity (Paget-Schroetter syndrome). Surg. Gynecol. Obstet., *88:* 89, 1949.

58. Hutchinson, J. H., and Howell, R. A. Cryoglobulinemia: report of a case associated with gangrene of the digits. Ann. Int. Med., *39:* 1953.

59. Jackson, B. B. *Surgery of Acquired Vascular Disorders.* Springfield, Charles C Thomas, 1969.

60. Jacobson, J.H., and Suarez, E.L. Microsurgery in anastomosis of small vessels. Surg. Forum, *11:* 243, 1960.

61. Judovich, B., Bates, W., and Drayton, W. Pain in the shoulder and upper extremity due to scalenus anticus syndrome. Am. J. Surg., *63:* 377, 1944.

62. Julian, O.C., Dye, W.S., Javid, H., and Hunter, J.A. *Cardiovascular Surgery.* Chicago, Year Book, 1962.

63. Kakkar, V.V., and Nocolades, A.N., Renney, J.T.G., *et al.* I¹²⁵ labelled fibrinogen test adapted for routine screening for deep vein thrombosis. Lancet, *1:* 540, 1970.

64. Kaufman, H.D. High pressure injection injuries, the problems, pathogenesis and management. Hand, *2:* 63, 1970.

65. Keil, H. The manifestations in the skin and mucous membranes in dermatomyositis. Ann. Int. Med., *21:* 828, 1942.

66. Kenney, F.R. Gangrene of the hand following treatment for pruritis of hepatotoxic origin. N. Engl. J. Med., *235:* 35, 1946.

67. Kinmouth, J.B., Rob, C.G., Simeone, F.A., *et al. Vascular Surgery.* Baltimore, Williams & Wilkins, 1963.

68. Kleinert, H.E., and Volianitis, G.J. Thrombosis of the palmar arterial arch and its tributaries. J. Trauma, *5:* 447, 1965.

69. Learmonth, J.R. Some sequels of abnormality at the thoracic outlet. Thorax, *2:* 1, 1947.

70. Leinward, I., Hinton, J.W., and Lord, J.W. Hypertensive vascular disease associated with quadrilateral Raynaud's disease treated by total sympathectomy. Surgery, *26:* 1034, 1949.

71. Lewis, T. and Pickering, G.W. Observations on maladies in which blood supply to digits ceases intermittently or permanently and upon bilateral gangrene of digits. Clin Sci., *1:* 327, 1943.

72. Lindstrom, L.J. A case report of fulminant occlusive arterial disease with gangrene of the extremities due to neoarsphenamine intoxication. Acta Chir. Scandinav., *100:* 509, 1950.

73. Lowenberg, E.L. Acute traumatic arterial thrombosis of the extremities. Va. Med. Mon., *67:* 630, 1940.

74. Luckey, E. H., Russ, E. M., and Barr, D. P. Cryoglobulinemia, etc. J. Lab. Clin. Med., *37:* 253, 1951.

75. Luke, J. C. Arterial trauma. In *Accident Surgery,* edited by H. F. Mosely. New York, Appleton, 1962.

76. McGowan, J.M. Cervical rib: The role of the clavicle in occlusion of the subclavian artery. Ann. Surg., *124:* 71, 1946.

77. McGowan, J.M., and Velinsky, M. Costoclavicular compression. Arch. Surg., *59:* 62, 1949.

78. McLoughlin, M.G. Ergotism causing peripheral vascular ischemia. Rocky Mt. Med. J., *69:* 45, 1972.

79. Mackey, W.A., Macfarlane, J.A., and Christian, M.S. *Arterial Surgery.* New York, Macmillan, 1964.

80. Malan, E., and Puglionsi, A. Congenital angiodysplasias of the extremities. J. Cardiovas. Surg., *6:* 255, 1965.

81. Mansfield, J.P.J. Traumatic thrombosis of the ulnar artery in the palm. J. Bone Joint Surg., *36B:* 438, 1954.

82. Maxwell, T.M., Blaisdell, F.W., and Olcott, C. Vascular complications of drug abuse. J.A.M.A., *221:* 343, 1972.

83. Middleton, D.S. Occupational aneurysm of palmar arteries. Br. J. Surg., *21:* 215, 1933.

84. Mostafavi, H., and Samimi, M. Accidental intra-arterial injection of promethazine HCl during general anesthesia. Anesthesiology, *35:* 645, 1971.

85. Mozersky, D.J., Hokanson, D.E., Baker, D.W., Sumner, D.S., and Strandness, D.E. Ultrasonic arteriography. Arch. Surg., *103:* 663, 1971.

86. Mullick, S.C., Wheeler, H.B., and Songster, G.F. Diagnosis of deep venous thrombosis by measurement of electrical impedance. Am. J. Surg., *119:* 417, 1970.

87. Nach, R.L., and Lohman, H. Gangrene of the hand fol-

lowing traumatic occlusion of the radial and ulnar arteries. N.Y. J. Med., *48:* 2173, 1948.

88. Naffziger, H. C., and Grant, W. T. Neuritis of the brachial plexus, mechanical in origin. Surg. Gynecol. Obstet., *67:* 722, 1938.

89. Orban, F. New trends in the treatment of thromboangliosis (Buerger's disease). Ann. R. Coll. Surg. Engl., *28:* 69, 1961.

90. Ouchi, H., and Warren, R. Detection of intravascular thrombi by means of I¹³¹ labelled plasmin. Surgery, *51:* 42, 1962.

91. Paaby, H., and Stadil, F. Thrombosis of the ulnar artery. Acta Ortho. Scandinav., *39:* 336, 1968.

92. Patten, B. M. *Human Embryology,* Ed. 3. New York, McGraw-Hill Book, 1968.

93. Paull, R. The neurovascular syndrome as manifested in the upper extremities. Am. Heart J., *32:* 32, 1946.

94. Pemberton, J. deJ., and Black, B.M. Surgical treatment of acquired aneurysm and arteriovenous fistula of peripheral vessels. Surg. Gynecol. Obstet., *77:* 462, 1943.

95. Peters, F.M. A disease resulting from the use of pneumatic tools. Occup. Med., *2:* 55, 1946.

96. Ponsdomenech, E.R., and Le Pere, R.H. Obstruction of the sub-clavian artery. Vasc. Surg., *3:* 211, 1969.

97. Pulvertaft, G. *Hand.* Philadelphia, Lippincott, 1970.

98. Reid, M. Studies in abnormal arteriovenous communications, acquired and congenital. Arch. Surg., *10:* 601, 1925; *11:* 996, 1925.

99. Richards, R.L. *Peripheral Arterial Disease.* Baltimore, Williams & Wilkins, 1970.

100. Rob, C.G., and Standeven, A. Arterial occlusion complicating thoracic outlet compression syndrome. Br. M. J., *2:* 709, 1958.

101. Robins, B., and Bernstein, A. Comparative studies of digital plethysmography and infra red thermography in peripheral vascular disease. Angiology, *21:* 349, 1970.

102. Roos, D.R., and Owens, J.C. Thoracic outlet syndrome. Arch. Surg., *93:* 71, 1966.

103. Russek, A.S. Diagnosis and treatment of scapulocostal syndrome. J.A.M.A., *150:* 25, 1952.

104. Scanlon, W.G. Successful treatment of hyperhidrosis with mephobarbital. J.A.M.A., *150:* 28, 1952.

105. Schneewind, J.H. Surgical emergencies of the hand. Surg. Clin. North Amer., *52:* 203, 1972.

106. Short, D.W. Occupational aneurysm of the palmar arch. Lancet, *255(2):* 217, 1948.

107. Shumacker, H. B., and Abramson, D. I. Posttraumatic vasomotor disorders. Surg. Gynecol. Obstet., *88:* 417, 1949.

108. Sigel, B., Felix, R., Jr., Popky, G. L., and Ipsen, J. Diagnosis of lower limb venous thrombosis by Doppler ultrasound technique. Arch. Surg., *104:* 174, 1972.

109. Singer, E. Embryological pattern persisting in the arteries of the arm. Anat. Rec., *55:* 403, 1933.

110. Strandness, D.E. *Collateral Circulation in Clinical Surgery.* Philadelphia, Saunders, 1969.

111. Strandness, D.E., Jr., and Sumner, D.S. Ultrasonic velocity detector in the diagnosis of thrombophlebitis. Arch. Surg., *104:* 180, 1972.

112. Taheri, S. Present state of surgical treatment of thoracic outlet syndrome.Vasc.Surg.,*4:* 217, 1970.

113. Teece, L.G. Thrombosis of the ulnar artery. Aust. N. Z. J. Surg., *19:* 156, 1949.

114. Teisinger, J. Vascular disease disorders resulting from vibrating tools. J. Occup. Med., *14:* 129, 1972.

115. Telford, E.D., and Stopford, J.S.B. The vascular complications of cervical rib. Br. J. Surg., *18:* 557, 1931.

116. Telford, E.D., and McCann, M.B., and MacCormack, D.H. "Dead hand" in users of vibrating tools. Lancet, *249(2):* 359, 1945.

117. Theis, F.V., O'Connor, W.R., and Wahl, F.J. Anticoagulants in acute frostbite. J.A.M.A.,*146:* 992, 1951.

118. Tsapogas, M.J.,*et at. Vascular Diseases.* Springfield, Charles C Thomas, 1968.

119. Ulmer, J.L., and Mayfield, F.H. Causalgia. Surg. Gynecol. Obstet., *83:* 789, 1946.

120. von Rosen, S. Ein fall von Thrombose in der Arteria Ulnaris nach Einwirkung von stumpfer Gewalt. Acta Chir. Scandinav. *73:* 500, 1934.

121. Warren R. *Procedures in Vascular Surgery.* Boston, Little, Brown, 1960.

122. White, J.C. Diagnostic blocking of sympathetic nerves to extremities with procaine. J.A.M.A., *94:* 1382, 1930.

123. White, J.C. Hyperhidrosis of nervous origin and its treatment by sympathectomy. N. Engl. J. Med., *200:* 181, 1939.

124. Wilkins, R.W., Doupe, J., and Newman, H.W. Rate of blood flow in normal fingers. Clin. Sci., *3:* 403, 1938.

125. Williams, C. Hysterical edema of hand and forearm. Ann. Surg., *111:* 1056, 1940.

126. Winsor, R., and Hyman, C. *Primer of Peripheral Vascular Diseases.* Philadelphia, Lea & Febiger, 1965.

127. Wiseheart, J.D. Patterns of reactive hypermia in the hand. Am. Heart J., *60:* 116, 1960.

128. Woollard, H. H. The development of the prinicpal arterial stems in the forelimb of the pig. Contrib. Embryol. Carnegie Inst., *14:* 141, 1922.

129. Woollard, H.H. Distribution of sympathetic fibers in extremities. J. Anat., *67:* 18, 1931.

130. Wright, I.S. The neurovascular syndrome produced by hyperabduction of the arms, etc. Am. Heart J., *29:* 1, 1945.

131. Wright, I. S. *Vascular Diseases in Clinical Practice,* Ed. 2. Chicago, Year Book, 1952.

132. Yao, S. T., Gourmos, C., Papthanasiou, K., and Irvine, W. T. A method for assessing ischemia of the hand and fingers. Surg. Gynecol. Obstet., *135,3:* 373, 1972.

133. Yee, J., Westdahl, P.R., and Wilson, J.L. Gangrene of the forearm and hand following use of radial artery for intra-arterial transfusion. Ann. Surg., *136:* 1019, 1952.

134. Zuckerman, I.C., and Proctor, S.E. Traumatic palmar aneurysm. Am. J. Surg., *72:* 52, 1946.

135. Zweig, J., Lie, K.K., Posch, J.L., *et al.* Thrombosis of the ulnar artery following blunt trauma to the hand. J. Bone Joint Surg., *51A:* 1191, 1969.

B.

Microsurgical Repair of Peripheral Nerves and Blood Vessels

James W. Smith, M.D.

NERVE REPAIR

Magnification is advantageous not only for the repair of the main branches of the peripheral nerves, but also for approximating smaller segments. However, its role must be limited to that of aiding the repair, for, if used continuously throughout the surgery, it could well prove to be more of a hindrance than a help. For example, it is usually easy enough to trace a nerve branch from a known site into an area of scar without magnification. Now, if one tries to do this under magnification, it can be laborious and time consuming. There is also a tendency to misjudge structures. For example, under the microscope, a thick band of scar tissue can easily be mistaken for a small nerve branch and a lot of time wasted dissecting it out, only eventually to discover the mistake. It is far better to use magnification to examine the surface of the nerve, remove excessive scar tissue from around it, dissect away the epineurium, and evaluate the degree of perineurial and interfascicular scarring.

Using magnification to its fullest advantage requires practice. The amount of practice needed seems to vary tremendously from individual to individual. This is perhaps related to an instinctive ability to use our hands in a way different than usual, when they are guided by the eye. With this technique, it is necessary to look in one direction and work with the hands at a slightly different direction, owing to the arrangement of lenses in the magnification system. The difficulties of most operators seems also related to the ability to appreciate depth perception, for learning to use micromicroscopy necessitates the development of a feeling for the position of the instruments in relation to the depth of the field. It is initially difficult to automatically realize the direction and angle needed to get to the right location and accomplish the task. Yet, some surgeons seem to be able to do it after one or two quick practices, while others need many sessions to learn to adapt their sight and alter their movements with sufficient automaticity to make worthwhile the potentially useful optical advantge of an aid for the work required.

At the time of any given nerve repair, the degree of magnification needed depends upon the size and condition of the nerves to be approximated. In some cases, the use of the loupe may prove adequate. In others, the dissecting microscope has distinct advantages. It is important, however, to understand that we seldom require magnification greater than 10 or 16 times.

The size of conventional surgical instruments makes them unsuitable for this technique. Locking implements of the ratchet type are also unsatisfactory because they necessitate excessive movement. The delicate instruments manufactured for ophthalmologists, jewelers, and diamond cutters have proved more satisfactory. Needle-holders and scissors of the spring-handled type can be opened and closed without changing the position of the fingers. The nonserrated instrument is preferable because it does not cause suture materials to slip, break, and fray.

Before suturing is begun, the ends of the nerve that has been identified by gross vision and dissected out must be properly prepared. Each is sectioned serially backward until a pattern of funiculi can be seen projecting slightly out from the ends of the nerve like wires extending from a section of cable. When the proper level has been found, the epineurium will slip back and forth over the bundles. Seddon and Medawen call this the prepuce test. The presence of scar, the condition of the funiculi, and the identification of the free margin of the epineurium can be more easily ascertained if a dilute solution of methylene blue is applied to the end. In a relatively bloodless field, there is little color contrast, and using a 2 per cent solution of methylene blue is an easy way to establish one quickly. A single drop is applied to the end of the nerve with the pointed end of a toothpick. Then, after several seconds, the excess can be washed away by liberal irrigation with saline solution. The connective tissues take up the stain more readily and so the light-blue-colored fasiculi will be ringed with a darker like margin of the perineurium. The epineurium will similarly be stained more darkly.

Before suturing, it is important to prepare each end of the nerve further, so the fascicular components make good contact with one another. Sometimes, in nerve repairs, the fascicular bundles seem small compared to the extensive amount of perineurium between them. The epineurim may further confuse the microsurgeon, for if it is thick and somewhat laminated, it can lessen the accuracy of the fascicular approximation. So, if it becomes a problem, any of this epineural or perineural connective tissue can be stripped away from the site for repair.

Only one or two sutures of 8-0 to 10-0 black silk or nylon (for color contrast) are needed to approximate a fasciculus or a complex of several small fasciculi. The size of the suture material to be used usually depends upon the size of the nerve filaments to be approximated. If microsurgical suture material is not available, then an ophthalmic suture with tiny taper needles will prove to be an excellent substitute. Careful hemostasis is needed at the site of nerve repair, for hematoma formation will delay revascularization and increase the amount of scar tissue. So will shielding of any type, and it is not advised. Ducker[6] reports he has recently limited nerve shielding to his cases of gunshot wounds, for on careful analysis of all of the others he found little or no difference in the rate of functional return.

When fascicular grafts are needed to eliminate any tension between the two ends of the nerve, donor sites to be considered include the sural nerve or one of the superficial sensory nerves such as the iliohypogastric. The important thing is to approximate fasciculi, and thus the epineurium and perineurium can be stripped back or removed from the graft because they only serve as the insulation between bundles. Fascicular ends of the graft should be matched up to the existing bundles of fasciculi so continuity is restored between corresponding ends of the nerve. Recall that fascicular grafts are revascularized along their entire length and not from the proximal and distal nerve junctions. Again shielding is not advised, but careful hemostasis is, because the bed for the graft must be a good vascular one. There should be a minimum of scarring and a ready source of blood supply to revascularize quickly the neural components throughout the course of the graft, as well as to the sites of nerve juncture.

Fascicular autografts of nerve should be considered any time there will be tension at the site of a repair. The amount of connective tissue proliferation and scar tissue formation at the site of repair are directly related to the degree of tension at the suture line.

Resecting a segment of epineurium from either side of the repair also helps to reduce scarring. Eliminating tension also reduces the amount of endoneural fibrosis that might subsequently develop in the proximal and distal nerve stumps. It also prevents the adverse effect of connective tissue proliferation and shrinkage at the suture line which affects regenerating axons in the distal stump long after they have crossed the gap. Millesi[16] has shown both experimentally and clinically that axons can more easily cross the two tensionless lines of a fascicular nerve graft than penetrate the scar which will form at a site of nerve repair carried out under tension.

Sometimes a simple suture or two will be sufficient to hold two nerve ends in proper approximation. In other instances, however, it will not produce a sufficiently accurate degree of alignment to satisfy the operating surgeon. In such cases, the usual problem is that the fasciculi kink and twist like limp pieces of well done spaghetti. To hold them in a more proper relation may require a "skewer" suture to lend stability to the site of intended juncture. A double armed monofilament nylon, placed into the perineurium of the interface on either side adjacent to the fasciculus to be stabilized and skewered back along the nerve parallel to the fasciculus for about 1 cm should help facilitate the approximation. When multiple fasciculi are being approximated, a second skewer suture may be advantageous. We find the use of these sutures cuts down tremendously on the need for marginal sutures to maintain accuracy of approximation (Fig. 13.2.1 A

and B). The skewer suture, once placed, can be tied or each of its ends passed separately out through the skin, to be tied loosely together at the completion of the surgery, after skin closure has been completed. When there are sufficient "simple" sutures to maintain approximation of the juncture, we cut one end of each skewer suture and pull them out after about seven days. This time has been chosen because it would seem that edema, the ingrowth of vascular buds, and the other components of early healing probably have fixed the ends in a relatively stable position. Even so, we discourage extensive movements or pressure at the site of repair along the course of a nerve graft from three to five weeks time.

BLOOD VESSEL REPAIR

There is still a great amount of controversy about the reapplication of the amputated parts. Nevertheless, we still have the problem of amputations, and in some instances there is great need for their reapplication. When all fingers have been amputated, except for the thumb, a finger can be replaced to serve as the other half of the pinch mechanism; it can be a very important thing. The literature suggests, at least theoretically, that without any cooling, we have between six and 12 hours to replace amputated parts. Experimental study has shown that, with cooling and the use of certain solutions, very possibly we can store an amputated part up to 24 hours.

When somebody comes into the emergency room bringing the amputated specimen with him, put it in a sterile basin of cool saline or Ringer's lactate solution. Do not wash it with phisohex or immerse it in a Betadine solution, for these antiseptic solutions are damaging to the tissues. Take the specimen to the operating room to debride it and keep it cool. In some instances, if the part is large enough, it can be placed on a profusion machine while the patient is being prepared in the emergency room and his blood work-up is being completed. Then he can be taken to the operating room for the repair.

Probably the most important thing to do in preparing to suture a vessel of the 1 mm size, (a digital vessel is that size) is not to introduce any instrument into the lumen that might damage the intima. Such a procedure will surely produce thrombosis. Employ the "no-touch" technique. If you do irrigate or profuse the specimen, touch only the more proximal part so that you can debride away that portion where you may have damaged the intima and remove it before you do the arterial repair.

While associates are working on the specimen in the operating room, here is what to do with the patient in the emergency room. Type and cross match the patient and prepare to heparinize him. Once in the operating room, irrigate the artery end again with heparinized Ringer's lactate solution through a tiny lacrimal cannula. While debriding, try to find an artery and perhaps two veins. At the same time coagulate or tie any small vessels that are bleeding.

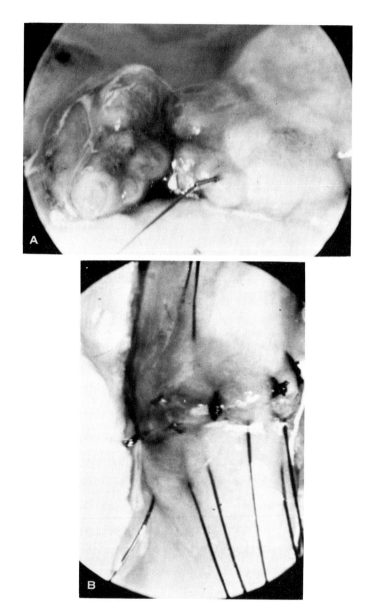

Figure 13.2.1 Nerve Repair. (A). The needle of a double armed microfilament black nylon suture is being passed through the perineural tissue to help stabilize the large fascicle adjacent to it. The other end of the suture will be inserted at a similar level into the perineural tissues of the opposing outer surface. (Note *small arrow*). *(B)*. After several (skewer) sutures are in place, only a few simple additional epineural sutures are needed to approximate the adjacent tissue. They complete the repair. They also will help to preserve the juncture and maintain nerve continuity after the nylon sutures are removed at 7 days.

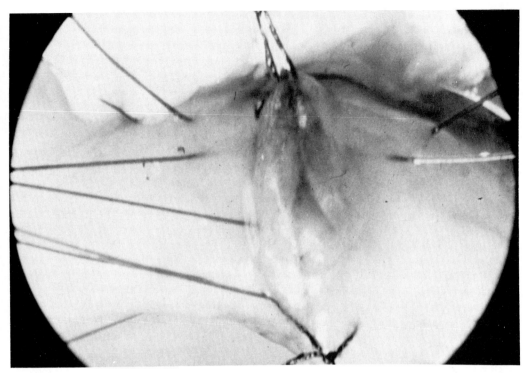

Figure 13.2.2. For the end-to-end suturing of small arteries, use the eccentric biangulation technique of Cobbett[4]. Place the first and second stay sutures about 120° apart. Then the posterior surface of the vessel juncture will remain lax and fall safely out of the way of the needle during the placement of the anterior suture line.

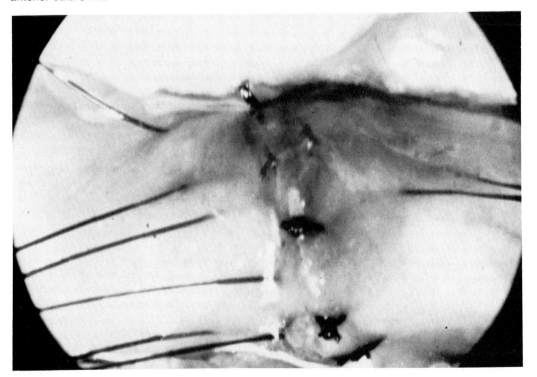

Figure 13.2.3. The anterior suture line is completed with interrupted sutures of 10-0 Nylon. Continuous sutures will invariably produce a dangerous narrowing of the lumen of the vessel. Place each of interrupted sutures about 0.5 mm from the edge of the juncture line.

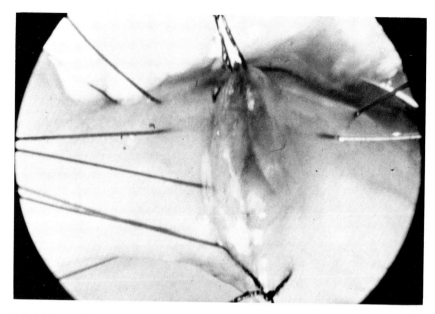

Figure 13.2.4. Venous Repair. The walls of the veins are thin and friable and careful approximation of the vessel edges is important. The slow, sluggish flow in the system is due to the low pressure so it is advisable to use an oblique suture line. This is a great help in preventing thrombosis.

It is important, at this point, to consider shortening the bones at the site of repair so there will not be a lack of soft tissue between the two ends or tension on the suture line. Insert a Kirschner pin between the proximal or distal bone ends. Drive it down the shaft of the bone so that it sticks into both ends and holds them together. As an additional aid, the extensor tendon should be quickly repaired to give two-point fixation. There is then less tendency for the amputated part to present any rotational problems.

If no Kirschner pin is available, use a 22-gage or 25-gage I.V. needle. It works very effectively in holding the two bone ends together.

Do the arterial repair first. Establish a free flow from the proximal arterial source and then apply a miniature Mayfield neurosurgical or a modified Scoville-Lewis clamp. Then use a lacrimal cannula to flush out the proximal and distal ends of the vessel with a heparinized Ringer's lactate solution, 10,000 units per 100 cc. But do not touch the intima of the vessels. Once the inflation of the pneumatic tourniquet has been accomplished, take off the clamps, for they cause more damage to the vessel wall if left in place. The use of an "eccentric biangulation" closure, allows better visibility to the posterior wall of the artery and more exacting insertion of the sutures. This means putting in stay sutures 120° apart rather than 180° (Fig. 13.2.2). Once the repair with interrupted sutures of 10/0 monofilament nylon is completed, the distal clamp is removed first, then the proximal one (Fig. 13.2.3). At the time that the clamps are removed

from the arterial repair, place a little piece of Saran wrap or some simular substance around the artery so that there is some compression at the point of the repair. Another technique is to apply some very gentle pressure to the site of anastomosis for two to three minutes if leakage is noted. In these arterial repairs strip back the adventitia as little as possible, for it may help to eliminate thrombosis (Fig. 13.2.4).

We did some vascular studies using silicone rubber. The vasovasorum runs in the adventitia to nourish the arterial wall. We observed that if one begins to strip it away, the little vessels going to the arterial walls are pulled away so there is no continuity between the external circulation and any remaining vessels with the arterial wall.

There are several things to relieve arterial spasm. Chemicals that may be helpful include: 2 per cent procaine cholorpromazine, 30 mg per cc of Ringer's solution or papaverine, 40 mg per cc. Sometimes the spasm can be relieved by carefully slitting the adventitia of the vessel wall longitudinally. Once the arterial inflow is established, it serves as a mean for identifying the best veins.

Venous anastomosis is next performed with similar technique, but, in the case of veins with an internal lumen diameter less than 0.8 mm, an oblique anastomosis is advocated, and sutures need not be as closely spaced as in the arterial repair.

Venous drainage is the keystone of success in reimplantation surgery. To prevent postoperative thrombosis, it is emphasized that pressure or longitudunal tension at the anastomosis site must be avoided. Tension at both venous or arterial anastomoses can be overcome either by bone shortening or the interposition of a free vein graft from the dorsum of the foot or the forearm.

REFERENCES

1. Buncke, H. J., and Blackfield, H. M. The vasoplegic effects of chlorpromazine. Plast. Reconstr. Surg., *31:* 353, 1963.
2. Buncke, H. J., Buncke, C. M., and Schulz, W. P. Immediate Nicoladoni procedure in the rhesus monkey or hallux to hand transplantation utilising microminiature vascular anastomoses. Br. J. Plast. Surg., *19:* 332, 1966.
3. Chase, R. A. The severely injured upper limb. Arch. Surg. *100:* 382, 1970.
4. Cobbett, J. R. Microvascular Surgery. Surg. Clin. North Am., *47:* 2, 521, 1967.
5. Cobbett, J. R. Free digital transfer. J. Bone Surg., *51B:* 4, 677, 1969.
6. Ducker, T. B., and Hayes, G. J. Experimental improvements in the use of Silastic cuff for peripheral nerve repair. Neurosurgery, *28:* 582, 1968.
7. Eiken, O., Mayer, R. F., Apastolou, K., and Deterling, R. A. Limb replacement, pathophysiological effects. Arch. Surg., *88:* 66, 1964.
8. Herbsman, H., and Lafer, D. (1966) Successful replantation of an amputated hand. Am. Surg., *163:* 137, 1966.
9. Herr, N., and Smith, J. W. (1967) *Microvascular Surgery. Report of First Conference, October 6-7, 1966.* Mary Fletcher Hospital, Burlington, Vermont, pp. 57-62.
10. Indue, T., and Fukusumi. Factors necessary for successful replantation of upper extremities. Am. Surg. *153:* 225, 1967.
11. Komatsu and Tamai. (1968) Successful replantation of a completely cut-off thumb. Plast. Reconstr. Surg., *42:* 374, 1968.
12. Lendvay, P. G. Anastomosis of digital vessels. Med. J. Aust., *2:* 723, 1968.
13. Lendvay, P. G., and Owen, E. R. (1970) Microvascular repair of completely severed digits. Med. J. Aust., *2:* 818, 1970.
14. Malt, R. A., and McKhann, D.F. Replantation of Severed Arms. J.A.M.A., *189:* 716, 1964.
15. McNeill and Wilson. (1970) The problems of limb replacement. Br. J. Surg., *57:* 365, 1970.
16. Millesi, H., Meissel, G., and Berger, U. A. The interfascicular nerve graft. Presented at the American Society for Surgery of the Hand, San Francisco, California, 1971.
17. Overton, J. H., and Owen, E. R. The successful replacement of minute arteries. Surgery, *68:* 713, 1970.
18. Paletta, F. X. Replantation of the amputated extremity. Am. Surg., *168:* 720, 1968.
19. Rank, B. K. (1963) Unique opportunities in the primary repair of hand injuries. In *Transaction of III International Congress of Plastic Surgery.* p. 995.
20. Rosenkrantz, Sullivan, and Welch. Replantation of an infant's arm. N. Engl. J. Med., *276:* 608-612, 1967.
21. Smith, J. W. Microsurgery of peripheral nerves. Plast. Reconstr. Surg., *33:* 317, 1964.
22. Smith, J. W. Microsurgery: Review of the literature and discussion of microtechniques. Plast. Reconstr. Surg., *37:* 227, 1966.
23. Smith, J. W. Factors influencing nerve repair. II. Collateral circulation of peripheral nerves. Arch. Surg., *93:* 433, 1966.
24. Smith, J. W. Factors influencing nerve repair. I. Blood supply of peripheral nerves. Arch. Surg., *93:* 335, 1966.
25. Smith, J. W. Injuries of the nerves. In Grabb, W. C. & Smith, J. W., *Plastic Surgery, A Concise Guide to Clinical Practice,* edited by W. C. Grabb and J. W. Smith. Boston, Little, Brown, 1968, p. 705.
26. Smith, J. W. "Peripheral nerves." *Microneurosurgery,* edited by R. W. Ran. St. Louis, Mosby, 1968.
27. Smith, J. W. "Surgical repair of peripheral nerves." In *Craft of Surgery,* edited by P. Cooper. Boston, Little, Brown, 1970.
28. Smith, J. W., and Jacobson, J. W. Microsurgical repair of blood vessels and peripheral nerves. In *Surgery of the Hand,* edited by J. E. Flynn. Baltimore, Williams & Wilkins, 1966, p. 729.

C.

Reflex Dystrophies of the Hand (The Causalgic States)

Frank H. Mayfield, M.D.

Injuries other than incised wounds that involve peripheral nerves often are followed by a condition of pain, vasomotor and sudomotor changes in the distal part of the extremity subserved by the injured nerve. For those that result from penetrating wounds, which are so common in war, the term causalgia, to describe the most common principal complaint, namely burning burning pain, is generally accepted.*

For those that follow closed injuries such as fracture or sprain of the wrist or ankle, which are more common in civilian life, a variety of titles have been used. Among these are Sudeck's atrophy, painful osteoporosis, post-traumatic dystrophy, minor causalgia, etc. It seems highly probable that these two groups are but variants (in degree) of the same disorder. Indeed, deTakats,[1] in a well documented, well reasoned argument, holds that the term "causalgic state" is a more accurate descriptive term.

In this chapter we are concerned with these disorders as they involve the hand, but it must be recognized that the problem is similar regardless of the part involved. It is important to emphasize that the causalgic states are often closely simulated by psychogenic disorders that also are post-traumatic in origin.

Another primary concern is that the causalgic states be recognized and dealt with before surgical correction of an injured part such as the hand be undertaken, for not only is wound healing poor in the presence of a reflex dystrophy, but surgery often is followed by an overwhelming ankylosis of the part and in addition emotional instability of sufficient degree to render rehabilitation impossible. Moreover, it is of profound importance that hysterical dystrophies be distinguished and dealt with by means other than surgery, for surgery upon a hysterical dystrophy not only fails to relieve the pain and dystrophic changes but almost invariably adds pain at the site of the new surgical incision and tends to fix the neurosis permanently.

The scope of this chapter does not permit a detailed discussion of pain mechanisms, but the reader is urged to review the work of Noordenbos,[13] who finds it necessary to hypothesize a new system, the multiple synaptic system (MAS) in order to explain the observation that he has made on many painful and/or dystrophic states. It is believed that a review of this volume will leave a few in doubt that the assessment of the dystrophies must as yet be made on the analysis of empirical clinical observations.

THE CAUSALGIC STATE

Although the syndrome now recognized as causalgia has been described previously, the description by Mitchell, Morehouse, and Keen[12] from their observations on the wounded of the War Between the States is a classic example of clinical writing.

"The seat of burning pain is very various, but it never attacks the trunk, rarely the arm or thigh, and not often the forearm or leg. Its favorite site is the foot or hand.

"The great mass of sufferers described this pain as superficial, but others said that it was also in the joints and deep in the palm. If it lasted long, it was referred finally to the skin alone.

"Its intensity varies from the most trivial burning to a state of torture, which hardly can be credited, but which reacts on the whole economy, until the general health is seriously affected.

"The part itself is not alone subject to an intense burning sensation but becomes exquisitely hyperaesthetic so that a touch or a tap of the finger increases the pain. Exposure to the air is avoided by the patient with a care which seems absurd, and most of the bad cases keep the hand constantly wet, finding relief in the moisture rather than the coldness of the application."

The term causalgia was actually introduced by Mitchell[11] in 1872.

"Perhaps few persons who are not physicians can appreciate the influence that long-continued and unendurable pain may have on both mind and body. Under such torments the temper changes, the most amiable grow irritable, the bravest soldier becomes a coward, and the strongest man is scarcely less nervous than the most hysterical girl. Nothing can better illustrate the extent to which these statements may be true than the cases of burning pain, or, as I prefer to term it, causalgia, the most terrible of all tortures which a nerve wound may inflict."

Subsequent to these reports by Mitchell et al., little was added to the literature in reference to causalgia until 1922, when Leriche,[7] from observations on the wounded of World War I, noted that interruption of the appropriate portion of the sympathetic nervous system would correct the disorder. Sudeck had in 1900 described peculiar vasomotor phenomena secondary to minor injuries. These cases resulted mostly from injuries that were closed and located at the wrist or ankle.

Pollock and Davis,[14] from their observations on the American wounded of World War I, confirmed the clinical observation of Mitchell and his co-workers and showed that the incidence of causalgia in patients suffering from peripheral nerve injuries was 2 per cent.

Leriche's observations in reference to causalgia were corroborated by several writers from experiences with sporadic cases between World War I and World War II. Among these were Spurling,[16] Ross,[15] Kwan,[6] White and Smithwick,[17] and Livingston.[8] During this interval also, numerous cases similar to those described by Sudeck were reported by Herrmann, Reineke, and Caldwell[4] by Homans,[5] and by Miller and deTakats. The latter had made searching studies on a large group of patients and were impressed with the fact that the blood flow in the injured extremity was increased in every case and concluded that the vasodilatation was related to and probably the cause of the pain.

The writer's first major experience with the causalgic state came during World War II with patients who suffered wounds of large peripheral nerves. Those with causalgia complained of severe pain, usually burning in character, in the distal part of the extremity, and often showed trophic, vasomotor, and sudomotor changes of the painful part. Some, however, were in a state of vasodilatation, while others noted to be in vasoconstriction, in contrast to the observations made by Miller and deTakats on their so-called minor causalgia cases, all of whom reportedly showed a state of vasodilatation. Interruption of the sympathetic chain would relieve the symptoms regardless of whether the patient was in vasodilatation or constriction. This was considered conclusive evidence that the alteration of blood flow was secondary and not the cause of the pain.

Originally it was difficult to correlate the observations of Miller and deTakats with those of the writer. However, since World War II many patients have been observed with a clinical picture similar to that described by these authors.

As observations on the war wounded continued, it became apparent that the alteration in blood flow varied, depending upon the duration of the illness. When seen early, most patients were in vasodilatation; if the disorder had been persistent for a prolonged period, vasoconstriction was apt to be observed.

DeTakats since has correlated his cases of minor causalgia with those seen as major injuries of the war wounded and has observed that they go through a similar three-stage course, namely vasodilatation, vasoconstriction, and subsequent atrophy. The writer's experience is similar to this.

CLINICAL COURSE AND DIFFERENTIAL DIAGNOSIS OF THE CAUSALGIC STATES

Many theories as to the underlying pathologic mechanism in the causalgic states have been advanced but none actually verified. The premise of Granit, Leksell, and Skoglund,[3] that a shunting of impulses from sympathetic to sensory fibers at the site of an injury due to fragmentation of myelin, is the most tenable hypothesis at the moment.

The onset of symptoms usually occurs immediately or within a few hours after the injury. At the outset, the pain, hyperesthesia, and trophic changes are confined to the tissues served by the injured nerve, and throughout the illness the symptoms and signs are most marked in that part, although they spread to involve the other parts of the extremity to some degree.

The median and sciatic nerves were the most frequent offenders. The principal symptom in most patients was that of burning pain, although many stated that it felt as if their hand were "squeezed in a vise" or the "flesh were being torn off". The pain always was continuous but varied in severity. In some it was mild but in others intense. The part was extremely hyperesthetic to touch.

Many were affected by emotional stimuli; some found the pain greatly increased by jarring of the bed or the slamming of a door. A draught of cool air sometimes induced severe pain. The squeaking of the wheels on a cart on the ward induced paroxysms of severe pain that were intolerable in one patient. Most kept themselves in a perpetual state of defense against such stimuli, and the facial expression usually reflected intense suffering (Fig. 13.3.1). Many learned to protect the part with makeshift coverings such as a soft cloth (Fig. 13.3.2). Others found relief by the immersion of the part in water. Usually if the part was swollen, hot, and dry, cool water was more comfortable. If the limb were in a state of vasoconstriction with soft, thin skin, excessive sweat, and loss of hair, the application of warm water was more apt to moderate the symptoms.

Emotional stimuli were usually accompanied by severe paroxysms of pain. Discipline by a ward nurse or a medical officer was sufficient to arouse anger and evoke horrible pain. The patients usually protected themselves throughout the day from environmental stimuli. After they once gained sleep, they would sleep soundly throughout the night and upon awakening would find the pain less intense. However, as the day progressed, the stress of the environment was again accompanied by marked exacerbation of pain.

Interruption of the sympathetic chain with a local anesthetic agent would, in cases of true causalgia, re-

sult in an immediate and complete relief of symptoms. This would persist for the duration of the anesthetic, only to be followed by their becoming intense again within a short time.

Until it was called to the writer's attention by deTakats, the three-stage course of causalgia had not been noted. There can be little doubt, however, that the disorder in its severe form does go through three stages. Pain, increased blood flow, hyperemia, pitting edema, dry scaly skin, increased temperature, particularly in the autonomous zone of the injured nerve, characterize the first stage. This may persist for several weeks or months. It is presumed that a vasodilator substance is released in the periphery to account for this phenomenon.

If the disorder is not arrested either spontaneously or by surgery, the character of the dystrophic phenomena gradually changes. The part becomes cold, the skin thin, hair growth lessens or ceases, the fingers become stiff and often ankylosed. Blood flow studies will, at this stage, show the part to be in vasoconstriction. Usually the entire extremity has become painful, and the patient is usually malnourished and emotionally distraught, with great danger of drug addiction. X-rays of the part usually will show osteoporosis of a spotty nature (Fig. 13.3.3). This deTakats considers the end of the second stage.

There is a gradual transition from this to a state of atrophy almost identical to that of Volkmann's ischemic paralysis, except that intractible pain usually persists.

All patients, however, do not reach this advanced stage. Some recover spontaneously. Review of the data gathered from World War II shows that approximately 20 per cent of all patients with wounds of peripheral nerves suffer causalgia of some degree, whereas only 5 per cent persisted in intractible form long enough to require that surgical interruption of the sympathetic chain be undertaken.

The nature of the author's practice rarely permits observation of patients with the minor causalgias at the outset of their illness, but analysis of a large number seen at varying stages after the onset supports deTakat's premise that the minor causalgias run essentially the same course. It also confirms his observation that if, after what appears to be mild trauma, there is pain, usually burning in nature, aggravated by jarring, air currents, noises, emotional upsets, and the like, even though the part is properly immobilized, uninfected, and seemingly on the way to normal repair, the suspicion that one is dealing with an early causalgic state should be realized.

Differential Diagnosis: The Psychogenic Dystrophies

The reflex dystrophies that arise from psychogenic causes, but secondary to trauma, are difficult to deal with. Because the intensity of symptoms with the causalgic state is greatly exaggerated by emotional stimuli, many have in the past been mistakenly consid-

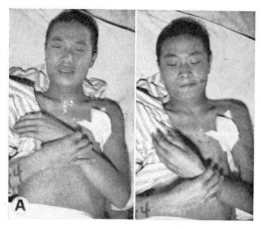

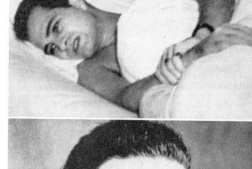

Figure 13.3.1. A. Photographs of Chinese soldier with causalgia due to bullet wound of left brachial plexus. Facial expression reflects intense suffering. Note also the defensive posture to prevent movement of painful part. (Reproduced from the Army Institute of Pathology, neg. no. A-4446-1, Washington 25, D.C.) *B.* Photographs showing facial expression and the patient immobilizing the painful member by holding it with the other hand, and the same patient following surgery. (Reproduced by permission from Surgery, Gynocology and Obstetrics, June, 1945.)

ered to be psychogenic in origin. This error is no longer justified. However, the clinical appearance of the dystrophic part in the hysterical state is so similar to that in the causalgic state that one must be extremely wary to avoid mistaking the psychogenic dystrophy for the causalgic state.

Careful analysis of the history and examination usually will permit accurate differential diagnosis. The onset of symptoms, for instance, is less likely to be immediately related to the trauma than with causalgia. In the majority of patients that the writer has seen, the onset of the dystrophic changes came later, usually at moments of stress, such as an interview with the legal representative or an altercation with an employer. The area of principal hyperesthesia and pain in never confined to the anatomic supply of one nerve, which is so characteristic of the causalgic state. The general health of the patient is rarely affected, even through advanced atrophy and ankylosis of the affected member may appear.

The response to chemical blockade of the sympathetic chain, however, is the most specific differential point in diagnosis. It is not unusual, for example, in a hysteric dystrophy to have the patient volunteer that the pain disappears simultaneously with the skin injec-

tion. The onset of relief is rarely coincidental with the signs of physiologic block, and oftentimes the pain returns before the signs of block disappear, or relief may project over a much longer period than the block can be expected to be effective. If one is in doubt, repeated injections should be made.

While each examiner must develop his own technique of establishing rapport with the patient suspected of hysterical dystrophy, the most effective method this writer has found involves the procedure of evoking the sympathy of the patient for the examiner by stating frankly that it is impossible to determine whether the disorder is organic or functional in origin. He is advised that, if it were functional and surgical correction were undertaken, the condition would be worsened rather than helped. Usually, for fear that error might be made, the patient accepts psychiatric evaluation as a favor to the examiner.

The underlying emotional factors may be as variable as human experience. Since many are industrial accidents or personal injury cases involved in litigation, the subconscious desire for gain or fear of injustice may be the cause. In others, hostility toward an employer or an immediate supervisor thought to be responsible for the patient's plight may be the issue.

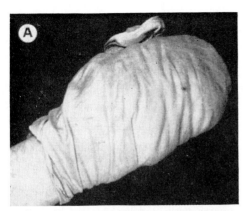

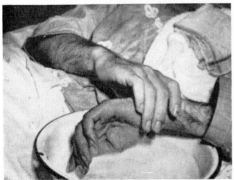

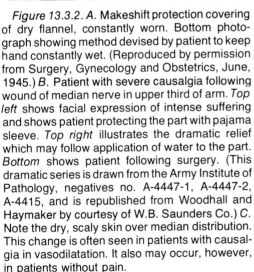

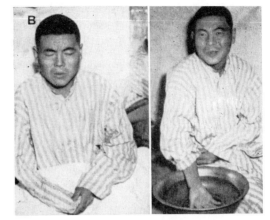

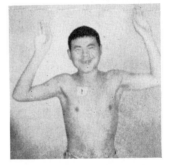

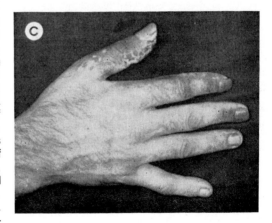

Figure 13.3.2. A. Makeshift protection covering of dry flannel, constantly worn. Bottom photograph showing method devised by patient to keep hand constantly wet. (Reproduced by permission from Surgery, Gynecology and Obstetrics, June, 1945.) *B.* Patient with severe causalgia following wound of median nerve in upper third of arm. *Top left* shows facial expression of intense suffering and shows patient protecting the part with pajama sleeve. *Top right* illustrates the dramatic relief which may follow application of water to the part. *Bottom* shows patient following surgery. (This dramatic series is drawn from the Army Institute of Pathology, negatives no. A-4447-1, A-4447-2, A-4415, and is republished from Woodhall and Haymaker by courtesy of W.B. Saunders Co.) *C.* Note the dry, scaly skin over median distribution. This change is often seen in patients with causalgia in vasodilatation. It also may occur, however, in patients without pain.

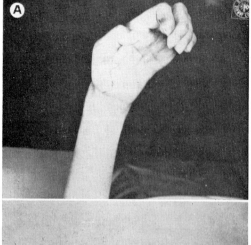
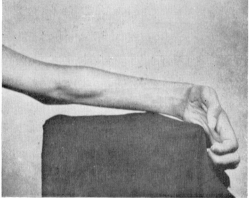
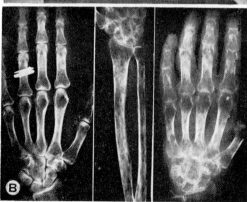

Figure 13.3.3. A. Combined median and ulnar nerve injury with causalgia. Pain prevented either active or passive movements. The atrophy, deformity, and rigid fixation of joints is apparent. Similar disabilities were frequently seen with less severe nerve injuries where causalgia went untreated for long periods, thereby precluding adequate physical therapy. *B.* X-ray photograph of hands and right forearm of patient with causalgia. *Left:* Normal left hand. *Center:* Marked spotty osteoporosis of bones of right forearm and wrist. *Right:* Osteoporosis of bones of right hand. Osteoporosis occurred in approximately 20 per cent of patients with causalgia.

Fear of loss of employment is a common cause in this disorder. Hostility toward a union who will not modify seniority rules to permit rehabilitation of the partially disabled has been found to be another cause. The desire for revenge upon the driver of the other car has been exposed as a factor. Indeed, any similar motive should be searched for in all cases.

OTHER REFLEX DYSTROPHIES

There is a miscellaneous group of patients who suffer with reflex dystrophies that are not hysteric in origin and cannot be classed as causalgia, but nevertheless run a somewhat similar course.

The Shoulder-Hand Syndrome.

This syndrome, which is often secondary to disease of the coronary arteries of the heart, is an example. There are many variations of this clinical picture and indeed many causes.

The most common course is the onset of pain within three to 16 weeks after myocardial infarction and often when recovery from the primary disease appears to be taking place. Mayfield and Newquist[9] have described the syndrome as follows: "Variations in the evolution of the clinical picture are many, but one may describe the events in a hypothetical 'typical' case thus: From three to 16 weeks after myocrdial infarction and often during recovery a patient may begin to notice the insidious onset of pain in elevating the shoulder, usually the left. Shortly thereafter he may complain of swelling, pain, and stiffness in the hand and fingers. The skin of the hand becomes smooth and a dusky pink. The grip becomes weak and the hand slightly warm to the touch. The shoulder is exquisitely tender to the touch, and the patient resists any passive or active movement of the extremity. X-ray at this time is usually negative.

"If untreated or unresponsive to treatment, the acute pain in the shoulder subsides in two to three months, but the shoulder becomes stiff and the range of motion limited. The hand becomes cool and cyanotic, and the palmar fascia thickens. In place of edema of the hand, there is substituted early atrophy of the subcutaneous tissue and intrinsic muscles. The hand and elbow assume a flexion posture. X-ray at this time may show diffuse or spotty osteoporosis of the hand and humerus.

"If totally refractory to treatment, in six to 12 months after the onset of symptoms the shoulder joint will have become 'frozen,' the musculature of the shoulder girdle atrophied and the hand flexed, contracted, and atrophied. The skin of the extremity will be cool, smooth, and blanched. X-ray may show severe osteoporosis, calcification in the tendons and bursae of the shoulder and possibly even subluxation.

"It must be remembered that, in addition to myocardial infarction, any disease of the cervical or upper thoracic spine, soft tissues of the neck, shoulder joint, arm, hand, or even the cerebrum may give rise to the clinical picture.

"Incidence of the syndrome following myocardial infarction is in the order of 10 to 20 per cent. Ernstene and Kinell in 1940 noted the occurrence of disabling shoulder pain in 17 out of 133 consecutive coronary occlusions. In 1943, Johnson reported that 39 out of 178 cases of myocardial infarction showed trophic hand changes and 34 of these also had shoulder disability. It is our experience that the incidence in cervical disc disease is less than 5 per cent. On the other hand, nearly 100 per cent of cases of cerebral thrombosis with hemiplegia will develop some manifestation of the picture. The incidence in bursitis, calcific tendinitis, hand and arm trauma is more difficult to assess because of the manifestations of the local lesions themselves.

"Treatment of the Shoulder-Hand Syndrome must be begun early to be effective. The most important step is prevention when possible. All who have dealt with surgical diseases of the upper extremities, including trauma, have recognized that elevation of the part and passive mobilization are essential to good healing and also to the prevention of ankylosis about the shoulder. It would appear that the severe pain, as well as the terrific anxiety that follows immediately upon a coronary occlusion, leads to immobilization that sets up tissue changes in the shoulder within the first few days. Passive exercise of the shoulder and elevation of the part from the outset and control of the pain by medication should avoid this complication.

"For the causalgic and vasomotor symptoms which may secondarily develop, procaine blockade of the sympathetic chain or long-acting ganglionic blockades such as tetraethylammonium salts, Etamon, or Priscoline, should be used. In the experience of the senior author, sympathectomy for coronary pain is frequently of value."

If one is to deal with this problem by sympathectomy, it must be remembered that the site of short circuit or shunt is in the thoracic cage and may involve sympathetic ganglia as low as D-4 or D-5.

The Carpal Tunnel Syndrome.

This syndrome, in its more exaggerated form, may produce a causalgic state, and the part may become severely dystrophic. It, of course, involves only the median nerve and the tissues this nerve subserves at the outset, but the dystrophic phenomena may spread to involve the entire limb, and diagnosis at the late stage is difficult. It should be suspected, however, when the dystrophy has been preceded by retention of fluid, tenosynovitis, fracture of the wrist, indeed, anything that increases the volume of tissues under the carpal tunnel or narrows the tunnel itself may initiate this disorder.

The part should be immobilized in a light cast for a time, for this usually will provide relief. Introduction of a local anesthetic agent into the nerve just proximal to the retinaculum will relieve the pain and the causalgia phenomena while rendering the paralysis of the nerve temporarily complete.

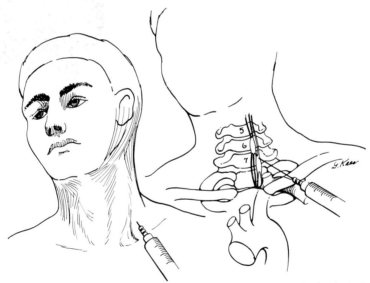

Figure 13.3.4. Technique for procaine block of cervico-dorsal sympathetic chain by anterior approach. A 3" or 4" 21-gauge intravenous needle attached to a 10 cc-syringe is passed through the scalenus anticus muscle till it encounters the transverse process of C-6 or C-7 vertebrae, where 20 cc of 1 per cent or 2 per cent procaine are instilled.

The scalenus anticus may be identified by palpation just above the clavicle and lateral to the sternocleidomastoid muscle. The needle is inserted at a point 1 to 2 cm above the clavicle to avoid the dome of the pleura and is directed slightly upward and medialward.

Prior to the injection of the solution, one should aspirate to insure that neither the lung nor a blood vessel has been entered.

If the roots or trunk of the brachial plexus are encountered, a slight deflection of the needle point up or down will permit passage through to the bony process sought.

When the needle point is in proper plane, the plunger meets little resistance as the solution is injected. If heavy resistance is encountered, it indicates that the fluid is being injected subperiosteally, and it should be withdrawn 1 or 2 mm.

A successful injection is indicated by the development of a Horner's syndrome and a rise of skin temperature of the part. If the patient has causalgia, relief of pain occurs immediately.

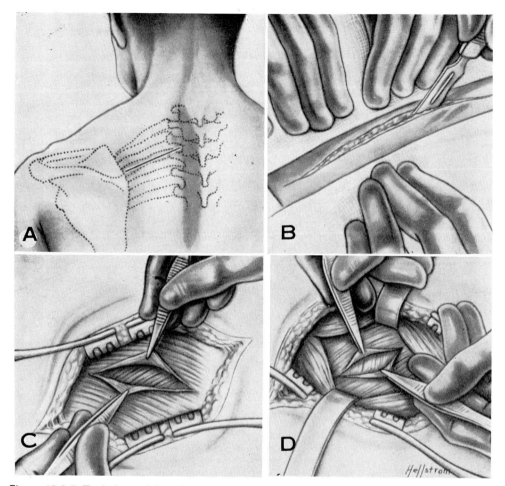

Figure 13.3.5. Technique of dorsal preganglionic ramisection. *A.* Position: May be face down or sitting. The arm should be so placed that the scapula is widely separated from the spine. *B.* Incision: Extends from a point 1 cm lateral to the spine of D-2 vertebra to the border of the scapula over the course of the third rib. A more oblique incision crossing the third rib is satisfactory. The skin is undermined to facilitate retraction. *C.* The fibers of the latissimus dorsi are split over the course of the third rib and retracted. *D.* The fibers of the rhomboid major are split and retracted. *E.* The serrations of the paravertebral muscles are detached from the third rib and transverse process. *F.* The paravertebral muscles have been retracted medially and a segment of the third rib and the transverse process of D-3 removed. Lateral retraction of the pleura then permits exposure of the second and third intercostal nerves being crossed by the sympathetic chain with communicating rami attaching the two. *G.* The sympathetic chain has been sectioned below D-3 ganglion and the two intercostal nerves sectioned proximal and distal to the ganglia. The proximal portion of the chain is sutured into the extrathoracic muscles to prevent regeneration. Simple detachment of the rami connecting D-2 and D-3 ganglia to the intercostal nerves and section of the chain below D-3 sympathectomizes the arm as completely but less permanently. White uses an impervious sac to encase the stump. *H.* Routine steps in closure.

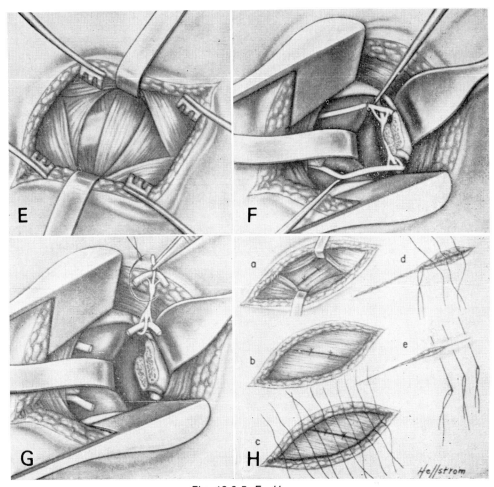

Fig. 13.3.5. E - H

Hyperpathia and Paresthesias.

As a final word of caution in making the differential diagnosis, the causalgic states must be distinguished from the hyperpathic or sensitive skin that commonly follows partial nerve injury in the recovery phase and which is evoked by touch or other stimuli to the part but which is not transmitted through the sympathetic chain.

THE CAUSALGIC STATES: DIAGNOSIS AND TREATMENT

The differential diagnosis depends almost entirely on local blockade of the appropriate portion of the sympathetic chain. In the case of the hand, this is easily done through an anterior approach to the region of the stellate ganglion (Fig. 13.3.4).

If the patient's symptoms are a reflection of a causalgic state, relief of pain will be immediate with the onset of anesthesia and will persist for the duration of that agent. The pain usually is not so intense immediately after the anesthesia has worn off, but return

of discomfort is without delay. In carrying out the injection procedure, It is important that the patient not be prompted or guided in any way as to the anticipated result. It should be noted whether the pain subsides before the block is effective. When this occurs, it is highly suggestive that the disorder is hysterical in origin.

Whether the surgical interruption of the sympathetic chain is indicated at this stage is necessarily determined by several factors. If there is, for example, urgent indication for surgical repair of the injured part (open reduction of fracture, skin grafts, etc.), the dystrophy should be corrected by sympathectomy promptly and before the other procedures are entered upon. If the symptoms are mild and subsiding and there is no urgent indication for reconstructive surgery on the part, a conservative course is justified and indeed indicated, for many will recover spontaneously. Sympathetic blocking agents which may be given systemically and certain tranquilizing agents appear to aid in the control of symptoms and to speed recovery.

Close observation should be maintained, however,

and if the dystrophy appears to progress despite conservative treatment, surgical interruption of the chain should be undertaken before the crippling effects of ankylosis and psychic trauma of prolonged pain are irrevocable.

Sympathetic Denervation of the Upper Extremity

The objective of the operation is to remove thoracic ganglia 2 and 3, thereby interrupting the chain below D-3 and removing the rami communicans from D-2 and D-3 to the intercostal nerves 2 and 3.

The upper portion of the thoracic sympathetic chain may be approached by any of four approaches. These are: (1) posterior; (2) supraclavicular; (3) standard transthoracic; (4) transaxillary. The selection of route obviously is determined by the surgeon's experience. The writer routinely uses the posterior approach (Fig. 13.3.5). The reader is referred to standard texts on Thoracic Surgery for technique of other approaches.[2]

Neurectomy and Neuroplasty

There are occasional cases in which resection of the injured segment is indicated in preference to sympathectomy. Pure sensory nerves such as the sensory branch of the radial or medial antebrachial cutaneous nerves which do not supply the palmar surface of the hands are examples. These may be sacrificed with less residual disability and risk than is incurred by sympathectomy.

Careful study and mature judgment are necessary when resection of the injured segment of a major mixed nerve that subserves the hand is being considered, for the residual disability is often substantial after resection, whereas the majority show little disability after the causalgic state is relieved by sympathectomy. It is an almost invariable rule that the severity of the causalgic state is in reverse ratio to the extent of the nerve lesion.

With ulnar nerve lesions accompanying fracture or fracture dislocation of the elbow, extensive partial laceration often produces motor and sensory paralysis of such severe degree that useful functional recovery cannot be expected, yet enough fibers may remain intact to permit the development of a mild causalgic state. It is better under these circumstances to resect, transpose, and resuture the nerve at the outset. A similar situation is seen at times with the radial nerve in fracture of the humerus or the fracture of the head of the radius. The median nerve is less likely to be so affected.

REFERENCES

1. deTakats, G. *Vascular Surgery.* Philadelphia, Saunders, 1959.
2. Gibbon, John H., Sabiston, David C., and Spencer, Frank C. *Surgery of the Chest.* Ed. 2. Philadelphia, Saunders, 1959, pp. 293-297.
3. Granit, R., Leksell, L., and Skoglund, C. R. *Fiber interaction in injured or compressed region of nerve.* Brain, *67:* 125, 1944.
4. Hermann, L. G., Reineke, H. G., and Caldwell, J.A. Post-traumatic painful osteoporosis: A clinical and roentgenological entity. Am. J. Roentgenol., *47:* 3, 1942.
5. Homans, J. Minor causalgia: A hyperesthetic neurovascular syndrome. N. Engl. J. Med., *222:* 870, 874, 1940.
6. Kwan, S. T. The treatment of causalgia by thoracic sympathetic ganglionectomy. Ann. Surg., *101:* 222, 1935.
7. Leriche, R. *La Chirurgia de la Douleur.* Paris, Masson et Cie., 1940.
8. Livingston, W. K. *Pain Mechanisms: A Physiological Interpretation of Causalgia and Its Related States.* New York, Macmillan, 1943.
9. Mayfield, F. H., and Newquist, R. E.: The shoulder-hand syndrome. Ohio State Med. J., 1959.
10. Medical Department, United States Army. *Surgery in World War II.* Neurosurgery, Vol. II. Washington, U.S. Government Printing Office, 1959.
11. Medical Department, United States Army. *War Surgery (Orthopedics). Hand Surgery; Foot Surgery.* Newsletter, Vol. I, No. 2, July, 1970.
12. Mitchell, Morehouse and Keen. *Gunshot Wounds and Other Injuries of the Nerve.* Philadelphia, Lippincott, 1864.
13. Noordenbos, W. *Some aspects of the anatomy and physiology of pain.* Chir. Belg. Brussels, *61:* 618, 1962.
14. Pollock , L.J., and Davis, L. *Peripheral Nerve Injuries.* Hoebers Surgical Monographs. New York, Hoeber, 1937.
15. Ross, J. P. Report of demonstrations of the results of sympathectomy for eleven median causalgias. St. Barth. Hosp. Rep. *66:* 39, 1933.
16. Spurling, G. Causalgia of the upper extremity; Treatment by dorsal sympathetic ganglionectomy. Arch. Neurol. Psychiatr., *23:* 784, 1930.
17. White, J. C., and Smithwick, R. H. *The Autonomic Nervous System: Anatomy, Physiology and Surgical Application.* Ed. 2. New York, Macmillan, 1941.

The author has reviewed his own material since the original publication and also has reviewed the literature dealing with the military operations in Vietnam and notes that there is no material which significantly changes the findings and opinions recorded in this chapter. He has, however, had the opportunity to follow up a few patients who had undergone sympathectomy for reflex dystrophy and who subsequently have had a recurrence of symptoms, either spontaneously or as the result of new trauma. In these, the usual methods of testing, such as sympathetic block and, indeed, the method of surgical treatment, are greatly modified, for the sympathetic fibers do regrow and grow very widely and are exceedingly difficult to identify and remove. It is true in the lumbar and thoracic also, but it is particularly difficult when the lesion involves the hand and therefore requires attack upon the cervicothoracic portion of the sympathetic chain.

chapter fourteen

Infections

A.

Bacteriology, Antibiotics, and Chemotherapy

Basil A. Pruitt, Jr., M.D., Colonel, MC
Robert B. Lindberg, Ph.D.
William F. McManus, M.D., Major, MC

Infection is the most devastating complication to occur after either injury or elective surgery of the hand. Major tissue loss, a nonfunctional limb, or even systemic toxicity and death can result from sepsis following a minor injury, a relatively small burn, or a technically satisfactory operative procedure.

An understanding of the pathogenesis of infection enables one to treat patients so as to minimize septic complications and to monitor wounds in a systematic fashion so that infections are recognized at the earliest possible moment and viable tissue is preserved. An appreciation of the characteristics of the common microorganisms causing hand infections assists in planning appropriate treatment, and knowledge of the characteristics of available antibacterial agents ensures prompt utilization of specific therapy. Lastly, an awareness of the special susceptibility to infection of certain groups of patients permits the attending surgeon to modify therapy or employ special treatment to enhance the protection afforded those individuals.

Both host and bacterial factors appears to be of significance in determining the incidence and severity of infection.[71] The interplay of these factors and the resulting balance may spell the difference between contamination and clinical sepsis. Patient factors of importance include the magnitude of injury, age of the patient, adequacy of the general circulation, adequacy of the local blood supply, the wound environment, past immunologic experience and the immunological competence of the patient, supervening complications, and pre-existing diseases. Microbial factors of importance include the bacterial density in the wound, bacterial virulence which may be strain variable, the invasive propensities of the organism, microbial competition, exogenous sources of bacterial seeding, and bacterial sensitivity to antibiotics.

HOST FACTORS OF IMPORTANCE IN SEPSIS

The susceptibility of a given patient to infection is directly related to the magnitude of the injury which he has sustained. Patients with extensive burns and patients with multiple injuries are more susceptible to septic complications than patients with lesser injuries, and infection, remains the most common cause of death in the severely injured who are successfully resuscitated.[20] The influence of age on infectious complications following a given injury is reflected in the greater susceptibility to septic complications of the neonate and the elderly as compared to that of a young adult patient.[47]

Prolonged hypotension increases the likelihood of subsequent infection by favoring bacterial proliferation even in superficial wounds. Invasion of a contaminated wound may occur with alarming rapidity in a hemodynamically unstable patient. Inadequacy of the local blood supply is perhaps more commonly related to subsequent infection. Local ischemia not only provides a pabulum for bacterial proliferation but prevents delivery of both protective inflammatory cells and an adequate concentration of antimicrobial agents to the site of microbial growth and proliferation. Such ischemia is of paramount importance in the burn patient where systemic antibiotics are ineffective in limiting bacterial growth in the nonviable avascular eschar and topical application of antibacterial medication is essential.[64] The predisposition to infection of traumatic or operative wounds containing nonviable tissue also reflects the importance of the local blood supply in limiting bacterial invasion and emphasizes the importance of adequate debridement.

The immunologic experience and competence of the host are also of consequence and explain in part the increased susceptibility to infection in the neonate as noted above. Alexander has shown that in burn patients the antibody response to a new antigen is diminished, although the ability to mount an anamnestic response is unimpaired.[2] Changes in circulating immunoglobulin levels have also been noted in patients with extensive burns in whom suppression of IgG may well relate to the increased susceptibility of such patients to bacterial invasion.[59] This suppression of the humoral component of host resistance has clinical relevance insofar as patients with burns of more than 30 per cent of the total body surface require more potent and more frequent doses of an antiPseudomonas vaccine than patients with lesser injuries.[4] Impairment of cellular defense mechanisms may also predispose patients to infection. Alexander has related fluctuation of intraneutrophil killing capacity to episodes of certain injured patients.[3] In our laboratory, Newsome and Eurenius, using a laboratory animal model of burn injury, have shown that sepsis suppresses not only the nondividing compartment of granulocytes but also bone marrow production of granulocytes.[61] The striking decrease in the dividing compartment of granulocytes due to sepsis occurs at a time when even more granulocytes than are normally present are needed for defense against invading microorganisms.

The injury-to-treatment interval is of both theoretical and practical significance since delay of therapy beyond the "golden period" of six to eight hours may change the injury from a contaminated to an infected wound requiring antibiotics for treatment rather than prophylaxis, and alteration of primary wound care to include delayed primary or even secondary closure. The presence of foreign bodies is a strong predisposing factor to bacterial survival and proliferation and is a common occurrence in traumatic wounds, especially those incurred in combat. Multiple, deeply imbedded, small foreign bodies defy removal and demand that delayed primary or secondary closure of such wounds be carried out, as well as the use of antibiotic therapy.[93] The predilection of microorganisms to take residence and proliferate on implanted foreign bodies must also be borne in mind when caring for patients with prosthetic heart valves or vessels who have sustained trauma or undergone elective surgery.

The wound environment *per se* also influences patient susceptibility to infections and the type of microorganisms present in the wound. The deleterious effect of excessive moisture is obvious to all who have seen infection develop in a macerated, superficial wound in constant contact with the bedclothes. A wound containing nonviable tissue is predisposed to Clostridial infection while viable tissue resists invasion of anaerobic organisms.[5] Moreover, wound invasion by some fungal organisms appears to be pH related, as indicated by the frighteningly rapid proliferation and invasion of Phycomycetes in uncontrolled diabetics with ketoacidosis.[1]

Pre-existing diseases or conditions which are known to increase the likelihood of sepsis include diabetes, leukemia and lymphoma, malnutrition, renal failure, previously implanted foreign bodies or burn injury, agammaglobulinemia and induced immunosuppression as seen in patients who have undergone organ transplantation. The increased susceptibility to infection in these patients results not only from alteration of the specific factors noted above but also from some general, as yet undefined, systemic effect of the disease processes.[67] Coexisting complications also increase the likelihood of subsequent infection by

further impairing host defense mechanisms and by direct seeding of distant sites from a primary focus of infection. Examples of the latter effect include seeding of a fracture hematoma by microorganisms from an infected burn wound, and hematogenous pneumonia occurring in the patient with suppurative thrombophlebitis.[72]

MICROBIAL FACTORS INFLUENCING SEPSIS

Microbial factors predisposing to clinical sepsis are the size of the initial microbial innoculum and the net rate of bacterial proliferation which determine the bacterial density in a wound. This density can be used as an index to determine the likelihood of bacterial invasion and also as an indication of the readiness of a given wound for closure.[75] Microbial virulence and invasiveness appear to be strain or type related in both bacteria and fungi. Marked variations of virulence exist between different Pseudomonas strains as tested in various laboratory models and the broad hyphal nonseptate fungi, with a predilection to vascular invasion, appear to be much more aggressive invaders than fungi with thin hyphae.[60] Local tissue ischemia secondary to bacterial or fungal vasculitis favors more rapid proliferation of the offending microorganisms and further extension of infection. The importance of microbial competition is indicated by the increasing frequency of clinical infections caused by uncommon opportunistic gram-negative bacteria, fungi, and viruses, which occupy the ecologic vacuum created by antibiotic control of the historically more common gram-negative bacteria.[73]

The source of microbial seeding may be either internal, as in the hematogenous spread of bacteria and fungi, or external, as in wound seeding by attending personnel who have come in contact with other patients, or by ward equipment such as ventilatory apparatus, sinks, and air-conditioning ducts.[94] In general, the gram-negative bacteria are poor air travelers and are spread by fomite or personnel contact, in contrast to the tubercle bacillus and some of the gram-positive organisms which are recognized as airborne pathogens.

The place of injury determines the initial microbial flora of the burn wound and specific geographic locations of injury should be noted, such as Southeast Asia where *Pseudomonas pseudomallei* is indigenous, or hospitals where resistant Staphylococci are commonly encountered. There are also microbial organisms more frequently encountered in certain occupational injuries, such as those which occur in slaughterhouse employees, animal handlers, workers who handle hair and hides, kitchen workers, and cooks.

Microbial resistance to therapeutic agents is also of critical importance and necessitates careful selection of specific antibiotics which will effectively control the offending microorganisms. The mixed microbial flora of traumatic wounds necessitates the selection of an antibiotic with the broadest possible spectrum and at times the use of multiple antibiotics.[22] Conversely, the recent identification of resistance transfer factors in bacteria which may impart resistance to several antibiotics speaks strongly for the use of single antibiotics of maximum specificity in the treatment of established infections.[24][76]

DIAGNOSIS OF INFECTION

The diagnostic criteria of infection are well known, but confirmation depends on identification of the causative organism by culture or other means. Wound monitoring involves not only appropriately frequent examination but culture of the wound when infection is suspected. For the best yield, cultures should be obtained from the tissue which is the site of bacterial growth and proliferation prior to the institution of antimicrobial therapy. Surface swabs may recover only surface contaminants from infected wounds and wound biopsies may be necessary to distinguish invading from colonizing organisms.

Wound biopsies are an essential component of present day burn care[74] and the technique may be used to enhance diagnostic specificity in order infections of soft tissue from which routine cultures have been unrewarding (Fig. 14.1.1). Obviously, the biopsy should avoid vital structures such as nerves, tendons, and vessels but should include the advancing edge of infection, so that adjacent viable tissue and the nonviable-viable tissue interface may be examined. One portion of the tissue sliver or fragment is quantitatively cultured in the microbiology laboratory. The specimen, if large enough, may be flamed to kill "surface contaminants," but small samples are cultured directly. Use of tissue slivers as opposed to tissue homogenates improves the culture yield of specimens suspected of harboring Clostridia or fungi.

The remainder of the biopsy specimen is processed immediately (standard slides can be prepared in about four hours) by the pathologist for histologic examination. A special stain developed at this Institute (a modified Giemsa-PAS technique) improves the light microscopic identification of both bacteria and fungi in a single slide (Fig. 14.1.2).[50]

Although infection can occur with fewer organisms, a bacterial density of 10^5 or more organisms per gram of tissue appears to be characteristic of overt clinical soft tissue sepsis. Bacterial populations below that density are often seen in contaminated wounds but can generally be defended against by the host. If serial quantitative cultures are obtained and a progressive increase in bacterial density is noted, some investigators have advocated that treatment be begun prior to the bacteria reaching a density of 10^5 organisms per gram of tissue. Delayed primary or secondary closure of wounds containing 10^5 or more organisms per milliliter of secretion has been associated with a high incidence of postclosure wound infection,[70] and this has been advanced as the rationale for serial monitoring of contaminated or infected wounds prior to attempted closure.

The histologic criteria of invasive sepsis are listed in Table 14.1.1. Of particular importance in the diagnosis of invasion is the involvement of previously viable tissue as indicated by the presence of an inflammatory response. Since the histologic changes indicative of invasive sepsis may be focal in nature, the physician should take care to biopsy that area of the wound which he considers most likely to be infected. The identification of vascular invasion, which is

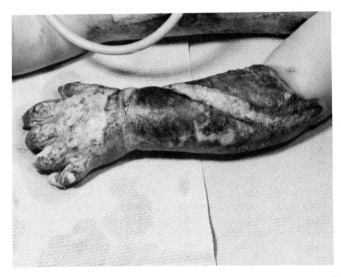

Figure 14.1.1. A mixed infection in the burn wound of the left hand and arm. Culture and biopsy examination were diagnostic of burn wound infection with Candida species and burn wound invasion with *Pseudomonas aeruginosa*. Note the hemorrhagic discoloration characteristic of bacterial invasion.

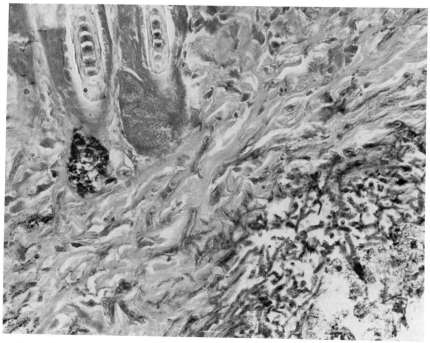

Figure 14.1.2. Photomicrograph of wound biopsy stained with PAS-Giemsa stain. Note fungal hyphae in the dermis and nidus of bacteria at the base of a hair follicle.

TABLE 14.1.1
Indications of invasive wound infection

A. Clinical
    1. Advancing soft tissue necrosis
    2. Skin discoloration
    3. Discoloration and/or liquifaction of fat
    4. Early seperation of eschar from burn wounds
B. Histologic
    1. Presence of microorganism in viable tissue
    2. Heavy microbial colonization throughout burn eschar or exposed non-viable tissues of traumatic wounds
    3. Accentuated suppurative tissue response
    4. Bacteria or fungal invasion of blood vessels

characteristic of both Pseudomonas species and many fungi, strongly suggests that hematogenous dissemination has occurred, and that systemic antimicrobial therapy should be employed.

In addition to this program of individual wound monitoring, bacteriologic surveillance of the entire hospital is recommended in order to identify prevalent organisms, clusters of operative infections, and the sensitivity patterns of the "resident flora" which influence housekeeping hygiene, attending personnel assignments, and initial choice of antibacterial medication prior to receipt of culture and sensitivity results in the early treatment of established infections as described below.

MICROORGANISMS OF SURGICAL IMPORTANCE IN THE HAND

Before the advent of chemotherapy and antibiotics, the most serious infections of the hand were caused by hemolytic Streptococci, Lancefield Group A. The sulfonamides and then the antibiotics reduced the incidence and complications of these infections. Today the Staphylococci are undoubtedly the most important organisms in hand infections (Fig. 14.1.3). Mixed bacterial populations characterize the contaminated hand wound soon after injury, but if infection is present, the causative organism usually predominates when cultured (Fig. 14.1.4). Quantitative cultures are of value, since the organism recovered in the highest dilution of the innoculum is unequivocally the predominant species. Such predominance can be masked by inhibitory action of other strains in a mixed culture, when only a qualitative technique is used. The initial infecting agent may be replaced, often during the second week, by other organisms which may arise from endogenous sources (skin, upper respiratory tract, feces, or external genitalia) or exogenously from the hospital environment, especially from adjacent patients. Pathogenic cocci, the most common primary invaders, may be combined with micrococci or with gram-negative bacilli, including Proteus-Providencia, Escherichia, Klebsiella, Enterobacter, or Pseudomonas species. In some instances actual

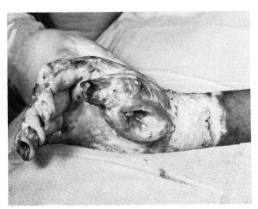

Figure 14.1.3. Thenar abscess of right hand and osteomyelitis of carpal bones of burned hand. Causative organism *Staphylococcus aureus*.

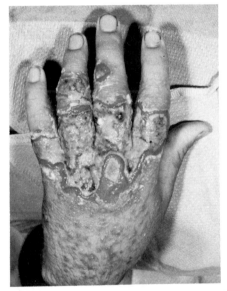

Figure 14.1.4. Mixed infection of hand after chemical injury. Note fibrinous membrane in base of wound and superficial infection of intact skin associated with macerating wet dressings.

synergistic action may occur, as seen in chronic progressive synergistic bacterial gangrene. The presence in some of the infecting flora of enzymes antagonistic to certain antibiotics may aid another segment of infecting flora by sparing them from such antibiotic action.

Gram-Positive Bacteria

Staphylococci

The Staphylococci are the most ubiquitous wound pathogens. It is difficult to designate sites from which they would not be recovered. Their classification,

which has a long and controversial history, will here be a current generally accepted schema. The genus is distinguished from other cocci by the formation of catalase.[96] The catalase reaction is a practical one which avoids the erroneous inclusion of other bacteria as presumptive Staphylococci. Pigment formation is typical but not constant, so that *Staphylococcus aureus*, the human pathogen, can include nonpigmented forms. The nonpathogenic species is *Staphylococcus epidermitis (Staphylococcus albus)*. The hemolytic, necrotizing, and leukocidal toxins of Staphylococcal infection are found in both pigmented and nonpigmented strains. The ability of pathogenic Staphylococci to clot plasma was first described by Loeb in 1904. This is now accepted as the most reliable single test for differentiating *Staphylococcus aureus*. This species also ferments mannitol. *Staphylococcus epidermitis* is, in contrast, coagulase negative and mannitol negative. *Staphylococcus aureus* is further distinctive in forming a DNAse and in tolerating 0.4 per cent NaC1. "Presumptive" media which select mannitolfermenting, DNAse producing strains aid in the prompt recognition of the Staphylococci.

Penicillin resistance has become an increasing problem in the control of Staphylococcal infections. Resistance is associated with the rate of formation of penicillinase, an enzyme which splits penicillin by destroying the beta-lactam nucleus which is the core of the penicillin structure.[81] The recently developed semisynthetic penicillins initially resisted penicillinase action, but subsequent exposure has permitted the rise of mutants which can again split the lactam ring, and a rise in forms resistant to the semisynthetic penicillin analogs has resulted.

Infections with a diffuse cellulitis are the most responsive to antibiotic therapy. When necrotic tissue or a fibrin barrier is present, the response to antibiotics is more likely to be equivocal. Staphylocoagulase, which is the species determinate for *Staphylococcus aureus*, causes deposition of fibrin around cocci in viable tissue, and thus aids the infecting activity of Staphylococci. The organisms also clump in tissue and this attribute, plus the action of coagulase, contributes largely to the tendency of Staphylococci to form abscesses in tissue. The organisms thus shielded and with a pabulum of necrotic tissue may persist for extended periods of time despite the highest blood concentrations attainable. Concentration of antibiotics in tissue is thus more important than blood levels.

Differentiation of strains of infecting bacteria is inherently helpful in understanding transmission patterns and mechanisms. Bacteriophage typing has been widely and successfully applied to the recognition of Staphylococcal strains.[95] Four broad groups of Staphylococci are recognized, with many types within each group. Typing is useful in recognizing potentially virulent types and in tracing cross infection sources. The most virulent type, which became known as the "hospital type," was for at least 10 years type 52, 52A, 80, 81. Since 1969, however, a sharp reversal has occurred and throughout the world the rise in types having factors 84, 85 has occurred. Penicillin resistance, which in the 1940's and early 1950's was the rule, increased markedly for the 80, 81 pattern, and in the past three years has been even more noticeable with the type 84, 85 strains. Penicillin resistance in 80 to 85 per cent of isolates has been observed in 1970 to 1972. The highest rate of resistance to this, and to other categories of antibiotics, is found in hospitals where penicillin and its analogs are extensively used. Restoration of susceptible flora to selected antibiotics in a given hospital has been achieved by totally withdrawing the antibiotic for a year or two; this experiment was convincingly conducted for erythromycin, but could well apply to other antibiotics. This result underscores the fact that the resistant flora in a given hospital is essentially created by that hospital. The resistance patterns are neither as specific nor as extensive in the flora of the normal population, and resistant strains do not persist in that population. However, the widespread use of penicillin has probably reduced the number of sensitive strains and allowed the penicillinase producers to become numerically prominent.

Streptococci

These organisms are classified broadly on the basis of their ability to hemolyze red blood cells in blood agar. Alpha-hemolysis displays a narrow zone of incomplete hemolysis, often with a green discoloration from breakdown products of hemoglobin. Beta-hemolytic Streptococci produce a clear zone of complete lysis with two separate lysins usually produced. Beta-lysin is oxygen labile and demonstrable only in deep colonies; S-lysin is oxygen stable and produces surface hemolysis. Gamma-hemolytic strains produce no lysis on blood agar. Infections are primarily due to beta-hemolytic Streptococci, which are more precisely classificed in antigenically distinct groups, designated groups A through S, on the basis of group specific carbohydrates. No group of bacteria causes a wider variety of disease in man than Group A Streptococci.[86] This phenomenon may be related to the wide variety of extracellular products that they form. Erythrogenic toxin, streptolysin, hyaluronidase, leukocidin, streptokinase, and deoxyribonuclease are prominent extracellular products. The erythrogenic toxin causes the rash in scarlet fever. Streptolysins, although lysing red blood cells *in vitro* probably principally act *in vivo* by damaging leukocytes and macrophages. Streptokinase dissolves fibrin and acts to lyse purulent exudates. Hyaluranidase has long been considered to act as a spreading factor in infection, lysing the ground substance of connective tissue. The hemolytic Streptococcus of Lancefield Group A is one of the few organisms capable of causing invasion even without the presence of devitalized tissue or blood

clot. Most other bacteria require devitalized tissue before infections can begin and these are frequently mixed infections. When Group A Streptococci colonize a granulating wound, they can elaborate enzymes which rapidly dissolve fibrin and thus can destroy the attachment of a skin graft. This process can be extremely rapid, and prophylaxis is necessary at the time of skin grafting.

Hemolytic Streptococci can cause a necrotizing fasciitis, or hemolytic Streptococcal gangrene. This subcutaneous or fascial necrosis produces extensive undermining of the skin, with later development of gangrene after circulatory compromise.

Anaerobic or more precisely microaerophilic Streptococci are associated with Meleney's ulcer. This lesion presents two forms; the first, a progressive undermining ulceration of the skin and subcutaneous tissue, is caused by a hemolytic, microaerophilic Streptococcus, the second form is designated "progressive synergistic gangrene" and is caused by a nonhemolytic, microaerophilic Streptococcus associated in a symbiotic manner with *Staphylococcus aureus*. Neither organism alone produces the infection, but it may be that Proteus strains can take the place of the Staphylococcus.

The importance of the role of anaerobic or microaerophilic Streptococci in a variety of infections such as human bite infections is widely appreciated. The morphology of these organisms resembles that of aerobic Streptococci. They are innocuous commensals in their normal habitat of the mouth, intestine, or female genitourinary tract, but trauma, necrosis, or ischemia alter the host tissue and they then behave as opportunistic pathogens.

The alpha-hemolytic Streptococci of which *Streptococcus salivarius* is a common member, and the nonhemolytic Streptococci are less prone to cause invasive infection. They do not produce infections with distinctive clinical features.

Clostridia

Anaerobic spore-forming bacilli belong to the genus *Clostridium*. Most species are strict anaerobes, with some so sensitive to oxygen that brief exposure of a culture to air is lethal; however, some will grow as microaerophiles. Most species are saprophytic, but toxigenic Clostridia produce serious human infections. Potent tissue destroying toxins and powerful endotoxins are the principal pathogenic agents formed by these bacilli. *Clostridium botulinum* forms the most potent bacterial toxin known; it is not, however, involved in infectious processes.

Clostridia are long, narrow, pleomorphic grampositive bacilli. Loss of the gram-positive staining reaction may occur after six to eight hours in culture or in tissue. Spores, although formed by all species, may require special conditions; in some important species (*i.e.*, *Clostridium perfringens*), spores are never formed in culture. Conversely, the relatively innocuus *Clostridium sporogenes* forms spores very readily. Organisms that cause tetanus and gas gangrene tend to remain relatively localized in the early stage of the infection; early extirpation of involved tissue is a necessary and effective form of treatment. Emergency excision or amputation may be necessary for the treatment of gas gangrene, but the disease can virtually always be avoided by careful initial wound management consisting of adequate debridement and intensive antibiotic therapy. Gas gangrene has become a rare entity. During the Korean War, estimates of total occurrence in American forces ranged from not more than 12 to as few as four.

Tetanus bacilli are ubiquitous, since they are commonly present in the feces of domestic animals. Tetanus is not an invasive infection and the organisms seldom extend far beyond the primary lesion. In culture the organism is a strict anaerobe. Its growth on most blood agar exhibits a characteristic thin film spreading over the surface. *Clostridium tetani* germinates only in tissue with very low oxygen tension. Thus spores may occasionally remain dormant in a healed wound for months, but later trauma with minute amounts of tissue necrosis can permit germination and elaboration of the toxin. Puncture wounds are especially dangerous when a minute foreign body is present. Two toxins, hemolysin and neurotoxin, are elaborated with the neurotoxin potency on the order of botulin toxin. The toxin has a strong affinity for neural tissue, and its main action is on the anterior horn cells of the spinal cord. Active immunization with tetanus toxoid prior to injury, is completely preventative in most patients. Re-injection with tetanus toxoid at the time of extensive wounding produces an anamnestic response in antibody titer in most patients and is mandatory in individuals whose last immunization was more than five years prior to injury.

The current recomendations for prophylaxis against tetanus by the Committee on Trauma, American College of Surgeons, are as follows. In previously immunized individuals who have received tetanus toxoid within six years of injury, 0.5 cc of fluid tetanus toxoid should be administered. If immunized more than six years prior to injury (including reinforcing dose) and the wound is tetanus prone, 250 units of tetanus human immune globulin should be administered in addition to a reinforcement injection of fluid toxoid. In those who have not been previously immunized and the wound is a clean, minor wound, primary immunization with 0.5 cc tetanus toxoid should be initiated. Previously unimmunized patients with other than clean, minor wounds should receive 0.5 cc fluid tetanus toxoid plus 250 units of human tetanus immune globulin with active immunization completed over the next three to six weeks. In wounds with an extensive area of devitalized tissue, in old or neglected wounds, 500 units of human tetanus immune globulin may be used.

Clostridial myositis or myonecrosis (gas gangrene) is a rapidly spreading infection usually originating in ischemic or traumatically devitalized muscle. The principal offending species include *Clostridium perfringens, Cl. novyi, Cl. septicum, Cl. histolyticum, Cl. tertium, Cl. bifermentans* and *Cl. sporogenes.*[45] Although the Clostridia are not highly invasive, their growth in damaged tissues may give rise to gas and by toxin action produce extensive destruction of muscle and connective tissue. Necrotizing, hemolytic, and lethal toxins are elaborated together with enzymes such as lecithinases, collagenases, proteinases, hyaluronidases, and deoxyribonucleases. The degradation products produced by these add further pathogenic potential to the Clostridia. Clostridia are divided into two major groups, the proteolytic and the saccharolytic. Proteolytic species, which include the most dangerous pathogenic forms, are most active in fermenting sugars. The splitting of lactose in milk produces the "stormy fermentation" which typifies *Clostridium perfringens*. Members of the proteolytic group, *e.g., Clostridium sporogenes,* liquefy coagulated serum and egg protein.

Clostridia cause several distinguishable infections including true gas gangrene, or Clostridial myonecrosis, a rapidly spreading infection of ischemic muscle, primarily caused by *Clostridium perfringens, Clostridium novyi,* and *Clostridium septicum.* Serotherapy with polyvalent antitoxins was historically recommended for the treatment of this entity, but extensive debridement, exteriorization, and delayed closure, plus protective action of sulfonamides, use of penicillin, the tetracyclines or erythromycin, is the treatment of choice. Treatment with hyperbaric oxygen as an adjunct to debridement has been reported as effective in arresting frank gas gangrene.

Anaerobic cellulitis is distinguished from myonecrosis by the fact that the offending organisms are less invasive and characteristically do not penetrate below the investing fascia unless the fascial barrier has been violated and there are subfascial areas of devitalized muscle. The causative organisms for anaerobic cellulitis are most often of the butyricium-tertium group. When *Clostridium sporogenes* or other proteolytic species are present, a putrefactive slough of the wound may occur. Various degrees of tissue involvement from simple wound contamination to extensive cellulitis can occur. Spread of anaerobes occurs in connective tissues deep in the wound. Gas may be present with either gas gangrene (myonecrosis) or cellulitis. Its presence is not, however, a reliable criterion for diagnosis of anaerobic infections since coliform bacilli, especially *E. coli* can also produce gas in devitalized tissue. Conversely, true Clostridial myonecrosis can exist without gas present in the involved tissues. Foreign bodies or sequestrae are a *sine qua non* for the establishment of Clostridial infection and adequate debridement and exteriorization of the wounds are the most important procedures to avoid this complication.

Acid-fast Bacilli

The principal infectious agent in this category is *Mycobacterium tuberculosis*. A significant number of cutaneous infections may be caused by other species, including *Mycobacterium balnei*. Mycobacteria are acid-fast bacilli varying in shape and texture. Granular or beaded forms occur as does branching. The characteristic cording growth in liquid medium typifies virulent strains. Mycobacteria contain a waxy substance in the cell wall which makes them resistant to many disinfecting agents. The lipid rich cell wall is responsible for the unique staining properties of this organism and also incites the tissue response which leads to an influx of monocytes, plugging of capillaries, and the necrosis which characterize acid-fast bacillus infections.

Three categories of Mycobacterium species have been classically recognized as pathogenic for man: *e.g.,* human, bovine, and avian. In the last decade a fourth species, *Mycobacterium balnei* has been shown to cause cutaneous infections when implanted in the skin by trauma.[31] Hand and arm infections have been traced to abrasians incurred in contaminated swimming pools. Most tubercular infections are of course caused by the human *Mycobacterium tuberculosis.*

Tuberculosis in the hand can occur in skin, tendon sheaths, bone, and joints. Tendon sheath infections are more common among people working with cattle, and suggest that the causative agent in bovine tuberculosis. When eradication of bovine tuberculosis is accomplished in the United States this preponderance may diminish.

Bone and joint tuberculosis is usually hematogenous in origin, from primary foci in either lung or the gastrointestinal tract. Such infection may occur without evidence of tuberculosis except for the secondary lesion. Single lesions in extremities are the usual form. Multiple lesions occur in about 15 per cent of cases. Joint tuberculosis may involve the periarticular soft tissue, the synovia, cartilage, bone, or all of these. Joint tuberculosis usually starts in the synovium at the point of its reflexion from the articular cartilage or the epiphyseal plate. Any person suspected of having tuberculosis infection of the hand should be screened thoroughly for other tuberculous foci including roentgenologic examination of the chest and bones, sputum cultures, and tuberculin (PPD) skin testing.

Since antibiotic-resistant strains of tubercle bacilli may appear during treatment, cultural monitoring of the lesion during treatment is indicated. Appearance of resistance may be delayed by the use of combined, concomitant therapy. The appearance of drug resistant mutants is thus prevented since variants simultaneously resistant to two or three antituberculous drugs are unlikely to appear.

Cultivation of *Mycobacterium tuberculosis* requires special media, and longer periods of incubation than other pathogenic bacteria. Coagulated egg media were long used, and Loewenstein-Jensen medium is still the basic substrate for the recovery of tubercle bacilli, but the Middlebrook 7H-10 agar substrate is now also widely used for the isolation and primary sensitivity testing.[54] Animal virulence testing utilizing the guinea pig is a classical procedure but this confirmatory reaction requires a lengthy test period and is uncommonly used today.

Bacillus Anthracis

Anthrax is still a significant disease in the population exposed to the organism, although modern agricultural practice has diminished its incidence. Since the organism is common on hair, hides, and feces of domestic animals, purulent lesions on individuals in contact with such materials may be caused by this organism. *Bacillus anthracis* is an aerobic spore-former and closely resembles *Bacillus cereus* which is commonly found in the soil. The latter is, however, nonpathogenic. The spores of the Bacillus species are highly resistant to disinfectants, drying, and moderate heat. The term "malignant pustule" correctly indicates the course of events in this cutaneous infection which begins as a small furuncle and advances rapidly to edema, inflammation, and multiple vesicles. The center of the lesion may become gangrenous forming a black eschar. Diagnosis may be made by the demonstration of capsulated gram-positive bacilli in the lesion. The bacillus is not culturally readily distinguished from nonpathogenic species but is rapidly lethal for mice with intraperitoneal injection of 0.01 ml of culture. The absence of motility, capsules in tissue, and marked susceptibility to penicillin are criteria which aid in its recognition. This disease may progress too rapidly to await cultural differentiation and presumptive identification should be followed by therapy with penicillin, the drug of choice.

Erysipilothrix Rhusiopathiae

This organism is a gram-positive, nonmotile microaerophilic bacillus, which tends to grow in long filaments and is the cause of human erysipeloid. This organism is closely related to *Listeria monocytogenes,* the latter being motile and beta-hemolytic while the nonmotile Erysipelothrix produces green hemolysis. The organism is pathogenic for many animals and birds. It infects man through minor abrasians following exposure to fish, shellfish, meat, or poultry.[87] The organism may be recovered from biopsy of the margin of the lesion. The infection remains localized to the skin, but bacteremia may develop and can be fatal. Recurrence or relapse of skin infection is common. Penicillin is effective in the treatment of this disease.

Corynebacterium Diphtheriae

Diphtheritic infection may appear in an open wound or can occur as a primary lesion in a minor puncture or laceration. Thus the hand is a likely site for such infection. Severe systemic manifestations may develop if the disease is not recognized and treated. Baceriologic diagnosis is by culture as is the case with pharyngeal diphtheria, Direct smear of diptheritic ulcers permits rapid presumptive diagnosis. During World War II biochemically distinctive strains of toxigenidiphtheria were recovered from ulcers on patients in the South Pacific. The existence of geographically localized variants must be borne in mind in the recognition of this infection.[16] The organism is a nonmotile, slender bacillus, growing with club-shaped swellings at the ends of the bacilli and densely staining metachromatic granules in the body of the cell.

Spirochaetes

The genera Treponemia, Borrelia, and Leptospira make up the family of Treponemas. Infections of the hand with these fastidious spiral-shaped organisms arise most often from human bites. Such infections are usually mixed with anaerobic and aerobic Streptococci. *Borrelia vincenti* is a spirochaete which is part of the normal flora of the mouth. It may appear in infected bites, together with the associated organism *Bacteriodes fusiformis*.

Gram-Negative bacteria

Enterobacteriaceae

This family includes the coliform or fecal flora with Klebsiella, Enterobacter, Serratia, Escherichia, Proteus, and Providence as the principal genera which may cause hand infections. Except for Klebsiella species which may be found in the throat as well as the colon, these bacteria are primarily intestinal in habitat.[18] They are prone to colonize and even invade in hand injuries in which the skin damage is extensive, *i.e.*, burns and avulsed wounds or multiple lacerations. In the typical sequence Staphylococci, Streptococci, and sometimes Corynebacteria are the first to colonize the injury, with coliform bacilli appearing in three to five days. (Klebsiella, Enterobacter and Escherichia species are the most commonly encountered forms.) Serratia species are less commonly encountered but may have greater invasive capability. Any member of the fecal flora may become the predominant flora of the wound especially in the immunologically deficient patient. Since 1967, an increasing incidence of Providencia species in wounds has been noted at this Institute. This genus, which is closely related to Proteus, had not previously been recovered from wounds. Proteus species may appear as soon as other fecal flora, but more typically enter the wound later. Of the four species of Proteus, *Proteus mirabilis* is the most commonly encountered.

Pseudomonas aeruginosa is a member of the group of oxidative bacteria, as opposed to the anaerobic fermentative enteric group of bacilli. *Pseudomonas aeruginosa* can be a major invasive organism in wounds in debilitated patients with such diseases as lymphoma, leukemia, and burns. Bacteremia can follow invasive infection in a relatively localized site such as the hand (Fig. 14.1.5), although in burn patients the entire burn wound is commonly infected. Septicemia from *Pseudomonas aeruginosa* often follows bacteremia from the Staphylococci or any of the common coliform bacilli in patients with polymicrobial wound flora. The clinical features of Pseudomonas septicemia include shock, leukopenia, hypothermia, and at times a characteristic skin lesion, ecthyma gangrenosum, a necrotizing hemorrhagic nodule which exhibits perivascular bacterial cuffing and consequent thrombosis.[55]

Organisms of the closely related genera, Mima and Herellea, are common inhabitants of the skin of the genitourinary area and may also be present on the oropharyngeal mucosa. They are also oxidative organisms, with limited biochemical activity. They are found on wounds soon after injury and may disappear within a few days or on occasion proliferate to penetrate the superficial tissues layers and cause infection. On rare occasions they have been the cause of generalized septicemia.[63] The bacteremia of gram negative bacilli is usually difficult to eradicate. Pseudomonas and Providencia bacteremias have been associated with an extremely high mortality. Antibiotic resistance of these organisms has, in recent years, also become extremely high. Resistance transfer factors offer a mechanism by which the population of resistant forms, in an environment in which antibiotics are being intensively used, is continuously enhanced. The only remedy thus far suggested for this situation is the restriction of use of certain antibiotics, so that in a given hospital environment, they will not be continuously active in the selection of resistant strains. Such intermittent proscription has been reported to result in the re-emergence of susceptible strains and thus restoration of the usefullness of an otherwise ineffective antibiotic.

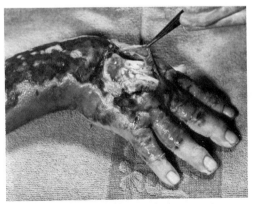

Figure 14.1.5. Subeschar abscess from which *Pseudomonas aeruginosa* was cultured, involving extensor tendons of right hand. Note black discoloration of eschar indicative of bacterial invasion.

Pasteurella Tularensis

This organism derived its name from Tulare County California, where it was discovered as a parasite in ground squirrels. It is a small gram-negative, non-motile aerobic bacillus which grows readily in routine culture media. It occurs in endemic fashion in small game, especially rabbits and squirrels, and in some game birds, so the infection is most often seen in hunters. Ticks and deer flies can carry the organism and transmit it by biting and it can also be acquired from the tissues of an infected animal. The lesion is initially a red, papular granuloma with surrounding inflammation. It develops a necrotic ulcer with raised borders. Diagnosis should be established by culture prior to starting treatment. The organism is hazardous to laboratory personnel.

Glanders is caused by *Malleomyces mallei,* a small nonmotile gram-negative bacillus often growing in filamentous form. It may be more properly classified as *Actinobacillus mallei,* primarily found in Asia but occurring rarely in the Western hemisphere. It is contracted through abrasions in the skin and may invade intact skin as well. Human infections most often occur in those handling horses or sheep. The guinea pig is useful in the diagnosis, since a characteristic ulcerating abscess develops with subcutaneous injection with resultant ulceration of the tunica vaginalis (Strauss reaction). This organism is hazardous in the laboratory and several laboratory infections have occurred. Although the infection is one in which the skin of the hand is a portal of entry, the disease is systemic.[32]

Brucella

Three species of Brucella, *Brucella abortus, Brucella melitensis,* and *Brucella suis* occur. This small nonmotile gram-negative coccobacillus is aerobic but difficult to cultivate. The natural reservoir of this organism is cattle, goats, and swine. Although infection usually occurs by ingestion of milk from an infected animal, the organism can penetrate the skin and contact with an infected animal may establish a hand infection. The lesion is a granuloma and rapid spread occurs via lymphatics. Regional lymph nodes are promptly involved in skin infections and the organism is not often recovered from the lesion unless it is suspected early. Serologic procedures are basic to the diagnosis and blood cultures the most frequent source of isolates.

Neisseriae

The Neisseriae are gram-negative diplococci. Neisseria meningitidis is an anaerobic organism which produces potent endotoxins. The usually portal of entry in man is the nasopharynx. Clinical infection has produced the Shawartzman phenomenon as evidence by cutaneous purpura (purpura fulminans) (Fig. 14.1.6), renal lesions, and the Waterhouse-Friderichsen syndrome with or without gross hemorrhage in the adrenal gland. Meningococci may be isolated from cutaneous purpuric lesions with wound

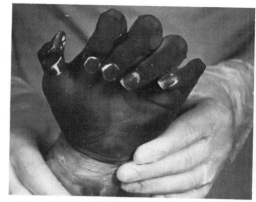

Figure 14.1.6. "Dry" gangrenous change in hand of patient with meningiococcemia and purpura fulminans. Amputation was required after patients general condition stabilized.

biopsy. The sulfonamides and penicillins are effective in treatment.

Viral Infections

Cat-Scratch Fever

This is a viral disease of the lymphogranuloma venereum (LGV) group. The primary lesion may be cutaneous and resembles a small pustule or furuncle with edema at the primary site and in regional lymph nodes. The infection is relatively benign and is manifested by fever and malaise. It is transmitted by bite or scratch from a feline carrier.

Herpes Simplex

An infection of the finger can occur with *Herpesvirus hominis,* manifested by a deep vesicle on a digit giving rise to other vesicles and superficial tissue destruction. When secondary infection with Staphylococcus occurs, it may obscure the primary lesion. Incision of herpetic lesions yield no purulence and ultimately tissue necrosis may occur with resultant tissue loss. The presence of herpetic vesicles is the important diagnostic criterion (Fig. 14.1.7). The infection occurs in personnel giving mouth or dental care to patients. The diagnosis may be made by identification of typical Cowdry type A intranuclear inclusion bodies in biopsy material.

Fungi

Trichophyton, Microsporum, Epidermophyton

Species of these dermatophytes may colonize a hand lesion especially a paronychia. Such infections may harbor bacteria as well and these contaminants must be differentiated. Direct examination of tissue or nail scrappings in potassium hydroxide and serial culture of scrappings are indicated to confirm or exclude the diagnosis of fungus infection in the hand. *Candida albicans* and other Candida species can also infect the ail bed causing paronychia and nail infections. Culture and direct microscopy identify yeast infections as well.

Sporotrichum Schenckii (Sporotrichosis)

This soil-inhabiting species is capable of invading the tissue through skin injuries and occurs in agriculture workers and gardeners. A primary lesion on the hand or wrist appears as an ulcer or abscess. A line of

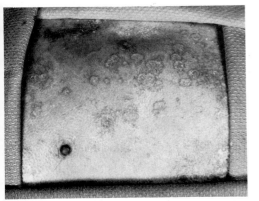

Figure 14.1.7. Herpesvirus hominus infection in healing partial thickness burn wound. Ruptured vesicles are rapidly secondarily colonized by bacteria and biopsy was necessary to establish viral etiology.

elevated subcutaneous nodules extends proximally from the initial lesion. Cultural confirmation of this infection is best accomplished by biopsy and culture on Sabouraud's agar. The organism grows readily. Direct microscopic examination of the lesion may reveal the organism in polymorphonuclear leucocytes.

North American Blastomycosis

This disease is caused by *Blastomyces dermatides* and is characterized by cutaneous lesions of the feet, hands, and extremities and by pulmonary involvement. It is most common in the southwestern United States and the Mississippi Valley. The skin lesions resemble tuberculous ulcers or epidermoid carcinoma. Blastomycin skin test antigen and complement fixation tests are the principal diagnostic tools. Biopsy of surface lesions with histology and culture, direct examination, and culture of purulence are additional techniques to aid in diagnosis. The organism is readily cultured when viable cells are present.

Actinomycosis

This is caused by *Actinomyces israelii*, an anaerobic, grampositive, nonacid-fast organism. The ray-like fungi can be seen in direct microscopic examination when the typical "sulfur granules" of the lesion are crushed (Fig. 14.1.8). The organism is difficult to grow in culture. It is found as a saprophyte in tonsillar crypts, tooth cavities, and under the gums. It occurs in nature on grains and grasses. The hand may

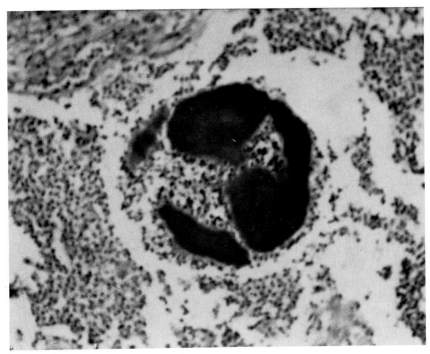

Figure 14.1.8. Basophillic colony of Actinomycetes surrounded by neutrophils, a typical "sulfur granule" noted on microscopic examination of resected tissue.

become infected from human bites or mouth contact. A similar organism, *Actinomyces bovis,* causes lumpy jaw in cattle but rarely invades humans. Actinomycosis produces a granuloma with destruction of tissue, extensive suppuration, and hypertrophy of fibrous connective tissue. The skin and subcutaneous tissue becomes swollen, hard or "woody," and dusky red. Eventually sinuses, which bleed easily, are formed.

Nocardia

Three species of *Nocardia asteroides, Nocardia madurae,* and *Nocardia mexicana* cause nocardiosis. This genus is closely related to Actinomyces. The organism occurs in soil and can enter the hand through an injury. The disease produces swelling, necrosis to include destruction of bone, and suppurating fistulas. "Sulfur granules" may be found in purulence on direct examination. The organism is usually acid-fast which aids in distinguishing it from Actinomyces. It is easier to grow than Actinomyces and positive cultures suggest the diagnosis of Nocardiosis.

Coccidioides Immitis

Coccidioidomycosis is typically a pulmonary disease resulting from the inhalation of the causative agen *Coccidioides immitis* in its endemic area. It was originally recognized in the arid area of southern California, but extends over much of the Southwest. The hand may, rarely, be infected through a break in the skin. The cutaneous manifestations of erythema nodosum may be accompanied by invasion of the small bones of the hand. The organism is dimorphic with a yeast and a mycelial phase. It is readily cultivated and merits caution in its handling since it is readily released from mycelia in culture. Diagnostic procedures include precipitin and skin test with coccidiodin. These reactions may be negative in mild infections.

Phycomycosis, Aspergillosis and Other Saprophytic Fungal Infections

The presence of severe dermal injury as in a partial or full thickness burn may pave the way for an extremely destructive lesion in the hand.[21] The burned tissue is frequently colonized by various saprophytes without invasion. However, for an unknown reason, an occasional patient will become infected with one of these fungi. The nonseptate, broad-hyphae fungi of the Phycomycetales, including Mucor, Rhizopus, Absides, and Basidiophilus are most prone to produce deep invasion of viable tissue, (Fig. 14.1.9 *A* to *D*), but Aspergillus, Fusarium and other saprophytes have been recovered also.[60] The infection proceeds with rapidity and may require excision or ablation to the level of viable tissue. Diagnosis is confirmed by quick section and stain of biopsy specimens since the rate of progression precludes a useful result from culture

(Table 14.1.2). Culture and definitive identification are indicated to document the precise etiologic agent.

Pneumocystis Carinii

This is an opportunitic protozoan which may cause pulmonary infections in debilitated patients who are immunologically deficient. Unexplained fever, with or without roentgenologic changes compatible with pneumonitis, especially in children with malignant disease receiving immunosuppression, should alert one to Pneumocystis pneumonia. Pentamidine, isethionate, a diamide active against protozoans with high rates of aerobic glycolysis, in dosage of 4 to 5 mg/kg of body weight per day, for 10 to 14 days, given intravenously or intramuscularly, has been reported effective in the treatment of this disease.[33] Side effects of this agent include transient hypotension following rapid intravenous administration, gastrointestinal irritation, hypoglycemia and hyperglycemia, and reversible nephrotoxicity.

THE PENICILLINS

Penicillin was the first antibiotic used in the treatment of clinical sepsis, and is today the most widely used antibiotic. Both natural and semisynthetic congeners of penicillin, including phenoxymethyl penicillin, phenethicillin, methicillin, oxacillin, cloxacillin, dicloxacillin, nacillin, ampicillin, and carbenicillin disodium, have been used and found to be effective against bacterial infections (Table 14.1.3).

Penicillin is produced by several fungi and is composed of interconnected beta-lactam and thiazolidine rings with a side chain which, when altered, changes the antibacterial properties of the drug. The penicillins are bactericidal and apparently act by interfering with the synthesis of the cell wall muramic acid peptide of growing bacteria.[65] This disturbance of cell wall metabolism renders such bacteria susceptible to osmotic injury with alteration of cell wall permeability persisting for several hours after removal of the penicillin.

The gastrointestinal absorption of orally administered penicillin varies with the congener given. The greatest part of an oral dose of penicillin G is inactivated by gastric juice or intestinal bacteria with only approximately one-third of the administered dose absorbed.[48] Absorption of penicillin after parenteral injection is quite rapid but the drug is excreted rapidly by the kidney and only minimal blood levels remain four hours after injection. The procaine and benzathine forms of penicillin G are more slowly absorbed and produce lower but more persistent blood levels, *i.e.,* two to five days. Probenecid may be administered concurrently to decrease the tubular secretion of penicillin, delaying its excretion and increasing its serum concentration.[23] Following administration of penicillin, its serum concentration exceeds that in the

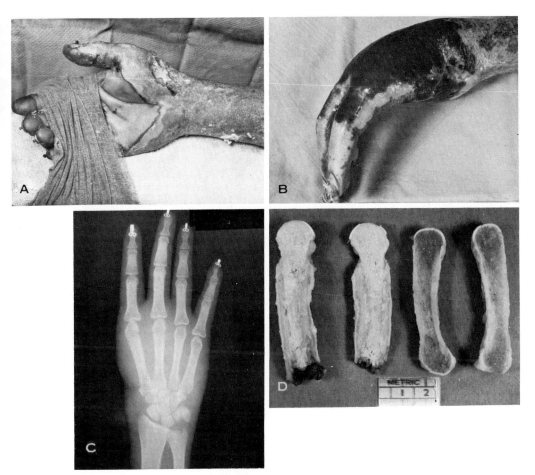

Figure 14.1.9 A. Indolent traumatic wound in patient with burns of upper limb. Persistent drainage from base of wound prompted biopsy which revealed mucor osteomyelitis necessitating amputation of thumb and first metacarpal. (Reproduced from Archives of Surgery, Vol. 102, May 1971.)

Figure 14.1.9 B. Persistent painful swelling of hand following amputation of thumb and first metacarpal suggested excision had been inadequate and that further fungal invasion had occurred.

Figure 14.1.9 C. Roentgenographic findings in first and second metacarpal bones of invasive Mucor. Note changes in marrow cavity and periosteal thickening. (Reproduced from Archives of Surgery, Vol. 102, May 1971.)

Figure 14.1.9 D. Sagittal section of metacarpal bones (shown in Figure 14.1.9 C) invaded by Mucor species. Note the replacement of marrow cavity by fungal hyphae.

tissues, but this agent does diffuse into most body tissues and fluids, including joint fluid when administered systemically. Since only the free antibiotic is active and all penicillins are bound to albumin, dosage should be adjusted to account for the congener-dependent protein binding which is greatest for cloxacillin and dicloxacillin and least for ampicillin and methicillin.[39]

Penicillins are effective against streptococci of groups A, C, G, H, L, and M, a variable but progressively smaller number of staphylococci, most gonococci and meningococci, virtually all pneumonococci, the majority of Corynebacterium diphtheriae and Bacillus anthracis, Pasteurella multocida, Streptobacillus moniliformis, Clostridia spp, Actinomyces bovis, Listeria monocytogenes and Treponema pallidum. They are ineffective against viruses, Rickettsieae, fungi, plasmodia, amoebae, and penicillinase producing staphylococci. Toxic reactions to penicillin are relatively rare and include hypersensitivity reactions (skin rash, fever, the Arthus phenomenon, serum sickness, and anaphylactoid

TABLE 14.1.2

Occurrence of fungi and yeasts in tissues of burn patients at U. S. Army Institute of Surgical Research in 1969

Genus	Number of Clinical Biopsies Positive	Number of Autopsy Specimens Positive
Candida	114	166
Geotrichum	63	75
Mucor	0	4
Aspergillus	12	4
Cephalosporium	7	7
Helminthosporium	3	2
Microsporum	1	1
Fusarium	5	1
Trichophyton	6	2
Penicillium	15	7
Rhodotorula	7	0
Rhizopus	7	0
Paecillomyces	1	0
Fonsecaea	0	8
Sporotrichum	0	1
Cladosporium	0	1
Trichothecium	1	0
Trichosporium	1	0
Fungi impertecti *	4	3
Total patients cultured	145	59
Total tissue samples	369	361
Total isolates	247	282

Fungi with hyphae resembling those of Phycomycetaceae but without fruiting bodies

shock), pain, sterile abscess formation, gastrointestinal irritation, phlebitis, CNS irritation with seizures[40] (most common in children receiving high doses), and alteration of the host bacterial flora with superinfection.

Penicillin G is available for administration orally and by all parenteral routes. Dosage is determined by the severity of the infection and the sensitivity of the causative organism, ranging from 200,000 units orally twice a day for Beta hemolytic streptococcus prophylaxis to several million units per day intravenously for bacterial endocarditis.

Phenoxymethyl penicillin and phenethicillin are more stable in an acid medium than penicillin G and are consequently better absorbed from the gastrointestinal tract. These congeners have virtually the same spectrum of action as penicillin G and are administered only orally.

SEMISYNTHETIC PENICILLINS[37]

Methicillin is a semisynthetic penicillin which is resistant to penicillinase cleavage and is administered only parenterally. This bactericidal agent is particularly useful in the treatment of infections caused by penicillinase-producing staphylococci,[26] but methicillin-resistant *Staphylococcus aureus* are frequently identified in hospital patients at the present time.[43] Methicillin is rapidly absorbed from an intramuscular site and rapidly excreted in the urine. The instability of this agent when in solution, its rapid excretion, and the fact that it should not be mixed with other antibiotics limits its intravenous usefulness. The pain associated with intramuscular injection is also limiting, since administration of 1 to 2 gm every two to four hours is required to maintain effective blood levels.

Oxacillin is resistant both to acid hydrolysis and penicillinase,[26] and may be given either orally or parenterally. Gastrointestinal absorption of this agent is rapid, as is its renal excretion, necessitating administration every four hours. Plasma protein binding of oxacillin is extensive but because of its greater effectiveness against penicillinase-producing staphylococci, the minimal inhibitory concentration of oxacillin is lower than that of methicillin and the necessary dosage of injectable sodium oxacillin is lower than that of methicillin. The recommended dosage of injectible sodium oxacillin is 1 gm or more every four to six hours for the adult and 100 mg/kg/day for children in divided doses. Less severe infections amenable to oral therapy can be treated with 500 mg every four to six hours for the adult, and 50 mg/kg/day for children in four divided doses.

Cloxacillin and *dicloxacillin* are acid-stable, penicillinase-resistant congeners of oxacillin. These agents are effective against organisms susceptible to penicillin G, and except for penicillinase-producing staphylococci, against which they are active, they are inactive against organisms insensitive to penicillin. Both agents are administered orally and are well absorbed from the gastrointestinal tract with detectable levels present in the plasma for up to six hours after administration of a single dose. The usual dosage of cloxacillin for adults is 250 to 500 mg every six hours, and 50 mg/kg/day in divided doses every six hours for children. The usual dosage of dicloxacillin is 250 mg or more every six hours for adults, and 25 mg/kg/day in divided doses every six hours for children.

Nafcillin is a semisynthetic penicillin, particularly resistant to penicillinase, available for both oral and parenteral administration.[36] This agent is subject to acid hydrolysis, making its enteric absorption unpredictable. Nafcillin diffuses into virtually all tissues and is primarily excreted in the bile, in which its concentration commonly exceeds that of the plasma. The route of administration is in part determined by the severity of the infection with 0.5 to 1.0 gm administered every four hours intravenously for the treatment of life threatening infections. The intramuscular dosage is 500 mg every four to six hours for adults, and 25 mg/kg twice daily for infants and children. Recommended oral dosage is 0.25 to 1.0 gm every four to six hours for adults, and 25-50 mg/kg/day in four divided doses for children.

Ampicillin, which is effective against both gram-positive and gram-negative organisms, has a broader spectrum of antibacterial action than the other semisythetic penicillins. This bactericidal agent which is stable in an acidic medium and well absorbed from the gastrointestinal tract is more slowly absorbed from muscle than the other penicillins. Ampicillin is rapidly excreted by the kidney, but is also concentrated and excreted in the bile.[15] This agent is available for both oral and parenteral use and has particular effectiveness against *Hemophilus influenzae* and *Streptococcus viridans*. Many strains of *Escherichia coli, Proteus mirabilis, Shigella,* and *Salmonella* are sensitive to this agent,[78] but a progressively greater number of resistant strains of these organisms has appeared with use of the agent. The amount administered is dependent upon the severity of the infection with dosage ranging from 2 to 8 gm per day in divided doses given every six hours for adults and from 50 to 200 mg/kg/day in divided doses for children.

Carbenicillin disodium is particularly effective against *Pseudomonas aeruginosa*[11] and some strains

TABLE 14.1.3
The penicillins

Agent	Mode of Action	Antibacterial Spectrum of Clinical Importance	Distribution	Excretion (Principal Route)	Routes of Administration
cillin G ium salt avail-e for patients h renal failure)	Bactericidal; interferes with bacterial cell wall synthesis	Streptococci, Pneumococci Clostridia, Neisseriae, Corynebacteria, *Pasteurella* Actinomyces, Treponema, Listeria	All body fluids, but little in CSF and anterior chamber of eye. 65% protein bound	Renal, delayed by probenacid	Oral and all parenteral
noxymethyl cillin ethicillin	Bactericidal; same as above.	Same as above	Same as above. 75% protein bound	Renal, same as above.	Oral
nicillin	Bactericidal; interferes with bacterial cell wall synthesis	Penicillinase producing Staphylococci	Same as above. 38% protein bound	*Renal* and hepatic	Intravenous and intramuscular
cillin	Bactericidal; same as above.	Penicillinase producing Staphylococci	Same as above. 80% protein bound	*Renal* and hepatic	Oral and parenteral
xacillin oxacillin	Bactericidal; same as above.	Penicillinase producing Staphylococci	Same as above. 95% protein bound	*Renal* and hepatic	Oral
cillin	Bactericidal; same as above.	Penicillinase producing Staphylococci useful against Methicillin-resistant Staphylococci	Same as above. 70% protein bound	*Hepatic* and renal	Oral and parenteral
picillin	Bactericidal; same as above.	*Hemophilus influenzae, Proteus mirabilis,* Salmonallae, Shigellae and some *E. Coli* Gram-positive same as with Penicillin G	Same as above. 25% protein bound	*Renal* and hepatic	Oral and parenteral
penicillin odium	Bactericidal; same as above.	*Pseudomonas aeruginosa,* Indole-producing Proteus	Same as above. 50% protein bound	*Renal* and hepatic	Parenteral

TABLE 14.1.3 — *continued*

			Side Effects			
Hypertensitivity	Nephrotoxicity	Ototoxicity	CNS toxicity	Gastrointestinal	Hematologic	Hostbiologic alterations
Atopy anaphylactoid reactions. "Autoimmune manifestations".			Convulsions with very high doses	Nausea and vomiting.		Jarisch-Herxheimer reaction in syphilitics. Superinfection uncommon
Same as above				Same as above		Same as above
Same as above					Bone marrow depression	Pain and abscess at injection site
Same as above				Nausea and vomiting with oral use		Same as above
Same as above				Same as above		
Same as above				Same as above		
Same as above			Convulsions with high doses	Same as above	Agranulocytosis and bone marrow histiocytosis	Superinfection
Same as above			Convulsions with high doses		Hemorrhagic Diathesis	Superinfection

of *Proteus* species, and shows some effectiveness against meningococci, pneumonococci, gonococci, group A streptococci, *Streptococcus viridans, Escherichia coli, Serratia, Aerobacter,* and *Salmonella* as well. This agent shows intermediate binding to plasma proteins and is rapidly and almost completely excreted in the urine.[80] Carbenicillin is not absorbed from the gastrointestinal tract and must therefore be given parenterally in doses ranging from 100-300 mg/kg/day for adults, and up to 400 mg/kg /day for children, as required by the severity of the infection and sensitivity of the causative organisms (doses of up to 30 gm per day have been administered to some patients). The frequently rapid emergence of carbenicillin-resistant *Pseudomonas* organisms[76] has been reported to be delayed by the concurrent administration of gentamicin.

ERYTHROMYCIN

Erythromycin is a metabolic product of *Streptomyces erythrus,* which is both bacteriostatic and bactericidal[27] (Table 14.1.4), as determined by the concentration of the drug and the microorganisms concerned. This agent is active against *Staphylococcus aureus,* Pneumococci, group A Streptococci, *Neisseria,* Enterococci, *Brucella, Pasteurella multocida, Rickettsiae, Treponema pallidum,* and Listeria. Erythromycin acts by inhibition of protein synthesis, and is apparently bound to the 50 S ribosomes of sensitive organisms with considerably greater binding occurring in gram-positive bacteria than in gram-negative bacteria.[92] The inactivation of erythromycin base by gastric juice can be avoided by use of enteric coated oral preparations or administration of the stearate form of the drug. Absorption of erythromycin takes place in the upper part of the small intestine, and is not imparied by the presence of food within the bowel when the estolate is given.[29] Erythromycin is distributed throughout total body water and higher concentrations are measurable in the tissues than in the blood. The active form of the antibiotic is excreted in the bile following concentration in the liver with only a small amount of the active antibiotic excreted in the urine.

The side effects of this agent include hypersensitivity reactions (fever, eosinophilia, and skin rashes), gastrointestinal irritation, and superinfection, particularly that due to Candida. No dosage reduction is necessary in patients with renal failure, since little of the drug is excreted by the kidney.

Erythromycin is effective in the treatment of a variety of bacterial infections, including those caused by *Staphylococcus aureus.*[28] However, staphylococcal resistance to this agent has increased significantly since its initial clinical use. The antibiotic is available in both oral and parenteral dosage forms with the usual oral dose for adults 1 to 4 gm per day in divided doses, given every six hours with dosage proportionately reduced for children, depending upon their weight. Intravenous administration is usually in the form of 1 gm every six hours until clinical symptoms relent.

LINCOMYCIN

Lincomycin (Table 14.1.4) and its congener, clindamycin, are antibiotics produced by *Streptomyces*

TABLE 14.1.4
Miscellaneous antibiotics

Agent	Mode of Action	Antibacterial Spectrum of Clinical Importance	Distribution	Excretion (Principal Route)	Route of Administration
ramphenicol	Bacteriostatic; inhibits protein synthesis	*Klebsiella pneumoniae, Aerobacter aerogenes, Bordetella pertussis, Escherichia coli,* Salmonella, Pasturella Brucella and some Rickettsiae	Body fluids, 50% protein bound	*Renal* and hepatic	Oral and parenteral
aromycin	Bacteriostatic and bactericidal: inhibits protein synthesis	*Staphylococcus aureus,* Pneumococci, Enterococci, Neisseria, *Treponema pallidum, Pasteurella multocida* and Streptococci, *Hemophilus pertussis*	All body fluids	Hepatic	Oral and parenteral
comycin	Bactericidal: inhibits bacterial cell wall synthesis	*Staphylococcus aureus, Corynebacterium diphtheria,* Streptococci, *Neisseria gonorrhea and Clostridia.*	Body fluids except spinal fluid 10% protein bound	Renal	Intravenous
omycin	Bactericial and bacteriostatic: inhibits protein synthesis	*Staphylococcus aureus,* Streptococci and Pneumococci	Total body water	Hepatic	Oral and parenteral
halosporins phalothin and phaloridine)	Bactericidal: interferes with bacterial cell wall synthesis	*Staphylococcus aureus,* Streptococci, Pneumococci, Clostridia, *E. coli,* Klebsiella, *Proteus mirabilis* and *Hemophilus influenza*	Water, low concentration in CSF. 50% protein bound	Renal	Parenteral
tracin	Bactericidal: inhibits cell wall synthesis	Stphyloccus, Streptococcus and Neisseriae	extracellular fluid	Renal	Topical and Intramuscular
stimethate	Bactericidal: alters cytoplasmic membrane allowing leakage of nucleosides	Pseudomonas, *E. coli, Aerobacter aerogenes, Klebsiella pneumoniae* and *Hemophilus influenza*	Body fluids	Renal	Oral and parenteral
mixin B	Bactericidal: alters bacterial lipoprotein membrane permeability	Pseudomonas, Shigella, Vibrio, Aerobacter, *E. coli,* Hemophilus Klebsiella, Salmonella and Shigella	Body fluids	Renal	Oral and parenteral

TABLE 14.1.4 — *Continued*

			Side Effects			
Hypertensitivity	Nephrotoxicity	Ototoxicity	CNS toxicity	Gastrointestinal	Hematologic	Hostbiologic alterations
Atopy				Nausea and vomiting	Bone marrow depression and aplastic anemia	Superinfection and gray syndrome in in neonates
Mild eosino- philia, atopy & fever				Cholestatic hepatitis		Superinfection especially by Candida
Atopy and anaphylactoid reactions	Azotemia	Auditory with blood level greater than 60 ug/ml		Nausea and vomiting		Superinfection
Atopy, serum sickness, and anaphylaxis		Vestibular		Diarrhea, naus- ea, and vomiting	Neutropenic, agranulocyto- sis thrombo- cytopenia	Superinfection
Atopy and anaphylaxis					Hemolytic anemia and neutropenia	Superinfection
Atopy	Preteinuria, hematuria, and azotemia			Nausea and vomiting		
Atopy	Azotemia, pro- teinuria, and hematuria	Vestibular				Superinfections
Atopy	Azotemia, pro- teinuria, and hematuria	Vestibular		Nausea and vomiting		Superinfections

lincolnensis, which bind to the 50 S ribosomes of bacteria and inhibit peptide bond synthesis.[92] These agents are both bacteriostatic and bactericidal, depending upon the drug concentration and the bacteria concerned. Clindamycin is more rapidly and completely absorbed from the gastrointestinal tract than is Lincomycin, and both are distributed in total body water appearing in virtually all tissues. The biologic half-life of clindamycin is shorter than that of lincomycin, which is in the neighborhood of six hours.[49] Both agents are excreted in the urine to only small extent and appear to be excreted in active form in the bile with hepatic dysfunction markedly prolonging their biologic half-life.

These agents are available for both oral and parenteral administration with the dosage employed depending upon the severity of the infection and the age of the patient. Lincomycin is reported to be effective in the treatment of infections, especially chronic osteomyelitis, due to *Staphylococcus aureus,* Streptococci and Pneumococci. Toxic effects of these agents include skin rashes, gastrointestinal irritation, leukopenia, neutropenia, thrombocytopenia, serum sickness, anaphylaxis, photosensitivity, and overgrowth of yeast in the gastrointestinal tract.

CHLORAMPHENICOL

Chloramphenicol, a derivative of dichloroacetic acid, containing a nitrobenzene moiety, is produced by the fungus *Streptomyces venzuelae.* Although this antibiotic is bactericidal to certain bacteria, it is principally bacteriostatic and is active against *Klebsiella pneumoniae, Aerobacter aerogenes, Bordetella pertusis, Escherichia coli, Hemophilus influenzae, Actinobacillus, Bacteroides, Salmonella typhosa, Pasteurella, Brucella, Shigella, Vibrio comma, Neisseria, Clostridia, Leptospira bartinella, Listeria, Corynebacterium diphtheriae, Bacillus anthracis,* and *Actinomyces.* This agent also has some rickettsia static properties and has been reported to be effective against the same nonbacterial diseases as the tetracyclines.

Chloramphenicol, (Table 14.1.4) which is both heat and pH stable, is available in both oral and parenteral dosage form. This agent exerts its antibacterial effect by inhibition of protein synthesis, interfering with the binding of messenger RNA to ribosomes.[7] The agent is rapidly absorbed from the gastrointestinal tract, has a biologic half-life of up to three and one-half hours, and approximately half of the drug is bound to plasma proteins. Chloramphenicol is conjugated in the liver and is rapidly excreted in the urine by both glomerular filtration and tubular secretions.

The side effects of chloramphenicol include hypersensitivity reactions, ranging from skin rashes and fever to profound bone marrow depression. Marrow depression, the most important side effect of this agent,[17] is initially manifested by leukopenia and thrombocytopenia, but may progress to pancytopenia, which has been associated with a high mortality. This toxic effect has generally occurred in patients receiving prolonged administration of chloramphenicol or repeated exposure to this drug, facts which necessitate frequent peripheral blood counts in patients receiving this drug. The most frequent manifestation of chloramphenicol's bone marrow depression is anemia, which appears to be dose related, but only rarely associated with the pancytopenia noted above. Patients receiving chloramphenicol who have coexisting hepatic dysfunction are more likely to manifest this anemia. Fatal chloramphenicol toxicity has been reported in neonates receiving this agent, and has been related to the hepatic and renal immaturity of such patients. Other toxic effects of the drug include optic neuritis, paresthesias, and chromosomal injury. Because of the severity of the toxic effects of chloramphenicol, the duration of treatment should be as brief as possible and it should be used only for the treatment of infections caused by organisms against which it is demonstratedly the most effective agent. Chloramphenicol therapy should be carried out only on patients in the hospital, should be stopped at the first sign of bone marrow depression, and should be avoided in patients who have previously received chloramphenicol.

Chloramphenicol is the agent of choice in the treatment of all three forms of typhus and Rocky Mountain spotted fever, with an initial dose of 50 mg/kg followed by 1 gm every eight hours in adults, and 75 mg/kg given in divided dosage every six to eight hours for children. Treatment should be continued until the patient has been afebrile for one to two days. Chloramphenicol is also the drug of choice in the treatment of typhoid fever, with doses of 1 gm every six hours continued for four weeks. Chloramphenicol is also effective in the treatment of psittacosis, granuloma inguinale, lymphogranuloma venereum, Brucellosis, atypical pneumonia and Klebsiela pneumoniae infections, but other antibiotics are preferred.

THE TETRACYCLINES

The tetracyclines (Table 14.1.5), which are produced by several species of Streptomycetes, are closely related naphthacenecarboxmide derivatives. Although these drugs may be bactericidal in sufficient concentration, the blood levels usually achieved in clinical practice exert only a bacteriostatic effect against rapidly multiplying organisms. The bacteria against which the tetracyclines are active include the Clostridia, *Diplococcus pneumoniae,* group A Streptococci, *Salmonellae, Escherichia coli, Klebsiella pneumoniae, Pasteurella tularensis, Borrelia* sp., and *Leptospira icterohaemorrhagiae.* The tetracyclines are also effective in the treatment of some rickettsial diseases, such as Rocky Mountain spotted fever, Q fever, rickettsial pox, and all forms of typhus, are inactive against yeast, fungi, and viruses, but have been reported to be effective in the treatment of lymphogranuloma venereum, psittacosis, and primary atypical pneumonia.[58]

The mechanism of action of these agents is incompletely defined, but is most likely due to specific binding of 30 S ribosomes, interfering with aminoacyl T-RNA metabolism.[92] The absorption of these agents, which occurs primarily in the upper gastrointestinal tract, is enhanced by fasting with effective levels maintained for six hours or longer following oral administration. The tetracyclines are distributed throughout total body water with plasma protein binding dependent upon the congener administered, ranging from 20 per cent oxytetracycline to 75 per cent for minocycline.[40] The excretion of the tetracyclines occurs mainly through the kidney but these agents are also excreted in the bile with hepatic concentration resulting in biliary levels several fold those in the plasma. Moreover, in the case of minocycline average tissue levels commonly exceed average serum levels.

Side effects of these agents include hypersensitivity reactions ranging from morbilliform rashes to exfoliative dermatitis and anaphylactoid reactions, gastrointestinal irritation, thrombophlebitis, leukocytosis, thrombocytopenic purpura, and phototoxicity. Acute hepatic necrosis (a particular threat to pregnant women), coagulopathies, brown discoloration of the teeth, and superinfections due to resistant yeast, fungi, or bacteria are also reported to occur. Staphylococcal enterocolitis is perhaps the most frequently encountered manifestation of bacterial overgrowth in surgical patients treated with tetracyclines. Smaller and less frequent doses of tetracyclines are indicated in patients with renal failure, since these agents have been reported to accentuate azotemia, hyperphosphotemia, acidosis, weight loss, nausea, and vomiting in such patients.

In the treatment of bacterial infections, the tetracyclines may be used either orally or intravenously, depending upon the severity of the disease, in a dosage of 2 gm per day for from one to six weeks, depending upon the disease. These antibiotics have been the most universally effective agents in the treatment of acute systemic melioidosis.[19] Intravenous dosage of 2 gm per day for the first seven days is followed by maintenance oral therapy of 2 gm per day for a total 30-day treatment period. As noted above treatment with tetracyclines has been reported to be effective in the treatment of *Mycoplasma pneumoniae* infections. In the treatment of rickettsial diseases, 2 to 3 gm of tetracycline for the initial 24 hours should be followed by

TABLE 14.1.5
The tetracyclines

Agent	Mode of Action	Antibacterial Spectrum of Clinical Importance	Distribution	Excretion (Principal Route)	Routes of Administratio
Chlortetracycline	Bacteriostatic: interference with bacterial ribosome metabolism	Clostridia, Pneumococci, Grp. A. Streptococci, Salmonellae, *Pasteurella tularensis,* Borrella sp., sp., *Leptospira icterohaemorrhagiae,* some Rickettsiae, *Entamoeba histolytica*	"Total body water," 50−70% protein bound	*Renal* and hepatic	Oral and parenter
Oxytetracycline	Bacteriostatic; same as above	Same as above	"Total body water," 20−25% protein bound	*Renal*	Oral and parenteral
Tetracycline hydrochloride	Bacteriostatic; same as above	Same as above plus *Pseudomonas pseudomallei*	"Total body water," 20−25% protein bound	*Renal*	Oral and parenteral
Demeclocycline	Bacteriostatic; same as above	Same as above plus *Mycoplasma penumoniae*	"Total body water," 40−50% protein bound	*Renal*	Oral only
Minocycline	Bacteriostatic; same as above	Same as above plus some "resistant" Staphylococci	"Total body water" with levels commonly exceeding serum levels, 70−75% protein bound	*Renal* and hepatic	Oral only at present patenteral form under study

				Side Effects			
Hypertensitivity	Nephrotoxicity	Ototoxicity	CNS toxicity	Gastrointestinal	Hematologic	Hostbiologic alterations
Skin rashes to anaphylactoid reactions	Elevation of BUN			Irritation; hepatic necrosis especially in pregnant women, staining of teeth in children	Thrombocytopenia	Superinfections
Same as above	Same as above			Same as above	Same as above	Same as above
Same as above	Same as above			Same as above	Same as above	Same as above
Same as above	Same as above			Same as above	Same as above	Same as above
Same as above	Same as above			Same as above	Same as above	Same as above

maintenance doses of up to 2 gm per day until the patient is asymptomatic. Although the tetracyclines are active against both the cysts and trophozoites of amoebae, they are usually administered in conjunction with another amoebicide for the treatment of amoebiasis.

CEPHALOSPORINS

The cephalosporins (Table 14.3.4) are a family of steroid antibiotics distinguished by their various side chains, derived from several fungi including Cephalosporium sp. This antibiotic is bactericidal and its mechanism of action, which resembles that of penicillin, is one of interference with bacterial cell wall synthesis. These agents are active against both gram-positive and gram-negative organisms[68] and have been used to treat *Staphylococcus aureus* infections, *Clostridium welchii* infections, pneumococcal pneumonia and group A Streptococcus pyogenes infections. The cephalosporins are also active against *Escherichia coli,* Klebsiella, and Proteus mirabilis, and cephaloridine has been used in the treatment of pulmonary infections due to *Hemophilus influenzae.*

The two cephalosporins which have been most widely used clinically are cephalothin and cephaloridine, with the former more resistant to penicillinase activity. Both agents are susceptible to hydrolysis by the cephalosporinase produced by some of the bacteria resistant to this antibiotic. Cephalothin is readily absorbed from muscle and poorly absorbed by the gastrointestinal tract, making parenteral administration necessary to achieve effective blood levels. Plasma proteins bind slightly more than half of the drug present in the blood, and excretion of the unchanged drug occurs primarily by renal tubular secretion. Cephaloridine, which is only inconsequentially bound to plasma protein, is poorly absorbed by the gastrointestinal tract and excreted rapidly by glomerular filtration. Both agents appear in all body tissues and fluids, but are present in the cerebrospinal fluid in extremely low concentration. The dosage of these agents is determined by the severity of the infection under treatment, and varies from 1 gm every six hours to 1 gm every two hours for cephalothin, and 0.5 gm every 6 hours to 1 gm every six hours for cephaloridine (a lesser dose because of its potential nephrotoxicity). Side effects of these agents include hypersensitivity reactions (skin rashes to anaphylaxis), neutropenia, hemolytic anemia,[25] renal failure (more commonly associated with cephaloridine administration[69]) chemical phlebitis, and superinfections.

AMINOGLYCOSIDIC ANTIBIOTICS

Streptomycin (Table 14.1.6) is an aminoglycosidic antibiotic produced by *Streptomyces griseus,* which is bactericidal in high concentration and bacteriostatic in lower concentrations. This antibiotic acts by inhibition of protein synthesis, disturbing ribosomal metabolism and genetic code translation.[92] This agent, which is poorly absorbed from the gastrointestinal tract, is well absorbed from either intramuscular or subcutaneous sites. Streptomycin distributes throughout extracellular fluid with about one-third of that present in the plasma bound to plasma proteins and is excreted unchanged by renal glomerular filtration.

The clinical use of streptomycin is today confined largely to the treatment of tuberculosis and plague, but in the past it was used with effectiveness in the treatment of a variety of bacterial infections, either singly or in combination with other antibiotics.[89] The rapid emergence of resistant strains of bacteria previously sensitive to streptomycin is the major disadvantage associated with the use of this drug. Side effects of streptomycin include hypersensitivity reactions (skin rashes, exfoliative dermatitis, angioedema, and anaphylactic shock), injury to the vestibular portion of the eighth cranial nerve, deafness, peripheral neuritis, injury of the optic nerve, respiratory arrest when administered intraperitoneally, albuminuria, and superinfections primarily due to Staphylococcus and Candida.

Streptomycin sulfate is usually administered parenterally, 0.5 to 1.0 gm every 12 hours, in the treatment of acute infections; and 1 gm per day as a single dose in the long-term treatment of tuberculosis.

Neomycin (Table 14.1.6), an aminoglycosidic antibiotic produced by Streptomyces fradiae, acts similarly to streptomycin interfering with 30 S ribosome metabolism and protein synthesis.[92] This agent, although poorly absorbed from the gastrointestinal tract, is well absorbed from intramuscular sites following which it is widely distributed throughout body tissues and rapidly excreted by the kidney. This agent, effective against both gram-positive and gram-negative bacteria,[88] is largely restricted today to use in preoperative bowel preparation. Side effects of neomycin include hypersensitivity reactions, eighth nerve injury, and nephrotoxicity. A toxic reaction of surgical importance is its curariform paralysis of respiration when applied to the peritoneum or pleura, especially in patients who have received a neuromuscular blocking drug. This type of respiratory arrest can be antagonized by either neostigmine or administration of calcium salts. Intestinal malabsorption and superinfections, particularly of the gastrointestinal tract, have also been reported during the use of neomycin.

This antibiotic is available in topical, oral, and parenteral dosage forms. Oral therapy, often employed for preoperative bowel preparation for the symptomatic treatment of hepatic coma, entails administration of 4 to 8 gm per day in divided doses. The topical form of neomycin has been used for the treatment of burns, dermatitis, and cutaneous ulcers, but the effectiveness of neomycin for such use remains undemonstrated.

Kanamycin (Table 14.1.6), an aminoglycosidic metabolic by-product of Streptomyces kanamyceticus, is either bacteriostatic or bactericidal, depending upon the concentration of the antibiotic and the organism considered. Because of its poor absorption from the gastrointestinal tract, oral kanamycin has been used for preoperative large bowel preparation, but is otherwise administered parenterally for the treatment of clinical infections. This antibiotic, which is not bound to plasma proteins, has a brief biologic half-life (only a few hours), and is excreted through

TABLE 14.1.6
The aminoglycosidic antibiotics

Agent	Mode of Action	Antibacterial Spectrum of Clinical Importance	Distribution	Excretion (Principal Route)	Routes of Administration
Streptomycin	Bacteriostatic: inhibition of bacterial protein synthesis	*Mycobacterium tuberculosis* and *Pasteurella pestis*	Extracellular fluid, 33% protein bound	Renal	Parenteral, primarily IM.
Neomycin	Bacteriostatic: same as above	*E. coli,* Aerobacter sp, *Klebsiella pneumoniae,* Salmonellae, Shigellae, *Vibrio comma, Streptococcus faecalis*	Extracellular fluid	Renal	Oral or intramuscular
Kanamycin	Bacteriostatic and bactericidal; same as above	*E. coli,* Aerobacter sp, Klebsiella sp, some methicillin-resistant Staphylococci, Salmonellae, Shigellae.	Extracellular fluid. No protein	Renal	Parenteral and oral
Gentamicin	Bacteriostatic and bactericidal; same as above	Klebsiella sp, Aerobacter sp., *Pseudomonas aeruginosa,* Serratia, indole-positive Proteus sp., some methicillin-resistant Staphylococci	Extracellular fluid. 30% protein bound	Renal	Parenteral only
Tobramycin (investigational)	Bactericidal	Enterobacteriaceae *Pseudomonas aeruginosa,* some methicillin-resistant Staphylococci	Extracellular fluid. No protein binding	Renal	Parenteral only

			Side Effects			
Hypertensitivity	Nephrotoxicity	Ototoxicity	CNS toxicity	Gastrointestinal	Hematologic	Hostbiologic alterations
Skin rashes to anaphylactoid		Vestibular and auditory	Central scotomata			Superinfections
Same as above	Azotemia and casts	Eighth nerve injury	Neuromuscular blockade			Superinfections
Same as above	Azotemia and proteinuria	Both portions of eighth nerve	Neuromuscular blockade			Superinfections
Same as above	Azotemia and proteinuria	Vesticular and auditory	Neuromuscular blockade			Superinfections
Same as above	Azotemia and proteinuria	Vesticular and auditory	Neurmuscular blockade			Superinfections

the kidney primarily by glomerular filtration, necessitating reduction of dosage in patients with renal insufficiency.[41] When administered parenterally, kanamycin appears in ascitic, peritoneal, synovial, and pleural fluids, but little diffusion into bile or feces occurs.

The side effects of kanamycin include hypersensitivity reactions, ototoxicity, and nephrotoxicity. Serial assessement of auditory acuity and renal function should be made in patients receiving kanamycin. Respiratory paralysis resembling that caused by neomycin has also been reported when the antibiotic has been instilled into the peritoneal cavity.[77] Paresthesias, blurring of vision, and superinfections have also been reported to occur during the use of this agent. Kanmycin has been found to be effective in the treatment of infections due to Aerobacter, Escherichia coli, Proteus and Klebsiella, as well as those caused by some methicillin resistant strains of Staphylococcus aureus. Parenteral dosage of 15 mg/kg/day with a maximum total dose of 1.5 gm per day has been recommended for adults, with a proportionately smaller dose for children. Oral dosage of 15 mg/kg/day up to 8 to 12 gm per day, administered in divided doses every six hours has been used for preoperative bowel preparation.

Gentamicin (Table 14.1.6) is a broad spectrum, aminoglycosidic antibiotic produced by Micromonospora purpurea, which is both bactericidal and bacteriostatic, depending upon the concentration employed. This antibiotic acts in a manner similar to that of the other aminoglycosidic agents — by interference with genetic translation. Gentamicin is poorly absorbed by the gastrointestinal tract but well absorbed from an intramuscular injection site with modest plasma protein binding and a biologic half-life of approximately four hours.[38] This drug is widely distributed throughout all body fluids, and is excreted principally by the kidney by glomerular filtration.

Side effects of this drug include gastrointestinal disturbances, nephrotoxicity, skin eruptions, and overgrowth of Candida in the intestinal tract following oral administration. Since the eighth cranial nerve toxicity, principally involving the vestibular segment of the nerve, is the most important toxic effect and occurs most frequently in patients with renal insufficiency, gentamicin dosage should be reduced in such patients.[12]

The most important clinical use of this antibiotic has been in the treatment of gram-negative infections, including those due to Klebsiella, Aerobacter, Pseudomonas aeruginosa, Serratia, indole-positive Proteus strains, and some Escherichia coli. This antibiotic is available for parenteral use in which the dosage employed is usually 0.8 to 5 mg/kg/day in equally divided doses, depending upon the severity of the infection. Gentamicin is also available as a 0.1 per cent ointment and cream, and it has been used topically in the treatment of burns, although its effectiveness in such use has been not statistically documented.

Tobramycin (Table 14.1.6) is a broad spectrum, aminoglycosidic antibiotic produced by Streptomyces tenebrarius which is bacteriostatic and currently is an investigational antibiotic available in the parenteral form only. This antibiotic is not bound to plasma proteins and is excreted through the kidney, primarily by glomerular filtration. The advantage of tobramycin is its potent bactericidal activity against Pseudomonas aeruginosa. The toxicity and side effects of this agent are currently being investigated but appear to be similar to those of gentamicin.

POLYMYXIN B

The polymyxins (Table 14.1.4) are cationic, polypeptide detergents produced by strains of Bacillus polymyxia. Polymyxin B, the only polymyxin available for clinical use, is poorly absorbed from the gastrointestinal tract and is slowly excreted, primarily by the kidney. This agent presumably acts by alteration of bacterial lipoprotein membrane permeability.[62] The development of bacterial resistance to this antibiotic is uncommon, but cross-resistance between polymyxin B and colistin is frequent.

The side effects of polymyxin B include hypersensitivity reactions (uncommon), flushing of the face, ataxia, paresthesias, external ophthalmoplegia, blurred vision, generalized areflexia, dysphagia, dyspnea, and acute tubular necrosis. Respiratory paralysis, different from that caused by neomycin and kanamycin, has also been reported, usually in patients with renal failure. Superinfections due to gram positive organisms, yeast, and fungi have also been reported.

Polymyxin B is available for topical oral and intramuscular administration and has been used in the treatment of infections caused by Escherichia coli, Aerobacter, Klebsiella, Hemophilus, Salmonella, Shigella, Vibrio, Pasteurella, and some strains of Pseudomonas aeruginoa.[82] The recommended oral dose is 75 to 100 mg three times daily for adults, with proportionately less for children. The recommended intramuscular dose ranges from 1.5 to 2.5 mg/kg in divided doses up to a total dose of 200 mg/day. This agent is also available as either a topical power or an otic solution, which have been used in the topical treatment of external otitis due to Pseudomonas sp.

COLISTIN

Colistin (Table 14.1.4) is a polypeptide metabolic by-product of Bacillus colistinus, active against gram-negative bacilli, especially Pseudomonas aeruginosa species. The structure and antibacterial activity of this agent is quite similar to that of polymyxin.[14] Colistin, which is unabsorbed from the gastrointestinal tract, is absorbed from an intramuscular injection site, and is excreted somewhat slowly by renal glomerular filtration.[44] Reported side effects of this antibiotic include skin rashes, paresthesias, gastrointestinal irritation, ototoxicity, bone marrow depression, nephrotoxicity, and respiratory paralysis, similar to that associated with polymyxin B.

Although available for oral administration in the treatment of diarrhea caused by sensitive bacteria, colistin is used primarily in its parenteral form for the treatment of gram-negative infections, particularly those due to Pseudomas, in a dosage of 2.5 to 5 mg/kg/day for the adult (depending upon the severity of the infection).

BACITRACIN

This polypeptide antibiotic (Table 14.1.4), whose mode of action remains undefined, is produced by a strain of *Bacillus subtilis*. The antibiotic is poorly absorbed from the gastrointestinal tract but rapidly absorbed from an intramuscular site.[51] It is apparently distributed throughout extracellular water after parenteral administration appearing in both peritoneal and pleural fluids, and is slowly excreted by glomerular filtration. Bacitracin is available for topical, oral, and intramuscular administration, but is used today primarily for topical treatment of external eye infections with little, if any, evidence available to confirm its effectiveness in the topical treatment of wounds. The side effects of bacitracin include skin rashes, pain and abscess formation at injection sites, gastrointestinal distress, and nephrotoxicity.

VANCOMYCIN

Vancomycin (Table 14.1.4), which is produced by *Streptomyces orientalis*, is a bactericidal antibiotic effective against a variety of bacteria, including Streptococci, Staphylococci,[35] *Corynebacterium diphtheriae, Neisseria gonorrhoeae, Diplococcus pneumoniae,* and several of the Clostridia. Vancomycin acts by inhibition of bacterial cell wall synthesis, and has a biologic half-life of approximately six hours. This agent is only slightly bound to plasma proteins and is excreted principally by the kidney.

Side effects of vancomycin include a variety of hypersensitivity reactions, chemical phlebitis, pain at injection sites, ototoxicity, and nephrotoxicity. Vancomycin is usually administered intravenously since it is unabsorbed by the gastrointestinal tract and is painful upon intramuscular injection. This drug has been reported to be useful in the treatment of methicillin-resistant staphylococcal infections, but has been supplanted by other, less toxic antibiotics for the treatment of other infections.

ANTIFUNGAL AGENTS

Nystatin

Nystatin is a fungicidal and fungistatic polyene antibiotic produced by *Streptomyces noursei* which has been reported as being effective against Candida, Cryptococcus, Blastomyces, Trichophyton, Histoplasma, *Microsporum audouini,* and Epidermophyton, but ineffective against viruses, bacteria, and protozoa. This agent exerts its antifungal activity by virtue of changing the permeability of the cell wall of the susceptible fungi due to its binding in the fungal membrane.[34] Nystatin is essentially unabsorbed from the gastrointestinal tract with virtually all of an orally administered dose excreted in the feces.

Nystatin is administered topically or orally as a treatment of Candida infections of the skin, mucous membranes and intestinal tract. The oral dose for adults is 500,000 to 1,000,000 units, three times a day, and up to 100,000 units three to four times a day for children. Nystatin is also used in the form of vaginal tablets as treatment for vaginal Candidiasis. Side effects are apparently uncommon and largely those of gastrointestinal irritation.

Amphotericin B

Amphotericin B is a fungistatic, fungicidal polyene antibiotic produced by *Streptomyces nodosus,* which is effective against a variety of fungi. Although incompletely defined, its mechanism of action appears to be similar to that of nystatin. Amphotericin B is poorly absorbed from the gastrointestinal tract with clinically effective blood levels achieved only by intravenous administration. The biologic half-life of amphotericin B is approximately 24 hours and it is distributed throughout extracellular fluid. Only a small percentage of administered amphotericin B appears in the urine in active form, but urinary excretion continues for many days following cessation of therapy. Side effects of this agent include hypersensitivity reactions, chills, fever, chemical phlebitis, anorexia, vomiting, anemia, and headache.[6] Acute hepatic failure has been associated with amphotericin B therapy, and most patients receiving amphotericin B show evidence of its nephrotoxic effect. Hypomagnesemia, ECG changes, and bacterial superinfections have also been associated with amphotericin B therapy.

Amphotericin B has been reported to be effective in the treatment of North American blastomycosis, coccidioidomycosis, pulmonary histoplasmosis, *Cryptococcus neoformans* infections, systemic candidiasis, mucormycosis, chromoblastomycosis, disseminated sporotrichosis, South American blastomycosis, and aspergillosis.[8] Amphotericin B is available as a powder for injection, which must be mixed with sterile water, since salt solutions precipitate this agent. For the treatment of severe systemic mycosis the authors prefer to initiate treatment with the administration of 0.25 mg/kg on the first day of therapy, increasing the dosage by 0.25 mg/kg each day until a total daily dose of 1.5 mg/kg is reached. Hospitalization of all patients receiving amphotericin B is essential, and therapy should be continued for six weeks or longer, depending upon clinical response. Amphotericin B lotions and creams are also available for the topical treatment of cutaneous mycoses.

Flucytosine

Flucytosine (5-Fluorocytosine) recently approved for clinical use, is reported to be effective against Candida species, *Torulopsis gladbrata,* and *Cryptococcus neoformans.*[84] This orally administered fungicide is well absorbed from the gastrointestinal tract and largely excreted by the kidney. Measurable serum concentrations persist for up to 10 hours after an oral dose and tissue levels equal or exceed those on the serum. Inherent fungal resistance is common and resistant strains may appear during therapy necessitating sensitivity testing prior to and during flucytosine therapy. Maximum recommended dosage is 150 mg/kg/day. The toxicity of this agent is less than that of Amphotericin B and includes nephrotoxicity, hepatotoxicity, bone marrow depression, and gastrointestinal irritation.

Other antifungal agents which are presently being evaluated include hamycin, kalafungin, endomycin, lomofungin, and rifampin but their clinical efficacy remains undefined.[85]

ANTIVIRAL AGENTS

Idoxuridine, which possesses, the ability to inhibit the growth of DNA viruses, such as *Herpesvirus hominis* and vaccinia, has shown effectiveness in the clinical treatment of *Herpesvirus hominis* infections. This agent has been used primarily for the treatment of Herpes keratitis as either a 0.5 per cent ophthalmic ointment or a 0.1 per cent ophthalmic solution. Systemic dosage of 0.5 mg/kg/day has also been reported of benefit in the treatment of systemic Herpesvirus hominis infections, principally encephalitis,[30] although conclusive proof as to its effectiveness for such use is lacking at the present time. The side effects of this agent are principally those of bone marrow depression and nephrotoxicity.

PROPHYLACTIC ANTIBIOTICS

Antibiotic prophylaxis should be employed with a high degree of selectivity and the antibiotic most effective against a given organism should be utilized rather than a broad spectrum antibiotic directed against a host of bacteria. In view of the side effects, rapid emergence of resistant organisms, the existence of transfer factors and the possibility of superinfections by bacteria and other microbial organisms, prophylactic antibiotics should be reserved for use in those surgical patients in whom postinjury or postoperative infection is likely to occur. The use of antibiotics in the treatment of patients in whom significant contamination exists at the time of initial emergency or elective treatment is perhaps best considered therapeutic rather than prophylactic. The effectiveness of antibiotics used prophylactically is determined by the susceptibility of the organism and its capability for reinfecting the host, the site of the organism, and the characteristics of the antibiotic.

Situations in which prophylactic antibiotics have been recommended, and some evidence exists to support their use are: (1) open fractures and open joint injury, (2) soft tissue injury with delayed treatment, (3) penetrating abdominal injury and penetrating chest in-

jury, (4) vascular injury in which prosthetic material must be used, (5) human and animal bites, (6) thermal trauma, including inhalation injury, (7) patients with preexisting diseases, such as rheumatic fever and tuberculosis, (8) patients with immunologic deficiencies either acquired or congenital, (9) patients with previously implanted foreign bodies, (10) wounds requiring skin grafting, and (11) wounds in which tissue of questionable viability must be left in place.

The selection of antibiotics should be based on the prevalent organisms recovered from similar wounds and the microbial flora of the hospital concerned. In order to select the antibiotic most likely to be effective in treatment of an infection prior to specific identification of the offending organism, it is helpful to continually monitor occurrence rates of bacteria in all patients encountered, as done by Boswick's group for hand infections.[83] Monitoring of wound bacterial populations as related to time in the hospital (Table 14.1.7), is also useful in the initial selection of antibiotics for treatment of infections. Monitoring antibiotic sensitivities of the microorganisms commonly causing infections in one's practice will further increase the likelihood of initially selecting (prior to reports of laboratory testing) the antimicrobial agents or agents most likely to be effective (Table 14.1.8). Wound cultures and wound biopsies should be employed as previously noted to monitor the effectiveness of antibiotic therapy in individual patients receiving such agents for the treatment of infections.

Prophylaxis should be initiated preoperatively in high risk patients or in the injured patient and continued during the intra-operative and postoperative period.[22] Duration of therapy should be limited to four to seven days to minimize the development of resistance in residual bacteria and emergence of insensitive opportunistic bacteria and fungi. It is to be emphasized that prophylactic antibiotics used even for specific indication in high risk patients for a limited period of time are in no way an excuse to abridge surgical asepsis or abandon meticulous surgical technique.

TOPICAL ANTIBIOTICS AND CHEMOTHERAPY

Topical application of antibacterial agents to control infection has documented usefulness in the treatment of certain wounds. Topical chemotherapy of burn wounds, the focal point of current postresuscitation burn care, has significantly improved survival of all patients with burns of up to 60 per cent of the total body surface by decreasing the incidence of invasive burn wound sepsis. Such topical therapy limits the proliferation of bacteria in the burn does not sterilize the wound. Agents which are currently available include Sulfamylon, 0.5 per cent AgNO3 soaks, and the investigational drugs 1 per cent silver sulfadiazine cream and 0.1 per cent gentamicin cream. Other silver-containing preparations have been used on

TABLE 14.1.7
Percentage of positive patients on admission at postburn time intervals

Organism	0-2	3-5	6-10	11-20	21 +
S. aureus	21.4	36.3	53.8	53.6	48.1
S. epidermidis	70.0	27.2			22.2
Micrococcus sp.	14.2				
S. faecalis (Gp.D)					
Corynebacterium sp.					
Bacillus sp.	32.1	36.4			
Candida albicans					
Candida sp.					
Mima Gp.					
H. vaginicola		18.1		19.5	18.5
A. faecalis					
Pseudomonas sp.		54.5		54.8	70.3
E. cloacae	25.0	54.5	23.0		
E. aerogenes					
Klebsiella sp.	21.4	54.5	30.5	40.2	44.4
E. coli	17.8	36.3	38.4	28.0	29.6
P. mirabilis			26.9	26.8	29.6
P. stuartii			26.9	41.4	48.1
Serratia				19.2	

Days Postburn — scale 0 → 80 %

TABLE 14.1.8
Staphylococcus aureus: cumulative inhibitory levels for strains isolated in the Institute of Surgical Research, 1969-1970

MIC g/ml	Antibiotics and Per Cent of Strains Inhibited						
	K	L	Ps	Sc	T	G	U
>25	100	100	100	100	100	100	100
25	38.7	58.6	51.0	47.1	22.7	72.6	63.0
6.25	18.2	37.9	26.9	21.5	7.7	36.9	36.4
3.12	11.2	24.1	17.0	7.9	5.5	15.4	25.3
1.5	6.9	14.9	8.7	1.1	2.7	7.1	16.2
0.78	3.8	7.4	3.2	1.1	2.2	7.1	7.7
<0.78	2.6	3.4	1.0	0	1.6	2.9	4.1
No. tested	186	174	182	176	180	168	166

K = Kanamycin, L = Lincocin, Ps = Prostaphlin, Sc = Staphcillin, T = Tetracycline, G = Gentamicin, U = Unipen.

small groups of burn patients but their value remains unverified.

The authors regard solubility and diffusibility of topical agents as critically important to permit absorption of the active agent into the eschar with maintenance of an effective concentration of antimicrobial drug at the viable-nonviable tissue interface, the characteristic locus of preinvasive bacterial proliferation. Application of nondiffusable agents such as the 0.5 per cent AgNO3 must be initiated immediately postburn prior to bacterial proliferation to be effective since such agents do most penetrate the eschar. The water soluble topical burn creams are usually applied to the entirety of the burn wound once each day and either left exposed or covered with a single layer gauze dressing with reapplication 12 hours later to areas from which the material has been abraded (more of-

ten, if necessary to maintain adequate coverage). The 0.5 per cent AgNO3 soaks are changed two times a day and moistened with AgNO3 solution as necessary between those times.[56]

Topical agents, both antibiotics and sulfonamides, have also been reported to decrease subsequent significant infection in traumatic wounds for which initial treatment must be for some reason be delayed.[46][52] Such is to be regarded as a seldom encountered situation and as no substitute for timely adequate surgical treatment.

Other studies have shown that intraperitoneal instillation of kanamycin is useful in decreasing postoperative peritonitis and intraperitoneal abscess formation in patients with perforated viscera.[10] Operative wound irrigation with kanamycin solution at the time of closure in patients with peritoneal contamination has also been reported to reduce the incidence of postoperative wound infection.[57][61]

Lastly, although application of antibiotic ointments to the skin at the site of cannulation has been reported to decrease cannula associated sepsis, recent studies at this Institute suggest that ordinary surgical hygiene and wound care without use of topical antibiotics is just as effective in the control of intravascular cannula related sepsis.

CHEMOTHERAPY

Chemotherapy, first employed for clinical infection in 1936, was soon overshadowed by the procession of antibiotics beginning with penicillin in 1941 but the recent development of effective sulfonamide topical treatment of burns has refocused attention on chemotherapy. Sulfonamides were the original chemotherapeutic agents and have been used for the treatment of a variety of infections because of their wide spectrum of activity against both gram-positive and gram-negative bacteria. Prontosil was the first sulfonamide-containing azo dye used to treat infection and, in 1936, Colebrook and Kenney reported that both it and sulfanilamide (its active radical) were effective in the treatment of bacterial infections.[9] Since then, many sulfonamide derivatives have been found to be clinically useful, including sulfadiazine, sulfisoxazole, succinylsulfathiazone, phthalylsulfathiazole, sulfacetamide, and mafenide, as well as combinations of the above, and other derivatives.[52,90]

Sulfonamides are characteristically bacteriostatic, less potent on a weight basis than antibiotics and, with the possible exception of mafenide, inhibited by blood, necrotic tissue, and purulent exudates. The principal antimicrobial action of the sulfonamides is felt to be due to their competitive antagonism of para-aminogenzoic acid (PABA), preventing its incorporation in bacterial Pteroylglutamic acid (PGA).[98] Bacteria which do not require PGA or can utilize PGA from other sources are of course insensitive to the sulfonamides. PABA and other materials containing PABA such as some local anesthetics antagonize the action of the sulfonamides.

Sulfonamides are almost always administered orally, and if absorbable, are rapidly absorbed from the gastrointestinal tract to produce effective blood levels. If oral administration is not possible, sodium salts of the sulfonamides can be given intravenously or even subcutaneously. Topical use of sulfonamides, previously condemned, is, in fact, effective in controlling the bacterial density of burn wounds.

The sulfonamides are bound to plasma proteins to a variable extent, depending on the specific derivative and the albumin concentration. This protein-binding reduces the amount of active agent available and accounts for the greater solubility of sulfonamides in plasma as compared to strictly aqueous solutions. These drugs rapidly diffuse into pleural and peritoneal fluids as well as synovial fluids where there exists a higher percentage of unbound active agent. Following absorption, acetylation, a metabolic process which renders the drug inactive, occurs to a variable extent. Sulfonamides are excreted principally in the urine, with small amounts measured in feces, bile, and milk.

Organisms against which sulfonamides have been shown to be effective include group A Streptococcus pyogenes, Hemophilus sp, *Corynebacterium diphtheriae, Bacillus anthracis, Pasteurella pestis,* Brucella spp., and some strains of *Escherichia coli.* Other susceptible microorganisms include Nocardia, Actinomyces, and *Donovania granulomatis.* Resistance can develop in organisms previously sensitive to the sulfonamides and such has indeed been noted clinically in Streptococci, Meningococci, Pneumococci, and Gonococci.

The rapidly absorbed and rapidly excreted sulfonamides include sulfadiazine, sulfamerazine, sulfamethazine, and sulfisoxazone, all of which have been used in the treatment of acute, systemic infections, utilizing an initial loading dose of between 2 and 4 gm in the adult, with supplemental dosage of 1 gm every four to eight hours depending upon the specific sulfonamide utilized. Rapidly absorbed but slowly excreted sulfonamides include methoxypyridazine and sulfadimethoxine, used primarily in the long-term treatment of urinary tract infection. The recommended dosage schedule of these agents includes an initial loading dose, with continued daily doses of 0.5 to 1 gm, depending upon the agent.

The poorly absorbed sulfonamides have been used for their suppressive effect on the bacterial flora of the gastrointestinal tract, and include succinylsulfathiazone, phthalylsulfathiazole, and sulfaguanidine. The dosage of each agent given for bowel preparation depends upon the weight of the patient and is given in divided doses over a five- to seven-day period following an initial priming dose. Sulfonamides for special uses include sulfisomidine sulfamethizone, and sulfacetamide, used for treatment for urinary tract infections, sodium sulfacetamide used in the treatment of eye infections, salicylazosulfapyridine used in the treatment of ulcerative colitis, and mafenide and silver sulfadiazine used in the topical treatment of burn wounds.

Side effects of the sulfonamides include hypersensitivity; crystalluria, which may lead to renal impairment; and injury to both white and red blood cells manifested by hemolytic anemia, agranulocytosis and thrombocytopenia. The hypersensitivity reactions include vasculitis, a variety of skin rashes, and anaphylactoid reactions. Hepatic necrosis has also been reported as associated with sulfonamide administration and the appearance of otherwise unexplained jaundice necessitates discontinuation of such therapy. Subsequent administration of a sulfonamide is contraindicated by the history of a previous significant reaction to its use, and it should be borne in mind that such a patient may show sensitivity to other sulfonamide compounds.

ISONIAZID

Isoniazid, a thiosemicarbazone, is an effective bacteriostatic agent against the tubercle bacillus, which is rapidly absorbed from the gastrointestinal tract and rapidly diffuses not only into all compartments of the extracellular fluid but also into cells. Isoniazid is inactivated primarily by acetylation with the acetyl derivative, being less toxic and considerably less bacteriostatic. The mechanism of action appears to involve inhibition of nucleic acid synthesis but remains incompletely defined.[97]

Isoniazid is commonly administered orally at a dosage level of 3 to 5 mg/kg/day in divided doses. Side effects of this drug include hypersensitivity skin reactions, seizures, and neurotoxic reactions, including optic neuritis. A pyridoxine deficiency-type anemia has been associated with isoniazid administration, and should be treated with large doses of pyridoxine.

AMINOSALICYLIC ACID

Aminosalicylic acid (PAS) is another chemotherapeutic agent possessing tuberculostatic properties. This compound, whose antimicrobial action is presumed to be related to PABA antagonism, as with the sulfonamides, is rapidly absorbed from the gastrointestinal tract and is distributed in total body water with the exception of the cerebrospinal fluid. The agent is rapidly excreted and is extensively acetylated in the blood. The acetyl form of the compound is relatively insoluble and alkalinization of the urine may be necessary to precent crystalluria. This drug is administered orally at a dosage level of 8 to 12 gm per day.

Side effects include gastrointestinal tract irritation, hypersensitivity skin reactions, hepatic injury, pancreatitis, nephritis, agranulocytosis, thrombocytopenia, and lymphocytosis. The direct effects of aminosalicylic acid on body metabolism include suppression of prothrombin production by the liver, production of goiter secondary to thyroid cell injury, and production of acidosis due to an obligatory excretion of bicarbonate in the urine.

ETHAMBUTOL

Ethambutol is another tuberculostatic chemotherapeutic agent which is rapidly absorbed from the gastrointestinal tract and appears to be selectively concenrated in the red blood cells. This agent is administered orally in a dosage of 15 to 25 mg/kg/day, and is more slowly excreted than the previously described chemotherapeutic agents. Anaphylaxis, leukopenia, and decrease in visual acuity are all described side effects.

SULFONES

The sulfones are derivatives of 4, 4[1]-diaminodiphylsulfone (DDS) which are bacteriostatic against *Mycobacterium leprae*. These agents are antagonized by para-aminobenzoic acid and are considered to have an action similar to that of the sulfonamides.[91] In general, the sulfones are incompletely absorbed from the gastrointestinal tract with a significant percentage of orally administered doses appearing in the feces. These agents distribute in total body water and are apparently concentrated in liver and kidney and to a lesser extent in skin and muscle. The preponderant route of excretion is through the kidney. Sulfone preparations which have been used clinically in the treatment of leprosy include glycosulfone sodium, sulfoxine sodium, sulfetrone sodium, thiazolsulfone, and dapsone, with the former administered intravenously and the latter four compounds

given orally. Side effects include hemolysis, methemoglobinemia, gastrointestinal disturbances, and a variety of neurologic changes ranging from headache to blurring of the vision and parasthesias.

FURAN DERIVATIVES

Compounds with a nitro group in the 5 position of the furan ring have been shown to be bacteriostatic against both gram-positive and gram-negative bacteria, and some fungi. Nitrofurantoin has been employed as a urinary antiseptic[66] but Proteus, Pseudomonas, and Alkaligenes species, common causative agents of urinary tract infection, are often insensitive to the agent. The usual oral dose of this compound is 7.5 mg/kg in four equal portions. Hypersensitivity reactions as well as gastrointestinal disturbances and polyneuropathy have been reported as well as hemolytic anemia.

Nitrofurazone has been used topically in the treatment of skin infections and wounds, but its lack of effectiveness against gram-negative opportunists limits its value. Furazolidone is employed as local treatment of the intestinal and reproductive tracts because of its effectiveness against *Trichomonas vaginalis* and *Giardia lamblia*. Nifurozime has been employed in the treatment of candidal vaginal infections.

REFERENCES

1. Abramson, E., Wilson, D., and Arky, R. A. Rhinocerebral phycomycosis in association with diabetic ketoacidosis. Report of two cases and a review of clinical and experimental experience with amphotericin B therapy. Ann. Int. Med., *66:* 735-742, 1967.
2. Alexander, J. W., and Moncrief, J. A. Alterations of the immune response following severe thermal injury. Arch. Surg., *93:* 75-83, 1966.
3. Alexander, J. W. Control of infection following burn injury. Arch. Surg., *103:* 435-441, 1971.
4. Alexander, J. W., Fisher, M. W., and MacMillan, B. G. Immunological control of Pseudomonas infection in burn patients: a clinical evaluation. Arch. Surg., *102:* 31-35, 1971.
5. Altemeier, W. A., and Furste, W. L. Collective review; gas gangrene. International Abstracts of Surgery. Surg. Gynecol. Obstet., *84:* 507-523, 1947.
6. Andriole, V. T., and Kravetz, H. M. The use of amphotericin B in man. J.A.M.A., *180:* 269-272, 1962.
7. Brock, T. D. Chloramphenicol. Bacteriol. Rev., *25:* 32-48, 1961.
8. Bruck, H. M., Nash, G., Foley, F. D., and Pruitt, B. A., Jr. Opportunistic fungal infections of the burn wound with phycomycetes and *Aspergillus.* Arch. Surg., *102:* 476-482, 1971.
9. Colebrook, L., and Kenny, M. Treatment of human puerperal infections, and of experimental infections in mice, with prontosil. Lancet, *1:* 1279-1286, 1936.
10. Cohn, I. Jr. Kanamycin as an intestinal antiseptic and in the treatment of peritonitis: resume of clinical experience. Ann. N.Y. Acad. Sci., *132:* 860-869, 1966.
11. Curreri, P. W., Lindberg, R. B., DiVincenti, F. C., and Pruitt, B. A., Jr. Intravenous administration of car-

benicillin for septicemia due to *Pseudomonas aeruginosa* following thermal injury. J. Infect. Dis. (Suppl.), *122:* s 40-43, 1970.

12. Cutler, R. E., Gyselynck, A-M, Fleet, W. P., and Forrey, A. W. Correlation of serum creatinine concentration and gentamicin half-life. J.A.M.A. *219:* 1037-1041, 1972.

13. Dienstag, J., and Neu, H. C. *In vitro* studies of Tobramycin, an aminoglycosidic antibiotic. Antimicrobial Agents and Chemotherapy, p. 41, Jan. 1972.

14. Eickhoff, T. C., and Finland, M. Polymyxin B and colistin: *in vitro* activity against *Pseudomonas aeruginosa*. Am. J. Med. Sci., *249:* 172-174, 1965.

15. Eickhoff, T. C., Kislak, J. W., and Finland, M. Sodium ampicillin absorption and excretion of intramuscular and intravenous doses of normal young men. Am. J. Med. Sci., *249:* 163-171, 1965.

16. Elek, S. D. Recongnition of toxigenic bacterial strains *in vitro*. Br. Med. J., *1:* 493-496, 1948.

17. Erslev, A. J., and Wintrobe, M. M. Detection and prevention of drug-induced blood dyscrasias. J.A.M.A., *181:* 114-119, 1962.

18. Ewing, W. H. The nomenclature and taxonomy of the proteus and providence groups. Int. Bull. Bacteriol. Nomen. and Taxon., *8:* 17-22, 1958.

19. Flemma, R. J., DiVincenti, F. C., Dotin, L. N., and Pruitt, B. A., Jr. Pulmonary melioidosis: a diagnostic dilemma and increasing threat. Ann. Thorac. Surg., *7:* 491-499, 1969.

20. Foley, F. D. The burn autopsy. Am. J. Clin. Path., *52:* 1-13, 1969.

21. Foley, F. D., and Shuck, J. M. Burn wound infection with phycomycetes requiring amputation of hand. J.A.M.A., *203:* 596, 1968.

22. Fullen, W. D., Hunt, J., and Altemeier, W. A. Prophylactic antibiotics in penetrating wounds of the abdomen. J. Trauma, *12:* 282-289, 1972.

23. Gibaldi, M., and Schwartz, M. A. Apparent effect of probenecid on the distribution of penicillins in man. Clin. Pharmacol. Ther., *9:* 345-349, 1968.

24. Gill, F. A., and Hook, E. W. Changing patterns of bacterial resistance to antimicrobial drugs. Am. J. Med., *39:* 780-795, 1965.

25. Gralnick, H. R., McGinniss, M., Elton, W., and McCurdy, P. Hemolytic anemia associated with cephalothin. J.A.M.A., *217:* 1193-1197, 1971.

26. Gravenkemper, C. F., Brodie, J. L., and Kirby, W. M. Resistance of coagulase-positive staphylococci to methicillin and oxacillin. J. Bacteriol., *89:* 1005-1010, 1965.

27. Greenwood, D., and O'Grady, F. Variety in the response of escherichia coli to erythromycin. J. Med. Microbiol., *5:* 321-326, 1972.

28. Griffith, R. S., and Black, H. R. Erythromycin. Pediatr. Clini. North Am., *8:* 1115-1131, 1961.

29. Griffith, R. S., and Black, H. R. Comparison of the blood levels obtained after single and multiple doses of erythromycin estolate and erythromycin stearate. Am. J. Med. Sci., *247:* 69-74, 1964.

30. Hanshaw, J. R. Idoxuridine in herpesvirus encephalitis. N. Eng.l. J. Med., *282:* 47, 1970.

31. Hellerstrom, S. Waterborne tuberculosis and similar infections of the skin in swimming pools. Acta Derm. Venereol., *32:* 449-461, 1952.

32. Howe, C., and Miller, W. R. Human glanders: report of six cases. Ann. Int. Med., *26:* 93-115, 1947.

33. Johnson, H. D., and Johnson, W. W. Pneumocystis carinii pneumonia in children with cancer: diagnosis and treatment. J.A.M.A., *214:* 1067-1072, 1970.

34. Kinsky, S. C. Nystatin binding by protoplasts and a particulate fraction of *Neurospora crassa*, and a basis for the selective toxicity of polyene antifungal antibiotics. Proc. Natl. Acad. Sci., *48:* 1049-1056, 1962.

35. Kirby, W. M., Perry, D. M., and Bauer, A. W. Treatment of staphylococcal septicemia with vancomycin. N. Engl. J. Med., *262:* 49-55, 1960.

36. Klein, J. O., and Finland, M. Nafcillin: antibacterial action *in vitro* and absorption and excretion in normal young men. Am. J. Med. Sci., *246:* 10-26, 1963.

37. Klein, J. O., and Finland, M. The new penicillins. N. Engl. J. Med., *269:* 1019-1025, 1963.

38. Klein, J. O., Eickhoff, T. C., and Finland, M. Gentamycin: activity *in vitro* and observations in 26 patients. Am. J. Med. Sci., *248:* 528-543, 1964.

39. Kunin, C. M. Clinical significance of protein binding of the penicillins. Ann. N.Y. Acad. Sci., *145:* 282-290, 1967.

40. Kunin, C. M., and Finland, M. Clinical pharmacology of the tetracycline antibiotics. Clin. Pharmacol. Ther., *2:* 51-69, 1961.

41. Kunin, C. M. Absorption, distribution, excretion and fate of kanamycin. Ann. N.Y. Acad. Sci., *132:* 811-818, 1966.

42. Kurtzman, N. A., Rogers, P. W., and Harter, H. R. Neurotoxic reaction to penicillin and carbenicillin. J.A.M.A., *214:* 1320-1321, 1970.

43. Lindberg, R. B., Latta, R. L., Thomas, E. T., and Pruitt, B. A., Jr. Emergence of methicillin-resistant *Staphylococcus aureus* type 84 in burn patients. U.S. Army Inst. of Surg. Res. Prog. Rept., Section 20, 30 Jun. 72, BAMC, Fort Sam Houston, Texas.

44. MacKay, D. N., and Kaye, D. Serum concentrations of colistin in patients with normal and impaired renal function. N. Engl. J. Med., *270:* 394-397, 1964.

45. MacLennan, J. D. The histoxic clostridial infections of man. Bacteriol. Rev., *26:* 177-276, 1962.

46. Mansberger, A. R., Ochsner, E. W. A., Jacob, S., Oppenheimer, J. H., and Gillette, R. W. A new preparation for the study of experimental shock from massive wounds. II. Evaluation of various therapeutic regimens with special reference to the role of antibiotics, fluid replacement and debridement. Surgery, *43:* 708-720, 1958.

47. Mason, A. D., Jr., Pruitt, B. A., Jr., Lindberg, R. B., Moncrief, J. A., and Foley, F. D. Topical sulfamylon chemotherapy in the treatment of patients with extensive thermal burns. In *Research in Burns. Transactions of the Third International Congress on Research in Burns*, Sept. 20-25, 1970, Prague. Bern, Huber Publishers, 1971, pp. 120-123.

48. McDermott, W., *et al*. The absorption, excretion and destruction of orally administered penicillin. J. Clin. Invest., *25:* 190-210, 1946.

49. McGehee, R. F., Jr., Smith, C. B., Wilcox, C., and Finland, M. Comparative studies of antibacterial activity in vitro and absorption and excretion of lincomycin and clinimycin. Am. J. Med. Sci., *256:* 279-292, 1968.

50. McKeel, D. W., Jr., Goodwin, M. N., Jr., Worley, B. L., Lindberg, R. B. Definitive identification of burn wound fungi in fatally burned military personnel by culture and by histopathology. U. S. Army Inst. of Surg. Res. Prog. Rept., Section 57, 30 Jun. 72,

BAMC, Fort Sam Houston, Texas.

51. Meleney, F. L., and Johnson, B. A. Bacitracin. Am. J. Med., 7: 794-806, 1949.

52. Mendelson, J. A., Lindsey, D.: Sulfamylon (Mafenide) and penicillin as expedient treatment of experimental massive open wounds with C. perfringens infection. J. Trauma, 2: 239-261, 1962.

53. Meyer, R. D., Young, L. S., and Armstrong, D. Tobramycin (Nebramycin Factor 6): In vitro activity against Pseudomonas aeruginosa. Appl. Microbiol., 22: 1147-1151, 1971.

54. Middlebrook, G., and Cohn, M. L. Bacteriology of tuberculosis: laboratory methods. Am. J. Pub. Health, 48: 844-853, 1958.

55. Moncrief, J. A., and Teplitz, C. Changing concepts in burn sepsis. J. Trauma, 4: 233-245, 1964.

56. Moyer, C. A., Brentano, L., Gravens, D. L., Margarf, H. W., and Monafo, W. W., Jr. Treatment of large human burns with 0.5 per cent silver nitrate solutions. Arch. Surg., 90: 812, 1965.

57. Moylan, J. A., Jr., and Brockenbrough, E. C. Antibiotic wound irrigation in the prevention of surgical wound infection. Surg. Forum, 19: 66-67, 1968.

58. Mufson, M. A., Bloom, H., Manko, M. A., Kingston, J. R., and Chanock, R. M. Acute respiratory diseases of viral etiology. V. Eaton agent: a review. Am. J. Pub. Health, 52: 925-932, 1962.

59. Munster, M., Hoagland, H. C., Pruitt, B. A., Jr. The effect of thermal injury on serum immunoglobulins. Ann. Surg., 172: 965-969, 1970.

60. Nash, G., Foley, F. D., Goodwin, M. N., Jr. Greenwald, K. A., and Pruitt, B. A., Jr. Fungal burn wound infection. J.A.M.A. 215: 1664-1666, 1971.

61. Newsome, T. W., and Eurenius, K. Suppression of granulocyte and platelet production by Pseudomonas burn wound infection. Surg. Gynecol. Obstet., in press.

62. Newton, B. A. The properties and mode of action of the polymyxins. Bacteriol, Rev., 20: 14-27, 1956.

63. Olafsson, M., Lee, Y. C., and Abernethy, T. J. Mima polymorpha meningitis: Report of a case in the review of the literature. N. Engl. J. Med., 258: 465-470, 1958.

64. Order, S. E., Mason, A. D., Jr., Switzer, W. E., and Moncrief, J. A. Arterial vascular occlusion and devitalization of burn wounds. Ann. Surg., 161: 502-508, 1965.

65. Park, J. T., and Strominger, J. L. Mode of action of penicillin. Science, 125: 99-101, 1957.

66. Paul, M. F., Bender, R. C., and Nohle, E. G. Renal excretion of nitrofurantoin (Furadantin). Am. J. Physiol., 197: 580-584, 1959.

67. Perillie, P. E., Nolan, J. P., and Finch, S. C. Studies of the resistance to infection in diabetes mellitus: local exudative cellular response. J. Lab. Clin. Med., 59: 1008-1015, 1962.

68. Perkins, R. L., Saslaw, S., Hackett, J. Cephaloridine and cephalothin comparative in vitro evaluation. Am. J. Med. Sci., 253: 293-299, 1967.

69. Perkins, R. L., Smith, E. J., and Saslaw, S. Cephalothin and cephaloridine: Comparative pharmacodynamics in chronic uremia. Am. J. Med. Sci., 257: 116-124, 1969.

70. Pruitt, B. A., Jr., and Baker, H. Bacterial populations as related to treatment and subsequent infection in war wounds. U.S. Army Medical Research Team (WRAIR) Vietnam and Institute Pasteur of Vietnam Annual Progress Report, 1967-1968, pp. 398-403.

71. Pruitt, B. A., Jr. Recent advances in burn treatment. Surgery, 68: 412-418, 1970.

72. Pruitt, B. A., Jr., Stein, J. M., Foley, F. D., Moncrief, J. A., and O'Neill, J. A., Jr. Intravenous therapy in burn patients. Arch. Surg., 100: 399-404, 1970.

73. Pruitt, B. A., Jr., and Curreri, P. W. The burn wound and its care. Arch. Surg., 103: 461-468, 1971.

74. Pruitt, B. A., Jr., and Moylan, J. A., Jr. Current management of thermal burns. In Advances in Surgery, edited by J. D. Hardy. Chicago, Year Book. In press.

75. Robson, M. C., Shaw, R. C., and Heggers, J. P. The reclosure of postoperative incisional abscesses based on bacterial quantification of the wound. Ann. Surg., 171: 279-282, 1970.

76. Roe, E., Jones, R. J., and Lowbury, E. J. L. Transfer of antibiotic resistance between Pseudomonas aeruginosa, Escherichia coli, and other gram-negative bacilli in burns. Lancet, 1: 149-152, 1971.

77. Rutenberg, A. M. Status of kanamycin in the treatment of surgical infections. Ann, N. Y. Acad. Sci., 132: 824-833, 1966.

78. Rutenberg, A. M., and Greenberg, H. L. Broad-spectrum penicillins and other antibiotics in the treatment of surgical infections. Ann. N. Y. Acad. Sci., 145: 451-463, 1967.

79. Seidenstein, M., Salomons, M. M., Herbsman, H., and Shaftan, G. W. Evaluation of local antibiotic instillation in extremity wounds. Surgery, 68: 809-812, 1970.

80. Smith, C. B., and Finland, M. Carbenicillin: activity in vitro and absorption and excretion in normal young men. Appl. Microbiol., 16: 1753-1760, 1968.

81. Spink, W. W., and Ferris, V. Penicillin-resistant staphylococci: mechanisms involved in the development of resistance. J. Clini. Invest., 26: 379-393, 1947.

82. Stansley, P. G. Polymyxins: a review and assessment. Am. J. Med., 7: 807-818, 1949.

83. Stone, N. H., Hursch, H., Humphrey, C. R., and Boswick, J. A., Jr. Emperical selection of antibiotics of hand infections. J. Bone Joint Surg., 51A: 899-903, 1969.

84. Tassel, D. A., and Madoff, M. A. Treatment of Candida sepsis and cryptococcus meningitis with 5-fluorocytosine. J. A.M.A., 206: 830-832, 1968.

85. Toala, P., Schroeder, S. A., Daly, A. K., and Finland, M. Candida at Boston City Hospital, clinical and epidemiological characteristics and susceptability to eight antimicrobial agents. Arch. Int. Med., 126: 983-989, 1970.

86. Topley, W. W. C. Principles of Bacteriology and Immunity, Ed. 5 Baltimore, Williams & Wilkins, 1964, p. 702.

87. VanEs, L. Swine erysipilas infections in man. Univ. Neb. Coll. Agr. Res. Bull., #130, 1942.

88. Waksman, S. A., and Lechevalier, H. A. Neomycin, a new antibiotic active against streptomycin-resistant bacteria, including tuberculosis organisms. Science, 109: 305-307, 1949.

89. Waksman, S. A. Streptomycin: Background, isolation, properties, and utilization. Science, 118: 259-266, 1953.

90. Weinstein, L., Madoff, M. A., and Samet, C. M. The sulfonamides. N. Engl. J. Med., 263: 793-800,

842-849, 900-907, 1960.

91. Weinstein, L. Drugs used in the chemotherapy of leprosy and tuberculosis. In *The Pharmacological Basis of Therapeutics,* Ed. 4, edited by Goodman and Gilman. New York, Macmillian, 1970, pp. 1311-1343.

92. Weisblum, B., and Davies, J. Antibiotic inhibitors of the bacterial ribosome. Bacteriol. Rev., *32:* 493-528, 1968.

93. Whelan, T. J., Jr., Burkhalter, W. E., and Gomez, A. Management of war wounds. In *Advances in Surgery,* Vol. 3. Chicago, Year Book, 1968, pp. 263-270.

94. Whitney, J. L., and Rampling, A. Pseudomonas aeruginosa contamination in domestic and hospital environments. Lancet, *1:* 15-17, 1972.

95. Williams, R. E. O., and Rippon, J. R. Bacteriophage typing of staphylococcus aureus. J. Hyg., *50:* 320-353, 1952.

96. Wilson, A. T., *et al. Diagnostic Procedures and Reagents: Techniques for the Laboratory Diagnosis and Control of the Communicable diseases,* Ed. 4. New York. American Public Health Association, 1963, p. 201.

97. Wimpenny, J. W. Effect of isoniazid on biosynthesis in mycobacterium tuberculosis var. bovis BCG. J. Gen. Microbiol., *47:* 379-388, 1967.

98. Woods, D. D. The biochemical mode of action of the sulfonamide drugs. J. Gen. Microbiol., *29:* 687-702, 1962.

B.

Lesser Infections of the Hand

John H. Crandon, M.D.

The fundamental contributions of Kanavel,[8] Koch,[10] and Mason[15][16] have established principles and guide-lines for treatment of infections of the hand from which there has been little deviation.

GENERAL PRINCIPLES

Elevation, immobilization, and heat to the part comprise the "sine qua non" in the conservative treatment of spreading infections of the extremity. The beneficial effect of bed rest, elevation of the part, and massive hot wet packs changed every two to four hours has remained over the years one of the major miracles of minor surgery. Exception should be made in case of vascular insufficiency. Immobilization of the hand should always be in a position of function. Infections localized to the hand are generally treated with hot soaks for 20 minutes at a time every four hours. Soaking can be overdone, resulting in a lymph stasis and a swollen boggy hand which impedes recovery.

An appropriate antibiotic may aid markedly in aborting the infection, but in some cases may only delay the formation of pus and thus prolong the course of the disease.

The signs of response to conservative treatment will be increased discomfort[12] with decreased tenderness, swelling, and shininess of the overlying skin.

In the treatment of even minor infections of the hand it is important to determine the presence of any systemic disease, such as diabetes or gout, which may jeopardize recovery or confuse the issue.[1,22]

An abscess, or localized collection of pus, should be drained promptly, particularly within a closed space.

In opening an abscess of the hand, two equally important considerations must be kept in mind: (1) adequate drainage of the pus; and (2) subsequent function of the hand. Poorly placed incisions may transect vital structures of the hand or may result in painful scars or crippling contractures. A tourniquet should be used to provide a clear dry operative field. In general, incisions of the palm or volar surfaces of the fingers should be transversely placed, parallel to flexion creases. Incisions should never violate flexion creases at right angles. Vertical incisions may be made only over the midlateral (midradio- or midulnar lateral) aspects of the fingers, over the dorsum of the hand, or over the midulnar or midradial aspects of the wrist. Where a long wound extending from a proximal to distal point is required in the palm or anterior wrist, the incisions should be S-shaped in course, parallel to flexion creases as much as possible, with gentle curves between. Inadequate incisions are often the product of inadequate anesthesia. We believe there is no place for use of "light gas" anesthesia in the adequate drainage of infections of the hand. Pus should always be cultured and sensitivity studies performed. Drains should generally be of rubber, the only exception being for the felon, for which a pack may be used advantageously. Through and through drainage should never be used in the hand.

PARONYCHIA

One of the most common infections of the hand is the paronychia, which involves the soft tissue directly beside and adjacent to the finger nail. A hangnail is frequently the cause, and the infecting organism is generally *Staphylococcus aureus.* Infection of the tissue overlying the base of the nail is termed an eponychia and generally results from direct extension of a paronychia. Extension of infections from paronychia on one side across eponychia to paronychial tissue on the other side of the nail is termed a runaround, and has become relatively uncommon except in children.

For practical purposes paronychia may be classified into three distinct types: superficial, deep, and chronic.

Superficial Type

Most amenable to treatment is the superficial type, which characteristically presents as a small gray-white intracuticular or subcuticular abscess, generally at the junction of paronychia and eponychia (Fig. 14.2.1). A physohex soak, preoperatively helps. This type can be incised without anesthesia, the point of the knife blade being passed into the abscess at an oblique angle (Fig. 14.2.2). A drop or two of pus exudes. A regimen of hot soaks may be instituted to promote drainage. An ointment dressing may be applied to keep the small drainage tract open until the abscess cavity has completely drained.

Deep Paronychia

This type of infection is more deep-seated and diffuse, and presents as a cellulitis with tender swelling which soon involves most of the paronychial tissue (Fig. 14.2.3). Early in its course, when there is no evidence of underlying pus, this type occasionally may be aborted by splint, local heat, and antibiotics. With this regimen, spontaneous drainage of two or three small beads of pus may occur from the sulcus along the lateral border of the nail on the second to fourth day, followed by rapid healing of the lesion. Liberal occlusive ointment dressings may aid in promoting such drainage by keeping the sulcus tissue soft and macerated. Spontaneous drainage of deep paronychia is always through the sulcus.

Where surgical drainage is necessary, proper incision involves: (1) adequate drainage of the sulcus formed by the paronychial tissue around the adjacent lateral border of the fingernail; and (2) adequate exposure and visualization of the most proximal corner of the fingernail. A vertical incision is therefore made with the knife blade so slanted that it is tangential to the dorsolateral curve of the fingernail, its point aimed at the sulcus at the lateral margin of the nail and its sweep parallel to the lateral margin of the nail and ex-

tending to its most proximal point (Fig. 14.2.4 A and B). The lateral margin of the nail is thus exposed over its entire extent. The adjacent eponychial tissue mesial to the incision should then be laid back. Thereby drainage is promoted, and the proximal corner of the nail can be adequately visualized to determine whether or not pus has extended under it (Fig. 14.2.4 C). If this has occurred, the nail, or at least its devitalized portion, must be removed before the infection will subside. Failure to recognize an early subungual abscess in conjunction with a deep paronychia is one of the most common errors in the treatment of the less severe hand infections, and may lead to a long, drawn out inflammatory process which is relieved only after the nail has been removed.

Chronic Paronychia

Suppurative

Chronic suppuration of the paronychial tissue, aside from being caused by devitalized fingernail or retained foreign bodies, may result from fusospirochetal or other specific, overlooked infection. Fusospirochetal infection, although rare, must be considered when the discharge is thin and foul-smelling. The specific organism should be identified by smear or culture.[2,5] In any chronic lesion the presence of osteomyelitis should be ruled out by x-ray. Tuberculosis and other granulomatous infections should also be considered, and, where the process is of long duration, biopsy may be advisable to rule out carcinoma.

Nonsuppurative

The commonest nonsuppurative type of chronic paronychia is caused by mycotic infection and presents as a low grade cellulitis frequently involving the eponychia as well. The delicate cuticle is generally missing in the involved area so that the tissue directly adjacent to the nail gives a slightly "rolled in" appearance.

An "ingrown nail" type of chronic nonsuppurative paronychia presents as a small area of very tender granulations directly adjacent to the lateral border of the fingernail (Fig. 14.2.5). This type may develop after infection, or trauma, or both. Here the problem is essentially mechanical: the lateral border of the nail irritates the granulations and stimulates their proliferation. A few applications of silver nitrate (in stick form) plus a tiny adhesive strapping aimed at pulling the affected paronychial tissue away from the nail border will generally affect a cure. The use of circularly placed, even slightly constrictive, dressings, such as a commercial adhesive bandage circularly placed around the finger, or the use of ointments or soaks will tend to perpetuate this lesion. Occasionally the lateral edge of the nail must be excised.

SUBUNGUAL ABSCESS

Subungual abscess often results from extension of a deep paronychia under one corner of the proximal nail. When this occurs, the portion of proximal nail

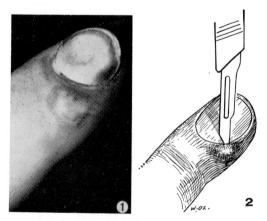

Figure 14.2.1. "Superficial" paronychia.

Figure 14.2.2. "Superficial" paronychia." Incision and drainage without anesthesia.

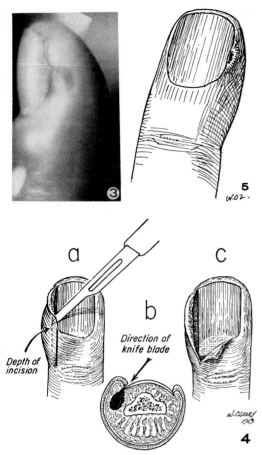

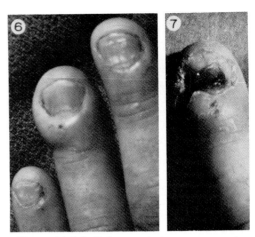

Figure 14.2.6. Subungual abscess secondary to "deep" paronychia.

Figure 14.2.7. Subungual abscess, secondary, 10 days after incision and drainage with removal of nail.

Figure 14.2.3. "Deep" paronychia arising from "hang-nail".

Figure 14.2.4. "Deep" paronychia. Incision and drainage.

Figure 14.2.5. "Ingrown nail" type paronychia.

involved becomes devitalized; devitalized nail plus infection combine to produce a persistent inflammatory process which will be eradicated only by removal of the offending, devitalized nail (Fig. 14.2.6). This may be accomplished by removing the proximal half of the nail, or even its proximal ipsilateral portion, but general over-all best results are attained by removing the entire nail (Fig. 14.2.7). Before removal of the nail, unilateral or bilateral, oblique or vertical incisions are made proximally from the paronychial-eponychial junction, laying back the eponychia to expose fully the offending portion of the nail and assure its removal.

Subungual abscess may also be primary, resulting from puncture wounds and foreign bodies extending under the nail. In these cases a "secondary" paronychia may develop. With infections of this type the paronychial involvement is usually less prominent, showing swelling, redness, and tenderness, and the response to removal of the nail is more rapid, than

in the type where the paronychia is primary and the subungual secondary. An adequately treated "primary" subungual abscess tends to heal more rapidly than a subungual abscess secondary to a "deep" paronychia.

Diagnosis of subungual abscess may be suspected, especially when a deep paronychia is present. Pressure on the base of the nail will generally cause the patient discomfort, and may allow the examiner to detect a slight floating sensation or abnormally increased anteroposterior excursion of the nail base. In neglected cases a subungual infection may progress to the volar aspect of the phalanx and cause a felon, but it is well to remember that marked swelling of the volar pulp may occur secondary to a subungual abscess.

Ancillary Measures of Treatment

The importance of adequate splinting of the finger with paronychial or subungual infection is not always appreciated. One has only to observe the color changes in his paronychial tissue on acute flexion of his finger to appreciate how much variation in tissue tension there is in these areas with movement of the digit. Such variation in tissue tension tends to perpetuate or aggravate any inflammatory process. Many patients are reluctant to have a digit immobilized in a splint for what seemingly is a trivial infection. Some patients have been observed to flex the digit repeatedly to determine for themselves whether the area is as painful as it was somewhat earlier. Such activity may occur subconsciously.

Elevation of the hand and hot soaks are also of value. For soaking before drainage, plain water is perfectly adequate; after drainage a solution containing nascent chlorine, such as Dakin's or Chlorazene, will help promote drainage by causing disintegration of fibrin and crusts.

After the incision has been made, in the early post-operative stage, an ointment dressing may be helpful by tending to prevent healing of the drainage tract and by protecting the sensitive part such as a nail bed from irritating contact with the overlying gauze dressing. Possibly certain antibiotic ointments are helpful.

Where infection is severe and the patient hospitalized, sterile wet saline dressings undoubtedly contitute the best method of promoting drainage of an open lesion between soaks.

FELON

The felon, or whitlow, a closed space infection in the pulp space of the terminal phalanx, is a most difficult problem, primarily because the drainage tract established by proper incision tends to seal off rapidly, before the infectious process has entirely subsided. The pulp space contains fat interspersed by numerous trabeculations of fascial strands, and the offending organism is Staphylococcus in almost every instance. The underlying pathologic anatomy is therefore not unlike that of a carbuncle.

Etiology

The felon most commonly results from a puncture wound of the fat pad on the volar aspect of the distal phalanx, and, not infrequently, especially in neglected cases, a drainage tract through this wound site may be seen (Fig. 14.2.8).

A felon may also develop from a neglected paronychia or subungual abscess (Fig. 14.2.9). On a rare occasion it may be seen after a severe contusion of the pulp without abrasion or break in the skin. Rarely, also, a felon my result from herpes, in which case incision and drainage may be contraindicated. History of exposure to herpes and the presence of vesicles or bullae may help in making this diagnosis.[24]

Diagnosis

Early diagnosis is mandatory, not only because a shorter course of the infection is brought about, but also because a progression of the process causes such tension within the closed space that the blood supply to the terminal phalanx is shut off, resulting in bony necrosis.

Constant, severe pain is an almost constant symptom, being alleviated only after the blood supply has been shut off. Swelling of the volar aspect of the phalanx is constant, but may go unnoticed unless the digit is compared with its contralateral member. Pressure over the volar aspect of the pulp space causes pain unless the condition has progressed to a point where the blood supply has been compromised. In doubtful cases transillumination of both the affected distal phalanx and its counterpart of the other hand over a flashlight in a darkened room will frequently show increased opacity from the infectious process (Fig.

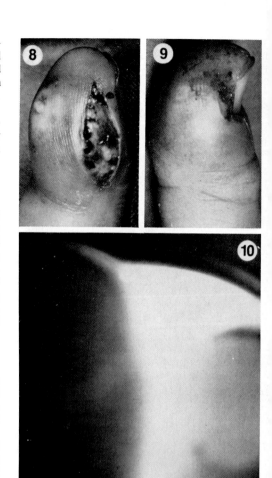

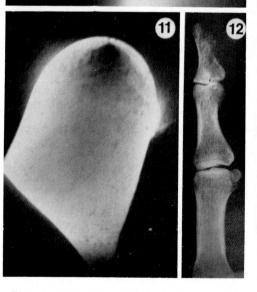

Figure 14.2.8. Felon with drainaging puncture wound of volar fat pad and lateral through-and-through drainage which proved inadequate.

14.2.10).[21] Transillumination will also differentiate a felon from an apical abscess (Fig. 14.2.11). An x-ray is advisable to detect early bony necrosis (Fig. 14.2.12).

Treatment

In certain early cases, where the diagnosis may still be doubtful, conservation therapy in the form of splinting, elevation, and antistaphylococcal antibiotics may be permissible. If favorable response is not evident within 24 hours, surgery is indicated.

The secret of proper surgical treatment lies in adequate drainage of the pulp space. This involves (1) a proper incision, and (2) keeping the wound packed open until the infection within the space has completely subsided. We agree with Louden et al.[11] that "the main concern must be not only to gain free exposure of the lesion but also to retain free blood supply to the skin and underlying tissues, and to secure good functional and cosmetic results."

Incision and drainage of a felon should be an inpatient procedure, with general anesthesia and an elastic-band tourniquet at the base of the digit. A fishmouth incision undoubtedly gives the most adequate drainage, but we have seen numerous instances where such an incision resulted in complete slough of the volar fat pad (Fig. 14.2.13). It is probable that the fishmouth incision, running on either side of the digit, may occasionally cause bilateral thrombosis of the closely adjacent volar digital arteries. This, in our opinion, is the most disastrous complication that may occur in treatment of a felon, far outweighing osteomyelitis of the distal bony phalanx which will generally regenerate if properly drained. For this reason the so-called hockey-stick incision is considered the incision of choice (Fig. 14.2.14 A).

A simple lateral incision or bilateral lateral incision with through and through drainage are totally inadequate in most cases (see Fig. 14.2.8), and a volar incision may leave a tender scar.[3,15,19]

A common error is to make the hockey-stick incision too far volarward. This results in inadequate drainage. Such an improper incision has been depicted as correct in several texts (Fig. 14.2.14 B). Incision

Figure 14.2.9. Felon secondary to paronychia and subungual abscess.

Figure 14.2.10. Transillumination of felon compared with contralateral distal phlanax.

Figure 14.2.11. Apical abscess demonstrated by transillumination. Treated by incision and drainage of finger-tip with wedge resection of distal nail.

Figure 14.2.12. Osteomyelitis of distal phalanx, thumb secondary to a felon.

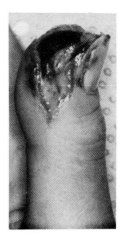

Figure 14.2.13. Gangrene of fat pad developing after "fish-mouth" incision.

should be made so that the knife tip comes down on the midlateral aspect of bony distal phalanx, the sweep of the wound curving around the tip of the finger about 2 mm anterior to the nail. It should commence about 0.5 cm distal to the distal flexion crease of the finger to avoid violation of the oblique septum of Wilkinson (Fig. 14.2.14 A and B). After the incision has been carried down to bony phalanx along its side and tip, as far as its other side but no further, the knife is carried through the lateral incision to bone, and then anteriorly into the pulp space (Fig. 14.2.14 C). By this incision, one is then able to break down all the fibrous trabeculations inserting onto the anterior aspect of bony phalanx within the pulp space (Fig. 14.2.14 D). An obviously necrotic tissue within the pulp space may be advantageously excised. The cavity is then packed open with gauze. We have found that if the cavity is merely drained with a piece of rubber, the wound is not adequately held apart and tends to seal over too quickly, so that reopening may be necessary. The idea of suturing the wound together rather than packing it open, as advanced by Louden et al.[11] and by Scott and Jones,[22] is foreign to our way of thinking. Carter[6] suggests that a polyethylene catheter be inserted deep in the wound for irrigation with antibiotics.

Finally, care must be taken to remove the fingernail with proper paronychial incisions should a subungual abscess and paronychia be present. Failure to recognize and properly treat a coexisting or causal and subungual abscess is an occasional, bad error.

Postoperative Care

Splinting is generally adequately accomplished by the bulky dressing required over the distal half of the finger during the first few postoperative days. Elevation of the hand on a pillow, with bed rest, is ordered.

Antibiotics may be used, but it is generally believed that they are of little value in adequately drained,

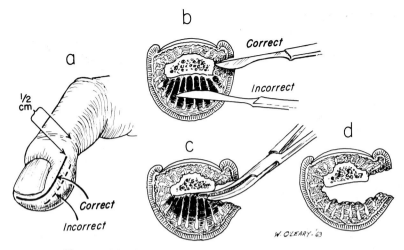

Figure 14.2.14. Proper incision and drainage of felon.

closed space infections unless there is evidence of spread.[25]

Hot soaks are commenced 24 hours after operation; earlier soaking may cause troublesome bleeding. It is recommended that for 24 hours the soaks be carried out with the original dressing in place. Forty-eight hours after incision and drainage, and immediately after a soak, the dressing should be changed and the pack removed. A pack, in contrast to a rubber drain, will leave a gaping wound. A dose of morphine before each early dressing will be greatly appreciated by the patient and facilitate reinsertion of another smaller pack, an important step in proper aftercare. Sterile technique is mandatory with dressing change. Only when the cavity appears clean and the infection subsiding should the patient be discharged from the hospital.

Complications

Necessity for reopening must be anticipated, marked by increased pain, swelling, and tenderness of the fat-pad and by evidence of increased bony necrosis by x-ray. It is our opinion that some severe felons will require reopening no matter how well they are incised primarily and watched postoperatively.

Bone necrosis of the distal phalanx, unless severe, is in itself no great cause for concern and is simply an indication for proper, adequate drainage. Under no circumstance should the bone be subjected to curetting since thereby the viable periosteum may be damaged and the entire bony phalanx lost. Loose spicules of bone may be picked out of the cavity with forceps. If adequate drainage is carried out, any sequestrum of bone will subsequently be extruded from the wound if allowed to do so.

Tenosynovitis may develop by direct extension from a felon. In certain rare, extreme cases, such as an aged arthritic with diabetes, development of tenosynovitis secondary to a severe felon may best be treated by amputation. Otherwise, convalescence may be so prolonged that stiffness of most of the joints of the hand may result.

Infection may extend proximally under the deep fascia of the proximal phalanges. This must be differentiated from tenosynovitis, and properly incised and drained through midlateral incisions extending to the most proximal edge of the process.

Lymphangitis may develop secondary to felon, and is treated with massive hot wet packs, bed rest, and elevation.

SUBFASCIAL INFECTIONS OF THE FINGER

Primary subfascial infection may occur on the volar aspects of either the middle or proximal phalanges. In the middle such an infection involves a closed space, and if neglected, may extend into the flexor tendon sheath or joint. In the proximal phalanx this infection frequently extends proximally into the lumbrical canal or web space (Fig. 14.2.15).

When no point of wounding is evident either by history or physical examination, subfascial infections of the middle and proximal phalanges may easily be confused with tenosynovitis or infection within the joint capsule. Acute gout may be a source of confusion. Treatment consists of a vertical incision over the mid-radiolateral or ulnarlateral aspect of the finger, with dissection medialward, or lateralward, into the involved space on a plane superficial to the flexor tendon sheath but deep to the neurovascular bundle. Drainage should be accomplished with small slips of rubber; splinting in a position of function is important.

WEB SPACE INFECTIONS

Web space or lumbrical space infections are not uncommon, most frequently arising from an infected callus of the palm over the metacarpal head. There is

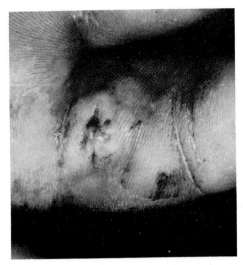

Figure 14.2.15. Subfascial infection, proximal phalanx with minimal but definite extension into web-space.

swelling and tenderness of the web space involved, and characteristically the fingers on either side of the web are held apart. Anterior-posterior pressure over the affected web elicits pain. There may be considerable lymphedema of the dorsum of the hand. In rare instances, a neglected infection in the web space between the index and middle fingers may progress medially to the other two web spaces (Fig. 14.2.16).

A proper approach for drainage of a web space infection consists of a curving incision in the distal palm commencing just proximal to the proximal flexion crease of the lateral finger on its medial aspect, and curving medialward to the distal flexion crease of the palm (Fig. 14.2.17). On the dorsum of the hand, a vertical incision may be made commencing about 1 cm proximal to the edge of the web and carried proximally for 2 cm, or a V-shaped incision proximal to the distal edge of the web may be used. Two small pieces of rubber drain are then inserted, one through each wound (Fig. 14.2.18). Violation of the most distal portion of the web should be avoided.

Complications

Neglected web space infections may extend into the flexor tendon sheath or into the adjacent midpalmar or thenar spaces. They may also dissect distally along the course of the lumbricals causing slough in some instances (Fig. 14.2.19). Rarely they may extend into the dorsal subaponeurotic space.

COLLAR BUTTON ABSCESS

Collar button abscess occurs most notably in the palm of the hand, frequently under a callus over the metacarpal head. Although it has been described in several texts as extending only subepithelially, it may

in fact extend more deeply between fibers of the palmar aponeurosis, from whence it readily extends into the web space. If an adequate incision, which should be transversely placed, is made into this abscess in a bloodless field, and the superficial pus is then wiped away, pressure over the adjacent palm will cause pus to exude through the narrow opening in the palmar fascia which serves as the constricting midportion of the "collar button." Proper extension of the incision may then be made.

DORSAL SUBAPONEUROTIC SPACE ABSCESS

Swelling of the dorsum of the infected hand is common, because of the drainage of lymphatics to this area. Care must be taken not to mistake such swelling for an abscess of the dorsal subaponeurotic space, which is rare. (There are actually three potential spaces on the dorsum of the hand; deep subcutaneous, intertendinous, and subtendinous. Their limitations are not very precise from a clinical viewpoint.[9]) Abscess of the dorsal subaponeurotic space is most often due to a direct extension of infection from the overlying skin. Swelling, tenderness, and occasionally frank fluctuation are present, and the patient is reluctant to flex the metacarpophalangeal joints (Fig. 14.2.20). Treatment consists of adequate incisions, vertically placed between the courses of the underlying extensor tendons.

CELLULITIS

Cellulitis of the hand, generally caused by a variety of hemolytic streptococcus, may cause diffuse and extreme swelling, frequently with marked associated ascending lymphangitis. There may or may not be any obvious point of origin. If no localizing signs of pus in the form of localized pain, swelling, tenderness, or

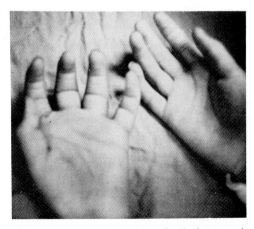

Figure 14.2.16. Infection of all three web-spaces secondary to "collar-button" abscess at base of index finger.

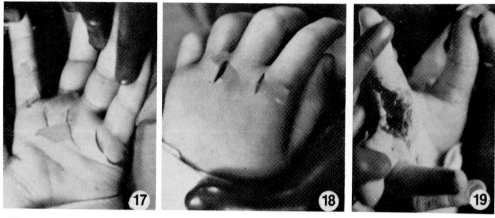

Figure 14.2.17. Proper palmar incisions for infected web-spaces.

Figure 14.2.18. Proper dorsal incisions for infected web-spaces.

Figure 14.2.19. Slough along course of lumbrical canal secondary to neglected web-space infection.

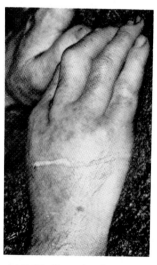

Figure 14.2.20. Dorsal subaponeurotic space abscess secondary to puncture wound.

fluctuation are present, treatment should be conservative, and consist of bed rest with massive hot wet packs, elevation, and immobilization of the hand and arm. Antibiotic therapy should be instituted if the patient's constitutional reaction is severe.[25] X-rays should be taken for question of retained foreign body, and, if there is no history consistent with infection, gout should be ruled out.

GRANULOMA PYOGENICUM

This small, red, easily bleeding, tumor-like projection of granulation tissue arising at the site of a subacute or chronic infection may give a startling appearance suggestive of a rapidly growing carcinoma. A history of a recent infectious process at the site of the "tumor" establishes the diagnosis. It is adequately treated by excision at its base, which is then cauterized with silver nitrate. One or two subsequent cauterizations will generally suffice to eradicate the process.

FURUNCLE AND CARBUNCLE

Furuncles commonly occur on the hair-bearing areas of the dorsum of the hand, particularly over the dorsum of the proximal phalanx. This area is particularly vulnerable to changes in tissue tension associated with active motion of the finger, as a result of which the infection may rapidly progress to become a carbuncle, with multiple heads and draining sinuses. Immobilization, with adequate incision and drainage, constitutes the most important treatment of this lesion. It should be remembered that all carbuncles extend down to deep fascia; adequate incision should carry to this level.

REASONABLE ERROR IN HAND INFECTIONS

Incision and drainage of cellulitis, in the absence of pus, is to be avoided wherever possible. However, where there is strong suspicion that a closed space lesion of the hand is infected, it is far better to open this space in error, and find no pus, than it is to delay opening until the process has become well established. This principle of aggressiveness is particularly wise in the treatment of tenosynovitis, felon, and subungual abscess.

HUMAN BITE

Human bite infection, like Vincent's angina, has become a much less severe problem since the advent of antibiotics. The potential of severe infection, however, remains. The causative wound most commonly occurs over the dorsum of a metacarpophalangeal joint as a result of an ill advised and poorly aimed blow of the clenched fist, which strikes an adversary's incisor tooth. The relatively small ensuing laceration may hide a partially divided extensor tendon or a violated joint capsule. Although a great variety of organisms may inoculate the wound, the most dangerous is the anaerobic streptococcus which grows in an anaerobic environment. Such an environment is readily established by the narrow penetrating nature of the wound, in the joint capsule, which is subcutaneous, and by the extensor tendon which glides laterally in making a fist, but seals off the wound on extension. If *Staphylococcus aureus* coagulase positive is present in addition, the complication rate approaches 100 per cent.[7] Because of the circumstances involved, patients frequently try to hide this injury or strongly deny its true cause. For this reason the infection is frequently well established when first seen (Fig. 14.2.21).

Before the advent of antibiotics, ankylosis of joints was common. The infection was often so severe that some authors recommended wide diathermy excision in early cases.[7] Today the operation is performed if the patient is seen within eight hours. The anaerobic state of the wound is converted into an aerobic state by adequate debridement; injured tendons are not repaired primarily; a violated joint capsule is drained through adequate incisions on either side; the injured hand is splinted in a position of function; wet dressings of hydrogen peroxide or zinc peroxide are used and the patient is hospitalized and kept in bed with the hand elevated on two pillows.[4] If seen after eight hours the wound is dressed, splinted, and the patient is given parenteral antibiotics. Using such a regimen, together with massive doses of penicillin, the Boston City Hospital Service has seen only three cases of ankylosis in the past 20 years.

MELENEY'S INFECTION

Meleney's infection, or progressive synergistic gangrene, is caused by the synergistic action of a microaerophilic nonhemolytic streptococcus and an aerobic hemolytic staphylococcus. It may be very refractory to treatment, especially if unrecognized for some time. The most characteristic feature of the infection is a progressively widening ulceration extending down to fascia, having at its edges undermined skin, the rim of which is gangrenous (Fig. 14.2.22).[18] The degree of surrounding cellulitis, and also the degree of constitutional symptoms, may be variable. A culture positive for the microaerophilic streptococcus may be difficult to obtain, and then only by removing some of the infected tissue at its periphery and placing this directly into an anaerobic medium.

The most important features of proper treatment are early recognition, wide excision of skin and subcutaneous tissue down to fascia on all sides of the infection, and local application of wet dressings contain-

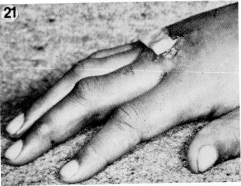

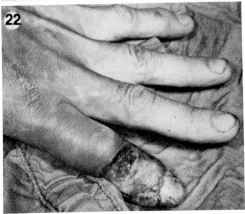

Figure 14.2.21. Human bite infection.

Figure 14.2.22. "Meleney's infection" of index finger.

ing either hydrogen peroxide or activated zinc peroxide.[17] Since the latter agent frequently cakes on the wound and forms a crust, we have found hydrogen peroxide solutions more satisfactory. Sensitivity tests are performed and the proper antibiotic is given. Meleney recommends bacitracin locally.[18]

REFERENCES

1. Bains, J. W. Care and treatment of hand infections. Va. Med. Mon., *95:* 601-606, 1968.
2. Bendeck, T. Fusospirochetal paronychia. Surgery, *11:* 75-80, 1942.
3. Bolton, H., Fowler, P. J., and Jepson, R. P. The natural history and treatment of pulp space infection and osteomyelitis of the terminal phalanx. J. Bone Joint Surg., *31B:* 499-504, 1949.
4. Boyce, F. F. Human bites: analysis of ninety cases. South. Med. J., *35:* 631-638, 1942.
5. Brand, C. Ulcerous paronychias due to fusospirochetosis. Arch. Dermatol., *188:* 181-187, 1949.
6. Carter, S. J., and Mersheimer, W. L. Infections of the hand. Orthop. Clin. North Am., *1, 2:* 455-466, 1970.
7. Farmer, C. B., and Mann, R. J. Human bite infections of the hand. South. Med. J., *59:* 515-518, 1966.
8. Kanavel, A. B. Study of acute phlegmons of the hand.

Surg. Gynecol. Obstet., *1:* 221-260, 1905.

9. Kaplan, E. B. *Functional and Surgical Anatomy of the Hand.* Philadelphia, Lippincott, 1953.

10. Koch, S. L. Editorial:Inflamed and injured tissues need rest. Surg. Gynecol. Obstet., *82:* 749, 1946.

11. Louden, J. B., Miniero, J. O., and Scott, J. C. Infections of the hand. J. Bone Joint Surg.,*30B:* 409-429, 1948.

12. Lowden, T. G. Infection of digital pulp space. Lancet, *1:* 196-199, 1951.

13. Lowden, T. G. Prevention and treatment of hand infections. Post. Grad. Med. J., *40:* 247-252, 1964.

14. Lowden, T. G. Severe infections of the hand. Physiotherapy, *54:* 128-130, 1968.

15. Mason, M. L. Fifty years' progress in surgery of the hand. Int. Abstr. Surg., *101:* 541-564, 1955.

16. Mason, M. L., and Koch, S. L. Human bite infections of the hand. Surg. Gynecol. Obstet., *51:* 591-625, 1930.

17. Meleney, F. L. Zinc peroxide in the treatment of microaerophibic and anaerobic infections. Ann. Surg., *101:* 997-1011, 1935.

18. Meleney, F. *Clinical Aspects and Treatment of Surgical Infections.* Philadelphia, Saunders, 1949.

19. Pilcher, R. S., Dawson, R. L. G., Milstein, B. B., and Riddle, A. G. Infections of the fingers and hand. Lancet, *1:* 777-783, 1949.

20. Rob, C., and Smith, R. In *Clinical Surgery,* Vol. 7, edited by G. Palvertaft. London, Butterworth, 1966.

21. Samuel, E. P. Transillumination of whitlows of terminal phalanx. Lancet, *1:* 763-765, 1950.

22. Scott, J. C., and Jones, B. V. Results of treatment of infections of the hand. J. Bone Joint Surg., *34B:* 581-587, 1952.

23. Sneddon, J. Dressings in hand sepsis. Br. Med. J., *1:* 372-373, 1969.

24. Stern, H., Elek, S. D., Miller, D. M., and Anderson, H. F. Herpetic whitlow: A form of cross-infection in hospitals. Lancet, *2:* 871-874, 1959.

25. Stone, N. H., Hursh, H., Humphrey, C. R., and Bostwick, J. A.: Empirical selection of antibiotics for hand infections. J. Bone Joint Surg.,*51A:* 899, 1969.

26. Trafford, H. S. Infections of hand. Practitioner, *201:* 723-729, 1968.

C.

The Grave Infections of the Hand

J. Edward Flynn, M.D.

Lymphangitis, deep fascial space abscesses, and acute suppurative tenosynovitis are major infections which are usually distinct, although the incidence of these infections has decreased to 25 per cent to 30 per cent of what it was before antibiotics, they present a most serious problem when encountered. A knowl-

edge of the anatomy involved is basic for a proper understanding of the clinical aspects and treatment of each of these entities.

LYMPHANGITIS

Lymphangitis is an inflammatory process of the lymphatic vessels. The two types of lymphangitis are superficial and deep. Superficial lymphangitis involves the superficial vessels that arise from plexuses in the skin. The collecting trunks of superficial lymphatics run in the subcuticular tissue. Deep lymphangitis involves the deep lymphatic vessels found in association with the arterial system. The superficial lymphatics of the fingers consist of volar and dorsal networks that converge into trunks at the sides of the fingers (Fig. 14.3.1). The digital trunks reach the bases of the fingers in the interdigital spaces and traverse the dorsal aspect of the hand to the wrist. The network of superficial lymphatics of the palm drain into trunklets that divide into external, internal, inferior, superior, and central (Fig. 14.3.2). In the forearm, the volar vessels divide into three groups, external, internal, and median, and the volar lymphatics are more numerous than the dorsal lymphatics. In the arm, the trunks unite into a single bundle on the external surface. The majority of collecting vessels terminate in the axilla in the humeral chain of axillary lymph nodes. Two or three of the most internal end in the epitrochlear lympth node, with efferent vessels that perforate the fascia to reach the deep vessels (Fig.

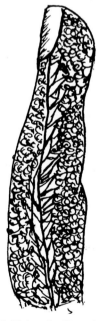

Figure 14.3.1. Network of lymphatics in the skin drain medially and laterally into trunklets in the subcutaneous tissue.

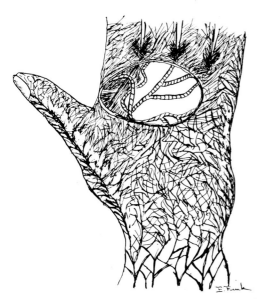

Figure 14.3.2. Superior, inferior, medial and lateral superficial lymphatics in palm extend from all borders to the dorsum. The central superficial lymphatics extend into the deep lymphatics along the palmar arch.

14.3.3). The most external trunk separates itself from other collecting vessels in the region of the humeral insertion of the deltoid and ascends in the deltopectoral groove, where it may traverse one or several lymph nodes. This trunk usually passes into a subclavian node placed at the spot where the cephalic joins the axillary vein (Fig. 14.3.4). The deep lymphatics follow the course of the brachial artery, usually with two lymphatics for each artery. The deep lymphatics of the upper extremity may be divided into radial, ulnar, anterior interosseous, posterior interosseous, and humeral. The radial trunks drain lymph from the part supplied by the deep volar arch and the deep palmar branch of the ulnar artery. The ulnar trunks drain lymph from the part supplied by the superficial volar arch and the superficial palmar branch of the radial artery. The anterior and posterior interosseous lymphatics follow the arteries of the same names. The humeral trunks are two or three in number. They run by the side of the brachial artery and terminate in the humeral chain of axillary lymph nodes.[3][15][17][18][21][22][27][31][33]

Symptomatology

Kanavel[21] stressed the importance of differentiating lymphangitis from other major infections of the hand and reiterated the need to distinguish superficial from deep lymphangitis. With superficial lymphangitis, there is usually a history of an abrasion or superficial wound of the hand. General signs of infection — fever, leukocytosis, nausea, vomiting, and tachycardia — may be present. Red streaks extend up the forearm and arm. Superficial lymphangitis usually

lacks the rapid and great swelling of the entire hand and forearm. With deep lymphangitis, there is a history of a deep infection, such as osteomyelitis. The general signs of infection are more pronounced than those found with superficial lymphangitis. Red streaks may or may not be seen. The outstanding differential point is that with deep lymphangitis, there is usually a rapid and striking increase in swelling of the entire hand and forearm. With lymphangitis there is voluntary movement of fingers without pain, absence of pain on hyperextension of fingers and thumb, absence of tenderness over tendon sheaths, absence of bulging of the palm, and absence of tenderness over the midpalmar and thenar spaces.[15][18][21]

Incidence

The incidence of lymphangitis has varied in three different eras. In the preantibiotic era, previous to penicillin, lymphangitis was common. Sufanilamide, sulfapyridine, sulfathiazole, and sulfadiazine in adequate blood concentration, although toxic, provided bacteriostasis of the hemolytic streptococcus which most often caused lymphangitis in the preantibotic era.

In the antibiotic-sensitive era (1942 to 1954), with the advent of penicillin and broad spectrum antibiotics, a sharp decrease in incidence to about 20 per cent that in the preantibiotic era was seen. This low incidence of 20 per cent was maintained until about 1954.

In the so-called antibiotic-resistant era (1954 to 1958), with the virulent *Staphylococcus aureus,* a sharp rise in incidence to about 45 per cent that in preantibiotic era has been noted. However, since 1959 there has been a decrease to about 30 per cent that seen before antibiotics (Graph 14.3.1).[18]

Treatment

Local measures to wall off and overcome infection together with procedures designed to support the system, increase its resisting power, eliminate toxins, and antibiotics are necessary. In cases of lymphangitis, until localization is present, warm saline dressings are used, together with cathartics, adequate electrolyte and fluid intake, sedatives, and antibiotics.

Warm saline dressings are used locally to produce hyperemia; their value in combination with antibiotics has been challenged.

Hospitalization, with local and systemic rest, is insisted on, especially in severe infections. Immobilization is necessary because every movement of the muscles of the fingers, hand, forearm, and arm favors lymphatic circulation and dissemination of infection. The hand should be elevated on pillows to allow proper lymphatic drainage. Seriously ill patients should be given adequate fluids and small amounts of easily digested food. Adequate quantities of fluids are important for diluting and eliminating toxins.[15][17][18][21]

When a wound is present a culture is taken and

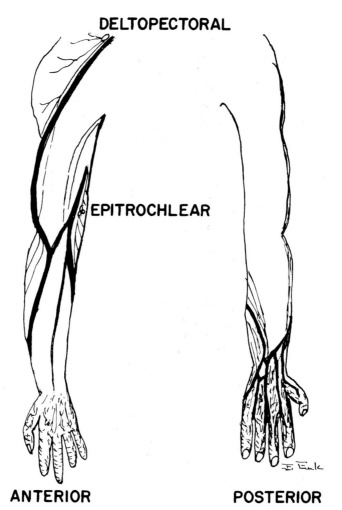

DELTOPECTORAL

EPITROCHLEAR

ANTERIOR

POSTERIOR

Figure 14.3.3. Lymphatic drainage of the thumb, index, and radial half of the middle finger is mainly by lymphatic vessels traveling with the cephalic vein. In the forearm the vessels are radial, median, and ulnar. Epitrochlear nodes may be by-passed by some lymphatic vessels.

sensitivity tests are performed. A specific antibiotic is given, if possible.

If the situation is urgent before organisms are identified, lincomycin, methicillin, erythromycin, and chloramphenicol are probably best for suspected gram-positive organisms, and kanomycin for gram-negative organisms.[32]

Complications

The complications of lymphangitis have been greatly decreased since the advent of antibiotics but still occur, often after antibiotic therapy has been discontinued.[17]

An understanding of the anatomy involved explains certain complications. The superficial lymphatics run in the subcutaneous tissue and may cause extensive subcutaneous destruction of connective tissue, with the formation of slough that is treated by incision and drainage usually on the dorsum. The superficial lymphatics especially, empty into the epitrochlear, axillary, deltopectoral, supraclavicular, and other lymph nodes. Abscesses arise from infected lymph nodes. Rarely a large quantity of pus fills the axilla and extends under the pectoral and subscapular muscles and must be drained. Subclavicular and shoulder abscesses are very rare and develop along the course of the lymphatics lying in the pectorodeltoid groove. Such infections have their origin most often in the long finger. The deep lymphatics are close to the tendon sheaths and may cause suppurative tenosynovitis. The humeral chain of axillary nodes eventually empty into the thoracic duct and general circulation, and may be the cause of septicemia or pyemia.[21] [27] [30] [31]

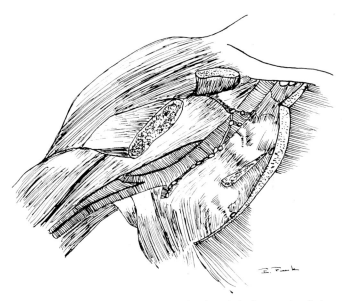

Figure 14.3.4. Superficial lymphatic drainage from the thumb, index, and radial one-half of the middle finger is mainly by way of lymphatics which follow the cephalic vein to the subclavian lymph nodes.

DEEP FASCIAL SPACE ABSCESS

A knowledge of the anatomy of the deep fascial spaces in necessary for the understanding of the signs and treatment of deep abscesses of the palm. Since Kanavel[21] described these surgically important spaces as the midpalmar and thenar, there has been some controversy about the anatomy. Brickel[8] stated that there is one common deep fascial space and not two. Anson and Ashley[1] described a fascial septum which separated the two spaces.

Kaplan[22] believes that there are two deep fascial spaces in the palm, separated by a fascial septum. In 100 anatomic specimens in which dissection was performed with special consideration of the fascial distributions, we found a defininte septum of fascia coming from the undersurface of the flexor tendons of the long finger, which was attached to the entire length of the long finger metacarpal bone (Fig. 14.3.5). This septum divides the palm into two fascial compartments, the midpalmar and thenar spaces.[13] [14] It is convenient to remember that the deep fascial spaces are deep to the flexor tendons. The midpalmar space extends from the middle metacarpal bone ulnarward to the radial side of the fifth metacarpal bone. Anteriorly this space is bounded by the flexor tendons of the long, ring, and little fingers, the third and fourth lumbrical muscles, and the thin fascia that connects these tendons and muscles. The posterior boundary or floor is formed by the fascia covering the second and third volar interosseous muscles, and the third, fourth, and fifth metacarpal bones. In the distal third of the floor, small compartments are formed, since septa coming

from the undersurface of the palmar aponeurosis are attached to the fascia of the volar interosseous muscles. These small compartments communicate with the midpalmar space. The medial boundary is the fascia on the radial side of the hypothenar muscles. The lateral boundary is the midpalmar septum, which extends from the undersurface of the flexor digitorum profundus tendon of the middle finger to the middle metacarpal bone (Fig. 14.3.6). Distally the midpalmar space extends to about 2 cm proximally to the webs. The distal boundary is composed mainly of fascial septa extending from the palmar aponeurosis to the floor of the space and to some transverse fasciculi. The proximal boundary is a thin fascial septum usually found at the level of the distal end of the transverse carpal ligament.[13] [14] [17]

The thenar space is bounded posteriorly by the adductor pollicis mescle. Medially, the boundary is the midpalmar septum, a thin fascia extending from beneath the flexor digitorum profundus tendon of the long finger to the third metacarpal bone (Fig. 14.3.7). Proximally, in all cases, this fascia, which is a part of the adductor fascia, forms the boundary. The proximal boundary is found at about the level of the distal end of transverse carpal ligament. The anterior boundary or roof is the thin layer of fascia formed as the midpalmar septum splits and courses laterally. In its lateral course this fascia ensheaths the flexor tendons of the index finger to form part of the anterior boundary. The lateral boundary of the thenar space is formed by the thin fascia as it extends over the lateral edge of the adductor pollicis muscle and is attached to the dorsal aspect of this muscle. This distribution of fascia

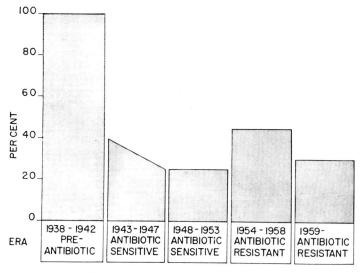

Graph 14.3.1 Lymphangitis incidence

over the anterior, lateral, and dorsal aspects of the adductor pollicis muscle clearly indicates why abscesses of the thenar space may extend to the posterior aspect of the muscle. The fact remains, however, that abscesses of the space tend to remain anterior to the adductor pollicis muscle.[13] [14] [17] [18] [21]

The midpalmar septum, which separates the midpalmar space from the thenar space, is a thin structure but is apparently adequate to keep an infection confined to one space. In a review of 100 cases of deep fascia space infection, both the thenar and midpalmar space were involved in only two cases, and in each case extensive local necrosis and osteomyelitis were found.[12] [13] [14]

Incidence

Infections of the deep fascial spaces have been less frequent since the advent of antibiotics. In 100 of the early cases studied at the Boston City Hospital, the thenar space was involved in 70, and the midpalmar in 30 cases.[15]

We have studied the incidence over three eras. Era I is the preantibiotic era, previous to 1942. There were 100 cases at the Boston City Hospital over a seven-year period from 1935 to 1942. Some sulfonamides were used in this era. Era II is the so-called antibiotic-sensitive era and extends over an 11-year period from 1943 through 1953. In Era II penicillin and other broad spectrum antibiotics were used and the predominant organism was hemolytic streptococcus. In the first five years of Era II, 25 cases were treated, an incidence of 35 per cent that in Era I. In the last six years of Era II, there were 18 cases, a drop to 19 per cent of the incidence in Era I.

Era III is the so-called antibiotic-resistant era. This era began in 1954 with the appearance of the virulent *Staphylococcus aureus*. From 1954 through 1958

there were 35 cases, an incidence of 49 per cent that of Era I. Since 1958 there has been a decrease to about four a year or an incidence of 28 per cent that of the preantibiotic era (Graph 14.3.2).[15] [17] [18]

Etiology

The commonest causes for thenar space abscesses are puncture wounds, acute suppurative tenosynovitis from index, thumb, and long fingers, septic abrasions, and blebs. The main cause for midpalmar space abscesses are lumbrical space infections from the lumbrical canal of the ring fingers, puncture wounds, septic abrasions, and acute suppurative tenosynovitis from the middle and ring fingers. Two of our cases of thenar space abscesses and two of midpalmar space abscesses developed from tenosynovitis of the long finger.[13] [15] [17] [18]

Differential Diagnosis

Tenderness is the most important sign. Swelling is of value.

With thenar space abscess there is tenderness over the thenar area on the palm. There is a rapid increase in swelling of the thenar area. The thenar area seems to balloon out from the radial longitudinal crease of the palm. Swelling over the dorsum of the hand is great. The index finger is usually flexed (Fig. 14.3.8*A* and *B*).

There is tenderness over the midpalmar space on the palm with midpalmar space abscess. With midpalmar space abscess swelling obliterates the palmar concavity, a bulge is seen over the palm, and swelling over the dorsum of th hand is great. The long and ring ringers are usually flexed. Temperature ranges from 100° to 104°F.(Fig. 14.3.9).[13] [15] [17] [18] [21]

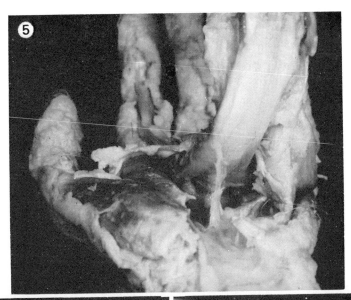

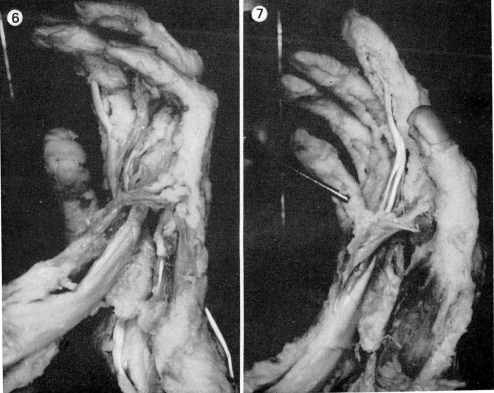

Figure 14.3.5. Middle palmar septum divides the palm into the thenar and midpalmar spaces
Figure 14.3.6. Middle palmar septum forms the lateral boundary of the midpalmar space
Figure 14.3.7. Middle palmar septum forms the medial boundary of the thenar space

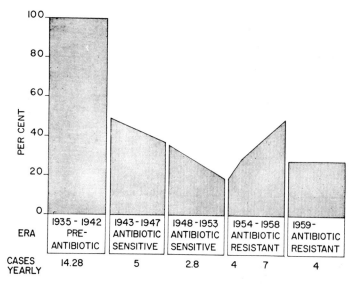

ERA	1935 - 1942 PRE- ANTIBIOTIC	1943-1947 ANTIBIOTIC SENSITIVE	1948-1953 ANTIBIOTIC SENSITIVE	1954 - 1958 ANTIBIOTIC RESISTANT	1959- ANTIBIOTIC RESISTANT
CASES YEARLY	14.28	5	2.8	4 7	4

Graph 14.3.2. Deep fascial space infection incidence (240 cases)

Mortality

There was a 3 per cent mortality in the preantibiotic era. The causes of death were bronchopneumonia, septicemia, and uncontrolled diabetes. Since the advent of antibiotics there has been no mortality in our series.[15][17][18]

Treatment

Thenar space abscess is best drained by an oblique incision over the dorsum of the thumb-index web, at the middle of a line drawn between the distal ends of the first and second metacarpals with the thumb hyperextended. The incision is carried through skin and deep fascia (Fig. 14.3.10). The thin subaponeurotic fascia that forms the lateral boundary of the thenar space and is attached to the dorsum of the adductor pollicis is then incised. Pus may be found dorsal to the adductor pollicis. A hemostat is then carried over the lateral edge of the adductor pollicis to the anterior surface of this muscle to drain the abscess. A rubber tissue drain is used for 24 hours.

Preferably a transverse incision is made for mid-palmar space abscess, parallel to the distal transverse crease and over the point of maximal tenderness. The transverse incision is carried through skin and palmar aponeurosis. The underlying thin subaponeurotic fascia, which is found between the flexor tendons, is incised longitudinally to enter the midpalmar space. A rubber tissue drain is used for 24 hours or longer if necessary. (Fig. 14.3.11).[15][17][18][21]

In the past few years, postincisional perfusion of the

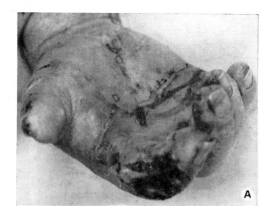

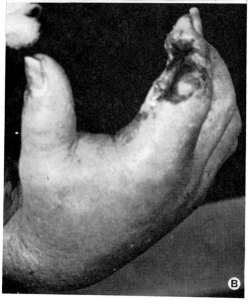

Figure 14.3.8. A. Thenar space abscess developed from acute suppurative tenosynovitis of right index finger. There is great swelling of thenar area. *B.* Swelling is greater over the dorsum than over the palm with thenar space abscess.

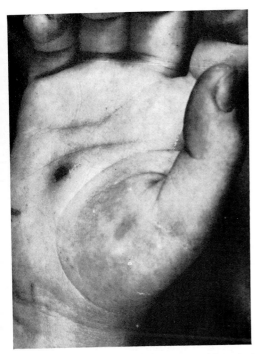

Figure 14.3.9. Palmar concavity is obliterated with midpalmar space abscess.

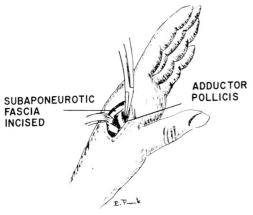

SUBAPONEUROTIC FASCIA INCISED

ADDUCTOR POLLICIS

E. Funk

Figure 14.3.10. Incision for thenar space abscess

abscess cavities with penicillin or some other broad spectrum antibiotic to which the organism is sensitive has been used. The incisions are the same, pus is evacuated, slough is removed. A 3-inch long and 3-mm wide polyethylene tube with perforations is inserted into the abscess cavity. A Rochester needle, 16 bore, is inserted with the tube. When the tube is in place the Rochester needle is removed. When penicillin is used, one million units of penicillin is added to one liter of saline solution every 24 hours. The infected hand is placed in a sterile pan and covered with a sterile towel. One of our associates[9] has had excel-

lent results with this method. It is a logical procedure, especially for early cases. Parenteral antibiotics are also used.

ACUTE SUPPURATIVE TENOSYNOVITIS

Suppurative inflammation of the flexor-tendon sheaths of the hand presents a controversial problem. A knowledge of the anatomy of the sheaths is basic for the proper treatment of suppurative tenosynovitis.

Before Sappey's[31] anatomic report a study of deep abscess of the hand was begun. Bauchet's[6] book on infections of the hand published in 1859 was a classic but lacked a treatise on the lymphatic vessels.

Early anatomists described accurately the synovial sheaths of the flexor tendons of the index, long, and ring fingers. These sheaths begin at the bases of the distal phalanges and extend about 2 cm proximal to the web.

Poirier and Cuneo[30] stated that in 19 of 20 cases the sheath of the flexor pollicis longus was continuous with the radial bursa. The tendon sheath of the flexor tendons of the little finger is continuous with the ulnar bursa in about half of all cases according to Poirier, but other authors disagree. We have seen infection of the flexor tendon sheath of the little finger clinically limited to the finger in only three cases. Poirier stated that the radial and ulnar bursas had no communication with each other, and cited Gosselin,[19] who had observed it only once. Kanavel[21] stated that clinically the communication between the two bursas is frequent. He found it in about half of his cases. Clinically, we have found a spread of infection from the radial to the ulnar bursa in 80 per cent of cases, and a spread from the ulnar to the radial bursa in 70 per cent (Fig. 14.3.12 *A* and *B*).[16] [17] Kanavel described an intermediary posterior palmar sheath connecting the radial and ulnar bursas in 80 per cent of dissections, and an

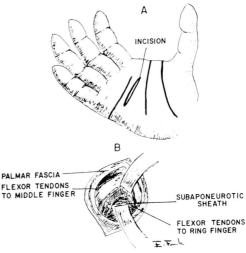

A

INCISION

B

PALMAR FASCIA
FLEXOR TENDONS
TO MIDDLE FINGER

SUBAPONEUROTIC SHEATH

FLEXOR TENDONS TO RING FINGER

E. Funk

Figure 14.3.11. Incision for midpalmar space abscess

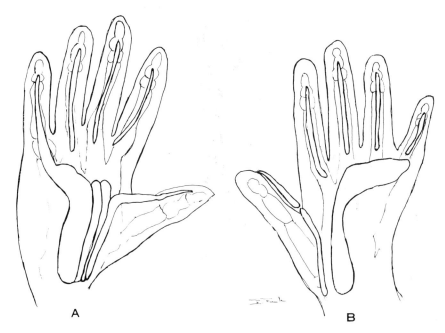

Figure 14.3.12. Diagram of two types of flexor tendon sheaths. *A.* The tendon sheath of the little finger is continuous with the ulnar bursa and that of the thumb with the radial bursa. There are communications between the radial and ulnar bursas in the wrist. *B.* The tendon sheaths of the thumb and little fingers are divided, and the radial and ulnar bursas do not communicate in the wrist.

anterior intermediary palmar sheath connecting the radial and ulnar bursas.[21]

Kanavel[21] stressed the four cardinal signs of suppurative tenosynovitis as follows: tenderness over the involved tendon sheath, pain on hyperextending the finger, flexion deformity, and swelling of the part involved. He also emphasized the need for differentiating acute suppurative tenosynovitis, lymphangitis, and deep fascial space abscess (Fig. 14.3.13*A* and *B*).

Incidence

Suppurative tenosynovitis has been less frequent since the advent of antibiotics.

The incidence has been studied in three eras. In Era I, there were 100 cases treated at the Boston City Hospital over a five-year period, 1938 through 1942.[16] In Era II, 1943 to 1953, 50 cases were seen, over the first six years (1943 to 1948), an incidence of 42 per cent of that seen in Era I. In the second half of the antibiotic-sensitive era, 1949-1953, a five-year period, 24 cases were encountered, an incidence of 24 per cent of the frequency before antibiotics. In Era III, 40 cases were encountered in the first five years, 1954 to 1958, a considerable increase to 40 per cent that before antibiotics. Since 1959 there has been an average of about five cases a year, a noticeable decrease to 25 per cent that found before antibiotics (Graph 14.3.3).[17]

Etiology

The origin of the infection is either a direct inoculation of the tendon sheath or a delayed inoculation in which infection spreads from a neighboring pathologic process. In our series at the Boston City Hospital, 59 per cent were of direct and 41 per cent were of delayed origin. Puncture wounds are the most common injuries causing suppurative tenosynovitis. In infections of direct origin, puncture wounds occurred in 27 per cent, lacerations in 18 per cent, and open dislocations and gunshot wounds in 2 per cent each. In infections of delayed inoculation, puncture wounds occurred in 5 per cent, lacerations in 12 per cent, abrasions in 8 per cent, human bite and felon in 6 per cent each, and blebs and callus in 1 per cent each.[15] [18]

Classification and Results

The cases were classified on the basis of functional results.

Group 1 (good)

Results were considered optimal in cases with normal or almost normal function of tendons and those with complete or almost complete motions of all finger joints. There was occasionally, slight limitation of extreme flexion. Active flexion in each interphalangeal joint was about 90 per cent. On flexion the tip of the finger touched or almost touched the palm.

Group 2 (Fair)

Cases with fair results included partial function of tendons, the limitation usually being caused by adhesions, and active but limited motion in the proximal or

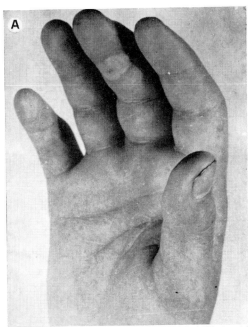

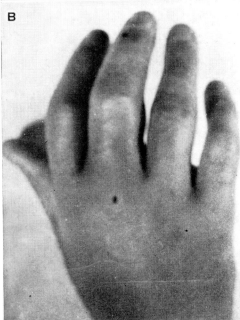

Figure 14.3.13. A. Flexion deformity of long finger with acute suppurative tenosynovitis. *B.* Swelling is greater on the dorsum than on the volar aspect with acute suppurative tenosynovitis of the long finger.

distal interphalangeal joints or both. Motion in the metacarpophalangeal joint was normal or slightly limited. A fist could be made actively. Active flexion in each interphalangeal joint was at least 45 per cent or the equivalent. Actively the digits could be flexed so

that the tips of the fingers reached to within 2 cm of touching the palm.

Group 3 (Poor)

Poor results included sloughed tendons with loss of flexion of the middle or distal phalanx, or both, and ankylosis of the proximal or distal interphalangeal joint. Motions in the metacarpophalangeal joint may not be present. Active flexion of each interphalangeal joint was less than 45 per cent or the equivalent. With active flexion the tip of the finger did not reach to within 2 cm of touching the palm. Amputations and deaths are in this group.[14] [15] [16] [17]

From 1943 to 1953, with antibiotics as an adjunct to surgery, optimal results more than doubled and poor results decreased to about one-third of what they were before the use of antibiotics. However, from 1954 to 1958, with *Staphylococcus aureus* the predominant bacteria, results reverted back to about 40 per cent those of the preantibiotic era. Since 1959 results have again improved to about those of the antibiotic-sensitive era (1943 to 1953) (Table 14.3.1).[15] [18]

Bacteriology

In the preantibiotic era (before 1942) and in the antibiotic sensitive era (1943 to 1953) *Streptococcus haemolyticus* was the predominant organism. Since 1954, hemolytic *Staphylococcus aureus* has been the predominant bacteria. In all eras, mixed infections were most noxious. *Staphylococcus aureus* was innocuous from 1938 to 1953, most virulent from 1954 to 1958, but less virulent since 1959 (Table 14.3.2).[15] [18]

The hemolytic streptococcus most prevalent in the preantibiotic era is most vulnerable to antibiotics and today is less threatening. *Staphylococcus aureus,* the leading offender today, produces a golden pigment on colonies grown on agar medium and thus is called *aureus*. Staphylococci that have the ability to coagulate citrated or oxalated plasma are reported by the laboratory as "*Staphylococcus aureus* coagulase positive."

The toxin of the *Staphylococcus aureus* causes a lysis of red and white blood cells, also a necrosis of living cells and tissues on which bacteria multiply and elaborate pus. In developing abscesses, the bacteria form clumps with a protective covering of fibrin. The surrounding blood vessels become thrombosed. Thus antibiotics in the circulating blood, even in high Titers cannot reach the bacteria within the abscess.

Staphylococci may become antibiotic-resistant. Some strains produce penicillinase, which destroys penicillin. Resistance to antibiotics reaches its peak on about the third day of bacterial invasion. Thus it is urgent to give large doses of the antibiotics prior to the third day of invasion.[11]

Complications

The incidence and severity of complications decreased in the antibiotic-sensitive era, increased in the

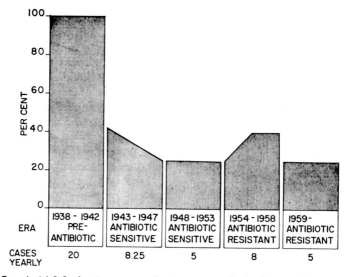

Graph 14.3.3. Acute suppurative tenosynovitis incidence (89 cases)

TABLE 14.3.1
*Acute suppurative tenosynovitis:
comparative end results*

Time	No. of Cases	Classification (%)		
		Good	Fair	Bad
Preantibiotic era (1938-1942)	100	33	20	47
Antibiotic sensitive era (1943-1953)	70	68	16	16
Antibiotic resistant era				
(1954-1958)	40	33	27	39
(1959-now)	98	71	14	14

TABLE 14.3.2
*Acute suppurative tenosynovitis results in three
epochs with hemolytic Staphylococcus aureus*

	Good Group	Fair Group	Bad Group
Preantibiotic era (1938-1942)	16	4	1
Antibiotic-sensitive era (1943-1953)	10	2	1
Antibiotic-resistant era			
(1954-1958)	7	4	8
(1959-now)	38	3	3

antibiotic-resistant era, and have decreased since 1959.

Previous to antibiotics or before 1942, tendon slough was the main cause for poor results. The incidence of this complication has decreased greatly since the advent of antibiotics (Table 14.3.3).[15] [18]

Treatment

Since the advent of antibiotics more investigations of acute suppurative tenosynovitis than of the other major hand infections have been reported.

Five types of treatment have been suggested for acute suppurative tenosynovitis since the use of antibiotics: antibiotic therapy alone in the early stages; intraarterial injection of antibiotics as an adjunct to surgery; removal of pus, with irrigation, application or instillation of an antibiotic locally; excision with suture technique (excision of slough and necrotic tissue and suture after incision); and adequate incision and drainage with antibiotic therapy parenterally.

Antibiotic therapy alone, and intraarterial injections of antibiotics have been generally discarded. Thus we have two main considerations: (1) Drainage of the abscess with small incisions and local irrigations with antibiotics. (2) Wide incision and drainage, with parenteral antibiotics, and with or without local irrigations with antibiotics.

Empirical Selection of Antibiotics

Antibiotics are used for infections which jeopardize important structures. The urgency of the situation usually requires that an antibiotic be selected before a culture and sensitivity tests can be reported. In such cases, reports of cultures and sensitivity tests are used to confirm that the empirical choice was correct or that a change is needed. Stone *et al.*[32] had as a basis for empirical selection of antibiotics the bacteriology of 656 cases and the antibiotic sensitivity of 569 organisms was analyzed from a series of 1077 patients hospitalized with infections. A single organism was isolated in 82.2 per cent of cultures. Multiple or-

TABLE 14.3.3
Acute suppurative tenosynovitis:
comparative end results

	Preanti-biotic Era 1938-1942 100 cases	Antibi-otic-Sensative Era 1943-1953 74 cases	Antibi-otic-Resistant Era 1954-1958 40 cases	Antibi-otic-Resistant Era 1959-now 98 cases
	%	%	%	%
Mortality	3	0	0	0
Amputations	10	8	12	6
Tendon slough	34	8	15	6
Osteomyelitis	10	10	18	10
Thenar space abscess	2	2	3	2
Midpalmar space abscess	2	2	6	0
Septic arthritis	2	2	12	2
Radial bursitis In palm	1	2	0	2
In wrist	1	0	0	0
Forearm inter muscular space	1	0	0	0

ganisms of the same gram-staining properties were isolated from 13.3 per cent of cultures. Only 4.5 per cent of cultures contained both gram-positive and gram-negative organisms. A gram-stained smear is a most useful guide to the empirical selection of antibiotics. Of all organisms cultured, 80 per cent were gram-positive and essentially all gram-positive organisms were sensitive to lincomycin, methicillin, erythromycin, and chloramphenicol. Among the gram-negative organisms, *Escherechia coli* and *Aerobacler aerogenes* accounted for more than half of the cultures. Kanamycin appears most effective for gram-negative organisms followed closely by cephalothin and chloramphenicol.

Our second consideration is wide incision and drainage with parenteral antibiotics, with or without local antibiotics. A wide incision and drainage of the involved tendon sheath, local irrigation of pus and slough, and large intramuscular doses of antibiotics are preferred. A bloodless field is obtained by constricting the arm with a pneumatic cuff inflated to 250 mm of mercury.

A knowledge of the underlying anatomy is basic for correct surgical treatment. The proper digital arteries are slightly posterior to the digital nerves, and are found at the level of the anterior third of the medial and lateral aspects of the fingers.

Auchincloss[3] has shown that the digital arteries give off branches that form an anastomotic arch of blood vessels in the anterior subtendinous space. This arch gives off vessels to supply the bone, the synovial membrane of the joint and the tendon sheath, and the tendon itself. The tendon receives its branches through the mesotendon or so-called "ligamenta brevis."

In our experience, the lateral incision has proved of the greatest value. It extends from the distal crease to the proximal volar crease. The incision is posterior to the lateral extensions of the volar transverse creases and posterior to the digital vessels and nerves (Fig. 14.3.14 *A* and *B*). The only objection to it is that it involves cutting the branch from the digital artery that makes up part of the anastomotic arch of blood vessels in the anterior subtendinous space, from which the mesotendon is supplied. This small cut branch, however, is not an end artery, and anastomotic circulation from the other side appears to be adequate to nourish the tendon sheath and tendon. In all cases of septic tenosynovitis of the flexor tendons of the index, long, and ring fingers it is also necessary to drain the palmar portion of the tendon sheath. This is accomplished by a longitudinal incision from the proximal digital crease, which is carried about 2 cm proximally into the palm. The incision is begun on the same side of the digital crease as the digital incision. The incision is made on the medial aspect of the index finger, and over the lateral aspect of the middle and ring fingers (Fig. 14.3.14 *A*).

In the surgical treatment of infections of the little finger tendon sheath and the palmar portion of the ulnar bursa we use the following steps: a longitudinal incision is made over the lateral aspect of the little finger, posterior to the digital vessels and nerves and to the lateral extensions of the volar digital creases. The palmar prolongation of the tendon sheath is drained by making an incision 2 cm long from the

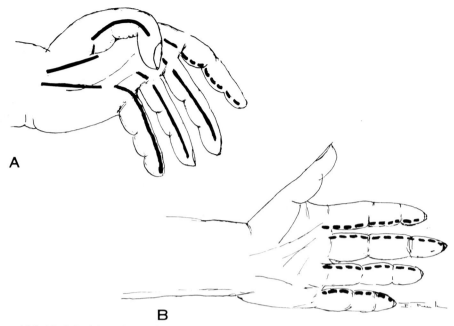

Figure 14.3.14. A. Incisions for tendon shealth infections of the thumb and little fingers are made over the lateral aspects. Palmar prolongations of all sheaths are incised in the palm. Incisions for radial and ulnar bursa infections in the palm are noted.*B*. Tendon sheath infections of the index finger are incised over the medial aspect. Tendon sheath infections of the middle, ring and little fingers are incised over the lateral aspects.

center of the volar aspect of the proximal digital crease into the palm. The palmar portion of the ulnar bursa is drained by an incision extending from a point just proximal to the distal transverse crease in the palm to about the apex of the triangle in the base of the palm. The incision is made over the lateral edge of the hypothenar eminence (Fig. 14.3.14 A). The digital branches of the ulnar nerve about 2 cm proximal to the metacarpophalangeal joint, the anastomotic branch of the ulnar nerve to the median nerve and the ulnar artery about 5 cm distal to the distal edge of the volar carpal ligament must be identified and retracted (Fig. 14.3.15).

In the surgical treatment of infections of the thumb, a position of extension of the thumb should be assumed to obviate anatomic distortion, particularly of nerves. We use a longitudinal incision from the base of the distal phalanx to the base of the thumb on the radial side. The palmar incision is a separate one that starts at about the middle of the proximal volar digital crease, just below the center of the volar aspect of the thumb. The incision is carried over the medial aspect of the thenar eminence, about two-thirds of the distance to its base (Fig. 14.3.14 A). The sensory and motor branches of the median nerve must be identified and retracted. At about the middle of the first metacarpal bone, a branch of the median nerve divides to send sensory branches to the medial and lateral aspects of the thumb. The important motor nerves to the opponens pollicis, abductor pollicis brevis, and lateral por-

tion of the flexor pollicis brevis, arise from the median nerve, usually about 1.5 cm proximal to the digital branches (Fig. 14.3.15). The portion of the radial bursa proximal to where the nerves to the thenar muscles are found is not drained unless the volar carpal ligament is cut. The entire volar carpal ligament may be incised.[15][18]

Auchincloss[3] stressed the fact that accumulations of pus in the radial and ulnar bursas in the wrist may rupture into the space bounded posteriorly by the pronator quadratus muscle and anteriorly by the flexor digitorum profundus and flexor pollicis longus tendons, Parona's space. From the wrist, pus spreads up the forearm into the space bounded anteriorly by the flexor digitorum superficialis and posteriorly by the flexor digitorum profundus and flexor pollicis longus (Fig. 14.3.16).[15][18]

Various anterior, medial, and lateral incisions have been described, but any incision into these spaces must be made with due regard for the underlying vessels and nerves. If both the ulnar and radial bursas are involved, or if pus has ruptured into Parona's space in the wrist, an incision on the ulnar side of the wrist is adequate. We prefer an incision 6 cm long over the anterior surface of the ulna about 2 cm above the styloid of the ulna (Fig. 14.3.17). The approach is behind the flexor carpi ulnaris muscle and ulnar vessels. When the deep fascia is incised, the bulging ulnar bursa may be seen in the wound.

If the radial bursa alone is involved, an incision

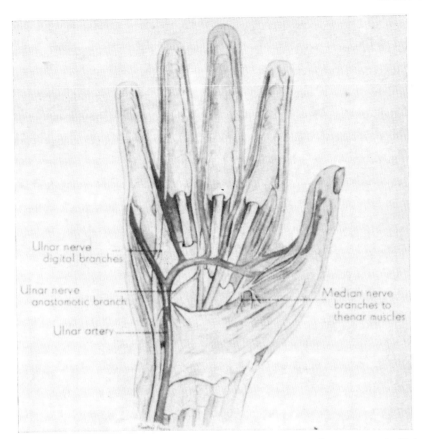

*Figure 14.3.15.*Superficial volar arch, ulnar and median nerves must be preserved with incisions in ulnar and radial bursas in palm.

over the radial side of the wrist is made. A 6-cm incision is made over the volar lateral aspect of the radius, as close to the bone as possible and posterior to the radial artery. When the deep fascia is incised, the bulging radial bursa may be seen in the wound (Fig. 14.3.17).

Most infections from the wrist tend to spread up the ulnar side of the forearm, where the flexors are found. With infections of the intermuscular space of the forearm, a 6-cm incision is made between the flexor carpi ulnaris and the ulnar margin of the flexor digitorum superficialis. The flexor digitorum superficialis is retracted laterally, and the space between it and the flexor digitorum profundus is entered by blunt dissection toward the latter. Great care should be taken not to injure the ulnar nerves and vessels that are adherent to the undersurface of the flexor digitorum superficialis (Figs. 14.3.16 and 14.3.17). Pus and slough are removed. Irrigation with saline or a specific antibiotic is performed. The specific antibiotic is used parenterally, with splinting in a position of function until infection subsides. Active motions are then instituted.[15][18]

One of our associates[9] has used a small transverse incision, just distal to the distal transverse crease in the palm, through which a small polyethylene catheter with multiple perforations is inserted into the tendon sheath with the aid of a Rochester needle. Another transverse incision is made just proximal to the distal transverse crease in the digit. The catheter is pushed the entire length of the digit. The sheath is flushed with a saline solution. A synthetic penicillin or cephalogen may be used until sensitivity studies are obtained. The drip is used as long as infection persists, as long as one week in some cases. Most infections are controlled within 48 hours. For the irrigation, one million units of penicillin in a liter of saline every 24 hours are used. The infected hand is placed in a sterile pan and is covered by a sterile towel. Brown's[9] results with a series of acute suppurative tenosynovitis have been excellent, and also with deep fascial space abscesses. He uses parenteral antibiotics as an adjunct (Fig. 14.3.18).

The local irrigation with an antibiotic is a rational procedure, as there would seem to be a better contact on the organisms than with parenteral antibiotics alone. However, with old cases with thick pus and slough, the more radical incisions should be used, with local irrigations and also parenteral antibiotics.

Meleney[28] and Bailey[4] have used ureteral cathe-

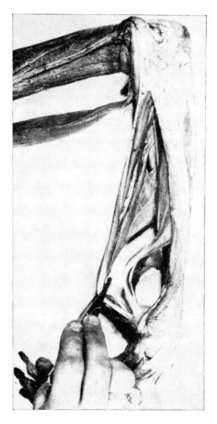

Figure 14.3.16. Dissection of Parona's space in wrist and interflexor space in forearm shows muscular boundaries.

jected locally; 15,000 units of penicillin are injected every three hours. He reports on 10 cases, with optimal results in five, fair results in three, and poor results in two.

Unonius,[34] in 1947, makes a small, curved incision into the sheath and introduces ureteral catheters proximally and distally. Penicillin solution is injected every six hours until the fluid contains no bacteria. In eight cases, Unonius reports the following results: optimal in five, fair in two, and poor in one.

Excision with suture technique has been suggested for treatment of suppurative tenosynovitis and deep fascial space infection.[2] All slough and necrotic tissue are excised, and the wound is sutured. Local and parenteral administration of antibiotics is recommended.

Loudon et al.,[24] in 1948, suggest a transverse incision over the distal end of the sheath. A needle is inserted proximally, and at times an incision is made proximally. First, 10,000 units of penicillin are injected through the needle, and the incisions are sutured; 20,000 units of sodium penicillin are injected intramuscularly twice a day for five days postopera-

ters. However, Carter and Mersheimer[11] believe that ureteral catheters are too rigid and that the use of fine, pliable plastic tubes has been a breakthrough in the treatment of hand infections.

Incision and drainage with local irrigations with antibiotics is apparently running in cycles.

Various types of local antibiotic therapy have been described. Five methods with local penicillin therapy are considered. In 1944, Florey and Williams[12] suggest the drainage of pus by a lateral incision. Daily, the wound is covered with calcium salt of penicillin and packed with gauze soaked with penicillin paste until cultures are negative. The results in 11 cases were optimal in five, fair in four, and poor in two.

Burt,[10] in 1946, advises lateral incisions over the proximal and middle phalanges, and the insertion of two fine rubber catheters into the tendon sheaths. Penicillin solution is injected through the tubes every three hours for five days. His results in three cases were optimal, fair and poor in one each.

Marsden,[26] in 1946, recommends the use of two small transverse incisions into the tendon sheath, one just proximal to the metacarpophalangeal crease and the other just proximal to the distal interphalangeal crease. Needles are inserted daily and penicillin is in-

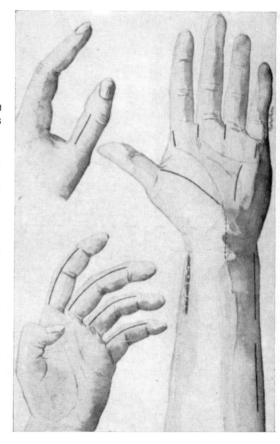

Figure 14.3.17. Incisions for infected radial and ulnar bursas, Parona's space in wrist and forearm space.

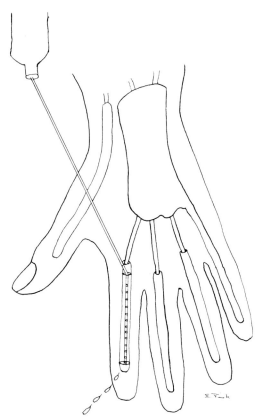

Figure 14.3.18. Polyethelene tube with multiple perforations is inserted into the entire length of tendon sheath. Proximal end of polyethelene tube is attached to a drip bottle for a continuous drip. Tube is inserted in proximal incision. Pus is flushed through distal incision.

tively. The results in seven cases were optimal in five, fair in none and poor in two. The authors also recommend this treatment for deep fascial space infection.

We have used excision with suture technique in only one case of subcuticular abscess, with a poor result.

Bingham,[7] 1960, suggests an incision over the lateral aspect of the middle phalanx. Pus is drained and the sheath is irrigated with a solution of 100,000 units of penicillin in 5 ml of physiologic saline. If pus is thick, an incision is made over the proximal cul-de-sac for more complete irrigation and drainage. The catheter may be left in the sheath for 24 to 48 hours with irrigations of penicillin solution every four hours.

More recently, 1970, Carter and Mersheimer[11] have suggested small incisions, followed by a continuous postoperative irrigation of the cavity. They use a fine pliable plastic tube to irrigate pus and necrotic tissue and to place a continuous drip of antibiotic solution directly into the cavity. They suggest two transverse incisions, one in the proximal part of the sheath, through which the catheter is inserted 2 cm;

the second transverse incision is into the distal part of the sheath, through which pus is evacuated.

REFERENCES

1. Anson, B. J., and Ashley, F. L. Midpalmar compartment, associated spaces and limiting layers. Anat. Rec., *78:* 389-407, 1940.
2. Arden, C. P., Kitchin, A. P., and Powell, H. D. S. Excision suture technique in infections of hand. Lancet, *2:* 188-190, 1949.
3. Auchincloss, H. Surgery of hand. In *Nelson's Loose-Leaf Living Surgery, Vol. 3.* New York, Thomas Nelson & Son, 1927, p. 459.
4. Bailey, D., *The Infected Hand.* London, H. K. Lewis, 1963.
5. Barber, M. Staphylococcal infection due to penicillin-resistant strains. Br. Med. J. *2:* 863-865, 1947.
6. Bauchet, L. J. *Du Panaris et des Inflammations de la Main.* Ed. 2. Paris, A. Delahaye, 1859.
7. Bingham, D. L. G. Acute infections of the hand. Surg. Clin. North Am., *40:* 1285, 1960.
8. Brickel, A. C. J. *Surgical Treatment of Hand and Forearm Infections.* St. Louis, Mosby, 1939.
9. Brown, H. Personal communication.
10. Burt, L. I. Treatment of suppurative tenosynovitis in fingers. Med. J. Aust., *1:* 299, 1946.
11. Carter, S. J., and Mersheimer, W. I. Infections of the hand. Orthop. Clin. North Am., *2:* 455, 1970.
12. Florey, M. E., and Williams, R. E. O. Hand infections treated with penicillin. Lancet, *1:* 74-81, 1944.
13. Flynn, J. E. Clinical and anatomical investigations of deep fascial space infections of hand. Am. J. Surg. *55:* 467-475, 1942.
14. Flynn, J. E. Surgical significance of middle palmar septum of hand. Surgery, *14:* 134-141, 1943.
15. Flynn, J. E. Grave infections of the hand. N. Engl. J. Med., *229:* 898-905, 1943.
16. Flynn, J. E. Suppurative tenosynovitis of hand. N. Engl. J. Med., *242:* 241-244, 1950.
17. Flynn, J. E. Modern considerations of major hand infections. N. Engl. J. Med., *252:* 605-612, 1955.
18. Flynn, J. E. *Hand Surgery.* Baltimore, Williams & Wilkins, 1966, pp. 815-832.
19. Gosselin, L. *Clinique Chirurgicale de l'Hospital de la Charite.* Paris, Bailliere, 1873.
20. Jepson, R. P., and Bolton, H. Modern trends in treatment of infections of hand. Postgrad. Med. J., *25:* 261-268, 1949.
21. Kanavel, A. B. *Infections of the Hand: a Guide to the Surgical Treatment of Acute and Chronic Suppurative Processes in the Fingers, Hand, and Forearm,* Ed. 7 Philadelphia, Lea & Febiger, 1939.
22. Kaplan, E. B. *Functional and Surgical Anatomy of the Hand,* Ed. 1. Philadelphia, Lippincott, 1953.
23. Lapidari, M. La terapia endoarteriosa pennicillino-novocainica nella cura delle flogosi acute delle extremita. Rass. indust., *19:* 88-94, 1950.
24. Loudon, J. B., Miniero, J. D., and Scott, J. C. Infections of hand. J. Bone Joint Surg., *30B:* 409-429, 1948.
25. Lowden, T. G. Severe infections of the hand. Physiotherapy, *54:* 128-130, 1968.
26. Marsden, J. A. Penicillin therapy for tendon sheath infections of hand. Med. J. Aust., *1:* 435, 1946.
27. Mascagni, P. *Vasorum Lymphaticorum Corporis Hu-*

mani Historia et Iconographia. Senis, P. Carli, 1787.

28. Meleney, F. *Clinical Aspects and Treatment of Surgical Infections.* Philadelphia, Saunders, 1949.
29. Pilcher, R. S., Dawson, R. L. G., Milstein, B. S., and Riddell, A. G., Infections of fingers and hand. Lancet, *1:* 777-783, 1948.
30. Poirier, P., and Cuneo, B. Lymphatics. Westminster, A. Constable & Co., 1903.
31. Sappey, M. P. C. *Anatomie, Physiologie, Pathologie de Vaisseux Lymphatiques Consideres Chez l'Homme et les Vertebres.* Paris, A. Delahaye and E. Lecrosnier, 1885.
32. Stone, N. H., Hursh, H., Humphrey, C. R., and Boswick, J. A. Empirical selection of antibiotics for hand infections. J. Bone Joint Surg., *51A:* 899-903, 1969.
33. Tillaux, P. J. *Traite d'Anatomie Topographique avec Applications a la Chirurgie.* Paris, P. Asselin, 1877.
34. Uuonius, E. Local penicillin treatment of suppurative infection in tendon sheath. Acta chir. scand., *95:* 532-540, 1947.

D.

Special Infections of the Hand

John M. Cahill, M.D.

Despite the fact that the overwhelming majority of hand infections, both major and minor, are due to staphylococcus and streptococcus, there are some unusual infections which are important.

Some of these infections are associated with certain occupations. Others are generally confined to certain geographic locations but, with current air travel, may be transported to an unusual area before symptoms arise. A few are frequently overlooked because the hand is not the usual site of the primary disease.

In the majority of cases, recognition of the condition will protect the patient from unnecessary surgery since only a few of these conditions require operative intervention. Early recognition, however, may be essential to prevent death or serious disability.

The following infections will be considered in this chapter:
A. Bacterial diseases
 1. Anthrax
 2. Erysipeloid
 3. Glanders
 4. Melioidosis
 5. Gonorrhea
 6. Pasteurellosis
 7. Tularemia
B. Viral diseases
 1. Herpes simplex
 2. Herpes zoster
 3. Cat scratch fever
 4. Warts
 5. Milker's nodule
C. Parasitic disease
 Leishmaniasis
D. Spirochetal disease
 Syphilis
E. Specific foreign body infections
 1. Barber's hand
 2. Milker's granuloma

BACTERIAL DISEASES

The diseases in this group are of major historic and clinical importance. Many of our present bacteriologic techniques were developed in studying them. Anthrax, glanders, melioidosis, and tularemia, and still may, carry a high mortality. Frequently the primary lesion is found on the hand, and delay in starting specific therapy may result in serious disability or a fatal result.

Anthrax

This is an acute infectious disease primarily seen in sheep and cattle. Although pneumococcal and typhoidal infections are not uncommon and frequently fatal,[6] [7] the hand is involved in the more common cutaneous type.

The disease has been recognized for centuries both in animals and man. Maret, in 1752, is credited with first describing the "malignant pustule" in man. This term is still commonly used and somewhat misleading since the lesion does not contain true pus and today is generally far from malignant. Rayer,[55] in 1850, demonstrated the bacterial forms in the blood of infected sheep and, in 1877, Koch[36] in a classic paper described the isolation and culture of the organism, demonstrated its ability to form spores, and experimentally reproduced the disease in animals from pure cultures of the organism. Perhaps best remembered is that Pasteur,[50] in 1881, publically demonstrated the production of immunity in animals from the injection of live attenuated strains of the organism.

Anthrax has been detected in nearly every country of the world but appears to be somewhat more common in warm climates. Despite the fact that it is primarily a disease of sheep and cattle, virtually all animals show varying degrees of susceptibility, ranging from marked in sheep to relative immunity in mature dogs. Man appears to be moderately susceptible. His infection usually develops after direct contact with infected animals or contaminated animal products.

In the United States, approximately 50 cases of cutaneous anthrax are reported each year. The disease is an occupational hazard for herdsmen, cattlemen, butchers, hide handlers, and wool workers. Sporadic cases appear in the general public from poorly sterilized animal products such as shaving brushes.

The cutaneous infection is believed to gain entry through a minor abrasion, most commonly on the hand, face, or neck. Incubation is generally 12 to 24 hours but may be four to five days on occasion. A pimple first appears which enlarges, vesiculates, and ruptures. Erythema and new vesicles appear about the periphery, and the center develops a black eschar (Fig. 14.4.1). The lesion discharges a serosanguinous fluid. Marked edema may develop locally or involve the entire extremity. Satellite lesions may occur. Despite its very angry appearance, pain is usually not severe. However, soreness along lymphatic pathways may be noted. Generalized symptoms of malaise, fever, and anorexia may accompany the early phase of the illness. The cutaneous form of the disease remains local, runs its course of necrosis, and heals spontaneously in

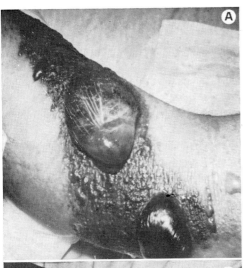
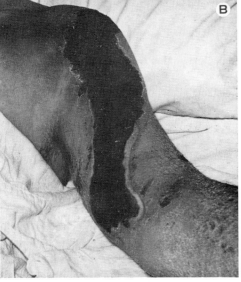

Figure 14.4.1. Large anthrax lesion showing *(A)* early vesicle formation, and *(B)* later development of black eschar. This case required a skin graft to close the area of necrosis. Courtesy C. Newton Peabody, M.D.

80 per cent of cases even without antibiotic therapy. Occasionally a more malignant course may ensue with rapid spread and blood stream invasion. High fever, vomiting, headache, prostration, shock, and death may result unless treatment is instituted. Some authors believe that a bacterial toxin is involved in the course of a fatal septicemia.[27,60]

The diagnosis of cutaneous anthrax should be immediately suspected in a typical case from the appearance of the lesion and the history. Only rarely is the appearance of the lesion nonspecific. The vesicular fluid generally teems with bacteria in the early stages of the disease. Later, they may be recovered by scraping the edge of the wound.

The organism is a large, nonmotile, grampositive rod and grows well on all regular laboratory media. Spores are readily formed in air, are smaller than the active bacillus, and stain with difficulty.

The treatment of cutaneous anthrax should result in close to a 100 per cent cure rate today since the bacillus is very sensitive to penicillin as well as the tetracyclines, erythromycin, and chloromycetin.[22] Although one author reported the use of excisional therapy for the primary lesions,[37] surgery probably has no place in the treatment of this disease. Rarely marked edema may spread to the neck and necessitate tracheostomy or a secondary infection may lead to abscess formation. Penicillin will usually sterilize the lesion in a matter of hours but will not effect its course of central necrosis and slough.

It should be remembered that the anthrax bacillus rapidly forms spores on exposure to air, and all dressings should be carefully disposed of by burning or suitable disinfection. Anthrax spores have remained viable for years under a variety of conditions.

Erysipeloid

This disease is caused by the organism, *Erysipelothrix insidiosa*, or *Erysipelothrix rhusiopathia*, also the cause of swine erysipelas. Isolated by Koch in 1880, it was studied by Pasteur[51] in 1883. It was first classified as a bacteria, later as a fungus. *E. insidiosa* is presently placed in the *Corynebacterium* family of bacteria.

The organism has a wide range of animal hosts on land, air, and sea. It may cause disease in these animals or remain commensal. The infection in man is largely occupational and is most often seen in workers of the meat and fish industries.[31] One large series of cases was reported among workers in a button plant.[43]

The portal of entry is usually a surface wound of the hand. The infection is low grade, and systemic symptoms are mild if present at all. Mild aching and itching are the local symptoms. Infection becomes manifest two to 15 days after injury.

A red or occasionally blue discoloration of the skin spreads slowly from the point of entry with moderate edema. When the infection starts in the hand, it rarely goes above the wrist. Even without specific therapy, the disease is self-limited and lasts about two to three weeks. Rare cases of fatal septicemia have been reported.[35]

Diagnosis is suggested from the history, appearance, and lack of constitutional symptoms that would accompany true erysipelas. A swab of the wound may not reveal the organism, but biopsy from the wound edge usually yields results.[56] The organism is a gram-positive rod which, in culture, may grow singly or in long filamentous chains.

The organism is very sensitive to penicillin, and resolution is rapid under this form of therapy. No surgery is required.

Glanders

Glanders, caused by the organism, *Pfeifferella mallei,* is primarily a disease of equine animals, and it is from such contact that the majority of cases in man have occurred.

In countries where rigid rules are enforced to prevent the spread of the disease in horses, cases of human glanders are practically unknown.[66] Despite this, the disease is so deadly when it occurs that it is worthy of mention.

Even in ancient times, this disease was recognized. Infected horses in the army of Constantine[28] were segregated, and in Book I of the *Iliad,* a disease which spread from the mules of the Greek army to the troops is mentioned. In 1837, Rayer[54] demonstrated that glanders was transmissable when he infected a horse with material from a human case. In 1884, Loeffler and Shutz first isolated and cultured the causative organism. The glanders or farcy order passed in Great Britain in 1907 practically eliminated a rather common disease from that country. In 1946, however, it was estimated that, in Russia, 5 per cent of all horses were infected.[31]

The disease in man has been largely an occupational hazard for those working with horses or a laboratory hazard for bacteriology workers.[45]

There are two forms of human glanders, acute and chronic, based on the severity of the disease and the rapidity of the course. The acute form is more common and, while it affects the body as a whole, respiratory symptoms predominate.[28] In cases, either acute or chronic, where skin and lymphatic involvement is outstanding, the disease is called farcy. When the hands are involved, local areas of induration occur, followed by nodule formation and later necrosis of the lesions. As the disease spreads, deep abscesses may develop, rupture, and form sinus tracts. An oily yellow discharge exudes from the lesions. Muscle, bone, and tendons may be involved. Lymphatics become thickened and ropelike and are called farcy pipes. Nodules form along lymphatics and are called farcy buds. The lesions are extremely painful and chronic disease may persist for years with periods of remission and exacerbation. The acute form of the disease may develop at any time, usually with rapid spread of the infection, high fever, vomiting, and diarrhea. Severe respiratory involvement is common, and bloody discharge with a fetid odor is present. The disease is difficult to recognize clinically, since it may resemble tuberculosis, actinomycosis, and other granulomatous diseases.[4] Secondary infection is common and may add to the diagnostic confusion. Some authors believe that misdiagnosis has accounted for the low incidence reported. Occasional cases have been recently reported in the United States.[45] [67]

Clinical suspicion should be aroused when chronic abscesses, ulcers, or fistulas develop on the hands or arms, especially when a history of exposure to horses is elicited. Definitive diagnosis may be made from smear and culture of the lesions. The organism is a small, nonmotile, gram-negative rod with rounded ends. It grows best in meat infusion media, on glycerin agar, or on potato. In late cases penicillin should be added to the media as gram-positive organisms may predominate. Guinea pigs and hamsters are very susceptible to infection intraperitoneally or subcutaneously. Serologic tests have not proven of much diagnostic value in man although a very high titer agglutination test may indicate the disease.[11] [45]

Successful treatment of laboratory-acquired infection has been reported with sulfadiazine.[11] [29] Although no organisms were recovered, agglutination titers rose markedly and clinical symptoms suggested the acute form. Variability in virulence of certain strains has been noted.[45] Initially most organisms reveal a sensitivity to streptomycin.[45] [67] Chloromycetin or one of the tetracyclines may also be effective. Surgically, conservative drainage of abscesses is reported to be helpful, and there is some evidence that wide excision of involved areas may obliterate the disease.[4]

Culture and sensitivity studies of all known antibiotics should be carried out. Good nursing care and general therapy is essential.

Melioidosis

This disease, like glanders, is rare in western countries. Only two recent cases have been reported in the English literature.[23] [42] Like glanders, it is a protean disease, and it may be that cases are frequently misdiagnosed. The disease first was described by Whitmore in 1912 and apparently resembles glanders in most respects. Both acute and chronic types have been reported.

The reservoir of this disease is believed to be the wild rat, and the infection is spread to man by way of the rat flea.

The organism is a gram-negative rod similar to *Pf. mallei* and is called *Pfeifferella pseudomallei* or *Pfeifferella whitmori.* Unlike *Pf. mallei,* the bacteria are motile.

Streptomycin may be used alone or in combination with a sulfa drug in the therapy of this condition.[45] More recently the tetracyclenes and chloromycetin have been found effective.[61]

Gonorrhea

With the advent of the antibiotic era, the treatment of acute gonorrhea has become so simple and effective that secondary complications are rarely seen. In hand surgery, the conditions which may come to our attention are arthritis, tenosynovitis, and keratoderma blennorrhagica, a rare skin disease.

These complications, when they occur, tend to do so during the second or third week of infection when the disease is relatively chronic. Gonorrhea, with its complications, formerly was more common in men.[65] However, the over-all incidence of chronic disease has been drastically reduced, and recent reports indicate that some complications are more frequently seen in women.[25] The acute disease in men is hard to miss and easier to treat effectively than in women. Homosexuals seem to have a somewhat higher complication rate, since the primary infection may occur in an unsuspected location and remain longer without treatment. Complications may increase with the present great increase in gonorrhea.

Gonorrheal arthritis affects several joints initially. However, severe symptoms rarely occur in more than one or two joints.[34] The onset of the condition is usually accompanied by fever and general malaise with mild involvement of several joints. Marked symptoms of heat, tenderness, redness, swelling, and severe pain on motion follow in one or two joints. In the upper extremity, the wrist, metacarpophalangeal, and shoulder joints are more commonly involved. Pain on motion is severe.

A high index of suspicion may be gained from the history and physical examination. Aspiration of the joint may yield a positive smear or culture.

The treatment is aimed at controlling the primary disease with penicillin, and the response is usually rapid. The affected joints should be immobilized and intermittently treated with hot soaks or compresses. Early active physiotherapy should follow subsidence of symptoms to prevent ankylosis, which may occur in any case if antibiotic therapy is delayed. Tetracycline, erythromycin, or kenemycin may be effective in penicillin-resistant cases or penicillin-sensitive patients.

Tenosynovitis may have a similar onset and may be associated with joint involvement.[5] Symptoms of pain on motion, tenderness, and swelling are similar to nonspecific tendon sheath infections.

Diagnosis is aided by the history, especially if no trauma is reported.[26] Aspirate of fluid from the tendon sheath frequently yields a positive smear and culture. In the flexor sheaths of the fingers, aspiration in the center of the crease of the proximal interphalangeal joint is the simplest method.[26]

When the diagnosis is doubtful, incision and drainage should be carried out since delay in pyogenic infection would invite disaster. However, if a positive smear is obtained, the finger should be splinted, and the patient treated with penicillin. The tendon itself is not usually destroyed by this infection. Physiotherapy should be instituted after subsidence of infection since adhesions are common. The degree of permanent disability usually corresponds to the duration of the untreated disease.

Keratoderma blennorrhagica is most common on the feet, but may affect the hands. Vesicular lesions are followed by horny crusting, with the skin taking on the appearance of a three-dimensional map. Lesions about the nail beds may resemble paronychia (Fig. 14.4.2). Although there are reports of the responsible organism being found in the lesions,[2] most investigators believe that this is an allergic reaction. The condition generally clears with treatment of the primary disease.

Pasteurellosis (cat bite infection)

Pasteurella multocida has been studied for centuries primarily because it is the source of disease in domestic livestock. It is the cause of swine and cattle plague, chicken cholera, and rabbit septicemia.[44] Epidemics have resulted in heavy losses in domestic herds. Pasteur[49] isolated it from chickens in 1880 during his early studies on immunity. Apparently many animals may be healthy carriers of *P. multocida* in their mouths and nasal passages.[9][17]

Human infection generally results from the bite of a household pet. After the injury, the wounded area becomes painful, red, and swollen. Abscess formation usually develops, and the regional lymphatics may become involved. Osteomyelitis has been frequently reported (Fig. 14.4.3), especially after cat bites of the hand. This is probably due to the needle-like fangs of the cat which easily inoculate the bones or joints in this area.[9] Veteran animal keepers are well aware that cat bites usually result in more serious infection than dog bites. This organism has been cultured from the mouth

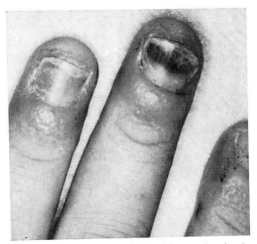

Figure 14.4.2. Keratoderma blennorrhagica involving the nail bed area and resembling paronychia. Courtesy Philip L. McCarthy, M.D.

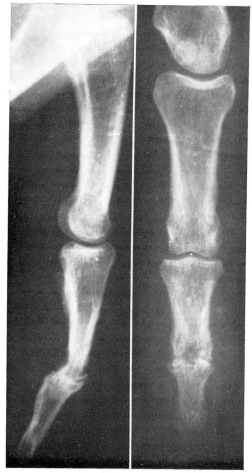

Figure 14.4.3. Osteomyelitis and arthritis of the index finger following a cat bite. Infection due to *P. multocida*. Courtesy C. Newton Peabody, M.D.

of over 50 per cent of healthy dogs and cats.[17][18][38] In general, hand infections tend to remain local and have not been a factor in the occasionally reported cases of systemic disease.[26][46][52][64]

The diagnosis should be suspected in any case of infection after a dog or cat bite. Wounds should be carefully cultured and careful notice given the bacteriologist to check for the presence of this organism. Confusion with other more common organisms has been reported,[9] and considering the number of animal bites, the number of documented cases of multocida infection is rather small. The organism may vary in appearance from short gram-negative rods to coccal forms which may be paired. Its characteristics[44] on culture have been well described.

Unlike the majority of gram-negative organisms, penicillin is the drug of choice and should be given to all deep dog and cat bites while awaiting the bacteriologic report. Occasional cases with penicillin-resistant organisms have been reported which re-

sponded to the broad spectrum antibiotics.[9] Whether or not primary excision of the wound should be carried out after dog or cat bites is a matter of judgmen.[9][33][38] All wounds should be left open, and ragged wounds should be debrided. Thorough cleansing of the wound with soap and water is, of course, mandatory. When the bite is penetrating and inoculation of tendon sheath, bone, or joint appears likely, excision of the wound edges and exploration should be the procedure of choice, just as in human bites. This organism, although very sensitive to penicillin, is not likely to be the only one present. When obvious infection is established, the decision must be based on the findings. Pure cellulitis should be treated conservatively; bone, joint, and tendon sheath infection should be drained. It should be stressed that cauterization of animal bites with phenol is a destructive and outmoded form of therapy, probably far less effective in preventing rabies than the use of soap and water.

Tularemia

Tularemia is a disease which is endemic and occasionally epidemic in wild animals. Man may be infected both by direct contact with these animals and indirectly by insect vectors or material contaminated by infected wild life.[21]

McCoy[39] first isolated the organism in 1911 and later named it *Bacterium tularense* after Tulare County, California, where he found it a plaguelike disease of squirrels. Most of our knowledge of etiology of the disease in man and animals results from the work of Francis,[21] who proved that two diseases of man, rabbit fever and deerfly fever, were actually one disease which he named tularemia. He demonstrated that the disease could be transmitted by a variety of methods besides direct contact with infected animals, including biting flies, ticks, and contaminated water and food. This organism has also been responsible for a large number of serious infections in bacteriology laboratories and should be handled with extreme care.[47]

Tularemia can manifest itself in a variety of ways. Oculoglandular, meningitic, pneumonic, and septicemic forms have been described. The ulceroglandular type, however, is the most common and is very likely to begin as a hand infection. The disease is generally contracted through breaks in the skin during handling of infected animals or transmitted by insect bites on exposed parts of the body. After contact, the incubation period is one to 10 days. Chills, fever, headache, and malaise may be the first noticeable symptoms. At the site of inoculation, a papule forms which undergoes central necrosis and sloughs, leaving a punched out ulcer with raised borders and a necrotic base. Lymphatic spread and bubo formation is the rule. Early apparent remission with later flare-up is common. When the blood stream is invaded, necrotic foci may occur in any organ accompanied with high fever and prostration.

Diagnosis is made from the history and physical findings plus identification of the organism, skin test, or serologic examination. *B. tularense* may be difficult to find on smear and is hard to culture on ordinary media. It is best grown in egg yolk, in guinea pigs, or on dextrose cystine agar. The Foshay skin test,[20] performed with a killed suspension of the organisms, should become positive in about one week, and a rising agglutinin titer on serologic examination is of help in differential diagnosis. Cat scratch fever is especially likely to be confused with this disease. However, a specific skin test for this condition is also available.[13]

At present, streptomycin appears to be the drug of choice in treating tularemia,[40 44] and usually cures the disease in five to eight days. The tetracyclines and chloromycetin are somewhat less effective but will control the disease.[40 47] Streptomycin-resistant strains are not rare, especially in laboratory-acquired infection.[47] Serum is available which has been shown to affect favorably the course of the disease but today is seldom required. Surgery is generally contraindicated except when glands suppurate or are greatly enlarged, but only after the disease is controlled. Tularemia is transmissable and care should be taken in dealing with the open wounds. Immunization vaccines have been developed which are used widely in Russia but seldom in this country. One infection usually confers the immunity.[44]

VIRAL DISEASES

Herpes Simplex

This viral disease most commonly affects the mucous membranes of the mouth, causing either a vesicular eruption or "cold sores." Although it is considered as contagious as chicken pox or measles, relatively few symptomatic infections result from contact. On the hands, it usually causes a vesicular lesion similar to herpes zoster. On the tips of the fingers, it may be confused with an early felon.

There appears to be a relatively high incidence of herpes of the hand in nurses caring for patients who have oral herpetic lesions.[16]

Unlike other similar viruses such as measles and varicella, one attack does not confer immunity.[66] Recurrent infection is common and the number of asymptomatic carriers is high.

Treatment is symptomatic. Secondary infection should receive antibiotics. 5-Iodo-2-desoxyuridine, an antiviral agent, has been effective in treating corneal infections, but its value in skin eruptions is probably slight.[8]

Herpes Zoster (Shingles).

This viral disease occurs primarily in adults. It is apparently related to chickenpox (varicella) and material from the skin lesions of shingles has caused chickenpox in children.[66] Whether there is a variation in the virus or in the immunity of the host is not clear. The virus that causes shingles, however, has a predilection for sensory nerve roots.

Approximately seven to 14 days (14 to 21 for chickenpox) after exposure, the disease appears with the onset of fever and general malaise, followed by severe pain in an area supplied by one or more sensory nerves. The upper extremity is not one of the more common areas involved, and thus a diagnosis of shingles may be missed when it involves this area. From three to four days after onset, vesicles form in the skin in the area supplied by the nerve, and these later may become purulent. (Figs. 14.4.4 and 14.4.5). Persistent neuralgia may occur in older people. Bilateral disease is rare.

Diagnosis is made from history and physical examination. The clinical picture is diagnostic if the disease is considered.

Treatment is largely expectant and symptomatic with sedatives. Cortisone has been reported to give some relief in shingles, but has been attended with fatalities in chickenpox. Antibiotics should be used for secondary infection. Isolation should be observed, especially for children where it has been associated with outbreaks of chickenpox. All patients with shingles should be carefully checked for the presence of a lymphoma, since there appears to be a high incidence of association between the two diseases.

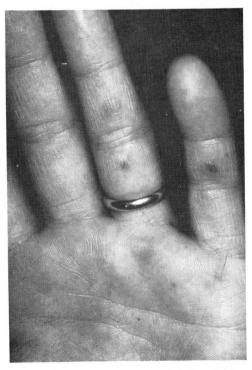

Figure 14.4.4. Herpes zoster of the hand. Ulnar distribution. Courtesy Philip L. McCarthy, M.D.

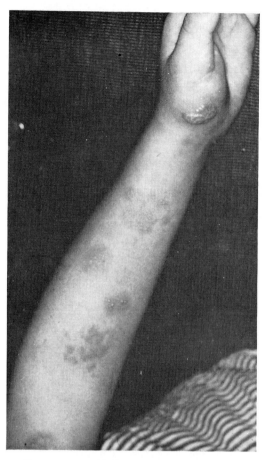

Figure 14.4.5. Herpes zoster involving the arm and hand with vesicle formation. Courtesy Philip L. McCarthy, M.D.

Cat Scratch Fever

This peculiar disease is probably viral in etiology, but definite proof is lacking at present.[13] The importance of the condition is the confusion it may cause in differential diagnosis. It is a self-limited disease and generally does not require specific therapy.

Foshay[20] and Debre apparently recognized the condition in about 1932[14] but the first report of cases did not appear until 1950.[14] Usually the disease follows a cat scratch, but infection from other agents has been described. The incubation period is one to two weeks, and, when the scratches are on the upper extremity, marked glandular swelling appears in the axillary area accompanied by malaise, headache, chills, and fever. Leukocyte count is usually normal or slightly elevated. Symptoms generally last one to three weeks. The adenopathy lasts longer, in the majority of cases subsiding in about six weeks, occasionally lasting several years.

Diagnosis should be suspect from the history and glandular enlargement. In most cases, however, a specific skin test is usually necessary to rule out other more serious conditions such as tularemia, infectious mononucleosis, Hodgkin's disease, lymphosarcoma, and tuberculosis.[24]

The antigen for the skin test is made from the aspirate of suppurative nodes.[13] Antigen made from the patient's nodes should also cause a positive test in known volunteer reactors.

Treatment is largely expectant. Excision of the enlarged nodes has been recommended with apparent good result[59] but in general seems unnecessary unless they cause a cosmetic problem or suppurate and develop a chronic secondary infection. If the diagnosis is in doubt, biopsy may be necessary to rule out a tumor. Some believe that the tetracyclines or chloromycetin may be of benefit.[13]

Warts

The common wart, verruca vulgaris, is a viral disease. They are most commonly seen on the hand where the lesions are frequently multiple and often located about the fingernail. The typical wart is a circular, papillary, painless growth with a hard top. Rarely, they may occur on the palm and be covered with a horny plate of skin.

Warts are best treated by electrodessication, liquid nitrogen, or applications of caustics. X-ray may be helpful when the nail bed is involved. The skin covering palmar warts should be removed and the underlying lesion removed by electrosurgery. When warts are excised by routine surgical methods, recurrence is frequent in the line of closure and suture holes.

Milker's Nodule

The characteristics of the virus responsible for this condition are not well identified. The disease differs from vaccinia in appearance. The lesion begins as an erythematous papule which develops slowly into a firm bluish-red nodule[10] varying in diameter from 2 to 4 cm. Slight pain may be present. Toxic symptoms are rare. Healing usually is spontaneous in four to six weeks. Treatment is symptomatic and to avoid contact with cows. These lesions may be confused with melanomas or pyogenic granulomas.[10]

PARASITIC DISEASE

Leishmaniasis

Leishmania tropica was recognized as the cause of "oriental sore" by Cunningham in 1885, but the first complete description of the organism was by J. H. Wright[69] in Boston in 1903. He found the organism in a recently emigrated Armenian patient undergoing treatment at the Massachusetts General Hospital.

Leishmania braziliensis, the causative organism of

espundia or American leishmaniasis, was identified somewhat later and at first confused with *L. tropica*.

Oriental sore is seen primarily in India, Asia Minor, parts of Africa, and the areas surrounding the Mediterranean Sea. Espundia is found in Central and South America (Fig. 14.4.6).

The initial lesion is similar in each disease. A reddish papule which is raised and indurated develops at the site of inoculation. Over a period of several months, it breaks down and forms an ulcer. This may last for years and, on healing, leaves a depressed scar. Sores may be single or multiple, and autoinoculation is possible. In the American type, metastatic lesions about the nose and mouth occur, and the disease has been called mucocutaneous leishmaniasis. These lesions may appear long after the original ulcer has healed. Direct transmission of the disease is possible, although the usual mode of transmission is the bite of the sand fly in both diseases[1] and exposed areas such as the hand and arm are likely to be the primary sites. Incubation is from a few days to several months.

In areas where the disease is endemic, it will immediately be suspected. In the United States, the patient will give a history of recent travel from an endemic area.[69]

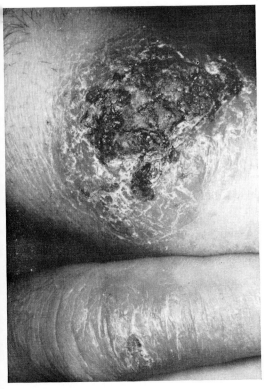

Figure 14.4.6. Ulceration in *Leishmania tropica* infection. Patient recently returned to the United States from the Middle East. Courtesy Philip L. McCarthy, M.D.

Needle punctures of the papule or about the edge of the ulcer will reveal the organism which may be stained with Wright's stain and cultured on N.N.N. media.

L. tropica and *L. braziliensis* cannot be distinguished from each other except by serologic test.

Antimony preparations may be useful in the treatment of both types; however, Amphotericin B is the treatment of choice if the disease is unresponsive or spreading.[57]

SPIROCHETAL DISEASE

Syphilis

Syphilis may affect the hand, either in the primary or chronic stages of the adult disease. It may also constitute a problem in children.

The primary lesion of syphilis, the chancre, occurs on the hands usually as a result of contact with the mouth or teeth of an infected person.[30][58] Infection of this type is an occupational hazard to dentists and physicians and may be transmitted during an examination.[30] When the nail bed area is the site of entry, the lesion may resemble a paronychia. Untreated, the nail is destroyed and later regrows. Healing usually takes place in several weeks if secondary infection is avoided. When the lesion occurs on other parts of the hand, the appearance may vary from a papule to the ulcerated form, with an indurated base. The chronicity of the lesion should arouse suspicion. Usually the regional lymph nodes become enlarged about the end of the first week.

Although the history and clinical findings may be suggestive, definitive diagnosis can only be made by dark field examination of the exudate from the lesion. One negative examination is not sufficient to rule out the disease. After several weeks, the serologic tests may become positive and lead to definitive diagnosis.

In the tertiary form of the disease, gummas may occur in any location, including the upper extremities. Skin, soft tissue, and bone may be involved. These usually develop as circumscribed subcutaneous nodules which enlarge slowly, erode the skin, and drain a thick material. Occasionally joints may be rapidly and painlessly destroyed by a neurotrophic disturbance. The involved area becomes abnormally mobile, and shortening may take place (Charcot joint). Rarely, firm, subcutaneous "juxtaarticular" nodules appear, especially on the palmar surface of the hands. These may be fixed to the tendons and do not cause damage to the skin or ulcerate.

Congenital syphilis may effect the bones and joints of infants in the form of osteitis, periostitis, and osteochondritis. The long bones are more commonly involved. Separation of epiphyses due to syphilitic involvement is occasionally misdiagnosed as a fracture. However, in the congenitally syphilitic infant, the constitutional symptoms are obvious enough so that the true condition is rearly missed. Wasting, pallor, skin rashes, bony deformity, and rhinitis (sniffles) are a few of the symptoms of this condition.[41] Deformity, pain, and pseudoparalysis may be present in the involved limb (pseudoparalysis of Parrot). X-ray changes at the epiphysial line are specific.

The diagnosis of tertiary and congenital syphilis is made by history and physical examination plus serologic test.

The treatment for all phases of syphilis is massive doses of penicillin. Tetracyclines of erythromycin may be useful in penicillin-sensitive patients. Most of the complications which involve the upper extremities will subside on this regimen. Occasionally, large gummas may have to be excised and flail joints fused. Separated epiphyses should be reduced and properly splinted.

SPECIFIC FOREIGN BODY INFECTIONS

Two infections should be mentioned that are related to penetration of the skin of the hands by foreign bodies. Both diseases are peculiar to specific occupations.

Barber's Hand

In 1946, Paity and Scariff[48] described an inflammatory process between the fingers of barbers caused by penetration of hair through the skin of the web space. Apparantly many barbers are now aware of this possibility and merely remove the hairs when they notice them. Occasionally if they remain long enough under the skin, an abscess or epithelialized fistulous tract may develop around the hair and be a source of recurrent infection.[15][62] Joseph[32] found 15 cases in 115 barbers that he examined. Eight were aware of the problem. Three had signs of inflammation.

Generally a pinpoint opening is noted in the web space with hairs protruding, or a cystlike nodule can be palpated from which hair may be expressed.[12] Occasionally severe infection may develop and, in one reported instance, a barber almost gave up work because of the unrecognized problem.[15]

The treatment is excision of the cyst after the inflammatory process has been controlled.[19][53] In early cases, simple removal of accessible hair may control the condition.

Milker's Granuloma

Milker's granuloma is a painful, red, granulating, discharging lesion found on the hands of milkers or those who work with cattle. The hairs of cattle are barbed and may work deeply under the skin, causing a foreign body reaction.

Treatment is removal of the hair and control of the inflammatory process. A persistent granuloma should be removed.

REFERENCES

1. Adler, S., and Theodore, O., Experimental transfer of cutaneous leishmaniasis to man from *Phlebotomus papatasii*. Ann. Trop. Med., *19:* 365, 1925.
2. Barrett, C. C. Keratoderma blennorrhagicum, report of two cases, gonococcus in the local lesion in one case. Arch. Dermatol., *22:* 627, 1930.
3. Bearn, H. J., Jacobs, K., and McCarty, M. *Pasteurella multocida* septicemia in man. Am. J. Med., *18:* 167, 1955.
4. Bernstein, J. M., and Carling, R. E. Observations on human glanders, with a study of six cases and a discussion of the methods of diagnosis. Br. Med. J., *2:* 319, 1909.
5. Birnbaum, V. Acute suppurative gonococcal tenosynovitis. J. A. M. A., *105:* 1025, 1938.
6. Brachman, P. S., and Fekerty, F. R. Industrial anthrax. Ann. N. Y. Acad. Sci., *70:* 574, 1958.
7. Brachman, P. S., Pagano, J. S., and Albrink, W. S. Two cases of fatal inhalation anthrax, one associated with sarcoidosis. N. Engl. J. Med., *265:* 203, 1961.
8. Burnett, J. W., and Katz, S. L. A study of the use of 5-iodo-2'-deoxyuridine in cutaneous herpes simplex. J. Invest. Dermatol., *40:* 7, 1963.
9. Byrne, J. J., Boyd, T. F., and Daley, A. K. *Pasteurella* infection from cats. Surg. Gynecol. Obstet., *103:* 57, 1958.
10. Cawley, E. P., Whitmore, C. W., and Wheeler, G. E. Milkers' nodules. South. Med. J., *46:* 21, 1953.
11. Cravitz, C., and Miller, W. R. Immunologic studies with *Malleomyces mallei* and *Malleomyces pseudomallei*. II. Agglutination and complement fixation tests in man and laboratory animals. J. Infect. Dis., *86:* 52, 1950.
12. Currie, A. R., Gibson, T., and Goodall, A. L. Interdigital sinuses of barbers' hands. Br. J. Surg. *41:* 278, 1953.
13. Daniels, W. B., and MacMurray, F. C. Cat scratch disease, a report of 160 cases. J. A. M. A., *154:* 1247, 1954.
14. Debre, R., Lamy, M., Jammet, M. L., Costil, L., and Mozziconacci, P. La maladie dies griffes de chat. Bull. mm. Soc. méd. hóp Paris, *66:* 76, 1950.
15. Downing, J. G. Barbers' pilonidal sinus. J. A. M. A., *148:* 1501, 1952.
16. Editorial. Herpetic whitlow. Br. Med. J., *2:* 696, 1961.
17. Emson, H. E. Local infection with *Pasteurella septica* after a dog bit. J. Clin. Path., *10:* 187, 1957.
18. Ericson, C., and Johlin, I. A case of *Pasteurella multocida* infection after cat bite. Acta. Pathol. microbiol. scand., *46:* 47, 1959.
19. Ewing, M. R. Hair bearing sinus. Lancet, *1:* 427, 1947.
20. Foshay, L. Tularemia: Accurate and earlier diagnosis by means of the intradermal reaction. J. Infect. Dis., *36:* 286, 1932.
21. Francis, E. Tularemia. In *The Oxford Medicine, Vol. 4,* Edited by H. A. Christian, New York, Oxford, 1948, p. 955.
22. Gold, H. Anthrax: A report of 117 cases. Arch. Int. Med., *96:* 387, 1955.
23. Grant, A., and Barwell, C. Chronic melioidosis. A case diagnosed in England. Lancet, *1:* 199, 1943.
24. Greer, W. E. R., and Keefer, C. S. Cat scratch fever. A disease entity. N. Engl. J. Med., *244:* 545, 1951.

25. Hagemann, P. O., Hendin, A., Lurie, H. H., and Stein, M. Therapy of gonococcal arthritis. Ann. Int. Med., 36: 77, 1952.

26. Hamlin, E., and Sarris, S. P. Acute gonococcal tenosynovitis: Report of 7 cases. N. Engl. J. Med., 221: 228, 1939.

27. Howe, C. Anthrax. In The Oxford Medicine, Vol. 5, Edited by H. A. Christian. New York, Oxford, 1950, p. 213.

28. Howe, C. Glanders. In The Oxford Medicine, Vol. 5, Edited by J. H. Christian. New York, Oxford, 1950, p. 185.

29. Howe, C., and Miller, W. R. Human glanders: Report of six cases. Ann. Int. Med., 26: 93, 1947.

30. Humphreys, H. F. Notes on three cases of specific infections of the hand in dental surgeons. Br. Dent. J., 80: 367, 1946.

31. Hunter, D. The Diseases of Occupations, Ed. 1. Boston, Little, Brown, 1955, (a) p. 639; (b) p. 650.

32. Joseph, H. L., and Gifford, H. Barbers' interdigital pilonidal sinus: Incidence, pathology and pathogenesis, Arch. Dermatol., 70: 616, 1954.

33. Kapel, I. Cat bite, pasteurellosis, halisteriesis. Acta chir. scand., 95: 27, 1947.

34. Keefer, C. S., and Spink, W. W. Gonococcus arthritis: Pathogenesis, mechanism of recovery and treatment. J. A. M. A., 109: 1448, 1937.

35. Klander, J. V., Kramer, D. W., and Nicholas, L. Erysipelothrix rhusiopathiae septicemia: Diagnosis and treatment. Report of a fatal case of erysipeloid. J. A. M. A., 122: 938, 1943.

36. Koch, R. Untersuchungen über Bacterien V. Die Aetiologie der Milzbrandkrankhiet begrundet auf die Entwicklungsgeshichte des Bacillus anthracis. Beitr. Biol. Pflanzen., 11: 277, 1877.

37. Lebowich, R. J., McKillip, B. G., and Conboy, J. R. Cutaneous anthrax: A pathologic study with a clinical correlation. Am. J. Clin. Path., 13: 505, 1943.

38. Lee, M. L., and Buhr, A. J. Dog bites and local infection with Pasteurella septica. Br. Med. J., 1: 169, 1960.

39. McCoy, G. W., and Chapin, C. W. Further observations a plague-like disease of rodents, with a preliminary note on the causative agent, Bacterium tularense. J. Infect. Dis., 10: 61, 1912.

40. McCrumb, F. R., Snyder, M. J., and Woodward, R. E. Studies on human infection with Pasteurella tularensis. Comparison of streptomycin and chloramphenicol in the prophylaxis of clinical disease. Am. Physicians, 70: 74, 1957.

41. McCune, J. D. Congenital syphilis. In Textbook of Orthopedics, Ed. 1, edited by M. B. Howorth. Philadelphia, Saunders, 1952, p. 540.

42. McDowell, F., and Varney, P. L. Melioidosis. Report of the first case from the western hemisphere. J.A.M.A., 134: 361, 1947.

43. McGinnis, G. F., and Spindle, F. Erysipeloid condition among workers in a bone button factory due to bacillus of swine erysipelas. Am. J. Pub. Health, 24: 32, 1934.

44. Meyer, K. F. Pasteurella. In Bacterial and Mycotic Infections of Man, Ed. 3, edited by R.J. Dubos, Philadelphia, Lippincott, 1958, (a) p. 400; (b) p. 425.

45. Miller, W. R., Pannell, L., and Ingalls, M. S. Experimental therapy in glanders and melioidosis. Am. J. Hyg., 47: 205, 1948.

46. Olson, A. M., and Needham, G. M. Pasteurella multocida in suppurative diseases of the respiratory tract. Am. J. Med Sci., 224: 77, 1952.

47. Overholt, E., Tigertt, W. D., Kadull, P. J., Ward, A. K., Charles, N. D., Rene, R. M., Salzman, T. W., and Stephens, M. An analysis of 42 cases of laboratory acquired tularemia. Am. J. Med., 30: 785, 1961.

48. Paitey, D. H., and Scharff, R. W. Pilonidal sinus in Barber's Hand with observations on post-natal pilonidal sinus. Lancet, 2: 13, 1948.

49. Pasteur, L. Sur les maladies virulentes, et en particulier sur la maladie appelée vulguirement, cholera des poules. Compt. rend. acad. sc. 90: 239, 1880.

50. Pasteur, L., Chamberland, C. E., and Roux, E. Compte vendu sommaide des experiences faites a Pouilly-le fort, pres Melun sur la vaccination charboneusie. Compt. rend Acad. Sc. 92: 1378, 1881.

51. Pasteur, L., and Thuillier, L. La vaccination de rouget des pores a l'aide du virus mortel attenuie de cette maladie. Compt. Rend. Acad. Sc. 97: 1163, 1883.

52. Pizey, N. C. D. Infection with Pasteurella septica in a child aged three weeks. Lancet, 2: 324, 1953.

53. Powell, H. D. W. Interdigital sinus in Barber's Hand. Br. J. Surg., 43: 520, 1956.

54. Rayer, P. De la morve et du farcin chez l'homme. Mem. Acad. Med., 2: 625, 1837.

55. Rayer, P. Inoculation du sang de Rate. Bull. Soc. Biol., 2: 141, 1850.

56. Reed, R. W. Listeria and Erysipelothrix In Bacterial and Mycotic Infections of Man, Ed. 3, R. J. Dubos, Philadelphia, Lippincott, 1958, p. 458.

57. Sampaio, S. A., Godoy, J. T., Paiva, L., Dillon, N. L., and Laaz, C. The treatment of American (mucocutaneous) leishmaniasis with Amphotericin B. Arch. Dermatal., 82: 627, 1960.

58. Sieff, B. Primary syphilis of the hand resulting from trauma sustained on striking an infected subject: A report of four cases. S. A. M. J., 20: 114, 1946.

59. Small, W. T., and Sniffen, R. C. Nonbacterial regional lymphadenitis ("cat scratch fever"). Evaluation of surgical treatment. N. Engl. J. Med., 255: 029, 1956.

60. Smith, H. J., Keppie, J. L., Harris-Smith, P., and Harris-Smith, S. The chemical basis of the virulence of bacillus anthracis. IV. Secondary shock as a major factor in the death of guinea pigs from anthrax. Br. J. Exp. Pathol., 36: 323, 1956.

61. Spotnitz, M., Rudnitzky, J. and Rambaud, J. J. Melioidosis pneumonitis. J. A. M. A., 202: 950, 1967.

62. Steele, J. H., and Helvig, R. J. Anthrax in the United States. Pub. Health Rep., 68: 616, 1953.

63. Stoip, A. Interdigital pilonidal sinus of both hands. Dermatol. Monatsschr., 156: 16, 1970.

64. Swartz, M. J., and Kung, L. J. Pasteurella multocida infections in man. Report of 2 cases: meningitis and infected cat bites. New Engl. J. Med. 261: 889, 1959.

65. Wehrbein, H. L. Gonococcus arthritis: A study of 610 cases. Surg. Gynec. Obst. 49: 105, 1929.

66. Wilson, G. S., and Miles, A. A. Topley and Wilson Principles of Bacteriology and Immunity, Vol. II, Ed. 4. Williams & Wilkins, Baltimore, 1955, (a) p.

1938, (b) p. 1606; (c) p. 2127; (d) p. 2132.

67. Womack, C. R., and Wells, E. G. Coexistent chronic glanders and multiple cystic osseous tuberculosis treated with streptomycin. Am. J. Med. 6: 267, 1949.

68. Wright, G. G. The Anthrax Bacillus in Bacterial and Mycotic Infections of Man, Ed. 3. R. J. Dubos, Editor. Lippincott, Philadelphia and Montreal, 1958, p. 330.

69. Wright, J. G. Protozoa in a case of tropical ulcer. J. M. Res. 10: 472, 1903.

70. Yater, W. M. Fundamentals of Internal Medicine, Ed. 2. Appleton, New York and London, 1944, p. 444.

E.

Tuberculosis of the Hand

Richard J. Smith, M.D.
Robert D. Leffert, M.D.

The clinical features of pulmonary tuberculosis were well known in eastern Europe as early as 1,000 B.C. The Greeks called the disease "phthisis" referring to the state of decay or emaciation of the more severely afflicted patients. Most probably, patients suffering from any severe fulminating pulmonary disease were all grouped under this diagnosis. In the early 19th century, postmortem pathologic findings and the patients' clinical course were compared and "tuberculosis" was defined as a disease quite separate from neoplasm, silicosis, fungal disease, and bronchiectasis. Indeed, many years before Koch identified the tubercle bacillis as the causative agent of the disease in 1882, it was well known that tuberculosis could be diagnosed through guinea pig inoculation of infected sputum.

BACTERIOLOGY AND PATHOGENESIS OF TUBERCULOSIS

Mycobacterium tuberculosis is "acid fast"; the bacillis does not decolorize with acid alcohol after being stained with steamed carbolfuchsin. Several other bacteria are also acid fast but only two others cause tuberculosis, Mycobacterium bovis and Mycobacterium avium. Among the acid fast bacilli which do not cause tuberculosis but may cause skin, nerve, tendon sheath infection in man are Mycobacterium leprae (Hansen's bacillis), Mycobacterium marinum (M. balnei) and the Battey bacilli. Each of these pathogens can be differentiated from each other by culture techniques. Their characteristics of growth on laboratory media and their animal virulence vary.

The three bacilli which cause tuberculosis also differ from each other as to their source, their mode of entry into the body, the tissues primarily involved in human infection, and their susceptibility to antimicrobial agents. Mycobacterium tuberculosis usually gains entry into the body through inhalation of droplet air-borne bacilli disseminated by a person with active pulmonary disease. The bacilli lodge within the alveoli and within 24 hours provoke an inflammatory response. Within one to two weeks macrophages appear and form epitheloid cells and giant cells. Local hilar lymph nodes are also involved and form the "primary complex" of tuberculosis. By the 15th to 30th day, necrosis may occur in the central portions of the pulmonary lesion, break into a blood or lymph vessel, and disseminate the bacilli throughout the body. Skeletal deposits will be most frequent in the areas of spongy, cancellous marrow and at the epiphyseal ends of the bone where blood flow is sluggish through vascular sinuses. Bone is the most common site of extrapulmonary tuberculosis and is involved in about 5 per cent of all cases. The spine and hip are the most common sites of osseous involvement. Of all cases of bone tuberculosis, the bones of the hand are affected in about 5 per cent of patients.

Mycobacterium bovis, ingested with the unboiled milk of diseased cows, and Mycobacterium avium, which gains entry to the gastrointestinal tract through eating diseased fowl and pork, are now rarely found in urban and industrial areas due to effective public health measures. Once gaining access to the gastrointestinal tract, however, these bacteria pass readily through the mucous membrane to the tonsils and through the lymphoid tissue of the lower ileum to regional lumph nodes. From here, they drain ultimately to the blood vascular system and may then disseminate throughout the body. Although there has been no documented case of avian tuberculosis of bone, bovine tuberculosis is clinically indistinguishable from infection by Mycobacterium tuberculosis.

Once the bacilli have lodged in bone they may lie dormant for a variable length of time, often for years, finally to become active once again inciting inflammation and infection.

Thus, with few exceptions, tuberculous osteomyelitis and synovitis of the hand are hematogenous in onset, almost always due to Mycobacterium tuberculosis and is secondary to pulmonary tuberculosis. On rare occasions, Mycobacterium tuberculosis can cause bone or joint infection as a result of a skin wound following a human bite.

INDIDENCE, AGE, SEX, AND ASSOCIATED LESIONS

The incidence of tuberculosis in the United States continues to decrease every decade. Nonetheless, in 1958, 63,000 new cases were reported. In 1967, there were 45,000 new cases in this country. Tuberculosis of the bone and joints is similarly decreasing. Involvement of the tendon sheaths, bones, and joints of he hand is so infrequent that even active clinical facilities see few cases. Patients with tenosynovitis tended to be older than those with tuberculous arthritis. Tenosynovitis appears most common in the 20 to 50-year age group. Males appear more frequently affected by tuberculosis of the bones, joints, and tendon sheaths of the hand than are females. Although history of antecedent trauma is frequently given, most authors feel that it is very rarely an important precipitating factor in the disease.

The presence of associated tuberculous foci often is sought as an aid in establishing the diagnosis of bone or joint tuberculosis. Robins[23] reported that, of 39 patients with tuberculosis of the wrist, 17 had tuberculous lesions elsewhere. Ten of these lesions were pulmonary. In a group of 36 cases of tubercular tenosynovitis of the hand, 11 had associated lesions elsewhere, eight of which were pulmonary. In 31 cases of tubercular compound palmar ganglion reported by Pinn and Waugh, 15 patients had other tuberculous lesions and six later developed tuberculosis of the wrist joint.

DIAGNOSIS

Tuberculosis of the hand is usually insidious in onset. It may provoke few complaints for many months or years. Later, when tenderness and swelling develop, interpretation of x-rays may be difficult and the correct diagnosis often is elusive. Other diseases which affect bone and which may be confused with tuberculosis include staphyloccocal osteomyelitis, sarcoidosis, fibrous dysplasia, rheumatoid arthritis, enchondromatosis, Ewings sarcoma, luetic osteitis, coccidioidomycosis, histoplasmosis, and blastomycosis. Several guidelines may be of help in establishing a diagnosis of a tuberculous infection about the hand:

A. Clinical
  1. Chronic course
  2. Little pain until late
  3. Doughy swollen area over the lesion is less tender, less hot and less red than with pyogenic infection
  4. Usually no lymphangitis
B. Radiologic
  1. Preservation of joint space long after joint involvement
  2. Loss of subchondral bone shadow
  3. Marked bone atrophy
  4. Spina ventosa in children
  5. Periostitis
  6. Bone erosion, "pseudocyst formation" and woolly cortical appearance at epiphyseal ends of bones in adults
  7. Primary complex of lung in child (often no longer visible in adults)
C. Laboratory
  1. Normal white count, occasional mild relative increase in mononuclear leukocytes
  2. Elevated sedimentation rate; may be 50 to 75 mm per hour during active phase
  3. Synovial fluid analysis; turbid fluid, leukocytosis (often 20,000 per cubic mm), increased protein, decreased mucin, marked decrease in sugar (often to 25 mg per cent)
  4. Positive skin test is virtually essential for diagnosis although may be negative during periods of severe illness, after measles, smallpox or smallpox vaccination.
D. Culture
  Two general methods of culture are available, animal innoculation and in vitro laboratory plating. Neither method is faultless although false negatives with guinea pig innoculation is probably less than 1 per cent and with culture as high as 14 per cent. Many authors recommended both means be used for speed of diagnosis and to insure against fewer missed cases. Sensitivity studies are also valuable. The specimen to be cultured may be taken from joint fluid but is best obtained from the tissues of the lesion in question. Lymph node biopsy, gastric washings and urine culture are usually unnecessary, as a diagnosis can best be made from a specimen removed from the hand.
E. Biopsy
  Despite potential dangers of introducing superimposed infection and of spreading local disease, biopsies are often of great value in securing a diagnosis. Although often difficult to interpret, many granulomatous lesions of the hand can be differentiated from tuberculous synovitis by histologic findings, presence or absence of caseation, and by acid fast stains.

PATHOLOGIC CHANGES WITH TUBERCULOUS LESIONS OF THE HAND

Tuberculous involvement of the hand may take different forms depending upon the site of involvement, the age of the patient, the treatment, and the patient's inherent resistance to disease.

Tuberculous Dactylitis in Children

Skeletal tuberculosis is considerably more frequent in children than in adults. Similarly, tuberculous dactylitis is uncommon after the age of ten. Typically, tuberculous involvement of the small tubular bones of the fingers, and to a much lesser extent of the toes, of the young child results in the development of "spina ventosa." This term means "spinelike projection" of the bone which appears as though it had been "puffed with wind." The tubercle bacillis, seeded within the medullary cavity of the phalanx provokes considerable edema and the proliferation of granulation tissue. Several fingers of one hand are frequently affected simultaneously. The tuberculous granulation tissue thins and expands the phalangeal cortex, occasionally perforating its bony shell to invade the adjacent soft tissue. The spongiosa is destroyed. Serous effusion through the cortex, and subperiosteal growth of tuberculous granulation tissue causes periosteal elevation and layering of new bone. Unless there is secondary abscess or sinus formation, healing is the rule and usually occurs with neither deformity nor shortening. Gradually, the expanded bone remodels and within a few years the only evidence of previous disease may be persistent moderate increase in the diameter of the bone (Fig. 14.5.1).

The x-ray appearance of the bones affected with spina ventosa closely reflect the pathologic processes. There is usually involvement of several of the proximal phalanges or metacarpals of the involved hand. During the active stages of the disease process the medullary cavity appears osteoporotic and has a "ground glass" or homogeneous texture. The cortex is expanded. Layers of periosteal new bone surround the expanding cortex and often a soft tissue density will lie adjacent to the site of cortical breakthrough where a small cold abscess has formed. With healing and remodeling the cortex may appear sclerotic and widening of the medullary cavity with increased radio-density of the diaphysis may remain as the scars of spina ventosa (Fig. 14.5.2).

Considering this benign course, treatment of spina ventosa should be conservative unless there is evidence of severe secondary infection from abscess or sinus formation. The digits must not be amputated despite a frightening appearance on x-ray of bony enlargement. Conservative treatment consisting of splinting and appropriate medication is all that is needed in most cases. Curettage of the medullary cavity is rarely necessary. If soft tissue abscess and sinus formation occurs, they should be excised and drained.

Tuberculous Dactylitis in Adults

Although considerably more frequent in children, tuberculous dactylitis can occur in adults as well. Indeed, a recent report reviewed 23 such cases in one medical center in New York City. There are several differences between the small tubular bones of the adult and those of the child. Unlike those of the child, the phalanges and metacarpals of the adult lack an epiphyseal plate and thus have no cartilagenous barrier between the articular cortex and the metaphysis of the bone. Tuberculous granulation tissue within the bone will therefore extend to the subchondral articular cortex which will gradually be replaced. There will be a loss of radiologic definition. If the epiphyseal end of the bone is affected, the joint is frequently violated and tuberculous arthritis may ensue.

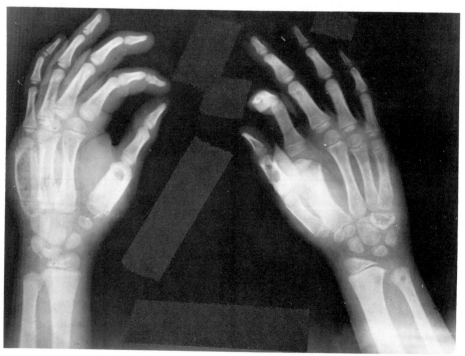

Figure 14.5.1. Diffuse tuberculous osteitis in a child. In the right hand, there is cavitation at the head of the ulna, the hamate, and the proximal phalanx of the thumb, spina ventosa in the second right metacarpal, and the first and fifth left metacarpals. Involvement of several rays in one hand is common in untreated tuberculosis. Tuberculosis of both hands simultaneously is rather rare. (X-ray courtesy of Alexander Norman, M.D., Department of Radiology, Hospital for Joint Diseases, New York.)

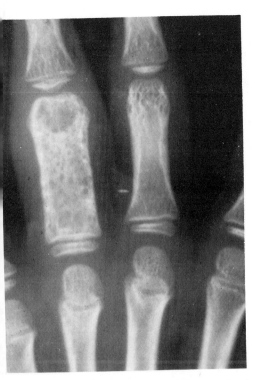

Figure 14.5.2. Spina ventosa of the proximal phalanx of a child. The cortex is expanded; there is mottling within the medullary cavity. The epiphyseal end of the bone is uninvolved. The joints do not appear involved.

The medullary cavity of the adult is less spongy than that of the child, and its cortex has a relatively poor blood supply. The periosteum of the adult is more fibrous and more firmly adherent to the shaft of the bone than is that of the child. Granulation tissue enveloping small areas of adult cortex may thus more readily absorb the bone and cause a punched out, woolly, or moth-eaten appearance to the osteoporotic bone. A localized region of periostitis may be noted at the site of cortical destruction but periosteal elevation is limited and the "blown up" appearance of these tubular bones which are seen in children is not seen in adults. With thinning of the cortex and poor periosteal response the bone is weakened and may frequently fracture. (Fracture is rare with spina ventosa.) Sequestra may form as a result of the periosteal stripping and the devascularization of cortical bone. Deformity may occur.

Tuberculous dactylitis in the adult may be restricted to one digit. Because of the frequent complications of secondary joint involvement with destruction of articular cartilage, the development of abscesses and of cortical fractures, and the ultimate stiffness and deformity of these fingers, dactylitis in the adult is much more serious than spina ventosa in a child. Curettage, splinting, and antitubercular therapy are indicated early. If the finger shows gross evidence of destruction and joint involvement it may require amputation (Fig. 14.5.3. A, B, C, D).

Carpal Tuberculosis

Tuberculosis about the wrist region usually begins at the carpometacarpal points, in the proximal metacarpals, and at the distal row of carpal bones. From there, infection extends proximally and frequently involves the radiocarpal and the radioulnar joints (Fig. 14.5.8). Tuberculosis about the proximal metacarpals and distal carpal row is clinically more apparent dorsally than volarly and may be accompanied by diffuse tenderness, swelling, and stiffness of the fingers and of the wrist. Bone resorption by tuberculous granulation tissue will cause mottling and atrophy about the proximal end of the metacarpal and marked atrophy about the carpal bones. Relatively early there will be a loss of joint space at the carpometacarpal and intercarpal joint areas. Sinus formation is frequent.

If tuberculous osteomyelitis of the carpal bones is treated prior to involvement of the radiocarpal joint, it can usually be successfully managed by splints, medication, and the drainage of any soft tissue abscesses. With more severe involvement, sequestra will require excision. Intercarpal synovectomy, occasionally with radiocarpal and radioulnar synovectomy will frequently be necessary. Severe deformity is infrequent following tuberculous involvement of the carpal bones (Fig. 14.5.4. A, B).

Tuberculosis of the Distal Radius and Ulna

As has been noted in the discussion of tuberculous dactylitis, tuberculous osteitis in the adult is most common at the epiphyseal ends of the bones. This is particularly true of involvement of the radius and ulna. Synovitis of the adjacent joint is frequently associated with epiphyseal disease. Whether it is the joint synovium or the epiphyseal end of the bone which is first involved is often impossible to determine. The tuberculous granulation tissue replaces the subchondral bone and soon the joint margins are difficult to detect radiographically. The tubercle bacilli produce no proteolytic enzymes and thus the joint space is usually preserved. Gradually, granulation tissue may separate cartilage from underlying bone and may advance over its free borders causing the articular cartilage to thin, to soften, and finally to die. Pieces of cartilage may fall freely from the joint. Sites of synovial attachment to bone are more severely involved with proliferating granulation tissue and deep grooves, cavities, and sequestra are formed at the joint margins. Most frequently both sides of the involved joint will show evidence of disease. If the tuberculosis is not arrested, cartilage is resorbed and granulation tissue at both sides of the wrist joint will coalesce gradually to form a bony ankylosis.

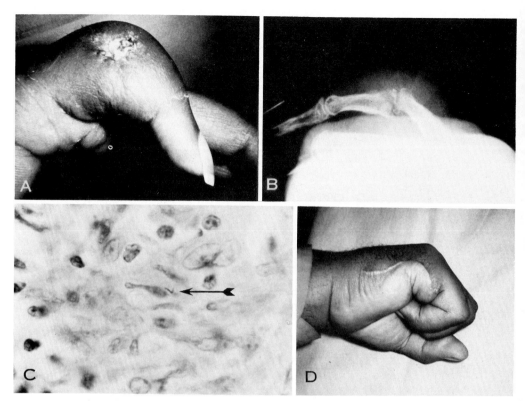

Figure 14.5.3A. Swelling, tenderness and a draining sinus in this adult with no previous history of tuberculosis had been misdiagnosed as rheumatoid synovitis.

Figure 14.5.3B. An x-ray reveals joint destruction and volar subluxation of the middle phalanx. There is soft tissue swelling.

Figure 14.5.3C. The microscopic slide reveals an acid-fast bacillis within the inflamed synovium.

Figure 14.5.3D. In view of draining, joint stiffness, and obvious osteomyelitis, the fifth ray was amputated. Full function was restored to the hand within a few weeks.

Tuberculous Synovitis, Arthritis, and Tenosynovitis

Intra-articular tuberculous synovitis of the wrist, of the small joints of the hand, and tuberculous tenosynovitis of the extrinsic tendons may either follow each other in sequence or may develop simultaneously. Although direct inoculation through cuts or bruises about the hand have been observed in those who worked with infected cattle, the control of *Mycobacterium bovis* has now essentially eliminated this mode of entry. Synovial tuberculosis is usually blood borne. Intra-articular tuberculosis may result either from primary involvement of its synovium, secondary involvement from adjacent tenosynovium or by direct extension of an osseus focus to the articular cartilage.

The pathologic changes associated with intra-articular synovitis vary considerably and are less severe when the infection has begun primarily within the joint than if it has spread to the joint from adjacent bone. With more severe involvement, the synovium is quite thickened and its surface is covered with a ragged layer of fibrin. Histologic examination will demonstrate vascular granulation tissue admixed with fibrin masses, caseation necrosis, leukocytes, and tubercles. Often, the tubercles may be difficult to identify. In many cases of tuberculous synovitis the changes are less pronounced and the synovium may be only slightly thickened and injected. Joint fluid may vary from a thick purulent coagulum to a thin opaque yellow fluid. Rice bodies, which may float within the joint, usually represent synovial villi which have undergone fibrinous transformation after long-standing mild infections.

Within tuberculous joints, the articular cartilage soon undergoes erosion and loosening as the vascular synovial granulation tissue proliferates both at the

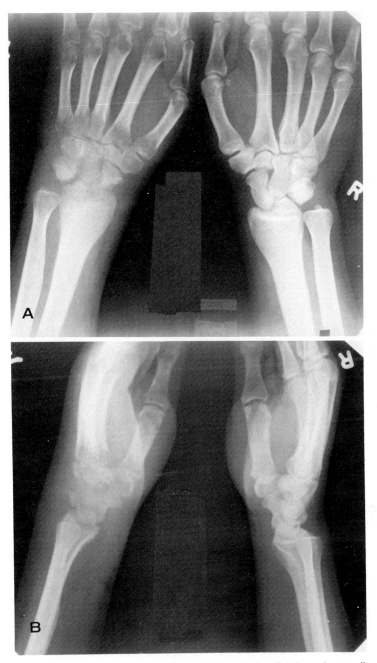

Figure 14.5.4A and B. With tuberculosis of the carpal bones the distal row is usually more severely involved. The bases of the metacarpals are also affected. Marked radiolucency probably represents medullary invasion with tuberculous granulation tissue. The uninvolved right wrist is shown for comparison. (X-rays courtesy of Radiology Department Teaching Collection; Massachusetts General Hospital, Boston, Massachusetts.)

joint surface and in the subchondral bone. Occasionally a superimposed pyogenic infection may cause further necrosis of the joint surfaces and total destruction of articular cartilage.

The pathologic changes associated with tuberculous tenosynovitis are similar to those of intra-articular synovitis. Initially, the tendon sheaths are swollen with serous fluid; later they may fill with a thick purulent material. The sheaths lose their luster and their walls thicken. Granulomatous changes, tubercle formation, necrosis, and fibrinous exudate may be seen about the shaggy synovium. If uncontrolled, the tendons become dull, adherent to each other and to the surrounding tissues, and are invaded by the synovium ultimately to rupture. Tuberculous tenosynovitis may be spread to adjacent bones and joints and to the deep spaces of the hand and the forearm (Fig. 14.5.5.A, B, C, D, and Fig. 14.5.7. A, B).

The term "compound palmar ganglion" is used today to describe flexor tenosynovitis of the hand and wrist not necessarily to tuberculous origin. Historically, however, this term refers to tuberculous tenosynovitis of the ulnar and radial bursae. The ulnar bursa alone, or in combination with the radial bursa, is involved more frequently than the radial bursa itself. Swelling, aching, and stiffness of the fingers are the usual complaints, and occasionally paresthesias are perceived. The flexor tendon sheaths of the index,

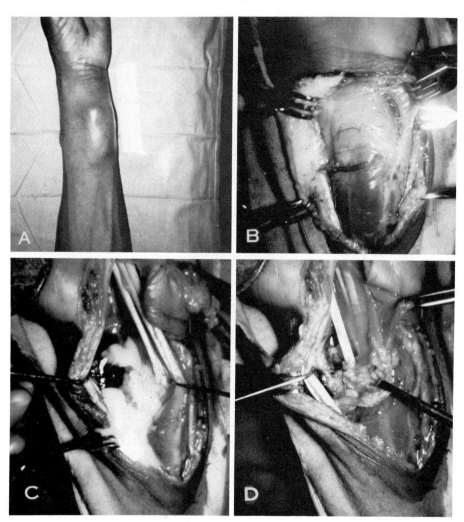

Figure 14.5.5A. Tuberculous abscess of the soft tissues of the forearm. The "cold abscess" of tuberculosis is neither as tender, as erythematous nor as warm to touch as would be a staphylococcal abscess.

Figure 14.5.5B. An incision through the skin and subcutaneous tissues reveals the pouting synovium of the flexor tendons.

Figure 14.5.5C. The synovium is opened and creamy pus exudes from about the flexor tendons.

Figure 14.5.5D. The carpal tunnel is opened and a tenosynovectomy is performed.

middle and ring fingers are sometimes involved with tuberculous infection and although swelling is common; pain is absent. The tendon sheath of the little finger often communicates with the ulnar bursa and thus forms part of the compound palmar ganglion. The extensor tendon sheaths of the hand are less frequently affected with tubercuous synovitis than are the flexors and the swelling which occurs is comparatively painless. (Fig. 14.5.6. A, B, C, D).

The radiographic changes associated with tuberculous arthritis reflect the pathologic changes within the joints. Early, x-rays may show evidence merely of effusion and involvement of the underlying bone may

not be appreciated. Later, there may be evidence of severe local and regional bone atrophy. Subchondral bone resorption by granulation tissue is reflected as loss of articular cortical definition with relatively late preservation of the joint space. Sequestration due to local subchondral bone infarction on either side of the joint may appear as rough, dense, wedge-shaped areas with preserved contacting articular margins — the so-called "kissing sequestra." Local cystic degeneration adjacent to the joint is often surrounded by a shell of sclerosis and has been termed "multiple pseudocystic tuberculosis of bone." Sometimes, the pace of joint destruction as noted on x-ray may be quite rapid,

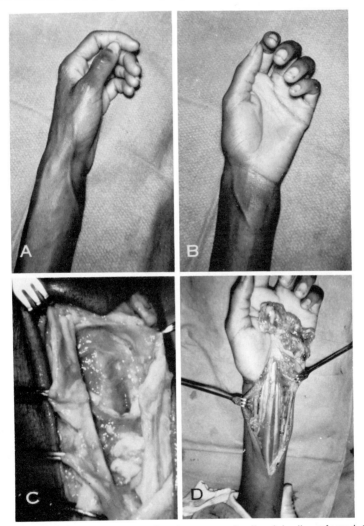

Figures 14.5.6A and B. The "compound palmar ganglion" originally referred to tuberculous tenosynovitis of the flexor tendons which extended from the proximal palm to the distal forearm. A compound ganglion is seen here.

Figure 14.5.6C. Shaggy, inflamed synovium is noted about the flexor tendons.

Figure 14.5.6D. Tenosynovectomy is performed.

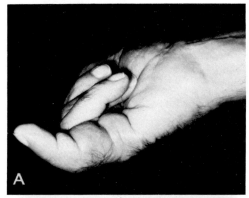

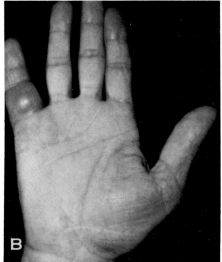

Figures 14.5.7A and B. Tuberculous flexor tenosynovitis of the little finger. This lesion may be difficult to differentiate from "atypical acid-fast" tenosynovitis without appropriate cultures. In either case, tenosynovectomy should be performed.

particularly if there is superimposition of pyogenic infection which further contributes to the bone sclerosis.

Successful treatment of tuberculous arthritis about the hand is more likely to preserve motion than is surgery upon the weight bearing joints of the lower limbs. Proper management includes surgical excision of infected tissues, prolonged and adequate administration of antimicrobial medication, and appropriate general measures to insure proper rest and nutrition of the patient.

To delay synovectomy until the disease becomes quiescent may result in fibrous ankylosis of the affected joints or rupture of the involved tendons. Early synovectomy is usually advisable. Although antimicrobial medication may not reach areas of ischemia, necrosis, and caseation, adequate blood levels of these drugs at the time of surgery may prevent dissemination of the bacillis through traumatized vascular chan-

nels. A course of antitubercular drugs is therefore given for two weeks preoperatively. Standard surgical approaches to the involved areas are used. Wide exposure of diseased and of nondiseased tissues is essential to preserve structures often enmeshed and concealed in fibrotic scar. Nerves and vessels should be identified before dissecting tendons; tendons should be visible before performing joint synovectomy. Necrotic segments of tendon should be excised and tendon stumps may be sutured to adjacent intact tendons to restore active motion. It is usually unwise to perform extensive tendon grafts or complex tendon transfers at the time of synovectomy. Abscesses and infected pockets of tissue should be exposed and cleaned by meticulous dissection. If there is no superimposed infection, the wounds may be thoroughly irrigated with saline or INH, then to be closed without a drain. With severe involvement of the single finger amputation must be considered.

The management of tubercular arthritis about the

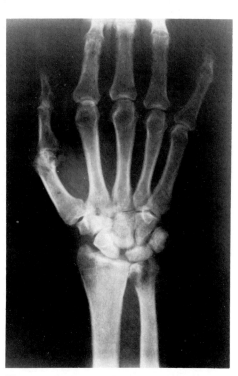

Figure 14.5.8. Tuberculous synovitis of the wrist. Synovial destruction of the radio-carpal ligament has allowed ulnar translocation of the hand. Synovitis in the region of the scapholunate ligament has resulted in scapholunate diastasis. The head of the ulna is also involved with tuberculous synovitis. The patient was treated with resection of the distal end of the ulna, synovectomy of the wrist joint, and subsequently a wrist arthrodesis. Antituberculous medication was continued for two years.

and depends a great deal upon the condition of the articular surfaces. With minor damage to the articular cartilage, joint synovectomy followed by external support and gradual resumption of motion under an umbrella of anti-tuberculous drugs may be expected to preserve motion and to eradicate the disease process in many cases. Carpectomy or arthrodesis should be performed in cases of severe joint destruction. In the event of serious uncontrolled pulmonary tuberculosis, or in the presence of a mixed superinfection within the joints of the hand, arthrodesis should be delayed and performed as a secondary procedure. Appropriate antimicrobial therapy should always be given both pre- and postoperatively.

ANTIMICROBIAL THERAPY

Many new drugs and combinations of drugs are presently being evaluated in the treatment of tuberculous infections. The three agents most commonly used include INH (isoniazid), PAS (para-aminosalicylic acid), and streptomycin.

INH is among the most effective and least toxic antitubercular drug in use today. It is frequently considered the "first line of defense." Although early elevation in serum transminase, due to hepatocellular damage has been noted in 10 per cent of patients, this rise is transient and the liver changes spontaneously revert to normal according to recent studies. INH should not be used alone in the treatment of bone or joint tuberculosis as there is a possibility of development of drug resistance by the organism. The usual adult dose is 4mg/kg, or 300 mg per day. Infrequently, peripheral neuropathy may develop in patients receiving INH due to their increased urinary excretion of pyridoxin (Vitamin B⁶). Thus, in patients who are in poor nutritional status, pyridoxin supplement of 10 mg per day may be a useful adjuvant to INH. Hypersensitivity or psychotic reactions with INH are rare.

A drug closely related to INH is iproniazid. This drug appears to have little antimicrobial advantage over INH and is potentially more toxic. Its use is limited.

Streptomycin is usually effective as an antituberculous drug especially given with INH. Usually it is given 1 gm per day for six to eight weeks and then 1 gm twice weekly for the remainder of therapy. Streptomycin is potentially dangerous to eighth nerve function and may be nephrotoxic. It should therefore be avoided in patients who have evidence of pre-existing auditory or vestibular deficits and in patients with evidence of impaired renal function. The toxic effects of streptomycin on eighth nerve function are dose related and may be irreversible. The drug should be stopped at the first sign of auditory nerve involvement.

PAS is a less effective antitubercular drug than either INH or streptomycin but is of value in preventing the development of bacterial resistance when given in combination with these two agents. The usual dose is 9 to 15 gm per day. PAS has been reported to produce gastrointestinal irritation in one third of those patients who receive it.

Other antimicrobial agents have been used for tuberculosis and other acid fast infections. These include cycloserine, ethionamide, ethambutal, viomycin, rifampin, and thiacetazone. Although "triple therapy" with ING, streptomycin, and PAS is effective in most cases of tuberculosis, there have been recent reports of drug resistance particularly in those personnel returning from the Far Eastern theaters of Korea and Viet Nam. Indeed, 25 to 70 per cent of tuberculous infections in these areas may be resistant to "triple therapy." It would thus seem wise to perform sensitivity studies of the bacillis in patients with tuberculosis. The results of such studies might be of considerable value in the event that one of the more standard drugs must be discontinued because of untoward reactions. Most patients developing tuberculosis of the bones and joints in this country, will respond to the triple therapy of INH, streptomycin, and PAS.

The duration of treatment in a patient with tuberculous infection of the hand will depend upon the presence and severity of associated active tuberculous lesions elsewhere, and the nature of the lesions about the hand. It is usually advised that drug therapy be continued for one year after the subsidance of signs and symptoms.

CONCLUSIONS

In years past, tuberculosis was endemic throughout most of the world, and was usually considered when joint or bone was diseased. The diagnosis was rarely missed, but the disease was rarely cured.

As the disease is now less frequently encountered, it is often not considered in the differential diagnosis of bone or joint pathology. To diagnosis a case of tuberculosis about the hand early is to gain an opportunity to treat it most effectively. Thus, with increased migration and travel to and from areas where tuberculosis is still endemic, we must be alert to its presence and prepared for its treatment.

REFERENCES

1. Adams, R., Jones, G., and Marble, H. C. Tubercular tenosynovitis. N. Engl. J. Med., 223: 706-708, 1940.
2. Beeson, P. B., and McDermott, W. In Cecil-Loeb Textbook of Medicine. Philadelphia, Saunders, 1967, pp. 259-295.
3. Bosworth, D. M. Modern concepts of treatment of tuberculosis of bones and joints. Ann. N.Y. Acad., 106: 98-105, 1963.
4. Committee on Division of Diagnosis Standards Diagnostic Standards and Classification of Tuberculosis. American Thoracic Society Medical Section of Material Tuberculosis and Respiratory Disease Association, N. Y., 1969.
5. Cowley, R. G., and Briney, R. R. Primary drug resistant tuberculosis in Viet Nam veterans. Am. Rev.

Resp. Dis., *101:* 703-705, 1970.

6. Cremin, B. J., Fisher, R. M., and Levinsohn, M. W. Multiple bone tuberculosis in the young. Br. J. Radiol., *43:* 638-645, 1970.

7. Davidson, Paul, T., and Horowitz, I. Skeletal tuberculosis. A review with patient presentations and discussions, Am. J. Med., *48:* 77-84, 1970.

8. Feldman, F., Auerbach, R., and Johnston, A. Tuberculosis dactylitis in the adult. Am. J. Roentgenol., *112:* 460.

9. Fellander, M. Tuberculosis tenosynovitis of the hand treated by combined surgery and chemotherapy. Acta Chir. Scand., *111:* 142, 150, 1956.

10. Flynn, J. E. *Hand Surgery.* 846-852, Baltimore, Williams & Wilkins, 1966.

11. Grunberg, E. Current status of tuberculosis. Ann. N.Y. Acad. Sci., *106:* 1-156, 1963.

12. Herzfeld, G., and Tod, M. C. Tuberculosis dactylitis in infancy. Arch. Dis. Child., *1:* 295-301, 1926.

13. Hollander, J. L., and McCarty, D. *Arthritis and Allied Conditions.* Philadelphia, Lea & Febiger, 1972, pp. 1242-1254.

14. Jaffe, H. J. *Metabolic, Degenerative and Inflammatory Diseases of Bones and Joints.* Philadelphia, Lea & Febiger, 1972, pg. 952-1004.

15. Johnson, J. E. *Rational Therapy and Control of Tuberculosis. A Symposium.* University of Florida Press, 1970.

16. Kelly, P. J., and Karlson, A. G. Musculoskeletal tuberculosis, Mayo Clin. Proc., *44:* 73-80, 1960.

17. Kelly, P. J., Weed, L. A., and Lipscomb, P. R. Infection of tendon sheaths, bursae, joints and soft tissues by acid fast bacilli other than tubercle bacilli. J. Bone Joint Surg., *45A:* 327, 1963.

18. Mathur, A. Letter to the Editor, N. Engl. J. Med., *285:* 410, 1971.

19. Phemister, D. B., and Hatcher, C. H. Correlation of pathological and roentgenological findings in the diagnosis of tuberculous arthritis. Am. J. Roentgenol., *29:* 736-752, 1932.

20. Pimm, L. H., and Wang, N. W. Tuberculous tenosynovitis of the hand treated by combined surgery and chemotherapy. Acta Chir. Scand., *111:* 142-150, 1956.

21. Pomeranz, M. M. Roentgenological diagnosis of bone and joint tuberculosis. Am. J. Roentgenol., *29:* 753-762, 1933.

22. Poppel, M. H., Lawrence, L. R., Jacobson, H. G., and Stein, J. Skeletal tuberculosis: A roentgenographic survey with reconsideration of diagnostic criteria. Am. J. Roentgenol., *70:* 936-963, 1953.

23. Robins, R. H. C. Tuberculosis of the wrist and hand. Br. J. Surg., *54:* 211-218, 1967.

24. Somowille, E. W., and Wilkinson, M. C. *Girdlestone's Tuberculosis of Bone and Joint.* New York, Oxford University Press, pp. 176-186, 1965.

25. Steiner, M., Chaues, A., Lyons, H., Steiner, P., and Portugaleza, C. Primary drug resistant tuberculosis: Report of an outbreak. Engl. J. Med., *283:* 1353-1385, 1970.

26. Stenstrom, B. Tuberculosis of the phalanges in older individuals. Acta Radiol., *16:* 471-477, 1935.

27. Umansky, A. L., Schlesinger, P. T., and Greenberg, B. B. Tuberculous dactylitis in the adult. Arch. Surg., *54:* 67–78, 1947.

28. Weed, L. A., and Macoy, N. E. Tuberculosis, problems in diagnosis and eradication. Am. J. Clin. Pathol., *53:* 136-140, 1970.

29. Wilkinson, M. C. Observations on the pathogenesis and treatment of skeletal tuberculosis. Ann. R. Coll. Surg., *41:* 168-192, 1949.

30. Wilkinson, M. C. Chemotherapy of tuberculosis of bones and joints. J. Bone Joint Surg., *36B:* 1954.

F.

Fungus Infections of the Hand

Henry Brown, M.D.

The infections are listed in three broad classes with examples of causative organisms of each.

I. Dermatomycoses or fungus infections of the skin
  A. *Trichophyton rubrum* (purpureum)
  B. *Trichophyton mentagrophytes*
  C. *Trichophyton schoenleini*
  D. *Epidermophyton floccosum*
  E. *Microsporum quickeanum*

II. Systemic mycotic infections, the hand being only one area involved
  A. Actinomycosis
  B. Blastomycosis
  C. Sporotrichosis
  D. Coccidioidomycosis

III. Yeast infections
  A. Candidiasis (formerly called Moniliasis)

DERMATOMYCOSES

Tinea capitis, ring worm, tinea manuum, tinea corporis, tinea cruris, tinea pedis, athlete's foot, and jungle rot are some terms listed for superficial fungus infections of the body in different geographic locations.[3] In addition, these organisms have a predilection for palms and soles, particularly *Trichophyton rubrum* (purpureum). *Trichophyton mentagrophytes* is also common in the toe webs. The term "tinea" refers to lesions of these infections.

Trichophyton rubrum is the commonest organism involving the nails. It affects the palms diffusely and may form a moccasin-like involvement of the soles. Since only one hand may be involved, some call the infection the "two-foot-one hand disease." In the differential diagnosis, the following are considered. *Epidermophyton floccosum* affects chiefly the groin. *Microsporum quinckeanum* causes mouse favus while ordinary favus characterized by horny plate-like scales or scutula is due to *Trichophyton schoenleini*. In addition, erythrasma causing organisms might be considered. Usually toe webs or axillary or groin folds are involved but palms might also be infected. Diagnosis is confirmed both by microscopic examination of skin scrapings digested with potassium hydroxide and by giving a reddish fluorescence under a Wood's (ultra-violet) light. This wavelength is also useful in localizing hair infected with fungi producing fluorescent substances. For completeness, the rare entity tinea nigra palmaris with its pigmented lesions occurring on the palms is pointed out.

The classic *onychomycosis* of the thumbnail may be associated with these palmar infections. In the differential diagnosis of causative organisms of onychomycosis, for example, the typical trichophyton rubrum of the palm demonstrates unilateral erythema and scaling (Fig. 14.6.1). More sharply defined lesions standing out in relief may be due to more exotic organisms as *Epidermophyton floccosum*. Keratotic lesions from this organism involving the nails as well, or bullae loaded with fungi in the web spaces may cause further infections, called tinea pedis, as well. In the tropics, more annular, less well defined lesions which may be in a lace-like pattern may be due to tinea imbricata. This is the clinical disease produced by Ticoncentricum.

Acute primary fungus infection of the hand is very unusual. Characteristically, vesicles occur singly or in patches on palmar surfaces as well as sides of fingers and palms in tinea rubrum infection. Dorsa are less often affected. On the other hand, *Trichophyton purpureum* infections cause thickened, sharply marginated, indurated dull red plaques with fine scaling but no vesiculation on either hands or feet. The infections are commoner in men than women, infrequent in children. Diagnosis depends strongly on location and character of the lesion. Even though a final diagnosis cannot be made on clinical findings alone, the examining physician must depend heavily on them.

For a more accurate diagnosis the fungus must be demonstrated microscopically. Skin scrapings or nail clippings are placed in 10 per cent potassium hydroxide for examination. Pathology of branching mycelia may be diagnostic, but identification is more certain by culturing scrapings or clippings on Sabouraud's medium. Success in identification depends not only on experience of examiners but also on stage of disease and repetition of examinations. More recently, an agar medium containing papaic digest of soya meal and dextrose, phenol red, and antibiotics has been used clinically to culture fungi. Termed "dermatophyte test medium" or DTM, it broadly identifies fungi by the change in color of phenol red from red to yellow. The color change is due to alkali produced by fungal proliferation in the high carbohydrate medium.[8] Success has been achieved with skin and hair, but not nail scrapings. *Candida albicans* also may not change the color. The method has the great advantage of being adaptable to an office procedure.

The extent and course of infection depends on the following factors: (1) The infecting organism; *Trichophyton rubrum* is the commonest offender. (2) Predisposing factors are important. These include (a) psychoneurogenic factors which exert an influence because of their effect on perspiration and circulation; (b) disturbed carbohydrate metabolism either from diabetes or (c) excessive alcohol intake is commonly associated with (d) fungus and intercurrent bacterial infections, and (e) decreased immune response. The latter may be due to a variety of causes, each probably due to a missing host factor. Examples are immune system defects as agammaglobulinemia or other congenital defects, as Wiskott-Aldrich syndrome or ataxia telangiectasia.[6] (f) The same is true of neoplasms as lymphoma, leukemia, or Letterer-Siwe disease. (g) Administration of corticosteroids, immunosuppressive drugs, and antibiotics also are associated with increased numbers of fungal diseases. (h) Respiratory or gastrointestinal viral infections may be equally important. (i) Allergic factors ranging from contact dermatitis to drug sensitivity play important roles. (j) Finally, local factors may aggravate the problem as excessive perspiration, particularly in hot,

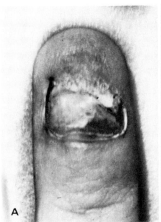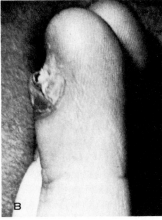

Figure 14.6.1. Two views of fungus infection of fingernail or onychomychosis. (From Flynn, J. E., by permission.)

humid weather, and increased acidity of sweat or maceration between fingers and toes from inability to separate them. Generally, fungus infections are worse in summer, better in winter.

Epidermophytid or "id" reactions occur from hematogenous spread and probably hypersensitivity to breakdown products of destroyed organisms. This classification of lesions was described by Jadassohn in 1912.[57] A vesicular eruption on the hand, particularly if the feet are infected, which improves when the feet improve, is usually an "id" reaction (Fig. 14.6.2). Isolation of organisms from the secondary site, in this case the hands, usually cannot be achieved. Further, the hands will not improve until the distant infection, which may be groin, perianal area, axillae, extremities, or center face as well as feet, is controlled. *Secondary infection* of this variety is usually a serious problem, leaving residual scaling crusts and even pustules with lymphangitis after fungi have been eradicated. Odorous hyperkeratotic plaques with sodden, moist scaling and fissures are characteristic of chronic secondary infection or "carrier" stage.

In a differential diagnosis of *chronic infections* consideration should be given to the following. Psoriasis particularly mimics tinea rubrum infection (Fig. 14.6.3). Dyshydrosis has a patchy, scaling, crusted eczema-like skin eruption and vesicles about and undermining the fingernails (Fig. 14.6.4). Familial epidermolysis bullosae is associated with large areas

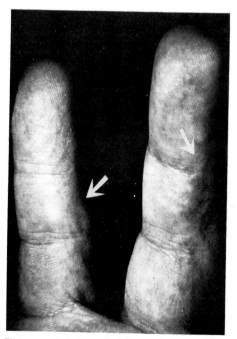

Figure 14.6.2. "ID" reaction of fingers secondary to fungus infection of feet. Note papules standing out as little mounds on lateral palmar surfaces of distal two phalanges. (From Flynn, J. E., by permission.)

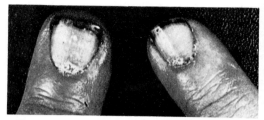

Figure 14.6.3. Stippling in a psoriatic nail resembling fungus infection. (From Woolridge,[11] by permission.)

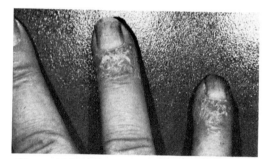

Figure 14.6.4. Subungual vesicles and nail undermining in dyshidrotic eczema. (From Woolridge,[11] by permission.)

of skin loss from bullous eruptions. These conditions as well as *Candida albicans* infection of finger webs and atopic dermatitis from contact or allergic reactions should alert one to look elsewhere for causes as intertrigenous areas (Fig. 14.6.5), paronychial areas, lips, and genitalia, particularly in women.

Treatment of Dermatomycoses

Most superficial fungal infections respond to griseofulvin.[4] This drug, which is fungistatic, rather than fungicidal in dosages administered, was isolated a generation ago but only used clinically since the 1950's. It is not effective, however, against candidiasis and tinea versicolor. The usual adult dosage is 125 mg of the powdered drug (micronized) four times daily orally. Dosage for children is 10 mg/kg divided into four equal dosages. Since absorption varies, two to four times these dosages may be required. Fatty meals may help absorption. Common side effects are diarrhea and headache. The drug is not used for pregnant patients or those with porphyria or liver failure. Necessity for prolonged administration of griseofulvin must be emphasized, particularly for tinea rubrum infection with nail involvement. Even after two to three years of therapy the disease frequently recurs when the drug is stopped.

For erythrasma, as mentioned in the differential diagnosis, erythromycin, 1 gm daily, in divided doses is administered for about three weeks.

Older treatments are still very helpful. Acutely, wet dressings, with 1/10,000 potassium permanganate

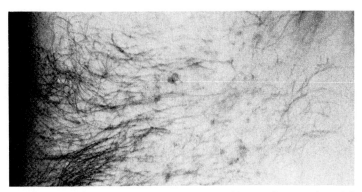

Figure 14.6.5. Axillary Candida infection causing moist skin erosions and pustules. (From Woolridge by permission.)

solution or 1/10 silver nitrate solution or boric acid, a teaspoon full to a pint of water are reliable in early states. Powdering with antifungicidal agents during symptom free periods is recommended, particularly for those who perspire much. Lamb's wool between the fingers acts as a wick and afterwards helps for aeration.

Tolfonate (Tinactin) locally applied either in cream, liquid, or powder is at times helpful in controlling these skin infections. It is ineffective agains nail infections. Adrenocorticoids may be administered topically for resistant infections and cautiously systemically. Antibiotics may be administered systemically for secondary infection. Topically, antibiotics may cause early drug resistance so that their usefulness applied in this manner is questionable.

In chronic hyperkeratotic stages keratolytic agents as Whitfield's ointment, which is salicylic acid 2 to 6 per cent in lanolin and petrolatum or Pragmatar are helpful. Actually, combinations of salicylic acid and sulfur ranging from 2 to 10 per cent in various bases are often used, keeping concentrations as low as is consistent with effective treatment.

Chronic paronychia may be associated with fungal infection. Removal of the lateral quarter of the nail under local anesthesia followed by packing the area with cotton pledgets wet with alcohol is probably most effective. Crooked or pitted nails are often due to skin infections of hands and feet. Nails improve as skin infections ae cured.

DEEP MYCOTIC INFECTIONS[2,4,9,10]

Chronic granulomatous forms of other primary fungal infections involving the hands as blastomycosis, sporotrichosis, actinomycosis, and coccidioidomycosis are relatively uncommon. The first three are seen more often in agricultural regions, particularly the Mid-west and Southern United States, while the last is seen in the West. To these infections, histoplasmosis, cryptococcosis, and nacardiosis may be added. Histoplasmosis and cryptococcosis as well as candidiasis, mucormycosis, and aspergillosis may

also be opportunistic or secondary invaders in very ill debilitated patients or complicate steroid, antimetabolite, or antibiotic therapy.

Blastomycosis forms papillomatous lesions with central contractual scars. They may be confused with epitheliomata because of epithelial hyperplasia. Lesions have miliary abscesses. Organisms from pus are double-contoured yeast, only budding forms being diagnostic. Currettage or excision of lesions is avoided because it may cause systemic spread. Amphotericin-B to be discussed below, is used for treatment.

Sporotrichosis occurs in two forms: (1) gumma-like lesions, rare in this country; (2) lymphatic infection. Organisms enter through an injury producing nodules with softening and discharge along lymphatics. The infection "metasticizes" to regional nodes. Organisms cannot be found on smears but may be cultured on glucose agar at room temperature. Here again, surgical excision of gummata and abscesses may only increase suppuration and spread infection. Sporotrichosis is best treated by saturated oral potassium iodide solution, five drops three times daily in water for adults. Proportionately, less is given to children. Dosage is increased one drop per dose per day to 30 or to tolerance, signified by ringing in the ears or skin eruption. Amphotericin-B and 2-hydroxy-stilbamidine may be considered in infections not responding to iodide.

Actinomycosis caused by *Actinomyces israelii* or *bovis* is characterized by sinus forming lesions of jaw, neck, face, and abdomen, rarely the hand. Thin yellow pus crushed on a slide shows "clubs" of the ray fungus. Deep induration with pus sinuses is characterized, but microscopic diagnosis is essential. Treatment is with penicillin intravenously in dosages of 10 to 20 million units daily for one to two weeks followed by one million units daily intramuscularly for six or more months. Erythromycin, tetracycline and other antibiotics are also effective. Antibiotic treatment has largely supplanted older treatment with iodides. General hygienic measures are important.

Coccidioidomycosis is not common and, again, is

treated by amphotericin-B. If not arrested it may end fatally with multiple ulcerating granulomata.

Histoplasmosis and cryptococcosis rarely involve the hand but also may be treated with amphotericin-B.

Amphotericin-B is potentially toxic. It must be used very carefully. It is administered intravenously in 5 per cent glucose solution, is light sensitive, *i.e.*, must be protected from light or will breakdown, and solution should not be used 24 hours after dissolving the drug. Daily dosage is 0.25 mg/kg of body weight, increasing dosage to 1.0 mg/kg until a total of 2 to 6 gm are given for adults. The drug is excreted slowly. Renal function is monitored by blood urea nitrogen, serum creatinine, and serum potassium every two days. Hematocrit and platelet counts and hepatic function must be similarly watched. Hydroxystilbamidine may be used for those developing toxicity to amphotericin-B.

CANDIDIASIS

Candidiasis is due to *Candida,* chiefly *Candida albicans.* Resulting paronychia and onychia are characterized by edema and redness with little tenderness. Discharge is scant and thin unless nails are secondarily infected. Nails often remain hard and retain their luster although they may become brownish and usually are thickened, ridged, distorted, and, at times, eroded. Erosio interdigitalis blastomycetica is the name applied when finger webs, usually between long and ring or ring and little fingers are involved. Most patients with this hand lesion are housewives, particularly those doing much hand washing (Fig. 14.6.5). This infection also occurs where skin folds upon itself as in the axilla.

For diagnosis, direct examination of scrapings as a rule is not helpful so that the organism must be identified by culture. *Candida albicans* is rarely found on normal skin even though it is very common in the throat, vagina, or stool of apparently healthy people. Finger infection is often secondary to mouth or anal involvement. The organisms are only weakly pathogenic. Infection usually results from predisposing factors listed under acute primary fungus infections of the hand. Unless these predisposing causes are controlled, monilial infection is almost incurable. Generalized systemic monilial infection may be fatal.[1] Following correction of local factors, treatment is similar to that outlined for fungus infections. Even though topical antibiotic administration is not generally recommended, local nystatin in solution or ointments or local amphotericin-B has been reported to be successful for some patients.

Acknowledgement

The author wishes to thank Dr. Robert F. Tilley of the Department of Dermatology, Harvard Medical School, for much helpful advice and constructive criticism during preparation of this chapter.

REFERENCES

1. Bernhardt, H. E., Orlando, J. C., Benfield, J. R., Hirose, F. M., and Foos, R. Y. Disseminated Candidiasis in surgical patients. Surg. Gynecol. Obstet., *134:* 819-825, 1972.
2. Conant, N. F., Smith, D. T., Baker, R. D., and Callaway, J. L. *Manual of Clinical Mycology,* Ed. 3, Philadelphia, Saunders, 1971.
3. Costello, M. J., and Gibbs, R. J. *The Palms and Soles in Medicine.* Springfield, Thomas, 1967.
4. Goldwin, L. Fungus diseases of the skin. In *Current Therapy,* edited by H. F. Conn. Philadelphia, Saunders, 1972, pp. 583-588.
5. Jadassohn, J. Korrespondenzblatt f. Schweitzer Aertze, *42:* 22, 1912. Jadassohn, Werner, and Peck, S. M. Arch. Dermatol. u. Syph., *158:* 16, 1929. Quoted by Stokes, J. *Handbook of Dermatology.* Philadelphia, 1942, p. 135.
6. Maibach, H., and Hildeck-Smith, G. *Skin Bacteria and Their Role in Infection.* New York, Blakiston, 1965.
7. Stokes, J. *Handbook of Dermatology.* Philadelphia, 1942.
8. Taplin, D., Zaias, N., Rebell, G., and Blank, H. Isolation and recognition of dermatophytes on a new medium (DTM). Arch. Dermatol., *99:* 203-209, 1969.
9. Tilley, R. F. Systemic mycotic infections. In *Current Pediatric Therapy,* Vol. 3, edited by Gellis and Kagan. Philadelphia, Saunders, 1968.
10. Tilley, R. F. Systemic mycotic infections. In *Pediatric Clinics of North America,* edited by N. B. Talbot. Philadelphia, Saunders, 1962.

G.

Tetanus

Louis Weinstein, Ph.D., M.D.

INTRODUCTION

The etiologic agent of tetanus is an anaerobic spore-forming organism, *Clostridium tetani.* None of the clinical manifestations of the disease are produced by tissue injury but result from the activity of a soluble exotoxin, *tetanospasmin,* which is elaborated at the site of injury by vegetative forms of the organism. Usually an uncommon disorder in the well developed parts of the world, the incidence of tetanus is often high in underdeveloped countries in which personal and community hygiene is poor, and during wars in which the combatants have not been immunized.

HISTORY

Tetanus has been known since ancient times. The first case was probably described by Hippocrates.[28] In the second century A.D., Aretaeus[2] wrote a complete clinical description of the course of this disorder to which very little has been added in the last 17 centuries. Carle and Rattone[10] were the first to demonstrate the transmissibility of the disease to animals in 1884. They infected the sciatic nerves of the rabbits with material from a pustule in a patient with tetanus. The animals developed tetanus two to three days later; suspensions of their nervous system tissue when injected into other rabbits reproduced the disease. In the same year, Nicolaier[42] induced tetanus in animals by inoculating them with soil; he observed the organism but was unable to isolate it. Two years later, Rosenbach[51] described a bacillus with a round terminal spore in the pus from a human case of tetanus; animals injected with this material developed the disease. Kitasato[32] was the first to isolate *Clostridium tetani* in pure culture and to fulfill Koch's postulates. A year later von Behring and Kitasato[60] reported that repeated injections of tetanus toxin in animals resulted in the appearance of specific antitoxin in their serum. Ramon and Zoeller[48] produced tetanus toxoid, the injection of which led to the development of active immunity.

ETIOLOGY AND EPIDEMIOLOGY

Clostridium tetani, in the vegetative form, is a gram positive, slender, motile rod. At the onset of sporulation, a bulge develops at one end of the organism; this contains the spore and produces the characteristic drumstick or tennis racquet appearance. With progression of spore formation, the rod shortens and the round spores, poorly stainable by the gram method, are extruded. Sporulation takes place in the tissues as well as *in vitro.* The organism is poorly saccharolytic and proteolytic. Although the vegetative forms of *Clostridium tetani* are as susceptible to heat and a variety of disinfectants as most nonsporulating bacteria, the spores are highly resistant to a number of injurious agents. They are not killed by boiling or by exposure to such disinfectants as phenol, cresol or 1:1000 mercury bichloride; autoclaving at 120°C for 15 to 20 minutes kills them, however. The spores are present in soil in which they may survive, if not exposed to sunlight, for months to years. They may be found in the feces of some horses, cows, guinea pigs, sheep, dogs, cats, rats, chickens, and humans. Three species of clostridia which resemble the tetanus bacillus morphologically but which are not pathogenic may also be present in soil, animals, and man and may cause diagnostic confusion; these are *Clostridium tertium, Clostridium tetanoides* and, *Clostridium tetanomorphum.* Cultivated soils are much more frequently contaminated with *Clostridium tetani* than virgin or uncultivated land. The incidence of carriage of this organism in man is variable, but is generally higher in rural dwellers and agricultural workers. The organism may be isolated from the skin and mouth as well as the intestinal tract of humans. It has also been found in house and street dust, in dirt from operating room floors, and in contaminated heroin solutions.

All of the clinical features of tetanus are produced by the activity of a neurotoxin, *tetanospasmin.* Although a hemolysin, *tetanolysin,* is also elaborated by the organism, it is not responsible for any of the manifestations of the disease. Purified crystalline tetanospasmin is a protein with a molecular weight of about 67,000.[46] With the exception of botulinum toxin, it is the most powerful poison known; 1 mg of purified material contains 6,400,000 lethal doses for mice and 0.00001 mg will kill a 20-gm mouse in two hours. Man is 2,500 times more susceptible to this agent than the cat and 350,000 more susceptible than the hen to equal quantities of this toxin.

Clostridium tetani is usually introduced into an area of injury as the spore, since this is the form in which the organism is present in soil and intestinal contents. Disease will not develop unless the spores are converted to the toxin-producing vegetative forms. This does not occur simple as a result of residence in tissue. If spores are injected into experimental animals with needles so sharp that they do not injure but merely separate tissues, tetanus will not develop. However, if a small amount of calcium chloride is added to a suspension of spores, typical disease follows. This is not related to any specific activity but is the result of necrosis produced by it which leads to a reduction of oxidation-reduction potential (Eh) and oxygen tension both of which are required for conversion of the spore to the toxin-producing vegetative form. This also is the course of events following trauma, introduction of a foreign body or the development of suppuration in the area where spores have gained entry.

PATHOGENESIS

There has been considerable controversy concerning the pathway over which toxin formed at the site of growth of *Clostridium tetani* reaches the central nervous system. It was first suggested that toxin is absorbed chiefly by motor nerve endings in the area of injury and then passes up axis cylinders to the anterior horn cells. Symptoms of tetanus are thought to appear only after toxin reaches the nervous system, the initial tetanic contractions occurring first in the injured extremity and then in the opposite limb and in all of the muscles as toxin diffused through the spinal cord. A small amount of toxin is thought to be absorbed into the lymph and carried to the blood stream from which it is taken up by motor nerve endings in various parts of the body.[38]

Abel[1] suggested that tetanus toxin reaches the nervous system by way of the arterial circulation and that the following series of events develops: Toxin diffusing from the wound into adjacent skeletal muscle acts on the neuromuscular organs to produce a state of maintained contraction, *local tetanus.* Some of the toxin also enters the lymphatics and blood stream from which a portion is taken up by specifically reactive cells in the spinal cord, medulla, and the motor end organs of muscle.

Because it was found that tetanus toxin did not pass the "blood-brain barrier", Friedemann and his co-workers[23] suggested that hematogenous transmission to the central nervous system was not involved. Recent attention has been focused on nerve transport of the toxin. Wright and his co-workers[64] noted that direct injection of toxin into the vagus, facial or hypoglossal nerves of rabbits was followed, within 24 hours, by a syndrome of brain stem tetanus with strabismus, immobility of the vibrissae, salivation, bradycardia, and torticollis. When the vagus was injected, there was successive development of these signs, those dependent on innervation from motor nuclei near the vagus tended to develop early. It has now been demonstrated that a wide variety of substances including India ink and radioactive compounds travel along peripheral nerves to the central nervous system after intraneural injection.[20] This fact, along with the demonstration by numerous investigators of the presence of toxin in the peripheral nerves closest to the site of inoculation, support the possibility of transport of tetanospasmin in nervous system tissue. Although knowledge of the exact mode of absorption of tetanus toxin and of its mechanism of action on body cells is incomplete, most of the presently available evidence suggests that some element of the peripheral nerve is involved; whether transport of toxin takes place in the axis cylinder, the perineural tissue spaces or in lymphatics is still unsettled. Roofe[50] has demonstrated that the neurofibrillae in axis cylinders can transport tetanus toxin to the neurones of the sciatic nerve at a rate of 3.35 mm per hour.

PATHOPHYSIOLOGY

Tetanospasmin exerts its effects on four parts of the nervous system; (a) the motor end plates in skeletal muscle, (b) the spinal cord, (c) the brain, and (d) the sympathetic nervous system in some cases.[5 6 7 9 16 30 31 37 55 61 65]

Motor End Plates in Skeletal Muscle

There is recent evidence that tetanospasmin interferes with neuromuscular transmission. The toxin inhibits the release of acetylcholine from the nerve terminals in muscle. Other observations indicate that the toxin is located in the transverse and terminal sacs of the longitudinal elements of the sarcotubular system of the skeletal muscles. This suggests that tetanospasmin acts by interfering with contraction coupling or mechanisms of contraction-relaxation. These phenomena are probably responsible for the manifestations of local tetanus.

Spinal Cord

The effects of tetanospasmin on the spinal cord are very similar to those of strychnine. The toxin does not act on reflex arcs that include only sensory and motor neurones (two-neuron or monosynaptic reflexes). However, it profoundly affects the more complex polysynoptic reflexes that involve interneurones. This effect leads to the inhibition of antagonists. Hyperpolarization of the nerve cell membranes which occurs normally when direct inhibitory pathways are stimulated is suppressed by the toxin. Depolarization associated with excitation is not affected. Whether tetanospasmin blocks inhibitory synapses by preventing release of the inhibitory transmitter substance or by preventing action of this substance on the membrane of the motor neurons is not known. The action of the toxin in selectively blocking inhibitory synapses in the central nervous system appears adequate to explain the primary phenomena of tetanus. Excitatory impulses multiply and run through reflex pathways unchecked and uncoordinated by inhibitory mechanisms to produce the muscular spasms characteristic of the disease.

Brain

Seizures that occur in the course of some cases of tetanus are possibly the result of the effects of tetanopasmin on the brain. There is evidence that the toxin is fixed by brain gangliosides. The antidromic inhibition of evoked cortical activity is reduced. The effects on the brain are similar to those on the spinal cord and those produced by strychnine.

Sympathetic Nervous System

In some instances, clinical features indicating an effect of tetanus on the sympathetic nervous system have been observed. The manifestations in such cases include labile hypertension, tachycardia, peripheral vasoconstriction, irregularities of cardiac rythms, profuse sweating, increased output of carbon dioxide, increase in urinary excretion of catecholamines and, in a few instances, late-appearing hypotension.

CLINICAL FEATURES

The incubation period in humans is usually three to 21 days. However, it may be as short as one day or as long as several months. There appears to be a relation between the site of injury and the interval before onset of disease; the longer the distance toxin has to travel along peripheral nerves to reach the central nervous system, the more prolonged the incubation period. The clinical features of the disease are due entirely to sustained or spasmodic contractions of isolated or multiple muscle groups. There are two forms of tetanus, *generalized* and *local*. The latter is uncommon in civilian life and may be easily overlooked. The characteristic manifestation of local tetanus is a persistent and unyielding rigidity of the group of muscles in close proximity to the site of the injury. It is frequently associated with the administration of a dose of antitoxin sufficient to neutralize circulating toxin but inadequate to prevent or inactivate significant local accumulations. Symptoms may persist for several weeks or even for a number of months, finally disappearing without residue. This form of the disease may precede the development of the generalized disorder. It is mild, the fatality rate being only about 1 per cent.[39]

Generalized tetanus is the most common form of the disease; it varies considerably in severity. The portal of entry in 80 per cent of cases is an insignificant wound.[47] Burns, blank cartridge wounds, embedded splinters, deep punctures, bed sores, hypodermic infections, dental extractions, furunculosis, and compound fractures with chronic osteomyelitis are typical examples of situations in which contaminations with tetanus spores may lead to active disease because the tissue environment is favorable for spore vegetation. Contaminated cow pox vaccine and surgical suture material have been incriminated as sources of iatrogenic infection. Cases of postoperative tetanus have been attributed to dust borne contamination in the operating room.[49 54] Umbilical infection of the newborn is the lesion most commonly associated with *tetanus neonatorum*, a particularly lethal form of the disease. Bee, scorpion, and chigger bites may serve as portals of entry for the organism. Infection has been recorded after induced abortion. Injuries to the scalp, eye, face, ear or neck, chronic otitis media, and, rarely, tonsillectomy may predispose to the development of cephalic tetanus, a particularly virulent form of the disease.

Trismus is the presenting symptom in over 50 per cent of the cases of generalized tetanus. It may be absent and replaced by restlessness, irritability, stiffness of the neck, rigidity of abdominal muscles, or difficulty in swallowing in some patients. The importance of trismus as the presenting sign cannot be overemphasized. If other causes for this condition, such as periapical dental abscess, measles encephalitis, trichinosis, parotitis, tender cervical adenopathy, ingestion of phenotheazine compounds, etc., can be excluded, tetanus must be considered. Local tetanus, characterized by rigidity of the muscles and increased reflexes at the site of inoculation of *Clostridium tetani*, is sometimes present prior to the development of the generalized disorder. Progression of the intoxication leads to involvement of other important muscle groups so that tonic contractions of the muscles of jaws, face, neck, back, and abdomen appear. Persistent trismus produces a characteristic facial expression, the so-called sardonic smile (risus sardonicus). The abdominal and lumbar muscles may become rigid. Vise-like constriction of the chest muscles and intense persistent spasm of the back musculature results in opisthotonus. This is usually associated with generalized seizures, so-called tonic tetanospasms, which are unique and peculiar to this disorder; characteristically, there is a sudden burst of tonic contraction of muscle groups causing opisthotonus, flexion and adduction of the arms, clenching of the fists on the thorax, and extension of the lower extremities. The patient is completely conscious during such episodes and experiences intense pain. Dysphagia occurs and leads to hydrophobia. The generalized seizures are often triggered by very slight external stimuli such as a breeze, talking, bumping into the bed, or touching the patient. The intense work and profuse sweating which accompany these seizures often result in elevation of temperature of from 2 to 5° above normal. Glottal or laryngeal spasm may develop and cause cyanosis and asphyxia if not promptly relieved by medical or surgical means. Dysuria or urinary retention may supervene. The intense suffering of the patient with tetanus and the utter frustration of the physician who often stands by helpless to alter the course of the disease has been described best by Aretaeus:[2] "An inhuman calamity! an unseemly sight! a spectacle painful even to the beholder! an incurable malady! owing to the distortion, not to be recognized by the dearest friends; and hence the prayer of the spectators, which formerly would have been reckoned not pious, now becomes good, that the patient may depart from life, as being a deliverance from the pains and unseemly evils attendant on it. But neither can the physician, though present and looking on, furnish any assistance, as regards life, relief from pain or from deformity. For if he should wish to straighten the limbs, he can only do so by cutting and breaking those of a living man. With them, then, who are overpowered by this disease, he can merely sympathize. This is the great misfortune of the physician."

The incubation period of cephalic tetanus is usually short, often only one or two days. The disease may follow injuries of the head or otitis media; the prognosis is extremely poor.[3] An outstanding feature of this form of tetanus are palsies of cranial nerves 3,4,7,9,10 and 12, singly or in any combination. The 7th nerve is affected most often. Dysfunction may persist for days or for many months; complete recovery is the rule, if the patient survives. Generalized tetanus follows the development of cephalic disease in some but not all cases.

DIAGNOSIS

The usual laboratory studies are of little value in the diagnosis of tetanus. Examination of the spinal fluid reveals no abnormalities. The peripheral white blood count may be elevated or normal. Gram stains of material obtained from the wound may show characteristic organisms in some instances. Culture of exudate or necrotic tissue in thioglycollate broth or chopped meat medium, may reveal typical sporulated forms; the yield of positive cultures has been found to be low in some studies.[13] The diagnosis of this disease is based on a history of injury followed by the development of any of the syndromes described above.

PROGNOSIS

The average death rate of tetanus is 45 to 55 per

cent. Two types of generalized tetanus have a particularly poor outlook. One of these is *tetanus neonatorum*. This occurs in infants as a result of infection of the umbilicus. It has become quite rare in civilized countries but is still observed frequently in less highly developed parts of the world where a variety of unclean agents are employed to sever the cord at birth and old rags, often contaminated with the feces, are used as dressings.[24] The fatality rate in one group of cases (5,794 patients) was 99.5 per cent.[27] Heroin addicts are especially prone to develop very severe tetanus and to exhibit a number of clinical features not common in nonaddicted individuals. The first complaint in such patients is often stiffness of the neck or back rather than trismus. The temperature is usually quite high and onset of coma early. Because the death rate from tetanus in heroin users is almost 100 per cent, they are usually given larger doses (two to three times) of antitoxin prophylactically than other persons; the standard dose (3,000 units of horse serum) has failed to protect in a significant number of instances.[34]

A number of other factors play an important role in determining the prognosis of tetanus. Survival is more frequent in the second and third decade of life and death more common in older age groups. The inverse relationship between the length of the incubation period and the fatality rate was first commented on by Hippocrates and has been well documented since. An interval of two to 10 days between injury and onset of disease has been found to be associated with a fatality rate of 58 per cent; when the incubation period was 11 to 22 days, death occurred in 35 per cent and when it was 22 days or longer, only 17 per cent of the group died. It has recently been suggested that the length of time elapsing between appearance of the first signs of tetanus and the onset of the first seizure or the development of maximal severity affects the ultimate outcome; the shorter this interval, the poorer the prognosis.[13] The administration of antitoxin (horse serum) prophylactically lowers the fatality rate from 53 to 22 per cent. The clinical characteristics of the disease are also of prognostic significance. Thus, cephalic tetanus and tetanus neonatorum are particularly severe; the outlook for recovery from local tetanus, on the other hand, is very good. The earlier the diagnosis is established and proper treatment instituted, the greater the possibility for survival.

TREATMENT

Treatment of tetanus has several goals: (a) Neutralization of any circulating toxin before it reaches the nervous system. This necessitates the administration of specific antitoxin as soon as the diagnosis is made.[5] It must be emphasized, however, that there is no evidence that toxin already fixed to tissues is neutralized by antitoxin. The role of antitoxin in reducing fatality rate has been questioned. (b) Eradication of the site at which the organisms are producing toxin. This can be accomplished by surgical excision of wound, in many cases. However, when this may be defacing or mutilating, parenteral administration of penicillin G or tetracycline is helpful in eradicating the organisms. (c) Intensive nursing care. (d) A very quiet environment with avoidance of even minor stimuli. (e) Maintenance of caloric, fluid, and electrolyte balance which are often disturbed by the hypermetabolic state associated with repeated severe seizures.

Since the slightest disturbance may precipitate spasms and/or generalized seizures, it is important that all necessary manipulations and treatment be performed in a well coordinated, thoughtfully scheduled fashion so that external stimuli are reduced to an absolute minimum. The patient must be placed in a quiet environment; a darkened room with padded doors, removed as far as is possible from the mainstream of hospital traffic is ideal.

The antitoxin presently recommended for treatment of tetanus is human hyperimmune globulin; the dose is 3,000 to 6,000 units given intramuscularly. There is no evidence that a second dose is necessary. In areas of the world where this material is not available, a dose of 100,000 units of horse serum antitoxin is recommended; half of this is given intramuscularly after appropriate tests to rule out sensitivity to horse serum have been carried out. If the intramuscular dose is well tolerated, the rest of the antitoxin is given in a slow drip intravenously. If the patient is sensitive to horse serum, he must be desensitized before treatment is given. Whenever possible, the use of horse serum should be avoided and human antitoxin given. An intramuscular injection of 80,000 units of tetanus antitoxin (horse serum) in man was found by Turner[58][59] to produce maximal quantities of antibody in the blood in 48 to 72 hours; very good levels were maintained for seven days. Intravenous administration of the same dose yielded serum concentrations of 40 units or more of antitoxin per ml after six hours; this persisted for about 48 hours. No difference was noted in the blood levels seven days after intramuscular or intravenous injection. Local instillation of antitoxin around the known or suspected wound is of value, if surgical excision is not possible. Omphalectomy has been performed with good results in cases of neonatal tetanus.[17] Hysterectomy has been advocated when tetanus has followed induced abortions; survivals have been recorded without surgical removal of the infected organ, however.

Penicillin kills the vegetative forms of *Clostridium tetani*. The administration of 1,200,000 units of procaine penicillin once daily, or 1,000,000 units of penicillin G parenterally every six hours for 10 days is recommended in all cases of tetanus. Tetracycline, 2 gm per day, may also be used.

Since the spasticity and seizures of tetanus appear to be due to exaggerated reflex responses to afferent stimuli as a result of suppression of balancing central inhibition, the possibility of controlling these manifestations by the use of drugs acting at different sites along the reflex pathway suggests itself. Agents which may be of value in treating this disease are: (a) *Hypnotics and sedatives;* these reduce sensory input and generalized excitability. (b) *General anesthetics;* these produce widespread depression of the central nervous system. (c) *Centrally-acting muscle relaxants or spinal depressants;* these lower reflex activity and decrease motor output from the spinal cord. (d) *Neuromuscular blocking agents;* these inhibit transmission of excess motor nerve activity to the effector muscles.

The ideal drug therapy of tetanus should control seizures and reduce spasticity without impairing respiration, voluntary movement, or consciousness. While the ability to control convulsions induced by strychnine has generally been used as a reliable guide for the prediction of activity of an agent in tetanus, this cannot always be relied upon. For example, phenothiazine derivatives which have been found to act as anticonvulsants in both naturally occurring and experimentally produced tetanus are ineffective in controlling strychnine-induced seizures. It has been pointed out by Creech[15] that "It may be concluded that any type of sedative or hypnotic agent when properly administered so as to avoid respiratory depression has the same effect or lack of effect upon the outcome of tetanus." The qualities desirable in such a drug are: (a) Ability to control reflex convulsions so that they occur infrequently, are of brief duration and do not arrest respiration. (b) Reduction of tonic muscle spasm, although helpful in reducing discomfort, is of secondary importance. (c) Rapid onset of action because patients may die of respiratory arrest during a seizure. (d) Some degree of depressive effect on consciousness; this is of value in dimishing the pain and extreme anxiety induced by the tonic muscle spasms. No single drug satisfies all of these requirements; the barbiturates and phenothiazine compounds come closest to meeting these criteria.

Seco-barbital (Seconal) sodium and pentobarbital (Nembutal) are highly useful drugs.[29][40] Their short action prevents long periods of over-depression while dosage is being adjusted. The initial dose is 3 to 5 mg per pound intramuscularly for children and 100 to 150 mg intramuscularly for adults. The daily requirement of these agents cannot be predicted and minute-to-minute administration of intravenous thiopental (Pentothal) sodium may be necessary to supplement the use of the other barbiturates, which may need to be given as frequently as every two hours if seizures are frequent and severe. The optimal level of sedation is one at which the undisturbed patient lies quietly without convulsions and very close to sleep, but, when stimulated, exhibits a definite response.

Chlorpromazine (Thorazine) is a highly effective anticonvulsant which controls tetanus convulsions when used alone; most reports suggest, however, that it is most effective when given together with barbiturates.[14] Tachyphylaxis, exaggeration of muscle spasm (usually due to an overdose) and failure to control severe seizures are the most untoward effects of the drug. Solutions of the drug may produce severe irritation when injected; this is especially so in neonates because of the small muscle mass into which the agent is instilled. The dose required to potentiate the hypnotics varies considerably. It ranges from 4 to 12 mg in the infant and 50 to 150 mg in adults; this quantity is administered parenterally every four to eight hours.

Meprobamate has been used with success in the management of tetanus.[45] It is relatively ineffective orally in this situation, and is usually given by intramuscular injection in polyethylene glycol solution. The dose is 400 mg every three to four hours in adults and 50 to 100 mg in children under two years. Chlorpromazine and, if necessary, a barbiturate may be added if meprobamate alone fails to produce the desired effects.

Diazepam (Valium) has been used successfully in prevention and control of seizures in tetanus.[12] It is given intravenously in a dose of 2 to 20 mg every two to eight hours, the single quantity and interval between injections depending on the severity of the disease.

Other drugs which have been employed for the treatment of tetanus but which are presently less commonly applied are methocarbamol, procaine, alcohol, tribromoethanol, paraldehyde, chloral hydrate, bromide, and magnesium sulfate. The latter was widely used but, because the therapeutic and toxic doses were little different, it has been discarded in most clinics. Opiates are contraindicated because they may produce respiratory depression and nervous system stimulation.

Neuromuscular blocking agents have been used for two purposes; (a) to control convulsions while sparing respiration, (b) to produce complete paralysis; in this case, artificial respiration is given. Since neuromuscular blocking agents paralyze diaphragmentic later than intercostal respiration, they control seizures but do not wholly abolish breathing. Such drugs together with artificial respiration should not be employed except in cases in which control of seizures is very difficult or in which respiratory failure has occurred. The technique of continuous artificial respiration requires adequate apparatus and the availability of personnel experienced in respiratory technics.[33] While there appears to be a greater margin of safety between the therapeutic and respiratory paralytic effects with gallamine (Flaxedil) than with curare or succinylcholine, facilities for artificial respiration must be available at the bedside when any of these agents is administered.

Tracheostomy should not be carried out as a routine procedure in tetanus. It should be performed, however, immediately after the onset of the first generalized seizure in order to prevent asphyxia due to the so-called respiratory convulsion which is the result of spasm of the glottis and larynx and which may develop suddenly and without warning. If such a seizure occurs in a patient without a tracheostomy, it must be terminated without delay by the administration of an agent such as succinylcholine, the action of which is rapid and short-lived.[22] Because this drug abolishes the most severe seizures, its administration allows time for tracheostomy to be performed; assisted respiration must be provided until the effects of the agent have disappeared. Tracheostomy is necessary in all instances of tetanus in heroin addicts because of the fulminant course frequently characterized by cardiorespiratory dysrythmia and hyperthermia.[45]

Rigid attention must be paid to care of the skin, bladder, mouth, and bowel of patients with tetanus. Maintenance of proper fluid and electrolyte balance is mandatory. An adequate caloric intake is recommended by some investigators who suggest that use of gavage feedings; this has been questioned by some observers because of the risks attendant on the introduction of material into the stomach of a heavily sedated patient. Hypostatic pneumonia may develop; it must be recognized promptly and treated appropriately.

Patients who have recovered from tetanus must be actively immunized since they do not have detectable antibody in the serum three months later.[59] Recurrent cases are rare.[8]

Animal studies indicate that adrenocortical steroids do not decrease the level of the activity of tetanus toxin. In mice injected with graded doses of toxin, Chang and Weinstein[11] found that, when clinical signs were present or when there was a significant delay between toxin injection and antitoxin prophylaxis, the administration of cortisone was not only without benefit but sharply decreased the efficacy of the antitoxin. Other studies have confirmed the lack of beneficial effects,[26][59] but have not demonstrated any deleterious effects associated with administration of corticoteroids. Critically evaluated clinical experiences have not established meaningful differences in mortality ascribable to the use of the adrenal steroids.[35]

CAUSES OF DEATH

The cause of death in clinical tetanus is often obscure because the course of illness may be prolonged and the therapy employed is complex and potentially dangerous. Animals may die after injection of tetanus toxin without developing recognizable signs of the disease.[21] Experiments in parabiotic rats have suggested that tetanus may exert a lethal effect on the respiratory center even in the absence of convulsions.[53] Evidence of medullary intoxication has been noted in both experimental and clinical situations and recurring attacks of respiratory failure, often without seizures, have been described in patients.[33][64] Cerebral intoxication has been thought to be responsible for hyperpyrexia, tachycardia with hypotension, bulbar palsy, and cardiac arrest.[41] Myocardial damage may also occur; both histologic and electrocardiographic abnormalities have been described.[44]

Death may occur during a convulsion; the mechanism for this is not always clear. Exhaustion, electrolyte disturbances, laryngospasm, and anoxia are probable contributory factors. Respiratory infection, resulting from aspiration because of inability to swallow and accidental oversedation, is a frequent complication. It may be directly responsible for death or may contribute to a fatal outcome by increasing the degree of respiratory center anoxia.

PREVENTION OF TETANUS

Tetanus is a preventable disease. Active immunization is readily achieved by means of either alum precipitated or fluid toxoid. Three injections of the alum precipitated preparation, preferably four weeks apart, are probably best for primary immunization. Antibody develops within one week after the second dose. It is demonstrable in the circulation one week after the third injection of fluid toxoid. However, this agent should not be given for primary immunization but employed only for booster doses when rapid protection is desirable. If no injury has occurred, it is now recommended that a booster dose of tetanus toxoid be given no more often than once every 10 years.[19] If an injury is incurred that may expose a patient to the risk of tetanus, but a booster injection of toxoid has been given within one year, another dose is not necessary. If, however, no toxoid has been administered for a period longer than one year before the injury, a booster dose should be given.[43] Turner[58] has demonstrated detectable antitoxin in the serum of patients five to 10 years after their last administration of toxoid. Booster doses have been noted to produce a rapid and significant increase in circulating levels of antitoxin when injected as long as 19 years after primary immunization.[63]

The effectiveness of active immunization against tetanus in man has been clearly proved by experience in wars. Of 217,000 wounded in the conflict between the states, 505 developed tetanus. In World War I there were 2,835 cases of the disease in 2,032,142 wounded British troops; 36 episodes were observed in 224,089 men in the American Army in the same conflict. No cases occurred among 100,000 British troops who suffered wounds at Dunkirk in World War II. Sixteen instances of tetanus were noted among 2,824,807 wounded in the U. S. Armed Forces during World War II; of these, only five had received a complete course of immunization.

The effectiveness of tetanus antitoxin titers achieved by active immunization has been demonstrated in animal studies which have indicated complete protection against exposure to large doses of tetanus spores. Animals with low levels of antitoxin were protected to a varying degree, some escaping the disease entirely while others developed only the localized form. Actively immunized animals developed a significant increase in serum antitoxin within a short time after a challenge inoculation of tetanus spores suggesting that infection had occurred despite the absence of any signs of tetanus. It is probable that the same phenomenon occurs in man. Animal studies have demonstrated that comparable blood levels of passively transferred antitoxin are significantly less protective than those achieved by active immunization.[59] This observation stresses the importance of active immunization and its advantages over passive protection. The simultaneous administration of antitoxin and toxoid in different sites has been recommended as prophylaxis in previously unimmunized individuals. This must always be followed by additional administration of toxoid in order to produce active immunity. Although the activity of the first dose of toxoid is somewhat suppressed, the second dose produces a typical rise in antitoxin titer. Reactions to toxoid occur occasionally but are generally not serious; a rare instance of anaphylaxis has been reported.

Immunization with tetanus toxoid should be carried out in *all* individuals, if possible. Persons with an allergic background or with known sensitivity to horse serum, farmers, hostlers, veterinarians, those working in environments where tetanus spores are apt to be present, and children in whom there is a high incidence of injuries into which tetanus spores may be introduced should be especially sought out for immunization. If human hyperimmune gamma globulin is not available, horse serum antitoxin should be given to individuals who have not been actively immunized and have incurred an injury which may expose them to the introduction of tetanus spores; the recommended dose is 3,000 units.[18]

While the establishment of active immunity against tetanus can be achieved with considerable ease and a high degree of efficiency, especially in a controlled group such as the military, large segments of the civilian population still fail to avail themselves of this protection. This is especially true of older women. Passive or combined passive-active prophylaxis in the nonimmune individual is a relatively poor but often necessary substitute for active immunization. Certain circumstances, deep puncture wounds with or without massive contamination and compound fractures for example, demand immediate protection. The administration of horse serum may be prohibited by a serious degree of hypersensitivity to this material. About 5 to 6 per cent of all patients given heterologous antitoxin develop serum sickness. Prior sensitization to horse serum or the development of serum sickness results in accelerated disappearance of the antibody.[7] [25] Antibiotic prophylaxis, without antitoxin administration, has not been proved to be an adequate substitute; failures have been recorded.[4] It is these observations that have prompted the development of human tetanus antitoxin.

The administration of tetanus-immune human globulin is effective prophylaxis and eliminates the hazards of the injection of heterologous substances such as horse serum. In addition, the half-life of human gamma globulin antitoxin is considerably longer than that of horse serum. The dose of human immune globulin required for effective prophylaxis is 250 to 350 units.[36] [52] The serum half-life of this material is from 3.5 to 4.5 weeks.[56] Following administration of 250 units of tetanus-immune human globulin, serum antibody levels of 0.01 units per ml or higher are present in 100 per cent of individuals for 28 days; protective concentrations are still demonstrable in 84 per cent after eight weeks and, in a few cases, after 14 weeks.[36] Human globulin may be given together with purified fluid toxoid (10 LF doses) for active passive immunization. If the materials are injected at different sites, the development of active immunity is not suppressed.

REFERENCES

1. Abel, J. J., Firor, W. M., and Chalain, W. Researches on tetanus. IX. Further evidence to show that tetanus toxin is not carried to central neurons by way of the axis cylinders of motor nerves. Bull. Johns Hopkins Hosp., *63:* 373-403, 1938.
2. Aretaeus. Tetanus. In *Classic Descriptions of Disease,* Ed. 2, edited by R. N. Major. Springfield, C. C Thomas, 1939, pp. 148-149.
3. Bagratuni, L. Cephalic tetanus. Br. Med. J., *1:* 461-463, 1952.
4. Botticelli, J. T., and Waisbren, B. A. Tetanus in an urban community. Am. J. Med. Sci., *242:* 44-50, 1961.
5. Bradley, K., Easton, D. M., and Eccles, J. C. Investigation of primary or direct inhibition. J. Physiol., *122:* 474-478, 1953.
6. Brooks, V. B., Curtis, D. R., and Eccles, J. C. Mode of action of tetanus toxin. Nature, *175:* 120-121, 1955.
7. Brooks, V. B., and Asanuma, H. Action of tetanus toxin in the cerebral cortex. Science, *137:* 674-676, 1962.
8. Cain, H. D., and Falco, F. G. Recurrent tetanus. Calif. Med., *97:* 31-33, 1962.
9. Carrea, R., and Lanari, A. Chronic effect of tetanus toxin applied locally to the cerebral cortex of the dog. Science, *137:* 342-343, 1962.
10. Carle and Rattone. Studio Esperimentale Sull'eziologia del Tetano. G. Accad. Med. Torino, *32:* 174-180, 1884.
11. Chang, T. W., and Weinstein, L. Effect of cortisone on treatment of tetanus with antitoxin. Proc. Soc. Exp. Biol. Med., *94:* 431-433, 1957.
12. Cordova, A. B. Control of the spasms of tetanus with Diazepam (Valium). Clin. Pediatr., *8:* 712-716, 1969.
13. Christensen, N. A., and Thurber, D. L. Clinical experience with tetanus: 91 cases. Mayo Clin. Proc., *32:* 146-157, 1957.
14. Cole, A. C. E., and Robertson, D. H. H. Chlorpromazine in the management of tetanus. Lancet, *2:* 1063-1064, 1955.
15. Creech, O., Glover, A., and Ochsner, A. Tetanus: Evaluation of treatment at Charity Hospital, New Or-

leans, Louisiana. Ann. Surg., *146:* 369, 1957.

16. Davis, J. R., Morgan, R. S., Wright, E. A., and Wright, G. P. The effect of local tetanus intoxication on the hind limb reflexes of the rabbit. Arch. Int. Physiol., *62:* 248-263, 1954.

17. Dietrich, H. F. Tetanus neonatorum. J.A.M.A., *147:* 1038-1040, 1951.

18. Edsall, G. Specific prophylaxis of tetanus. J.A.M.A., *171:* 417-427, 1959.

19. Edsall, G., Elliott, M. W., Peebles, T. C., Levine, L., and Eldred, M. C. Excessive use of tetanus boosters. J.A.M.A., *202:* 17-19, 1967.

20. Fedinec, A. A., and Matzke, H. A. The role of tissue spaces and nerve fibers in the spread of tetanus toxin in the rat. Univ. Kans. Sci. Bull., *38:* 1439-1498, 1958.

21. Firor, W. M., Lamont, A., and Shumacker, H. B. Studies on the cause of death in tetanus. Ann. Surg., *111:* 246, 1940.

22. Forresester, A. T. T. Treatment of tetanus with succinylcholine. Br. Med. J., *2:* 342-344, 1954.

23. Friedemann, U., Zuger, B., and Hollander, A. Investigations on the pathogenesis of tetanus, I and II. J. Immunol., *36:* 473-484, 485-488, 1939.

24. Friedlander, F. C. Tetanus neonatorum. J. Pediatr., *39:* 448-454, 1951.

25. Godfrey, M. P., Parsons, V., and Rawstron, J. R. Rapid destruction of antitetanus serum in a patient previously sensitized to horse serum. Lancet, *2:* 1229-1230, 1960.

26. Green, A. E., Ambrus, J. L., and Gershenfeld, L. Effect of cortisone and desoxycorticosterone on infection with tetanus spores and on toxicity of tetanus toxin. Antibiot. Chemother., *3:* 1221, 1953.

27. Hines, E. A., Jr. Tetanus neonatorum: Report of a case with recovery. Am. J. Dis. Child., *39:* 560-572, 1930.

28. Hippocrates. Tetanus. In *Classic Descriptions of Disease,* Ed. 2, edited by H. H. Major, Springfield, C. C Thomas, 1939, pp. 148-149.

29. Jenkins, M. T., and Luhn, N. R. Active management of tetanus. Anaesthesiology, *23:* 690-709, 1962.

30. Kaeser, H. E., and Saner, A. Tetanus toxin, a neuromuscular blocking agent. Nature (Lond.), *223:* 842, 1969.

31. Kerr, J. H., Corbett, J. L., Prys-Roberts, Smith, A. C., and Spalding, J. M. K. Involvement of the sympathetic nervous system in tetanus. Lancet, *2:* 236-241, 1968.

32. Kitasato, S. Ueber den Tetanus bacillus. Z. Hyg. Infektkr., *7:* 225-234, 1889.

33. Laurence, D. R., and Webster, R. A. Pathologic physiology, pharmacology and therapeutics of tetanus. Clin. Pharmacol. Ther., *4:* 36-72, 1963.

34. Levinson, A., Marske, R. L., and Shein, M. K. Tetanus in heroin addicts. J.A.M.A., *157:* 658-660, 1955.

35. Lewis, R. A., Satoskar, R. S., Joag, C. G., Dave, B. T., and Patel, J. C. Cortisone and hydrocortisone given parenterally and orally in severe tetanus. J.A.M.A., *156:* 479, 1954.

36. McComb, J. A., and Dwyer, R. C. Passive-active immunization with tetanus immune globulin (human). N. Engl. J. Med., *268:* 857-862, 1963.

37. Mellanby, J., Van Heyningen, W. E., and Whitaker, V. P. Fixation of tetanus toxin by subcellular fractions of

brain. J. Neurochem., *12:* 77-79, 1965.

38. Meyer, H., and Ransom, F. Untersuchungen uber den Tetanus. Arch. Exp. Path. Pharmakol., *49:* 369-416, 1903.

39. Millard, A. H. Local tetanus. Lancet, *2:* 844-846, 1954.

40. Miller, C. L., and Stoelting, V. K. Recent evaluation of the treatment of tetanus. J.A.M.A., *168:* 393-394, 1958.

41. Montgomery, R. D. The cause of death in tetanus. West Indian Med. J., *10:* 84, 1961.

42. Nicolaier, A. Ueber Infectiosen Tetanus. Dtsch. Med. Wochenschr., *10:* 842-884, 1884.

43. Peebles, T. C., Levine, L., Eldred, M. C., and Edsall, G. Tetanus-toxoid emergency boosters. N. Engl. J. Med., *280:* 575-581, 1969.

44. Perez, L. R. The electrocardiogram in tetanus. Rev. Clin. Esp., *75:* 20, 1959.

45. Perlstein, M. A., Stein, M. D., and Elam, H. Routine treatment of tetanus. J.A.M.A., *173:* 1536-1541, 1960.

46. Pillemer, L., Wittler, R. G., and Grossberg, D. B. The isolation and crystallization of tetanal toxin. Science, *103:* 615-616, 1946.

47. Pratt, E. L. Clinical tetanus: A study of 56 cases, with special reference to methods of prevention and a plan for evaluating treatment. J.A.M.A., *129:* 1243-1247, 1945.

48. Ramon, G., and Zoeller, C. L'immunité antitetanque par l'anatoxine chez l'homme. Presse Méd., *34:* 485, 1926.

49. Robinson, D. T., McLeod, J. S., and Downie, A. W. Dust in surgical theatres. Lancet, *1:* 152-154, 1946.

50. Roofe, P. G. Role of the axis cylinder in transport of tetanus toxin Science, *105:* 180-181, 1947.

51. Rosenbach. Arch. Klin. Chir., *34:* 306, 1887.

52. Rubbo, S. D., and Suri, J. C. Passive immunization against tetanus with human immune globulin. Br. Med. J., *2:* 79-81, 1962.

53. Schellenberg, D. B., and Matzke, H. A. The development of tetanus in parabiotic rats. J. Immunol., *80:* 367, 1958.

54. Sevitt, S. Source of two hospital-infected cases of tetanus. Lancet, *2:* 1075-1078, 1949.

55. Sherrington, C. S. *The Integrative Action of the Nervous System.* New York, Yale University Press, 1906, pp. 303 and 112.

56. Smolens, J., Vogt, A. B., Crawford, M. N., and Stokes, J., Jr. The Persistence in the human circulation of horse and human tetanus antitoxins. J. Pediatr., *59:* 899-902, 1961.

57. Talmage, D. W., Dixon, F. J., Bukantz, S. C., and Dammin, G. J. Antigen Elimination from the blood as an early manifestation of the immune response. J. Immunol., *67:* 243-255, 1951.

58. Turner, T. B., Stafford, E. S., and Goldman, L. Studies on the duration of protection afforded by active immunization against tetanus. Bull. Johns Hopkins Hosp., *94:* 204-217, 1954.

59. Turner, T. B., Velasco-Joven, E. A., and Prudovsky, S. Studies on the prophylaxis and treatment of tetanus. Bull. Johns Hopkins Hosp., *102:* 71-84, 1958.

60. Von Behring, E., and Kitasato, S. Ueber des Zustandekommen der Diphterie-Immunitat und der Tetanus Immunitat bei Teiren. Dtsch. Med. Wochenschr., *16:* 1113-1114, 1890.

61. Van Heyningen, W. E., and Miller, P. A. The fixation of tetanus toxin by ganglioside. J. Gen. Microbiol., *24:* 107-119, 1961.

62. Young, L. S., LaForre, F. M., and Bennett, J. V. An evaluation of serologic and antimicrobial therapy in the treatment of tetanus in the United States. J. Infect. Dis., *120:* 153-159, 1969.

63. Worman, R. K., Kiss, Z., Camp, F. A., McDonald, K. E., and Schenk, W. G. Residual antitetanus protection 17 to 19 years after active immunization. Surg. Gynecol. Obstet., *116:* 576-578, 1963.

64. Wright, E. A., Morgan, R. S., and Wright, G. P. Tetanus intoxication of the brain-stem in rabbits. J. Pathol. Bacteriol., *62:* 569-583, 1950.

65. Zacks, S. I., and Shef, M. F. Tetanus toxin: Fine structure localization of binding sites in striated muscle. Science, *159:* 643-644, 1968.

chapter fifteen

Contractures

A.

Splinting

Elden C. Weckesser, M.D.

GENERAL

A splint is an appliance rigid in one or more planes used either internally or externally to preserve form, maintain balance, promote rest, or mobilize stiffened joints. It is also used to maintain balance when certain muscles or tendons are either malfunctioning or non-functioning due to metabolic disease, paralysis, or trauma. When substituting for paralyzed muscles, the use of elastic or spring pull (dynamic splinting) is highly desirable as it allows exercise of opposing muscles and prevents joint stiffness, the calculated risk of all rigid splinting.

Stiffened joints may be mobilized by spring or elastic tension in addition to exercise.

Purpose of Splints

Skeletal Substitution. (1) Broken bones; (2) congenital absence of bones; (3) diseased bones and joints.

Muscle Balance. (4) Weakened muscles (dystrophy); (5) paralyzed muscles; (6) divided tendons or muscles.

Joint Motion. (7) To preserve joint motion; (8) to increase joint motion (both require dynamic splinting).

Rest. (9) To promote wound healing; (10) treatment of infection; (11) healing of certain metabolic diseases; (12) relief of pain.

Special Uses. (13) The restoration of prehension to the paralyzed hand by the flexor hinge splint, which may be powered by the finger, wrist, or artificial muscle.

Since immobilization leads to joint stiffening, the following precautions should be observed whenever possible: (1) immobilize in the position of function; (2) immobilize the least number of joints; (3) immobilize for the shortest period of time; (4) allow slight movement, if possible.

It is far easier to prevent joint stiffness than to overcome it once it has occurred.

MATERIALS

These should be light, sufficiently strong, durable, and malleable enough to be properly fitted. The more commonly used materials are:

Plaster of Paris. Named for the gypsum found at Montemarte, a district of that city, it is readily available, inexpensive, and simple to use. It is easily applied and can be molded to shape readily before setting. It is heavy, not water-resistant, and nonpliable after setting has taken place.

Aluminum. This material is light, strong, malleable, and available in various shapes, forms, and thicknesses.

Stainless Steel. Stronger than aluminum but more difficult to fit because it is less malleable.

Wood. Light, inexpensive, but not malleable.

Cramer Wire. Light and readily molded. Excellent for temporary splinting of finger, hand, wrist, or forearm.

Plastics. These materials are light, strong, water-resistant and durable. The thermoplastic materials are most practical since they can be molded when heated. The high temperature thermoplastics such as alloys of acrylic, synthetic rubber and styrene, and copolymers of polyvinyl chloride and acrylic are examples which require heating to 250 to 350°F. They must be molded on a model because of the high temperatures involved but are more durable than those molded at lower temperatures. The low temperature thermoplastics which are molded at 140 to 170°F such as isoprenes (Orthoplast, Johnson & Johnson(and neoprene are of more practical use since they can be molded directly on the body. These materials are available in sheets which are semirigid at room temperature, but become completely limp and pliable when heated in hot water or hot air. They can be readily cut by scissors when heated. The properties of these materials, indications for their use, sources of supply, and methods of fabrication are outlined by Malick.[13]

EMERGENCY SPLINTING MATERIALS

Figure 15.1.1 shows some materials used for emergency splinting of the hand and upper extremity. Cardboard, plaster of Paris, flexible Cramer wire, a magazine, inflatable plastic splint, and wood are each satisfactory. In fact, any material with rigidity can be used. A pillow folded about the forearm and hand should be remembered as a satisfactory emergency splint.

The inflatable splint devised by Gardner[7] (Figs. 15.1.1E and 15.1.2) is excellent in many ways. It is compact to carry when collapsed, readily inflatable by mouth, and exerts uniform pressure over the entire surface that it encases.

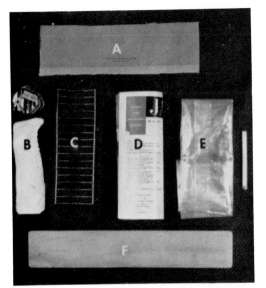

Figure 15.1.1. Some materials suitable for emergency splints for the hand and forearm. *A.* Cardboard. *B.* Plaster of Paris. *C.* Cramer wire. *D.* Magazine. *E.* Inflatable plastic splint. See Figure 15.1.2. *F.* Wood.

INTERNAL SPLINTING

This type of splinting is particularly suited for fractures about the hand, and for fixing hand position, for the application of pedicles and for wound healing. Stainless steel Kirschner wires can fix the small fractured bones of the hand, either longitudinally or trans-

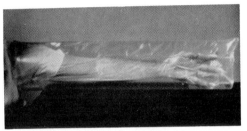

Figure 15.1.2. Inflatable emergency splint for the upper extremity developed by W. James Gardner, M. D. This splint is very compact to carry. It is inflated by mouth with a small piece of tubing (Fig. 15.1.1E) and immobilizes the upper extremity with uniform pressure. (Courtesy of W. James Gardner, M.D.).

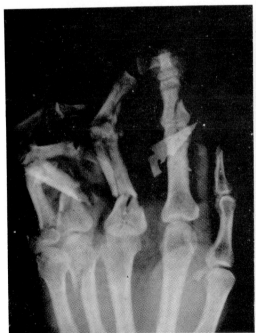

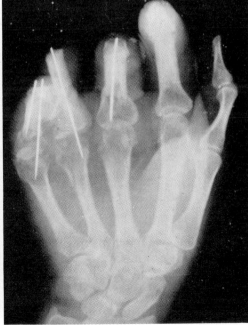

Figure 15.1.3. Multiple fractures of phalanges immobilized by internal splinting with longitudinal Kirschner wires.

versely at angles, as shown in Figures 15.1.3, 15.1.4, and 15.1.5, so that adjacent joints can be kept moving and joint stiffness avoided. The Kirschner wires may be applied at open operation or, if, reduction is adequate, percutaneously.

Metacarpal fractures may be immobilized by longitudinal Kirschner wires introduced through the dorsal portion of the metacarpophalangeal joint to span the fracture site, or by transverse wires into adjacent metacarpals as shown in Figure 15.1.5. The latter technique takes advantage of the unique anatomy in the metacarpal area with four parallel bones closely adjacent to one another. It carries less risk of disturb-

ing the metacarpophalangeal joint. This technique is not suitable, of course, when the adjacent metacarpals are also broken.

WRIST SPLINTS

The wrist has been described as the key joint of the hand just as the metacarpophalangeal joint has been described as the key joint of the finger (Bunnell[6]). For optimal function, the hand should be in the position of function (Fig. 15.1.8). This involves 30 to 35° of dorsiflexion of the wrist. As the fingers close in grasp, the wrist normally dorsiflexes. Whenever possible, the

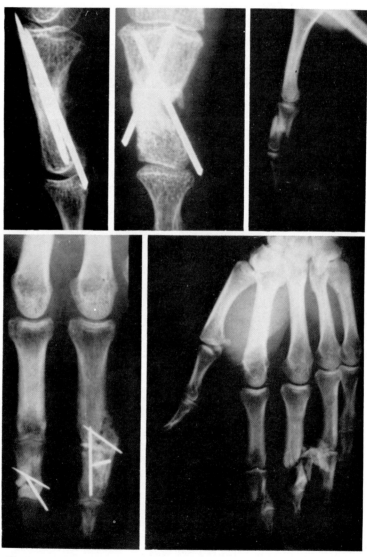

Figure 15.1.4. Phalangeal fractures immobilized by internal splinting with oblique Kirschner wires cut off beneath the skin. The wires are removed after the fractures are healed.

wrist should be immobilized in the position of function.

Figure 15.1.6 shows several kinds of wrist splints that hold the wrist in the position of function. The aluminum cock-up splint (A) has the advantage that it can be heat-sterilized as can the universal splint of Allen (B). The Oppenheimer splint (C) applies spring dorsiflexion to the wrist joint and is most useful in paralysis of the wrist extensors. The small light Stern splints (D) are very useful especially after casts or larger splints are removed. The aluminum rod held in canvas can be molded by hand to hold the wrist in any desired position.

Low temperature thermoplastics such as isoprene and neoprene[9] are also excellent.

FINGER SPLINTS

Figure 15.1.7 shows some of the more useful types of splints for immobilization of digits. It is desirable to immobilize the fingers in flexion just as it is important to immobilize the wrist in dorsiflexion.

OPPOSITION OR ABDUCTION SPLINTS

When the opponens muscle of the thumb is paralyzed for any reason, the thumb tends to fall in adjacent to the index finger which is an ineffective position for grasp. To avoid this, the thumb may be blocked in abduction as shown in Figure 15.1.8 with a light plastic splint or by elastic outrigger pull as shown in Figure 15.1.9 A. Although these splints hold the thumb in abduction, the opponens muscle can function effectively from this position when nerve regeneration occurs. The thumb may also be held in this

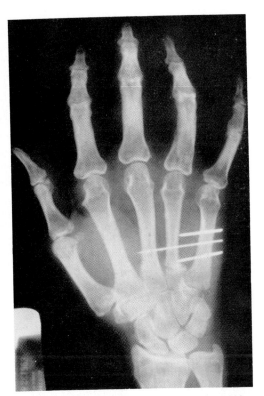

Figure 15.1.5. Fracture of metacarpal immobilized by internal splinting with transverse Kirschner wires cut off beneath the skin. This allows immediate finger movement which prevents joint stiffness.

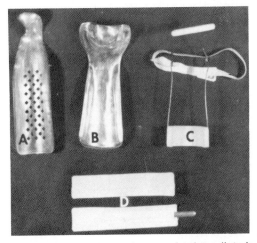

Figure 15.1.6. Several types of wrist splints in addition to plaster of Paris. *A.* Aluminum cock-up splint. *B.* Universal splint (Allen-molded aluminum). *C.* Oppenheimer (spring dorsiflexion). *D.* Aluninum rod in canvas (Stern). (Courtesy of G. A. Guilford and Sons, Cleveland.)

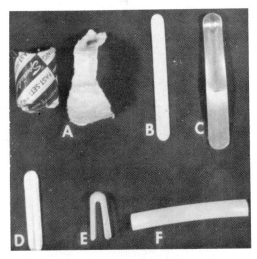

Figure 15.1.7. Finger splints. *A.* Molded plaster of Paris. *B.* Tongue blade. *C* and *D.* Malleable aluminum. *E* and *F.* Plastic.

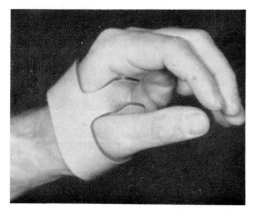

Figure 15.1.8. The position of function of the hand. Abduction of the thumb is prevented by a light plastic splint. This type of splint is useful for paralysis of the opponens muscle. (Courtesy of G. A. Guilford and Sons, Cleveland.)

position by bandages and gauze placed between the thumb and index finger.

Dynamic Splinting of the Metacarpophalangeal Joints

Stiffening of the metacarpophalangeal joints is prone to occur when these joints are held immobile in extension. The knuckle bender splint (Fig. 15.1.9 B), which applies elastic pull-in flexion to these joints, is most useful in restoring flexion. Alternative methods are outrigger flexion either by splint (Fig. 15.1.10) or by cast (Fig. 15.1.11 C).

The reverse knuckle bender splint (Fig. 15.1.9 A) is an effective means of applying elastic extension traction to the metacarpophalangeal joints when desired. An alternative method is outrigger extension as shown in Figure 15.1.11 A.

DYNAMIC SPLINTING OF THE INTERPHALANGEAL JOINTS

Figure 15.1.12 shows methods of increasing motion of stiffened interphalangeal joints by means of several types of dynamic splints.

Figure 15.1.12 A and B shows examples of splints which straighten both interphalangeal joints of the finger. Glove traction as shown in Figure 15.1.12 C is a good method of applying flexion to all three finger joints. It is a particularly good night splint. The finger knuckle bender, a very useful splint which flexes the middle joint of the finger, is shown in Figure 15.1.12 D. Gentle flexion traction can also be applied to the middle joints of the fingers by the "belt and buckle" method. Figure 15.1.13 shows this simple but effective technique applied with a Velcro strap flat tourniquet. A small ace bandage can also be wrapped in this manner. The constant gentle pull of the elastic traction is particularly beneficial when joint stiffness is of recent origin. In late cases, adhesions and liga-

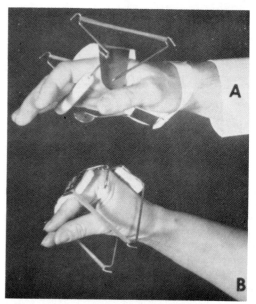

Figure 15.1.9. A. Reverse knuckle bender splint. B. The knuckle bender splint. These useful splints apply elastic pull flexion or extension to the metacarpophalangeal finger joints as required.

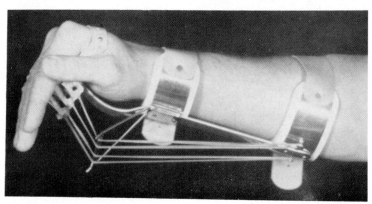

Figure 15.1.10. Elastic outrigger flexion for metacarpophalangeal joints. An alternative to the knuckle bender splint. (Courtesy of G. A. Guilford and Sons, Cleveland.)

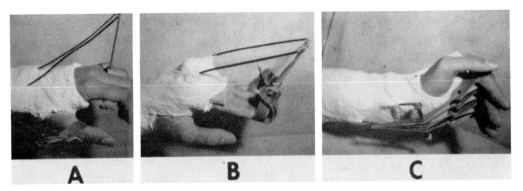

Figure 15.1.11. Outrigger elastic traction applied to plaster casts. *A.* Elastic extension of metacarpophalangeal joints and elastic thumb opposition. *B.* Elastic extension of the interphalangeal joints. Note the felt padding over the proximal phalanges. *C.* Elastic metacarpophalangeal joint flexion.

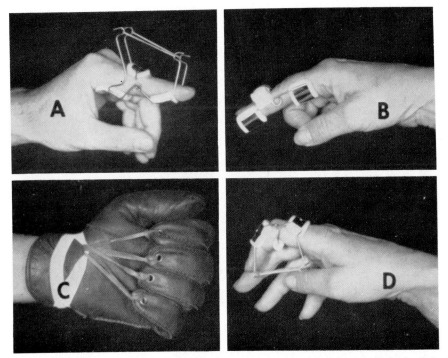

Figure 15.1.12. Methods of dynamic extension and flexion of the interphalangeal joints of the finger. *A.* Reverse finger knuckle bender splint. Extension of both interphalangeal joints. *B.* Safety pin splint. Extension of both interphalangeal joints. *C.* Glove traction. Flexion of all finger joints. *D.* Finger knuckle bender. Flexion to middle joint of finger. (Courtesy of G. A. Guilford and Sons, Cleveland.) See also Figure 15.1.15.

ment shortening may be too great to yield. The elastic pull should be gentle and allow active motion in the opposite direction. This type of pull is less likely to become uncomfortable or produce pressure necrosis.

SPLINTS FOR FRACTURES

The type of splint suitable for a fracture depends on the location of the break and whether the fracture is stable or unstable. Some incomplete transverse fractures may require only a curved finger splint. However, if the fracture is complete or the line is oblique (unstable fracture), internal fixation is often the best procedure so that adjacent joints can be kept moving.

Figure 15.1.13 shows an effective method of splinting stable fractures of metacarpals and phalanges after they have been reduced. Skin traction is usually sufficient, although skeletal traction may be used as well as pulp traction in some instances.

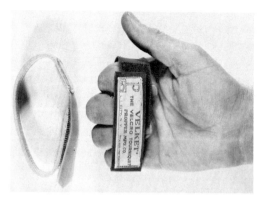

Figure 15.1.13. A simple method of applying flexion traction to the middle joint of the fingers. A webb strap with buckle can be used. The velcro buckle and elastic band such as that of a flat tourniquet is a good alternative.

SPLINTS FOR RADIAL NERVE PALSY

Splinting in this condition should supply wrist, finger, and thumb extension, if the lesion is complete. Of these, wrist extension is most important to supplement.

Figure 15.1.11 *A* shows one means of supplying these forces with a plaster cast and outrigger elastic traction. This allows motion and also corrects the lack of active extension of wrist, fingers, and thumb. The Oppenheimer splint (Fig. 15.1.6 *C*) supplies elastic wrist dorsiflexion which is adequate for partial lesions. Rigid splints can be used but these are awkward to wear and lead to joint stiffness.

SPLINTS FOR ULNAR NERVE PALSY

The clawing of the ring and small fingers in ulnar nerve palsy is well controlled temporarily by the knuckle bender splint (Fig. 15.1.9 *B*). An alternative method is rubber band flexion with finger slings over the clawed fingers (Figs. 15.1.10 and 15.1.11 *C*). This type of splinting is advisable during the period of regeneration after surgical nerve repair.

SPLINTS FOR MEDIAN NERVE PALSY

Opponens paralysis in median nerve palsy is adequately splinted by a light plastic block splint as shown in Figure 15.1.8. It also can be splinted by outrigger traction (Fig. 15.1.11 *A*).

SPLINTS FOR MEDIAN AND ULNAR NERVE PALSY

The complete claw hand of combined median and ulnar paralysis requires flexion of the metacarpophalangeal joints and "opponens" splinting of the thumb. This can be done by an elastic outrigger pull. When the knuckle bender splint is used, a bar to preserve abduction of the thumb should be added.

SPLINTS FOR ARTHRITIS

Light splints to maintain form and prevent deformity and pain during the acute phase of arthritis are highly desirable. In this disease, structures become so weakened that the hand is deformed, not only by outside forces as the hand is used, but also by the internal mechanical forces of tendon and muscle action. It is particularly important to hold the wrist in dorsiflexion during the acute phase of the disease and to maintain the normal relationships of the metacarpophalangeal joints by preventing subluxation and ulnar deviation of the proximal phalanges of the fingers. The normal curve of the fingers should also be preserved by light splints to prevent swan neck and boutonniere deformities which are very prone to occur.

Figure 15.1.14 shows a light splint readily molded

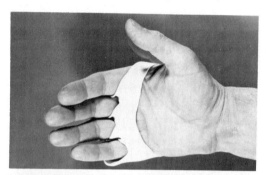

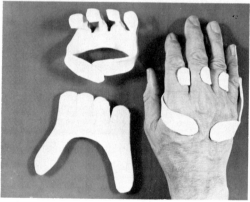

Figure 15.1.14. Splint to prevent ulnar drift in arthritis. This light weight plastic splint, made of an isoprene type of material, gives support on the ulnar borders of the fingers and yet allows movement. The material is available from Johnson & Johnson dealers as "Orthoplast" in sheets ⅛ inch thick. It is readily cut to pattern and molded to the hand, when softened by heat at approximately 140°F.

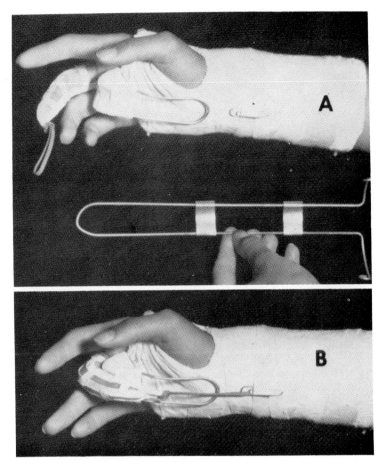

Figure 15.1.15. A. and *B.* Method of splinting fractures of metacarpals and phalanges. Traction is applied with the finger in the flexed position (*B*). To avoid overlapping, the fingers are made to converge to the base of the thenar eminence to avoid rotation at the fracture site.

to the hand to prevent ulnar drift. Hammond[9] has reported favorable results with this splint in the prevention of progression of ulnar drift of the fingers in patients with rheumatoid arthritis.

SPLINTS TO RESTORE PINCH GRASP TO THE SEVERELY PARALYZED HAND

The extended use of appliances to aid paralyzed patients has been a recent development of much interest and usefulness. The work of Nickel[14] has been outstanding in the development of the "flexor hinge splint" which can be motored by a residual finger flexor, a wrist extensor, or by an artificial muscle. Figure 15.1.16 shows the flexor hinge splint motorized by a residual wrist dorsiflexor. When the patient extends the wrist with his wrist extensor, the index and long fingers flex against the thumb by reciprocal action as shown. This allows fingertip-to-thumb prehension in a hand that actually has only active wrist dorsi-

flexion. Usually sensation is present in the fingertips making the grasp more useful. This type of mechanical hand acts similarly to an automatic hand with tenodesis of the finger flexors. The latter has the advantage of requiring no mechanical appliance. Figure 15.1.17 shows the flexor hinge splint motorized by an "artificial muscle." When the patient wishes to close the index and long fingertips against the tip of the thumb, a valve is opened which allows compressed gas from a small pressure tank to enter the woven cylinder shown in the photograph. The expansion of the woven cylinder, due to the pressure of the gas within it, closes the grasp by reciprocal action and holds it there until the pressure is released. Very firm grasp between these three digit tips is possible by this means. Grasp and release depend upon the opening and the closing of a valve which the patient must be able to control in some way. The development of this type of apparatus offers great help to persons seriously paralyzed.

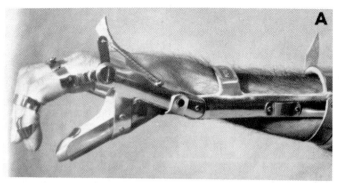

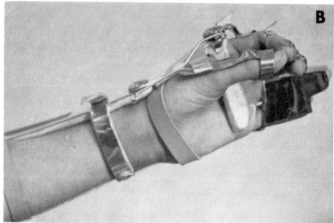

Figure 15.1.16. The flexor hinge splint motorized by a wrist extensor. When the patient dorsiflexes the wrist, the thumb, index, and long fingers automatically oppose. The patient's sensation is present in this pinch grip (*B*). (Courtesy of Vernon L. Nickel, M.D.)

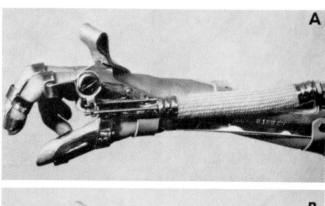

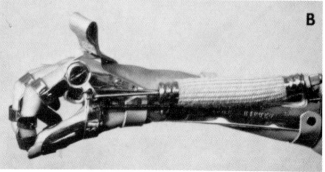

Figure 15.1.17. The flexor hinge splint motorized by an artificial muscle. Expansion of the woven cylinder by gas from a small pressure tank causes the wrist to dorsiflex and the index and long fingers to oppose the thumb by reciprocal action (*B*).

THE BRACE MAKER (ORTHOTIST)

The field of the brace maker (orthotist) has advanced greatly in recent years.[2][3][4][8][10][11][12][16][17] The training of the brace marker has advanced concomitantly. He now must have four years of experience and undergo examination before certification.

Acknowledgment

The author has drawn freely on all the references listed below. Special thanks are due Mrs. Marjorie Herring and Miss Virginia Allen for their help with the plastic splint materials.

REFERENCES

1. Anderson, M. H. *Functional Bracing of the Upper Extremities,* edited by R. E. Sollars. Springfield, C. C Thomas, 1958.
2. Anderson, M. H. *Functional Bracing of the Upper Extremities.* Springfield, C. C Thomas, 1965.
3. Anderson, M. H. *Upper Extremities Orthotics.* Springfield, C. C Thomas, 1965
4. Bender, L. F. Prevention of deformities through orthotics. J.A.M.A., *183:* 946-948, 1963.
5. Bunnell, S. Illustration, p. 279. In *Orthopaedic Appliances Atlas,* Vol. 1. Ann Arbor, Edwards, 1952.
6. Bunnell, S. *Surgery of the Hand,* Ed. 3. Philadelphia, Lippincott, 1956, p. 113.
7. Gardner, W. J. An inflatable emergency splint. Cleve. Clin. Q., *29:* 54-56, 1962.
8. Glancy, J. J. Technical responsibility of the orthotist. J.A.M.A., *183:* 936-938, 1963.
9. Hammond, J. Abraham Lincoln Memorial Hospital, Lincoln, Ill. Personal communication.
10. Leavitt, L. A. Orthotic devices for patients with chronic physical handicap. J.A.M.A., *183:* 939-941, 1963.
11. Licht, S. *Orthotics.* Springfield, C. C Thomas, 1965.
12. Lowman, E. W. Orthotics in musculoskeletal disease. J.A.M.A., *183:* 942-945, 1963.
13. Malick, M. H. *Manual on Static Hand Splinting.* Pittsburgh, Harmarville Rehabilitation Center 1974.
14. Nickel, V. L. Development of function in the severely paralyzed hand. J. Bone Joint Surg., to be published.
15. Pease, C. N., Editor. *The American Academy of Orthopaedic Surgeons Instructional Course Lecture,* Vol. 9. Ann Arbor, Edwards, 1952.
16. Rancho Los Amigos Hospital. *Handbook on Hand Splints.* Downy, 1973.
17. Rotstein J. *Simple Splinting.* Philadelphia, Saunders, 1965.
18. Skinner, H. A. *The Origin of Medical Terms,* Ed. 2 Baltimore, Williams & Wilkins, 1961, p. 329.

B.

Surface Flexion Contractures
Franklin L. Ashley, M.D.
George V. Webster, M.D.
Dennis P. Thompson, M.D.

INTRODUCTION

Flexion is the dominant function of the hand. Of the many uses of the hand and fingers, only a few require full extension of the hand and digits for their performance. The "intrinsic plus" position of the hand, as assumed when putting a hand through a coat sleeve or holding it flat for slapping or striking an object, requires full extension, but needs very little power from the extensors. Merely enough strength is needed for full extension of the hands to overcome the dominant flexor power. In actual power, the flexors exert many times the amount of force on the hand and fingers that the extensors do.

It is small wonder that disabilities affecting the hand result more commonly in flexion contractures than in extension contractures.

ANATOMY

Although the skin covering the hand is continuous, each small area of the integument is highly specialized. A review of the specialized character of the contiguous skin segments helps in the better understanding of problems of skin contracture and functional correction. On the dorsum, the most conspicuous highly specialized structure is, of course, the fingernail, which originates at the nail bed, grows distally to cover the distal terminal phalanx with heavily cornified and insensitive chitinous structure and to splint smoothly the pulp of the finger, and finally grows beyond the finger itself for scratching and digging. The delicate and highly specialized skin over the distal phalanx, just proximal to the nail, provides a smooth transition from the nail to the intact skin on the dorsum of the hand. The elasticity of the skin over the dorsum of the fingers allows unrestricted flexion and yet resiliently recoils upon extension of the fingers, producing only slight folds over the dorsum of the joints. The slippery areolar tissue underlying the dorsal skin allows its maximal elasticity to function well; fixation of the skin to the underlying structures is mainly at the lateral aspect of the joints. The webs between the fingers, and between the thumb and index finger, are delicately designed folds of skin, which accommodate flexion, extension, separation, or stretching of the fingers or thumb in any direction. The amount of skin necessary to replace a web which has been destroyed is much greater than it would appear, and cannot be imagined until one tries to reconstruct and replace a web which has been lost. Bunnell's emphasis on the use of transposition flaps from dorsal and volar surface to reconstruct the base of the web further points out the need for maximal flexibility of a digital web if finger function is to approach normal.

The skin on the dorsum of the hand and wrist is loose enough so that it can be picked up easily between the thumb and forefinger of the other hand and has a "two-way stretch," both laterally and over the long axis of the hand. In this area also the areolar subcutaneous tissue and lack of significant amounts of fat contribute to the highly specialized function of this skin. It is interesting that the newborn has a well developed cherubic subcutaneous dorsal fat pad, which disappears almost entirely by the age of four years as it undergoes metaplasia to adult slippery areolar tissue. Dorsal skin must essentially provide cover during full expansion and recoil. It is also subject especially to thermal injury in burns. The skin is thin, and thermal damage, which would scarcely more than blister the well calloused palm of the hand, may cause destruction of the full thickness of the dorsal skin.

The specialized character of mature volar skin is evident on simple inspection. This interesting tissue acts as a protective armor, and is extremely tough, yet soft and pliable. It is extremely sensitive to stimuli of pain, touch, and temperature, and via the superficial blood vessels in the dermis aids in maintenance of body temperature. Variations in temperature are quite accurately measured, even as low as 1°C. As much as 1,500 to 2,000 ml of sweat may be excreted through the hyperactive sweat glands in an hour and also sebum which forms vitamin D when activated by the sun. The fingertips, with their whorls and delicate tactile sensation, are protected by a heavy cornified layer, and there may be callus formation which is normal response to repeated trauma of this specialized area of skin. Such calluses are seen in players of stringed instruments, for example.

The palm of the hand is built to absorb shock and the heavily trabeculated fat pads can protect it against severe impacts. A baseball player or the operator of a jackhammer absorbs terrific palmar blows with little or no apparent damage. Callus formation is usually noted over the margins of the palm, while the central portion of palmar skin remains thin by comparison. The abrupt junction of the callused skin of the proximal palm with the thin, elastic, transparent skin of the flexor aspect of the wrist is another example of the need for resilience in flexion and extension to accommodate for almost 180° of change between extreme volar fixation and extreme dorsiflexion, at the wrist.

The palmar surface varies markedly with the dorsal, being much thicker, less pliable, and more sensitive. The palmar skin is also less mobile in that it is attached to the underlying bones by fibrous septa, forming so-called functional and protective tunnels for the pas-

sage of tendons, nerves and blood vessels. The dorsal skin is thin, pliable, and loosely attached to the underlying fascia by a fibrofatty layer simulating paratenon.

The fat pads beneath the palmar skin cause the formation of creases when the fingers are flexed and a fist is made.

It is important to remember that all the skin of the hand is needed and the loss of even 1 sq cm should be promptly replaced. This is especially true over the dorsum because of its great flexibility and excursion with stretching from flexion to extension of the digits (over 4 cm). The dorsal skin should therefore be replaced either by a split graft or flap and the hand splinted in complete flexion.

The volar surface of the tips of the fingers is extremely sensitive to stimuli. The limit of two-point discrimination on the tips of the fingers is 2.5 mm, whereas on the dorsum it is 6.9 mm.

TYPES OF CONTRACTURES

Cicatricial Scarring

Cicatrix, or contracted scar tissue, is the cause of the majority of flexion contractures in the hand and fingers, both on the volar and dorsal surfaces. It should be completely eliminated by excision and replacement with good skin, either a free graft or pedicle flap, before it has an opportunity to deform the hand.

When deeper structures are involved beneath or within the cicatricial scarring, a free graft is not sufficient covering, especially when some of the deeper structures must be replaced, such as a damaged tendon with a tendon graft. In this case a pedicle flap is necessary with its subcutaneous fat to provide a gliding surface and new blood supply for healing tendons, bone, and nerves.

Trauma

Trauma is responsible for most flexion contractures of the hand. Lacerations, crush injuries, and fractures in the hand carry with them various potentialities for contracture. Should infection ensue, the late fibroblastic response to infection is often so great as to produce irreparable destruction of volar soft tissue. Burns of the volar aspect of the hand, whether due to heat, friction. chemical injury, or freezing, can produce contracture so severe that one sometimes sees a mere club of scar projecting from the wrist, and only by x-ray can it be determined that stumps of digits are still present.

Fractures may produce flexion contractures, due to a shortening at the fracture site, or secondarily due to prolonged flexion during treatment. Stabilization of bone fragments by modern internal fixation has allowed for earlier mobilization of the fingers during treatment of fractures in the hand, and has prevented much in the way of latent contracture.

Before the enlightened teachings of Kanavel and Bunnell a major cause of flexion contractures of the hand was the surgeon's scalpel. Arbitrary incisions

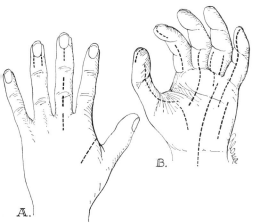

Figure 15.2.1. Adapted from Bunnell, showing incorrect "pernicious" incisions crossing skin lines and in areas endangering deeper structures. *A.* Dorsal. *B.* Volar.

into the palmar skin for repair of underlying injury or treatment of infection, if made at right angles to the normal flexion creases of the hand, unless closed with a Z-plasty, create disastrous and unyielding contractures which respond only partially, if at all, to the plastic surgeon's attempt to restore full motion and extension to the fingers and hand (Fig. 15.2.1).

Infection

Another principal cause of flexion contractures in the hand and fingers is infection. Infections are becoming more prevalent as the antibiotics are encountering increasingly resistant organisms. It is therefore necessary to revert to fundamental surgical principles in the treatment of some of these resistant infections and provide adequate drainage, elevation, heat, and splinting to prevent contractures.

Infections involving the synovial sheaths and fascial spaces are devastating in that they cause cicatricial contracture of the surrounding deeper structures and therefore require much more extensive reconstruction. It is important to keep in mind that drainage incisions should be elective and never cross flexion creases and thus cause further cicatricial scarring (Fig. 15.2.2). During the healing phase, adequate splinting in the position of function is most important to prevent contraction as the wounds heal with proper scar tissue.

Another infection that is deforming because of formation of cicatricial scarring and subsequent contractures in the hand is that following deep second or third degree burns, to be discussed in more detail later.

Burns

Burns of the hand deserve especial consideration as there is considerable controversy among the various centers, at this time, concerning the primary treatment of these injuries. If it is possible to ascertain the exact extent of the third degree burn of the hand, primary excision and grafting should be performed within the

first 24 to 48 hours. It is difficult, however, to distinguish between deep second degree burns and third degree burns in most instances. In these doubtful cases a period of watchful waiting is best, with early debridement and skin grafting in less than 14 days, that is, before contractures develop. Contraction of tendons should be avoided, and meticulous observation of all burns is imperative to prevent hyperextended metacarpophalangeal joints and hyperextended wrist, especially in burns of the dorsum of the hand.

Severe burns of the palm, especially in children, may cause flexion contracture primarily by fibrous contracture of the bed beneath the burned surface (Fig. 15.2.3*A*). This occurs in the ungrafted deep burn, but also to a lesser degree in the burned palm which has been promptly grafted, since the graft and its underlying bed continues to contract unless stretched by splinting. The loss of surface covering of the palm is dramatically apparent when surgery for secondary release of contracture is performed. One often sees large surface defects open up when the hand is fully extended by mere incision of contracted areas and without any excision of scar (Fig. 15.2.4).

Incorrect Incisions

Incorrect incisions in the hand are another of the principal causes of flexion contractures. Incisions that cross skin lines in a perpendicular fashion should always be avoided; if the incisions are elective they should parallel the skin lines or cross them at a small, oblique angle. If the incisions are involuntary, such as are made by trauma, it may be necessary to change the direction of the scars, either with a Z-plasty or by the use of local flaps.

Incisions on the fingers should always be made

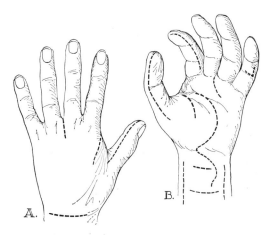

Figure 15.2.2. Adapted from Bunnell, showing correct incisions. *A*, dorsal view, and *B*, volar view parallel to skin lines or crossing them at gentle angles. Midlateral incision on finger, dorsal to neurovascular bundle; also emphasizing incision carried from palm into wrist, with S at wrist flexion creases.

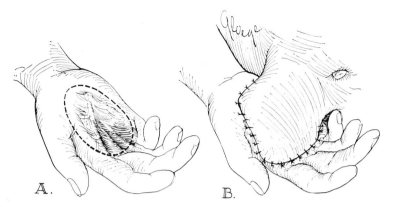

Figure 15.2.3. Damage to volar palmar skin. *A.* Involving underlying structures with cicatrix. *B.* Excision and replacement with direct abdominal flap. Note dart breaking up web between thumb and index finger.

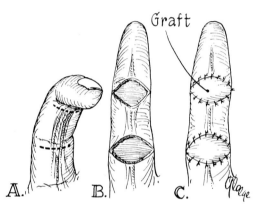

Figure 15.2.4. Longitudinal contracture of volar surface of finger. *A.* Incised at interphalangeal flexion creases. *B.* Allowed to retract. *C.* Defects covered with full thickness skin graft.

either parallel to the flexion creases, or along the mid-lateral line of the finger, never along the volar or dorsal surfaces (Fig. 15.2.2).

Keloids

In our more recent studies of keloids and hypertrophic scars, we have found that when incisions are closed under tension or when incisions cross flexion creases at a perpendicular angle, the chance of keloids forming is great. In our experience the best treatment for keloids or recurrent hypertrophic scars has been excision and suture, followed by immediate roentgen therapy consisting of a total of 1,500 units in divided doses. This may be calibrated to avoid damaging deeper structures in children. The patient is taken directly from the operating room to the roentgenologic theater, where the first prophylactic dose of roentgen therapy is administered.

A distinction between keloids and hypertrophic scars should be made. It is known from histologic studies that the keloid extends past the area of scar into the normal tissue, whereas the hypertrophic scar is limited to the area of the scar itself. If watchful waiting is adopted, the hypertrophic scar usually subsides but the keloid will subside only rarely without proper therapy.

Congenital Conditions

One primary type of contracture of the flexor aspect of the hand is found in congenital contractures. These shortenings of the soft tissues on the flexor aspect of the hand, wrist, and elbow are of unknown origin. They may involve isolated areas, such as the common congenital flexion contractures of the little finger affecting chiefly the proximal interphalangeal joint, or they may involve all the skin and soft tissues on the flexor aspect of the hand, wrist, elbow, and shoulder. Such contractures are often associated with other congenital anomalies. Congenital flexion contractures of the fingers seem to be caused by shortening and congenital absence of adequate skin covering in the majority of instances. The fingers resist passive extension and weblike bands of otherwise perfectly normal volar skin restrict movement. Correction by Z-plasty is often possible in the minor degrees of congenital contracture, but more often actual skin grafts to lengthen the volar cutaneous covering are necessary to relieve the congenital condition. Adduction and flexion contractures of the thumb and thumb web are seen occasionally. Partial correction by traction extension splints usually must be accompanied by Z-plasty and the addition of volar skin grafts to accomplish release of the contracture. Contraction bands constricting the fingers or wrist may be corrected by Z-plasties in two or more stages (Fig. 15.2.5).

Nerve Injuries

Injuries to peripheral nerves can produce marked flexion contractures of the hand and fingers. Such contractures occur from the muscular atrophy and contraction, from the upset in the delicate balance bet-

veen extensors and flexors, and from imbalance bet-
veen small muscles of the hand and the long motors of
he hand. Atrophy and scarring of the small muscles of
he hand with secondary shortening and contracture
an result in the commonly known "intrinsic plus"
nd "intrinsic minus" deformities of the hand. Loss
f sensation can produce trophic ulceration of the hand
vith secondary infection or contracture.

pecialized Types

Specialized types of contracture of the hand are
ound in such conditions as scleroderma and in Volk-
nann's contracture, both local and in the forearm.
ccleroderma may be treated by excision and contrac-
ure release with replacement of the involved skin by a
plit thickness skin graft. Volkmann's contracture, ar-
hritis, and Dupuytren's contracture will be discussed

elsewhere. However, a two-stage operation and a reverse flap technique, found useful by us, will be described.

Two-stage operation for Dupuytren's Contracture

First Stage. Under general anesthesia and with an
inflated sphygmomanometer arm cuff on the arm, an
incision (Fig. 15.2.6 A) is made overlying and approximating the course of the flexor tendons of the little finger from the distal border of the transverse carpal ligament to the distal palmar flexion crease, where
the incision is curved gently toward the radius along
the distal, or proximal, margin of this crease to a point
opposite the web between the long and ring fingers as
recommended by Bunnell. The flap is dissected from
the underlying aponeurosis, leaving all subcutaneous
fat attached to the skin flap. The dissection is then car-

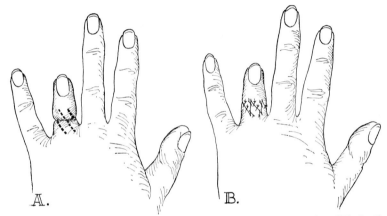

Figure 15.2.5. Congenital contraction band around ring finger. *A.* Incised and Z-plasties outlined. *B.*
Closed with multiple Z-plasties in stages: dorsal surface, then volar surface at a later date.

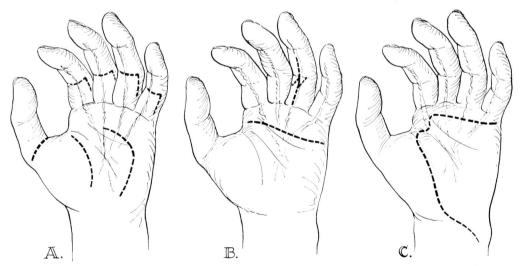

Figure 15.2.6. *A.* Two stage incisions in palm and fingers for palmar fasciectomy in definitive treatment of Dupuytren's contracture (Ashley modification of Bunnell's technique). *B.* McIndoe-Skoog incisions for radical fasciectomy in one stage. *C.* Webster flap for approach to palmar fascia.

ried proximally to the point of aponeurotic narrowing that becomes the palmaris longus tendon. This tendon is severed. The fibrotic aponeurosis is dissected, subcutaneously, distally to the bases of the long, ring, and little fingers, with the deep septa carefully removed from their attachment to the metacarpal bones. The digital bands are then dissected free of their attachments to the skin and vaginal ligaments with small, narrow, moderately blunt, Stevens type scissors. Next, the digital bands are severed from their attachments to the palmar aponeurosis. An incision is then made along the median line of the ulnar or radial surface of the proximal phalanx of the little finger and curved gently along the proximal flexion crease, thus making an angle of approximately 100°. This small flap is elevated, care being taken to isolate and retract the digital vessels and nerves. The digital band from the palm is then grasped and drawn distally through this new incision on the finger, dissected free of its attachments, and removed. Care should be taken to remove the three fanlike divisions of this digital band. The process is repeated on the ring and long fingers. The tourniquet is then released and a warm pack applied for 10 min. Any active bleeding on removal of the pack is controlled by accurate ligation with 4-0 plain catgut. Finally the wounds are irrigated gently with warm saline and the skin is closed with interrupted 5-0 Dermalon. A pressure dressing of cotton mechanic's waste is applied and the hand is fixed in the position of function. A dorsal plaster splint may then be applied if deemed necessary.

Second Stage. The second stage may be performed at any subsequent time after complete healing of the first stage, although this second procedure is usually unnecessary unless the first two fingers are involved by the disease process. If they are primarily involved or if they become involved at a later date, the procedure is repeated. An incision is made just distal to, or proximal to, and parallel with the thenar flexion crease from the transverse carpal ligament to the radial margin of the palm. Through this approach the digital bands to the thumb and index finger may be dissected free and removed through the curvilinear incisions on the proximal phalanges as in the first stage. This procedure also may be completed fairly rapidly, so that release and reapplication of the tourniquet is unnecessary. The dressing is removed on the seventh or eighth postoperative day. Most of the sutures are removed at this time and mild exercise of the distal interphalangeal joints is instituted. A splint and a lighter pressure dressing are left in place during the second week. In the third postoperative week full active motion is begun.

Another method for the total removal of the palmar fascia has been advocated by McIndoe, Bunnell, and Skoog and has been widely accepted and utilized. This involves a transverse palmar incision parallel to the distal flexion crease and gives good exposure for all of the palmar fascia to the base of the fingers. (Fig.

15.2.6 *B*). The digital bands are then excised through midline longitudinal incisions which are closed with Z-plasties to prevent contracture. Sometimes this procedure is followed by marginal loss of the skin especially along the distal margin of the palmar incision, but generally is very convenient and successful.

Webster has advocated a reverse flap technique (Fig. 15.2.6 *C*), which allows good exposure and removal of the palmar fascia, followed by excision of the digital bands by the conventional incisions in the skin of the proximal finger.

RECONSTRUCTIVE PRINCIPLES

When cicatricial scars are small and the surrounding skin is adequate and flexible, the scars may be excised and the surrounding skin undermined and closed without tension. However, if the scar is contracted a Z-plasty or similar procedure must be performed; that is, tissue from the surrounding area must be shifted into the scarred area to relieve the contracture (Fig. 15.2.7). If the surrounding skin is inadequate, a Z-plasty is dangerous, and the pedicle flap should be substituted for this procedure. Z-plasties are especially good for web contractures if the tissue involved is pliable and free of scarring (Fig. 15.2.8). If the entire web is scarred, however, it should be incised and good tissue placed across it, either in the form of a flap or a skin graft.

Longitudinal contractures along the volar surface of the fingers, if accompanied by loss of tissue, should be completely excised and replaced with skin grafts along the entire length of the finger or a pedicle flap extending to the midlateral line. If the contractures are limited to the interphalangeal flexion creases, or just along the median line of the finger, they can be incised at the flexion creases and allowed to retract, and diamond shaped grafts are placed into the defects (Fig. 15.2.4).

If the cicatricial area in the finger is localized, such

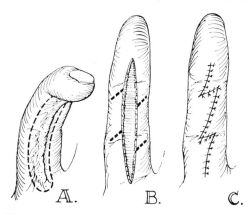

Figure 15.2.7. A. Longitudinal contracture of volar surface of finger localized to midline. *B.* Excised. *C.* Closed with Z-plasties.

as from a burn or a penetrating wound, and the underlying structures are involved, a flap from an adjoining finger may be more efficient than a skin graft since it brings its own blood supply and subcutaneous tissue. The donor site is covered with a split thickness skin graft (Fig. 15.2.9).

Cicatricial scarring that involves the fingertip may be excised and replaced with a skin graft from a toe or may be covered by a flap from an adjoining finger.

Sometimes island flap procedures may be used. A

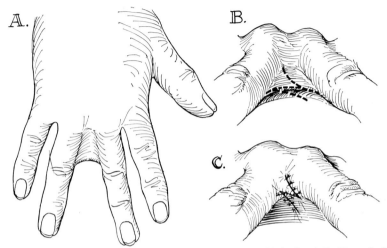

Figure 15.2.8. A. Web contracture, either congenital or acquired. *B.* Incised. *C.* Closed with Z-plasty.

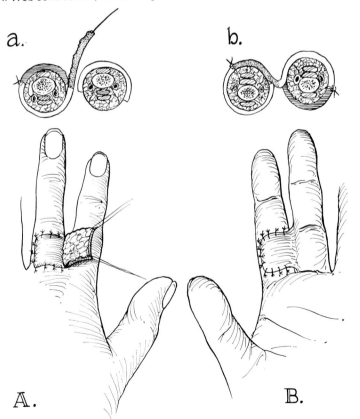

Figure 15.2.9. A. Defect on volar surface of finger involving small area of skin and deeper structures. *B.* Closed with cross-finger flap. *a* and *b.* Donor site covered with split thickness skin graft.

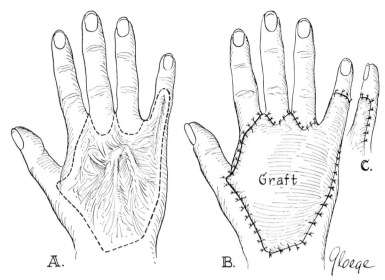

Figure 15.2.10. Cicatricial contracture on dorsum of hand after burn or abrasive trauma involving skin only. *A.* Lines of excision. *B.* Covered with split thickness skin graft with appropriate darts in webs and where necessary carrying grafts out to finger, with *(C)* edge of graft along midlateral line.

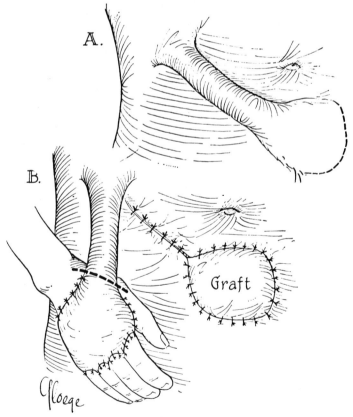

Figure 15.2.11. A. Formation of thoracabdominal tube with primary closure of underlying donor defect (if tube is large, then this area may have to be skin grafted) and tube transferred to defect on hand involving skin and underlying tissues. *B.* Flap inset with appropriate darts into webs, and donor site of pedicle on abdomen covered with skin graft.

flap of skin is carried from a distant area of the hand so that it is isolated except for its blood and nerve supply, to supply a tactile surface where the skin has been destroyed. Its advantage is that it retains its nerve supply and good tactile function results.

The volar surface of the hand usually is covered by a pedicle flap (Fig. 15.2.3 B) either from the abdomen or lateral thoracic region, especially when deeper structures are involved or after infections. The split thickness skin graft is usually the preferred procedure in the reconstruction of the burned hand, as the burn usually does not involve the deeper structures (Fig. 15.2.10).

When a pedicle flap is utilized, it is most important to leave no raw areas, that is, the unused portion of the pedicle should be skin grafted as should the donor site on the abdomen or thorax at the time of transfer.

It is important to remember also that the skin and subcutaneous tissues in pedicle flaps always retract, and therefore it is imperative that they be at least one-fourth larger than the area to be covered.

The tube pedicle flap is one of the preferred methods of reconstructing areas of the hand that require deeper repair, as it is long and pliable and thus very comfortable for the patient (Fig. 15.2.11). Also, if the donor site on the abdomen is closed primarily, either by skin graft or by primary suture, the wound is well healed and closed at the time of transfer with very little chance of infection.

When free skin grafts are used, it is important to remember that the chance of success with a split thickness skin graft is much better than with a full thickness. However, the functional result when the full thickness does "take" is much better than with the split thickness. The size of a full thickness graft must be limited by the fact that the donor site must be closed, either by skin grafting or primary suture, and the reduction of chances of a good take with a larger full thickness graft. In most cases we use a thick split graft, about 20/1000 inch, taken usually from the upper buttocks area or the lower back where the skin is the thickest, but from a hairless area.

When these grafts are placed over areas of flexion, such as on the dorsum of the hand at the metacarpophalangeal joints, the hands should be splinted in flexion to allow for the contracture of the split thickness grafts (Fig. 15.2.10). When these grafts are placed on the volar surface of the hand, as following a burn, the hand should be splinted in full extension, or even hyperextension to compensate for the contracture, and this extension should be maintained for a period longer than would ordinarily be necessary for a skin graft.

REFERENCES

1. Anson, B. J., and Ashley, F. L. Mid-palmar compartments, associated spaces and limiting layers. Anat. Rec., *78:* 389, 1940.
2. Ashley, F. L. A two-stage operation for Dupuytren's contracture. Plast. Reconstruct. Surg., *12:* 79, 1953.
3. Bunnell, S. *Surgery of the Hand,* Ed. 3. Philadelphia, Lippincott, 1956.
4. Clarkson, P., and Pelly, A. *The General and Plastic Surgery of the Hand.* Oxford, Blackwell, 1962.
5. Davis, J. S., and Finesilver, E. M. Dupuytren's contracture; with note on incidence of contraction in diabetes. Arch. Surg., *24:* 933, 1932.
6. Dupuytren, G. Permanent retraction of the fingers produced by an affection of the palmar fascia. Lancet, *2:* 222, 1834.
7. Gill, A. B. Dupuytren's contracture. Ann. Surg., *70:* 221, 1919.
8. Jackson, I. T., *et al.* A method of treating chronic flexion contractures of the fingers. Br. J. Plast. Surg., *23:* 373-379, 1970.
9. Johnson, R. K., *et al.* Cross-finger pedicle flaps in the hand. J. Bone Joint Surg., *53A:* 913-919, 1971.
10. Hamlin, E., Jr. Limited excision of Dupuytren's contracture. Ann. Surg., *135:* 94, 1952.
11. Kanavel, A. B. *Infections of the Hand.* Philadelphia, Lea & Febiger, 1939.
12. Kanavel, A. B., Koch, S. L., and Mason, M. L. Dupuytren's contracture. Surg. Gynecol. Obstet., *48:* 145, 1929.
13. Kelleher, J. C., *et al.* Use of tailored abdominal pedicle flap for surgical reconstruction of hand. J. Bone Joint Surg., *52A:* 1552-1562, 1970.
14. Marble, H. C. *The Hand. A Manual and Atlas for the General Surgeon.* Philadelphia, Saunders, 1961.
15. Myerding, H. W. Dupuytren's contracture. Arch. Surg., *32:* 320, 1936.
16. Myerding, H. W., Black, J. R., and Broders, A. C. Etiology and pathology of Dupuytren's contracture. Surg. Gynecol. Obstol., *72:* 582, 1941.
17. Nichols, H. M. *Manual of Hand Injuries.* Chicago, Year Book, 1957.
18. Palmer, L. A., and Southworth, J. L. Bridge operation for Dupuytren's contracture. Am. J. Surg., *68:* 351, 1945.
19. Pulvertaft, R. G. Reconstruction of the severely mutilated hand. Rheumatol. Phys. Med., *11:* 90, 1971.
20. Ryan, R. F. Plastic and reconstructive surgery including burns. Surg. Gynecol. Obstet., *132:* 231-234, 1971.
21. Skinner, H. L. Dupuytren's contracture; operative correction by use of tunnel skin graft. Surgery, *10:* 313, 1941.
22. Skoog, T. Dupuytren's contracture. Acta chir. scand., *96:* suppl. 139, 1948.
23. Takara, K. Two point discrimination on various types of skin grafts to hand and foot. J. Kumamoto Med. Soc., *45:* 94-121, 1971.
24. Webster, G. V. A useful incision in Dupuytren's contracture. Plast. Reconstruct. Surg., *19:* 514, 1957.
25. Webster, G. V. Reappraisal of radical fasciectomy for Dupuytren's contracture. Am. J. Surg., *100:* 372, 1960.
26. Webster, G. V. Skin grafting of the hand. West. J. Surg. Gynecol. Obstet., *70:* 279, 1962.

C.

Adduction Contracture of the Thumb

Paul W. Brown, M.D.

INTRODUCTION

The most useful part of hand function is prehension, the ability of the thumb to approximate any or all of the fingers to form a pincers of varying gap and strength. Control of this function depends on the range of motion of the three joints of the thumb, the strength of the muscles acting on the thumb and fingers, and coordination and control of their motor function by sensory feedback from sensory end organs in the tactile pads of the involved digits. Proprioceptive sense in the thumb and fingers also contributes to control.

Prehension is accomplished in two phases: first is a preliminary positioning in which circumduction of the first ray, *i.e.*, (the thumb and its metacarpal) places the thumb in a position which then secondly allows subsequent flexion of the thumb and fingers to meet each other or to meet on an interposed object.

Our concern here is with those conditions which prevent the preliminary positioning of the thumb, those positions which tether the thumb to the remainder of the hand and thereby prevent circumduction.

FUNCTIONAL ANATOMY

The skin of the thumb web is extremely supple and its mobility on the dorsal side allows extremes of circumduction before the slack is taken up. The extensor pollicis longus and extensor pollicis brevis are very mobile under the skin and move readily over the first metacarpal as they are only loosely affixed with filmy paratenon.

All three joints of the thumb, the trapeziometacarpal (carpometacarpal), metacarpophalangeal, and interphalangeal, contribute to the first phase of prehension, *i.e.*, positioning, and also to the second which is the actual prehension or pinch. The more proximal the joint, the greater is its contribution and importance. Stiffness of the IP joint gives little disability and stiffness of the MP joint only moderate disability if both IP and trapeziometacarpal joints are normal. Loss of motion of the first ray on the carpus severely limits positioning and prehension. The trapeziometacarpal joint, a saddle joint, allows a wide arc of motion of the first metacarpal on the carpus.

The position of the first ray is controlled by both intrinsic and extrinsic muscles and all three motor nerves of the forearm exercise control of some of these muscles. The radial governs the extensor pollicis lon-

gus, extensor pollicis brevis and abductor pollicis longus, the median governs the flexor pollicis longus and most of the thenar intrinsics, the opponens pollicis, the abductor pollicis brevis, the palmaris brevis and one-half of the flexor pollicis brevis. The motor branch of the ulnar nerve controls the adductor pollicis, the deep head of the flexor pollicis brevis and the first dorsal interosseous. Thus, there are four extrinsic motors, muscle tendon units which cross the wrist and six intrinsic motors which must be coordinated to give prehension (Fig. 15.3.1).

As the thumb is positioned there must be coordination of all these muscles with a graduated and reciprocal contraction and relaxation of each muscle and its opponent. Coordination and integration of these varying forces varies with position and intensity or strength of effort and is very complex. The various positions are extension, flexion, abduction, and adduction. Combinations of these give rotation, circumduction, opposition, and apposition. Extension moves the thumb radialward while it remains in the same plane as the palm. Flexion of the MP and IP joints is obvious enough but flexion of the first metacarpal moves it toward the ulnar side of the hand and is closely allied to adduction. Adduction moves the first metacarpal toward metacarpals two and three, whereas abduction moves the first metacarpal away from them in a plane volar to the palm.

In circumduction the first metacarpal swings in an arc pivoting on the trapeziometacarpal joint. As it swings from a position of extension it passes into abduction and the flexion and finally adduction, the latter two causing apposition with opposing digits. The total movement through this arc constitutes opposition and the net result is to have the thumb clear the palm, span the object to be grasped, and to end up with the tactile pulp of the thumb facing that of the opposing finger of fingers.

TYPES OF ADDUCTION CONTRACTURE

Contracture in the web space tethering the first to the second metacarpal is a pure adduction deformity and is generally caused by scarring between metacarpals one and two. When flexion forces are added to this, a combined adduction-flexion deformity occurs and this is inevitably more crippling, as the thumb is pulled into the palm and interferes with clearance of the fingers in the actions of hook and grasp. The adduction-flexion combination not only is more serious but also more difficult to correct than a pure adduction deformity, and in this type both the MP and IP joints of the thumb are generally held in flexion so that the thumb is curled across the palm. A further complication is the intrinsic plus contracture deformity in which not only the first metacarpal is adducted and flexed into the palm but there is a flexion of the MP joint and hyperextension of the IP joint (Fig. 15.3.2*A*, *B*, *C*).

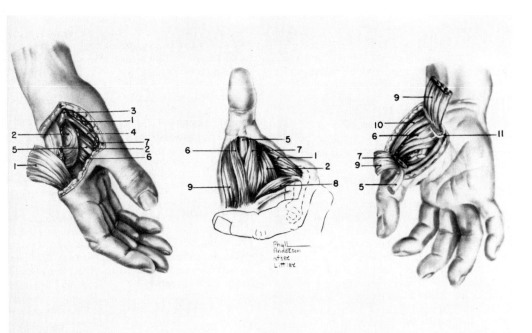

Figure 15.3.1. Thenar anatomy. 1. First dorsal interosseous muscle: origin from first metatarsal. 2. Adductor pollicis. 3. Radial artery. 4. Princeps pollicis artery. 5. Flexor policis longus. 6. Flexor pollicis brevis: superficial (lateral) head. 7. Flexor pollicis brevis: deep (medial) head. 8. First dorsal interosseous muscle: origin from second metatarsal. 9. Abductor pollicis brevis. 10. Opponens pollicis. 11. Recurrent branch of median nerve.

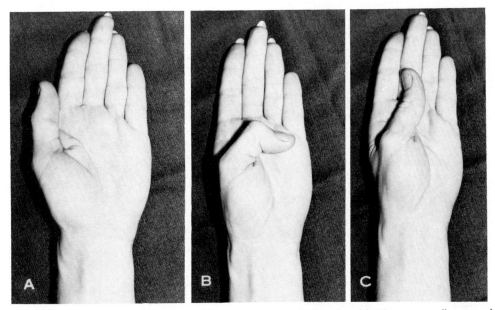

Figure 15.3.2. The three types of adduction contracture: *A.* Simple adduction: generally caused by scar in thumb web space. *B.* Combined adduction-flexion contracture. Not only is the first metacarpal adducted to the second, there is also flexion at the carpometacarpal and metacarpophalangeal joints of the thumb and frequently interphalangeal flexion as well. *C.* Intrinsic plus contracture: adduction of the first metacarpal plus flexion of carpometacarpal and metacarpophalangeal joints and hyperextension of the interphalangeal joint.

CAUSES

Fractures of the proximal half of the first metacarpal may cause a slight adduction deformity as the distal fragment is pulled into some flexion and adduction by the adductor pollicis and flexor pollicis brevis, but generally this deformity is more apparent on x-ray than in gross appearance and function is seldom impaired. When fractures of the base of the first metacarpal extend into the trapeziometacarpal joint and the joint is allowed to become stiff in adduction there may be some loss in the span of grasp and the arc of circumduction. If active motion is started early in these cases, seldom will the decreased range of motion be enough to interfere with function (Fig. 15.3.3).

The most common cause of adduction contracture of the thumb is the formation of scar in the first web space as a result of burns and such trauma as crush and avulsion injuries and gunshot wounds. Scarring may also be the result of infection of the thenar space or of the tendon sheaths. Dupuytren's contracture may occasionally pull the first metacarpal toward the palm and second metacarpal (Fig. 15.3.4).

Fibrosis of the thenar intrinsics due to infection, traumatic scarring, or to ischemia is particularly per-

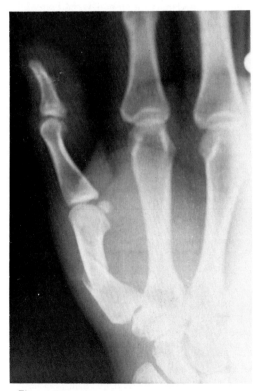

Figure 15.3.3. A fracture of the first metacarpal shaft tends to assume a position of adduction and flexion. Easily correctable by internal fixation and opens reduction. If uncorrected only mild disability results.

nicious and is the cause of those contractures which are most difficult to correct. Ischemic contracture may result from arterial damage itself or more commonly to the persistent edema associated with tight plaster casts and dressings.

Paralysis resulting in the unopposed pull of antagonists may be a cause. In this group the spastic type of cerebral palsy is the most difficult to treat. The combined median and ulnar palsy frequently causes the deformity and almost always there is a large element of flexion combined with the adduction.

Although most rheumatoid thumb problems involve the MP and IP joints with flexion of the former and extension of the latter, the occasional rheumatoid patient with demonstrate the opposite position of MP hyperextension and IP flexion. In this type the trouble starts with dislocation of the trapeziometacarpal joint which allows the first metacarpal to fall in toward the second metacarpal giving an adduction deformity, due not to tightness of the soft tissues, but to instability at the base of the thumb (Fig. 15.3.5 A and B).

Congenital flexion and adduction contracture of the thumb occurs and may be due to anomalies of the thenar muscles or absence of the thumb extensors. It may be isolated or may occur in conjunction with arthrogryposis or congenital spasticity. When isolated it is easily correctable early, but if left untreated, the contracture will become fixed.

PREVENTION

Although some adduction contractures may not be preventable due to extensive scarring or loss of various structures, most need never reach the crippling stage if early preventive measures are applied. If early in the development of scar and fibrosis the first metacarpal is maintained in a position midway between abduction and extension the contracture, if it develops, will generally not be severe. This can be done with a static splint such as a volar plaster slab molded closely to the palm and thumb and into the maintained web space, or better yet with a circular plaster thumb spica (Fig. 15.3.6 A and B). Dynamic splinting with an outrigger, thumb sling, and rubber band is more difficult to maintain but allows the options of easily changing the direction of pull and also allows some active motion of the thumb. Correction of the mature or long established contracture by splinting is time consuming and frequently results in failure but may help simplify subsequent corrective surgery (Fig. 15.3.7 A, B, and C).

CORRECTION OF DEFORMITY

If primary or preventive splinting has not been applied or has failed to prevent the contracture, surgical release of the deforming structures will be necessary. The simplest is a thumb web contracture where a skin contracture alone prevents abduction. Z-plasty of the contracted web is often enough to correct the de-

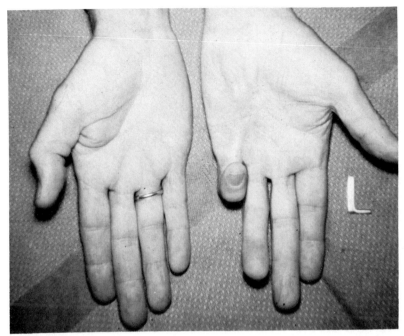

Figure 15.3.4. Mild adduction contracture of the thumb in Dupuytren's contracture. There is a tight fascial band contracting the right thumb. This is far less common than the contracture demonstrated in the small finger of the left hand.

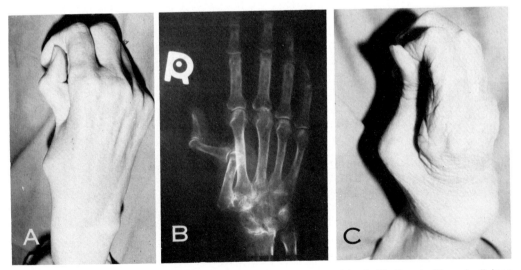

Figure 15.3.5.A, B, and *C.* Adduction deformity of the rheumatoid arthritic thumb. There is dislocation at the trapeziometacarpal joint with adduction of the first metacarpal, hyperextension of the metacarpophalangeal joint and flexion at the interphalangeal joint. This is the exact opposite of the much more common deformity in Figure 15.3.5 *C.*

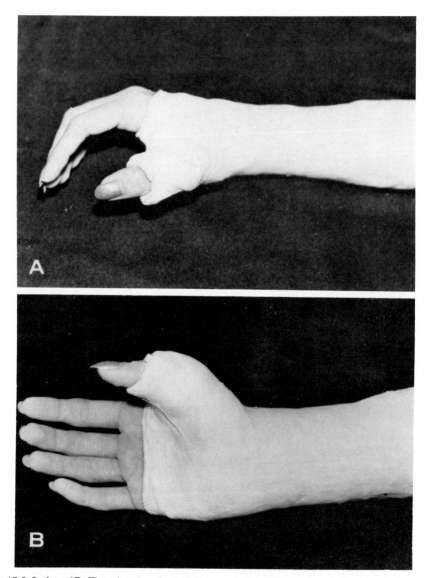

Figure 15.3.6. A and*B.* Thumb spica. Immobilizes wrist and holds thumb in moderate abduction and extension, *i.e.,* the position of function.

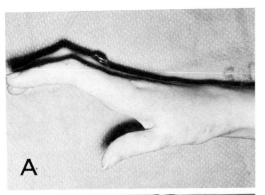

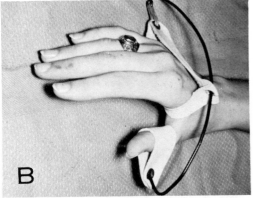

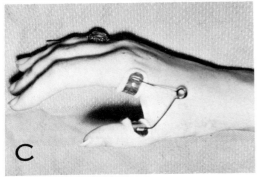

Figure 15.3.7. A. Mild adduction contracture due to scarring in thumb web space. *B.* Contracture successfully overcome dynamic splint worn constantly for four month period. The splint is powered by the rubber band over the fifth metacarpal. *C.* Correction maintained by a simple and more convenient spring-powered dynamic splint used at night for a year after contracture had been corrected by the previous splint. Five years later there is still a tendency for the contracture to recur and patient must use this night splint intermittently to control this.

formity. If skin loss is extensive and the cicatrix very dense, the Z may not give enough release in which case a longitudinal incision and AP incision in line with the long axis of the forearm between the first and second metacarpals will allow abduction of the first metacarpal. This will result in a diamond shaped skin defect which can be satisfactorily covered with a free, full thickness (Wolfe) graft or a split thickness skin graft approximately 0.0015 inches thick.

Only the simplest type of contractures will respond to release of the skin alone. The surgeon must release all contracted structures before the thumb can be moved to a more functional position and in the severest form of adduction flexion contractures, all structures attaching to the first metacarpal may have to be released. This becomes a formidable task when it is realized that this includes not just a severence of the adductor tendon but also the origins in whole or part of the first dorsal interosseous, the opponens, and the short abductor and short flexor muscles. It may also require a capsulotomy of the trapeziometacarpal joint. To accomplish this and still identify and preserve the arterial and sensory supply to the thumb, as well as the flexor pollicis longus, requires a longitudinal incision on the ulnar aspect of the dorsum of the first metacarpal as well as a volar longitudinal incision (Fig. 15.3.8 *A* and *F*).

The majority of contractures can be released through the dorsal incision. After the skin is released the origin of the first dorsal interosseous muscle is easily stripped off the first metacarpal taking care to avoid the radial artery as it turns volarward from the snuff box. Following the muscle distally along its radial border allows one to identify and protect the princeps pollicis artery. After this the tendinous portion of the adductor pollicis is encountered, and, as this usually contributes to the contracture, it must be transsected. Various planes of fascia and intermuscular septa may also be felt while attempting to force the thumb into abduction: these should be severed if tight. Usually at this point the first metacarpal will start to move toward abduction if manual traction is maintained. In cutting the adductor tendon the tendinous part of the deep head of the flexor pollicis brevis must also be severed. If release is not yet obtained the ulnar aspect of the trapeziometacarpal joint can be opened through this dorsal incision, thereby completing release of all elements which would contribute to the adduction deformity. Flexion deformity may persist, however, in which case the volar incision must be used and it will then be possible to detach the thenar intrinsics originating on the first metacarpal as well as to perform a capsulotomy on the radial side of the trapeziometacarpal joint.

The thumb can then be moved into a position of abduction and extension and should be thus maintained with two nonparallel Kirschner wires transfixing metacarpals one and two (Fig. 15.3.9).

When the release is complete the resulting skin defect may be quite large and will have to be covered by skin from elsewhere. Large split thickness grafts are not very satisfactory in the thumb web and, therefore, pedicle transfer is usually required. A pedicle from the trunk or opposite arm may be used but has the usual

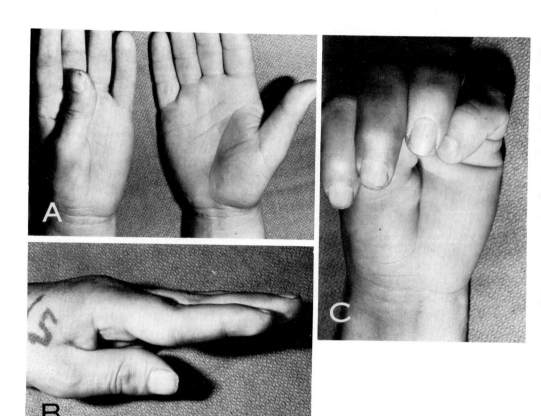

Figure 15.3.8. A. Adduction contracture of the left thumb due to ischemic contracture of the thenar muscles. The ischemia resulted from sustained pressure by a heavy object on the forearm while the patient was unconscious. There is both adduction and flexion deformity in this thumb. *B.* Patient is unable to abduct first metacarpal and prehension is seriously impaired. *C.* The thumb cannot be extended and therefore cannot be cleared from the palm. In attempting to make a fist the fingers must flex over the thumb. *D.* Release of the adductor and first dorsal interosseous muscle allows a significant gain in abduction. *E.* Release of the skin, fascia and flexor pollicis brevis from the volar side then allows thumb extension. No skin graft required. Surgical release followed by thumb spica for two months and then a dynamic splint for another three months. *F.* The end result one year later. Patient now has prehension and can flex fingers into palm. He has retained active adduction and flexion of the thumb.

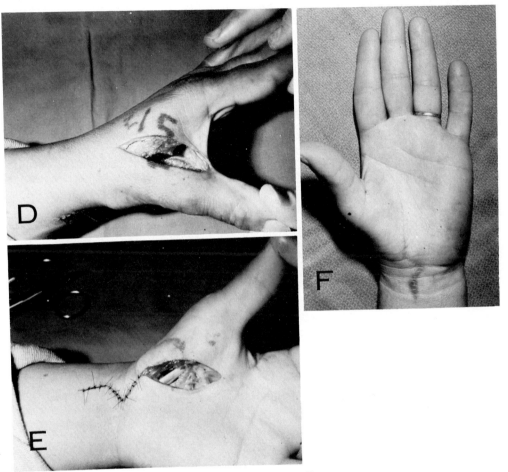

Figure 15.3.8. D—F

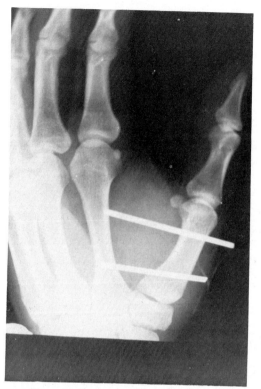

disadvantages of a pedicle transfered from a distance: it will have poor sensibility and a tendency to be too bulky and it may be lost in the process of transfer. Much more effective is the use of a flap rotated from the dorsum of the hand, a technique devised by Dr. Raymond Curtis and adopted by many of his students (Fig. 15.3.10 *A* and *B*). This flap is of ideal thickness, carries with it its own sensibility and presents far fewer complications than does a pedicle from a distance. If fashioned and handled properly, its failure rate is extremely low and the donor defect is not only easily covered by a split thickness graft but presents an acceptable appearance once healing is complete (Fig. 15.3.11).

After cutting the dorsal rotation flap the tourniquet should be released and hemostasis obtained. The K wires are removed after six weeks and active exercise begun. A night splint should be used to maintain the thumb in its corrected position until it is certain that there will be no recurrence of the contracture. The released thenar muscles may be somewhat impaired in function but usually not appreciably so, although it may be necessary to later add a tendon transfer for opposition and adduction if these muscles were beyond salvage (Fig. 15.3.12).

Figure 15.3.9. K-wire fixation between metacarpals I and II after surgical release. The wires should be nonparallel and can be removed after two to three months.

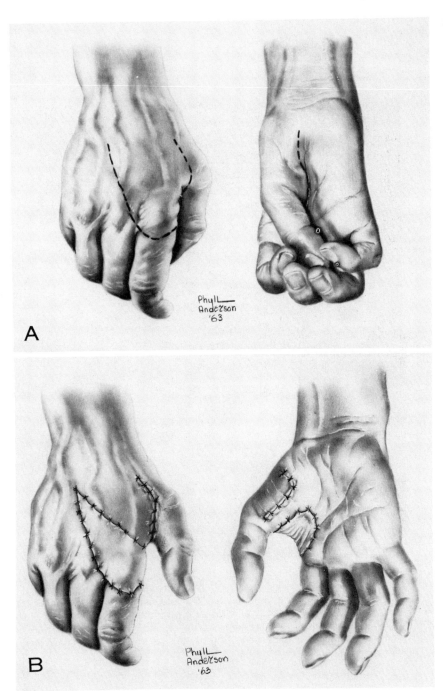

Figure 15.3.10. A. The adducted-flexed thumb deformity. The dotted lines show the incisions required for release of a severe contracture where rotation of a dorsal flap will be required. *B.* After surgical release of the adduction-flexion deformity through both dorsal and volar approaches and after rotation of the dorsal flap and skin grafting of the resultant skin defect over the second and third metacarpals.

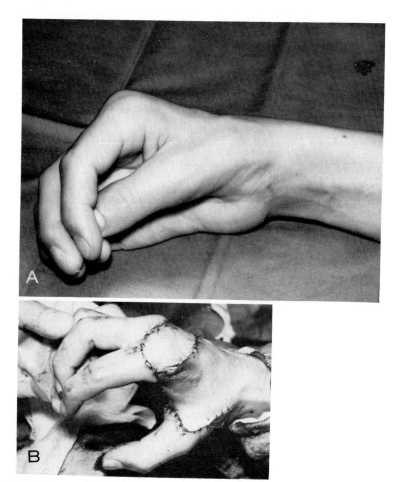

Figure 15.3.11. A. Severe adduction-flexion deformity secondary to a combined median and ulnar nerve palsy, infection in the hand, sloughing of the then muscles and massive scar formation. Hand function is markedly impaired by rigid fixation of the thumb in adduction and flexion. *B.* Surgical release of all structures inserting on the first metacarpal, capsulotomy of the trapeziometacarpal joint, K-wire fixation between metacarpals I and II and rotation of a dorsal flap. *C.* The correction 75 days after surgery. *D.* The correction one year after surgery. Active adduction and opposition have been supplied by tendon transfers and the correction has been maintained.

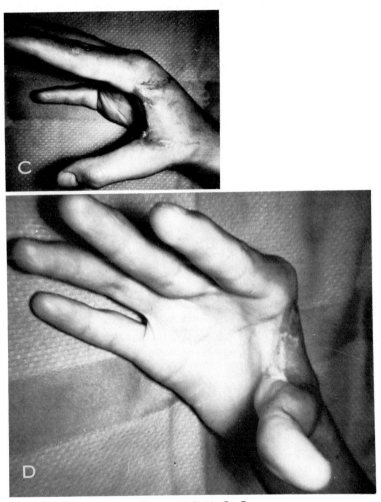

Figure 15.3.11. C–D

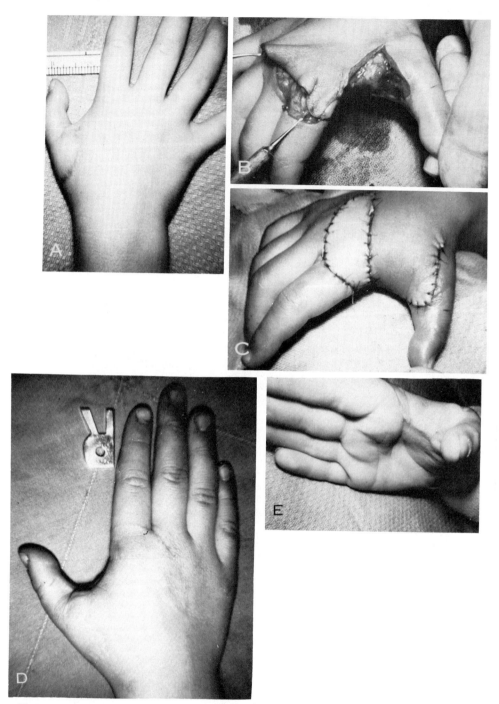

Figure 15.3.12. *A.* Child's thumb with moderate limitation of abduction and extension secondary to extensive laceration and crush injury. Deformity was progressive in nature as child grew. *B.* and *C.* Surgical release of all structures inserting on first metacarpal. Release of trapeziometacarpal joint was not necessary. Resulting skin defect in thumb web space filled in with dorsal rotation flap. Corrected position maintained by thumb spica for one month followed by dynamic splint for several months. *D* and *E.* A good functional result one and one-half years after surgery. The split thickness skin graft on the dorsum of the hand is barely noticeable.

REFERENCES

1. Brand, P. W. In *Leprosy in Theory and Practice,* 2nd Ed. 2, Edited by R. G. Cochrane. Bristol, John Wright, 1964, p. 485.
2. Brown, P. W. Adduction-flexion contracture of the thumb. Clin. Orthop., *88:* 161-168, 1972.
3. Bunnell, S. *Surgery of the Hand,* Ed. 4. Philadelphia, Lippinoctt, 1964, pp. 196-231, 248, 531.
4. Converse, J. M. *Reconstructive Plastic Surgery,* Vol. IV., edited by J. W. Littler. Philadelphia, Saunders, 1964, pp. 1598-1599, 1620.
5. Curtis, R. M. Personal communication.
6. Flatt, A. E., and Wood, V. E. Multiple dorsal rotation flaps from the hand for thumb web contractures, Plast. Reconstr. Surg., *45:* 258, 1970.
7. Flynn, J. E. Adduction contracture of the thumb. N. Engl. J. Med., *254:* 677, 1956.
8. Howard, L. B. Contracture of the thumb web. J. Bone Joint Surg., *32A:* 267, 1950.
9. Littler, J. W. The prevention and correction of adduction contractures of the thumb Clin. Orthop., *13:* 182, 1959.
10. Weekesser, E. C. Congenital flexion-adduction deformity of the thumb. (Congenital "clasped thumb") J. Bone Joint Surg., *37A:* 944, 1955.
11. Youngelson, J. H. The management of the contracted first web space. S. Afr. Med. J., *39:* 716, 1965.

D.

Dupuytren's Contracture

Robert D. Larsen, M.D.

Dupuytren's contracture is a progressive disease which involves the palmar fascia and the digital extensions of the palmar fascia. The disease usually begins with a small nodular thickening in the palm. In its most advanced form, the disease causes a severe and crippling contracture of the palm and one or more of the digits. Less frequently, the condition is encountered in the foot, but contracture of the toes does not occur.

HISTORY

Dupuytren's contracture seems to have been with mankind for a very long time. The apostolic blessing may have been originated by some long forgotten cleric who was unable to extend his ring and little fingers because of Dupuytren's contracture. The earliest mention of this contracture in medical literature, however, appears to be that of Plater in 1614.[108] Henry Clive also described a contracture of this type in his lectures in 1808.[15] In 1823, Sir Astley Cooper[22] described a contracture of the palmar fascia and differen-

tiated it from contractures caused by involvement of the flexor tendons and their sheaths. Some have argued that the disease should, therefore, be called Cooper's contracture. Cooper's brief mention of the contracture, however, does not contain a record of an actual dissection of a hand afflicted with the contracture, nor is there a record of an operation for relief of the contracture.

On December 5, 1831, Dupuytren[30] showed the hands of a coachman to his students. The patient had a contracture of the palmar fascia in the ring finger. Dupuytren felt that the contracture was due to the repeated palmar trauma sustained by the coachman when using his whip. In 1832, Dupuytren[31] published an article describing this condition. The article contains the first definite description of an operation for relief of the contracture. Dupuytren operated upon the coachmen whom he had shown to the students and also upon a wine merchant. In each patient, the operation was a multiple fasciotomy performed through several incisions. Dupuytren also described dissection of the hand of a cadaver with the contracture. His description of the gross pathologic changes has been improved upon only slightly in the past 140 years.

Since 1832, a great volume of literature about this disease has been published. There is not general agreement about the cause, pathogenesis, and pathologic changes of the contracture. Most, but not all, authors believe that the treatment of the contracture is surgical.

Guillaume Dupuytren, made Baron in 1816, was born on October 5, 1777, at Pierre-Buffiére near Limoges. At the age of 17, he was appointed prosector at Ecole de Medicine in Paris, and became surgeon second class at the Hotel Dieu at the age of 27. In 1814, at the age of 37, he was appointed chief surgeon at the Hotel Dieu. Dupuytren died in 1835 at the age of 58 after having had apoplexy at the age of 56. The many excellent biographic sketches of Dupuytren lead us to conclude that he was universally respected as a surgeon and teacher, but personally disliked by almost all who knew him.[63]

ANATOMY

The following description is meant to be an aid to the surgeon operating for Dupuytren's contracture, and is not intended to be a complete description of all details of the anatomy of the palmar fascia. The palmar aponeurosis is a triangular sheet of fibrous tissue which lies immediately beneath the subcutaneous fat of the palm. The apex of the triangle, in the proximal palm, receives the insertion of the palmaris longus tendon, when this tendon is present. The superficial surface of the palmar aponeurosis is attached to skin and subcutaneous flap by numerous, small vertical projections of fibrous tissue. On its deep surface, the palmar aponeurosis is separated from the flexor tendon sheaths and neurovascular bundles by a thin layer of fat and areolar tissue. Several small vertical fibrous septa, which are important surgically, pass from the deep surface of the palmar aponeurosis between the flexor tendon sheaths and neurovascular bundles, and attach to the preosseous fascia overlying the metacarpals and interosseous muscles deep in the palm. The palmar aponeurosis is made up of longitudinal and transverse bundles of fibrous tissue. The longitudinal fibers lie superficial to the transverse fibers. Only the longitudinal fibers are involved in Dupuytren's contracture. Skoog[123,124] considers that the transverse elements of the palmar aponeurosis make up a separate structure which he has called the superficial transverse palmar ligament.

From the palmar aponeurosis, a fibrous layer extends into the fingers forming the superficial digital fascia. From the vertical septa of the palmar aponeurosis, digital projections also pass into the fingers forming the deep digital fascia. These layers lie superficial and deep to the neurovascular bundles, respectively. In the normal, the layers of digital fascia are thin and pliable. In a finger afflicted with Dupuytren's contracture, the digital fascia layers are often very thick, fibrotic, and contracted. In the finger web are several small fibers of palmar aponeurosis called the natatory ligaments or interdigital ligaments. This structure may also be involved in the disease, producing a marked contracture of the finger webs.

ETIOLOGY

The exact cause of Dupuytren's contracture is unknown. Dupuytren[30,31] and Cooper[22] believed that the contracture was caused by repeated trauma to the palm. This concept has been supported and denied by many authors. Disagreement over whether or not Dupuytren's contracture is caused by trauma represents the main point of dispute among those who are especially interested in this disease. Certain predisposing factors, however, have found almost universal acceptance.

Age

Dupuytren's contracture appears most frequently in the fifth, sixth, and seventh decades of life.[33,57,78,79,86,121] In one series of 99 patients reported by Larsen and Posch,[78] only 12 were under 40 years of age. In a group of 154 patients reported by Luck,[86] there was no patient younger than 21 years of age. The average age was 56.5 years for men and 61.1 years for women. There are occasional reports of patients in their twenties and thirties with Dupuytren's contracture, and very rarely, a teenage patient will be found to have the disease.[33,94]

Sex

Dupuytren's contracture is predominantly a disease of men. Most reported series indicate that the disease occurs seven to eight times more frequently in men than in women. Hueston,[57] however, found that there was no increase in the incidence of Dupuytren's contracture in men over women. Bunnell states that Dupuytren's contractures occurs in perhaps 1 to 2 per cent of the population.[15] Early[33] found an over-all average of 4.2 per cent men and 1.4 per cent women over the age of 15 years to have some degree of Dupuytren's contracture. Certainly, however, such a large percentage of the population of the United States do not have Dupuytren's contracture in the stage which requires surgery.

Race

Dupuytren's contracture is primarily a disease of the Caucasian race. The existence of this condition in the Negro has often been questioned. Certainly it does occur in the American Negro. A review of the literature[138] and personal communication with surgeons working in Africa has left me in doubt about whether or not Dupuytren's contracture occurs in the presumably pure African Negro. The contracture does occur in the Oriental, but much less commonly than in the Caucasian.[131]

Heredity

There is a definite hereditary tendency toward the development of Dupuytren's contracture. European writers frequently report that as many as one-third of their patients with Dupuytren's contracture have a positive familial history of the disease.[27,94,119,121] The incidence of a positive familial history in most series reported in the United States is somewhat lower than this.[78,86,147] I, and other writers, have felt that the lower incidence of a positive familial history in this country is because so many of our population are first and second generation Americans and really have no accurate knowledge of the medical history of their ancestors.

Except for the four predisposing factors of age, sex, race, and heredity, there is no general agreement about the cause of Dupuytren's contracture. Krogius[74,75] in 1920 advanced the idea that Dupuytren's contracture is due to the presence of a primitive flexor brevis manus superficialis muscle within the palm. This theory has found more recent support,[139] but, in general, has not been accepted. Lund[87] in 1941 first called attention to the high incidence of Dupuytren's contracture in patients with epilepsy. This has been confirmed by several other authors.[6,33,43,57,121] Arieff and Bell[6] were unable to find any correlation between the development of Dupuytren's contracture in the epileptic and the type of medication, type of seizure, or changes in electroencephalographic records. The high incidence of Dupuytren's contracture in patients with epilepsy is an interesting, but poorly understood observation. Epilepsy, however, is not common in patients with Dupuytren's contracture.

Dupuytren's contracture has been regarded as a form of primary fibrositis but this concept has not found general acceptance.[128,129] The appearance of coronary artery disease in patients with Dupuytren's contracture[35] seems to be simply a fortuitous occurrence of two diseases of advancing years in the same person.[6][43] Diabetes, neurocirculatory dystrophy, shoulder-hand syndrome, alcoholism, and/or cirrhosis of the liver, and many other conditions have been associated with Dupuytren's contracture by various authors.[12,25,57,109,113,116,117,130,143,146]

There is no general agreement in the literature which would indicate that any of these conditions are uniformly related to the development of Dupuytren's contracture.

Nezelhof and Tubiana[103] have listed several popular etiologic theories and rejected each of these theories on the basis that none of them can explain gross or microscopic changes noted in Dupuytren's contracture. Cooper[22] and Dupuytren[30,31] both believed that the contracture arose as a response to repeated palmar trauma. Whether or not trauma plays a role in development of the contractures is the main point of disagreement among persons interested in this disease. Moorhead,[100] McIndoe,[94] and Gordon[43] believe that there is no relationship between trauma and Dupuytren's contracture. Luck[86] believes that trauma may hasten or aggravate the contracture, but feels that the same degree of contracture would have occurred without any trauma to the palm. Clarkson[16] stated that trauma, a single major injury, or repeated minor trauma, maybe a causative or aggravating factor in the development of Dupuytren's contracture. Gordon[44] has reported one case of a hyperextension injury of the long finger which was followed by the development of a nodule in the distal palm that was histologically like Dupuytren's contracture. In 1948, Skoog[121] published a most exhaustive review of Dupuytren's contracture. In this review, Skoog reported his observations on the microscopic pathology of the contracture. On the basis of this very careful study, Skoog[121,122] concluded that trauma may play a role in the development of the disease. Larsen and Posch[78,80] have supported this hypothesis. This support is based upon observations of the microscopic changes of the palmar aponeurosis of patients with Dupuytren's contracture and also upon certain experimental work on the palmar aponeurosis of a monkey.

A recent report from London[34] states that the frequency of the condition is much higher than usually realized, particularly when thickening in the palm is taken as the only criterion for diagnosis. Over the age of 60 as much as 20 per cent of the population may have it;[57] the usual and considerable male preponderance disappears in the older age-groups. The disease is virtually confined to peoples of European descent and runs in families.[85] Probably a single gene behaving as an autosomal dominant is involved.

The frequency of Dupuytren's disease seems to be increased in a number of chronic diseases, particularly pulmonary tuberculosis,[61] but it is the association with alcoholic cirrhosis which is perhaps the best known.[146] The original patient was a brewer, but Dupuytren did not think of alcohol as a possible cause. Occupational trauma was believed to be a likely explanation. Any thoughts, however, that our latter-day cirrhotics may acquire the disease from overfrequent clasping of the bottle must be dismissed. No relation to manual occupation exists,[33][50] nor can the occurrence of Dupuytren's disease be related to the degree of liver impairment in patients with cirrhosis.[102] The incidence is increased in patients with chronic alcoholism who have no evidence of significant liver disease, although the deformity starts at an earlier age and is more frequent in alcoholics who have cirrhosis as well.[146] Thus the drug, alcohol, may be more important than the disease, cirrhosis, and this may also be relevant to the situation in epileptics on long-continued phenobarbitone and other anticonvulsants, in whom Dupuytren's disease is common.[33][88] Such drugs, as well as alcohol, are known to induce hepatic microsomal enzymes and produce hypertrophy of the smooth endoplasmic reticulum in the liver. Is a disturbance of liver function the common factor? This question has been examined in more detail by Pojer and colleagues.[110] In addition to 60 men with chronic alcoholism, of whom a quarter had Dupuytren's disease, they examined 65 epileptic patients who had all been treated with phenobarbitone and often other anticonvulsants for many years. Remarkably, 55 per cent of the epileptic group had evidence of Dupuytren's disease.

Abnormalities in the serum-levels of "hepatic excretory enzymes" were frequently present in both groups, although evidence of hepatic cellular dysfunction was lacking in the epileptics. A raised alkaline phosphatase was common, particularly in the epileptics, but was not related to the presence or absence of Dupuytren's disease. Gamma-glutamyl-transpeptidase was often raised in both groups, and in the alcoholics the enzyme level correlated with the presence of palmar abnormality. Glutamic-oxaloacetic transaminase was normal in the epileptics, but glutamicpyruvic transaminase and creatine phosphokinase were frequently abnormal in epileptic males with Dupuytren's disease. Pojer et al.[110] take their findings to indicate the development of abnormal liver function in some epileptics on phenobarbitone. But their work certainly requires further amplification since these enzymes are not liver-specific, and gamma-glutamyl-transpeptidase, one of the most significantly and frequently abnormal in this study, may be raised in pathologic conditions not involving the liver.[64] Moreover, an important hepatic excretory defect is unlikely in epileptic patients on phenobarbitone, since they commonly have low plasma-bilirubin levels.[133]

How far events in the liver influence normal collagen metabolism in the peripery is unknown, and the possiblity that peripheral enzyme systems themselves may be disturbed by inducing agents has not been investigated. The presence of a muscle abnormality is suggested by the increase in glutamic pyruvic trans-aminase and creatine phosphokinase in some epilep-tics. Whatever the mechanism, it seems that environ-mental agents, including drugs, may determine the development of Dupuytren's disease, perhaps in genetically predisposed individuals. It seems, too, that Dupuytren's disease should be added to the grow-ing list of possible complications of long-term an-ticonvulsant therapy, which includes osteomalacia[62] and folate deficiency.[92]

Bruner[14] has suggested that the mechanical stresses on the ulnar side of the hand may play a part in the de-velopment of Dupyytren's contracture in otherwise predisposed individuals.

The chief arguement used to disprove any relation-ship between trauma and the development of Dupuyt-ren's contracture is that, in most published series, there are slightly more nonmanual workers than there ure manual workers.[15 33 57 68 78 86] This finding has been used by many authors to rule out occupational trauma as the cause of Dupuytren's contracture. The evidence has then been expanded to rule out all forms of trauma to the palm as a possible cause of the con-tracture. It has certainly not been finally determined whether or not trauma does play a part in the develop-ment of Dupuytren's contracture, since the many ex-cellent studies disagree so markedly. I support the concept of Skoog, and believe that repeated minor trauma of the palm may be, at least, one of the inciting factors that cause the palmar aponeurosis to develop this disease.

In summary, Dupuytren's contracture seems to de-velop in predisposed persons as a response to some in-citing agent, drug, or incident. The separate predis-posing factors are age, race, sex, and heredity: others, as yet unknown, may be operative also. I believe that repeated minor trauma to the palm is one means by which the development of the contracture can be pro-voked in predisposed persons. The reader should re-member, however, that not all who have an authorita-tive opinion share this concept.

DIAGNOSIS

The earliest recognizable stage of Dupuytren's con-tracture usually begins in the palm, but may rarely

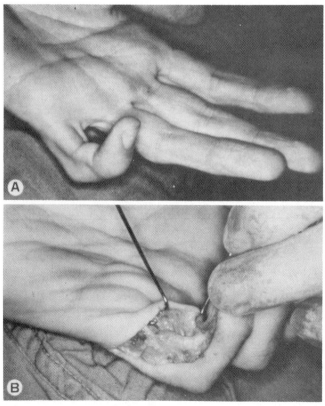

Figure 15.4.1 A. Dupuytren's contracture manifested entirely by nodules and contracted band in the little finger. Usually the contracture occurs first in the palm and involves the finger secondarily, but an occasional patient will be encountered with the contracture occurring only in one or more of the fingers, and no disease in the palm. *B.* Operative exposure of the contracture in the little finger. Same patient as *A.*

occur first in one of the digits (Fig. 15.4.1). The disease begins as a small nodular area in the palmar fascia, usually at the level of the distal palmar crease and, most commonly, in line with the ring finger. The nodule is usually painless and nontender.

Because of this, the patient often cannot accurately recall when the disease began. During progression, other nodules appear, either in line with the original nodule or at other points (Fig. 15.4.2). The skin is usually adherent to the nodules. This is the proliferative phase according to the classification of Luck.[86]

During the involutional stage, the size of the fibrous nodules decreases and they become firmer in consistency. At this time, contracted longitudinal bands of palmar fascia may appear beneath the skin (Fig. 15.4.3). When the digital projections of the palmar fascia to the superficial and deep layers of the digital fascia become involved in this process, the metacarpophalangeal joints or proximal interphalangeal joints, or both, will be gradually drawn into a fixed flexion deformity (Fig. 15.4.4 A). The contracted bands of palmar and digital fascia may become greatly thickened and firmly resist all attempts at passive extension of the metacarpophalangeal and proximal interphalangeal joints. Only rarely will the distal interphalangeal joint be involved in the flexion contracture (Fig. 15.4.4 B). Usually, the distal joint is held in the

extended position. Not infrequently, this joint will be markedly hyperextended or have even developed a dorsal subluxation (Fig. 15.4.5).

In the final form of the contracture, designated by Luck[86] as the residual stage, only the contracted fibrous bands are present. Small nodular thickenings may be palpable within the bands. The length of the contracted bands varies greatly. Not infrequently, however, one or more bands will be observed passing from the proximal portion of the palm to the mid portion of the middle phalanx, uninterrupted.

Dupuytren's contracture is more apt to involve the ulnar side of the palmar aponeurosis than any other part of the hand. Skoog[121 122] reported the ring finger to be involved in the contracture 1451 times in 2277 hands, the little finger 1217 times, the long finger 536 times, the index finger 123 times, and the thumb only 73 times. It is more common to find the contracture in both hands, but the right hand will be involved more frequently than the left, when the condition is unilateral. Boyes[10] found that, in right handed persons, the contracture was apt to appear first in either hand with about equal frequency, but in 44 per cent of his patients, the contracture developed in both hands simultaneously.

Differential Diagnosis

It is not difficult to differentiate Dupuytren's contracture from other deformities of the hand. Arthritis of the hand limits flexion as well as extension. In Dupuytren's contracture, flexion is unimparied, except in those contractures where the distal interphalangeal joint is drawn into hyperextension. Flexion deformities due to flexor tendon injuries or suppurative tenosynovitis usually involve the distal interphalangeal joint as well as the proximal interphalangeal and metacarpophalangeal joints. In Dupuytren's contracture, the distal interphalangeal joint is uninvolved or is held in the hyperextended position. Congenital contractures of the ring or little fingers, most often seen in the proximal interphalangeal joint, lack the characteristic nodule and band formation of Dupuytren's contracture. Longitudinal scars and burn scars should be easily differentiated by careful examination and history and the same is true for extensor tendon injuries producing flexion deformities of the fingers.

Related Conditions

The Foot

A small percentage of patients with Dupuytren's contracture in the hand will also have the contracture in the plantar aponeurosis (Fig. 15.4.6), (5 per cent in my experience).[24 40 64 78 86 94 107 147] Histologically, the lesion in the foot is the same as that encountered in the hand. The nodules tend to be larger and somewhat more cellular. The lesion in the foot undergoes the same stages of maturation as does the lesion in the

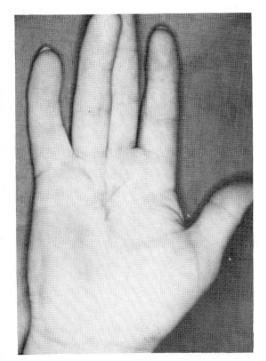

Figure 15.4.2. Early Dupuytren's contracture manifested primarily by two nodules in the palm in line with the ring finger. Minimal limitation of extension of the metacarpophalangeal joint of the ring finger is just beginning to occur.

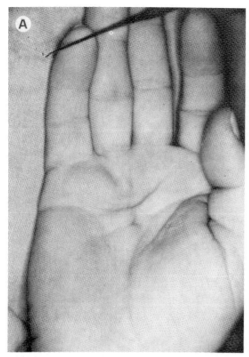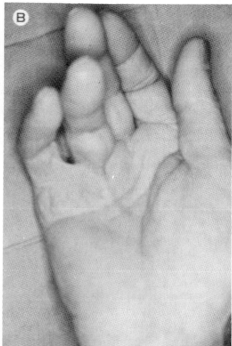

Figure 15.4.3. A. Slightly more advanced stage of Dupuytren's contracture than illustrated in Figure 15.4.2. The skin at the level of the distal palmar crease is just beginning to be drawn into a crescentic fold. A prominent contracted band in line with the ring finger is forming beneath the palmar skin. There is as yet no limitation of extension of the digits. This patient, when first seen, had only a solitary nodule at the level of the distal flexion crease of the palm. He developed this degree of contracture during a one year period of observation. *B.* More advanced stage of Dupuytren's contracture with a prominent band beneath the skin in line with the ring finger. There is a large proliferating nodule overlying the proximal finger segment. Limitation of extension of the metacarpophalangeal joint is pronounced. Limitation of extension of the proximal interphalangeal joint is just beginning.

hand, but this seems to occur more slowly.[86] Contracture of the toes does not occur in Dupuytren's disease of the foot because the plantar aponeurosis does not send pretendinous bands into the toes, as does the palmar aponeurosis into the fingers.[69]

Knuckle Pads

Patients with Dupuytren's contracture may have a nodular thickening over the dorsal aspect of one or more proximal interphalangeal joints. Skoog[121] has reported knuckle pads to be present in as many as 44% of patients with Dupuytren's contracture. Hofmeister[52] found the same histologic changes in knuckle pads as was encountered in the palmar aponeurosis in patients with Dupuytren's contracture.

Peyronie's Disease

Peyronie's disease has been considered to be another form of hereditary fascial contracture in the penis.[121] [137] The relationship between Dupuytren's contracture and Peyronie's disease was first described by Kirby in 1850.[70] McIndoe[94] has challenged this concept and believes that the relationship between Peyronie's disease and Dupuytren's contracture cannot be proved. In several hundred patients with Dupuytren's contracture, I have encountered only one patient with Peyronie's disease.

PATHOLOGY

Gross Pathology

The primary gross morbid changes of Dupuytren's contracture lie entirely within the palmar aponeurosis and its various septa and digital projections. The borders of the early nodules are ill defined and blend insensibly into the surrounding palmar fascia. The nodule itself is pale grayish-white and lacks the slightly yellow color of the normal fibers of the palmar fascia. The nodule is attached to the deep surface of the skin with little or no intervening subcutaneous fat. One cannot demonstrate an actual cleavage plane between the nodule and the skin. The skin over the nodule is often drawn into crescentic folds with the concave surface of the crescent pointed proximally. Luck[86] be-

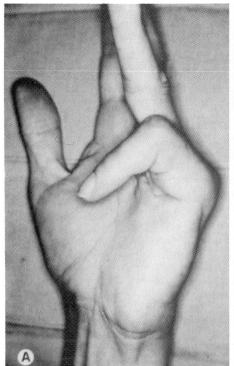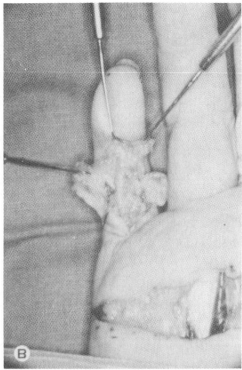

Figure 15.4.4. A. Quite advanced stage of Dupuytren's contracture involving the palm and the little finger. There is slight maceration of the opposed skin surfaces in the distal palm. When a contracture has reached this stage, secondary changes in the skin and in the joints will often preclude a completely normal return of extension. *B.* Operative exposure of the patient illustrated in *A*. Note the band in the little finger extending to the distal phalanx. This is an uncommon finding. Ordinarily the contracture does not extend beyond the midportion of the middle phalanx, and the distal interphalangeal joint remains uninvolved.

lieves that all of the contracture occurs within the nodular areas while the formation of the contracted cords represents hypertrophy of the palmar fascia in response to repeated stress.

Later, thick bands of palmar aponeurosis may tent up the overlying skin. These contracted bands may not be attached as intimately to the skin as are the nodular areas. The contracted bands may occur anywhere there is palmar fascia or one of the projections of the palmar fascia. Thus, the vertical fibrous septa may become involved in the contracture. At the level of the metacarpophalangeal joints, as the septa pass into the digits to communciate with the deep digital fascia, extremely thick bands of contracture may be encountered.

The superficial and thus more clinically noticeable contracture of the pretendinous bands pass from the base of the palmar aponeurosis beneath the skin to enter the digits. The bands of contracture formed in the pretendinous bands tend to be somewhat more centrally located over the volar aspect of the metacarpophalangeal joint in contrast to the lateral position of the bands formed within the small vertical fibrous septa. The contracted pretendinous bands tend to be adherent to the skin without intervening subcutaneous fat. Often separation of the contracted pretendinous bands from the deep surface of the skin can only be accomplished artifically with a scalpel.

The contracture formed within the pretendinous bands and superficial digital fascia tends to lie more in the midline of the digit. In the advanced form, these bands attach quite deeply along the sides of the flexor tendon sheath at the base of the middle phalanx. The contracted bands formed in the deep layer of the digital fascia attach more to the sides of the proximal and middle phalanges. An attachment of these deeper bands to the free edge of the lateral band of the extensor apparatus may account for the tendency for the distal phalanx to be drawn into hyperextension in advanced cases of Dupuytren's contracture (Fig. 15.4.5).

In the late stages of the disease, little, if any, nodule formation is present. The contracted bands at this stage often appear grossly to have undergone hyalini-

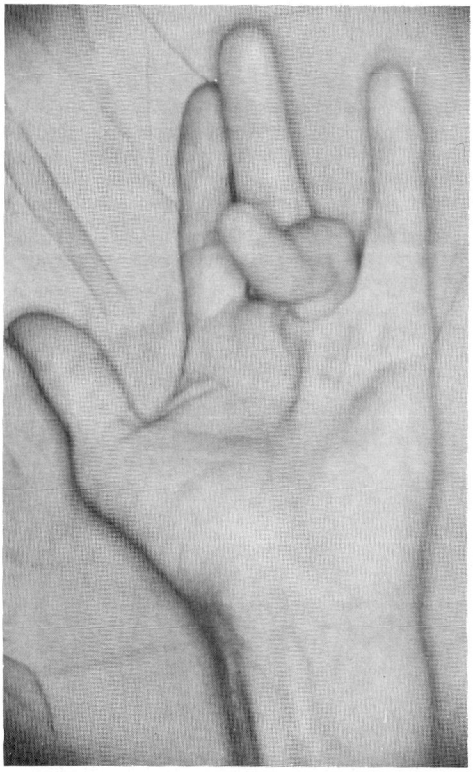

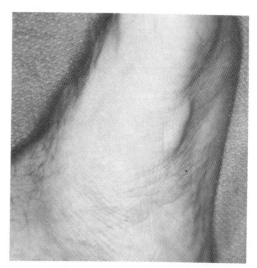

Figure 15.4.5. Advanced stage of Dupuytren's contracture with limitation of extension of the metacarpophalangeal and proximal interphalangeal joints. The hyperextension deformity of the distal interphalangeal joint has extended to the point of dorsal subluxation of this joint. The hyperextension deformity of the distal interphalangeal joint probably occurs as a result of contraction of the digital fascial attachments to the lateral bands, drawing these bands forward much as in a boutonnière deformity. Production of the hyperextension deformity of the distal phalanx may at times be assisted by the repeated effort to push the handle of a tool into the palm.

zation, with a yellowish, almost translucent appearance.

One will occasionally encounter areas of contracture, either in the distal palm or in the digits, where a digital nerve appears to pass directly through a nodule of contracture. This is caused by involvement of both the superficial and deep layers of the palmar or digital fascia on each side of the digital nerve. Careful dissection will always reveal that the digital nerve is surrounded by, but not actually involved in, the contracture.

When the palmar aponeurosis and its deep vertical projections are severely involved in Dupuytren's contracture, it may appear that the contracture is attached to the flexor tendon sheath. However, the flexor tendon synovial sheaths always remain uninvolved and are not attached to nor invaded by the contracture. By careful dissection, the synovial layer can be maintained over the flexor tendons, intact.

As pointed out by Skoog,[123][124] the transverse fibers of the palmar aponeurosis are not involved in the contracture. These fibers are deep to the longitudinal fibers which are involved in the contracture. They pass transversely across the palm at the level of, and a short distance proximal and distal to the distal flexion crease of the palm.

Secondary Changes in Other Tissues of the Hand

In moderately advanced and later stages of the Dupuytren's contracture, the overlying skin may be intimately adherent to the palmar fascia over long distances. Contracture and shortening of the skin at this stage often makes wound closure a difficult problem. In addition, the necessity for creating an artificial cleavage plane between the palmar skin and the contracture often leaves very thin skin flaps which show a poor tendency to heal.

Secondary joint contracture in the metacarpophalangeal or proximal interphalangeal joint, or both, occurs quite commonly in the advanced stages of Dupuytren's contracture. This appears to be due to shortening of the anterior capsular and ligamentous structures of the joints. The secondary changes are particularly prone to occur in the proximal interphalangeal joint and less in the metacarpophalangeal joint. Once an established joint contracture has occurred, removal of the contracted palmar fascia will not result in complete release of the flexion deformity.

Figure 15.4.6. Dupuytren's contracture of the foot. The location of the nodule in this patient was quite characteristic.

Microscopic Pathology

In 1887, Langhans[77] published the first detailed account of the microscopic changes encountered in Dupuytren's contracture. Since that time, a great number of authors have reported their observations on the microscopic changes encountered in Dupuytren's contracture.[4 5 7 9 12 18 19 25 38 54 63 67 74 81 103 105 122 139 140] Advanced techniques of tissue preparation, staining and histochemistry have been included in these reports as these techniques became available. There is little disagreement about the microscopic changes in the palmar aponeurosis, but there is considerable disagreement about the interpretation that should be placed upon these various changes.

In the nodular or proliferative stage of the contracture, the primary lesion is one of marked fibroblastic proliferation. The early nodule of Dupuytren's contracture is primarily made up of many immature fibroblasts. There is marked capillary vascularity of the nodule. Small collagen fibers, and, perhaps, precollagen fibers, are scattered irregularly throughout the nodule. These areas are not encapsulated. Rather, they blend insensibly into the surrounding and normal palmar aponeurosis (Fig. 15.4.7 A and B). Small granules of iron pigment deposits, presumeably hemosiderin, may be found scattered throughout the proliferating area, particularly when the tissues are stained with Prussian Blue (Fig. 15.4.7 C and D). Metachromasia is present almost uniformly in the early nodules of Dupuytren's contracture. The fibers formed in the proliferative stage of the disease are entirely collagen. No elastic fibers are present (Fig. 15.4.8 A).

Perivascular accumulation of inflammatory cells, almost entirely lymphocytes, is a common finding. This inflammatory response, however, is almost uniformly confined to the fat (Fig. 15.4.8.B.). Perivascular inflammation within the aponeurosis itself occurs rarely (Fig. 15.4.8 C).

Some authors have noted the appearance of both capillary and arteriolar proliferation in the early lesions of Dupuytren's contracture, and have felt that fibroblastic proliferation arises from fibrocytes clustered about the small vessels of the palmar aponeurosis (Fig. 15.4.8 D and 15.4.9 A).

Skoog, in 1948,[121] and Larsen et al. in 1960[80] have noted that the fibers of the palmar aponeurosis at the margins of the proliferating nodules appear to have been ruptured. These fibers approach the margins of the proliferating nodule in an undulating fashion, where they terminate abruptly.

The undulating course of the aponeurotic fibers gives these fibers the appearance of having been released from tension (Fig. 15.4.9 B and C). This finding, together with the hemosiderin of the proliferating nodule, which has been interpreted as evidence of previous microhemorrhage, and the fibroblastic and angioblastic proliferation within the early nodule of Dupuytren's contracture, has led the above authors to conclude that the primary lesion of the contracture is a response to microrupture of portions of the palmar aponeurosis. According to this hypothesis, the fibers of the palmar aponeurosis are ruptured. The intervening defect is first filled with a small hemorrhage, and this area is subsequently invaded by proliferating fibroblasts and capillary buds. The reader should remember that although I favor this hypothesis, it has not found universal acceptance, and indeed, has been vigorously denied by others.

Between the early nodules of fibroblastic proliferation and the mature collagen fibers of the residual stage, there is a steady and gradual transition of maturation of fibrous tissue. The plump, irregularly arranged nuclei of the early nodule become elongated and oval, and assume a regular pattern with the long axes of the nuclei lying roughly parallel to each other (Fig. 15.4.9D). The collagen fiber content of the contracting area increases and the nuclei become more widely separated. The capillary vascularity steadily decreases. Iron pigment is not found in the later stages. The ultimate fate of the maturing fibrous tissue is a very dense band of collagen fibers (Fig. 15.4.10). The nuclei are pyknotic and are seen as flattened, densely stained structures which are separated by dense collagen fiber, with little or no nuclear detail visible.

In the most advanced state of the contracture, the collagen of the contracted band may undergo hyalinization.[76 80] The hyalinized collagen tissue within the contracted band takes the blue stain of hematoxylin and eosin and stains red or reddish-blue with Mallory's connective tissue stain.

In 1960, Larsen et al.[80] reported an experiment on the palmar aponeurosis of the monkey (Fig. 15.4.11). The fibers of the palmar aponeurosis were partially torn (Fig. 15.4.12A and B) and the areas of partial rupture of the palmar aponeurosis removed in intervals of one to nine months. The histologic changes which occurred within the area of partial rupture of the monkey's palmar aponeurosis were felt to be identical with the various stages of Dupuytren's contracture (Fig. 15.4.13 A and B). On the basic of this experimental evidence, it was concluded that partial or microrupture of the fibers of the palmar aponeurosis was at least one method by which the lesion encountered histologically in human Dupuytren's contracture could be produced.

Summary

Dupuytren's contracture begins as a proliferating vascular nodule of young fibrous tissue. Many of these fibers contain hemosiderin. Gradually, the nodules mature with increasing regularity of the arrangement of the nuclei and increasing collagen fiber content. As the maturation of the fibrous tissue proceeds, the vascularity of the area decreases. Finally, a

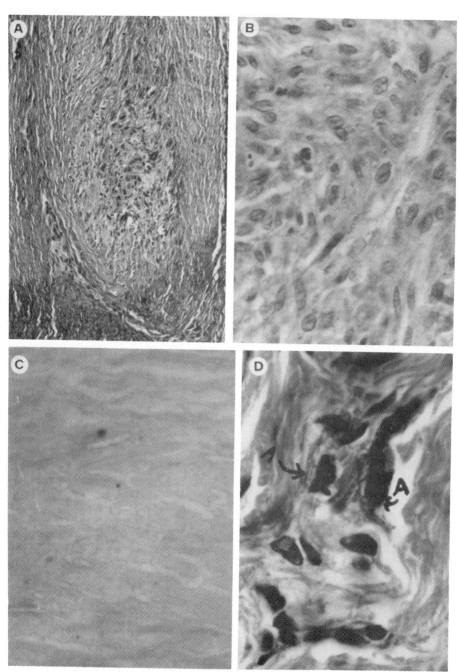

Figure 15.4.7. A. Low power photomicrograph of an early nodule of Dupuytren's contracture. Note that the cellular nodule in the center of the field blends insensibly into the surrounding normal palmar aponeurosis. The nodule is not encapsulated. Hematoxylin and eosin. × 135. *B.* High power photomicrograph of the early, proliferative, stage of Dupuytren's contracture. The fine black granules scattered throughout the area are hemosiderin, which appears yellow-brown in this preparation. Hematoxylin and eosin. × 400. (*A* and *B* are reproduced from Larsen *et al.*[80] by permission of the *Journal of Bone and Joint Surgery.) C.* Prussian blue stain, × 600, of an early nodule of Dupuytren's contracture. The dark granules are hemosiderin. They stain a deep blue, and are readily recognizable with this stain. Eosin counterstain. *D.* High power photomicrograph of a very early area of fibrous tissue proliferation in Dupuytren's contracture. The dark granules at A are hemosiderin granules, and stain a dense blue in this preparation. Prussian blue, hematoxylin and eosin counterstain. × 1100. (*C* and *D* are reproduced from Larsen and Posch[78] by permission of *Journal of Bone and Joint Surgery.*)

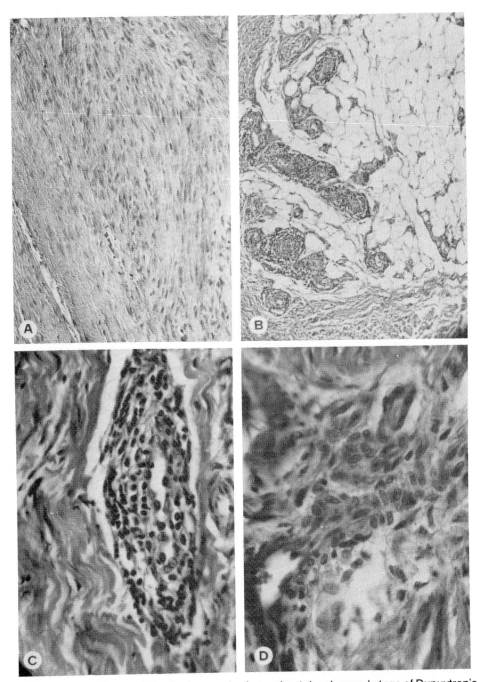

Figure 15.4.8. A. Low power photomicrograph of a moderately advanced stage of Dupuytren's contracture. This preparation is made with Verhoeff's elastic tissue stain and illustrates that there is no formation of new elastic tissue in Dupuytren's contracture. If elastic tissue were present in this preparation, it would be visible as very dark prominent undulating bands. × 135. *B.* Perivascular accumulation of inflammatory cells in the palm of a patient afflicted with Dupuytren's contracture. The location of these inflammatory cells is quite characteristic. The inflammatory cells are perivascular in location and are almost always encountered in the subcutaneous fat of the palm, rather than within the aponeurosis itself. Hematoxylin and eosin. × 135. *C.* Perivascular accumulation of inflammatory cells within the palmar aponeurosis of a patient with Dupuytren's contracture. This is an uncommon finding. If perivascular inflammation is present, it is almost uniformly confined to the subcutaneous fat. Hematoxylin and eosin. × 400. *D.* Thick walled blood vessels in the palmar aponeurosis of a patient with Dupuytren's contracture, showing early proliferation of perivascular fibrocytes. Hematoxylin and eosin. × 400. *(A, B, C,* and *D* reproduced from Larsen and Posch[78] by permission of the *Journal of Bone and Joint Surgery.)*

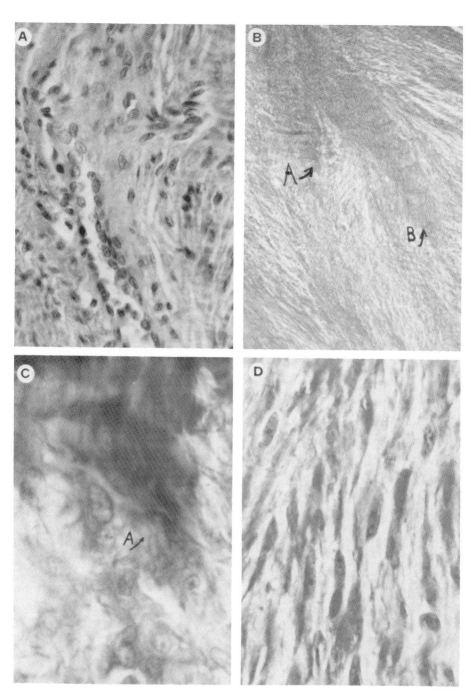

Figure 15.4.9.A. Section through an early nodule in the palmar aponeurosis of a patient with Dupuytren's contracture. Note the apparent, "streaming" of immature fibrocytes along the wall of the small blood vessel. It is probable that the perivascular fibrocytes are the site of origin of the proliferating tissue of Dupuytren's contracture. (Reproduced by permission of the *Journal of Bone and Joint Surgery.*[78])*B.* Section through a proliferating nodule of Dupuytren's contracture, illustrating the abrupt termination of fibers of the aponeurosis at the margin of the nodule (*A, B*). Mallory's connective tissue stain. × 135. *C.* High power view of the margin of an early nodule of Dupuytren's contracture illustrating the abrupt termination of the fibers of the aponeurosis at the margin of the nodule. The fibers at *A* are the same as those at *A* in *B*. Mallory connective stain. × 1100. *D.* This photomicrograph illustrates the increase in the collagen fiber content of the nodule as it matures. The nuclei are more elongated, with their long axes arranged parallel to each other. Hematoxylin and cosin. × 400.

Figure 15.4.10. Mature scarlike stage of Dupuytren's contracture. This is a very dense, scarlike stage, with only a few blood vessels visible. The nuclei are widely separated by the collagen fibers and are quite pyknotic. Hematoxylin and eosin. × 135. (Reproduced from Larsen *et al.*[80] by permission of the *Journal of Bone and Joint Surgery.*)

mature scar like stage is reached. At this time, the contracted band is almost avascular, and there are a great number of collagen fibers widely separating very dense, pyknotic nuclei. Nezelhof and Tubiana[103] have listed seven popular etiologic surveys: (1) inflammatory disease; (2) rheumatic disease; (3) congenital malformation; (4) traumatic and occupational disease; (5) collagen disease; (6) trophic or dystrophic disease; (7) tumor. These authors have concluded that none of these theories can explain the clinical and histologic findings encountered in Dupuytren's contracture.

It must be said, therefore, that there is no unanimity of opinion regarding the interpretation to be placed upon the histologic changes observed in Dupuytren's contracture. The exact nature of these changes, and thus the etiology of Dupuytren's contracture, therefore, remain unknown.

TREATMENT

Nonoperative Treatment

Attempts to treat Dupuytren's contracture by the injection of pancreatic extract,[115] pepsin,[51] fibrinolysin,[83] copper sulfate,[53] cortisone,[8] and hydrocortisone[148] have all been found to be without value. Vit-

amin E and compounds with Vitamin E activity may temporarily soften the contracture, but do not cure the disease nor has the progress been halted.[78 79 128 129]

Irradiation of the palm[36 37 141] may have some effect upon the early stages of the contracture but has no effect whatever on the more advanced stages of the disease. The published results of radiation therapy appear to be inferior to those obtained with a properly selected and carefully executed operation.

Operative treatment

It is generally agreed that the only consistently efficacious treatment for Dupuytren's contracture is excision of the diseased palmar aponeurosis.[10 15 17 20 29 41 42 46 68 72 78 79 96 121 123 124 134 135 149] The surgeon confronted with a patient with Dupuytren's contracture has two important decisions to make. The first of these is to decide when surgery becomes necessary. Many patients with one or two early nodules of Dupuytren's contracture spontaneously arrest their disease at this point and never progress further. The nodules are painless and cause no disability. Surgery for this minor degree of Dupuytren's contracture is not indicated. On the other hand, one should not wait until a severe, advanced stage of Dupuytren's contracture has developed. Secondary changes in the skin and finger joints, which are so commonly associated with the advanced stage of the disease, may preclude an entirely satisfactory surgical result. In general, the earlier the stage of the contracture when the operation is

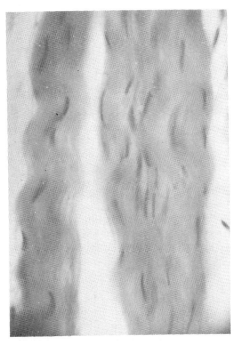

Figure 15.4.11. Photomicrograph of the normal palmar aponeurosis of the Rhesus monkey. Hematoxylin and eosin. × 400.

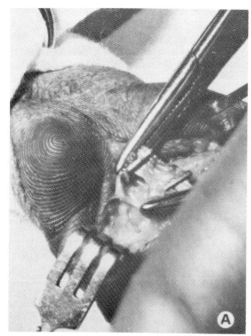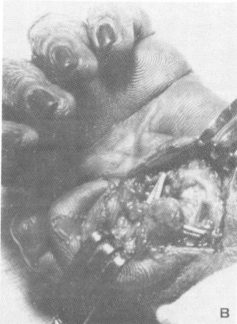

Figure 15.4.12. A. Experiment to test the effect of partial rupture of the palmar aponeurosis of the Rhesus monkey. The area to be tested is identified between small silver clips. The fascia on each side of the clips is grasped with hemostats. The segment of palmar aponeurosis between the clips is then gently pulled apart until a small degree of tearing of the aponeurosis is noted. *B.* Nodule lesion produced in the palmar aponeurosis of the monkey by the technique described in *A.* This nodule occurs only in the area of fascia between the clips. Control studies indicate that the nodule would not form unless the fibers were partially torn.

performed, the better will be the operative result.[94] [95] Once it has been decided that surgery for Dupuytren's contracture is necessary, the surgeon must make the second major decision. What type of operation is to be performed?

There are, in general, three types of operations performed for Dupuytren's contracture. In order of increasing magnitude they are: fasciotomy, partial or limited fasciectomy, and radical or total fasciectomy.

Fasciotomy is the simplest of the operative procedures performed for Dupuytren's contracture. The operation of fasciotomy may be performed by the blind or subcutaneous route, or by an open technique under direct vision. Fasciotomy performed by the subcutaneous or blind technique is accomplished with a thin, narrow-bladed knife. This is usually introduced at the ulnar border of the palm, and passed in a radial direction until the contracted bands of the disease are encountered. The knife is then gently pressed through the contracted bands until the entire band has been sectioned. Open fasciotomy is usually performed by making small skin incisions directly over the contracted bands. The bands of the contraction are then divided under direct vision.

Fasciotomy was the procedure describer by Cooper[22] and by Dupuytren.[30] [31] Apparently these pioneers

performed the fasciotomy by the open technique. Boyes,[10] Bunnell,[15] and Luck[86] have performed the closed fasciotomy in the palm, but cautioned that this is a dangerous procedure in the fingers. The advantage of the direct or open fasciotomy over the blind or closed fasciotomy is the lessening of the danger of injury to the neurovascular bundles at the time of division of the contracted bands. We have had no experience with the subcutaneous technique of fasciotomy, but have occasionally performed the procedure of open fasciotomy under direct vision.

Fasciotomy maybe performed either as a definitive procedure or as a preliminary procedure preparatory to more radical procedures. As a definitive procedure, the technique of fasciotomy will not infrequently be efficacious in patients who have a single mature contracted band passing from the palm into one or two of the fingers. This is particularly true in patients of advanced age. This procedure may also be efficacious in patients with concomitant diseases which preclude the more extensive procedures (Fig. 15.4.14).

Occasionally, in patients with quite advanced stage of Dupuytren's contracture, Fasciotomy will be of advantage as a preliminary procedure. Partial relief of an advanced contracture will frequently allow some recovery of skin length and may allow some improve-

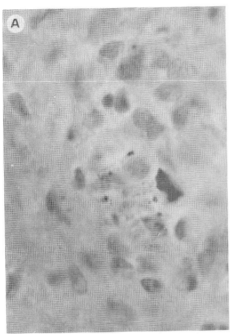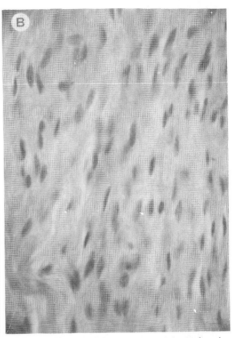

Figure 15.4.13. A. Photomicrograph of the proliferating nodule obtained in the palmar fascia of the monkey by partial rupture of the fascia. Hematoxylin and eosin. × 400. The dark granules visible in the field are hemosiderin granules. Note the marked similarity between this photomicrograph and Figure 15.4.7 B. Photomicrograph of the proliferating nodule in the monkey's palmar fascia produced by experimental partial rupture of the fascia, five months after the experimental operation. The tissue here has undergone maturation. The collagen fiber content has increased. The nuclei are oval in shape with their long axes arranged parallel to each other. Note the similarity between the photomicrogragh and Figure 15.4.9 D. Hematoxylin and eosin. × 400. (A and B reproduced from Larsen et al. [70] by permission of the Journal of Bone and Joint Surgery.)

ment of secondary joint contractures prior to the definitive excision of the contracture (Fig. 15.4.15).

It is my practice to limit fasciotomy to a preliminary operation preparatory to more radical procedures later on or to a definitive operation for patients of advanced age or those who have concomitant diseases which would preclude a more complete operation. It should be emphasized that Tubiana[134] found that age, in itself, is not a factor which influences the postoperative result of surgery for Dupuytren's contracture.

Partial or Limited Fasciectomy

There are many factors that influence the result of surgery for Dupuytren's contracture. The stage of the contracture before surgery is perhaps the most important single consideration.[94] [134] [136] The earlier the disease is operated upon, the more satisfactory will be the operative result. The patients own tendency toward the development of joint stiffness, together with the strength of his diathesis for the development of the contracture, are also important factors which adversely effect the outcome of an operation for Dupuytren's contracture.[57] These are factors over which the surgeon has little, if any, control. One of the factors over which the surgeon has direct control, however, is

the magnitude of the operation. Conway,[20] Hamlin,[47] [48] Hueston,[58] and Riordan[112] were prominent among contemporary surgeons who have popularized the procedure of partial or limited fasciectomy for the treatment of Dupuytren's contracture. The literature on the treatment of Dupuytren's contracture has, during the past 20 years, shown a definite trend toward more limited operations and a trend away from the radical or total excision of the palmar aponeurosis.[17] [42] [123] [124] [135] [149] The limited procedure was practiced by Kocher[73] in the later part of the 19th century. Conway,[20] Hamlin,[47] [48] and Hueston[58] have all concluded that the degree of postoperative morbidity increases as the extend of the operation increases.

The incisions for limited fasciectomy are, in general, oriented longitudinally (Fig. 15.4.16). A sinuous longitudinal incision was described by Hamlin.[47] [48] In making this incision, care was taken to avoid crossing any flexion crease at a right angle. Multiple z-incisions with transposition of the triangular flaps have been described. A straight longitudinal incision, centered directly over a contracted band, will often give the best exposure for removal of a contracture which is limited to one prominent band passing into only one digit. Such an incision must be converted

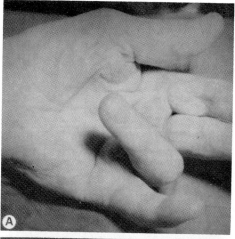

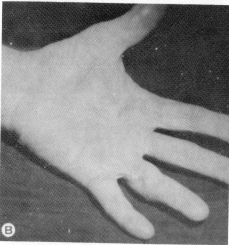

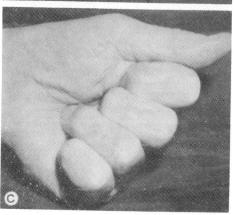

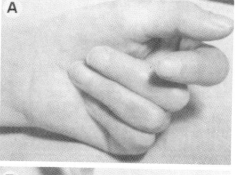

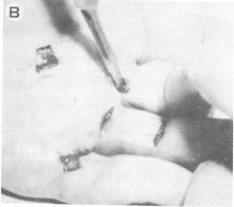

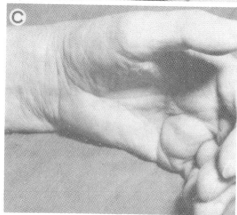

Figure 15.4.15. A. Preoperative photograph of a 48-year-old housewife with a severe and advanced stage of Dupuytren's contracture, showing the maximal possible preoperative extension. *B.* Same patient as *A.* Operative view illustrating multiple fasciotomy under direct vision. *C.* Patient's postoperative ability to extend after multiple fasciotomy as illustrated in *B.* The procedure in this instance was done as a preliminary operation, preparatory to more radical excision of the diseased palmar fascia. *(A, B,* and *C* reproduced from Larsen and Posch[78] by permission of *Journal of Bone and Joint Surgery.*

Figure 15.4.14. A. Preoperative photograph of a 78-year-old male office worker. It was felt that the patient's age and concomitant diseases precluded a more extensive operation for Dupuytren's contracture. Patient treated by simple fasciotomy under direct vision. *B.* Same patient's postoperative ability to extend after simple fasciotomy. *C.* Same patient's postoperative ability to flex following simple fasciotomy. *(A, B,* and *C*

reproduced from Larsen and Posch[78] by permission of the *Journal of Bone and Joint Surgery.)*

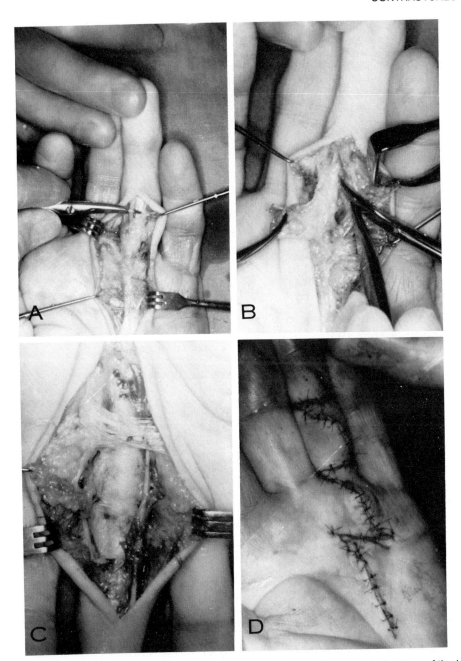

Figure 15.4.16. The left hand of a 63-year-old dentist with a troublesome contracture of the left ring finger and early contracture of the left thumb. *A.* A straight longitudinal incision over the contracture of the ring finger. The contracted band is visible. A digital nerve can be visualized running over the point of the scissors. *B.* The contracted band has been dissected from the palm and is being removed from its attachment within the ring finger. *C.* The contracted band has been removed. The digital sheath is completely intact. Both digital nerves can be visualized and are intact. The superficial transverse palmar ligament of Skoog is visible at the level of the distal flexion crease of the palm. *D.* The stright longitudinal incision has been converted to multiple Z-plasties prior to wound closure. A small band of contracture has been removed from the thumb through a midlateral incision.

into multiple Z-plasties at the time of wound closure. Tubiana[135] describes combinations of sinuous longitudinal incisions in the palm combined with one or more Z-plasties in the digits. Skoog[123] [124] illustrates a combination of transverse and vertical incisions, without and with or without Z-plasty. Luck[86] describes a very limited fasciectomy which involves excision of the ''nodule-cord'' unit. This procedure is slightly more radical than a simple fasciotomy but more limited than the usual partial fasciectomy.

It is apparent that, in the operation of limited fasciectomy, the choice of incision or incisions will be influenced primarily by the configuration of the contracture which is to be removed. As a general principle, the incision will have a longitudinal orientation, but must be of a type which will either not cross flexion creases at right angles or of a type which can be converted to meet this requirement at the time of wound closure.

The operation of limited fasciectomy has the following advantages: (1) The diseased area of fascia is more completely removed than with a simple fasciotomy. (2) Postoperative morbidity after limited fasciectomy is less than that after radical fasciectomy. (3) If recurrence or appearance of the disease in unremoved portions of the fascia does occur, it may again be dealt with a simpler, more limited type of operation.

Although the limited fasciectomy has enjoyed increasing popularity during the past 20 years, care must be taken lest the pendulum swing too far in the other direction. As has been pointed out by Tubiana,[135] dissatisfaction with the results of limited fasciectomy led to the development of the more radical procedures at about the beginning of this century.

The author, in his own practice, has, to some degree, followed the trend toward the more limited operations. The radical operation has not, however, been abandoned. The radical operation is still a good operation when the operation is properly performed upon an individual whose contracture requires such a procedure.

Radical Fasciectomy

The term, radical fasciectomy, implies removal of not only the diseased portions of the palmar fascia but also all of the uninvolved portion of the palmar aponeurosis together with its vertical septa as completely as possible. Nodules or contracted bands within the figures are removed through appropriate incisions which may or may not be in direct continuity with the major incision in the palm. The tendency toward development of the contracture in those portions of the palmar aponeurosis which are not removed in the more limited operations lead to the development of the radical fasciectomy. The increased morbidity of the more radical operation, however, lead Hamlin[47] [48] and others to favor the more restricted fasciectomy.

A great variety of incisions for radical removal of the palmar aponeurosis has been described. The single, long, transverse incision at the level of the distal flexion crease of the palm is the incision which is used most commonly and is the one which I prefer. When it is necessary to make additional incisions in the digits, the appropriate incision will usually be dictated by the configuration of the contracture within each individual digit. The digital incisions may or may not have to be extended into direct continuity with the major palmar wound.

Operative Technique

It is essential that excision of the palmar fascia be performed in a completely bloodless field. Wherever subcutaneous fat remains between the palmar fascia and the skin, it is essential that the fat remain attached to the skin. In those areas where the skin is intermittently adherent to the nodules or bands of the contracture, subcutaneous fat may be absent. It is then necessary to create an artifical dissection plane between the derma and the adherent contracture. This portion of the skin is then, in reality, converted to a free full thickness skin graft. No difficulty in healing of this area will be encountered, however, if every detail of the operation is performed

Fasciotomy. The author has no experience with the blind or subcutaneous fasciotomy technique. In the technique of open fasciotomy, one or more skin incisions are made directly over contracted bands. There is usually little, if any, subcutaneous fat between the skin and the contracted band. Small skin hooks will supply some exposure of the contracted band. The band is then divided under direct vision until there is noticeable release of the contracture as evidenced by increased ability to extend the involved joint or joints. Digital nerves may be found in abnormal positions in patients with advanced Dupuytren's contracture. This is quite common in the fingers, fairly frequent in the distal palm at the base of a finger, and unusual in the midpalm. Care must be taken that the structure which is being divided is only the contracted band of fascia and that a digital nerve is not included. The skin can usually be closed providing one does not insist upon maintaining the digit in full extension immediately. Within a few days, gentle elastic traction can be applied to maintain the improved extension of the digit without producing disruption of the small wounds. When it is not possible to close a fasciotomy wound completely the wound may be left open to heal secondarily.

Limited Fasciectomy (Figs. 15.4.16 and 15.4.17). After the appropriate longitudinally oriented incision has been selected and made, the skin and subcutaneous fat, which are present, are elevated from the superficial portion of the diseased palmar aponeurosis and any digital extensions of the disease. The longitudinal band is then divided at the proximal limit of the incision, which extends slightly proximal to the contracture itself. The contracted band is then dissected dis-

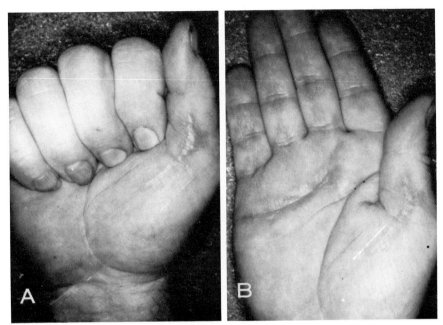

Figure 15.4.17. Postoperative flexion and extension 39 days after limited fasciectomy on the radial side of the palm and the radial side of the thumb.

tally by sharp dissection. At a level slightly proximal to the distal flexion crease of the palm, the transverse fibers of the palmar aponeurosis will be observed deep to the longitudinal contracted band. The transverse fibers are not involved in the contracture. The longitudinal contracted band can be separated from the transverse element of the aponeurosis (the transverse palmar ligament of Skoog) (Fig. 15.4.16). This maneuver will leave a thin covering of transverse fascial fibers over the neurovascular bundles and flexor tendon sheaths at the level of the distal flexion crease of the palm. As the dissection is continued distally, one may or may not encounter involvement of the vertical septa. If this portion of the palmar aponeurosis is involved in the contracture, this element must be removed before the flexion deformity of the metacarpophalangeal joint can be corrected. In the distal palm, great care must be taken to identify and preserve the digital nerves. The nerves maybe found to run superficial to (Fig. 15.4.18), deep to and apparently through areas of the palmar aponeurosis which are involved in the contracture.

In the operation of limited fasciectomy, the digital incision is usually continuous with the palmar incision. The configuration of the contracture within each digit is widely variable. The digital contracture is

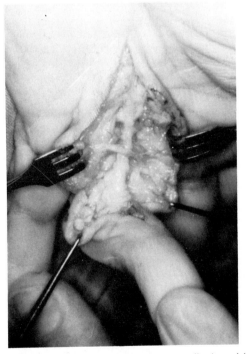

Figure 15.4.18. In the dissection of this Dupuytren's contracture, a digital nerve was encountered passing superficial to the band of the contracture. The nerve can be seen crossing the contracture in the distal palm. A nerve displaced in this manner can be divided during the surgery if the possibility of abnormal relationships of the digital nerves is not constantly kept in mind during the operation.

completely exposed with preservation of subcutaneous fat on the skin and positive identification and protection of digital nerves. The most superficial digital contracture will usually be found attached quite firmly to the flexor surface of the base of the middle phalanx on one or more sides of the flexor tendon sheaths. The deeper digital contracture may be found attached to the sides of the middle or proximal phalanges or to the free edge of the lateral band of the extensor tendon apparatus. Following complete removal of the digital contracture, whatever its attachments may be, the metacarpophalangeal and proximal interphalangeal joints will be capable of full passive extension unless secondary joint contracture has occurred. This is much more common at the proximal interphalangeal joint than it is at the metacarpophalangeal joint. In those patients who have a marked secondary contracture of a proximal interphalangeal joint, some authorities will proceed immediately with surgical mobilization of the joint, arthrodesis of the joint, or amputation of the finger. The author's preference is to accept the secondary contracture and to hopefully deal with this by appropriate splinting during the postoperative period. Secondary procedures upon the joint itself or amputation of the finger are then the subject of a second operation. It is surprising how seldom a second operation for joint contracture is required.

After all of the diseased palmar aponeurosis and its digital extensions have been removed, attention is turned to wound closure. The details to be attended to prior to wound closure are described in the section on radical fasciectomy and need not be repeated here. The incision of limited fasciectomy will, in general, be a longitudinal type of incision. If such an incision crosses a flexion crease at or near a right angle, a Z-plasty must be constructed at this point in order to avoid a scar contracture which maybe as bad as or worse than the original contracture. Such a maneuver is particularly important at the proximal and middle flexion creases of the digit and at the distal flexion crease of the palm. If an incision has been chosen which does not cross any flexion crease at a right angle, simple closure of the original wound may be possible.

Radical Fasciectomy. The term radical fasciectomy implies a removal of all of the palmar aponeurosis together with the vertical septa which extends from the deep surface of the aponeurosis to the preosseous fascia. A transverse incision at the distal flexion crease of the palm is usually the most satisfactory. It is usually easier to dissect proximally first. The subcutaneous fat is preserved and remains attached to the skin. As the dissection progresses proximally, small arteries will be encountered (Fig. 15.4.20). These arteries perforate the palmar fascia from below and pass into subcutaneous fat of the palm. Preservation of these small arteries will greatly improve the circulation of the skin and subcutaneous tissue which has been elevated from the superficial surface of the palmar fascia. Although careful attention to this detail of the operation was re-

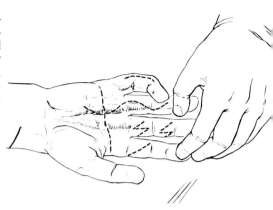

Figure 15.4.19. Some of the commonly used incisions for excision of Dupuytren's contracture. In the little finger the midlateral incision is illustrated. In the ring finger the sinuous longitudinal incision described by Hamlin and others for partial or limited fasciectomy is illustrated. In the long finger, multiple Z-incisions as popularized by McIndoe are illustrated. The incision of Mason, obliquely across the proximal finger segment, is illustrated in the index finger. The transverse incision in the distal palm at the level of the distal flexion crease is the incision most commonly used for radical fasciectomy.

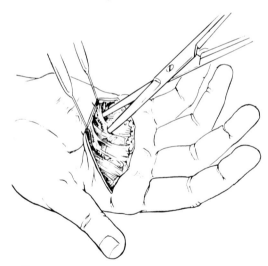

Figure 15.4.20. Preservation of the small arteries passing from the neurovascular bundles to the subcutaneous fat and skin of the palm. Preservation of these small vessels is important for satisfactory wound healing in radical excision of the palmar aponeurosis. The relative size of the arteries is somewhat exaggerated by the drawing.

peatedly emphasized by the late Doctor Michael L. Mason,[91] it was never published by him.

The superficial dissection is carried as far proximalward as possible. Usually, it will be possible to dissect as far as the junction of the proximal and middle one-thirds of the palm. It is seldom necessary to dissect more proximally, since the most proximal portion of the palmar aponeurosis is not frequently involved in the contracture. If more proximal dissection is necessary, a curved incision in the thenar flexion crease maybe made. Exposure of the borders of the triangular sheet of palmar aponeurosis ordinarily constitute adequate dissection on the radial and ulnar sides of the fascia, unless a band is present passing into the thumb. The distal dissection is then begun. Approximately 1.0 cm distal to the distal flexion crease of the palm, the base of the triangle of palmar fascia will be encountered. From this point on, the palmar fascia is represented only by the pretendinous bands passing into the digits. Where the pretendinous bands are not involved in the contracture, they are small and difficult to identify. When the pretendinous bands are involved in the contracture, they are often greatly thickened and hypertrophied. Intimate attachment to the deep surface of the skin, with complete absence of subcutaneous fat, over a long distance is common. Again, an artificial dissection plane must be created.

Once the entire palmar fascia, together with the contracted bands has been exposed, the deep dissection is begun. This dissection begins at the most proximal point and proceeds distalward in an orderly fashion. There is a small layer of fat lying between the deep surfaces of the palmar fascia and the neurovascular structures. The small layer of fat is present even in the most advanced contractures. The proximal portion of the palmar aponeurosis may be transversely divided without injury to the nerves and arteries if care is taken not to penetrate this small fat layer. The deep attachments of the palmar fascia are then sectioned in an orderly fashion. At approximately the midpalm, the vertical fibrous septa will be noted passing from the deep surface of the palmar aponeurosis to the preosseous fascia. These vertical septa are removed in the radical operation (Fig. 15.4.21). Three prominent septa are encountered separating the four groups of digital flexors. Secondary septa, however, are also present. These separate the neurovascular structures from the flexor tendons. In complete excision of the palmar fascia both the major and secondary septa are removed. This can be most conveniently accomplished by proceeding in an orderly manner from the radial to the ulnar side of the hand, retracting the neurovascular bundles and flexor tendons as the deep attachments of the vertical septa are divided. At no point is the synovial sheath of the flexor tendons involved in the contracture. With careful dissection, it is always possible to leave the synovial sheath intact. The involvement of the septa and the distortion of the normal relationships of the digital nerves has been described in the section on limited fasciectomy. This must be borne in mind during the radical operation as well.

Once all superficial and deep attachments of the palmar fascia have been sectioned, attention is turned

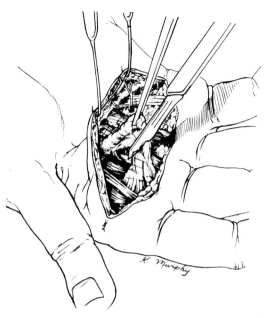

Figure 15.4.21. One step in the procedure of radical palmar fasciectomy. The scalpel is shown dividing one of the vertical septa of the palmar aponeurosis. The septa may become involved in Dupuytren's contracture and require removal at the time of the radical fasciectomy, or may lead to recurrence if they are not removed.

to the fingers. In those digits which have a palpable contracture, an appropriate incision is required. The incision will depend upon the configuration of the contracture in each finger. Several possible incisions are illustrated by Figure 15.4.19. The digital incisions may not be continuous with the main palmar incision. Excision of the band passing from the palm into the digits is then accomplished by creating a subcutaneous tunnel between the two incisions. When this becomes necessary, it is necessary to be aware constantly of the possibility of displacement of the digital nerves from their normal position. The details of removal of the digital contracture are the same as those described under limited fasciectomy.

When a band is present passing into the thumb, the incision must be selected to conform to the location of the band (Figs. 15.4.16 to 15.4.24 C). Often these bands may be removed at the time of the excision of the palmar portion of the palmar fascia and no incision in the thumb will be required. When incisions in the thumb are necessary, a mid lateral incision placed on the radial or ulnar side of the thumb, as indicated, will ordinarily produce adequate exposure of the contracture (Fig. 15.4.16 D). Occasionally, transverse, oblique or Z-incisions placed directly over the thumb contracture will be required.

It is the author's practice to perform as much of the operation as possible with a scalpel. Almost the entire procedure can be performed by careful sharp dissec-

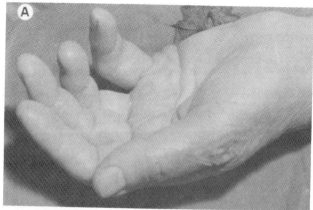

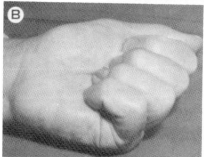
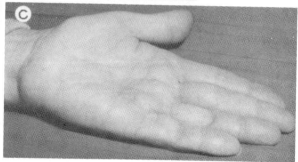

Figure 15.4.22. A. Preoperative view of the hand of a 75-year-old retired factory worker with moderately advanced Dupuytren's contracture involving the palm and the little finger. Patient was treated by total excision of the palmar aponeurosis. *B.* Postoperative flexion of the fingers of the patient illustrated in *A.* Photograph taken two months after surgery. *C.* Postoperative extension of the fingers of the patient illustrated in *A.* This photograph taken two months after surgery. The surgical procedure was total excision of the palmar aponeurosis.

tion. The surgeon who excises the palmar fascia in this way will be rewarded during the postoperative period by less postoperative edema, less likelihood of hematoma formation, better wound healing, and diminished postoperative morbidity. I am convinced that the technique of radical removal of the palmar fascia by the method of spread, cut and tear with scissors and hemostats, leads to many of the complications which have caused this procedure to be condemned.

Once all necessary dissection has been completed, attention is turned to hemostasis. The hand is wrapped in several large moistened sponges and the tourniquet is released. Five minutes of quite firm compression of the wounds by the operator's hands will control the vast majority of bleeding. If the dissection has been performed carefully and with a scalpel, very few bleeding vessels of any consequence will be encountered. Absolute hemostasis is an important feature of a successful radical excision of the palmar aponeurosis.

Once hemostasis has been secured, the tourniquet is again inflated. The bloodless field is maintained during the period of wound closure, and until the compression dressing and splint have been applied. Small

rubber tissue drains are ordinarily employed. A heavy silk suture tied about the free end of the drain and let out through the dressing will allow removal of the drain within a day or two without disturbing the original dressing. Actual wound suction should rarely, if ever, be required. Almost all authors recommend a voluminous dressing to which mild compression is applied by one of several types of elastic bandages. Splinting of the hand in the position of function is recommended by most authorities.

Wound Closure

After most operations for Dupuytren's contracture, whether performed by limited or radical fasciectomy, the wound or wounds can be directly closed. After excision of Dupuytren's contracture in an advanced case, one may find that there is insufficient skin remaining for wound closure (Fig. 15.4.25). This may be due to irreparable damage to adherent overlying skin during excision of the contracture. More commonly, however, the palmar skin has become so contractured over an area of advanced Dupuytren's contracture that it will no longer stretch to cover the palm

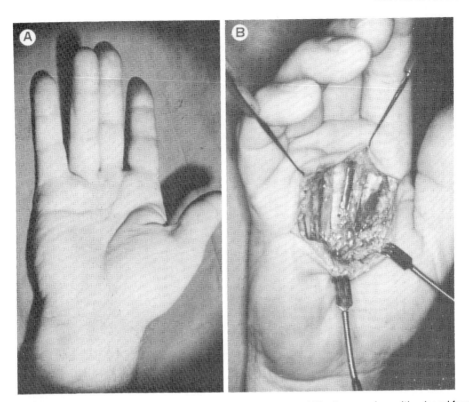

Figure 15.4.23. A. Preoperative view of the hand of a 48-year-old factory worker with a band forming in line with the ring finger and early limitation of extension of the ring finger. *B.* Operative exposure after excision of the palmar aponeurosis. Note the preservation of the synovial sheaths of the flexor tendons. In this instance, no finger incisions were necessary for relief of the contracture. Same patient as *A.*

where the fingers are extended. In such a situation the wound edges can often be closed if the finger joints were allowed to assume a position of moderate flexion. Such skin will often stretch postoperatively and recover normal or nearly normal length thus allowed progressive improvement of extension of the digits during the early postoperative period.

In a small percentage of cases, it may be absolutely impossible to close completely one or more wounds. In such cases, a thick split thickness skin graft will provide wound closure and satisfactory substitute for palmar skin. If careful attention has been paid to every detail of the operation and if the flexor tendons have not been stripped of their sheaths, such skin grafts will take without difficulty. Rotation flaps[13] or distant flaps for coverage of the palm are not unusually required.

Rarely, a finger may be so badly contracted and prove to be so refractory to attempts at improvement of extension that it will require amputation. If the decision for amputation is made during the operation for Dupuytren's contracture, some of the skin and the amputated digit maybe used as a flap to help wound closure.

About ten years ago, McCash[93] described the "open palm" technique of wound management following surgery for Dupuytren's contracture. This is a technique with which the author has had no personal experience. Apparently, the palmar wound can be left open and allowed to heal secondarily in difficult cases of completely closed wounds even if one or more small free skin grafts were required to complete wound closure.

Postoperative Care

A voluminous compression dressing with a splint to maintain the hand in the position of function is used by most authors. Almost all patients operated upon for Dupuytren's contracture will show some tendency to swelling of the hand in the immediate postoperative period. Elevation of the hand will assist in control of postoperative edema. A sling is worn with the hand held high on the chest when the patient is ambulatory. Pendulum exercises of the shoulders should be instituted on the first postoperative day to prevent the complication of frozen shoulder.

The postoperative care varies with different authors. It is our practice to change the dressing on the fourth postoperative day. Drains, if they have been used, are removed at this time. If the wounds are doing

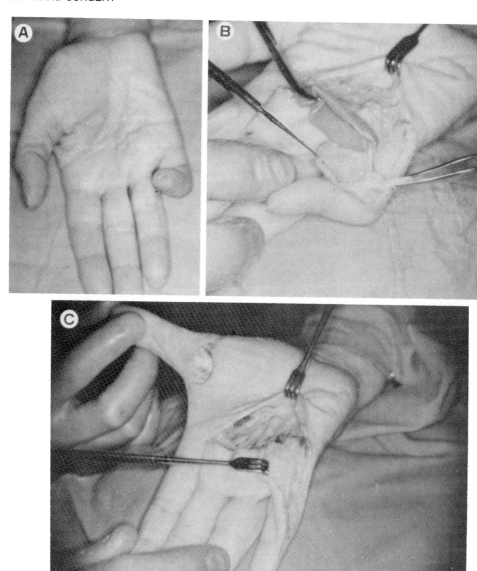

Figure 15.4.24. A. Preoperative view of moderately advanced Dupuytren's contracture involving the palm, the little finger, and the thumb. *B.* Same patient as *A.* Operative exposure of the digital sensory nerve on the ulnar side of the little finger. Note that the nerve appears completely surrounded by a nodule of contracted digital fascia. *C.* Operative view, illustrating radical excision of the palmar fascia. A transverse incision at the metacarpophalangeal joint of the thumb for removal of the contracted band to the thumb, and a distally based L-flap type incision for excision of the contracture in the little finger. Note the preservation of the digital sensory nerve on the ulnar side of the little finger. Same patient as *A.*

quite well, splinting can be discontinued and a lighter dressing and warm hand baths with beginning active exercise can be instituted as early as the fourth day. If the wound or wounds appear to be healing slowly, it maybe preferable to resume the bulky dressing and splint for an additional week. Early finger motion is encouraged, particularly when digital incisions were not required at the time of surgery.

COMPLICATIONS

Complications after surgery for Dupuytren's contracture are not infrequent. Ordinarily, the more radi-

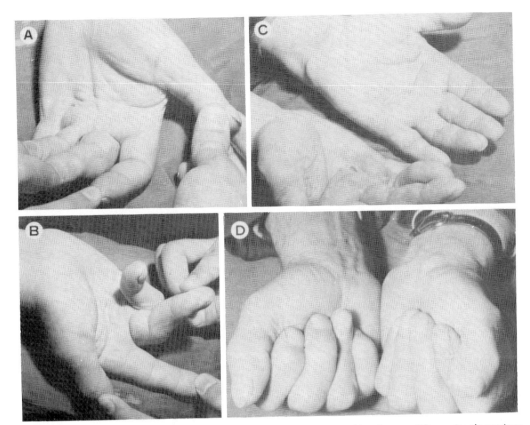

Figure 15.4.25. A. Preoperative view of the left hand of a patient with advanced Dupuytren's contracture. *B.* Preoperative view of the right hand of the patient illustrated in *A.* Note the hyperextension deformity of the distal interphalangeal joint of the ring finger. This patient was a common laborer and attributed the hyperextension of the distal joint of the ring finger to the repeated pushing of a tool handle into the palm. *C.* Postoperative extension of the patient illustrated in *A* and *B,* three and one-half months after surgery. Note the skin graft in the palm of the left hand. This hand was treated by total excision of the palmar aponeurosis, and was continuing to do well when the patient was last seen three years after surgery. The right hand was treated by multiple fasciotomy and limited excision of the contracted band to the ring finger in the palm. Together with a small split thickness skin graft which is visible in the photograph. When last seen three years after surgery, this patient was beginning to develop recurrence in the right hand. *D.* Postoperative flexion of the patient illustrated in *A* and *B,* three and one-half months after surgery. Patient returned to his work as a common laborer approximately two months after surgery.

cal the procedure, the more likely complications are to occur. It is to lessen the incidence of postoperative complications that Hamlin[47][48] and others have advocated the more restricted procedure of the limited fasciectomy.

A wound infection in an elective procedure of this type is a devastating complication. This complication has been reported quite infrequently. In our own experience, wound infections occur in approximately 0.5 per cent of operated cases.[78]

Wound hematoma is caused by faulty wound hemostasis. This complication should be virtually eliminated by careful attention to control of bleeding

at the time of surgery, and to the proper application of a compression dressing in the immediate postoperative period.

Skin loss in the postoperative period is a serious complication. Careful dissection with preservation of the small arteries to the skin, careful hemostasis and careful aseptic technique will do much to minimize the frequency of this complication.

Some edema of the hand is almost always encountered after radical excision of the palmar fascia. There are wide individual variations in the tendency to edema formation after excision of the palmar fascia. Compression dressings and elevation of the hand in the immediate postoperative period will help to minimize edema formation. Use of one of the proteolytic enzymes may help limit edema formation. Allaben[3] and associates have experimental evidence that intramuscular chymotrypsin assists in the reduction of edema.

Almost all patients operated upon for Dupuytren's contracture will show some tendency of swelling of the hand in the immediate postoperative period. An elastic bandage applied at the time of the operation is ordinarily too tight on the first postoperative day and requires loosening. Olesen and Zachariae[106] found that oxyphenbutazone had no effect upon edema following surgery for Dupuytren's contracture.

Postoperative stiffness is the most frequent complication after a radical excision of the palmar fascia. The prevention of edema and hematoma formation will do a great deal of minimize the frequency of the postoperative status. When stiffness has occurred, warm hand baths several times daily together with active exercise within the limits of pain are helpful. Physiotherapy should ordinarily be avoided at this time. Pushing the stiffen joints beyond the limits of pain only produces a reactive edema which ultimately makes the stiffness worse and delays recovery.

McIndoe[94] has listed vascular spasm as a postoperative complication. He found that no type of therapy except stellate ganglion block was of value in the treatment of this condition and warned that further surgery on such a hand should be avoided.

RESULTS OF TREATMENT

The results after surgery for Dupuytren's contracture vary with the magnitude of the operation performed,[17 28 47 48 58 81 95 112 145] with the degree of advancement of the contracture at the time of the surgical treatment and with many individual factors adherent within the patient himself.[58] Some of these individual factors are age, sex, tendency to develop joint stiffness after minor insults, and the presence or absence of arthritis. Indeed, the presence of rheumatoid arthritis has been regarded as an absolute counterindication to surgery for Dupuytren's contracture.[94]

Dupuytren's contracture is a disease which exhibits a fairly marked tendency toward recurrence. It has been assumed by most authors that the more limited the surgical procedure performed, the more likely one is to encounter recurrence of the disease. Hueston[58] has questioned whether or not this is true.[58] Recurrence does not occur beneath a free full thickness skin graft.[59 60]

Tubiana[134] found 43 per cent very good and 39 per cent good results after excision of the palmar fascia in his patients. Local factors and particularly the stage of the contracture at the time of surgery had a great influence on the prognosis in Tubiana's cases. Previous injuries did not seem to influence the operative result.

The age of the patient has no influence on the operative result. The presence or absence of knuckle pads has no prognostic significance. The stage of advancement of the contracture and such problems as secondary joint contracture do unfavorably influence the prognosis following surgery for Dupuytren's contracture.

SUMMARY

Dupuytren's contracture is a disease of the palmar fascia, which in its advanced stages is capable of producing a crippling flexion contracture of one or more of the digits. The fundamental change within the palmar aponeurosis is that of a pronounced proliferation of fibrous tissue. The exact cause of this fibrous tissue proliferation, and thus the etiology of the contracture, is still not well understood. The only consistently efficacious therapy for the disease is surgical excision. Three operations were performed: in order of increasing magnitude, fasciotomy, limited fasciectomy, and radical fasciectomy. Many local and systemic factors influence the choice of operation in each individual patient. In 80 to 90 per cent, good to excellent results can be expected after surgical treatment of Dupuytren's contracture, provided that the operation has been properly selected, carefully performed, and that complication have been avoided.

REFERENCES

1. Acklecker. Cited by Tubiana.[134]
2. Adams, W. Cited by Tubiana.[134]
3. Allaben, R. D., Posch, J. L., and Larsen, R. D. The efficacy of chymotrypsin in the control of edema in crushed extremities. J. Bone Joint Surg., *44A:* 41-48, 1962.
4. Anderson, W. Contractures of the fingers and toes; their varieties, pathology, and treatment. Lancet, *2:1:* 57, 1891.
5. Anderson, W. Deformities of the fingers and toes. Cited by Nichols.[104]
6. Arieff, A. J., and Bell, J. L. Epilepsy and Dupuytren's contracture. Neurology, *6:* 115, 1956.
7. Banfield, W. G. Aging of connective tissue. In *Connective Tissue in Health and Disease,* edited by G. Asboe-Hansen. Copenhagen, Munksgaard, 1954, p. 151.
8. Baxter, H., Schiller, C., Johnson, L. H., Whiteside, J. H., and Randall, R. E. Cortisone therapy in Dupuytren's contracture. Plast. Reconstr. Surg., *9:* 261, 1952.
9. Böhme, H. *Zur Aetiologie der Dupuytren'schen Fingerkontraktur.* Gluckstadt-Holstein, H. Kock, 1933.
10. Boyes, J. H. Dupuytren's contracture: Notes on the age at onset and the relationship to handedness. Am. J. Surg., *88:* 147, 1954.
11. Boyes, J. H. Discussion of Article by Larsen and Posch.[78]
12. Broadbent, T. R. Dupuytren's contractures Observations on the pathology. Rocky Mt. Med. J., *52:* 1087, 1955.
13. Bruner, J. M. The use of dorsal skin flap for the coverage of palmar defects after aponeurectomy for

Dupuytren's contracture. Plast. Reconstr. Surg., *4:* 559, 1949.

14. Bruner, J. M. The dynamics of Dupuytren's disease. Hand, *2:* 172-127, 1970.

15. Bunnell, S. *Surgery of the Hand,* Ed. 3. Philadelphia, Lippincott, 1956, 229.

16. Clarkson, P. The aetiology of Dupuytren's disease. Guy Hosp. Rep., *110:* 52, 1961.

17. Clarkson, P. The radical fasciectomy operation for Dupuytren's disease: a condemnation. Br. J. Plast. Surg., *16:* 273-9, 1963.

18. Clay, R. C. Dupuytren's contracture: fibroma of the palmar fascia. Ann. Surg., *120:* 224, 1944.

19. Coenen, H. Die Dupuytren'schen Fingerkontraktur. Ergeb. Chir. Orthop., *10:* 1170, 1918.

20. Conway, H. Dupuytren's contracture. Am. J. Surg., *87:* 101, 1954.

21. Conway, H., and Fieury, A. F. Indications for skin grafting in primary treatment. Plast. Reconstr. Surg., *16:* 264, 1955.

22. Cooper, A. *A Treatise on Dislocations, and on Fractures of the Joint,* Ed. 2. London, Longman Hurst, Rees, Orme, and Browne, 1823, p. 524.

23. Crawford, H. R. Surgical correction of Dupuytren's contracture. S. Clin. North Am., *36:* 793, 1956.

24. Curtin, J. W. Surgical therapy for Dupuytren's disease of the foot. Plast. Reconstr. Surg., *30:* 568, 1962.

25. Davis, J. S., and Finesilver, E. M. Dupuytren's contraction, with a note on the incidence of the contraction in diabetes. Arch. Surg., *24:* 933, 1932.

26. Deckner, K. Cited by Wang *et al.*[139]

27. Demers, R., and Blais, J. A. The familial and hereditary character of Dupuytren's contracture. Union Med. Can., *89:* 1238, 1960 (Fr.).

28. Deming, E. G. Y-V advancement pedicles in surgery for Dupuytren's contracture. Plast. Reconstr. Surg., *29:* 581, 1962.

29. Dickie, W. R., and Hughes, N. C. Dupuytren's contracture: A review of the late results of radical fasciectomy. Br. J. Plast. Surg., *20:* 311-4, 1967.

30. Dupuytren, G. *Lecons Orales de Clinique Chirurgicale, Faites a l'Hotel-Dieu de Paris.* Paris, Germer-Bailliere, 1832-1834.

31. Dupuytren, G. De la retraction des doigts par suite d'une affection de l'apponevrose palmaire, description de la maladie, operation chirurgicale qui convient dans de cas. J. Univ. Med. Chir. Paris, *5:* 352, 1831-1832. Also Eng. transl. in Lancet, *2:* 222, 1834. Reprinted in Med. Classics, *4:* 86, 1939.

32. Durel, L. Essai sur la maladie de Dupuytren. Paris, 1888. Cited by Skoog.[121]

33. Early, P. F. Population studies in Dupuytren's contracture. J. Bone Joint Surg., *44B:* 602, 1962.

34. Editorial. The puzzle of Dupuytren's Contracture. Lancet. July 22, 1972, 170-171.

35. Fauteux, M., and Ripstein, C. B. Dupuytren's contracture associated with coronary artery disease. Can. Med. Assoc. J., *58:* 502, 1948.

36. Finney, R. Dupuytren's contracture, a radiotherapeutic approach. Lancet, *2:* 1064, 1953.

37. Finney, R. Dupuytren's contracture. Br. J. Radiol., *28:* 610, 1955.

38. Fremont-Smith, F. In *Effect of ACTH and Cortisone on Connective Tissue.* Tr. First Conf. Josiah Macy, Jr. Foundation New York, The Foundation, 1950.

39. Garrod, A. E. On the unusual form of nodule upon the joints of the fingers. St. Bartholomew's Hosp. Rep., *29:* 157, 1893.

40. Galfarb, M., and Michaelides, P. Plantar fibromatosis. Arch. Dermatol., *85:* 278, 1962.

41. Gill, A. B. Dupuytren's contracture. Ann. Surg., *107:* 122, 1938.

42. Gonzalez, R. I. Dupuytren's contracture of the fingers: a simplified approach to the surgical treatment. Calif. Med., *115:* 25-31, 1971.

43. Gordon, S. Dupuytren's contracture; the significance of various factors in etiology. Ann. Surg., *140:* 683, 1954.

44. Gordon, S., and Anderson, W. Dupuytren's contracture following injury. Bri. J. Plast. Surg., *14:* 129, 1961.

45. Graubard, D. J. Dupuytren's contracture, an etiologic study. J. Int. Coll. Surg., *21:* 15, 1954.

46. Halliday, D. R., Lipscomb, P. R., and Seldon, T. H. Fasciectomy and controlled hypotension in treatment of Dupuytren's contracture. Am. J. Surg., *3:* 282-285, 1966.

47. Hamlin, E., Jr. Limited excision of Dupuytren's contracture. Ann. Surg., *135:* 94, 1952.

48. Hamlin, E., Jr. Limited excision of Dupuytren's contracture: A follow-up study. Ann. Surg., *155:* 454, 1962.

49. Harper, W. F. The distribution of the palmar aponeurosis in relation to Dupuytren's contraction of the thumb. J. Anat., *69:* 193, 1935.

50. Herzog, E. G. Aetiology of Dupuytren's contracture. Lancet, *1:* 1305-13011, 1951.

51. Hesse, E. Zur Behandlung der Dupuytren'schen Kontraktur. Zentralbl. Chir., *58:* 1532, 1931.

52. Hofmeister, F. The knuckle padding, a special form of Dupuytren's contracture. Chirurg, *28:* 35, 1957.

53. Horodynski, M. Morbus Dupuytreni. Gaz. Lek., 1917. Cited by Skoog.[121]

54. Horwitz, T. Dupuytren's contracture; a consideration of the anatomy of the fibrous structures of the hand in relation to this condition, with an interpretation of the histology. Arch. Surg., *44:* 687, 1942.

55. Howard, L. D., Pratt, D. R., and Bunnell, S. The use of compound F (Hydrocortone) in operative and nonoperative conditions of the hand. J. Bone Joint Surg., *35A:* 994, 1953.

56. Howes, E. L. The connective tissues in wound healing. In *Connective Tissue in Health and Disease.* edited by G. Asboe-Hansen. Copenhagen, Munksgaard, 1954, p. 159.

57. Hueston, J. T. The incidence of Dupuytren's contracture. Med. J. Aust., *47 (2):* 999, 1960.

58. Hueston, J. T. Limited fasciectomy for Dupuytren's contracture. Plast. Reconstr. Surg., *27:* 569, 1961.

59. Hueston, J. T. Digital Wolfe grafts in recurrent Dupuytren's contracture. Plast. Reconstr. Surg., *29:* 342-4, April 1962.

60. Hueston, J. T. Further studies on the incidence of Dupuytren's constracture. Med. J. Aust., *1:* 586-588, 1962.

61. Hueston, J. T. The control of recurrent Dupuytren's contracture by skin replacement. Br. J. Plast. Surg., *22:* 152-156, 1969.

62. Hunter, J. D., *et al.* Altered calcium metabolism in epileptic children on anticonvulsants. Br. Med. J., *4:* 202-204, 1971.

63. Ikle, C. Zur Histologie and Pathogenese der Dupuytren'schen Kontraktur. Dtsch. Z. Chir., *212:* 106. 1928.

64. Jacobs, W. L. W. Glutamyl-transpeptidase in diseases of the liver, cardiovascular system and diabetes mellitus. Clinics Chim. Acta, *38:* 419, 1972.

65. Jahnke, A. Electron microscopic research on Dupuytren's contracture. Zentralbl. Chir., *85:* 2295, 1960 (Ger.).

66. James, J. I. P. and Tubiana R. La maladie de Dupuytren. Rev. Chir. Orthop. Paris, *38:* 352, 1952.

67. Janssen, P. Zur Lehre von der Dupuytren'schen Fingerkontraktur mit besonderer Berucksichtigung dkr operativen Beseitigung und der pathologischen Anatomie des Leidens. Arch. Klin. Chir., *67:* 761, 1902.

68. Kanavel, A. B., Koch, S. L., and Mason, M. L. Dupuytren's contraction: With a description of the palmar fascia, a review of the literature, and a report of twenty-nine surgically treated cases. Surg. Gynecol. Obstet., *48:* 145, 1929.

69. Kaplan, E. B. The palmar fascia in connection with Dupuytren's contracture. Surgery, *4:* 415, 1938.

70. Kirby, J. Ann. mal. org. genitourin., 1849-1850. Cited by Waller and Dreese.[137]

71. Kirby, J. Dublin Med. J., *22:* 210, 1885. Cited by Waller and Dresse.[137]

72. Koch, S. L. Dupuytren's contracture. J. A. M. A., *100:* 878, 1933.

73. Kocher, T. Behandlung der Retraktion der Palmaraponeurose. Zentralbl. Chir., *14:* 481, 1887.

74. Krogius, A. Neue Gesichtspunkte zur Aetiologie der Dupuytren'schen Fingerkontraktur. Zentralbl. Chir., *47:* 914, 1920.

75. Krogius, A. Studien und Betrachtungen uber die Pathogenese der Dupuytren'schen Fingerkontraktur. Acta Chir. scand., *54:* 33, 1921.

76. Lagier, R., and Rutishauser, E. Anatomie pathologique et pathogenie de la maladie de Dupuytren. Presse med., *64:* 1212, 1956.

77. Langhans, L. Cited by Kocher.[73]

78. Larsen, R. D., and Posch, J. L. Dupuytren's contracture with special reference to pathology. J. Bone Joint Surg., *40A:* 773, 1958.

79. Larsen, R. D., and Posch, J. L. Dupuytren's contracture. A collective review. Inter. Abstr. Surg. Surg. Gynecol. Obstet., *115:* 1, 1962.

80. Larsen, R. D., Takagishi, N., and Posch, J. L. The pathogenesis of Dupuytren's contracture, experimental and further clinical observations. J. Bone Joint Surg., *42A:* 993, 1960.

81. Ledderhose, G. Zur Pathologie der Aponeurose des Fusses und der Hand. Arch. klin. Chir., *55:* 694, 1897.

82. Ledderhose, G. Die Aetiologie der Fasciitis Palmaris, Dupuytren'schen Kontraktur. Munch. med. Wochenschr., *67:* 1254, 1920.

83. Lengemann, P. Zur Thiosinaminbehandlung von Kontrakturen. Dtsche. med. Wochenschr., *30:* 463, 1904.

84. Lexer, E. *General Reconstructive Surgery,* Ed. 2. Leipzig, J. A. Barth, 1931.

85. Ling, R. S. M. The genetic factor in Dupuytren's disease. J. Bone Joint Surg., *45B:* 709-718, 1963.

86. Luck, J. V. Dupuytren's contracture, new concept of the pathogenesis correlated with surgical management. J. Bone Joint Surg., *41A:* 635, 1959.

87. Lund, M. Clinical connection between Dupuytren's contracture, fibroma plantae, periarthrosis humeri, helodermia, induration penis plastica and epilepsy, with attempt at pathogenetic valuation. Acta Psychiatr. Neurol., *16:* 465, 1941.

88. Lund, M. On epilepsy in Sturge-Weber's disease. Acta psychiat. Neurol., *24:* 569, 1949.

89. MacMahon, H. E. Baron Guillaume Dupuytren and the palmar contracture that bears his name. Bull. Tufts-N. Engl. Med. Center, *5:* 2, 1959.

90. Mason, M. L. Syposium on recent advances in surgery. Dupuytren's contracture. Surg. Clin. North Am., *32:* 233, 1952.

91. Mason, M. L. Personal communication, 1956.

92. Maxwell, J. D., Hunter, J. Stewart, D. A. Ardeman, S., and Williams R. Folate deficiency after anticonvulsant drugs: an effect of hepatic enzyme induction? Br. Med. J., 1972, *1:* 297-299, 1972.

93. McCash, C. R. The open palm technique in Dupuytren's contracture. Br. J. Plast. Surg., *17:* 271-80, 1964.

94. McIndoe, A., and Bear, R. L. Surgical management of Dupuytren's contracture. Am. J. Surg., *95:* 197, 1958.

95. Meagher, S. W. The Dupuytren contracture controversy. A presentation of the facts. J.A.M.A., *180:* 140, 1962.

96. Meyerding, H. W. Dupuytren's contracture, treatment. Am. J. Surg., *49:* 94, 1940.

97. Meyerding, H. W. In discussion of article by Larsen and Posch.[78]

98. Meyerding, H. W., Black, J. R., and Broders, A. C. The etiology and pathology of Dupuytren's contracture. Surg. Gynecol. Obstet., *72:* 582, 1941.

99. Miskalczy: Cited by Wang *et al.*[139]

100. Moorhead, J. J. Trauma and Dupuytren's contracture. Am. J. Surg., *85:* 352, 1953.

101. Moorhead, J. J. Dupuytren's contracture: review of disputed etiology, 1831-1956. N. Y. J. Med., *56:* 3686, 1956.

102. Nazari, B. Dupuytren's contracture associated with liver disease. J. Mt. Sinai Hosp., *33:* 69-72, 1966.

103. Nezelhof, C., and Tubiana, R. La maladie de Dupuytren, etude histologique. Sem. Hop. Paris, *34:* 1102, 1958.

104. Nichols, J. B. A clinical study of Dupuytren's contraction of the palmar and digital fascia. Am. J. Sci., *117:* 285, 1899.

105. Nichols, J. B. The histology of Dupuytren's contraction of the palmar fascia, report of microscopic examination in two additional cases. Med. News, *75:* 491, 1899.

106. Olesen, E., and Zachariae, L. Absent effect of oxyphenbutazone (Tanderil) upon oedema following operation for Dupuytren's contracture. Acta Chir. Scand., *129:* 352-358, 1965.

107. Pedersen, H. E., and Day, A. J. Dupuytren's disease, fibromatosis of plantar fascia, of feet, J.A.M.A., *154:* 33, 1954.

108. Plater, F. Observationum liber, *1:* 140, 1614. Cited by Durel.[32]

109. Pojer, J., and Jedlickova, J. Enzymatic pattern of liver injury in Dupuytren's contracture. Acta med. scand., *187:* 101-104, 1970.

110. Pojer, J., Radivojeric, M. and Williams, T. F. Dupuytren's disease. Its association with abnormal liver function in alcoholism and epilespy. Arch. Intern. Med., *1:* 561-566, 1972.

111. Richer, P. Retraction de l'aponeurose palmaire. Bull.

Soc. Anat. Paris, *2:* 124, 1877.

112. Riordan, D. C. Dupuytren's contracture. South. Med. J., *54:* 1391, 1961.

113. Roodenberg, A. I. Hyperplasia of the palmar aponeurosis, Dupuytren's contracture. Arch. Int. Med., *101:* 551, 1958.

114. Rutishauser, E., and Lagier, R. Dupuytren's disease. Schweiz. Z. Allg. Pathol., *18:* 1262, 1955.

115. Sachs, O. L. Beitrag zur Spontanheilung der plastischen Induration der Corpora cavernosa penis. Arch. Dermat. Syphilol., *139:* 121, 1922.

116. San Martino, A. Lineamenti di patologia della malattia di Dupuytren; rilievi istologici, oscillografici, fotopletismografici. Chir. Organi. Mov., *45:* 59, 1957.

117. Schaumann: In discussion. Trans. Swedish Dermatol. Soc., 1944. Acta dermatal. venereol., *27:* 68, 1947.

118. Schink, W. Surgical treatment of Dupuytren's contracture. A report on 100 surgically treated hands. Langenbecks Arch. Chir., *299:* 118, 1961 (Ger.).

119. Schroeder, C. H. Berufsarbeit und Trauma bei der Dupuytren'schen Kontraktur. Dtsche. Z. Chir., *244:* 140, 1935.

120. Schroeder, C. H. Cited by Wang et al.[139]

121. Skoog, T. Dupuytren's contraction, with special reference to aetiology and improved surgical treatment. Its occurrence in epileptics. Note on knuckle pads. Acta chir. scand., *96:* Suppl. 139, 1948.

122. Skoog, T. Dupuytren's contracture. Postgrad. Med., *21:* 91, 1957.

123. Skoog, T. Dupuytren's contracture: pathogenesis and surgical treatment. Surg. Clin. North Am., *47:* 433-444, 1967.

124. Skoog, T. The transverse elements of the palmar aponeurosis in Dupuytren's contracture. Scand. J. Plast. Reconstr. Surg., *1:* 51-63, 1967.

125. Smith, N. Cited by Wang et al.[139]

126. Sproges. Cited by Davis and Finesilver.[25]

127. Stahnke, E. Zur Behandlung der Dupuytren'schen Fingerkontraktur. Zentralbl. Chir., *54:* 2438, 1927.

128. Steinberg, C. LeR. A new method of treatment of Dupuytren's contracture, a form of fibrositis. Med. Clin. North Am., *30:* 221, 1946.

129. Steinberg, C. LeR. Fibrositis, muscular rheumatism, including Dupuytren's contracture; a new method of treatment. N. Y. J. Med., *47:* 1679, 1947.

130. Su, C. K., and Patek, A. J., Jr. Dupuytren's contracture. Arch. Intern. Med., *126:* 278, 1970.

131. Takagishi, N. Personal communications, 1959.

132. Tanzer, R. C. Dupuytren's contracture, with a note on the use of the "compression suture." N. Engl. J. Med., *246:* 807, 1952.

133. Thompson, R. P. H. Eddleston, A. L. W. F., and Williams, R. Low plasma bilirubin in epileptics on phenobarbitone. Lancet, *I:* 21-22, 1969.

134. Tubiana, R. Prognosis and treatment of Dupuytren's contracture. J. Bone Joint Surg., *37A:* 1155, 1955.

135. Tubiana, R. Limited and extensive operations in Dupuytren's contracture. Surg. Clin. North Am., *44:* 1071-1080, 1964.

136. Tubiana, R., Michon, J., and Thomine, J. M. Scheme for the assessment of deformities in Dupuytren's disease. Surg. Clin. North Am., *48:* 979-984, 1968.

137. Waller, J. I., and Dreese, W. C. Peyronie's disease, associated with Dupuytren's contracture. J. Urol., *68:* 623, 1952.

138. Walters, J. H., and Zahra, A. Etiology of Dupuytren's contracture in Eastern Nigeria. Trans. R. Soc. Trop. Med. Hyg., *51:* 346, 1957.

139. Wang, M. K. H., Macomber, W. B., Stein, A., Rajpal, R., and Heffernan, A. Dupuytren's contracture, an analytic and etiologic study. Plast. Reconstr. Surg., *25:* 323, 1960.

140. Warren, R. F. The pathology of Dupuytren's contracture. Br. J. Plast. Surg., *6:* 224, 1953.

141. Wasserburger, K. Therapy of Dupuytren's contracture. Strahlentherapie, *100:* 546, 1956.

142. Webster, G. V. A useful incision in Dupuytren's contracture. Plast. Reconstr. Surg., *19:* 514, 1957.

143. Wegmann, T., and Geiser, W. Frequent occurrence of Dupuytren's contracture in chronic alcholism. Schweiz. Med. Wochenschr., *91:* 719, 1961 (Ger.).

144. Weese, K. On Surgery of Dupuytren's contracture. Bruns Beitr. Klin. Chir., *203:* 57, 1961 (Ger.).

145. Wilson, J. N. Correction of Dupuytren's contracture. Plast. Reconstr. Surg., *29:* 332, 1962.

146. Wolfe, S. J., Summerskill, W. H. J., and Davidson, C. S. Thickening and contraction of the palmar fascia, Dupuytren's contracture, associated with alcoholism and hepatic cirrhosis. N. Engl. J. Med., *255:* 559, 1956.

147. Yost, J., Winters, T., and Fett, H. C. Dupuytren's contracture, statistical study. Am. J. Surg., *90:* 568, 1956.

148. Zachariae, L., and Zachariae, F. Hydrocortisone acetate in the treatment of Dupuytren's contraction and allied conditions. Acta chir. scandi., *109:* 421, 1955.

149. Zachariae, L. Dupuytren's contracture. Scand. J. Plast. Reconstr. Surg., *3:* 145-149, 1969.

E.

Volkmann's Ischemic Contracture

J. Leonard Goldner, M.D.

ETIOLOGY AND TREATMENT DURING ACUTE PHASE

Volkmann's ischemia connotes primary insufficient arterial blood supply to forearm muscles, nerves, vascular tree, and even bone. Volkmann's contracture implies subsequent necrosis and contracture of these muscles as well as motor weakness, sensory disturbance, and contracture of the elbow, wrist, and hand. The primary arterial deficit may be compounded by venostasis, accumulation of harmful metabolites, and extra- and intracellular edema. Also, there may be direct soft tissue injury from bone fragments, compression by fascial bands, and, finally, multiple tissue necrosis and fibrosis. Observations at the time of emergency surgery have shown contusion, spasm, or a combination of changes in the arterial tree but minimal alteration in the venous system. The primary arterial injury has been observed by several investigators and myself, yet recognition must be given to the accumulated evidence, which shows that massive venous occlusion, as seen in phlegmasia cerulea dolens, does result in gangrene of a portion of an involved extremity. Concomitant constriction of the artery and mechanical compression of the venous tree may result in segmental muscle damage.

Comparison of the Volkmann's ischemia to phlegmasia cerulea dolens does not appear entirely justified: (1) In typical early Volkmann's ischemia, improvement usually results after direct treatment to the brachial artery and collateral circulation. (2) Improvement usually occurs without anticoagulation or venous thrombectomy or other treatment directed toward the venous system other than relief of the external mechanical blockage. (3) Thrombophlebitis, in the usual sense, does not result in gangrene or necrosis *per se,* although fibrosis may occur. (4) Peripheral changes accompanying venous thrombosis usually show mottling, cyanosis, minimal sensory change, venous dilation superficially, and engorgement of the extremity at its periphery. The arterial injury, as seen in the early stage of Volkmann's usually shows minimal swelling, pallor, paresthesia, hypesthesia, and varying degrees of paralysis, pain, and pulselessness.

Certainly the venous factor in the chronic phase of Volkmann's may play a part in subsequent fibrosis, and certain factors are associated with this: (1) Vasoconstrictive action of serotonin produced by platelet breakdown with vasospasm producing edema, pallor, and ischemia. (2) Mechanical obstruction of the venous system by chronic venous occlusion in the presence of a patent arterial system allows the vascular bed to fill to its limit with subsequent edema. The effect of this circulatory arrest and increase in reduced hemoglobin is noted by cyanosis and ischemia. External compression from edema may cause arterial constriction or compression secondarily. This is similar to the mechanisms of the anterior tibial compartment syndrome when that condition is caused from direct trauma leading to a tamponade. Fasciotomy, if done early for the treatment of anterior compartment, usually allows increased arterial blood supply, improved venous outflow, and maintenance of viable muscle. Extraction of a clot from the venous system has not been necessary and recovery has occurred.

Currently, there is abundant evidence to prove that arterial insufficiency is the primary cause of Volkmann's ischemia although a combination of arterial and venous change does occur with the condition being made more serious because of the venous factor.

The muscle change caused by infarct or ischemia should be considered as a spectrum. On one side there is total death of all muscle fibers, necrosis, fatty degeneration, fibrosis; or, necrosis and fatty degeneration with minimal fibrosis, but total loss of all viable muscle. On the other side of the spectrum is the change that occurs with tourniquet ischemia during an operative procedure. After two hours there are measurable changes in pH, pCO_2, pO_2, and alterations in enzymes, glycogenesis, membrane potential, and membrane permeability. These are, in general, reversible changes if they are not present too long. Four hours of ischemia are usually considered as a maximum period of arterial insufficiency. This period of total ischemia may not result in complete loss of muscle fibers, but will affect not only the muscle fibers, but also the neural elements as well.

Muscle biopsy may show groups of muscle fibers with necrosis of all fibers and phagocytosis, or several fibers with a group that show spotty necrosis. Special staining may show some of the fibers to be rich in RNA and indicative of a possibility of regeneration. Structural occlusion may be found in some of the small arterials and in the main artery, or external occlusion of the arteries and capillaries may occur by pressure without actual embolization.

Selye has shown that large doses of serotonin gave focal necrosis. The same findings have been noted with norepinephrine and other vasoconstrictors.

The arterial damage includes the following elements either singly or in combination: (1) Arterial thrombosis at the site of direct trauma caused by intimal damage, or thrombosis at a distance from the site of the original trauma, with the trauma occurring to the brachial artery and the thrombosis possibly occurring in radial and ulnar arteries. (2) External compression of the artery resulting from bone fragments, from edema of surrounding tissue, or closed space compression under intact skin. Intra- and extracellular edema, if they persist, aggravate the compression. (3) Arterial vasospasm does occur and recur from serotonin expulsion, direct trauma from bone fragments, or repeated manipulation. The arterial spasm is considered as protective in some instances, if the venous portion of the vascular tree is engorged. With spasm, the diminished arterial supply decreases the load on the venous side.

If extensive muscle cell death occurs as a result of irreversible injury to the forearm tissues, all or some of the known elements of Volkmann's contracture will result. Prolonged ischemia of the forearm muscles, regardless of the cause, will result in partial or complete fibrosis and paralysis of the wrist and digit flexors. Also, direct contusion and ischemia of the median nerve and, frequently, injury to the ulnar and radial nerves will complicate the situation by increasing the degree of paralysis in the hand because of loss of intrinsic muscle function and by causing pain and trophic change associated with single or multiple nerve compression. The addition of pain and paralysis to the existing muscle necrosis diminishes function of a hand that is already greatly incapacitated.

Treatment of Severe Elbow Injury with Arterial Insufficiency Acute Phase, 2 to 24 to 48 hours.

A brief review of the principles involved in managing severe elbow injuries in children and adults demands an understanding of acute arterial injuries, roller or compression injuries of the forearm and elbow, and venous blockage, as well as nerve contusion. The patient with a severe elbow injury must be examined carefully to determine the presence of motor weakness of the digits, sensory impairment, or circulatory deficiency that might affect either the radial or ulnar arteries or the nail bed circulation. Paleness of the skin, diminution of the peripheral pulses, slow capillary flushing, excessive skin coolness, pain with extension of the digits, and evidence of motor paralysis all suggest severe involvement of the arterial tree at the elbow level. Closed manipulation of the fractured elbow in certain situations is *harmful* because the median nerve and brachial artery and vein are impaled on the distal end of the proximal humeral bone segment. An example of this problem was illustrated by a six-year-old boy who was seen four hours after severe elbow fracture with an impending Volkmann's. No manipulation was done. After general anesthesia was given, a faint radial pulse was palpable with the forearm angulated laterally 50°, and with the elbow in extension. Gentle flexion of the elbow through 30°, without manipulation of the bone fragments, caused the radial pulse to disappear. The skin and fascia were opened but this did not affect the diminished volume of the peripheral pulses. The brachial vein had not dilated, even four hours after the initial injury, indicating little evidence of venous congestion or venous thrombosis. Arterial spasm did exist and a 1-cm segment of the artery was discolored and irregular. Swelling about the elbow was caused primarily by hemorrhage from the open bone ends and soft tissue edema. Relief of arterial spasm was attempted in several ways. These are listed to indicate the various things that should be done to reestablish arterial flow.

The neurovascular bundle was elevated from the humeral spike and the fracture was gently manipulated under direct vision. It was evident that if a closed manipulation had been done additional damage to the nerve and the artery would have been inevitable. Treatment of the arterial contusion and spasm included: (1) Irrigation of the involved artery segment, as well as artery above and below, with 1 per cent lidocaine (Xylocaine), but no change occurred in size of the vessel or in peripheral blood flow. (2) Infiltration of the median nerve with 1 per cent Xylocaine three inches proximal to the site of injury, without relief of arterial spasm after 5 min. (3) Local use of papaverine gave no improvement. (4) Injection of 0.1 cc or 1 mg of heparin solution with a total volume of 1 cc just proximal to the contused area and obliteration of the distal segment resulted in intra-arterial dilatation that rapidly diminished arterial spasm and improved peripheral blood flow.

A fixation pin was used to maintain stability of the fracture, skin closure was done, a posterior plaster splint was applied over a compression dressing, and the extremity was tied to a pillow with about 5° of elevation of the hand in relation to the body. Circulation continued to be good with no loss of volume of the ra-

dial pulse. Sensation and distal motor weakness continued to improve but, even six months after the injury, there was partial weakness of the intrinsic muscles of the thumb supplied by the median nerve. Sensation, however, was excellent. Functional recovery occurred gradually. The muscle paralysis was due to denervation and not to muscle necrosis. The latter was prevented by restoration of arterial flow. A closed supracondylar fracture accompanied by diminished or absent radial pulse, good capillary circulation, good motor power, and little or no sensory change, may be treated by brachial plexus block and stellate ganglion injection, and by traction and/or manipulation. If the peripheral circulation remains intact and if the radial pulse improves, then the extremity can be treated in Dunlop's traction. Absence of the radial pulse is not necessarily an indication for decompression of the elbow region, but if the hand shows immediate evidence of nerve and circulatory impairment then operation is indicated.

Other efforts at relieving arterial spasm might include incision of the involved artery and dilatation by using a probe; also, Fogarty Catheters are inserted to determine if there is intimal blockage or clots that can be removed. Excision of an involved area of the artery can be done and direct suture accomplished. then resection and insertion of a vein graft or plastic graft; or resection and resuture or ligation of the artery may show that the peripheral circulation is satisfactory.

The use of intravenous heparin postoperatively, and a large dose of intra-arterial heparin at surgery is justified.

Delayed Treatment (One to Four Weeks)

If early treatment has not been available or completed during the 48 hours after injury, or if vascular injury has been so extensive that the forearm muscles are crushed to a point beyond regeneration, then the findings as described by Volkmann will occur (Fig. 15.5.1 A). These include muscle fibrosis, muscle shortening, nerve ischemia, venous stasis, and joint fixation. During this period, median nerve involvement may be the most serious problem and early release of the median nerve is essential. Release of the median nerve will decrease the possibility of permanent nerve damage, diminish pain, and avoid additional motor loss of the intrinsic muscles and the forearm flexor muscle mass.

The major limiting factor in treatment at this stage is the condition of the skin. Edema is usually evident, crusts of epidermis are present, and these may be serous or purulent. Multiple blisters do occur and the skin condition implies that any surgical procedure would lead to secondary infection. The fracture *per se* is not the major limiting factor.

Frequently, the treatment requires maintenance of the fracture by external plaster, outrigger traction to the fingers, direct attention toward diminution of edema, and prevention of additional contracture. During a four-week period, the condition of the extremity

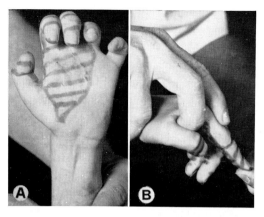

Figure 15.5.1. A. Ischemic contracture of the forearm and hand of a 5-year-old boy that resulted from external constriction at elbow region after manipulation and reduction of a supracondylar fracture of the humerus. This photograph was taken three weeks after the injury when there was hypesthesia and paresthesia of the median nerve zone. Trophic skin changes had occurred, constant pain was present, and there was flexion deformity of the thumb, fingers, and wrist. The intrinsic muscles supplied by the median nerve were paralyzed, and the radial pulse was palpable but weaker than the opposite radial pulse. *B.* Lateral view of the same hand showing almost complete passive extension of the digits when the wrist was held in flexion. This indicates contracture of the flexor sublimis and profundus muscles proximal to the wrist joint. The thumb web had already contracted moderately. Early clawing of the fingers existed because of intrinsic muscle paralysis and forearm muscle contracture.

usually improves to such a degree that surgical intervention can be done without danger of complications.

Muscle and Nerve Ischemia and Compression

Interference with arterial blood supply to the soft tissues in the elbow region affects the flexor muscles and also the median nerve. This nerve does not receive as much collateral circulation as the ulnar and the radial nerves. Constriction of the nerve by fibrosis interferes with nutrition, axon plasm flow, and axon conduction. By clinical examination nerve change secondary to direct contusion is difficult to differentiate from that which is caused by ischemia. Nevertheless, the fate of the median nerve is important. Release of the median nerve compression, next to the primary establishment of arterial blood supply, is the most important factor in decreasing pain, saving sensation, and assuring recovery of motor power of the hand.

The contracture, once present, may be partially reversible if the forearm muscles are decompressed. Nerves are affected by pressure, also, but they have

the ability to sustained compression longer than muscle and still recover at least partially. Direct contusion and ischemia of the median nerve and partial involvement of the radial and ulnar nerves will aggravate the forearm contracture. The combination of direct muscle necrosis and denervation cause the most severe form of deformity. The compressed nerve causes hand pain, weakness, and progressive loss of function in the hand that is already greatly incapacited (Fig. 15.5.1).

Peripheral nerve compression syndromes occur at crucial points where nerves enter or leave a closed space or small rigid foreamens. Compression of the median nerve occurs at the wrist by the transverse retinacular ligament and the contents of the carpal canal, in the hand by extension of the attachment of the palmaris longus and the palmar fascia; in the forearm by the pronator and flexores digitorum sublimes; and in the supracondylar area by the supracondyloid process and/or an aberrant origin of the pronator teres. Compression of the ulnar nerve also occurs at several points along its course, including a point proximal to the ulnar groove at the elbow, intermittently over the medial epicondyle, distal to the ulnar groove at the entrance of the nerve into the flexor carpi ulnaris, at the wrist, and in the hand. Compression syndromes of the radial nerve have been described due to involvement of the nerve where it passes near the radial groove, in the area of the radial neck where the nerve enters the supinator muscle, and at the point where the superficial branch of the radial nerve emerges in the distal forearm. Clinical examples of all of these compression problems have been recognized and treated with relief of pain.

Compression of mixed nerve roots occurs as a result of intervertebral disc compression.

Interference with the conducting mechanism of a peripheral nerve does occur at a point near the origin of the flexor digitorum sublimis or flexor pollicis longus. Constriction here will diminish conducting ability of the nerve and also interfere with blood flow through the median artery. Interference with the nerve in this way affects the circulation of the nerve and causes local nerve damage secondary to ischemia and the compressing force.

In addition to ischemia and external pressure, acute angulation of a nerve results in structural change. The pathologic changes that take place in compression neuropathy, as seen in the carpal tunnel syndrome, are usually of the "first degree." In this degree of injury there is no actual loss of continuity or degeneration of nerve fibers other than localized vacuolization of the myelin, local edema, and cellular infiltration. Proprioceptive and motor functions are more vulnerable in first degree injury than are functions of pain, touch, and sympathetic activity. These "first degree" nerve changes are readily reversible. If the mechanism causing these alterations is unrelieved for several weeks or months, then "second degree" nerve change may occur. The axonal injury will then progress, leading to Wallerian degeneration distally, as well as changes proximally for a short distance. If nerve compression has been prolonged and severe, recovery will be slow and incomplete after the compression is released.

The experimental and clinical findings are that pain, sensory disturbance, and interference with motor function of the end organ will occur as the results of external compression of a nerve. As in the "carpal tunnel syndrome," the symptoms, even though present for several weeks or months, may be relieved rapidly and recovery may occur gradually if the nerve is freed of external compression. This same principle applies to treatment of the compressed median nerve in the forearm and the elbow if there is evidence that external compression exists or that internal compression of the nerve persists after an original injury.

Injury to the median nerve occurs in many ways and the degree of injury may be directly related to the mechanism of injury. Direct contusion of the nerve, compression by swollen forearm muscles, constriction by fibrous bands, and ischemic necrosis of the median nerve may occur individually or in combination. The severity of the final contracture of the hand is partially dependent on the extent of interruption of motor and sensory components of the three major nerves of the forearm. Forearm muscle ischemia alone could be tolerated and a substitute could be provided, but when nerve damage is included the seriousness of the problem is magnified immensely.

The critical points of median nerve injury are: (1) opposite the fracture site, and (2) the point where the median nerve courses through the pronator radii teres and under the origin of the flexores digitorum sublimes as the nerve enters the forearm.

Secondary and delayed constriction associated with fibrosis may occur by the flexor pollicis longus because of its anatomic relationship to the median nerve and by the transverse carpal ligament at the wrist.

At the point where the median nerve is initially covered by the superficial head of the pronator there is very little room for expansion of a swollen nerve, and compression by swollen muscle tissue indirectly affects the nerve. Secondly, the point where the nerve and artery pass behind the sublimis muscle origin is an area that allows very little tissue expansion. The relationship of the median nerve and the flexor sublimis at this point (Fig. 15.5.2) is similar, in certain respects, to that of the median nerve and the volar carpal ligament. The pronator radii teres superficially and the flexores sublimes, condensed by a fascial band at its upper border, cover the nerve like a belt or band. As supination occurs, the "belt" tightens and, as fibrosis occurs later, the "belt" constricts. The importance of this closed space in the upper portion of the forearm is obvious when one realizes that intermittent compression of the median nerve and its nutrient artery occur in this area, without direct trauma but spontaneously by tenosynovitis or prolonged excessive pronation and supination by a tennis player with abnormally large forearm muscles that rotate frequently. The nerve may

be compressed by forced supination in the patient with a spastic extremity secondary to cerebral palsy where one attempts to stretch or elongate a spastic or contracted pronator and flexor muscle mass.

Figure 15.5.3 shows the flat, pale segment of the median nerve after incision of the pronator teres and part of the origin of the flexores sublimes during exploration of the forearm for treatment of an established Volkmann's contracture. There was improvement in sensory perception of the hand and diminution of pain within 24 hours after the soft tissue release. The relief of pain was comparable to that in degree and time to

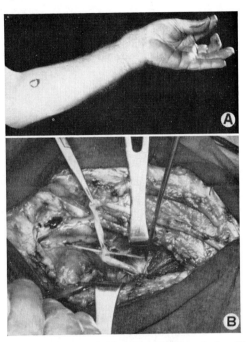

Figure 15.5.2. A. The arm and hand of a 60-year-old man with symptoms and signs of median nerve compression in the forearm. Local tenderness was present at the point where the median nerve courses through the pronator muscle and under the flexor sublimis muscle. Hypesthesia was present in the median nerve distribution of the hand. Neurolysis in the upper forearm gave relief of symptoms. Compression of the median nerve by the forearm muscles at this particular point without trauma emphasizes the importance of the nerve-muscle relationship and the likelihood of compression of the nerve at the same place in Volkmann's contracture. *B.* Surgery of the forearm shown in Figure 15.5.2 A. The pronator has already been partially separated and the main point of constriction of the median nerve was at the site of origin of the flexor sublimis from the radius. A fascial band was present here and constricted the nerve as it passed under the fascia. The entrance to the forearm is on the right and the dark pointer is over the muscle origin.

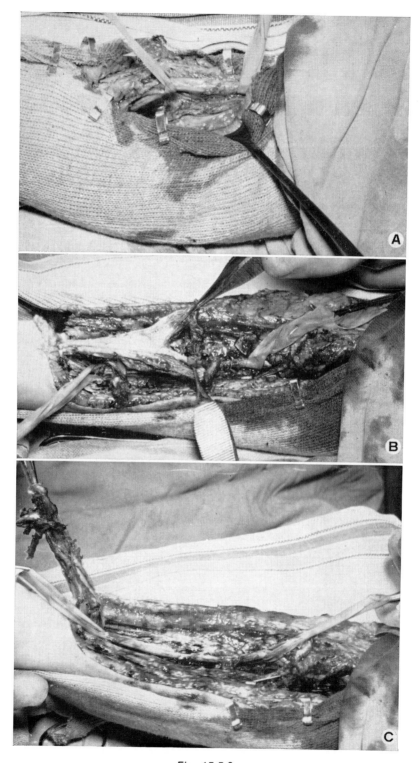

Fig. 15.5.3.

the improvement that occurs after removal of a large fragment of a ruptured intervertebral disc or by incision of the transverse retinacular ligament at the wrist. Compression of the proximal segment of the median nerve by the flexores digitorum sublimes and the pronator muscle may be compared to an "internal tourniquet" (Fig. 15.5.4).

Treatment during the Recovery Period after Volkmann's Ischemia (One to 12 Months)

Operative treatment is carried out as early as possible once arterial insufficiency and nerve compression have occurred. A delay in the surgical therapy may be necessary for several weeks, however, because of skin lesions and superficial infection. If the compression is in the midforearm or distal to the muscle mass, then spontaneous recovery of axonal conduction and relief of contracture by splinting and stretching may occur over a period of several months.

Maximal spontaneous recovery may occur in 12 to 18 months. Improvement of digit contractures in most instances, is slow, with minimal change occuring after elastic traction. The Tinel's sign over the median nerve may advance slowly, and hand sensation may be incomplete and accompanied by hyperesthesias and paresthesias. Motor power of the forearm muscles may be absent and the intrinsic muscles of the hand supplied by the median nerve may recover only a part of their strength (Fig. 15.5.5).

Thus, a policy of "watchful waiting" is not justified when this situation exists and, in the subacute phase, decompression of the median nerve should be done as soon as the condition of the extremity will alow the operation. The forearm is opened through an anterior medial incision extending from 1 inch above the elbow joint to the musculotendinous junction of the forearm flexors. The median nerve is isolated proximal to the point of injury and a neurolysis is carried out (Fig. 15.5.6). An electrical nerve stimulator is used to identify small motor branches, and the

stimulator should be available throughout the operative procedure.

After the median nerve and its motor branches are identified, and the decompression is carried down to the musculotendinous junction in the midforearm, the decision must be made regarding exploration of the wrist and hand. This depends on the appearance of the nerve, the amount of fibrosis distally, and the degree of pain. In most instances, the transverse retinacular ligament at the wrist is incised in order to avoid localized constriction at that time or in the future.

The ulnar nerve should be examined during the same elbow-forearm exploration; managent of this nerve depends on the preoperative clinical findings and the condition of the flexor carpi ulnaris at the time of the operation. The ulnar nerve should be released from the constricting fascia that envelopes the flexor carpi ulnaris and, if necessary, the nerve should be transplanted anteriorly. If there is clinical evidence of ulnar nerve involvement, the nerve should be followed into the forearm to a point where it is free from fibrous compression or constriction.

The radial nerve may be involved in the same process, depending on the mechanism of injury and the degree of external compression or internal displacement of the bone fragments. The decision to explore this nerve will depend on the clinical findings and the possibilities of nerve laceration or nerve compression. Pure radial nerve injury associated with supracondylar fracture does occur without ischemia and without nerve laceration and the presence of paralysis of the extensor musculature may require operative treatment, but only after repeated examination using progression of the Tinel's sign and electromyography.

Contracture of the Elbow, Wrist and Digits

Flexion deformity of the elbow may be associated with the fracture and with capsular injury to the joint as well as to fibrosis of the forearm muscles originat-

Figure 15.5.3. A. First operation on arm shown in Figure 15.5.1 A, six weeks after injury. The median nerve was isolated at the elbow and is seen from the radial side. The nerve was edematous proximal to the pronator and sublimis muscles, but became flat and pale as it passed under these muscles. B. The pronator radii teres was severed and the nerve isolated in the midforearm. The rubber dam retractors on the right and left are around the proximal and distal segments of the median nerve. All finger flexor muscles and wrist flexor muscles were fibrous and contracted. These are being held by the forceps. The muscle bellies were released from the lower humerus proximally for advancement, and this aided in wrist extension but did not affect the finger contractures. The median nerve was severely constricted in the mid and upper forearm and was moderately swollen opposite the fracture site. The radial pulse was good. All contracted, useless, fibrous tissue was excised to correct finger and wrist deformities and to free nerves and blood vessels. Tenotomy was necessary in order to extend the digits and the wrist. C. The long ischemic segment of median nerve is isolated between the pieces of rubber dam. The nerve had been partially ischemic and constricted for several weeks and the pronator radii teres and the flexor sublimis muscles compressed it, similar to an internal tourniquet. Sensation was improved dramatically within 48 hours after the operation and discomfort in the hand rapidly disappeared during the first three days after the surgery. The diminution of pain within the first 72 hours after surgery, as compared with the persistent paresthesias that had occurred for six weeks, was more than coincidental.

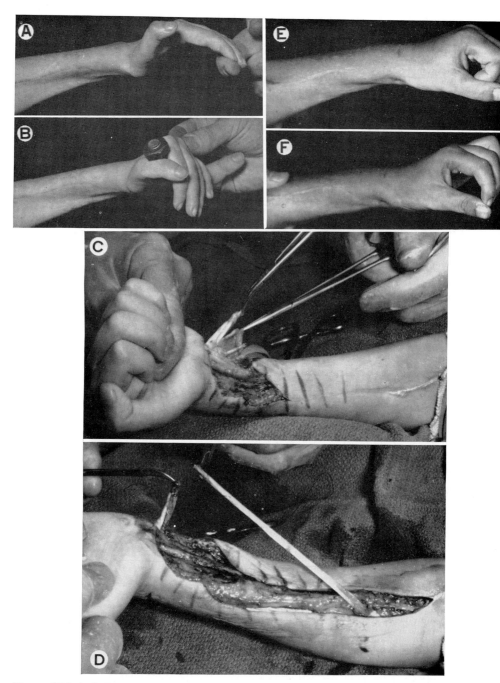

Figure 15.5.4. *A.* Postoperative view of the hand seen in Figure 15.5.1 and Figure 15.5.3, four months after the first operative procedure. Minimal contractures of the fingers and wrist are present. The nutrition of the hand is excellent and sensation is good. There is still paralysis of the thumb intrinsic muscles and the extrinsic finger flexor. *B.* Interosseous muscle function of the fingers is evident. The pinch is not good, grasp is fair, and the hook is poor because of weakness of the finger flexors. This hand is ready for replacement of thumb intrinsic muscles and finger flexors. *C.* The second operative procedure consisted of isolation of the flexores sublimis and profundi at the wrist and excision of the sublimis tendons from the wrist area to decrease fibrous adhesions. The flexores profundi were released completely from the forearm ischemic muscles. *D.* The median nerve was inspected, the trans-

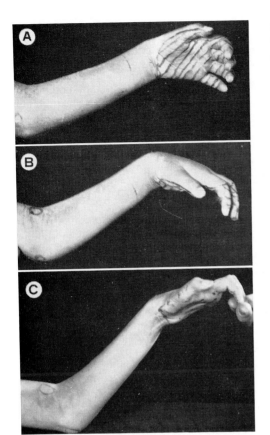

ing from the medial and lateral epicondyles and condyles of the humerus. Flexion deformity at the wrist joint usually is caused by shortening and fibrosis of the wrist, finger, and thumb flexors; the degree of deformity depends on the seriousness of the muscle and nerve involvement. The flexed position of the interphalangeal joints and extension at the metacarpophalangeal joints is related directly to the complete or partial paralysis of the intrinsic muscles and fibrosis and contracture of the flexores digitorum sublimes and profundi.

When the forearm nerves are inspected and freed from constriction, the existing contracture can be improved by release of muscle origins from the lower end of the humerus and from the upper segments of the radius and ulna. The palmaris longus, the flexor carpi radialis, and the flexor carpi ulnaris can be released at the elbow region by sharp dissection and the muscle origins advance distally. The motor branches of the median and ulnar nerves are identified and spared during this muscle advancement (Figs. 15.5.6 and 15.5.7. If there is minimal fibrosis of the wrist flexors, release of the origins will allow improvement of wrist extension. If the wrist improves by advancement of those muscles, the same process should be considered

Figure 15.5.5. A. The hand and forearm of an 8-year-old child first seen three weeks after supracondylar fracture of the elbow treated by manipulation and acute flexion. A weak radial pulse was present. There was pain, hyperesthesia, and paresthesia over the entire hand, and no active motion was present in the fingers or the wrist. Forearm skin was in poor condition and the general nutrition of the tissues of the entire forearm was unhealthy. A "traction" plaster cast was applied and immediately after application was bivalved so that the fingers could be gently stretched during daily soaking and removal of the cast. B. Preoperative lateral view of the hand shows flexion deformity of the wrist and fingers and adduction contracture of the thumb web. Positive Tinel's sign was present at the elbow over both median and ulnar nerves, implying injury at these areas. Radial sensation and muscles supplied by the radial nerve were intact. C. The same extremity two months after application of plaster traction splints, daily soaks, adequate skin care, and gentle finger stretching on an outpatient basis showed general improvement. The radial pulse had regained almost full volume, sensation improved slightly over the ulnar distribution but practically none over the median distribution. The hand was extremely painful to manipulation and the child had a pain reaction similar to that seen in causalgia. The position of the digits indicates that contractures of the flexor sublimis muscles and flexor pollicis longus existed. The opponens muscle was paralysed but the adductor pollicis brevis was functioning. The forearm was held in pronation and the elbow was limited in extension.

verse carpal ligament incised, and the extensor carpi radialis longus tendon was removed from the dorsum of the wrist and rerouted toward the volar surface of the lower forearm. This muscle was used as the motor for the finger flexors. The extensor carpi ulnaris and a free tendon graft from the foot were used to replace the opponens of the thumb. No bone surgery was necessary to correct the hand or finger contractures. E. Six months postoperative illustration of the hand showed that the child had ability to flex the proximal and distal interphalangeal joints actively. The wrist could be voluntarily bent and elevated, and this assisted finger function. Sensation had returned except for recognition of two point pressure. Strength was diminished noticeably but the hand was useful. F. An opponens transfer activated the thumb satisfactorily. Pinch and opposition were present. The first dorsal interosseous was functioning and controlled the index finger. The wrist was stable. Deformity did not occur as the child became older, and during the several years of follow-up there has been only minimal evidence of recurrence of a tendency to wrist flexion contracture.

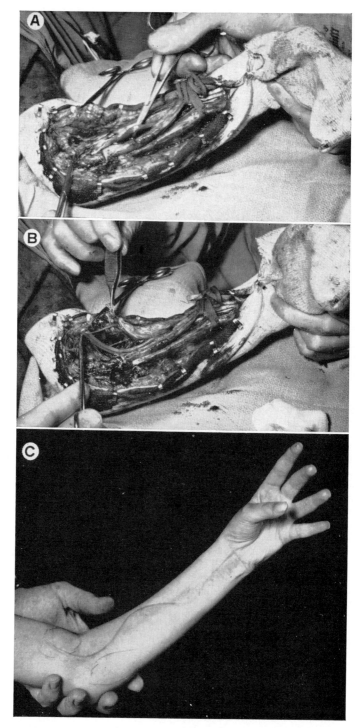

Figure 15.5.6. A. Photograph taken at time of surgical treatment of the hand shown in Figure 15.5.5. The full arm and elbow region were opened approximately four months after injury. Circulation and nutrition of the skin were adequate. The first step included advancement and release of the muscle bellies from the humerus and ulna. This allowed full view of the upper portion of the median nerve with its motor branches. The wrist contracture improved about 25 per cent after the proximal release but no

for the thumb and finger flexors, both superficial and deep. The motor branches should be spared. Postoperative traction, directed toward improving hand extension and thumb extension, should be carried out diligently for several weeks.

The muscle advancement or "sliding" operation will not be beneficial in proving wrist and finger flexion contracture if the deformity is of long duration and if fibrosis is extensive.

Neurolysis and release of the muscle origins may be sufficient to allow rapid improvement of the contracture by splinting, traction, and exercise. If the muscle advancement operation does not allow noticeable improvement in wrist or finger extension, each unit is lengthened at the musculotendinous junction. The tendon lengthening incision for the flexores profundi should be made far enough proximal to the transverse carpal ligament to allow 2 cm of tendon between the suture line and the ligament when the digits are in full extension. The amount of lengthening will depend on the condition of the muscle mass. Lengthening, as a rule, should be sufficient to allow the digits to extend to 0° when the wrist and finger joints are held at 0°. The flexor pollicis longus should be lengthened at its musculotendinous function proximal to the annular ligament at the wrist. This digit should be released enough to allow the tip of the thumb to be brought to a straight line when the metacarpal is in extension and external rotation. The flexores digitorum sublimis may prevent the digits from being completely extended after the profundus tendons are lengthened; the superficial flexors should be lengthened at the musculotendinous junction. The decision to remove the distal segments of the sublimis tendons rather than lengthen them depends upon the extent of fibrosis in the forearm, the degree of contracture of the fingers, and the likelihood of recovery of the forearm musculature. The more extensive the contracture, the more indication there is for removal of the distal segments of the sublimis tendons in the palm.

Preoperative examination will determine whether or not tendon lengthenings will result in adequate correction of the wrist and interphalangeal joint contractures. Flexion of the wrist and flexion of the metacarpophalangeal joints should allow complete extension of the digits if the primary cause of the contracture is in the extrinsic finger flexors. Volkmann's contracture of long standing shows shortening of the volar ligaments of the wrist and fingers, contracture of the interosseous membrane, and shortening of all the deep volar connective tissue. These contractures are managed by ligamentous release of the fingers, joint arthrodesis, or other appropriate local therapy in addition to forearm surgery already mentioned. The purpose of these initial operative procedures is: (1) Decompression of the entire median nerve to improve sensation, protect motor power, and diminish pain. Other involved nerves are treated in a similar manner. (2) Rapid correction of the flexion deformity of the fingers and wrists to prevent fixed contractures within the digits. (3) Excision of large segments of nonviable muscle, as these tend to cause fibrosis of the adjacent musculature and do not stretch during rapid growth of the forearm bones.

Substitution muscles and tendons are available for reinforcement and are useful at the appropriate time. These tendon transfers done for substitution of intrinsic or extrinsic muscles are not done at the time of the initial release operation. Tendon transfer surgery is postponed until there is an indication of the degree of nerve recovery, and until finger and wrist contractures have been corrected by plaster appliction and elastic extension traction. Also, traction is used to increase the width of the thumb web and to provide resistance for the weakened intrinsic muscles of the hand. The cast may be bivalved and removed daily for cleansing of the skin. Active assistive exercise with traction apparatus should be done several hours each day.

The permanent status of the intrinsic muscles of the hand cannot always be determined during the first few

change was noted in the finger or thumb flexors. The midsegment of the nerve is identified by the hemostat in this photograph and the area proximal to this was the point of greatest nerve constriction. To correct the digit contractures, the sublimis and profundus tendons, as well as the flexor pollicis longus and pronator teres, were tenotomized at the musculotendinous junction and a Z lengthening was completed. Sensation of the thumb and fingers improved rapidly after the neurolysis and release of the "internal tourniquet." B. The median and ulnar nerves showed compression in the upper third of the forearm, constriction by fibrous tissues in the midforearm, and compression by the transverse carpal ligament at the wrist. Pain was rapidly relieved within a few days after the surgery and correction of the contracture progressed quickly after the tenotomies. Minimal fibrous tissue was excised and there was no indication here for removal of any specific large infarct. C. Postoperative hand one year after injury shows recovery of thumb (median nerve) intrinsic muscles and good function of the intrinsic muscles supplied by the ulnar nerve. Sensation of the index finger improved but was not yet normal for two point discrimination. Nutrition of the hand was excellent. Minimal tenderness existed at the elbow at the site of the old injury, and paresthesias could still be elicited when the ulnar and median nerves were percussed at the elbow region and in the upper forearm. Finger flexors did not function and it was necessary to supplement them by transfer of the extensor carpi radialis longus to the distal segment of the profundus tendons. A seven-year followup showed good sensation, good strength, adequate coordination, and no increase of contracture during the adolescent growth spurt.

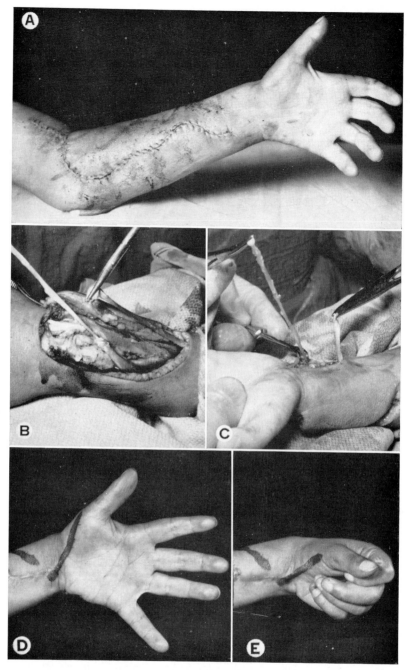

Figure 15.5.7. A. Forearm and hand of a child, age five, whose median and ulnar nerves had been released and whose wrist and finger flexors had been tenotomized 10 days before this photograph was made. The operation had been done three months after treatment for a supracondylar fracture which resulted in Volkmann's ischemia and contracture. Median nerve sensation was impaired, ulnar nerve sensation was diminished slightly, and the thumb intrinsic muscles supplied by the median nerve were not functioning. Burning pain was a major problem preoperatively and this was relieved within 48 hours after surgery. B. Eight months after injury and four months after the first operative procedure. The intrinsic thumb muscles had not shown evidence of recovery and the finger and thumb flexors were not functioning. The extensor carpi ulnaris was lengthened by a toe extensor tendon, rerouted toward the volar surface of the wrist from the ulnar side, passed subcutaneously over the thenar eminence, and

weeks after the initial injury. Forearm decompression and a waiting period, will give an indication of the potential of the intrinsic thumb muscles (Fig. 15.5.7 A). Decompression of the median nerve will allow maximal regeneration of the sensory and motor axons in an unimpeded way.

Late Treatment (Tendon Transfers)

Neurolysis, release of specific contractures, excision of large segments of nonviable tissue followed by elastic traction on the fingers and wrist, and active and passive exercise will allow maximal improvement of the extremity. Figure 15.5. 4 A and B represents the hand of a child who has had the treatment mentioned; improvement in sensation allowed detection of pin point, recognition of light touch and temperature change, but lack of detection of two-point discrimination. The intrinsic muscles of the thumb have recovered completely but the flexores digitorum profundi, which had been ischemic initially, did not recover. A substitute for these motors was necessary, and this was obtained by transfer of the extensor carpi radialis longus around the radial side of the forearm into the distal ends of the flexor tendons (Fig. 15.5. 4 C and D). These flexor tendons had originally been lengthened at the time of the median neurolysis, and these completely severed at the time of the second stage operative procedure because the flexor profundus muscle mass was not functioning. The flexor tendons were isolated on the volar surface of the lower forearm and separated from the fibrous ischemic muscle mass by sharp dissection, by tendon strippers, and manual traction to obtain full extension of the digits and freedom of gliding of the flexor tendons. The extensor carpi radialis longus tendon was severed from its attachment into the second metacarpal, and the muscle and tendon were mobilized freely on the dorsum of the forearm. The muscle was then rerouted under the brachioradialis and inserted into the flexores profundi by splitting the extensor tendon into two segments, and passing each of these through small slits in the flexor tendons in such a way that appropriate tension could be obtained. The final tension must be adequate to hold the digits in 45° flexion at the metacarpophalangeal joints and 45° at each of the interphalangeal joints. A firm suture is obtained by the use of medium braided wire or synthetic polyester suture, and the hand and digits are immobilized in 20° of flexion. Plaster splints are placed on the dorsum of the hand and forearm and include the elbow. Active exercise is started in three weeks and gentle extension is obtained by use of molded plaster splints at night, mild manual stretching each hour, and, at the end of six weeks, elastic traction and outriggers if necessary. Full extension may not be possible because of the limited excursion of the wrist extensor muscles and persistent fibrosis of the digits. In this instance, the result at the end of six months is evident in Figure 15.5.4 E and F.

If the flexor pollicis longus tendon has been severed because of extensive ischemia of its muscle mass, the extensor carpi radialis longus may be added to this digit tendon also. If a paucity of transfer motors exists, the thumb should be included with the finger flexors.

In certain instances, the intrinsic muscles of the thumb may not recover and muscle power must be added as a substitute. The extensor carpi ulnaris plus a free tendon graft may be used as a motor for providing opposition. The tendon is detached about 5 cm proximal to its insertion and elongated by a free tendon graft from the second or third segment of the extensor digitorum communis of the foot. The suture line bet-

---

attached to the proximal phalanx of the thumb as a substitute for muscles of opposition. The extensor carpi radialis longus, which is seen in the hemostat in the illustration, was detached and passed around the radial side of the distal forearm into the flexor profundus muscles. Fibrosis in the interosseous area made it inadvisable to pass the tendon through the interosseous membrane. C. The extensor carpi radialis longus, which is the short tendon in the illustration, has been rerouted toward the volar surface and is ready for attachment to the flexor digitorum profundus muscles. The extensor carpi ulnaris and its graft are ready for passage subcutaneously into the thumb as a subcutaneous substitute for the muscles of opposition. In general, the opponens attachment is carried out by drilling a hole in the proximal portion of the proximal phalanx and knuckling the tendon in the hole and fixing it with a stainless steel wire that will be removed. D. Here is the hand several weeks after surgery; the markings are in line with the tendon transfers. The child is able to open the hand completely whereas before the first operative procedure the typical "claw digits" were present. Sensation had improved rapidly and there was satisfactory, although incomplete, extension of the wrist because two wrist extensors had been removed to replace the ischemic flexor tendons and the remaining extensor digitorum communis and extensor carpi radialis brevis were not normal in strength, and therefore not able to stabilize the hand fully. E. This shows the ability of the fingers to be flexed and the thumb to be moved about six months after the tendon transfers. Active flexion at the interphalangeal joints was possible, functional opposition of the thumb existed, and reasonably good stability of the wrist was present. Because of weakness of the extensor musculature, arthrodesis of the wrist was contemplated when the child became older. She moved from this area in 1953 and was not heard from until 1963, when Dr. William Frackelton of Milwaukee saw her for examination, as she had moved to that city. He described normal sensation, good finger flexion, adequate stability but incomplete hand extension at the wrist, and suggested to her that arthrodesis of the wrist should be done.

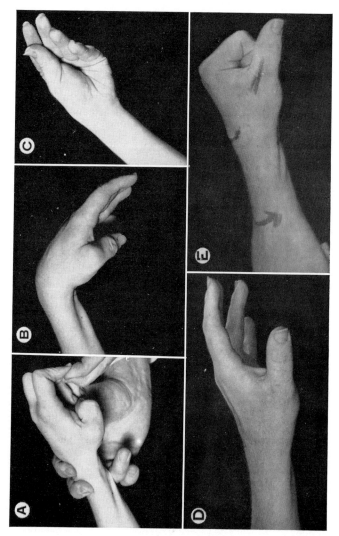

Figure 15.5.8. A. Hand of a 19-year-old youth with Volkmann's contracture present for 12 years after a supracondylar fracture. No surgery had been done to the forearm at any time. Median nerve sensation was protective throughout the median nerve zone. The patient had no recognition of light touch, had difficulty in differentiating large coins, and had no discrimination for two point pressure. The flexor digitorum sublimis muscles were contracted and there was limited active and passive extension of the digits except when the wrist was in flexion. A tenodesis effect compromised the major means whereby the hand was used for grasp and hook. The flexor pollicis longus was contracted and pulled the thumb into the palm when the wrist was in neutral position. The thumb was voluntarily active with adequate intrinsic muscles but the stability was unsatisfactory because of hypermobility of the metacarpophalangeal joint and overpull of the flexor pollicis brevis. The wrist could be forced to 0° with considerable difficulty. Malformation of the distal end of the radius had occurred as a result of the prolonged flexed position of the wrist. A positive Tinel's sign was still present in the region of the sublimis and pronator teres. *B.* The fingers could be completely extended passively and actively with intact interossei and tenodesis of extensors when the wrist was in flexion. With the wrist in full flexion, however, the thumb could not be extended adequately to allow grasp of small or large objects. The extensor pollicis longus and abductor pollicis longus were normal in strength but could not extend the thumb against the firm flexion contracture of the flexor pollicis longus. The position of the hand as illustrated was the way the hand was placed when grasp or hook were initiated. The thumb in the palm was one of the major handicaps. *C.* There was no active flexion of the proximal or distal interphalangeal joints or the distal joint of the thumb because of muscle injury and nerve ischemia at the time of the original injury. The

ween the free tendon graft and the motor should be about 5 cm proximal to the natural insertion of the extensor carpi ulnaris. The extensor carpi ulnaris used as an opponens muscle and the extensor carpi radialis longus as a digital flexor will not deprive the wrist of controlled dorsiflexion if the extensor carpi radialis brevis, the extensor digitorum communis, and the extensors of the thumb are within functional level (Fig. 15.5. 7 *B* and *E*). If both extensors are utilized for flexor muscle power in a growing child, a protective night splint, or occasional plaster wedging, or even tendon lengthening are necessary to prevent flexion contracture during rapid growth periods.

Other tendon transfers include use of the brachioradialis as a thumb flexor by mobilizing the muscle belly and tendon high in the forearm and rerouting the musculotendinous unit to the volar aspect of the distal forearm; the brachioradialis tendon is attached to the distal segment of the flexor pollicis longus about 4 cm proximal to the transverse retinacular ligament.

The biceps humerus muscle may be utilized as a digital flexor if the muscles supplied by the radial nerve have been partially damaged and are not available for transfer to the volar forearm muscles. The biceps insertion is detached from the radius through a horizontal incision in the elbow crease. The muscle is elongated by a toe extensor, or plantaris or a forearm tendon, which is passed subcutaneously from the elbow to the junction of the middle and distal forearm. The distal forearm segments of the thumb and finger flexors are isolated and sutured with firm tension into the prolongation of the biceps humerus muscle. Segments of the flexores digitorum sublimis may be removed from the distal forearm and hand and used to reinforce the point of suture at both the elbow and the lower forearm region. After this procedure, several patients have obtained sufficient improvement to flex the digits when the elbow is in extension and the wrist is in dorsiflexion. They have a hook and a weak pinch and are able to use the hand for carrying light objects.

Carpalectomy and Digital Joint Arthrodesis for Old Contractures

Removal of the proximal and/or distal row of carpal bones may be the most desirable way of bringing the hand to a neutral position and, at the same time, maintaining enough flexibility to activate a tenodesis action of flexors and extensors of the digits. In the treatment of contractures of long standing with severe enough deformities to justify carpalectomy, removal of the carpal bones should be done before tendon transfer is done. If the extensors are not strong enough for transfer but rate poor plus (25 per cent) to fair minus (40 per cent), then the carpalectomy can be followed by arthrodesis of the interphalangeal joints of the fingers and arthrodesis of the metacarpophalangeal joint of the thumb. The relief of contracture afforded by removal of the carpal bones will allow a hand with protective sensation and stable digits to function as a hook and an assistive unit which, in many ways, is superior to a prosthesis.

Carpalectomy in an adult who has had an ischemic episode as a child will provide improvement in hand and finger function and offers a method of treatment that will maintain reasonable joint motion, relative lengthening of the forearm flexor muscle mass, and diminution of finger contractures. Figure 15.5. 8 *A* to *C* shows an extremity that had been injured 15 years before the time this examination and photograph were made. The finger flexors were irreparably damaged by ischemia but the intrinsic muscles of the hand were functioning and adequate sensation had returned. A wrist flexion deformity had occurred and pinch and grasp were limited when the hand was at 10° of flexion because of excessive tension by the extensor

pinch was weak and the grasp for large objects was absent. *D.* This postoperative appearance of the hand was possible after proximal and distal carpalectomy, leaving the pisiform and the greater multangular. In addition to the carpalectomy, arthrodesis of the metacarpophalangeal joint was utilized to stabilize the thumb and obtain moderate shortening of this digit, to correct the severe flexion deformity at the joint. Tendon transfers were not done during this first stage reconstruction. Thumb extension and digit extension were performed adequately within a few weeks after these "shortening" operations. Active motion at the metacarpophalangeal joints of the fingers improved as the tension on the extensors was relieved, and thumb motion was considerably better after stabilization of the metacarpophalangeal joint. Internal fixation with several crossed Kirschner wires allowed early mobilization of the thumb and made it possible to do tendon transfers within several weeks after wrist arthroplasty. *E.* Four months after carpalectomy, the extensor carpi radialis longus tendon was transferred to the volar aspect of the wrist and sutured into the flexor digitorum profundus muscles, leaving these tendons attached to the fibrotic muscle mass. This assured maintenance of the tenodesis effect of the profundus tendons and supplemented their strength with the wrist extensor. Active flexion of the interphalangeal joints through a functional range was possible after the tendon transfer. The wrist was stable and strong, and active motion was maintained at the wrist joint although limited considerably when compared with normal. Even limited motion was important in assisting voluntary finger flexion and flexor tenodesis. Cosmetic improvement was obvious, and pinch, grasp, and hook were established, along with individualized flexion of the digits. This patient was examined 13 years after the reconstructive surgery and the muscle strength had persisted, the sensation had not changed, the wrist was not painful, and the thumb-to-index pinch was strong.

mechanism of the digits. The fingers could not be forcibly flexed because of weakness of the finger and thumb flexors and because of the firm wrist contracture. Structural bone change involved the wrist joint and contractures of the volar capsule of the wrist were of such severity that tenotomy of the wrist and finger flexor tendons was not sufficient to elevate the hand to neutral or dorsiflexed position. Wrist joint arthrodesis was not advisable, as this would eliminate the dynamic affect of wrist motion on tenodesis action of the digits. A partial proximal and distal carpalectomy was done, leaving the pisiform and the trapezium. This allowed elevation of the wrist to 15° beyond the straight line and placed the fingers in an optimal position for grasp and pinch. Also, a flexion deformity of the metacarpophalangeal joint of the thumb had resulted from prolonged contracture of the flexor pollicis longus, hypermobility of the joint, and subsequent contracture of the anterior capsule and collateral ligaments. Soft tissue release was not sufficient to obtain stability because of deficiencies in the flexor and extensor mechanisms. Arthrodesis of the metacarpophalangeal joint positioned the thumb out of the palm and provided a stable base for the thumb intrinsic muscle. The initial operative procedure included carpalectomy and thumb joint arthrodesis. The second operation consisted of transfer of the extensor carpi radialis longus tendon, subcutaneously around the radial border of the distal forearm and suture of the tendon into the flexores digitorum profundi tendons. The suture was done proximal to the transverse retinacular ligament. With the hand in neutral position, with wrist position improved and the contracture diminished, active flexion at the interphalangeal joints was possible by the wrist extensor tendon to the volar forearm tendons (Fig. 15.8.8 E).

SPECIAL CONSIDERATIONS OF RECONSTRUCTION AFTER VOLKMANN'S CONTRACTURE

1. Split skin graft or abdominal flap.
2. Thumb adduction contracture release including interosseous stripping, adductor lengthening or excision, excision of trapezium, and new skin in the thumb web.
3. Nerve graft or nerve transfer; median, ulnar, or superficial radial to distal median nerve.
4. Arthrodesis of interphalangeal joints of the fingers.
5. Distal amputation.

Split Skin Graft

Use of split skin grafting may be an essential step in the early or late reconstructive program. Occasionally, skin must be incised from above the elbow to the midpalm to obtain full relief of the internal tamponade during the acute phase of the ischemic syndrome. This is particularly necessary when the circulation to both the hand and forearm muscles is diminished. Once the blood supply has improved in these critical areas, closure of the skin is not always desirable because of recurrent vascular and nerve compression. The wound may be left open to granulate for five days. As soon as a dry, firm, base occurs, split skin is used to fill the defect.

Split skin grafting is used to cover small areas of ulceration from skin ischemia in the region of the elbow, forearm, or hand. This may be done within several days after the forearm muscles and nerve tissue have been decompressed. Split skin may be used also to open the thumb web and to replace areas of fibrosis in the palm in the salvage hand before doing any final tendon surgery.

Abdominal Skin Flap

Figure 15.5.9 A shows an extremity several months after a severe roller injury. The skin on the forearm has healed by keloid but surgical entry for decompression of the median nerve, tendon lengthening, and excision of excessive fibrosis was not advisable until an abdominal flap had been applied.

Carpalectomy

Removal of the proximal and distal carpal bones is a useful salvage operation if tendon transfer and tendon lengthening operations are not possible. If limited active flexion and extension of the fingers and wrist do exist, even though these functions are less than normal, carpalectomy will allow the digits to close by a combination of active flexion and extension, as well as tenodesis (Fig. 15.5.9 B).

Ischemia of the volar surface of the forearm and direct trauma to the extensor surface of the forearm may co-exist. This combination of injuries eliminates the early use of supplementary motors and makes any tendon transfer unlikely. If flexion contracture of the wrist develops, carpalectomy is done to improve the range of wrist joint motion and enhance the tenodesis effect. The hand may then function as a hook with moderate grasp and pinch (Fig. 15.5.10).

Occasionally, the vascular damage is of such severity and the time after injury so long that repair of the median nerve will not result in satisfactory sensory recovery (Fig. 15.5.11 A). Carpalectomy is then a salvage operation done to increase the range of motion of the hand and to improve the pinch and hook. The patient is taught to use visual cues with hand action.

Excision of Trapezium

Arthroplasty at the base of the thumb is useful in severe contractures of the hand when the thumb web has been partially obliterated by skin, muscle, and joint change, and particularly by extensive fibrosis of the intrinsic hand muscles. Also, this procedure is useful when sensation has recovered for protective use, but not sufficient to warrant reconstructive surgery except for positioning of the thumb, and arthroplasty or ar-

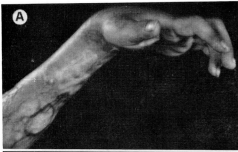
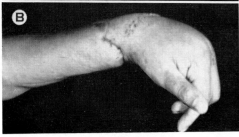

Figure 15.5.9. A. Muscle and skin ischemia and deep contracture resulted from direct trauma to the forearm and elbow when the extremity was pulled into a heavy roller. The brachial artery and adjacent nerves were compressed. Contracture of the wrist occurred within the first few weeks after injury, associated with adduction contracture of the thumb, hyperextension of the metacarpophalangeal joints and flexion contracture of the fingers. The intrinsic muscles of the thumb maintained activity. The extensor muscles were damaged severely and were not available for use as tendon transfers. The goal was directed toward mobilization of the wrist, coverage of the forearm with healthy skin, improvement in sensation, and establishment of a digital hook. *B.* The initial procedure included a direct abdominal flap to the forearm, followed in several weeks by proximal and distal carpalectomy. The thumb web was opened at the time of the carpalectomy, the adductor muscle was lengthened, and the fascia was incised. The collateral ligaments of the metacarpophalangeal joints were excised and the extensor apparatus was released from the dorsum of the hand. Active wrist motion occurred in flexion and extension. The tenodesis effect was enhanced by improving function of the metacarpophalangeal joints and providing extension at the wrist joint. Tendon transfers in this hand were not practical but the patient maintained a good grasp and pinch. Shortening of the forearm bones should not be considered in most of these extremities because of precarious condition of soft tissues.

throdesis of other digits. Adduction contracture is released by removing the interosseous muscle mass from the first and second metacarpals, lengthening the

adductor pollicis muscle at the musculotendinous junction, incising the heavy deep fibrous bands that have formed after ischemia and local edema, and capsulotomy of the first metacarpal-carpal joint. Stability is usually no problem fibrosis has been severe. Mobilization of the thumb is superior to arthrodesis or intermetacarpal or bone block if function of the hand is already limited. Silicone Dacron implants have been used for the trapezium in two instances in hands with ischemic forearm necrosis and good stability and fair mobility have occurred.

Arthrodesis of the Interphalangeal Joints of the Fingers

Arthrodesis of the interphalangeal joints of digits, deformed by severe flexion deformity at the proximal and distal interphalangeal joints secondary to extensive forearm fibrosis and ischemia of the hand,

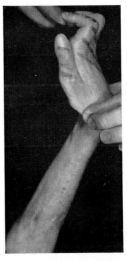

Figure 15.5.10. Hand of a 13-year-old boy who had a mild supracondylar fracture 18 months before examination. Manipulation and flexion were recorded as the initial treatment. Median and ulnar nerve sensations were completely absent immediately after the accident but radial nerve function was fair. Trophic changes were present on the fingertips and extensive dermatitis and pyodermia were present on the forearm skin. The nutrition of the hand and forearm was poor and the radial pulse was weak. This is a "preamputation hand" suitable only for salvage procedures. Skin attention and healing required several weeks of treatment. Traction splinting does no good in such a situation. Carpalectomy was done to get the wrist up and relieve tension on the extensor tendons. Median and ulnar nerve anastomoses were considered but have not yet been done. Ultimate function will be limited to hook and weak thumb-to-side-of-index pinch.

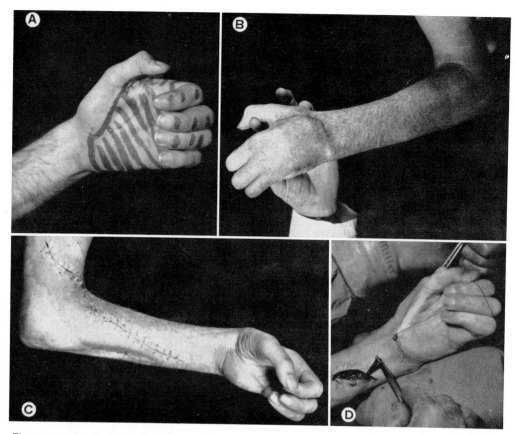

Figure 15.5.11. A. Hand of a 25-year-old man examined 16 months after repair of a small herniation of the flexor muscles of the forearm had been attempted. Volkmann's ischemia and contracture resulted. There was minimal sensation present over the median nerve zone and no sensation along ulnar nerve distribution. The radial nerve muscles were severely damaged. The thumb was in external rotation, the web space was contracted, and there were fixed contractures at the proximal interphalangeal joints. Wrist flexion deformity was also present. The hand was useless for pinch, grasp, or hook. Reshaping the digits and establishing even slight sensory recovery was worthwhile before considering amputation. *B.* Initial procedures included: (1) excision of the contracted adductor muscles and fascia; (2) excision of greater multangular to diminish adduction contracture of the thumb and mobilize thumb; (3) excision of proximal and distal carpal bones, except the pisiform, to correct wrist flexion contracture and to remove tension on the median nerve when the hand was brought up to neutral; and (4) amputation of fifth ray because of irreparable ulnar nerve lesion. *C.* The second stage reconstruction included exploration of the forearm. The nerve was ischemic over a long segment starting at the pronator radii teres and extending to the lower portion of the forearm. A large neuroma that had resulted just distal to the pronator muscle was resected, and resuture of the nerve was accomplished by transplantation over the pronator teres. Deep sensation improved but there was little change in epicritic sensation. The thumb did have protective sensation on the radial aspect from the superficial radial nerve branches, and this important overlap assures protection for this digit. *D.* Final procedures included transfer of the extensor carpi ulnaris tendon prolonged by a tendon graft from toe extensors as an opponens, and arthrodesis of the proximal and distal interphalangeal joints of the fingers in a position of function. The patient developed a good grasp, pinch, and hook. Several years later, the function of the hand proved that this salvage unit was superior to a prothesis in most activities.

can be done in order to provide digits used for hook and grasp even though a good range of motion may not be obtained by mobilization of the forearm muscles or the metacarpophalangeal joints. Figure 15.5.11 *C* and 15.5.11 *D* represents a situation where tendon transfers to the thumb and arthrodesis of the proximal interphalangeal joints of the digits were done to improve grasp and hook even though minimial sensation was present. The combination of mobilization of the thumb by release of the adduction contracture, excision of the os trapezium, transfer of tendons to the thumb, and arthrodesis of the interphalangeal joints (Fig. 15.5.11 C and 15.5.11 D) will give a helping hand that should be protected by a glove and that will require visual cues while it is used. Frequently this kind of hand is superior to a prosthesis, if wrist motion has been partially recovered by carpalectomy and if there are enough arm or forearm motors available to provide a few degrees of digit motion.

Nerve Graft or Nerve Transfer

Median or ulnar nerve grafting was not done in any of the 60 patients included in this review. In most instances, neurolysis was sufficient to aid in the recovery of protective sensation or in some instances, sensation that approached normal. Bulb suture, followed by a second or even a third suture, is usually superior to substitution by long segments of free nerve graft, particularly in the presence of extensive ischemia. On one occasion, a large superficial branch of the radial nerve was sutured into the distal segment of the median when the defect in the midforearm was several centimeters long and the duration of the ischemic process had been several months. This was an appropriate solution in a young person, in the presence of moderate fibrosis in the elbow area and more extensive damage at the midforearm area, and was a satisfactory alternate to suturing the median and ulnar nerves together and advancing the distal segment of the ulnar to the distal segment of the median. We have examined or treated 60 patients during various phases of the ischemic process, and protective sensation has been obtained in 56 without utilizing nerve grafting. Two nerve sutures showed no improvement, and two patients had injuries thought to be irreparable by any reconstructive surgery.

Axillary or brachial artery trauma secondary to intimal damage associated with percutaneous arteriography may cause ischemia of three major nerves of the arm and forearm and peri-articular fibrosis of the forearm and hand. In even more severe instances, injury to the axillary or brachial artery may result in insufficient blood supply to the forearm and hand with resulting gangrene and tissue necrosis. In the latter instance, there is little question about the necessity for amputation.

Hand deletion, even in the most severe form of Volkmann's, is usually not desirable, as the hand, even without sensation, provided with pinch and hook and moderate wrist motion, will be superior to that with a prosthesis in many instances.

SUMMARY

1. Once the primary arterial embarrassment has been relieved, decompression of the median and other nerves is the most essential treatment that can be done either early or in the late phases of the established Volkmann's ischemic syndrome.

2. The relationship of the median nerve to the pronator radii teres and the flexores digitorum sublimis has been emphasized and details have been presented describing decompression of the median nerve in the upper forearm region.

3. The evidence supplied by the group of patients included in this review indicates that primary arterial insufficiency is the major cause of Volkmann's ischemia. Secondary factors such as venous congestion, accumulation of metabolites and other biochemical, and cellular alterations play a part in aggravating the initial process or, occasionally, are primarily responsible for the tissue damage.

4. Correction of the flexion contractures of the wrist and fingers should be accomplished as rapidly and as early as possible. The discreet use of outrigger traction will allow moderate improvement during the early phase, but several months of traction and splinting will not provide total correction. Lengthening of the muscle unit at the musculotendinous junction may be done at the same time that neurolysis is carried out. Tenotomy without lengthening may be necessary in the late cases.

5. Excision of the muscle infarct, or ischemic myositis, is not essential for restoration of function; if indicated, however, it should be done at the time of neurolysis to diminish the possibilities of future contracture during rapid growth period. Muscle tissue that is not obviously completely fibrotic should not be removed. Some regeneration has been observed.

6. Voluntary flexion of the digits and opposition of the thumb may be restored by using the wrist extensor tendons as finger or thumb flexors. If the ulnar innervated muscles are spared, the flexor carpi ulnaris may be used as a thumb or finger motor. The brachioradialis may be used as a thumb flexor if other motors are not available. The biceps humerus will give moderate active finger flexion that is usually functionally more beneficial than flexor tenodesis.

7. Supplementary skin may be useful in the overall reconstructive program. An abdominal pedicle flap is used to replace badly damaged forearm skin. Split skin graft is used to cover cutaneous ulcerations that have occurred as a result of the initial trauma. Split skin may also be used in the adductor web space to assist in mobilizing the thumb and in diminishing the adduction contracture.

8. Carpalectomy is a useful procedure for diminishing flexion contracture of the wrist in adults who have an old contracture. Carpalectomy is usually not necessary or advisable in children.

9. Excision of the trapezium is useful in mobilizing the base of the thumb and diminishing the adduction contracture. Arthrodesis of the metacarpophalangeal joint is helpful when severe flexion contracture of the thumb exists and tendon lengthening and other soft tissue operations have neither established continuity of the extensor mechanism nor relieved the contracted volar capsule.

10. Volkmann's ischemia in the early phase and Volkmann's contracture in a later stage both should be

treated actively and vigorously by a combination of restoration of arterial and venous blood flow, neurolysis, muscle and tendon lengthening, muscle and tendon substitutions, active splinting, and active exercise. Prevention must be emphasized. The attending physician must be alert always to the possibility of arterial insufficiency regardless of the cause of the original injury. This is true after trauma to the extremity or specific trauma to the arterial tree such as might occur with arteriography.

REFERENCES

1. Adams, J. P. Personal communication, January, 1957.
2. Beaton, L. E., and Anson, B. J. The relation of the median nerve to the pronator teres muscle. Anat. Rec., 75: 23-26, 1939.
3. Bell, G. E., and Goldner, J. L. Compression neuropathy of the median nerve. South. Med. J., 49: 966, 1956.
4. Blount, W. P. Fractures in Children. Baltimore, Williams & Wilkins, 1954.
5. Brooks, B. Experimental study of Volkmann's paralysis. Arch. Surg., 5: 188-216, 1922.
6. Bunnell, S. Surgery of the Hand, Ed. 3 Philadelphia, Lippincott, 1956.
7. Console, A. D. Segmental arterial spasm associated with supracondylar fracture of the elbow. S. Clin. North Am., 28: 467-472, 1948.
8. Crystal, D. K., Burgess, E., and Wangeman, C. Thrombectomy in Volkmann's contracture. N. Engl. J. Med., 247: 10-15, 1952.
9. Cywes, S., and Louw, J. H. Phlegmasia cerulea dolens; successful treatment by relieving fasciotomy. Surgery, 51: 161-176, 1962.
10. Denny-Brown, D., and Brenner, C. Paralysis of nerve induced by direct pressure and by tourniquet. Arch. Neurol. Psychiatr., 51: Jan.-June, 1944.
11. Deverell, W. Median nerve compression secondary to forced supination of forearm of jet pilots. Piedmont Orthopeadic Society Letter, 1971.
12. Dunlop, J. Transcondylar fractures of the humerus in children, J. Bone Joint Surg., 21: 59, 1939.
13. Eaton, R. C., and Green, W. T. Volkmann's contracture in children. American academy of Orthopedie Surgeons, New York, 1965.
14. Fletcher, V. Abdominal pain due to compression of nerve or vessel by fascia of the abdominal wall. South. M. J., 48: 644, 1955.
15. Goldner, J. L. Volkmann's contracture. J. Bone Joint Surg., 37A: 621, 1955.
16. Griffiths, D. L. The management of acute circulatory failure in an injured limb. J. Bone Joint Surg., 30B: 280-289, 1948.
17. Hamiovici, H. Gangrene of extremities of venous origin. Circulation, 1: 225-240, 1950.
18. Jones, R. Volkmann's ischemic contracture with special reference to treatment. Br. Med. J., 2: 639, 1928.
19. Jones, S. G. Volkmann's contracture. J. Bone Joint Surg., 17: 649, 1935.
20. Kulowski, J. Segmental arterial spasm of the brachial artery (report of case treated by procaine into median nerve). Surgery, 38: 1087-1089, 1955.
21. Leriche, R. Surgery of Pain (Translated from the French and edited by Archibald Young.) Baltimore, Williams & Wilkins, 1939, p. 310-311.
22. Lipscomb, P. R., and Burleson, R. J. Vascular and neural complications in supracondylar fractures of the humerus in children. J. Bone Joint Surg., 37A: 487-492, 1955.
23. Littler, W. Personal communication, 1957.
24. McNab, I. Personal communication. Anterior compartment Syndrome. Biodynamics and different classifications of anterior compartment syndrome.
25. Meyerding, H. W. Volkmann's ischaemic contracture associated with supracondylar fracture of the humerus. J.A.M.A., 106: 1139, 1936.
26. Mitchell, W. J., and Adams, J. P. Effective management for supracondylar fractures of humerus in children. Clinical Orthop., 23: 197, 1962.
27. Ochsner, J. L., and Knudson, R. J. Phlegmasia cerulea dolens after aorto-iliac operations. J.A.M.A., 182: 942-943, 1962.
28. Parkes, A. R. Traumatic ischaemia of peripheral nerves with some observations on Volkmann's ischaemic contracture. Br. J. Surg., 32: 403, 1945.
29. Seddon, H. J. Volkmann's contracture: treatment by excision of the infarct. J. Bone Joint Surg., 38B: 152-174, 1956.
30. Steindler, A. Orthopaedic Operations. Springfield, C. C Thomas, 1940.
31. Sunderland, S. Classification of peripheral nerve injuries producing loss of function. Brain, 74: 491-516, 1951.
32. Sunderland, S. Blood supply of the nerves of the upper limb in man. Arch. Neurol. Psychiatr., 53: 91, 1945.
33. Surls, J. K. Extension in Volkmann's ischaemic contracture. N. Y. J. Med., 3227-3234, 1962.
34. Sutton, H. J. Volkmann's Ischemia, British Medical Journal, 1: 1587, 1964.
35. Volkmann, R. V., Die Ischamischen Muskellahmungen und Kontracturen. Zentralbl. Chir., 8: 801-803, 1881.
36. Wartenburg, R. Digitalgia parestheticagonyalgia. Neurology, 4: 106, 1954.
37. White, J. W., and Stubbins, S. G. Carpectomy for intractable flexion deformities of the wrist. J. Bone Joint Surg., 26: 131, 1944.
38. Wissinger, A. Personl communication. Measurement of subfascial pressure of forearm after trauma with water manometer.
39. Woodhall, B., and Davis, C., Jr. Changes in the arteries nervorum in peripheral nerve injuries in man. J. Neuropathol. Exp. Neurol., 9: 335-343, 1950.
40. Woodhall, B. Personal communication, 1955.

F.

Intrinsic and Extensor Contracture of the Hand due to Ischemic and Nonischemic Causes

J. Leonard Goldner

GENERAL CONSIDERATIONS

Fibrous or ischemic changes occur in the intrinsic muscles or their tendinous extensions into the thumb or fingers resulting in mild, moderate, or severe contractures of the metacarpophalangeal or the interphalangeal joints, or the thumb web. Arterial insufficiency may occur from wrist, forearm, or elbow injuries causing intimal damage or excessive external pressure on the vessel that prevents arterial input. Chemical injections of the arteries at the wrist or in the hand may result in ischemia of the intereossei or lumbricals with fibrosis and contracture. Massive venous occlusion, excessive external compression caused by roller injuries may indirectly result in contracture of the intrinsic muscles. The diagnosis should be suspected whenever severe trauma has occurred to the hand or the more proximal parts of the extremity.

The usual appearance of the hand or of an isolated digit is one of flexion at the metacarpophalangeal joint and extension at the proximal interphalangeal joint. Figure 15.6.2 demonstrates the method of doing the intrinsic contracture test.

INTRINSIC CONTRACTURE OR DEFORMITY NOT DUE TO ISCHEMIA

Several conditions result in contracture or imbalance of the intrinsic muscles or tendons and cause the digits to assume a position of flexion at the metacarpophalangeal joints and extension at the proximal interphalangeal joints. Before appropriate treatment is determined, individualization of deformity must be done.

Flexor Tendon Injuries or Lacerations

A digit in which a laceration of the flexor digitorum profundus and sublimis has occurred may develop gradually an extension contracture of the interphalangeal joints because of adhesions and contractures of the oblique or transverse fibers of the lateral band mechanism. The fibrous adhesions aggravate shortening of the tendinous prolongations of the interossei and lumbrical muscles and subsequently limit passive flexion of the interphalangeal joints of the involved digit when the proximal phalanx is forced into extension. This may occur in spite of seemingly adequate splinting in the functional position unless special effort is made to extend the metacarpophalangeal joint and forcibly flex the interphalangeal joints several hours of each day.

Primary involvement of the lumbrical muscle tendon unit tightens the radial lateral band of the digit because of retraction of the flexor profundus tendon. If this deformity exists for a brief period time, the imbalance between the lumbrical and the remainder of the extensor mechanism can be overcome by splinting and positioning.

Flexor tendon grafting or repair may fail if the contracture of the radial lateral band caused by a pathologic condition in the lumbrical units is not recognized. The deformity can be treated by either resection of the lumbrical or of the distal oblique fibers and this can be done at the time that the tendon surgery is accomplished. This observation was emphasized when causes for failure of tendon graft were being analyzed.

The tendon graft will only function when the wrist, metacarpophalangeal joint, and proximal interphalangeal joint are in maximum extension during the first few weeks after immobilization.

If a *flexor graft is too loose,* the lumbrical will contract first when the proximal part of the flexor profundus moves and the paradoxical action of flexion of the digit at the metacarpophalangeal and extension at the proximal interphalangeal joint will occur. The oblique fibers of the radial and ulnar lateral bands will usually have to be released in order to correct the deformity. If this is recognized after the graft has been done, the lateral band release will not be beneficial unless the graft is tightened or shortened.

If a sufficient contracture of the digit is recognized by the intrinsic contracture test, both the radial and the ulnar oblique fibers should be released rather than radial alone.

Contracture of the lumbrical and the radial lateral band may occur during the time that a silicone rod is being used in preparation for insertion of a free tendon graft at a later time. The profundus tendon may be amputated both at the base of the palm and again at the wrist level and the intervening segment left in place. If this is done, the lumbrical has a proximal attachment. This may result in fibrosis of the lumbrical and subsequent intrinsic contracture. Splinting and stretching during the time that the rod is in place should include splinting in the position of claw hand, a few hours each day. This provides stretch of the lateral band mechanism by extension of the metacarpophalangeal joint and flexion of the interphalanageal joints. When the free tendon graft is inserted neither to the wrist or to the palm, the intrinsic test should be done prior to final fixation of the tendon graft proximally. If a contracture is recognized, it can be managed by release of the radial and ulnar oblique fibers at the level of the proximal phalanx, or by excision of a lumbrical in the palm.

The *lumbrical should not be wrapped* around a flexor tendon repair in the palm because of the alteration of the extrinsic, intrinsic relationship. If the lumbrical is fixed to the tendon and not allowed to glide, a contracture will occur and a paradoxical affect on the interphalangeal joint will result. If the surgeon wants to use the lumbrical muscle as an insulator against adhesions, then the lumbrical tendon distally should be incised.

Direct trauma to the lumbrical caused by puncture wounds in the palm may result in fibrosis of the muscle, secondary adhesions between the lumbrical and the profundus, and shortening of the lumbrical tendon. Excision of the lumbrical muscle and fibrous tissue surrounding the tendon or excision of the oblique fibers of the lateral band distally will eliminate the contracture if the condition has not existed for a long time.

Watson has described *injury to the lumbrical muscle tendon unit as it crosses the transverse metacarpal ligament* on the radial side. This condition may be associated with intrinsic contracture or may be recognized only by pain and weakness. Release of the tendon at the site of involvement will relieve the condition.

Rheumatoid Arthritis

Rheumatoid arthritis may result in contracture of the intrinsic muscles of the hand and these changes are not caused primarily by muscle ischemia.

Pain at the metacarpophalangeal joint may cause increased intrinsic muscle tension with subsequent ulnar deviation due to overactivity of the ulnar interossei and the concurrent changes resulting from synovitis, cartilage damage, and collateral ligament involvement on the radial side. Volar subluxation of the proximal phalanx and thickening of the tendon sheath of the flexor profundus contribute indirectly to limited flexion of the proximal interphalangeal joint. This mechanical distortion as well as the erosion of the intrinsic insertions causes flexion of the metacarpophalangeal joints and extension of the interphalangeal joints. *Vasculitis affects the muscle* mass of the interossei just as it does many other tissues in patients with rheumatoid arthritis. Shortening of the muscle fibers and fibrosis may be sufficient to aggravate the intrinisic contracture but certainly this pathology is not the primary cause. Figure 15.6.5 shows an intrinsic deformity of the hand of a patient with rheumatoid arthritis with flexed metacarpophalangeal joints and extended interphalangeal joints. In this instance, the major pathologic condition is at the proximal interphalangeal joint where there is contracture of the dorsal capsule, shortening of the collateral ligaments, and tightness of the extensor tendons. Also, the synovial swellings of the metacarpophalangeal joints, the subluxation of the phalanges and alterations

of the dorsal hood and extensor tendon add to the "intrinsic plus" position of the hand. Incision or excision of the oblique fibers alone will *not* correct this intrinsic contracture because the changes are multiple and intra-articular in origin. There are many gradations of deformity of the rheumatoid hand, and *most of these do not respond to isolated release of the lateral band mechanism.* The intrinsic contracture in a rheumatoid hand usually requires detachment of the insertion of the interossei from the proximal phalanges, excision of the oblique fibers of the lateral bands, centralization of the entire extensor mechanism, definitive treatment to the metacarpophalangeal joints themselves, and lengthening of the extensor tendon over the proximal or middle phalanges.

Intrinsic and Extension Contracture

Intrinsic contracture alone is not the main reason that the digit cannot be flexed passively several weeks after injury although it is a contributing factor. Figure 15.6.1 shows the hand of a young male with lacerations of both digital flexor tendons. Passive flexion was limited during the first few months after injury for these reasons: (1) loss of the smooth gliding surface of

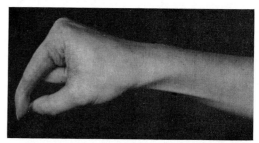

Figure 15.6.1. This patient's index finger had been severely damaged by volar laceration that included both flexor tendons and one digital nerve and vessel opposite the middle phalanx. Primary repair had been attempted and failed. Contracture resulted and the position of the digit implies contracture of the intrinsic mechanism including the lumbrical in the palm, the oblique fibers in the area of the metacarpophalangeal joint, and the proximal end of the phalanx, and contracture of the collateral ligaments at the proximal interphalangeal joint. Flexor tendon replacement in the digit such as this will fail unless the intrinsic contracture is released and unless the interphalangeal joints are mobilized. This is not primarily an ischemic process but one of local fibrosis compounded by absence of flexor tendons and inability of the patient to move the digit actively. Mobilization of this digit must be accomplished by release of the lateral band oblique fibers, tenolysis of the extensor tendon over the proximal and middle phalanges, and excision of the collateral ligaments at the proximal interphalangeal joint level.

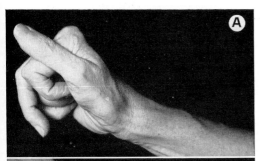

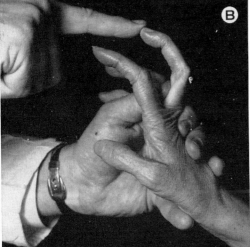

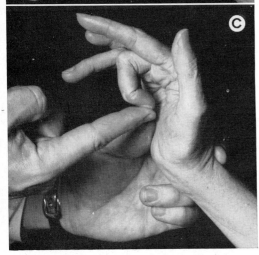

the flexor profundus tendon; (2) adhesions of the collateral ligaments of the proximal interphalangeal joints due to fibrosis secondary to edema; (3) adhesions and contracture of the lateral band mechanism due to abnormal pull of the contracted lumbrical; (4) contracture of the entire extensor mechanism over the proximal and middle phalanges.

Differential Tests to Determine Intrinsic Contracture and Contracture of the Extensor Tendons

Figure 15.6.2 demonstrates the method of determining intrinsic contracture.[2] This test requires extension of the wrist in order to apply tension to the flexor profundus and the lumbrical extension of the proximal phalanges at the metacarpophalangeal joints as this maneuver also adds tension on the volar intrinsic muscles and tendons, and passive effort to flex the proximal interphalangeal joint. In this position, maximal tension is placed on the entire intrinsic mechanism. The range of motion at the proximal interphalangeal joint depends on the degree of gliding of the intrinsic tendons. The second part of the test requires passive flexion of the metacarpophalangeal joint as this will

limited gliding of the flexor tendons are the major causes for limited motion when the hand is in this position. Note the patient's ability to flex the proximal interphalangeal joint actively through 70° when the metacarpophalangeal joint is flexed. *B.* This test detects contracture of the lateral band mechanism someplace along its course. With the proximal phalanx held in hyperextension, there is increased tension on the proximal portion of the intrinsic mechanism. Downward pressure applied to the dorsal tip of the involved finger will bring out limited flexion at the proximal interphalangeal joint due to the bowstring effect of the oblique fibers of the lateral band mechanism in the area of the proximal phalanx. Actual ischemia of the intrinsic muscles is not present although ischemic contracture simulates the appearance of this digit. The syndrome in this digit resulted from fibrosis, limited flexor tendon activity, and mild collateral ligament fibrosis as well as adhensions along the extensor mechanism. *C.* The last step of the intrinsic test is done by obtaining full flexion of the metacarpophalangeal joint followed by passive flexion of the interphalangeal joints. The lateral band mechanism is now relaxed and not affecting the proximal and distal interphalangeal joints. The improved range of flexion of the distal interphalangeal joint indicates that contracture is present within the extensor mechanism covering the finger as well as the portion in the palm. The contracture is primarily outside of the collateral ligament mechanism and is dependent on changes in the central slip of the extensor, as well as the oblique fibers. True contracture of the central slip does not exist here because the digit can be passively placed in flexion.

Figure 15.6.2. A. The long finger shows limited flexion at the interphalangeal joints. Previous injury to the flexor tendons in the palm has caused fibrosis of the lumbrical muscle and lateral band mechanism with subsequent contracture now acting as a check-rein through the lateral band mechanism which, in turn, limits flexion at the proximal interphalangeal joint when the digit is extended. The diminished activity of the digit with mild contracture of the collateral ligaments and

automatically relax the tension on the intrinsics and in turn will allow improved passive flexion of the proximal interphalangeal joint provided that the extensor communis is not contracted and the collateral ligaments of the proximal joint are not affected. If flexion of the proximal joint occurs when the metacarpophalangeal joint is flexed, proximal interphalangeal joint contracture is not present. This improvement indicates that surgical release of the intrinsic mechanism either within the muscle belly itself, at the insertion of the interosseous tendon into the proximal phalanx, or within the oblique intrinsic tendons, depending on where the primary condition is located, will result in diminution of the intrinsic deformity. Figures 15.6.3 and 15.6.4 show excision of the triangular ligament on both the radial and ulnar aspects of the digit after which immobilization of the digits was carried out with the metacarpophalangeal joints in extension and the proximal interphalangeal joints in flexion. The dorsal incision was made over the proximal phalanx with enough exposure to allow localization and excision of the distal and proximal expansions of each lateral band. Immobilization was used for 14 days and this was followed by application of an outrigger brace with elastic traction that held the proximal phalanx extended and the interphalangeal joints could be flexed actively and voluntarily. Splinting and voluntary exercise and supervised care on a home program for at least six weeks is essential if maximum range of motion is to be obtained after an intrinsic contracture release.

The test for contracture will differentiate a simple intrinsic contracture from a complex one. The latter may include fixed flexion deformity of the metacarpophalangeal joint, in addition to extension deformity of the interphalangeal joint. The existence of a contracture of the *extensor digitorum communis* can also be detected by systematically testing the position of each joint with the wrist in maximum dorsiflexion and then in complete volar flexion. If the wrist is held in neutral position and the metacarpophalangeal joints are positioned in full flexion then passive flexion of the interphalangeal joints, even in the presence of intrinsic contracture, should allow the fingertips to come to the palm if there is no extension contracture of the extensor communis. However, if the wrist is at zero degrees and the metacarpophalangeal joints are in flexion and the interphalangeal joints cannot be flexed passively then a contracture of the extensor digitorum communis at some point throughout its course does exist. The base-line for contracture of the extensor tendon cen be determined by completely flexing the wrist, flexing the metacarpophalangeal joints and then attempting to flex passively the proximal interphalangeal joint. In the normal hand without contracture, the fingertip can be flexed to the palm. If the extensor digitorum communis is contracted the interphalangeal joints can be flexed only if the metacarpophalangeal joint is extended and vice versa.

Figure 15.6.6 shows the position of the hand after the intrinsic muscles and fascia are shortened and deformity had occurred. The axis of rotation of the metacarpophalangeal joints is toward their volar surface and the tendons of the lumbricales and the interossei now pull on the volar side of the phalanges. The proximal interphalangeal joints are hyperextended by the strong pull of the intrinsic muscle mass and the lateral bands of the interphalangeal joints displace gradually toward the dorsum of this joint. As volar subluxation occurs, hyperextension at the proximal interphalangeal joint causes pressure on the flexor digitorum profundus which, in turn, flexes the distal phalanx. The interphalangeal joint alteration is primary and migration of the extensor mechanism is secondary. The degree of alteration at the proximal joint affects the ultimate position of the distal joint. If the intrinsic muscle is functioning and not acting through a contracture, the distal phalanx may hyperextend.

Other Causes of Intrinsic Contracture

Direct trauma to the dorsum or volar surface of the hand with either edema, fibrosis, or subsequent infection will directly affect the relationship between the interossei and the lateral bands and cause flexion of the metacarpophalangeal joint, if nerve damage has not occurred and extension of the interphalangeal joints. Protective splinting during the acute stage is essential. Decompression of massive swelling may be necessary.

Fractures in severe malposition such as excessive volar angulation cause increased tension on the intrin-

Figure 15.6.3. A. The radial approach to the lateral band mechanism of the index finger. A small segment of the oblique fibers detached distally is being held in the forceps. The extensor mechanism has not been incised. These triangular fibers on the radial side of the index finger were partially responsible for the deformity even though tickness in size of the fibrous tissue was not great. The bone attachments of the dorsal and volar interosseous muscles were not disturbed. After removal of this segmen of tissue, 30° of passive flexion at the proximal interphalangeal joint was possible, whereas before excising this tissue there was no passive flexive flexion when the knuckle joint was held in extension. *B.* The lateral band oblique fibers on the ulnar side of the index finger were wider, thicker, and heavier than those on the radial side, and had more contracture influence on the extensor mechanism. The extensor mechanism is visible and has been separated from the oblique fibers. *C.* An additional 60° of flexion were possible after the ulnar fibers had been excised. The vertical fibers were not incised or disturbed. The tissue removed has been placed on the skin over the middle phalanx, illustrating the side of the fibrous tissue removed from this area.

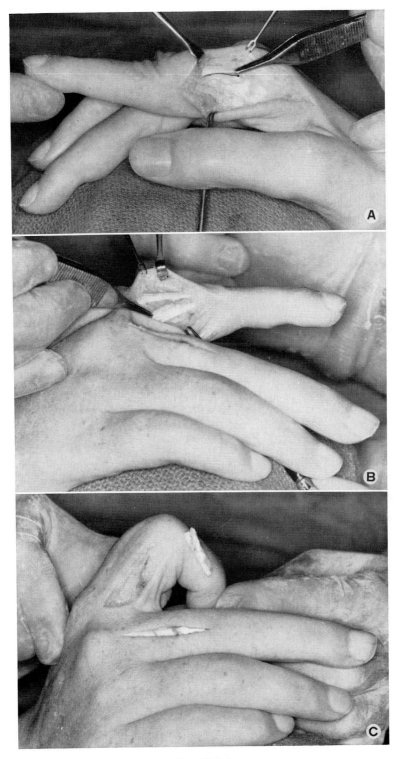

Fig. 15.6.3.

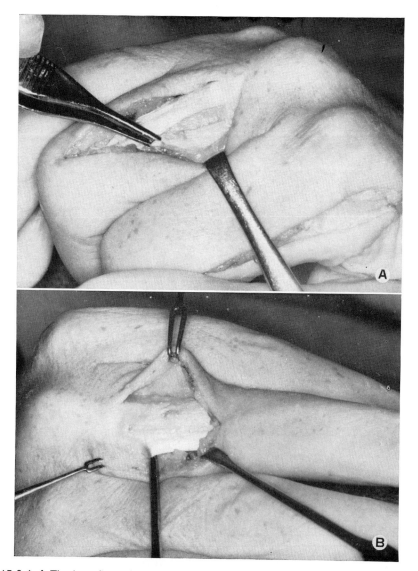

Figure 15.6.4. A. The long finger has been opened through a midcentral dorsal incision rather than ulnar and radial incisions. This incision is used if the preoperative condition of the finger implies that the central slip of the extensor tendon may have to be lengthened. The lateral incisions are desired, as these can be extended forward for exposure of the interphalangeal joint and removal of collateral ligaments if necessary. The radial fibers of the long finger are heavier than those of the index. The ulnar fibers are in the forceps and have been separated from the central slip of the entensor tendon. If the interphalangeal joints were to be opened, these oblique fibers could be left attached distally and separated only proximally and used as reinforcements over the interphalangeal joints. *B.* The oblique fibers on the ulnar side of the long finger are heavier and thicker than those on the radial side. The distal attachment of this tendon has been incised; immediately after this the degree of contracture diminished. Notice how the underlying gliding mechanism can be separated easily from the oblique fibers and the extensor. Occasionally, if the contracture is mild, this intrinsic tendon can be lengthened and not actually excised. *C.* The extensor digitorum communis of the long finger rests on the dorsum of the proximal phalanx. The oblique fibers and the tendinous insertion of the lateral band mechanism have been excised and are seen at the lower flap of the incision. The vertical fibers are intact and their attachment to the extensor mechanism is evident. It is through this unit that continued extension of the interphalangeal joints is actively done. If the range of flexion, after release of the oblique fibers on both sides of the digit, is not sufficient for functional use, then the extensor tendon would be lengthened after

sic muscles and subsequent intrinsic digit deformity. Angulation is more dangerous than overlap.

Intrinsic contracture resulting from surgical procedure. A *lateral band* tendon transfer for treatment of "claw hand" and for improvement of strength of grip can result in an intrinsic contracture if the tension of the transferred tendon is excessive, or if localized fibrosis occurs between the oblique fibers of the lateral band and the phalanx. When a lateral band transfer is being done, the tension on each digit should be tested after the transferred tendon has been fixed with a single suture. The object of an active intrinsic transfer is to obtain increased strength of flexion and a reasonable degree of active interphalangeal extension. The tension of the tendon should be too little rather than too much. Once the contracture occurs, however, a release of the oblique fibers of the intrinsic tendon distal to the point of suture will diminish the contracture. The oblique fibers on both sides of the extensor mechanism should be released, as both usually tighten even though the tendon transfer is only on one side.

Bow stringing of the flexor tendons has been recommended as a method of diminishing "claw hand." If the flexor annular ligament over the metacarpophalangeal joint is incised completely, the flexor tendons will bow string and affect the range of flexion of the proximal interphalangeal joints. This may provide temporary improvement of the claw hand position, but, eventually, will lead to ulnar deviation of the phalanges and interphalangeal joint extension.

If the *intrinsic transfer is inserted into bone* on the radial side, there may be less chance of developing extension contracture of the proximal interphalangeal joint. However, that deformity is not completely eliminated because the fibrosis that occurs from elevating the oblique fibers, drilling the hole, and inserting the tendon may very well be sufficient to cause localized contracture of the lateral bands and result in static intrinsic contracture.

Spasticity is one cause of intrinsic contracture. The interossei and the lumbricals may be affected by overaction associated with such conditions as cerebral palsy or spasticity resulting from stroke. The most common area of spasticity in the patient with cerebral palsy is in the first dorsal interosseous and the adductor. The management of the spastic intrinsics depends on the age of the patients, the severity of the deformity, and the function of the extrinsic musculature as well as other neuromuscular units of the extremity.

In the adult patient with spasticity resulting from stroke, management is even more difficult because the extent of motor involvement is usually severe. Occasionally, however, the patient with spasticity of the intrinsics resulting from cerebral trauma can be improved by releasing the muscle bellies from the metacarpals, by releasing the interossei origins from the phalanges, or merely by excision of the oblique fibers from the radial and ulnar sides of the proximal phalanx. Improvement may occur but optimism is not encouraged.

Intrinsic contracture secondary to aging collagen (Fig. 15.6.12A) shows the ulnar deviation of the extensor tendons when the fingers were flexed half way to the palm. She did not have rheumatoid arthritis, and the cartilage surfaces were not involved.

Figure 15.6.12B shows a dorsal view of the same hand with the uncovered metacarpal head of the long finger and the extensor tendon deviated into the intermetacarpal groove. Deviation of the adjacent extensors existed but was less severe. Minimal ulnar deviation was present, but as the fingers were flexed completely deviation of the phalanges did occur. The intrinsic test on the long finger (Fig. 15.6.12C) showed flexion of the middle phalanx through 60° when the metacarpophalangeal joint was extended and the extensor tendon was centralized over the metacarpal head. As the metacarpophalangeal joint was flexed, the range of flexion at the proximal interphalangeal joint increased (Fig. 15.6.7).

Treatment included exposure of all the metacarpal heads through a transverse incision, plication of the stretched radial collateral ligament in each digit and plication of the radial retinaculum after the dorsal capsule had been isolated and sutured into the undersurface of the extensor tendon. This maintained an upward (dorsal) position of the phalanx and assisted in

the collateral ligaments of the proximal interphalangeal joints had been excised, depending on the location of the primary contracture. Release of the bony attachment of the interossei is done only when fixed contracture of the metacarpophalangeal joint exists and when this contracture is in flexion and not due to changes in the volar capsule. *D.* The ulnar side of the index finger, after the triangular fibers have been excised and the vertical fibers are isolated. The extensor mechanism is seen at the top of the incision and the forceps are under the point of attachment of the vertical fibers to the extensor communis. If the contracture is severe and if it does not respond to the releases already mentioned, then the oblique fibers should be left attached to the distal segment of the extensor mechanism and the transverse fibers incised and insertion of interossei released. *E.* With the metacarpophalangeal joint in maximal extension and after the oblique fibers of both the radial and ulnar aspects of the intrinsic extensor mechanism have been excised, the proximal interphalangeal joint can be placed passively to a position of 90° of flexion. While the patient is under anesthesia, the digit should not be manually forced at any of the joint areas involved. The correction obtained must be without force or it will not be maintained. Both middle phalanges can now be flexed to 90° when the metacarpophalangeal joints are in the extended position. The ring and little fingers have not yet been corrected, and these show no passive flexion at the proximal joints, when the metacarpophalangeal joints are placed in a similar position.

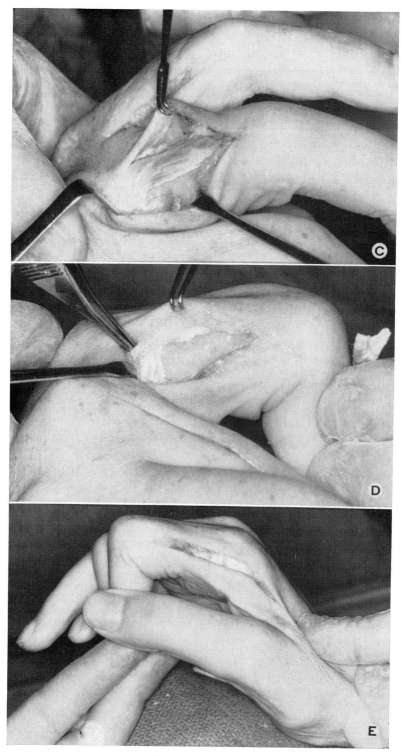

Fig. 15.6.4. C to E.

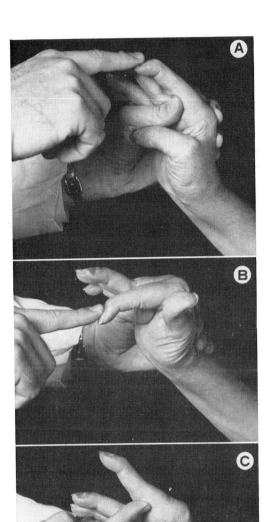

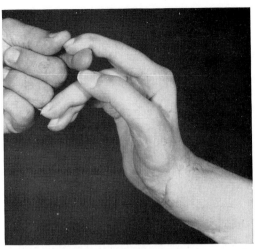

Figure 15.6.6. A hand involved by trauma to both the forearm and the hand, with primary intrinsic contracture. This should be compared to the rheumatoid hand shown in Figure 15.6.5. Appearance only would imply that both hands are deformed by the same tissue changes but manipulation and testing of the various joints in the positions indicated show that this hand is contracted primarily by the lateral band tendons which, in turn, are shortened from ischemia of the small muscles of the hand and a slowly developing contracture resulting from injury to the flexor muscle mass.

re-centralizing the extensor tendon. The oblique fibers of the radial and ulnar lateral bands were lengthened but not excised. After this was done, the interphalangeal joints could be flexed completely when the metacarpophalangeal joint was in extension. Figure 15.6.12D shows the range of flexion during which time the extensor tendons remained centralized. The intrinsic contracture test was negative.

Figure 15.6.5. A. The digits have the appearance of ischemic contracture. The patient has rheumatoid arthritis. Every digit with the appearance of ischemic contracture is not necessarily the result of ischemia. The Bunnell test is being done with forcible extension of the proximal phalanx accompanied by direct pressure downward to the dorsum of the distal phalanx in an effort to produce flexion of the proximal interphalangeal joint. No active flexion occurs, indicating that fixed contracture of the intrinsic mechanism and, because of complete absence of motion at the proximal interphalangeal joint, probable involvement of the dorsal capsule, the collateral ligaments and the entire extensor mechanism. B. Flexion of the metacarpophalangeal joint should give relaxation of the lateral band mechanism. No noticeable change in the range of motion at the proximal interphalangeal joint occurs in spite of the change of joint motion. The metacarpophalangeal joint flexes to 90° and the distal joint can be carried through 45°. This lack of motion in the proximal joint is positive evidence that the limitation is within the digit and within the joint rather than in the intrinsic muscles and the lateral band mechanism. C. Forced extension of the proximal phalanx implies changes in the metacarpophalangeal joints, contracture of the volar capsule and shortening of the interossei. The rheumatoid digits do have an element of contracture of the intrinsic muscles and intrinsic tendons, but the joint change is the major deforming cause.

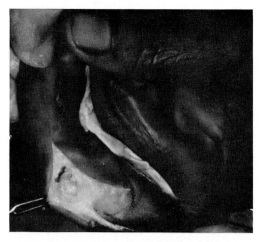

Figure 15.6.7. Intrinsic contracture of a digit plus involvement of the extensor mechanism and contracture of the collateral ligaments of the interphalangeal joints. Release of the lateral band mechanism alone did not allow full extension of the metacarpophalangeal joints or adequate flexion of the interphalangeal joints. Small joints must be opened to allow the flexor tendons to mobilize the joints rather than by-pass them. The index finger was exposed by a long incision extending from the radial aspect, bypassing the transverse creases over the proximal interphalangeal joint, and extending to the ulnar side of the digit. The long finger was opened by separate radial and ulnar incisions on either side of the interphalangeal joints. A vertical incision in the retinaculum has been made and the collateral ligaments have been excised. The oblique fibers of the lateral band mechanism have been detached proximally and will be swung over the retinaculum of the proximal joint and used as a reinforcement. This was done on both sides of the proximal interphalangeal joint.

THUMB WEB CONTRACTURE — INTRINSICS

Not only are the fingers involved in an extensor and intrinsic contracture, but also the thumb web becomes contracted and limits the use of the entire hand. A narrow thumb web space lessens the size of grasp, limits dexterity, and results in inability to hold large objects. Thumb web contracture is a combination of many factors, but one condition of great importance is muscle and fibrous shortening of the adductor pollicis and first dorsal and volar interossei muscles. This may be due to *ischemic* or may be the result of *nonischemic* contracture.

Fibrosis of the extensor pollicis longus sheath and shortening of this tendon holds the first metacarpal in an adducted position and limits the width of the web. Contracture of the carpometacarpal joint is a late effect of soft tissue shortening of the thumb.

PREVENTION OF FIBROUS AND ISCHEMIC CONTRACTURE OF THE HAND

External forces that cause arterial insufficiency, venous congestion, lymphatic stasis, or limitation of finger motion because of malposition of the digits must be avoided. Ischemia and local fibrosis of the hand that cause contracture of the intrinsic muscles can be lessened if arterial insufficiency is avoided. Tight external elastic wrappings or tight plaster casts that hold the palm in a compressed cupped position diminish input of arterial blood and outflow of venous blood and exaggerate the changes associated with ischemia. Rigid dressings covering the interphalangeal joints encourage periarticular fibrosis and subsequent contracture of the extensor mechanism. The intrinsic muscles are affected indirectly.

Dressing applied to postoperative extremity wounds in a circumferential fashion become saturated with blood and act as external constrictors and diminish both venous and lymphatic flow. The first layer of the dressing should be fluffed gauze, mechanics waste or fluffed cotton, or an absorbable synthetic material. The soft underdressing should extend from the fingertips to above the elbow so that localized segmental constriction does not occur. Cotton wadding that tears easily and is nonelastic should then be wrapped over the fluffed dressing. All bony prominences and subcutaneous nerves are padded and protected from external compression. After the circumferential wrapping has been applied it is cut throughout its entire length and a second layer of wrapping is applied over the basic layer. Four-thickness dorsal plaster splints are then placed over the soft dressings and wrapped in place by bias-cut stockinette. Most hand dressings should be applied proximal to the elbow for three to four days in order to avoid dependent edema and provide comfort. Elevation is mandatory. A sling is not used if the patient has enough strength to elevate the arm.

If plaster is used on an extremity in order to manage a fracture or to provide immobilization, the underlying sheet cotton should be cut in order to provide for swelling and the plaster should be wrapped on in such a way that it is not constricting at any location. A plaster cast can be split immediately after it is applied with little risk of interfering with healing or positioning of osseous tissue or soft tissue.

External *compression* is necessary to prevent edema, but excessive pressure is to be avoided. If there is evidence of circulatory involvement, either venous or arterial, all external compression should be split and if improvement does not occur, then skin and fascia should be incised.

Dependent edema must be avoided. The upper extremity should be immobilized with the elbow at right angles. If possible, a sling should not be used but the patient should be encouraged to maintain elevation of the extremity with the arm away from the side. This seems awkward initially, but most patients adapt to this position without difficulty.

The thumb should be positioned in full abduction, slight external rotation with the tip of the thumb toward the radial side of the hand so that full flexion of the index finger is possible. If the thumb is positioned in full opposition, flexion of the fingers is limited.

TREATMENT OF INTRINSIC CONTRACTURE

Each deformity must be treated after the pathologic state has been determined and the cause of the contracture recognized. The details may include a single procedure or combination of procedures and these are listed numerically. Clinical material is presented that demonstrates patient problems that have been partially of completely solved by adhering to these principles.

1. Adherent or contracted intrinsic tendons are managed by excision of the triangular segment of the oblique fibers of the lateral band mechanism on the radial and ulnar sides. Usually, both wings must be excised. Where the contracture is mild, the dense segment of the oblique fibers can be lengthened or merely tenotomized without actually excising a triangular segment with good relief of the contracture. Figure 15.6.3 shows complete excision.

2. The interossei attachments to bone are released, the triangular segments are excised, and the transverse fibers remain intact so that the intrinsic muscles will have an effect on extension of the interphalangeal joints. If the flexion deformity at the metacarpalphalangeal joint is severe, and the interphalangeal joints contracted, the transverse fibers also may have to be released even though a mild flexion deformity of the interphalangeal joints may result.

3. After the triangular lateral bands of the intrinsics have been released but the vertical fibers are intact, and if the interphalangeal joint range of motion improves but is not complete the proximal joint must be released. If there is evidence of periarticular fibrosis of the proximal joint, then this joint should be opened, the collateral ligaments excised from the radial and ulnar sides, and the dorsal capsule released (Figure 15.6.7).

4. Collateral ligament contractures of the interphalangeal joints are managed in one of two ways. (a) If a mild contracture exists, a vertical incision is made through the retinaculum and the collateral ligament is excised completely by removing both the upper and the lower fibers. Separate radial and ulnar incisions are used through which the dorsal capsule can be released and the volar capsule freed from the distal end of the proximal phalanx. The extensor tendon must be examined after the joint contracture is released. Occasionally, adhesions of the extensor to an old fracture of the phalanx or to the periosteum may require lengthening of that tendon proximally and/or tenotomy of the extensor tendon distally.

If release of the collateral ligaments of the interphalangeal joint does not provide adequate flexion, then the extensor tendon is lengthened over the proximal phalanx and the oblique fibers of the lateral band

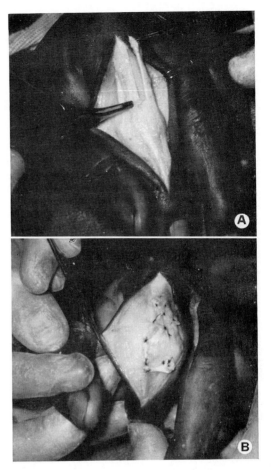

Figure 15.6.8. A. Adequate flexion of the index finger was not possible after the proximal interphalangeal joints had been opened and after the oblique fibers of the intrinsic mechanism had been released. The central slip of the extensor tendon was obviously the limiting factor in obtaining adequate flexion and this unit was lengthened by Z-plasty. The two arms of the lengthened extensor are visible in the forceps. The oblique fibers of the lateral band mechanism were saved to reinforce the retinacula of the proximal interphalangeal joints on both the medial and lateral sides of the extensor tendon. These are sutured in place with 4-0 white silk. The oblique fibers are placed under the retinaculum and reinforced in this position in order to replace the excised collateral ligaments. This allows adequate stability. *B.* The lengthened extensor tendon had been resutured in its new position. The oblique fibers have been placed under the retinaculum and sutured proximally and distally. One end of the oblique fibers has been attached to the central slip over the middle phalanx to avoid the development of a buttonhole deformity.

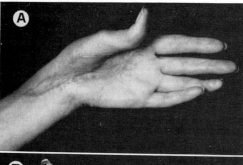

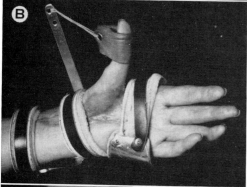

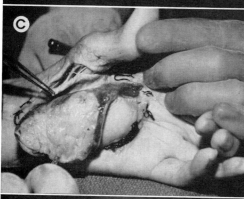

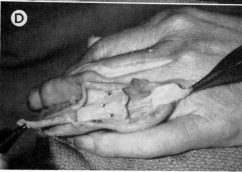

are saved in order to reinforce the extensor tendon. The triangular fibers are left attached distally and used to supplement the extensor proximally (Fig. 15.6.8).

(b) A more extensive release of the collateral ligaments and the extensor mechanism is accomplished by raising the entire extensor unit through a horizontal incision excising dorsal capsule, collateral ligaments, and lengthening the extensor tendon. A dorsal skin incision is a disadvantage because tension is placed on the incision when the finger is immobilized in flexion.

5. Arthrodesis of the proximal interphalangeal joints and soft tissue release of the attachment of the intrinsic tendons to the proximal phalanges will restore the contour of the digits, enlarge the grasp, and give good stability. This procedure is reserved for the most severe deformities (Figure 15.6.9) .

6. Advancement or excision of the muscle bellies of the interossei is used as a corrective procedure occasionally. In the spastic hand, the adductor is released from the third metacarpal through the web space and the tendon is lengthened. The first dorsal interosseous is removed from the first and the second metacarpals and is advanced. The radial artery is isolated. Patients with intrinsic deformity but without contracture and with spastic interossei such as those seen with cerebral trauma or spasticity secondary to spinal cord injury may be improved by release of the intrinsic muscle bellies.

7. Thumb web contracture may require: (a) Split graft or pedicle skin flap; (b) fascial release; (c) lengthening of the adductor muscle and release of the origin of the adductor from the third metacarpal; (d)

Figure 15.6.9. A. The hand has been severely damaged by a roller. A web contracture occurred between thumb and index and a palmar contracture affected the intrinsic muscle area in the base of the first metacarpal. The digital nerves to the index finger, as well as to the thumb, were both affected by ischemia and resulted in pares-

thesias. Interphalangeal joints of the long, ring, and little fingers were limited in both flexion and extension. The initial step included opening of the thumb web, neurolysis of the involved nerves and placement of a split skin graft. An abdominal flap was elevated during the same period. Intrinsic contracture involves all of the digits, the cause being fibrosis as well as ischemia. B. A thumb splint was applied to maintain abduction and extension of the thumb. This stretching is of some help but will not persist unless the basic contracture has been completely eliminated and flexible skin used to fill the web. C. An abdominal flap has been transferred to the palm and the thumb web. The split skin graft was excised, the digital nerves were identified and the entire area was covered with the flap. Improved circulation resulted and correction of the contracture was maintained. D. This same hand required individual treatment to each digit. The index finger was mobilized by release of the oblique fibers of the lateral band mechanism, the long finger required release of the oblique fibers, collateral ligament excision at the proximal interphalangeal joint and lengthening of the extensor tendon. The ring finger would not respond to mobilization and joint arthrodesis and shortening of the digit were necessary.

release of the interosseous muscle bellies from the first and second metacarpals; (e) capsulotomy of the carpal metacarpal joints; (f) Excision of the trapezium or the base of the first metacarpal depending on the side of the joint that is most severely involved. Dacron silicone prosthetic replacement has been done in order to provide increased stability and maintain length.

CLINICAL MATERIAL

Figure 15.6.10 *A* shows the less serious form of intrinsic contracture caused by fibrosis of the lateral bands and retraction of the lumbrical muscle attached to the proximal end of the lacerated flexor profundus. Flexion of the interphalangeal joints is usually firm and limited when the proximal phalanx is extended, but flexion is possible when the metacarpal phalangeal joints are flexed. Release of the lumbrical or excision of the lumbrical at the time of flexor tendon grafting is usually sufficient to correct moderate extension contractures of interphalangeal joints. If the contracture is severe, however, as was the situation in this particular patient, the triangular fibers of the lateral band should be excised a few weeks prior to the flexor tendon grafting, and exercise and splinting done. This observation has been verified not only in hands damaged by direct trauma but also hyperextension deformities of the interphalangeal joints in the hand in cerebral palsy.

Figure 15.6.10 *B* shows a combination of contractures caused by minimal change within the inter-

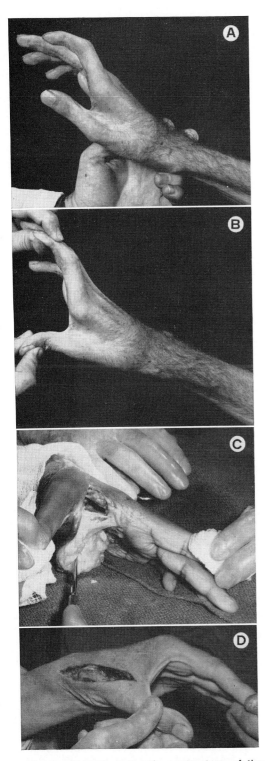

added to the ischemic fibrosis. The index, long, ring, and little fingers show interphalangeal joint contractures and contracture of the lateral band mechanism caused by local changes within the digits and contractures from the extensor mechanism as well as the intrinsic muscles and tendons. *B.* The skin in the web is limiting movement of the metacarpals even though the digits can be spread. Release of the adductor and first dorsal interosscous muscle are necessary and either split skin graft or abdominal flap, depending on the particular situation, are needed to maintain width of the thumb web. *C.* In this instance the web contracture was released and the abdominal flap that had been previously placed in the palm was mobilized and used to fill in the web. *D.* Ischemic contracture of the thumb web can involve the deeper structures primarily with minimal change in the skin. If direct trauma to the carpometacarpal joints has occurred, the correction of contracture will depend on soft tissue excision and arthroplasty. In this instance the adductor pollicis brevis was lengthened, the first dorsal interosseous was removed from the first metacarpal and the superficial fascia was excised. Excision of the greater multangular was necessary to obtain adequate correction of the final degrees of the tight web. The abductor pollicis longus has been advanced up the shaft of the metacarpal, to prevent hyperextension.

Figure 15.6.10. Ischemic contracture of the thumb web may involve the deeper stuctures primarily and not affect the skin severely. Atrophy of the interossei due to ulnar nerve injury has

phalangeal joints, but maximal contracture of the lateral bands and changes in the extensor tendon proper. These digits had been immobilized in flexion at the metacarpal phalangeal joints and extension at the interphalangeal joints for several months after median and ulnar nerve injury at the wrist. In addition to median nerve decompression at the wrist and opening of the thumb web, the fingers were treated by (1) release of the triangular intrinsic fibers opposite the proximal phalanx on both the radial sides of the fingers, (2) collateral ligament excision of the interphalangeal joints, and finally (3) lengthening of the extensor communis over the proximal phalanges. Each of these corrections allowed about 30° of improvement and the combination brought the interphalangeal joints to 90° and the metacarpalphalangeal joints up to neutral.

Figure 15.6.10 C shows a combination of ischemic contracture of the hand, thumb web space contracture, and digital nerve injury. These deformities resulted from a heavy roller injury causing loss of skin, damage to digital nerves in the palm, and crushing injury to the interphalangeal joints. Severe contractures developed in the early weeks after injury and these involved primarily the interphalangeal joints; also, the thumb web contracted because of skin damage, ischemic fibrosis and pain. Maximal web release required removal of the interossei from the first and second metacarpals, lengthening of the adductor pollicis, capsulotomy of the carpometacarpal joint of the thumb, and an abdominal pedicle skin flap.

Specific deformities of each finger were treated surgically with moderate improvement. The index finger showed contracture of the metacarpophalangeal joint in flexion, a fixed extension deformity of the proximal interphalangeal joint and diminished sensation. The collateral ligaments of the proximal interphalangeal joints were excised, and the triangular fibers of the lateral band mechanism were removed from the proximal phalangeal region. This was sufficient to improve the range of flexion of the small joints and extension of the metacarpophalangeal joints.

The long finger showed an uncomplicated contracture of the lateral band mechanism that improved by excision of the triangular ligament from both the radial and ulnar sides of the phalanx, as well as excision of the collateral ligaments from the proximal interphalangeal joint. The little finger showed severe flexion deformity at the proximal joint, irreparable change of the extensor mechanism, fixed changes in the volar capsule of the proximal joint, and moderate diminution of sensation. Arthrodesis and shortening of the little finger through the proximal interphalangeal joint resulted in sufficient improvement to maintain the digit out of the palm and yet provide enough stability to allow it to function with the adjacent digits in performaning grasp. The ring finger showed no small muscle contracture, but did have a firm flexion deformity at the proximal interphalangeal joint at 90 degrees. Arthrodesis and shortening were done without complication.

The hand in Figure 15.6.9 was accidentally injured when caught in a hot press. This kind of injury leads frequently to fibrosis and temporary ischemia of the small muscles. The contractures that develop are of the usual pattern of extension of the fingers and adduction contracture of the thumb. The initial loss of motion improved gradually, but flattening of the thumb and loss of the thumb web persisted because of ischemic contracture of the interossei and adductor, as well as a fracture at the base of the first metacarpal and fibrosis of the skin and fascia. Mobilization of the thumb web was the major goal. This contracture was partially due to intrinsic deformity. Treatment included: (1) incision of the thumb web from the base to the end of the web without opening the volar aspect; (2) lengthening of the adductor muscle and excision of the contracted fascia; (3) release of the interossei from the first and second matacarpals and of the adductor from the third metacarpal; (4) capsulectomy of the carpometacarpal joint and excision of part of the base of the first metacarpal (Figure 15.6.10D). The thumb was repositioned in abduction and opposition after this release. Five days later a split thickness skin graft closed the dorsal defect. The thumb web was stretched for two weeks with steel pins between the first and second metacarpal bones. After this, several weeks of external splinting and mobilization were done in order to obtain a maximum range of motion. An opponens transfer with a flexor digitorum sublimis tendon of the ring finger replaced the paralyzed intrinsic muscles usually innervated by the median nerve and provided an active neutralizer of web contraction.

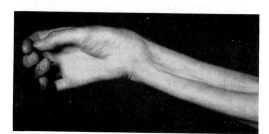

Figure 15.6.11. Ischemic contracture of the intrinsic muscles of the digits of the hand without the typical position of the fingers. Ischemia of the small hand muscles does not necessarily lead to hyperextension of the interphalangeal joints if the involvement of the flexor muscle mass causes severe flexion of the fingers. The contracture of the flexor mass was strong enough to prevent extension at the interphalangeal joints by the lumbricales and interossei even though they were severely ischemic. Carpalectomy, opening of the thumb web, and arthrodesis of the interphalangeal joints of the fingers all were necessary to maintain pinch. Volkmann's ischemia of the forearm does not necessarily lead to ischemic changes in the hand, but in severe situations both segments of the extremity may be involved.

Figure 15.6.11 shows the typical changes of primary arterial insufficiency associated with Volkman's ischemia of the forearm with changes occurring secondarily in the hand. The injury was a Colles fracture with subsequent localized external compression extending from the elbow to the mid forearm. Infarction of the forearm muscles developed and ischemia of the median and ulnar nerves occurred, with circulatory and neural defects affecting the hand. A severe thumb web contracture and partial paralysis of the intrinsic muscles of the thumb and fingers resulted. The interphalangeal joints were fibrosed in flexion because of contracture of the forearm muscles. Treatment included decompression of the entire median nerve in the forearm and at the wrist and removal of the necrotic muscle mass from the forearm. This tissue was re-

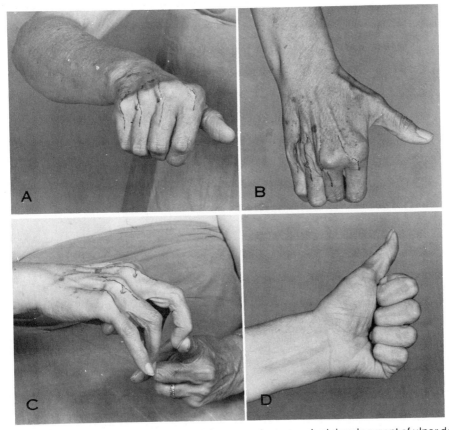

Figure 15.6.12. A. This hand in a 62-year-old woman shows gradual development of ulnar deviation of the proximal phalanges and lateral displacement of the common extensor tendons. This occurs when the patient clenches the fingers. Trauma has not been the major cause of this difficulty. The dotted lines coincide with the extensor digitorum communis tendons. The metacarpal heads are partially uncovered. The interossei on the ulnar side contract forcibly and flex the phalanges, as well as rotate them externally. All tissues on the radial side undergo moderate stretch. B. When the patient extends the digit, the long finger lags because of impingement of the common extensor on the ulnar side of the metacarpal head. The connective tissue making up the extensor mechanism has undergone noticeable stretch. This is primarily related to the patient's age and to a lesser degree, her occupation or any special trauma. C. A test is being done to the long finger in order to determine contracture of the intrinsic muscles. The intrinsic test was positive when the extensor tendon was centralized. As the proximal phalanx was flexed the range of flexion at the proximal interphalangeal joint increased. When the proximal phalanx was extended and the proximal interphalangeal joint flexed, the range of motion was limited noticeably. Treatment consisted of tenotomy of the oblique fibers of the lateral band on both the radial and the ulnar sides, plication of the dorsal retinaculum on the radial side, and insertion of the dorsal capsule into the extensor hood. D. The patient could make a full fist without limitation, and could claw the fingers when the proximal phalanges were extended. This indicated that intrinsic contracture had been released by the lengthening of the lateral band fibers on the radial and ulnar sides and that the extensor tendons were centralized and stable.

sponsible for persistent drainage. Later, treatment included: (1) carpalectomy, (2) opening of the thumb web without addition of abdominal flap or split skin graft, (3) interphalangeal joint arthrodeses, and (4) minor tendon transfers. Histologic appearance of the muscles of the hand were the same as those seen with any localized ischemia. The deformities seen in this hand, however, were not typical of those with the usual intrinsic contracture involving the hand because of the combination of forearm contracture and alteration of the deep tissues of the hand.

Figure 15.6.12A to D demonstrates a problem with combined deformities that responded to intrinsic release and reconstrustion of the extensor band.

REFERENCES

1. Amick, L. D. Muscle atrophy in rheumatoid arthritis: An electrodiagnostic study. Arthritis Rheum., 3: 54-63, 1960.
2. Backhouse, K. M., and Catton, W. T. An experimental study of the functions of the lumbrical muscles in the human hand. J. Anat., 88: 133-141, 1954.
3. Braithwaite, F., Channell, G. D., Moore, F. T., and Whillis, J. The applied anatomy of the lumbrical and interosseous muscles of the hand. Guy's Hosp. Rep., 97: 185-195, 1948.
4. Bunnell, S. Surgery of the intrinsic muscles of the hand other than those producing opposition of the thumb. J. Bone Joint Surg., 24: 1-31, 1942.
5. Bunnell, S., Doherty, E. W., and Curtis, R. M. Ischemic contracture, local, in the hand. Plast. Reconstr. Surg., 3: 424-433, 1948.
6. Bunnell, S. Ischemic contracture, local, in the hand. J. Bone Joint Surg., 35A: 88-101, 1953.
7. Curtis, R. M. Capsulectomy of the interphalangeal joints of the fingers. J. Bone Joint Surg., 36A: 1219-1232, 1954.
8. Eyler, D. L., and Markee, J. E. The Anatomy and function of the intrinsic musculature of the fingers. J. Bone Joint Surg;, 36A: 1-9, 18-20, 1954.
9. Goldner, J. L. Deformities of the hand incidental to pathological changes of the extensor and intrinsic muscle mechanisms. J. Bone Joint Surg., 35A: 115-131, 1953.
10. Goldner, J. L. Intrinsic and extensor contracture of the hand due to ischemia and other conditions. In Hand Surgery, edited by J. E. Flynn. Williams & Wilkins, Baltimore, pp. 978-992, 1966.
11. Goldner, J. L. Surgery of the hand. In Practice of Surgery, Orthopedics (2). Hagerstown, Harper & Row, 1970, pp. 71-73.
12. Kestler, O. C. Histopathology of the intrinsic muscles of the hand in rheumatoid arthritis: A Clinico-Pathological Study. Ann. Rheum. Dis., 8: 42-58, 1949.
13. Landsmeer, J. M. F. Anatomical and functional investigations on the articulations of the human fingers. Acta Anat., 24 (Supplement): 1955.
14. Milford, L. W. Retaining Ligaments of the Digits of the Hand; Gross and Microscopic Anatomic Study. Philadelphia, Saunders, 1968, p.31.
15. Parks, A. R. Traumatic ischaemia of peripheral nerves with some observations on Volkmann's ischaemic contracture. Br. J. Surg., 32: 403-414, 1945.
16. Parkes, A. R. The "lumbrical" finger. J. Bone Joint Surg., 53B: 236-239, 1971.
17. Riordan, D. C., and Harris, C. Jr., Intrinsic contracture in the hand and its surgical treatment. J. Bone Joint Surg., 36A: 10-20, 1954.
18. Smith, R. J. Non-ischemic contractures of the intrinsic muscles. J. Bone Joint Surg., 53A: 1313-1331, 1971.
19. Stack, H. G. Muscle function in the fingers. J. Bone Joint Surg., 44B: 899-909, 1962.
20. Watson, K. Saddle deformity of intrinsics. American Society for Surgery of the Hand, Washington, D. C., January 1972.

chapter sixteen

Disability Evaluations

J. Edward Flynn, M.D.

Statistics of the National Safety Council and State Industrial Commissions show that trauma to the hand is of great importance economically. In 1971, there were 11,200,000 disabling injuries in the United States of which about 2,300,000 were occupational accidents. The estimated cost of all accidents was about $29,500,000,000, or which $9,300,000,000 or about one third represents the cost of occupational accidents (Table 16.1). Of the 2,300,000 occupational accidents in 1971, 760,000 involved the upper extremity, about one-third of all occupational accidents. Averages for other years are similar.

Movements for safety in industry are well established by Federal, State, and City laws. The National Safety Council, local councils, and associations are very active. Heinrich[8] has shown that for every accident there is an unsafe personal act or a mechanical hazard or both. The best surgical treatment, performed within six hours, is the cheapest in the end. A report of the accident should include an accurate history, the time of the injury, detailed description of the injury, a diagnosis, witnesses to the accident, past history, other disabilities, details of treatment, prognosis, and an estimate of disability. An early return to work improves patient's morale and hand function.

WORKMEN'S COMPENSATION

Workmen's compensation was started in the United States in 1911, when 10 states enacted compensation laws. It was previously adopted in Germany in 1884, England in 1897, and in all of Europe by 1910. The cost is written off similar to any cost in industry. The injured is treated medically and compensated financially for temporary or permanent disability. All states have a waiting period of three days to three weeks, most seven to 10 days, before compensation starts. For temporary disability, compensation is from 50 to 67 per cent of the employee's salary up to a maximal wage for a period of from 50 weeks to eight years, averaging about 300 weeks.

In 1958 "A Guide to the Evaluation of Permanent Impairment of the Extremities and Back"[7] was pub-

TABLE 16.1
Accident incidence and costs, 1971

Number of accidents	11,200,000
Accident incidence at work	2,300,000
Cost of all accidents	$29,500,000,000
Cost of industrial accidents	$ 9,300,000,000

lished by the Committee on Medical Rating of Physical Impairment of the American Medical Association. This guide provides an excellent reference for evaluating permanent loss of part or function. This Committee stressed the importance in distinghishing between "impairment" and "disability."

The Committee of the American Medical Association estimated that a loss of the entire upper extremity constitutes a loss of 60 per cent of the whole man. Estimates for other losses in the extremity are also made (Table 16.2) (Figs. 16.1–16.3).

For loss of:

Extremity at elbow	95% of entire extremity
Extremity at wrist	90% of entire extremity
Thumb	40% of hand
Index finger	25% of hand
Middle finger	20% of hand
Ring finger	10% of hand
Little finger	5% of hand
One phalanx of thumb	75% of entire thumb
One phalanx of any finger	45% of entire finger
Two phalanges of any finger	80% of said finger

The Disability Evaluation Committee of the American Society for Surgery of the Hand considers motor and sensory losses (Figs. 16.1–16.4).

In Massachusetts, compensation is paid on the basis of loss of function or specific loss, and disfigurement also.

For loss by severance of the right or major hand at the wrist, $6,750 are paid. For loss by severance of the left or minor hand at the wrist, $4,500 are paid. The estimated loss of function in the hand or digits is

635

TABLE 16.2*
Amputations

	Digit	Hand	Upper Extremity	Whole Man
			Impairment of (%)	
Forequarter amputation.....................................				70
Disarticulation at shoulder joint...........................			100	60
Amputation of arm above deltoid insertion............................			100	60
Amputation of arm between deltoid insertion and elbow joint..			95	57
Disarticulation at elbow joint..............................			95	57
Amputation of forearm below elbow joint proximal to insertion of biceps tendon			95	57
Amputation of forearm below elbow joint distal to insertion of biceps tendon		100	90	
Disarticulation at wrist joint..............................		100	90	
Midcarpal or midmetacarpal amputation of hand.....................		100	90	
Amputation of all fingers except thumb at metacarpophalangeal joints		60	54	
Amputation of thumb				
At metacarpophalangeal joint or with resection of carpometacarpal bone	100	40		
At interphalangeal joint................................	75	30		
Amputation of index finger				
At metacarpophalangeal joint or with resection of metacarpal bone................................	100	25		
At proximal interphalangeal joint.....................................	80	20		
At distal interphalangeal joint	45	11		
Amputation of middle finger				
At metacarpophalangeal joint or with resection of metacarpal bone................................	100	20		
At proximal interphalangeal joint.....................................	80	16		
At distal interphalangeal joint	45	9		
Amputation of ring finger				
At metacarpophalangeal joint or with resection of metacarpal bone................................	100	10		
At proximal interphalangeal joint.....................................	80	8		
At distal interphalangeal joint	45	5		
Amputation of little finger				
At metacarpophalangeal joint or with resection of metacarpal bone................................	100	5		
At proximal interphalangeal joint.....................................	80	4		
At distal interphalangeal joint	45	2		

*Table 16.2 and legend are reproduced with permission of The Committee on Medical Rating of Physical Impairment of the American Medical Association.

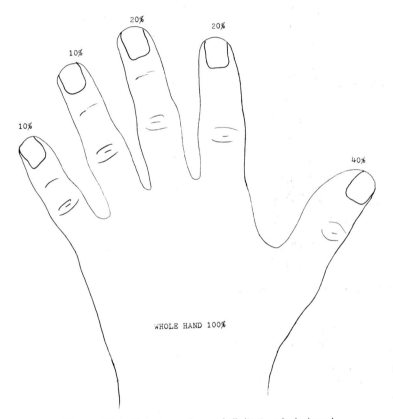

Figure 16.1. Relative values of digits to whole hand.

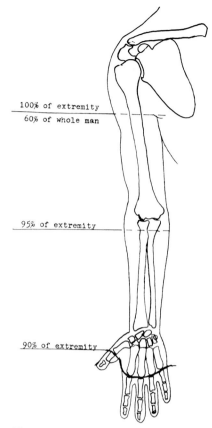

100% of extremity
60% of whole man

95% of extremity

90% of extremity

Figure 16.2. Amputation level, arm 7

comparable to the loss estimated by the Committee on Medical Rating of Physical Impairment of the American Medical Association.

In Massachusetts compensation is paid for the loss of different members according to the following percentages (Fig. 16.5).

For the loss of:

Thumb	36%
Index finger	24%
Middle finger	18%
Ring finger	12%
Little finger	10%
One phalanx of the thumb	75% of entire thumb
One phalanx of any finger	50% of entire finger
Two phalanges of any finger	90% of said finger

In Massachusetts, compensation is paid for bodily disfigurement as well as specific loss of function. In determining what is equitable and proper compensation, the Industrial Accident Board endeavors to classify the disfigurement as follows, and the percentages set forth are in proportion to the total of $6,600 as

TABLE 16.3
Schedule of payments for disfugurement for the amputation of a hand, or its fingers or parts thereof

The numerals 1, 2, 3, 4, 5, shall designate, respectively, the following: 1, thumb; 2, second or index; 3, third or middle; 4, fourth or ring; 5, fifth or little. Applicable to injuries occurring on and after November 1, 1962.

						No. of Weeks	Total Amount
1		Hand				150	$3000
		Fingers and Combinations					
2	1	2	3	4	5	125	2500
3	1	2	3	4		108.25	2165
4	1	2	3		5	101.25	2025
5	1	2		4	5	101.25	2025
6	1		3	4	5	101.25	2025
7	1	2	3			86.25	1725
8	1	2		4		86.25	1725
9	1	2			5	77.25	1545
10	1		3	4		86.25	1725
11	1		3		5	79.25	1585
12	1			4	5	79.25	1585
13	1	2				63.25	1265
14	1		3			63.25	1265
15	1			4		63.25	1265
16	1				5	54.25	1085
17	1					31.25	625
18	1 (Distal)					20	400
19		2	3	4	5	102	2040
20		2	3	4		84	1680
21		2	3		5	74	1480
22		2		4	5	74	1480
23		2	3			53	1060
24		2		4		53	1060
25		2			5	46	920
26		2				24	480
27			3	4	5	74	1480
28			3	4		55	1100
29			3		5	45	900
30			3			24	480
31				4	5	43	860
32				4		24	480
33					5	15	300

provided by the Workmen's Compensation Act.

1. Slight	0 to 10%
2. Moderate	11 to 30%
3. Severe	30 to 75%
4. Very severe	75 to 100%

Disfigurement may range from scars to major amputations.

A schedule of payments for disfigurement for the amputation of a hand, or its fingers or parts thereof has been established (Table 16.3).

In the analysis of loss of function, charts indicating percentages of specific loss are valuable. However, one must consider the hand in all its functions, *i.e.* grasp, pinch, and stereognosis, also strength of grip in the final estimate of loss of function.

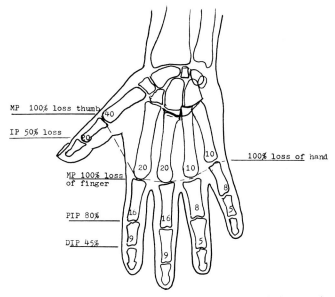

Figure 16.3. Amputation levels, percentage loss of digit, or to hand.

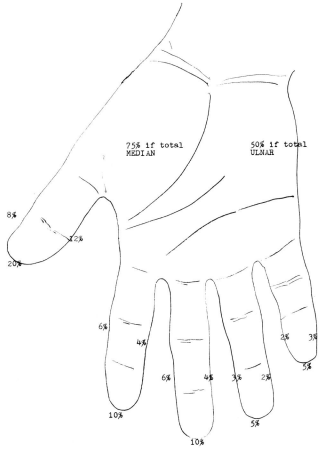

Figure 16.4. Sensory loss exclusive of tendon and joint damage. Relative value to whole hand for total sensory loss of digit and comparative loss of radial to ulnar sides.

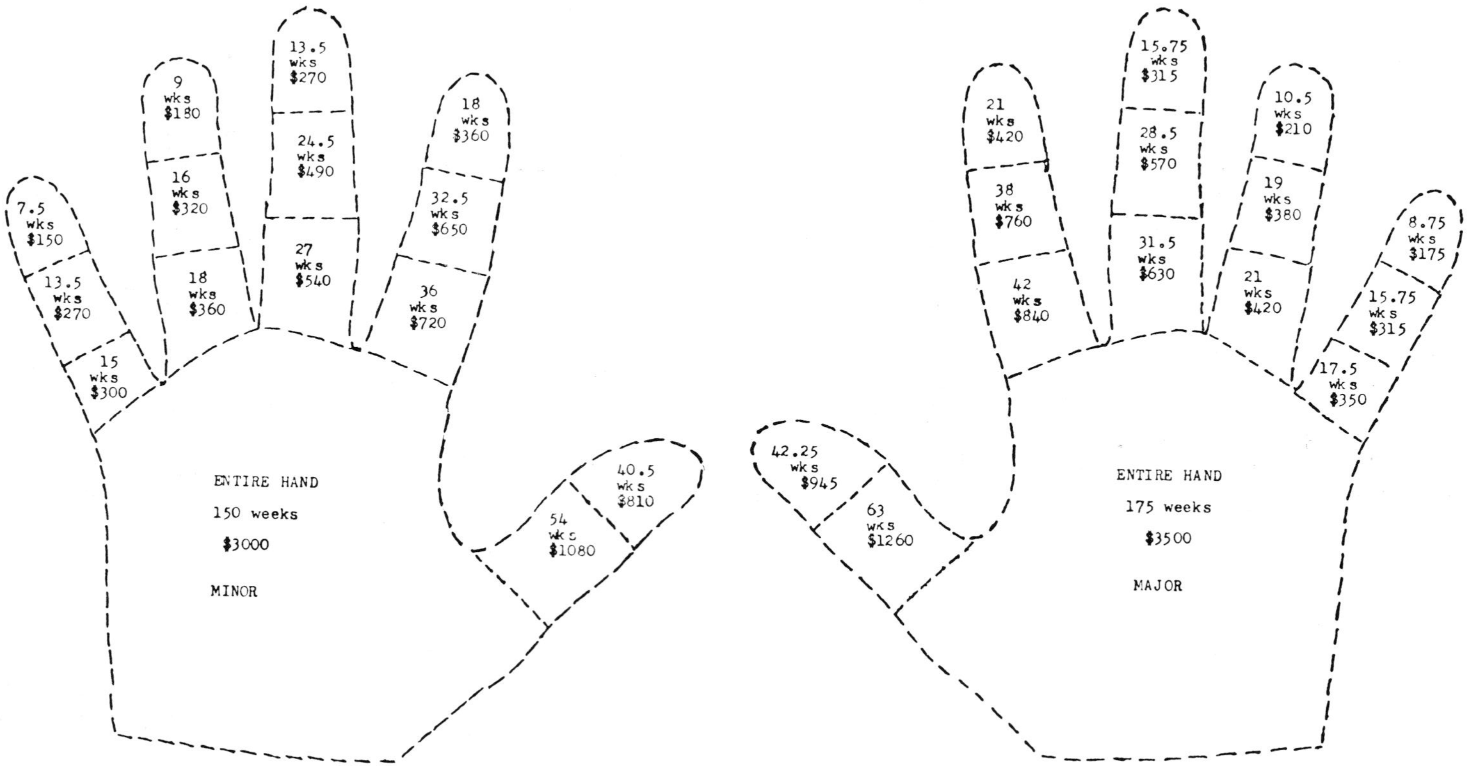

Figure 16.5. Chapter 471, effective and applicable to injuries occuring on or after November 1, 1962. Thumb, 36 per cent of hand; index, 24 per cent of hand; long, 18 per cent of hand; ring, 12 per cent of hand; little, 10 per cent of hand; one phalanx of thumb, approximately 75 per cent of thumb; one phalanx of finger, approximately 50 per cent of finger; two phalanges of finger, approximately 90 per cent of finger.

REFERENCES

1. Accidents Facts: The National Safety Council, 425 N. Michigan Ave., Chcago, Ill., 1972.

2. American Society for Surgery of the Hand Disability Evaluation Committee, Adams, J. P., Swanson, A. B., and Riordan, D.C. Jan. 10, 1966.

3. Bulletin of U. S. Bureau of Labor Statistics No. 333, 72−150; Bulletin No. 359 Standard Permanent Disability Schedules 17−30.

4. Couch, J. H. *Surgery of the Hand*. Toronto, University of Toronto Press, 1939.

5. Dublin, L. I., and Vane, R. J.: Occupation hazards and diagnostic signs, guide to impairments to be looked for in hazardous occupations. U. S. Dept. of Labor Standards Div. Bull. No. 41 (Div. of Labor Statistics Bureau Bull. No. 582), Washington, D.C., Supt. of Doc., Government Printing Office, 1941.

6. Fay, B. J. Evaluation of compensation injuries. Indust. Med., *10:* 244−246, 1941.

7. *A Guide to the Evaluation of Permanent Impairment.* A. M. A., 15, 1971.

8. Heinrich, H. W. *Industrial Accident Prevention*, Ed. 2. New York, McGraw-Hill, 1941.

9. Hobbs, C. W. *Workmen's Compensation Insurance,* Ed. 2. New York, McGraw-Hill, 1939.

10 Insurance Statistical Service of North America: *Standard Body Parts Adjustment Guide: Traumatic Cases, Occupational Diseases, Disability Evaluations, Medical Fees, Statutory Digests.* Chicago, Ill., 1941.

11. Kessler, H. H. *Accidental Injuries: The Medico-legal Aspects of Workmen's Compensation and Public Liability,* Ed. 2. Philadelphia, Lea & Febiger, 1941.

12. Lasher, W. W. Causal relationships, disability periods, and schedule losses. S. Clin. N. Am. *22:* 1251−1260, 1942.

13. Magnuson, P. B. Evaluation of disability. Indust. Med., *11:* 133, 1942.

14. McBride, E. D. *Disability Evaluation,* Ed. 4. Philadelphia, Lippincott, 1948.

15. Standard Permanent Disability Schedule Internat. Assn. Indust. Acc. Boards and Commissions. U. S. Dept. of Labor, Bur. Labor Statistics, *359:* 16−30, 1924.

16. Workman's Compensation Charts 2, 3, 7, 8, of June 1946, Division of Labor Standards, U.S. Dept. of Labor.

17. The Workmen's Compensation Act, Commonwealth of Massachusetts General Laws. Ch. 152: Sec. 36 (r.) Compensation for Loss of Fingers and Toes. Sec. 36 (h.), Bodily Disfigurement. 1961. Rates for incapacity, Nov. 1, 1972. Ch. 741 f, 1972, Compensation for amputations. Bodily disfugurement, add. Ch. 741, k, 1972.

18. Guides to the evaluation of permanent impairment. American Medical Association, 535 North Dearborn St., Chicago, Illinois, 1971.

chapter seventeen

Tumors

A.

Soft Tissue Tumors of the Hand

Joseph L. Posch, M.D.

Soft tissue tumors of the hand present many interesting and varied problems. They may arise from the skin, the subcutaneous tissue, the tendons, nerves, and blood vessels. In addition to primary tumors, metastatic tumors, although rare, may also be found. The majority of metastatic tumors to the hand are metastases to bone arising from carcinoma of the lung.

Many of the soft tissue tumors of the hand and wrist arise from local structures, although many times a swelling may indicate a generalized disorder, such as a disturbance in fat metabolism, as is found in xanthomatosis, or, in gout, a disturbance in protein metabolism. Injuries of the hand also may give rise to soft tissue swelling. This is seen in foreign body granulomas arising from the injection of grease under high pressure.

The neoplasms of the hand may, in themselves, be benign and cause local disturbances, such as interference with the tendons and nerves going to the digits (Figs. 17.1.1 and 17.1.2). On the other hand, a small soft tissue tumor that causes no inconvenience whatsoever may even be malignant, eventually leading to death.

These soft tissue tumors of the hand may occur at any age. An infant may be born with a tumor that will require surgery soon after birth.

The taking of an adequate history and a routine physical examination is always performed. One can learn from the history whether or not pain is present with the tumor and whether numbness has resulted from pressure on the nerves by the tumor, and with a careful examination, one can often determine the type of tumor present.

In potentially malignant lesions, the epitrochlear and axillary nodes should be palpated. Roentgen ray examination of the chest is extremely important. In addition, a roentgen ray examination of the hand or wrist should be done almost routinely to rule out the possibility of encroachment of the bone by the soft tissue mass. Occasionally, calcification is seen in tumors (Fig. 17.1.3).

Routine blood examination and urinalysis are always indicated.

Adequate anesthesia is important. We prefer the utilization of general anesthesia whenever possible. However, brachial block, axillary block, and local digital block without adrenalin may also be utilized.

Removal of these tumor masses is routinely performed in a bloodless field with the use of a pneumatic tourniquet inflated to 280 mm of mercury. The pneumatic cuff is never left on for more than 1½ hours. If one is desirous of having a bloodless field in a digit, we would recommend the utilization of a relatively large Penrose drain or a relatively large catheter.

Table 17.1.1 lists the tumors encountered on our service during the past 25 years. The majority of these, of course, are ganglions, but benign tumors and malignant tumors of all types are encountered.

The same general principles that apply to surgery of the hand apply here also. Care must be taken to protect the small digital vessels and nerves as they often lie adherent to the tumor. We find that a nerve stimulator is very useful when working about the motor branch of the median nerve and the deep branch of the ulnar nerve.

Adequate follow-up is essential, especially in potentially malignant tumors where recurrence may occur rapidly. Occasionally, benign tumors also have a tendency to recur. "Once a hand patient, always a hand patient."

TUMORS ARISING FROM THE EPITHELIUM

The most common tumors arising from the skin are wart, verruca vulgaris, or molluscum contagiosum. Frequently these disappear spontaneously, but occasionally it is necessary to excise the entire growth and close the wound with sutures. Cautery and dessication is often used with good results also. Occasionally the wart may be so large that skin grafting is necessary to replace the area excised. Recurrence of the wart, however, is frequent. Occasionally warts are seen that arise from under the nail, and, in that case, the nail itself must be removed along with the wart. The defect can be replace with a skin graft.

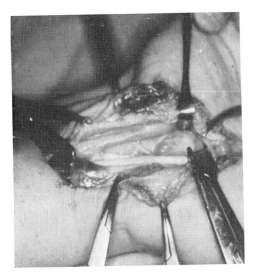

Figure 17.1.1. Ganglion in carpal tunnel caus-ing pressure on the median nerve leading to signs and symptoms of a carpal tunnel syndrome. The ganglion is at the end of the hemostat at the distal portion of the operative site.

Keratotic Lesions

Keratotic lesions are found in the older age group, golfers, farmers, and others who have been exposed to the sun and weather a good deal. They usually appear on the dorsum of the hand and should be watched for malignant changes. Excision can be done without any difficulty, and should be done if malignancy is sus-pected.

Epidermoid Cysts

Epidermoid cysts or inclusion cysts are frequently found on the hand, especially on the volar aspect of the fingers and palm. Carpenters and men who do a con-siderable amount of manual labor frequently drive skin deep into the palm, and cysts form about this skin giving rise to a nodule that is hard and firmly fixed. The mass can be readily excised and usually consists of a cavity filled with debris and cholesterol and sur-rounded by a wall of epithelium resembling normal skin (Fig. 17.1.4).

Treatment consists of surgical removal of the tumor mass, dissecting it free from the surrounding area and removing it entirely.

We have encountered four cases of epidermoid or epithelial cysts that have involved the distal phalanges of the thumb. These are manifested by partial destruc-tion of the nail with swelling under the nail and roentgen ray examination reveals a depression in the distal phalanx (Fig. 17.1.5A, B, C, D). Careful surgi-cal excision results in relief of symptoms, and the nail regenerates uneventfully.

Keratoacanthomas

In 1954, keratoacanthoma was described in the American literature for the first time. Usually these le-

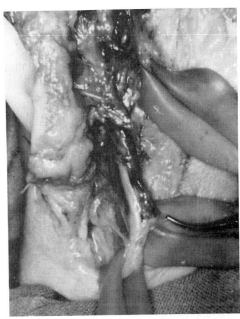

Figure 17.1.2. Hemangioma causing pressure on the deep branch of the ulnar resulting in signs and symptoms of weakness of the ulnar nerve and numbness in the little finger and ulnar aspect of the ring finger. Excision of the hemangioma re-sulted in relief of symptoms.

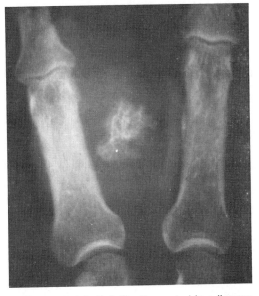

Figure 17.1.3. Calcification noted in a lipoma. Calcification is also seen in hemangiomas and liposarcomas.

TABLE 17.1.1

Type of Tumor	Number of Cases
Ganglia	801
Giant cell tumor an xanthoma	196
Epidermoid inclusion cyst	70
Verruca vulgaris, molluscum, contagiosum, senile keratosis, and sebaceous cyst	41
Hemangioma	68
Glomus tumor	29
Lipoma	46
Pyogenic granuloma	31
Aneurysm, arteriovenous malformation	9
Osteochondroma	12
Enchondroma	18
Fibroma	17
Osteoid osteoma	5
Synovioma	3
Gout	4
Boeck sarcoid	1
Tumors of the peripheral nerve, neurilemoma, Bowler's thumb	25
Malignant tumors of various types	
Fibrosarcoma	3
Squamous cell carcinoma	12
Keratoacanthoma	6
Malignant melanoma	3
Kaposi's cell sarcoma	1
Malignant variant giant cell tumor	3
Malignant schwannoma	1
Synovial cell sarcoma	1
Liposarcoma	3
Hemangioendothelioma	1
Basal cell carcinoma	6
Granular cell myoblastoma	1
Mucous cyst	72
Lymphangioma	3
Myxoma	2
Myxolipoma	1
Leiomyoma	1
Nodular fascitis	2
Myositis ossificans	1
Total	1499

involution is usually complete in four to six months, leaving a deep scar. The epidermis extends like a lip or buttress over the sides of the crater, and the proliferations appear somewhat atypical. (Histogenises is not clear. However, it is certain that the epidermal proliferation represents a pseudocarcinomatous hyperplasia. Several authors believe that the lesion starts by hyperplased hair follicles and squamous metaplasia of the sebaceous glands.) Bruner feels that keratoacanthoma is a genuine squamous cell carcinoma of very low malignancy but with a very high potential for production of keratin. This keratin plug acts as a foreign body causing inflammatory changes in the tissues under and around the lesion, which, in

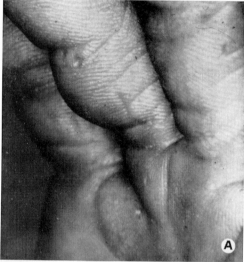

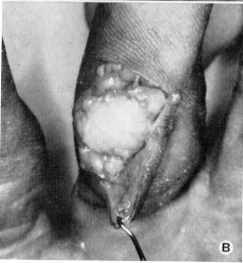

Figure 17.1.4. A. Inclusion cyst; volar aspect proximal joint of left ring finger. B. Inclusion cyst at the time of surgery. Notice right angle type of incision.

sions involve the face, but there have been cases involving the hand, and, more recently, Lamp and his associates have reported three cases involving the subungual area of the thumb. We have encountered lesions involving this area, and also we have seen several involving the dorsal aspect of the hand. Usually these lesions are treated as blisters or some type of benign reaction.

The maximal size is about 2 cm, and it takes about eight weeks to reach this size. The surrounding skin is often inflamed. Spontaneous regression can occur and

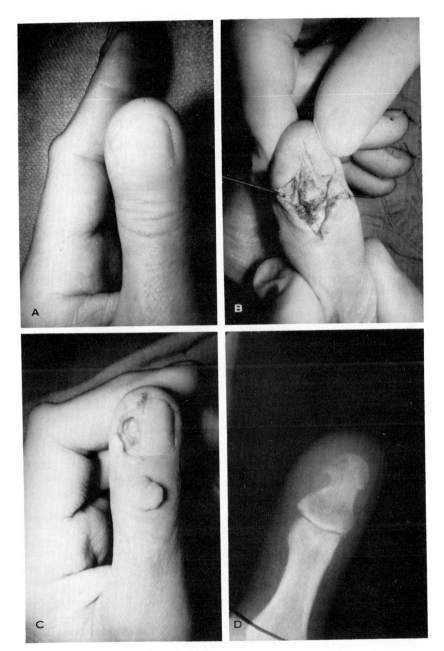

Figure 17.1.5. A 57-year-old man with a three-week history of partial loss of left thumb nail. *A.* This figure shows the relatively minor depression in the nail. *B.* Shows the nail incised and a rather large tumor mass encountered. *C.* Shows the tumor mass excised. The microscopic diagnosis was verruca vulgaris. Similar deformities have been caused by epithelial and carotene cysts.

turn, causes extrusion of the tumor before there is time for metastatic spread (Fig. 17.1.6).

Carcinoma

Trauma and infections play important roles in the etiology of carcinoma of the hand. In addition, malignancies can arise from previous skin tumors and also from normal skin. It is said that 5 to 10 per cent of all carcinomas occur in the hand and foot. Squamous cell and basal cell carcinomas comprise 90 per cent of all malignancies in the hand. Squamous cell carcinoma is, by far, the most common and is usually located on the dorsal aspect of the hand, but occasionally it is also seen in the palm.

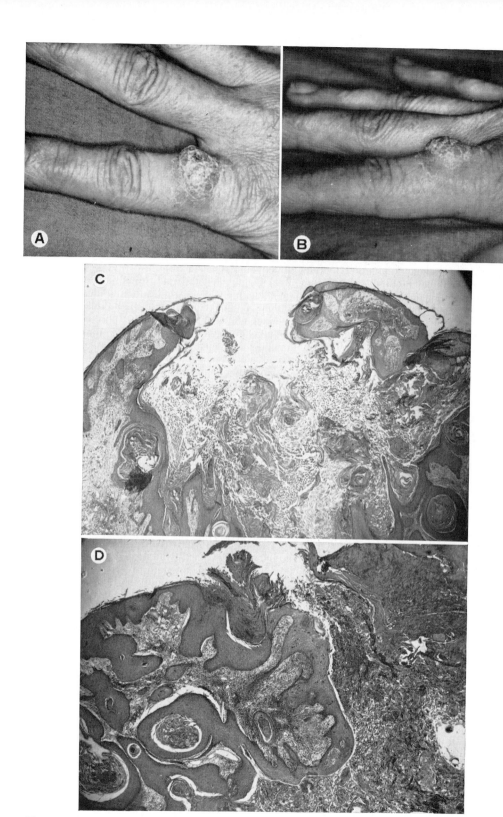

Figure 17.1.6. A and B. Keratoacanthoma in a 48-year-old woman. The lesion started as a blister. Healing developed only on top and subsequent inflammation took place. The lesion was present for approximately eight weeks when the patient was first seen. C and D. Keratoacanthoma, high powered view. Note stratified squamous epithelium with marked acanthosis. Laminated keratin is also present.

Treatment consists of wide excision of the lesion and skin grafting, if necessary, to cover the open area. If palpable nodes are present in the epitrochlear area or axillary region, they are removed approximately two weeks after the original tumor is removed. Prophylatic dissection may be done six weeks later, where the patient may be observed and the axillary and epitrochlear nodes removed if necessary.

The gross appearance of a squamous cell carcinoma is usually that of an ulcerated area that has a regular line and a hard border. Microscopically, the lesions are composed of columns of squamous epithelial cells, producing epithelial pearls (Fig. 17.1.7).

Basal cell carcinoma is also found in the hand; it has the typical appearance of the rolled-up, indurated area of a rodent ulcer. Metastases to lymph nodes are quite rare.

An example of carcinoma arising from a chronic infection of the nail is presented. These usually arise where infections have not healed over a long period of time and will eventually reveal a squamous cell carcinoma. Amputation of the involved digit must be done, and a secondary dissection of the epitrochlear and axillary nodes is performed. This malignancy is

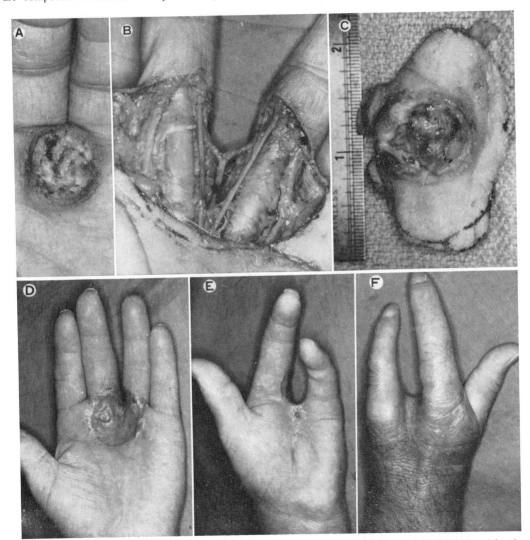

Figure 17.1.7. A. A 60-year-old patient had a small wart on the volar aspect of his left hand for the past two years. Biopsy revealed the presence of squamous cell carcinoma. B. The tumor was widely excised and the tendon sheath was unroofed. Note the preservation of the digital nerves and arterial blood supply. C. Gross specimen with surrounding skin margin removed. D. Recurrence developed within a few months and amputation of the long and ring fingers including removal of the metacarpal bone. was carried out. E. There was some delayed healing on the volar aspect of the palm of the left hand, but this eventually healed. F. Dorsal view.

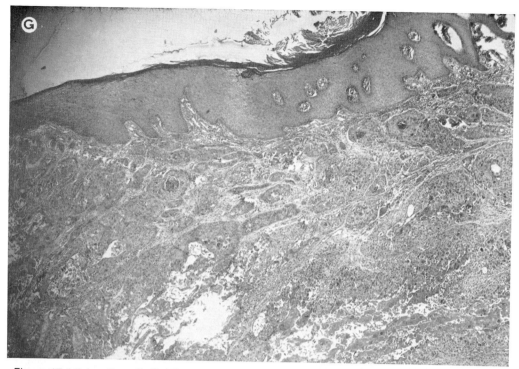

Figure 17.1.7 (continued). G. Microscopic view of squamous cell carcinoma excised at the time of the original surgery. The patient subsequently had an axillary and epitrochlear node dissection. However, none of the lymph nodes were involved.

quite rare. Until 1939 only 19 cases were reported in the literature. We had one case occurring in a 50-year-old dentist who had a chronic paronychia for 19 months (Fig. 17.1.8).

Benign moles or nevi are found in the hand rather frequently. If subject to irritation, or if they do appear to be increasing in size, they should be removed. Biopsy should not be done, but the mole and surrounding area must be removed. Cautery, electrodissection, and irradiation is contraindicated.

Those in the subungual area may give rise to malignant melanoma, and these must be removed. In malignant melanomas (Hutchinson's melanotic whitlow), 50 per cent arise from an area that has been traumatized. The most common location of these malignant tumors is on the thumb. The infection appears first and sparates the nail and nail bed. An ulcer-like growth begins to occur with or without pigmentation. Many times pigmentation is noted at the periphery of the ulcer. Microscopically, evidence of inflammation is present in addition to the ulcerating mass. The tumor is composed of fusiform spindle-like cells with frequent mitoses, hyperchromatic nuclei, and both intra-and extracellular pigment. Treatment consists of early amputation of the digit and, either immediately or approximately two weeks later, removal of the regional lymph nodes. In regard to prognosis, the subungual types present the best possible

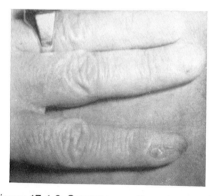

Figure 17.1.8. Squamous cell carcinoma of the nail in a chronic infection. Treated by amputation of the digit and subsequent epitrochlear and axillary node dissection. Although axillary nodes were palpable, they were lymphadenitis and there was no spread of the tumor. The patient has had no recurrence.

chance or cure. Pack reports a five-year survival rate of 18.75 per cent with no evidence of recurrence for all subungual melanomas (Fig. 17.1.9). Melanotic melanoma profusion with appropriate chemicals is also indicated.

Rarely, lentigo maligna has been encountered. This

type of melanotic freckle or precancerous melanosis is contrasted to the superficial spreading malignant melanoma. However, these lesions can involve not only the epidermis but also the nail matrix, nail bed, and nail plate (Fig. 17.1.10 A, B).

TUMORS ARISING FROM CONNECTIVE TISSUE

Fibromas

Fibromas of the hand are quite rare. Two types are noted: the deep type, arising from the joint capsule, and the superficial type. The etiology is unknown. Grossly, these tumors are well encapsulated, and microscopically, dense fibrous tissue in sheets or whorls is noted. These tumors are located on either the palmar or dorsal aspect of the fingers. The differential diagnosis is neurogenic tumor, epidermoid cyst, gangloin, or xanthoma. Treatment consists of removal of the entire structure, and prognosis for cure is good. Calcification, cartilage, and bone formation may occur. They may be connected with the deeper tissue or ligaments. They have been described as tumors of the tendon sheath and also the tendon proper. A subungual fibroma may cause distortion of the nail and pressure atrophy of the distal phalanx. Diagnosis is made on the basis of the firmness of the tumor (Fig. 17.1.11 A, B, C).

Lipomas

Lipomas may also be found in the hand, and actually their presence is not too rare. They resemble lipomas elsewhere. The etiology is unknown. Grossly, they are soft, well encapsulated tumors, and microscopically, fatty tissue and fibrous tissue are noted. They are frequently found on both the volar and dorsal aspect of the hand; in our series of cases, they were most common on the volar aspect. Mason states that they can be divided into groups, the superficial or subcutaneous and a subfascial group. This latter is also divided into two groups, the epivaginal and endovaginal. Treatment is excision with preservation of the vessels and nerves. The prognosis for cure is good. Occasionally it is rather difficult to distinguish clinically a lipoma from a xanthoma or tuberculous tenosynovitis. Symptoms produced are those caused by mechanical disturbances (Figs. 17.1.12 and 17.1.13).

Ganglia

Ganglion is the most common tumor found in the hand. Trauma as the etiologic factor was seen in about 15 per cent of the patients. Although many individuals do give a history of trauma, it is thought that the traumatic episode merely called the individual's attention to the ganglion cyst already present. The etiology of these cysts is said to be unknown, although extensive research has shown that these ganglia are composed of a main cyst with a pedicle going from the

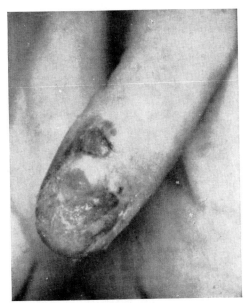

Figure 17.1.9. Melanotic melanoma in a 40-year-old factory employee seen for examination in February 1953. She had suffered an injury to the nail of her right thumb on a drill press in August 1948, and chronic infection had ensued. Repeated biopsies made at yearly intervals had been reported as being negative, and treatment had consisted of removal of the nail, incision and drainage, x-ray and ultaviolet ray treatments, and the injection of penicillin, locally and systemically. When first seen by the author, the lesion appeared to be a melanoma. Wide excision was recommended and carried out, and a malignant melanoma was encountered. Subsequently, on March 13, 1953, amputation of the thumb along with epitrochlear and axillary lymph node dissection, was carried out. The patient worked at intervals but eventually, on April 30, 1955, died as a result of widespread metastasis.

deep part of the cyst to the underlying joint capsule. It has been found that the joint capsule is involved in the structure of the ganglion, and communication between the pedicle and the joint has been shown on microscopic studies. If contrast material is injected into the ganglion, it does not communicate with the joint, but if a contrast material is injected into the wrist joint, it does communicate with the ganglion. It was thought that this may be due to a valve phenomena in the duct.

The cysts are located on the dorsoradial aspect of the wrist joint, the volar radial aspect of the wrist joint, and the flexor tendon sheaths of the fingers. In addition, they may be intratendinous. They, actually, can arise anywhere in the hand, on the dorsal ulnar aspect of the wrist joint, the metacarpophalangeal joints, the proximal interphalangeal joints, and the distal interphalangeal joints (Fig. 17.1.14 A through C).

The most common location for these ganglions is on

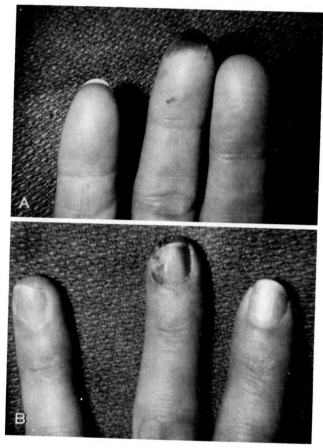

Figure 17.1.10. A and *B*. A 50-year-old white woman. Note the dark discoloration at the tip of the left middle finger eight years previously. The dark area had spread gradually. After the diagnosis of lentigo maligna was made by biopsy, the entire third ray including the metacarpal was excised.

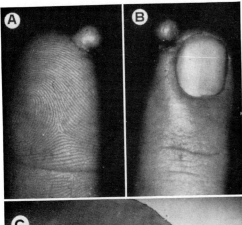

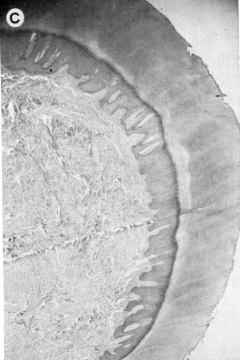

Figure 17.1.11. A and *B*. Anterior and dorsal view of a fibroma on the tip of the right index finger. This growth had been present for approximately 11 years. Surgery consisted of wide excision of the base of the tumor and primary closure of the skin. The pathologic diagnosis was fibroma of the skin. *C*. Microscopic view showing dense fibrous tissue in the fibroma.

the dorsoradial aspect of the wrist joint, where they appear to arise from the articulation of the trapezium and trapezoid bones and from the navicular-lunate articulation. They present between the extensor carpi radialis longus and brevis and the extensor digitorum communis tendons to the fingers.

The next most frequent site is the volar radial aspect of the wrist joint between the tendons of the brachial

radialis and the flexor carpi radialis from the same joints mentioned above. The superficial branch of the radial nerve and the radial artery usually have to be retracted to one side. The cyst here appears to arise from the volar aspect of the wrist joint, and the cyst and the underlying joint capsule must be completely removed.

The next most common site is the flexor tendon sheath of the fingers on the volar aspect of the metacarpophalangeal joint over the proximal phalanx. Here, the tumor, on palpation, is quite hard and is often thought to be involved with bone. X-ray examinations are negative.

The ganglion cysts also are often found to be intratendinous, especially involving the extensor tendons on the dorsal aspect of the hand, where they must be carefully dissected from the tendons themselves.

In addition, a ganglion cysts can involve an entire tendon itself. For example, a flexor carpi radialis or an extensor carpi ulnaris will occasionally be the site of a large ganglion cyst surrounding the entire tendon.

The ganglion cysts on the dorsal ulnar aspect of the wrist joint can be traced to their origin on the dorsoradial aspect of the wrist.

Treatment of these ganglion cysts is usually surgical. On the volar radial aspect of the wrist joint, we make a longitudinal, semi-curved incision since this does seem to cut down on the recurrence rate.

On the dorsoradial aspect of the wrist joint, either a transverse or a lazy "S" type of incision can be made. The transverse incision gives a better cosmetic result, but occasionally small sensory branches of the radial nerve are disturbed and will cause some difficulty.

Cysts involving the flexor tendon sheaths on the fingers can be excised with the underlying tendon sheath.

Ganglion cysts may cause erosion into carpal bones. They may cause carpal tunnel syndrome symptoms when they are located in the floor of the carpal canal, and they may give rise to snapping thumb or trigger fingers when they involve the tendon sheath.

Mucous Cysts

Frequently, in a middle-aged patient, one encounters small ganglion-like cysts on the dorsal aspect of the distal interphalangeal joints of the fingers. These are located to either side of the extensor tendon. These cysts are white, hard, occasionally break, ooze clear fluid, and may even become ulcerated. Occasionally they become infected and can cause severe septic arthritis involving the distal interphalangeal joint.

The cyst does press upon the nail bed and nail matrix and frequently causes a longitudinal striation in the nail itself. (This fact serves as a differential diagnosis from giant cell tumors.) Underlying this cyst we frequently find an osteoarthritic process (Fig. 17.1.15*A*, *B*).

Treatment consists of wide excision of the cyst and surrounding skin and replacement of the area with a free full thickness skin graft. The cyst may be excised

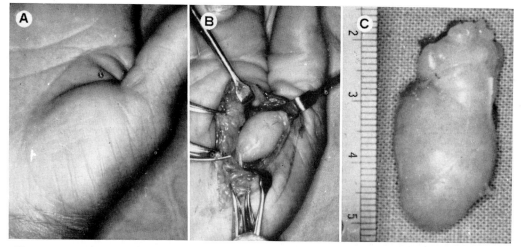

Figure 17.1.12. A. Lipoma of thenar eminence of the right thumb. *B.* Operative findings. *C.* Gross specimen.

and closed with a right angle sliding pedicle flap or it may be excised and closed with a rotational skin flap also. Recurrences are rare when the area is excised and replaced with a skin graft or adequately excised and replaced with a sliding pedicle graft (Fig. 17.1.16).

Although a diagnosis of ganglion cyst is readily made, occasionally rather diffuse swellings on the dorsal aspect of the wrist, which do appear to be ganglions, on operation prove to be rather diffuse tenosynovitis involving the extensor tendons. This is usually rheumatoid in nature (Fig. 17.1.17). On the volar aspect of the wrist, one has, in the past, encountered a tuberculous tenosynovitis rather than a ganglion although a diagnosis of ganglion or compound ganglion had been made. However, on opening the cyst, straw-colored fluid and rice bodies are encountered. Destruction of tendons can result from this type of lesion (Fig. 17.1.18).

A ganglion cyst has occasionally been seen overlying a bony protuberance. Diagnosis of this entity is confirmed by lateral roentgen ray, especially with the wrist acutely flexed. Conservative treatment is preferred unless the area becomes quite painful or unless there is a history of trauma. Then, a radical excision of the bony protuberance is indicated.

Knuckle pads seen in Dupuytren's contracture are occasionally identified as ganglion cysts, but the hardness and the fact that they are usually located in more than one finger will aid in the differential diagnosis. In addition, Dupuytren's contracture, which is usually, although not always, present, aids in the identification of these knuckle pads (Fig. 17.1.19 *A, B*).

Bowlar's thumb neuroma of the ulnar digital nerve to the thumb is occasionally mistaken for a ganglion cyst. However, the fact that this tumor mass is rather elongated and painful on palpation aids in the differential diagnosis (Fig. 17.1.19).

In the final analysis, if a ganglion cyst is not in its usual location, that is, the dorsoradial aspect or volar radial aspect of the wrist joint or directly connected with the tendon or tendon sheath, it is usually not a ganglion cyst (Fig. 17.1.20).

Giant Cell Tumors

Giant cell tumors are one of the more common tumors of the hand. The etiology is unknown, although it is thought that trauma may be an exciting cause.

Grossly, the tumors are yellow or yellow-brown with streaks of grey. Microscopically, one sees the characteristic foam cells, the foreign body giant cells, and the spindle cells. These tumors are located in either the volar or dorsal aspect of the hand; in our series of cases, they were more prominent on the volar aspect. The diagnosis can be made by palpating a hard, irregular mass that is not movable. At times there may be some difficulty in differentiating this from a lipoma or a ganglion. In surgery the tumor is found to arise from the tendon sheath. If the tumor presents on the volar aspect, it is often found to extend behind the tendon. Occasionally they can invade bone. The treatment consists of excision of the tumor. The growth itself is a benign one and, if all of the tumor is removed, recurrence will not occur. The recurrence rate is said to be 10 per cent, but this is usually those involving the distal phalanx.

In the past, the terms xanthoma and giant cell tumor have been rather loosely exchanged. Stevenson, in reviewing xanthoma and giant cell tumors occurring in 50 patients in a 20-year period, stated that there is a definite difference in the two. The xanthoma tissue infiltrates widely, while the giant cell tumor is encapsulated. Xanthomas are found symmetrically in the fingers, elbow, buttocks, knees, ankles, heels, and toes. In addition, xanthomatosis is associated with a high cholesterol level. One of our tumors on the dorsal aspect of the wrist eroded into the capitate and hamate bones (Figs. 17.1.21, 17.1.22, 17.1.23).

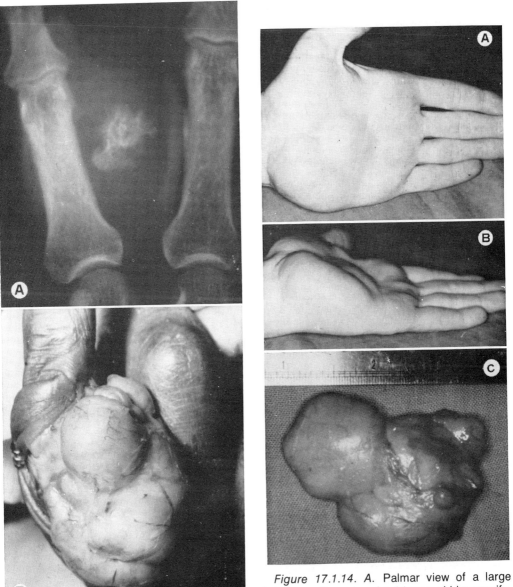

Figure 17.1.13. A. Roentgen ray examination of a soft tissue mass of the right index finger showing calcification. B. Operative findings showing a large lipoma which was readily shelled out after the digital vessels and nerves were retracted.

Figure 17.1.14. A. Palmar view of a large lipoma on the palm of a 24-year-old housewife. The only thing that bothered her was the growth in the palm of the left hand. There were no other complaints. B. View from the side of the hand. C. Gross specimen.

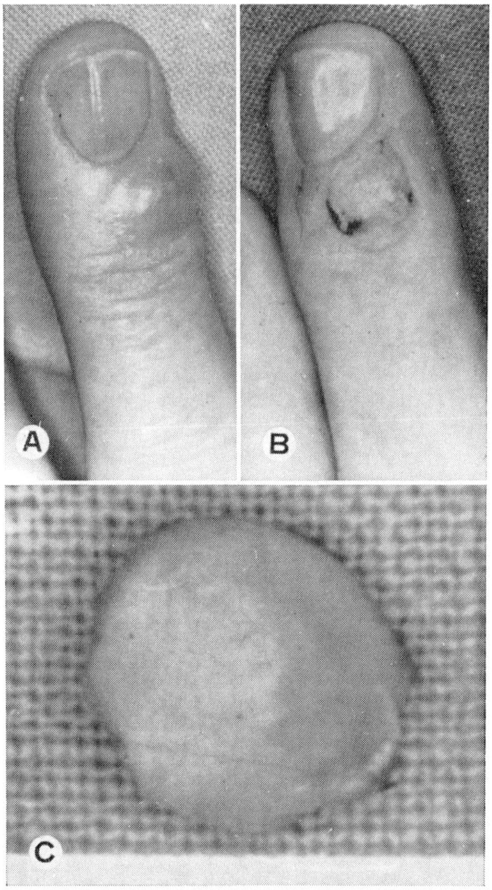

Figure 17.1.15. A. Mucous cyst on the dorsal ulnar aspect of the distal interphalangeal joint of the right long finger in a 60-year-old woman with osteoarthritis. Note changes in the nail from pressure by the cyst. *B.* The cyst widely excised; this defect is then covered with a skin graft. *C.* Gross specimen.

Glomus Tumors

Although these tumors may be found in almost any part of the body, the most common place is the fingers, especially in the subungual areas. The tumor itself arises from the normal glomus which is present throughout the skin structures of the body and aids in heat regulation by the vasomotor system. Trauma is thought to be an exciting factor in some of the cases. Pathologically, on gross inspection, the tumor is a small, encapsulated and ranges from several millimeters to 1 cm in diameter. The color is deep red or purple. Microscopically, increased number of glomal cells and nonmyelinated fibers are noted. These tumors are made up of blood vessels with thickened walls, the media is replaced by epithelial cells interspersed with smooth muscle cells and myelinated and nonmyelinated nerve fibers. The tumor is found more commonly in men than women, and has been found at all ages. In about one-half of the cases it is subungual. The predominant symptom is pain which becomes worse in changes in weather. The diagnosis is made upon noting that the tumor itself is extremely painful. In addition, a bluish or cyanotic coloration may be seen under the fingernail. The treatment is surgical removal, and the prognosis for cure is good once this has been carried out. Multiple glomus tumors are rare, but may occur (Figs. 17.1.24, 17.1.25, 17.1.26).

Pyogenic Granuloma

Pyogenic granulomas are red, mushroom-like growths that appear on the volar aspect of the fingers and the palmar surface of the hand. There is usually an antecedent history of trauma or infection of the involved area. The area bleeds readily and, sometimes, that is the presenting complaint. The diagnosis is made on the gross appearance and the history of the injury. Treatment consists of excision or cauterization. The prognosis for cure is good once the entire base has been irradicated (Fig. 17.1.27).

Foreign Body Granulomas

Foreign body granulomas are found in the hand. They are due to foreign bodies accidentally introduced into the hand. Paraffin injected for cosmetic reasons or grease accidentally injected under high pressure by a working man also give rise to foreign body reactions. Microscopically, the foreign body is surrounded by indolent granulation tissue with a dense fibrous tissue capsule. Numerous foreign body giant cells are found (Fig. 17.1.28).

Boeck's Sarcoid

Boeck's sarcoid is very rare in the hand. It is a tumor of the reticuloendothelial system, composed of epithelial and giant cells. Bone changes may occur. Treatment is supportive.

Sebaceous Cysts

Sebaceous cysts are seen on the dorsal aspect of the hand; however, these are quite rare. They are similar to sebaceous cysts found elsewhere and can be readily removed without difficulty.

Fibrosarcoma

Fibrosarcomas are thought to arise from connective tissue elements or from benign tumors of fibrous tissue origin. Their appearance may vary considerably; however, they usually are a rather large, diffuse mass, soft in consistency, infiltrating the nerves, tendons, and vessels without limiting motion to any great degree.

Clinically they may appear to be benign tumors, but microscopically one encounters a malignant picture.

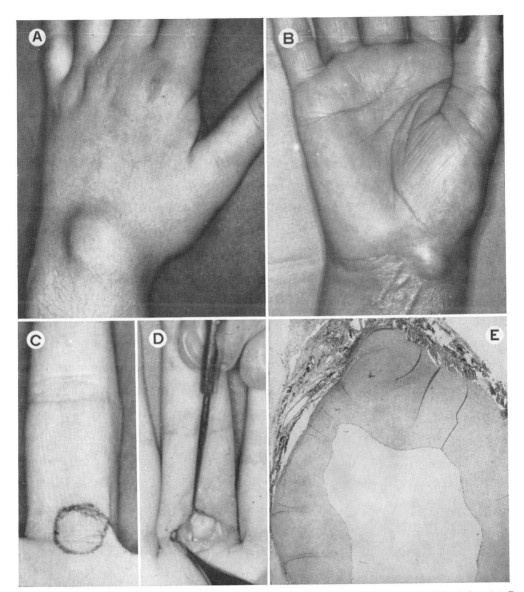

Figure 17.1.16. A. Typical location of ganglion cyst, on the dorsal radial aspect of the left wrist. *B.* Ganglion on the volar radial aspect of the right hand. Ganglions in this area are rather difficult to remove, and the recurrence rate is often quite high. *C.* Ganglion on the tendon sheath of the right long finger. *D.* Operative findings showing a small ganglion cyst as removed through a small transverse incision. The underlying tendon sheath is removed with the cyst. *E.* High powered microscopic view showing the rather thick cyst wall.

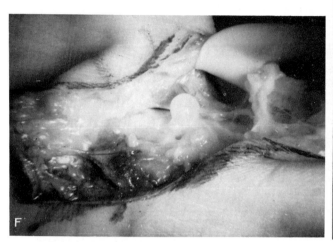
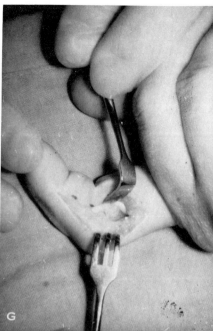

Figure 17.1.16. (continued). F. A large ganglion cyst encountered in the flexor tendon sheath. The flexor pollicis longus tendon of the thumb. The digital nerves retracted to one side with a rubber drain. A large hard mass clinically. Thought to be a neuroma and found to be a ganglion cyst involving the flexor tendon sheath. *G.* A ganglion cyst encountered under the flexor digitorum superficialis tendon of the index finger of a 28-year-old dental hygenist. Patient presented limitation of flexion with slight swelling of the finger. Exploration of the flexor tendons in the palm was negative; however, exploration of the digit revealed a large ganglion cyst on the flexor tendon sheath excision of the cyst resulted in complete normal range of motion.

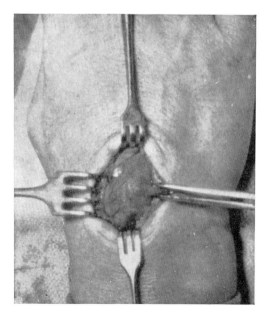

Figure 17.1.17. Chronic tenosynovitis, involving the extensor tendons of the dorsal aspect of the right wrist. The involved tendons were dissected free from the tumor mass. There has been no recurrence of the tumor in the year since this surgery was done.

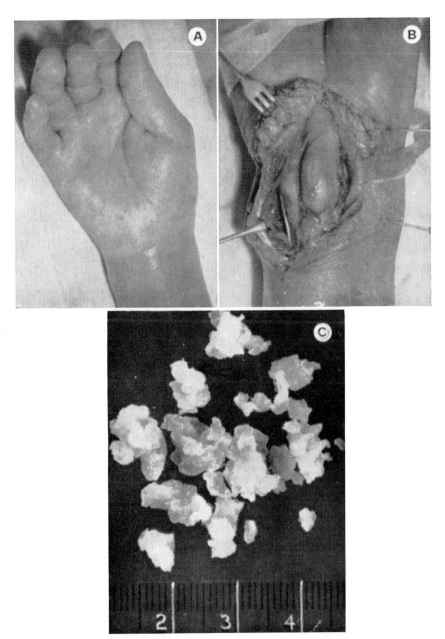

Figure 17.1.18. *A.* A large swelling on the palm and wrist of the right hand. *B.* Chronic tuberculous tenosynovitis. *C.* Rice bodies obtained at the time of surgery. The lesion has not recurred since the operation, but flexion of the ring and little fingers has remained limited.

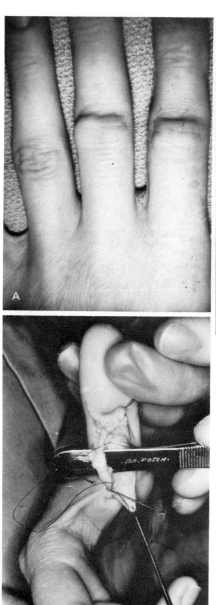
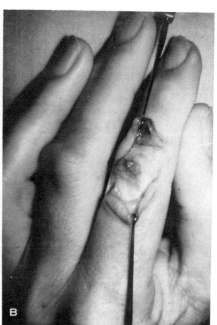

Figure 17.1.19. A and *B*. A 51-year-old housewife with no evidence of Dupuytren's contracture but rather markedly enlarged knuckle pads on the dorsal aspect of the middle, ring, and little fingers of the left hand and on the dorsal aspect of the index, middle, and ring fingers of the right hand. *A*. Shows the markedly enlarged knuckle pads on the dorsal aspect of the left index and middle fingers. *B*. is the operative photograph showing the marked fibromatosis encountered. *C*. Bowler's thumb. A 38-year-old female noticed a palpable mass at the base of the right thumb approximately three months previously. This slowly increased in size and tenderness. A diagnosis of neuroma was made, now known as Bowler's thumb. More recent literature indicates that a neurolysis, internal and external, is the procedure of choice. Originally, these areas were excised and a secondary anastamosis was carried out usually with good results.

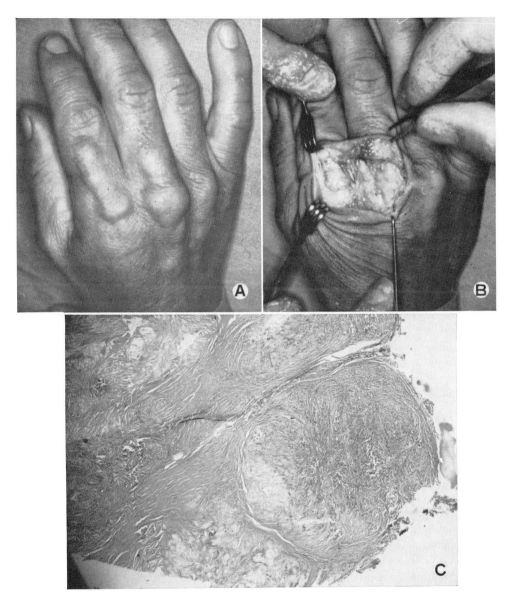

Figure 17.1.20. A. Xanthomatosis of a 55-year-old man. He had nodules on the dorsal aspect of the metacarpophalangeal joints of both hands without any complaints of pain. Gradual increase in size had been noted for the past 10 years. *B.* Findings at surgery. *C.* Microscopic findings.

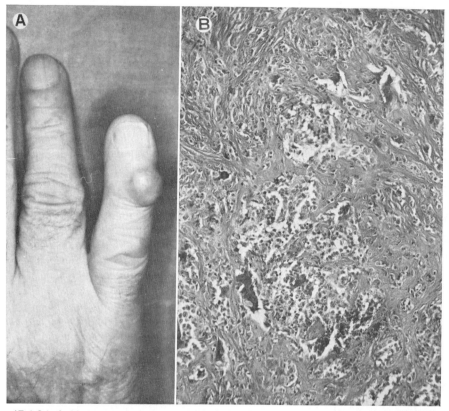

Figure 17.1.21. A. Mass on the dorsal ulnar aspect of the right little finger. This was thought to be a mucous cyst; however, at the time of surgery, it was found to be a giant cell tumor. This was carefully excised. No recurrence was noted 18 months after surgery. B. Microscopic view of the giant cell tumor reveals multiple giant cells.

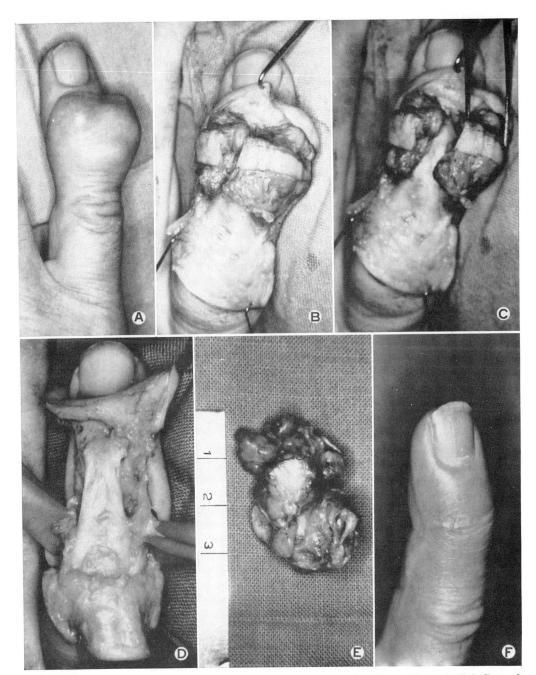

Figure 17.1.22. A. A 56-year-old man with swelling on the distal phalanx of his right little finger for approximately 2 to 3 years. There was no pain. *B.* At the time of surgery, a large giant cell tumor was encountered that extended under the extensor tendon to the flexor tendon underneath. *C.* Shows the separation of the tumor mass and exposed extensor tendon. *D.* Findings at the conclusion of the procedure, the extensor intact, small Penrose drains have been placed about the digital nerves. *E.* Gross specimen. *F.* The finger six months after surgery. No evidence of recurrence with a good range of motion.

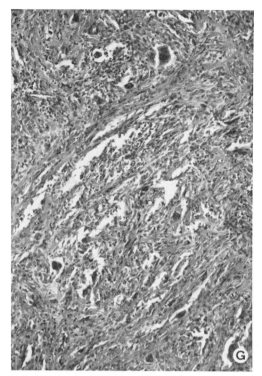

Figure 17.1.22 (continued). G. Microscopic section of the numerous giant cells present.

These are usually located in the superficial tissues rather than the deep tissues, and the tumor is present for quite some time. The best evidence, of course, is a local recurrence within a short time after removal.

If recurrence does occur, wide radical excision must be carried out, and in the highly malignant tumor, amputation should be done without hesitation. However, low grade types of fibrosarcomas can occur. In children, we find a juvenile type of fibromatosis, or so-called benign fibrosarcoma, in which local recurrences occur. However, wide excision, preserving the intricate structures of the hand and wrist, can result in a good functioning extremity without resorting to amputation, and metastases do not occur. In about one-third of our cases of fibrosarcoma, there is a history of trauma.

Synovioma

Synoviomas are very rare in the hand. They may arise from either the lining of the joints or tendon sheaths. This tumor may be benign or malignant. If malignancy is encountered, many times heroic measures must be taken to save the individual's life.

Other Malignant Tumors

One encounters many other variations of malignant tumors in the upper extremity and hand, such as malignant schwannomas, liposarcomas, synovial cell

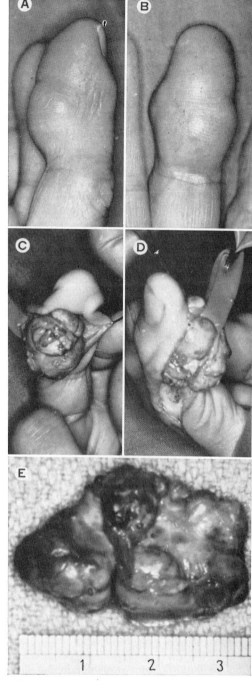

Figure 17.1.23. A and *B.* A 60-year-old woman with a large mass involving the middle and distal phalanx of her right long finger. It has been present for approximately 8 years. There was some numbness in the finger. *C* and *D.* Operative findings. Note the tumor mass completely surrounds the digital nerve. This must be retracted to one side. *E.* Gross specimen.

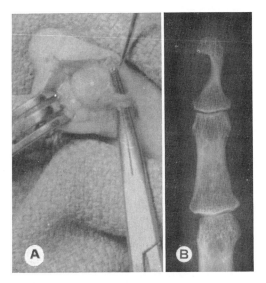

Figure 17.1.24. A. Large glomus tumor on the radial volar aspect of the right ring finger. Specimen is being removed in a bloodless field. Attempts to remove it after taking off the nail were unsuccessful, so a counter incision had to be made here where the large tumor was identified and removed. B. Erosion caused on the distal phalanx by this glomus tumor of many years standing.

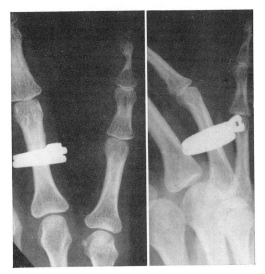

Figure 17.1.25. Compression of distal phalanx of little finger caused by glomus tumor in a 30-year-old nurse.

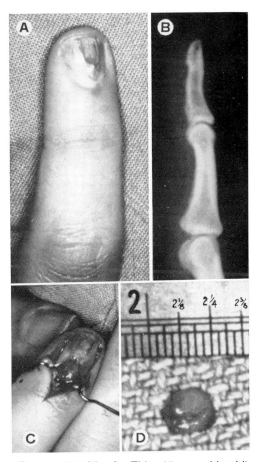

Figure 17.1.26. A. This 45-year-old white housewife had intermittent pain on the tip of her right index finger for the past 25 years. The base of the nail was very sensitive. In addition, the nail was deformed. There was tenderness in the center of the nailbed. Note the bluish discoloration at the base of the nail and the area of the nail distal to that which is deformed. B. Questionable pressure on the dorsal aspect of the distal phalanx of the right index finger by the tumor. C. The nail has been removed, the nailbed has been incised, and a large glomus tumor was encountered. D. Gross specimen.

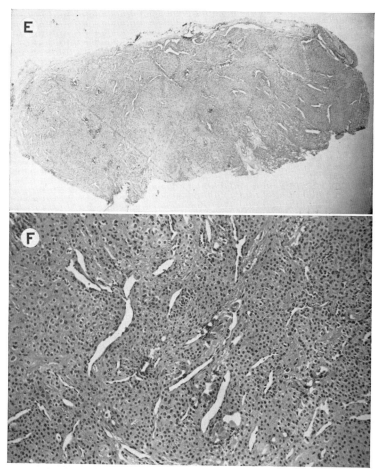

Figure 17.1.26 (continued). *E.* Reveals endothelial-like lumen surrounded by some irregularly ar-ranged muscular coat. *F.* Microscopic view. Note the large number of glomal cells.

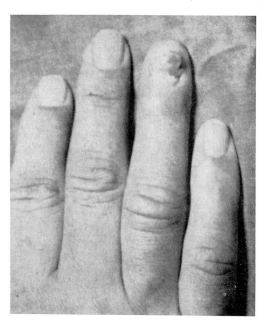

Figure 17.1.27. Pyogenic granuloma, excised, and closed primarily without any difficulty.

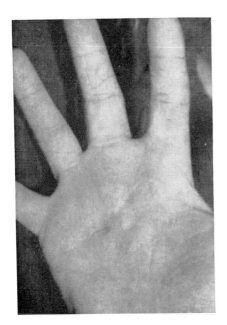

Figure 17.1.28. Foreign body granuloma in the palm of the right hand. The patient was an employee in a gasoline station, and the tumor had developed after the injection of grease under high pressure. A previous attempt to remove the tumor had been made elsewhere, but this attempt had failed and the nodules had recurred. I cleaned the entire involved area in the palm and also the dorsal aspect of the right long finger where further nodules had appeared. Subsequently the ring finger became involved and another operation was necessary.

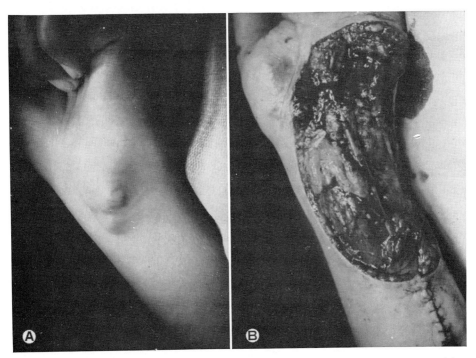

Figure 17.1.29. A. Synovial cell sarcoma in a 29-year old white man. The patient gave a history of falling from a vehicle. He developed bluish and purplish discoloration of the hand. He was given stellate ganglion blocks and clinically it was felt that he had a large ganglion on the volar surface of the wrist. This was excised and proved to by a synovial cell sarcoma. *B.* Excision at the time of surgery.

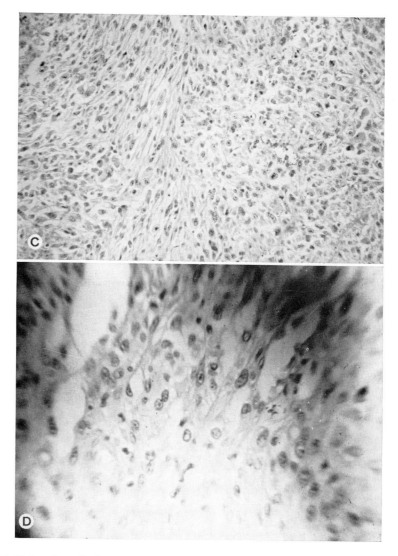

Figure 17.1.29 (continued). C and *D.* Synovial cell sarcoma. Patient alive and well four years after onset of symptoms, although he has had x-ray therapy, perfusion of the upper extremity, and tendon transplants.

sarcomas, and malignant fibrous xanthomas. One can classify all of these, including the fibrosarcomas, as an epitheloid sarcoma. It is pointed out that these grow in a nodular manner along the tendons, often with an ulceration of overlying skin. These may grow slowly and have repeated surgical excisions. Microscopically, the tumor consists of irregular nodular masses of large deeply acidophilic polygonal cells merging with spindle cells frequently associated with large amounts of hyalin and collagen. Since these are slow-growing, a wide excision is indicated early. If recurrences occur, amputation of the involved member is definitely indicated. In a series of cases reported by Enzinger, 85 per cent had recurrence with metastasis in 30 per cent.

The main difficulty in this type of lesion, which is encountered by all surgeons, is that the benign process originally is deceptive. However, with recurrence and further investigation one can readily see that this is a highly malignant tumor (Figs. 17.1.29, 17.1.30).

When one encounters this type of lesion, one must consider amputation, even fore quarter if necessary. Radiation therapy, when indicated, is occasionally life saving. Profusion of the extremity with appropriate chemotherapeutic drugs has been used to good advantage. Recently, chemotherapy with a combination of adriamycin and dimethyl triazeno imidazole carboxamide, a good response rate of 41 per cent has been obtained, where metastasis had occurred.

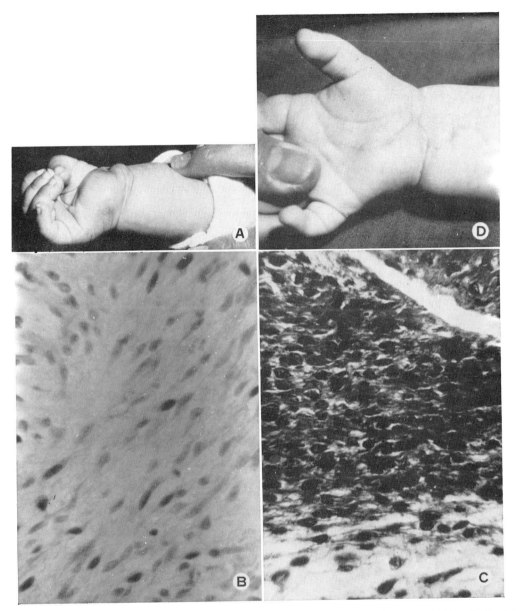

Figure 17.1.30. A. A four-month-old child with a large swelling on the volar aspect of his right wrist and palm. *B* and *C.* Excision revealed a differentiated fibrosarcoma cross-indexed as juvenile aponeurotic fibroma. Probably should be listed as a juvenile fibromatosis. *D.* One year later, no sign of recurrence. Good function of the hand.

B.

Tumors of the Hand Skeleton

Robert E. Carroll, M.D.

Tumors arising or situated in the bony structure of the hand are exceedingly rare. They are almost always benign and are readily accessible. Because the hand skeleton can be seen on roentgenograms, more information is obtained than in the soft tissue tumors. This aids greatly in arriving at an early diagnosis and deciding on a course of treatment.

In general, the literature consists of isolated case reports rather than presentation of any collections of this type of tumor. This would preclude a general evaluation of most tumors by percentage. The experience here presented is based on the material that I have collected and treated. It is set forth as the best course of diagnosis and treatment of tumors at the present time.

Classification of tumors is important as it furnishes a framework for the understanding of tumorous growths. The deductive evaluation of a pathologic finding is helped by consideration of the types of tumors that evolve from basic tissues. There is a recognized systematic classification started in 1920 by The Registry of Bone Sarcoma of The American College of Surgeons. Started by Ewing, Codman, and Bloodgood, this classification was used in the original and modified form specifically for bone tumors. With the change of pathology concepts, new groups of tumors were presented and old group were revised. Today, it is best to consider each type of lesion in view of its own entity based just as much on clinical factors as on tissue pathology.

This chapter is not based on the general classification of bone tumors but on the frequency that one encounters tumors in the care of the hand. In this way, the clinician may better know what to expect when he finds a pathologic entity in the skeleton of the hand. The diagnosis can be more easily considered and the treatment more apparent.

ENCHONDROMA

Solitary enchondroma and multiple enchondroma together comprise 90 per cent of the tumors arising in the skeleton of the hand. The ability to recognize this tumor gives any clinician a marked advantage in making his diagnosis. Fortunately these tumors rarely become malignant. It is well known that a solitary enchondroma may undergo malignant transformation but this is most unusual. The multiple enchondroma cause swelling and often deformities of the digits.

These are noticed from a very early age. The discovery of the solitary enchondroma takes a different pattern.

Seventy-five per cent of the cases of single enchondroma are discovered by the occurrence of a pathologic fracture. The grasping or twisting motion may be slight but the sudden pain and swelling thereafter leads to a roentgenogram and finding of the bone defect (Fig. 17.2.1).

Twenty per cent of the cases of enchondroma are discovered by chance. There is never a hint that prior existence is known. An x-ray of the hand for soft tissue injury or suspected fracture is a common path to the revealing of a bone lesion (Fig. 17.2.2). The alarm at finding such a defect usually causes the patient to seek consultation.

Five per cent of enchondromas must be kept for a rather nebulous group. Occasionally a patient claims that he has noticed a vague ache in a digit. There are

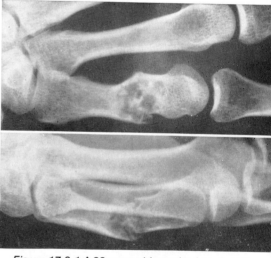

Figure 17.2.1 A 28-year-old man had no disability in the function of his right hand before the present episode. While hand wrestling, he felt a snap. The next day pain and some swelling lead to roentgenographic examination. The film shows an expansile lesion in the midshaft of the right fifth metacarpal. The borders are smooth and slightly sclerotic. The central lucency has blotches of radiopaque material. A fracture line can easily be seen involving both cortices. This is a typical example of an enchondroma identified after a fracture. Care consisted of immobilization in the correct alignment of the metacarpal and phalanges until the fracture had healed. The lesion was then curetted from the metacarpal and the defect filled with cancellous bone. The pathology report was benign enchondroma. Complete obliteration of the surgical intervention was found on review five years later.

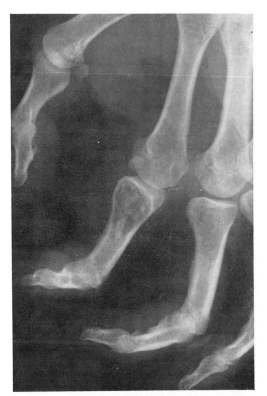

Figure 17.2.2. A 42-year-old woman had no disability in the function of her left hand. Soft tissue damage lead to an examination that included a roentgenogram. This film showed a typical enchondroma in the base of the proximal phalanx of the index finger. The lesion is central and expands the cortex which is in continuity. The margins of the lesion are sclerotic indicating a benign process of long standing. In the center, the lucent area has stippling of opaque islands which represent calcification in the cartilaginous cells. The enchondroma was excised and found to be benign. Cancellous bone was used to fill the defect. Both biopsy and complete irradication of the lesion was accomplished by this operation.

some who think that they feel a swelling in the finger. One case was discovered in a person seeking advice for spasms in the hand while writing.

Age and Sex

These have not been significant in the enchondroma. There have been cases reported with initial identification of the lesion from age 10 to 60. The highest group of patients does fall into the third and fourth decades of life from the 20's to the 40,s. As many men have been treated as women.

In reviewing the great number of enchondroma, a racial difference has been noted. It would be possible to ascribe this to location of practice, hospital, or type of practice. However, most of these variations can be accounted for in each instance. The enchondroma were rarely found in Negroes. We do have some but the number is low. Since one of our hand services is located in Harlem Hospital, New York City, it would seem likely that one would be able to evaluate the occurrence in the Negro. No cases were found in the brown or yellow races.

Location

The solitary enchondroma is found in the phalanges most commonly. Of the phalanges, the greatest numbers are found in the proximal phalanx. The next most frequent site is the middle phalanx or the metacarpal shaft. Lesions of the distal phalanx occur in the lowest frequency. None are found in the carpal bones. No enchondroma in our collection has been found in the carpal bones. Takigawa[4] has reported the operative finding of material compatible with a cartilagenous tumor in the right carpal navicular and lunate bones.

The position of the enchondroma in the shaft of the skeleton is not necessarily near the metaphysial region. In the metacarpal, this is rarely seen at the base. The cartilaginous lesion causes an expansion of the cortex in the majority of the cases. The tumor generally is centrally located but also may be found involving the cortex of one side of the bone.

Roentgenogram

The most common defect seen in the phalanx or metacarpal is an ovoid lytic pattern that resembles a bubble. This may have several round expansions. It is usually eccentrically placed and thins the cortex on one side. The border has a thin margin of sclerotic bone that may only be seen in one region. The central area may appear lytic, shaded, or stippled. When there are small patches of calcific stippling within the bone defect, it is much easier to make the diagnosis of enchondroma.

Differential Diagnosis

Since the enchondroma is the most frequently seen lesion in the hand, it would seem that it would be easily identified. This has most always been the case. There are several valid considerations, however, in making a diagnosis on x-ray. In the terminal phalanx, an epidermoid or epithelium-lined inclusion cyst may show a similar picture. The more proximal phalanges and the metacarpal occasionally contain an eccentrically shaped lytic area with gross trabeculation that is a bone cyst or fibrocystic defect of bone. This may look very much like an enchondroma. Multiple enchondroma rarely give any trouble in diagnosis.

Treatment

Should the enchondroma be discovered by a pathologic fracture, the digit should be treated as a fracture and properly aligned (Fig. 17.2.3). The fractured bone will heal leaving the enchondroma in its

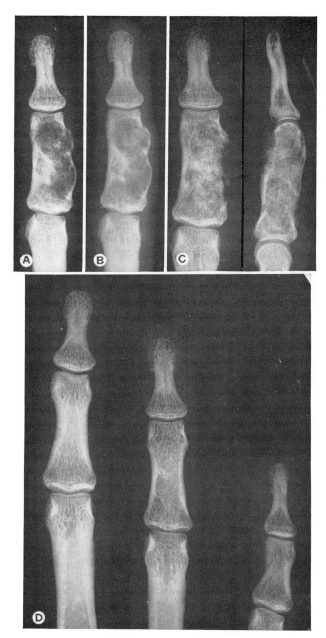

Figure 17.2.3.A. A 31-year-old governess grasped the collar of a struggling child and felt a snap in the fourth digit of her right hand. No previous defect had ever been noted in this finger by the patient. The roentgenogram revealed a fracture through a benign enchondroma of the middle phalanx of the ring finger. *B.* The fracture was protected and allowed to heal in proper alignment. The present film shows the finger 3 months after the accident. The cortical supporting bone has healed. *C.* At a time convenient to the patient, an operation was carried out to remove the tumor which was found to be benign. The defect was packed with cancellous autogenous bone and only a small bandage was necessary. Early motion of the operated finger was encouraged. *D.* Films taken 2 years after the operation show no sign of the tumor. The bone graft has been incorporated and almost normal phalangeal trabeculation is present. This patient was followed more than 10 years from the time of her accident.

original state. Roentgenograms will show the healed defect on subsequent films. An attempt at excision of the enchondroma when identified by fracture further disturbs the mechanical support of the cortex and has been seen to result in shortening and gross angulation of the healing bone.

All single enchondromas should be excised to prevent recurrent fractures and to remove a potentially malignant source. A window is made in the cortex and the contents carefully curetted. The cavity can be mechanically cleaned by surgical instruments. No advantage has ever been seen from chemical cleansing with phenol or zinc chloride. The cavity should be filled by firmly packed small fragments of cancellous bone. This may be obtained from the patient or a bone bank. With this technique, there should be no problem of recurrence.

Rarely is it necessary to excise a single lesion in multiple enchondroma. The major problem in this type of involvement is the skeletal deformity of a single digit. This deformity may assume such disabling proportions that amputation of a phalanx or even the entire ray is best for the patient.

Pathology

The surgeon must be the most efficient gross pathologist. He will see the lesion at the time of initial exposure. The bulging cortex will be almost like thin parchment in places. Upon unroofing the affected area, one will see a pearl-grey granular material. If a fracture has taken place, yellow or orange shading will be present. The material itself somewhat resembles tapioca as it is excised.

Ordinarily, the microscopic pathologist should have no difficulty in identifying the material as benign enchondroma. More latitude can be used here in evaluating the cellular structures than in sections from another skeletal area, such as the femur. Should a question of malignant trasformation arise in a specimen from a clinically benign lesion, it would be well to have confirmation from pathologists with great experience in this field. So rare is the malignant occurrence in an enchondroma in the hand that the existence or discovery must be weighed exceedingly well before surgical treatment is performed.

MAFFUCCI SYNDROME

With multiple enchondroma, another aberration may occur. This is extraskeletal and consists of multiple hemangiomas. The vascular changes involve the soft tissues adjacent to the bone and give a bluish tint to the digits or hand when abundant. On the roentgenogram, the tissues surrouding the skeletal changes of multiple enchondroma show this vascular pattern by the multiple round opacities of phleboliths. There are, however, a number of cases in which the vascular pattern has not yet formed the calcified clot and these are not as apparent unless the soft tissue outline of a digit is well shown.

As in multiple enchondroma, the only treatment needed is in case of a major skeletal deformity of the hand.

OSTEOCHONDROMA

The majority of these tumors are solitary. They are the cartilaginous growths which protrude or grow out of the bone of the hand and can thus be called ecchondroma. They constitute the second most frequently found tumor in the hand skeleton. These are generally noticed by a prominence from early age but are not alarming as no pain accompanies them. The single lesion occurs near the metaphysial region of the bone except for one type. This is the osteochondroma arising from the tuft of the distal phalanx (Fig. 17.2.4).

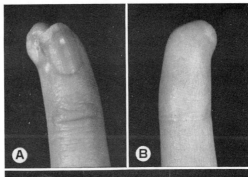
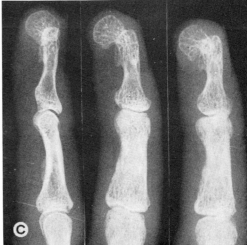

Figure 17.2.4.A. and *B.* Posterior and anterior views of the distal phalanx, fifth finger, of a 38-year-old woman. This growth had been noted by slow enlargement over a period of 3 years. The only pain existed after striking it directly. *C.* The roentgenogram of the finger reveals the osteochondroma of the distal phalanx to be of the pedunculated variety. Covering the crown of the tumor is a thin, sclerotic area representing cartilaginous cells. The remaining section of the tumor consists of regular bony elements of cancellous and cortical bone.

Osteochondroma of the hand is either pedunculated or sessile. It is extremely rare to find a case of malignant transformation but it can occur. Where there are many osteochondromas in the hand, the finding is a local manifestation of the general skeletal problem of hereditary multiple exostosis.

Ninety per cent of the cases of osteochondromas are discovered by the patient who feels a mass in his hand. Curiosity may being him to seek medical advice. If the mass projects in a contact surface and causes a disability, he will usually ask for help at an early age.

Ten per cent of the ecchondroma cases are found by chance. A roentgenogram of the hand when involved in trauma leads to the disclosure of a small mass. There are examples where the findings of an osteochondroma in the hand will lead to the location of similar lesions in the humerus and femur.

Age and Sex

It would be difficult to state at exactly what age a mass was noticed in the hand. The patients will usually have a consultation at about the age of 10 if the mass gives pain with grasp. Parental anxiety may also cause an early visit. There are, however, some stoic people who do not investigate this problem until the age of 40 or 50. About this time, a small question of cancer is planted in the back of the mind by a friend's illness or an article in the press.

While there is no marked difference in the sex incidence, in my series, there are a few more men than women. This is probably due to chance.

In the problem of multiple exostoses, there is no significance to age incidence. The skeletal deformities are noted at an early age. There is a noted sex difference. The percentage of men is just double that of women.

Locations

The exostosis usually appears near a zone of growth or previous cartilaginous activity. In the phalanx, it is found near the base or proximal third. In the metacarpal, it appears near the distal third of the bone. These do not appear in the carpal bones. The one exception to this rule is the subungual exotosis. This is a true osteochondroma projecting from beneath the nail and arising from the terminal tuft of the distal phalanx.

Roentgenogram

The bony mass is easily seen projecting from the outline of the cortex. The stalk of the pedunculated variety is not easily seen. The flatter sessile mass may not be as apparent. When the projecting bone has a lobular cap with some adjacent stippling, this represents the cartilaginous mass which tips the osteochondroma.

Differential Diagnosis

It would be hard to consider another diagnosis when such a lesion is seen. The major difficulty comes in viewing the roentgenographic projection. Should the base of the cone face the viewer, it may give the appearance of a lytic lesion.

Treatment

The growing mass should be removed in the hand. In such a delicately balanced skelton, a growing lesion gives a deformity that causes painful pressures and is readily apparent. When this lesion is excised, the bone must be exposed by incising the periosteum and a generous segment of bone removed. The periosteum never should be elevated over the mass with an elevator. This leaves cartilaginous cells which may be the nidus for further tumors. When excising a lesion from the terminal tuft of the distal phalanx, I generally like to remove the nail at the time of surgery. This permits easier handling of the soft tissues and the nail will grow again.

Pathology

On exposure of the osteochondroma, the cap is not adherent to the adjacent tissues. Often the cartilaginous formation is easily seen. In the hand, it does not form the overlying bursa that one may find in the long bones.

A sagittal section of a lesion, removed intact from the shaft of the bone, will show a cartilaginous portion at the top resting on a cone of cancellous bone with walls of cortical bone covered by a periosteal sleeve.

The microscopic picture is not of special significance.

OTHER LESIONS

The remaining categories of lesions found in the hand skeleton constitute an exceedingly small percentage of all hand tumors. They are presented in the order of dimishing occurence in my series. Many lesions will not be included because they are so rarely seen.

Solitary Bone Cyst

This term is used to describe a defect found in the phalanges and metacarpals which contains some fibrous connetive tissue segments and a small amount of brown or yellow fluid. They are quite similar to defects found in the humerus of children. Another term might be used, such as fibrocystic defects of bone. The defects cause a swelling of the cortex where it can be seen in many cases. The distal half of a metacarpal or the lateral aspect of a phalanx is an obvious spot. In this series of cases about half are found by chance in a roentgenogram of the hand. The other half is found by a palpable swelling.

These cysts are not to be confused with the cysts produced by the parathyroid adenoma. The metabolic changes which cause demineralization and cystic changes in the skeleton are not specific to the hand. When they do occur in the hand, there are many changes in all of the bony framework making the metabolic defect more apparent.

Age and Sex

The patients with cysts found by chance are, in general, younger than those found by swelling. The growth of the cyst is slow and the age that it can be noticed by a palpable swelling is in the third or fourth decades of life.

No sex difference is thought to be significant. There are a few more women than men in this series.

Location

When the cyst is found in the metacarpals, it has been located in the distal third. This would be in keeping with a similar juxtaepiphysial site of a bone cyst in a humerus. In the phalanges, it has usually been found in the midshaft. No cyst has so far been found in the distal phalanx.

Cysts may fill the medullary cavity and cause expansion of the cortex. More frequently they are eccentrically located and cause a bulging of the cortex on one side. This cortex may be expanded to an exceedingly thin shell (Fig. 17.2.5).

In discussing the bone cyst of the hand skeleton, the cystic defects seen in the carpal bones are not included. These are of a different nature and are found at a later age. I feel that they represent a degenerative cyst resultant to decreased blood supply and avascular necrosis.

Roentgenogram

The lesion is usually unicameral. It may be ovoid or round. More commonly found with an eccentric development, it expands the cortex to a thin shell on one side. The inner aspect is smooth with a sclerotic margin. There are several cysts that have multiple protrusions that give it a multicamerate effect. The trabeculae that appear are well demarcated and not of delicate tracing.

Differential Diagnosis

By far, the most frequently used diagnosis when this lesion is first seen is that of enchondroma. When the lesion is of unicamerate nature and large with expanded cortex, the confusion should not exist. There is a distinct similarity, however, between the enchondroma and the multicamerate cyst.

Treatment

Only one case has been seen in which a pathologic fracture took place. This was treated just like an enchondroma. Usually the discovery of a swelling causes the patient to seek advice regarding his tumor. He does not like the swelling and does not want to keep a pathologic entity. In such a case, the lesion is excised and the defect filled with bone. Should a question arise as to the type and nature of the tumor present, a biopsy would settle the question. In this tumor,

excision of the whole lesion would identify the tumor and remove the problem from the patient.

Pathology

On exposing the bone, a swelling of the cortex is readily apparent. The periosteum is intact. Beneath the periosteum, the cortex may be very thin and resemble a shell. When the cortex is opened, some thin fluid will be found. This is generally yellowish tending towards brown. A true membrane is not found. There may be patches of fibrous connective tissue present.

Microscopic examination of the removed soft tissue reveals it to be mainly connective tissue with an occasional multinuclear giant cell.

Osteoid Osteoma

This is an unusual lesion found in the skeleton of the hand, as well as other sites, which is listed among the

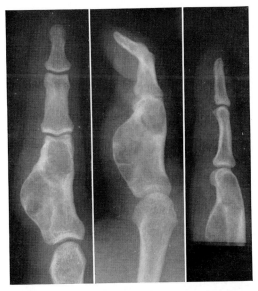

Figure 17.2.5. This 23-year-old man had been aware of a painless swelling in the proximal phalanx of his right hand for at least five years. In using his hand, pressure caused minor discomfort. Urged by his family, he sought medical attention. The roentgenogram readily demonstrated the expansile lesion causing the distortion of the cortex with resultant thinning and is typical of a solitary bone cyst. The periosteum is eccentric to the main axis of the phalanx. A smooth, sclerotic margin indicated a benign nature. This particular lesion has two large chambers and only a few trabeculae. Compare it to *Fig. 17.2.3.A.* to note the similarity and difference between this lesion and an enchondroma. The lesion was removed by curettage and filled by a bone graft. Complete replacement resulted.

tumors of bone. It would not be included among the infections causing bone manifestations. The clinical history is unique in that there is a long history of aching pain which is greater at night. Moreover, this pain can readily be relieved by the ingestion of aspirin (Fig. 17.2.6). In the hand, there is a finding that is not seen elsewhere in the body, *i.e.* the noticeable swelling of the surrounding soft tissue when a member is involved.

Age and Sex

This is a tumor of young people. It is found in the second and third decades of life. The distribution between men and women has been about equal in the hand. This is somewhat different from the ratio of two men to one woman, as reported by others.

Location

This tumor occurs in all short tubular bones of the hand and in some carpal bones. The proximal phalanx is the most frequently involved site. It is in this bone that the rarely seen subperiosteal nidus is found. The next bone most involved is the metacarpal. After that the incidence in the middle and distal phalanges is about the same. Finally there are some carpal bones with nidus formation. Of these, the navicular is most frequently involved.

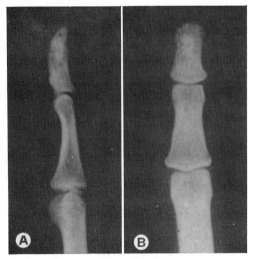

Figure 17.2.6. Pain and gradual swelling was present in the distal phalanx of the right index finger of a 24-year-old man over a period of one year. The pain was relieved by aspirin. A film of the finger shows the finding of an osteoid osteoma in the distal phalanx. The central nidus is seen to be sclerotic. Surrounding this is a ring of lesser opacity. The adjacent bone shows the usual sclerotic changes. The nidus was excised and pain promptly subsides. No bone graft was used and the surgical defect filled in during the ensuing year. *A.* Lateral. *B.* Anteroposterior.

The actual nidus of the lesion can be found in three difinite locations. It may be located in the central or medullary portion of the bone. A second common location is within the very substance of the cortex. Some lesions are hard to locate accurately since they seem to arise from the endosteum where the medullary cavity joins the cortex. The rarest location is between the outer cortex and the periosteum.

The soft tissue swelling is readily apparent when the hand skeleton is a location for osteoid osteoma. By finding the part most sensitive to external pressure, the nidus can frequently be located.

Roentgenogram

The most helpful laboratory aid is the film of the hand. On this, the location of the osteoid osteoma and the nidus should be made. Commonly the nidus is a lytic patch with an area the size of a match head. It should never be larger than 1 cm. Around this, there is a great area of bone sclerosis. The nidus in the cortical area will generally have a granular appearance. Surrounding this is a perimeter of radiolucency which will separate the nidus from the surrounding sclerotic bone. This has frequently been called a ring sequestrum. The rare cases of subperiosteal osteoid osteoma will cause a sclerotic reaction of adjacent bone with the cortex showing a pressure defect only on a certain oblique view of the area.

Differential Diagnosis

The most usual diagnosis raised in these cases is that of a bone infection or abscess. Here the clinical history should be of great help. The radiographic picture of a bone abscess would not contain the round nidus typical of the osteoid osteoma.

Among other diagnoses that have been considered is syphilis which is a great imitator. Examples of syphilitic dactylitis can produce diffuse sclerosis of the shaft with just a suggestion of a nidus. Tuberculosis of the phalanx or metacarpal may appear similar to the osteoid osteoma. Very little difficulty arises with most roentgenograms of osteoid osteoma, as these findings are quite typical of the correct diagnosis.

Treatment

After the nidus has been localized clinically by the point of maximal pain, it must be located roentgenologically. The treatment consists of excising the nidus. Only this relieves the pain. In the problem of a nidus located intracortically, it is frequently a problem mainly of location to excise. Help may be obtained by a roentgenogram taken on the operating table. An excised block of bone as the specimen may show the nidus on a film. When cutting the bone affected by this tumor, a surgeon is impressed by the dense, sclerotic qualities. Once the nidus is excised, the bone appears normal on follow-up roentgenograms. This may take several years, however, in some cases. The patient is pleased with the immediate relief of pain.

Pathology

In the midst of the dense bone of the areas surrounding the nidus can be found a tiny area that can resemble a loose pearl. The color is frequently darker than the surrounding bone. This is the nidus that is sought. Under the microscope, this nidus consists of osteoid tissue set among trabeculae or islands of newly formed bone. This area of developing bone tissue rests in an area where formalized bony construction is readily apparent.

Epidermoid (Epithelial Inclusion) Cyst

Although epidermoid cysts are commonly seen in the soft tissues of the hand, the osseous lesion is rarely seen. Since this tumor results from antecedent trauma of a crushing or penetrating type, it is, therefore, the only tumor which can name trauma as the etiologic factor (Fig. 17.2.7). Because the lesion is not frequently encountered, the preoperative diagnosis is not often made.

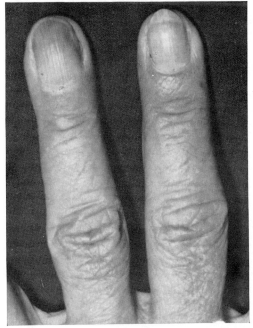

Figure 17.2.7. In a 47-year-old woman, the terminal phalanx of the right long finger had gradually enlarged over the previous five years. About 12 years before examination, this finger nail had been crushed by a closing door. No roentgenogram had been made at the time of the accident or subsequently. While using the finger tips to lift a heavy table, the patient felt a snap in the swollen finger and this lead to an examination.

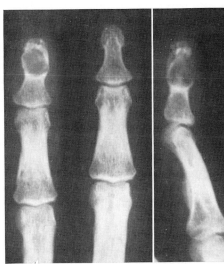

Figure 17.2.8 In the distal phalanx of the third digit (see Figure 17.2.7), a lytic area was found. This was centrally placed and expanded the surrounding cortex causing it to be thin. The bone surrounding the lesion had a sclerotic margin. An irregularity could be seen in the cortices, and it was felt that a fracture was present which accounted for the recent snap. The central area of the lesion was of a uniform light ocpacity. The diagnosis of an epidermoid cyst should immediately come to mind. About the only other lesion presenting the same appearance would be an enchondroma.

This tumor is a lesion lying within the confines of the bone of the phalanx. In many case reports, it is frequently confused with defects that occur in the soft tissue of the digit and cause extraosseous pressure. The tumor is always located in the terminal phalanx of the digit (Fig. 17.2.8). In an early case report, the terminal digit was the middle phalanx as the distal phalanx had been previously amputated.

Age and Sex

With so few recorded cases, there is no significance as to sex difference. It does happen that there are twice as many men as women. This would not help in making a diagnosis, however. The age distribution is quite wide. It ranges from ages 12 to 55 at the age of discovery.

Location

In each case, the trauma is located in the terminal phalanx of the digit. Here the nail appears to be enlarged and the phalanx appears to be swollen. In each case, a history of prior trauma can be found. This may have occurred many years before examination and could be easily forgotten. The precipitating factor that causes the patient to seek medical care is the pain of a recent fracture through the already thin cortex.

Roentgenogram

The lesion is a lytic area in the terminal phalanx. It is usually round but may be ovoid. This is found in the area of the tuft or midshaft of the distal phalanx. This lesion is expansive and may replace all but the very base of the phalanx on occasion. The cortex is expanded and very thin but there is no evidence of periosteal reaction. A fracture line may frequently be seen in the thinned area of the cortex. The lytic pattern may rarely be eccentrically placed within the phalanx but a cortical pattern should be seen surrounding the defect.

Differential Diagnosis

The lesion has commonly been called an enchondroma. This is a sound observation as the enchondroma is the most frequently found tumor causing a centrally located defect in the osseous skeleton of the hand. Another tumor that has been diagnosed is a cyst, but the fibrocystic defects found in the hand would not give this neat round pattern. It would certainly not be in the same family as the juvenile bone cyst seen in the long bones of the skeleton. The use of the term cyst would not be a thoughful diagnosis.

Treatment

When the epidermoid cyst has expanded to the extent that the terminal phalanx is replaced, the best treatment consists of amputation. It is certainly the most definite treatment. Curettage should be used when the cyst is relatively small. The defect can be filled with cancellous bone fragments. Since the cyst will recur if any epidermoid cells are left within, the patient should be carefully followed and warned of the potentiality of recurrence. These epidermoid cysts are hard to eradicate and the patient should be informed of the possibility of a phalangeal amputation.

Pathology

On opening the soft tissues, a thin shell of cortex may be present. The capsule of the cyst itself is quite easily identified. It is a tough, firm membrane which adheres to the bone. The contents of the cyst is a white caseous material that has a typical odor of cellular debris.

Aneurysmal Bone Cyst

The benign tumors of bone cannot be left without considering the unusual tumor which was called for many years a giant cell tumor of bone. As the pathologists formulated a basis for making the diagnosis of aneurysmal bone cyst, many of the cases of giant cell tumor were switched to the more current diagnosis. There are some cases which still give difficulty in that the surgical material reviewed could be either tumor.

In the light of the present standards for diagnosis, the aneurysmal bone cyst is more frequently found in the hand skeleton than a grant cell tumor. Both tumors have the same history and clinical findings. The roentgenograms give little help in distinguishing between them. The method of treatment is the same.

The usual history is one of an awareness of a vague ache in the hand. A swelling of one area is next noticed. It is not unusual to have a patient relate the history and findings to trauma. This may not be of significance. It is believed that a slight blow may really lead to an awareness of the existing condition. The affected bone enlarges rapidly in several months. When seen at six months from onset, the swelling of the bone is most prominent (Fig. 17.2.9). Pressure on the area will produce a crackling similar to compressing a celluloid ball. The vessels in the area are prominent as well.

Age and Sex

There is no statistical significance in the number of men and women. Both are represented just about equally. The age grouping starts in the later half of the second decade and extends through the third decade.

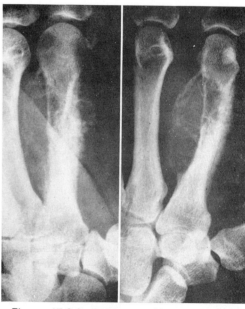

Figure 17.2.9. A 27-year-old woman noticed that her left hand had increased in size during the previous five months. No trauma had occurred and pain was minimal. The roentgenogram showed the shaft of the second metacarpal to be expanded markedly. The cortex existed as a very thin line. Throughout the area of the lesion, a faint lacy pattern was seen. The tumor involved the entire bone, but an outline of the metacarpal could still be seen. At a most vascular operation, the abnormal tissue was removed and a bone graft inserted between the distal and proximal segments of the metacarpal. Over the period of two years, the metacarpal reformed and no further evidence of tumor was present.

Location

The aneurysmal bone cysts are to be found in the distal half of the metacarpals and the proximal half of the phalanx. When the epiphysis is closed the lesion involves the whole metaphysis. An extremely rare case is one involving the carpal bones.

Roentgenogram

The findings on the roentgenogram are easily pathognomonic of the aneurysmal bone cyst in the later stages. The cortex is found to be greatly expanded so that it can barely be seen as a faint outline. The contents of the lytic area may have a faint lacy pattern throughout. The whole circumference of the bone is frequently affected. There are, however, examples where only one side of the shaft is involved. In the earlier stages, the cortical expansion is not as great. As the lesion has not caused the degree of distension later found, the trabeculae are more definite and lattice the area of expansion.

Differential Diagnosis

Neither on clinical examination nor on roentgenogram can a distinction be made between an aneurysmal bone cyst and a giant cell tumor of bone. Even the field of pathology has had difficulty in making the distinction. Knowledge of the findings at operation may help a little.

The picture presented by a benign chondroblastoma can be similar. In one known instance both the pathology diagnosis and the roentgenologic diagnosis were that of giant cell tumor, and would have been aneurysmal bone cyst if that diagnosis were currently popular when the tumor was first seen.

This is a vascular lesion, but I have never seen a true hemangioma of the bone of the hand present a similar picture. It could conceivably happen.

A metastatic lesion to the phalanx or metacarpal might give some similarities. In general, the metastatic lesions do not show the large bubble or blown-out lesion that characterizes the aneurysmal bone cyst. The metastatic lesions are invasive and destructive. They also give more pain clinically.

Treatment

A surgeon embarking on the treatment of an aneurysmal bone cyst is to expect a most vascular experience. These tumors can be healed by curettage and packing with bone chips. The shell of expanded cortex may resemble parchment on exposure. The contents of the cavity is mostly blood interspersed by strands of reddish brown soft tissue. The blood spaces are lakes and not masses of vessels. Blood seems to ooze from everywhere. The only solution is a thorough and complete extirpation of all vascular tissue. When this is done, the bleeding stops. Such cases must be done with tourniquet control. A limited biopsy will produce a problem in controlling the great residual bleeding. Therefore, the biopsy should consist of eradicating the whole lesion. Failure to curette out all tissue completely will result in a recurrence of the lesion. This recurrence does not indicate malignant transformation. A recurrence may be easily handled by a relatively low amount of roentgen therapy in the range of 800 r to 1000r.

Pathology

Grossly, the picture of blood spaces with small amounts of soft brownish or reddish tissue is typical.

In the microscopic section, one should see abundant vascular spaces. The strands of soft tissue adjacent contain many multinuclear giant cells. Occasionally, narrow strands or trabeculae of bone are encountered.

Giant Cell Tumors of Bone

This tumor does occur in the phalanges and the metacarpals of the hand. It has not been seen in a carpal bone. Fewer such tumors are now described with the recognition of the aneurysmal bone cyst. This tumor does, however, exist in the hand in both the benign and the malignant types.

The history, physical findings, roentgenograms, and even the gross pathologic findings are about the same as the aneurysmal bone cyst. The microscopic findings have been such that pathologists have given identical diagnoses on different tissues and different diagnoses on the same tissue.

At operation, the substance of the giant cell tumor bleeds profusely until all fragments are excised. Recurrence here is more alarming than in the aneurysmal bone cyst. It is well to obtain tissue from a recurrent tumor site before considering roentgen therapy.

Metastatic Tumors to the Hand

Although exceedingly rare, lesions are found in the hand representing spread from a soft tissue malignancy or even a bone tumor located at a distant area in the body. About the only primary bone tumor that has been known to shed metastases reaching the hand is the chondrosarcoma. The mechanism of spread in this case would be to the lung and thence by blood to the end arterioles of the hand.

Metastatic tumors to the hand skeleton occur from the lung most frequently. In many instances, the advent of a lesion in the hand was the first sign of the presence of the lung tumor. With an established knowledge of a lung tumor present, single metastasis has shown up in the hand skeleton. All cases follow a similar pattern which helps in the diagnosis.

Usually pain of an aching nature, present night and day, directs attention to a phalanx or metacarpal. In the phalanx, swelling is seen within six to eight weeks. The metacarpals have more soft tissue adjacent so that the swelling is marked for a longer period of time. Upon roentgenogram, there is a lytic area of destruction which does not cross articular outlines. An aspiration biopsy with a needle may be all that is necessary to obtain a diagnosis. Treatment by roentgen therapy has not been satisfactory in the hand. There has been little control of the growth and it has caused secondary painful radiation burns of the digit or entire hand. I favor a limited radical excision of the ray whenever the lesion is first demonstrated.

Metastatic tumors from the breast (Fig. 17.2.10) constitute the second largest group. These respond more favorably to roentgen therapy. The primary tumor in this case has already been identified. Recognition of the nature of pain in the hand skeleton is the factor of importance.

The tumors of the gastrointestinal tract are third in frequency, with representation from thyroid, kidney, prostate, and uterus, as well.

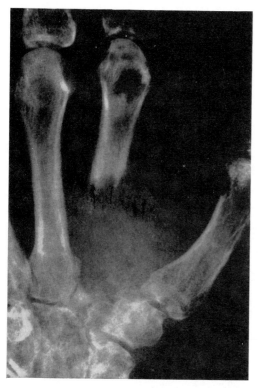

Figure 17.2.10. This roentgenogram reveals complete, aggressive destruction of bone in the base of the second metacarpal. There is no evidence of a benign, slow growth found with sclerotic margins. Pain is a constant factor. When knowledge of a previous malignancy is present, the diagnosis should immediately point to a metastatic tumor. This photograph is typical of metastatic tumors in the bone of the hand. It does happen to be unusual in that it represents a metastasis from a carcinoma of the male breast.

Chondrosarcoma

The majority of this type of tumor develops from a known area of enchondroma. Occasionally, a tumor does grow from a bone when there is no evidence of a previously existing enchondroma. This is most rare. More malignant transformations occur in a hand when multiple enchondromas exist. There are cases when a single enchondroma was known to exist and later malignant transformation did occur. Extremely rare is a transformation from a benign osteochondroma into a malignant lesion.

It is indeed fortunate that the skeleton of the hand is superficial. This allows early visualization of the tumor. The wealth of sensory perception accentuates the pain at an early stage. These combine to cause a patient to seek help while reasonable corrective surgery can be done. Rarely is there need to amputate the whole hand. In general, a limited radical resection will give adequate margin for corrective surgery and yet leave a useful mechanism.

Osteogenic Sarcoma

This is rare but can be encountered. The phalanges are about as equally involved as the metacarpals. When such a diagnosis is considered, the roentgenogram and a biopsy will confirm the supposition. If the lesion is a new growth with no other complicating factor, a local radical resection will give the best treatment. Although the number of this area of involvement is low, the prognosis seems to be markedly different than any other area involved by osteogenic sarcoma.

The bone changes that occur after prolonged area irradiation or general exposure to ingested radium salts can produce an osteogenic tumor in the hand. Because of exposure of all tissues in the hand by the radiation, the prognosis is not the same. Other foci can develop.

A single case is known to exist where the hand was the site of a metastatic focus from an osteogenic sarcoma in another area of the body. This may be true hematogenous spread or it may be related to a condition of changing bone metabolism, such as Paget's disease. We do not know that in such a case the appearance of osteogenic sarcoma can affect many bones and it does occur in the hand skeleton.

REFERENCES

1. Coley, B. L. *Neoplasms of Bone,* Ed. 2. New York, Hoeber, 1960.
2. Jaffe, H. L. *Tumors and Tumorous Conditions of the Bone and Joints.* Philadelphia, Lea & Febiger, 1958.
3. Stringa, G. *Condromi delle Ossa della Mano.* Firenze, Instituto Ortopedico Toscano, 1957.
4. Takigawa, K. Carpal chondroma: Report of a case. J. Bone Joint Surg., *53A:* 1601-1604, 1971.

C.

Tumors of the Blood and Lymphatic Vessels

Raymond M. Curtis, M.D.

INTRODUCTION

Tumors of both the blood and lymphatic vessels are common in the hand. Watson and McCarthy,[48] in a series of 1056 cases of blood and lymph vessel tumors, found 26 per cent of these in the extremities. Stout,[42] in reporting 921 cases of patients with superficial capillary, cavernous, and venous hemangiomas, found 142 of these cases in the upper extremity.

The great majority of these tumors of the upper extremity are benign.

HEMANGIOMAS

Ewing[13] has defined a hemangioma as a benign tumor composed of newly formed blood vessels. Pack and Ariel[30] have stated that these tumors comprise 22 per cent of all benign tumors and 46 per cent of the tumors of the soft tissues of the body. Chamberlain and Pendergrass[8] found that 5 per cent of all cavernous hemangiomas occurred in the hand.

Classification

The hemangiomas of the extremities have been classified in several ways. Goidanich and Campanacci[16] prefer to classify this as follows: (1) localized angiomas; (2) multiple or diffuse angiomas; (3) angiomas with arteriovenous fistulas; (4) angiomas with skeletal hyperplasia. Goidanich and Campanacci, in a study of 94 cases of angiomatous lesions of the extremities, have preferred to call these tumors hamartomas to indicate that they are tumors caused by a new growth of blood vessels. In their series these were discovered at birth or early in life and did not seem to grow after the age of 20. They describe this hamartoma as characterized microscopically by a tissue composed almost exclusively of angioblastic cells and capillaries or cavernous sinuses with pseudoarterioles and pseudoveins but benign in character. This term, they feel, distinguishes these tumors from those caused by secondary vascular hyperplasia and the true neoplasms. Stout[45] prefers to classify these tumors on the basis of their microscopic appearance. Byars[7] uses the gross and microscopic appearance as a method of classification and to decide how the lesion should be treated.

Etiology

In most instances the hemangiomas are congenital. Watson and McCarthy[48] in their large series found that 75 per cent were present at birth and that 85 per cent had appeared within the first year.

If we remember that the vascular system originates from a disconnected group of cells which become canalized and later join to form a common capillary plexus, it is possible to visualize how readily remnants of this embryonic plexus can remain behind to produce these angiomatous lesions in the various tissues of the body.

Diagnosis

The simple angioma of a localized character which presents itself beneath the skin in the subcutaneous tissue is readily diagnosed inasmuch as it is compressible (Fig. 17.3.1). It may enlarge when the venous return is obstructed and may empty itself partially with the extremity elevated. These tumors are characterized by a bluish discoloration beneath the skin. The hemangioma which lies deep within muscle may be more difficult to diagnose (Fig. 17.3.2). This may present itself merely as a tumor of the hand which grossly may be difficult to distinguish from other tumors, other than the fact that there may be some compressibility to the tumor itself. Roentgenograms may be helpful in some of the hemangiomas involving muscle, for in some longstanding cases, areas of calcification caused by phleboliths may be visualized on the roentgenogram (Fig. 17.3.3.). The diagnosis of hemangiomas with arteriovenous communications will be discussed more thoroughly under congenital arteriovenous fistulas.

Symptoms

The patient usually presents himself for treatment because of the tumor mass. However, there may be pain in the area of the tumor, particularly if it is located in one of the muscles of the hand or forearm. In addition there may be spontaneous thrombosis in the tumor itself giving rise to local tender areas in the lesion.

Treatment

Surgical excision of the localized hemangioma when it lies in the subcutaneous tissue or even when it involves the muscle of the hand or forearm can be accomplished without much difficulty. The dissection must be carried out under tourniquet technique so that the entire tumor mass is removed and so that one can identify all the important structures of the hand that appear in the operative field. It is helpful in using the tourniquet not to compress the hand so completely as to empty the lesion of all of its blood, for if the operator can leave some blood in the hemangioma and still carry out the surgery under tourniquet technique, the dissection will be much easier. Where the angioma involves the skin itself, in addition to the

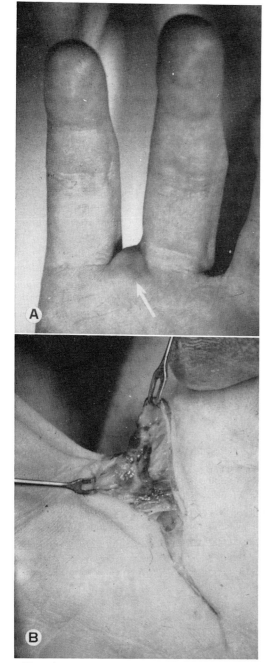

extensive lesions that before removing the blood pressure cuff completely, one should release the cuff slightly allowing some blood to enter the arm and then reinflate the cuff. With local pressure about the wound, one can demonstrate the openings of the various cut vessels and ligate these before complete release of the tourniquet. By repeating this several times one can obtain almost complete hemostasis to prevent the profuse hemorrage that frequently occurs in these patients once the tourniquie is released. In the diffuse hemangioma involving interosseus muscles or involving muscles of the forearm, a complete surgical removal may be difficult to carry out without interfering with function. It is important in this type of patient to be certain that one is not dealing with an angiosarcoma that would necessitate radical resection. Such a diagnosis, however, would best be

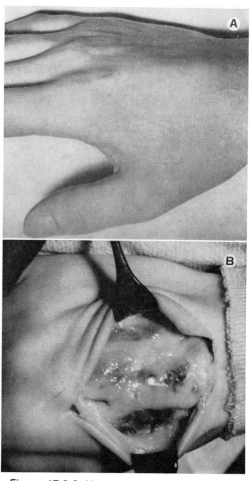

Figure 17.3.1.A. Simple hemangioma in the subcutaneous tissue presenting in the web between index and long fingers. *B.* Gross appearance of tumor consisting of a network of dilated but normal appearing thin walled blood vessels.

Figure 17.3.2. Hemangioma involving interosseous muscle between index and long finger metacarpals. *A.* Gross appearance of swelling on dorsum of hand between index and long finger metacarpals. *B.* Operative exposure of tumor within the interosseous muscle.

subcutaneous tissue, it may be necessary to excise the skin along with the underlying tumor and cover the defect by a partial thickness skin graft or pedicle flap. Bunnell has recommended in some of the difficult and

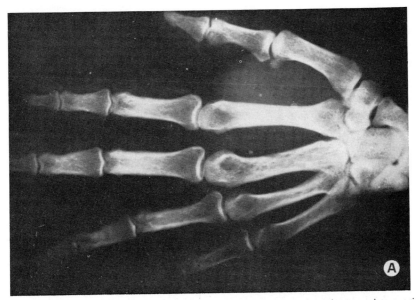

Figure 17.3.3. A. Roentgenographic appearance of an extensive deep hemangioma arising within the muscles. Moth-eaten appearance of long finger metacarpal suggests that the tumor involves the diaphysis. Phleboliths are present in the tumor mass. Arteriovenous communications were suspected.

made on permanent sections after a local resection had been carried out. The prognosis must be guarded in both the benign and in the malignant form. In the benign form, it is very difficult to remove completely all of the tumor as a rule and there may be some recurrence after local excision. The complete removal of the tumor is the ideal treatment but this is not always possible since some of these tumors involve muscles and nerves, the loss of which would be disastrous. If tumor is benign, it is better judgment to accept incomplete removal to avoid destroying a useful hand. Frequently the feasibility of complete excision of the hemangioma can only be determined by surgical explorations since the external appearance may be deceptive.

Cryotherapy

Cryotherapy or freezing with carbon dioxide ice, as recommended by Pack and Ariel,[30] may be a useful method of treating some of the superficial hemangiomas involving the skin. This treatment produces a frostbite, which causes thrombosis, which is followed by organization and obliteration. Pack and Ariel report that this method is particularly useful in infants.

Injection Treatment

Injection treatment in which a sclerosing agent, such as a 5 per cent solution of sodium morrhuate, is injected into the tumor has been used in some of the extensive tumors; however, it is rarely used in the extremities since the extensive hemangioma may involve a nerve[26] and here the result might be

disastrous. There are some instances in which surgery may be combined with injection therapy.

Radiation Therapy

Radiation therapy offers another method of treatment since the henangiomas of infancy and early childhood may be very sensitive to irradiation. There are, however, certain complications to this therapy in the growing hand, in that the therapy may arrest skeletal growth or produce atrophic changes in the skin and subcutaneous tissue. For these reasons it seems applicable in the extremities to only the very superficial hemangiomas. Byars[7] has emphasized the fact that it is the highly undifferentiated hemangioma in infants and children (Fig. 17.3.4.) that will respond to radiation therapy. The hemangioma composed of mature blood vessels in not radiosensitive (Fig. 17.3.5). Pack and Ariel[30] have used gold radon seeds successfully in the treatment of cavernous hemangiomas of the tongue.

CONGENITAL ARTERIOVENOUS FISTULAS

Introduction

The surgical treatment of congenital arteriovenous fistulas of the extremities has been extremely unsatisfactory in the past. This has been due to the very nature of the anomaly, with multiple communications between artery and vein, many of them minute.

History

The first reported case of a congenital arteriovenous

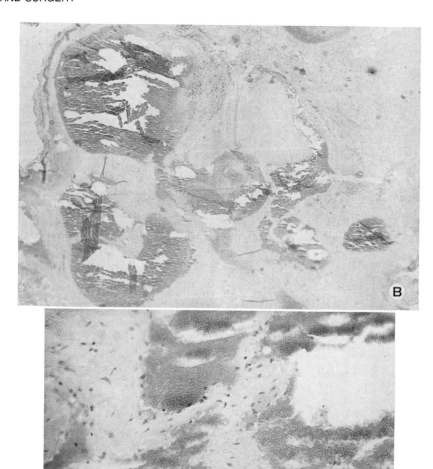

Figure 17.3.3. (continued). B. Photomicrograph of tumor. × 6. *C.* Photomicrograph of tumor. × 125. Courtesy of Lt. Col. George Omer, United States Army Medical Corps.

fistula of the hand seems to be that described in 1867 by Gherini[15] of Milan, in a girl 9½ years old. This was treated by proximal ligation of the ulnar and radial arteries. Although it did not progress after operation, it was not cured, since the veins remained dilated. Horton and Ghormley[20] in 1935 reported two cases of congenital arteriovenous fistulas of the hand. In one, only the index finger was involved and it was treated by amputation of that finger. In the other patient, there was involvement of the long and ring fingers, and it was necessary to amputate both fingers as well as to perform a wedge resection of the palm for complete eradication. Lewis[24] found only 30 cases of

arteriovenous fistula of the extremities recorded in the literature up to 1930.

Curtis[10] described three personal cases of arteriovenous fistula of the hand treated surgically in 1953. One patient with involvement of the long finger responded to amputation when conservative surgery failed. Two patients responded to radical excision (Fig. 17.3.6).

Etiology

The findings of Sabin[36] and Willard[49] indicate that in the embryo, arteries and veins differentiate from a common capillary plexus and that certain embryonic vessels function as arteries at one stage and as veins at another. Congenital arteriovenous fistulas result from a failure in differentiation of the common embryonic anlage into true artery and vein, and the persistence of a communication between them, producing a shortcircuiting of blood. This process may persist in a limited area, such as a finger, or it may be so extensive as to involve the entire extremity.

In some instances the abnormal communications seem to reopen, becoming active shunts, after trauma to the part. While most of these arise from congenital remnants, it may be possible for such an abnormal communication to develop from the normal arteriovenous communications in the neuromyoarterial glomus, which occur in the hand proximal to the capillary bed. Popoff,[33] in 1934, described such an uncontrolled arteriovenous anastomosis which developed after cellulitis of a finger; the Sucquet-Hoyer[46] canal of the glomus became inefficient as a result of the inflammatory process and acted as an arteriovenous fistula.

Clinical Manifestations and Diagnosis

Varicose veins are always associated with congenital arteriovenous fistulas. One must always suspect an anomaly such as congenital arteriovenous fistula of the hand in a patient who presents himself with varicose veins of the upper extremity and a wound which fails to heal. Such a wound may follow even a trivial injury. Chronic ulceration of a finger may be followed by gangrene. The extremity or the part of an extremity that is involved may be either hypertrophied or normal in size. The skin temperature of the affected part is usually higher than that of the normal member. As a rule, neither a bruit nor a thrill can be elicited due to the small caliber of the anastomotic channels, but in some instances these channels may be large enough to produce both clinical signs. Bradycardia or a decrease in the heart rate, usually of from four to eight beats per minute, can sometimes be demonstrated when the artery above the

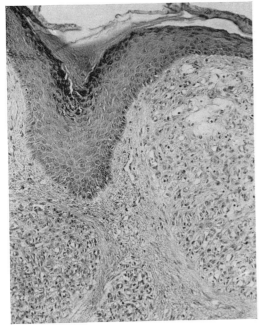

Figure 17.3.4. Photomicrograph of the highly undifferentiated hemangioma of childhood characterized by nests of cells beneath normal epithelium. × 150.

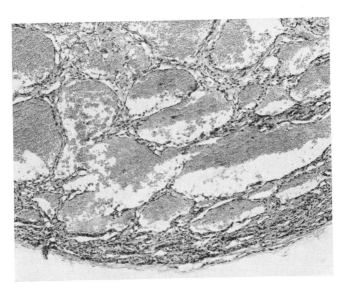

Figure 17.3.5. Photomicrographic appearance of the capillary hemangioma composed of normal appearing capillaries. × 100.

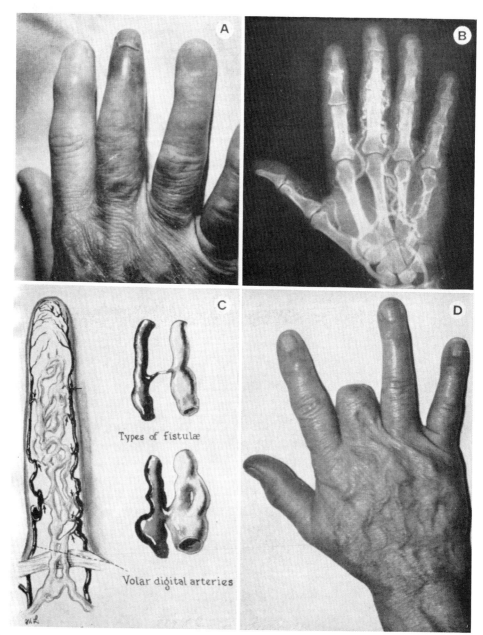

Figure 17.3.6. A. Atrophy of terminal portion of long finger and fingernail, with discoloration in a woman who 20 years previously had had an infected finger following a burn. *B.* Arteriogram demonstrates that the arterial tree is well outlined. Pudding of Diodrast in region of proximal interphalangeal joint points out area of arteriovenous communications. *C.* Schematic diagram showing sites of the fistulas and types of communications found at operation. *D.* Amputation was necessary despite radial excision of all communications because of persistent pain in fingertip. (Reproduced from an article by Curtis[10] by permission of the *Journal of Bone and Joint Surgery.)*

site of the fistula is compressed. As a result of the shunt of arterial blood to the venous side, the oxygen saturation of the venous blood can be used as a diagnostic sign of the presence and location of the anomaly, as proposed by Veal and McCord,[47] and postoperatively to determine if the eradication has been complete, as advocated by Horton and Ghormley.[20] Cardiac enlargement is not, as a rule, a complication of congenital arteriovenous fistulas, because of the small caliber of the communications. However, occasionally the channels will be large enough to produce a change in the heart size as in acquired arteriovenous fistulas. The systolic and diastolic blood pressure in some instances is elevated in the involved arm when compared to the opposite normal extremity.

Arteriogram

The actual area where the communications exist and the completeness of the surgical eradication can best be demonstrated by the arteriogram.

The characteristic findings of the arteriogram in congenital arteriovenous fistulae as previously reported by Allen and Camp[4] are: (1) dilatation of the arteries leading to the fistulas; (2) absence of normal filling of the arteries distal to the fistulas; (3) pooling of the arteriographic medium in the region of the fistulas: the pattern made by the contrast medium is suggestive of snowflakes in the region of the communications; (4) appearance of the contrast medium in the veins distal to the point of injection in the first roentgenogram, while the proximal arteries are still occluded, indicates an arteriovenous fistula.

Treatment

The treatment of congenital arteriovenous fistulas is complicated and the treatment varies with each patient. The complaints of the patient and the magnitude of the lesion are two of the most important considerations.

When the lesion is localized or where there are only a few communications, surgical excision is successful and can be carried out with no difficulty.

Proximal artery ligation alone is of little value. In 34 cases reported by Lewis[24] in which this was the method of treatment, amputation was necessary in spite of ligation and in seven instances it was performed because of gangrene.

When the arteriovenous fistula appears in the young child before the epiphysis have closed, surgical excision is indicated when possible to prevent the hypertrophy of the fingers which otherwise will occur.

When the process is extensive, with numerous communications, the treatment is best planned after an arteriogram and clinical examination. With these two aids, one can map out the major communications and plan the surgical steps necessary to eradicate the major shunts; however, one must be certain to preserve enough circulation to have survival of the part.

It is possible with this approach to reduce the number of shunts to obtain healing of ulcerated areas and prevent spontaneous hemorrhage even though the lesion has not been completely removed. With this approach, one is less likely to have secondary gangrene in the hand and fingers after surgery, a complication which may follow a very radical procedure.

Amputation may have to be resorted to when more conservative surgical procedures fail.

Where the patient's main complaint is one of pain, local excisions and ligation of some of the dilated veins and arteries with their arteriovenous communications will give relief even though the entire lesion is not completely excised. This is a satisfactory approach when one feels that a more radical procedure might cause circulatory embarrassment and gangrene.

Once ulceration of a funger has occurred, healing will not occur nor relief of pain be obtained unless a major portion of the arteriovenous communications are excised.

Partial thickness skin grafts or pedicle skin flaps may be needed as cover in some instances after excision, for the angiomatous tissue may so involve the skin as to make its excision necessary.

In several patients that I have seen, pain still persisted after multiple local excisions. A stellate ganglion block gave temporary pain relief and this was followed by permanent relief of pain after sympathectomy.

TUMORS OF LYMPH VESSELS

These tumors do occur in the hand and upper extremity, although they are rare. The tumors may occur as small localized lesions. The lymphangioma may involve an entire finger, the entire hand, or the upper extremity.

Allen, Barker, and Hines[3] prefer Wegner's classification in which he divided these into three types: the simple, the cavernous, and the cystic or cystic hygroma. Watson and McCarthy[48] have added another type which they call the diffuse systemic lymphangioma which is a lesion involving the entire extremity and probably representing a congenital type of lymphedema.

Simple Lymphangioma

The simple lymphangioma is almost always congenital and appears soon after birth.[18 35] The lesion is small and circumscribed. It has an elastic consistency. Microscopic examination of the specimen after excision reveals an anastomosing network of spaces and vessels of small and medium caliber, with rather thin cellular septal strands. The endothelial lining of the spaces is flat or cuboidal. Projecting endothelial buds, layering of endothelium, and proliferation of fibrous tissues are rarely seen. The treatment is local excision.

Cavernous Lymphangioma

These tumors also are congenital and appear soon after birth and grow slowly. It is felt that they represent abnormal mesodermal rests which develop into isolated, imperfect lymph vessels, with a slight tendency to abnormal growth (Fig. 17.3.7). Mixed hemangioma and lymphangioma tumors are apt to be

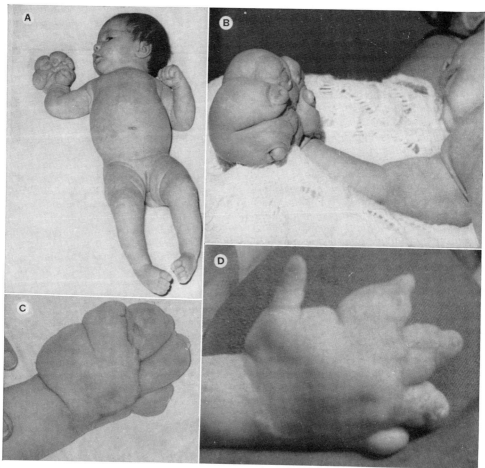

Figure 17.3.7. A and *B.* Clinical appearance of a child 50 days old with extensive lymphangioma of dorsum and volar aspect of entire hand. *C.* Hand after first operation which was performed soon after photograph in *A* and *B.* This consisted of an exploration of the volar arch and volar aspect of wrist where no constricting bands were found, and an excision of part of the tumor mass in continuity with skin on the dorsum of the hand. *D.* Hand after second operation which consisted of the removal of almost all the mass from dorsum of hand and fingers. On the fingers quadrilateral flaps were used and turned so as to depend on the palmar circulation of the fingers for survival. *(Continued on p. 0000.)*

more common than pure lymphangiomas.[34] The cavernous lymphangiomas are composed of numerous dilated lymphatic sinuses filled with lymph or mixtures of blood and lymph. The vessels are relatively thin, but there may be budding and proliferation of the endothelium and proliferation of the fibrous tissue between the spaces. Watson and McCarthy[48] describe a cellular or hypertrophic lymphangioma as a more active and growing type, with smaller sinuses and more solid endothelium. Cavernous lymphangiomas, as Allen, Barker, and Hines[4] state, are susceptible to infection from rather trivial trauma.

Treatment

Surgical excision is the best treatment, although unsightly scars and keloids may follow the excision through this lymphangiomatous tissue. There may be

constricting amputation-like bands at the base of a finger or circumferentially about a hand in the presence of these lymphangiomatous lesions which will need multiple Z-plasties in addition to the surgery for resection of the lymphangiomatous tissue. This amputation band has almost seemed in some instances to play a role in the production of the lymphangiectasis. In some instances the multiple Z-plasties through the amputation band has led to a great deal of improvement in the lymphatic stasis, greatly minimizing the amount of resection that was subsequently necessary. For this reason, if the lesion is essentially one caused by a congenital band defect, the Z-plasty to the band should be the first procedure to be carried out. Resection of the involved skin, with skin grafts for replacement or using the skin itself as full thickness skin graft removing all of the underlying lymphangiomatous tis-

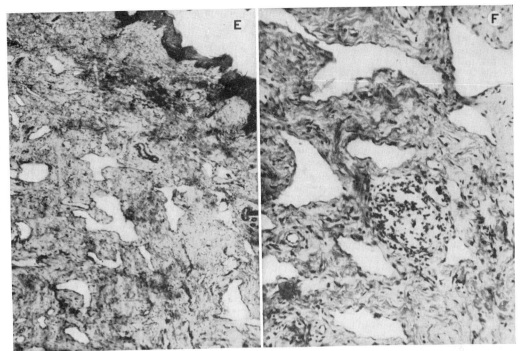

Figure 17.3.7. (continued). E. Low power photomicrograph showing tumor and overlying skin. *F.* High power photomicrograph shows lymphatic sinuses surrounded by fibrous tissue. Courtesy of Dr. Ivo Pitanguy, Rio de Janeiro, Brazil.

sue, may be necessary in correcting some of the extensive lesions. The acquired dilatation of the lymphatics which occurs as a result of the chronic lymphatic obstruction leads to dilatation of the lymphatics rather than new growth formation.

GLOMUS TUMOR

Introduction

The glomus tumor, also called by some glomangioma, angioneuromyoma, "Popoff" tumor, or Barré-Masson[5] tumor·is a rare but not uncommon tumor in the hand.

The tumor arises from the normal peripheral arteriovenous anastomosis called a glomus. This normal structure was described in detail by Sucquet[46] and Hoyer.[21] The tumor is thought to be an enlargement or hypertrophy of the normal glomus. Popoff[33] has demonstrated that the normal glomus has two functions: (1) a regulation of blood pressure; and (2) a local and general regulation of heat.

The normal glomus, as described by Popoff,[33] consists of an efferent arteriole which connects to an adjacent vein by way of a neuromyoarterial canal system called the Sucquet-Hoyer canal. The glomera are not present at birth, but, according to Popoff, develop in the first few months of life. This canal system consists of an endothelial lined tube surrounded by longitudinal and circular smooth muscle cells. Scattered among these muscle cells are epithelioid-like cells which have been called glomal cells or pericytes. Stout[43][44] gives Margaret Murray the credit for having proved by tissue culture that these glomal cells were true pericytes found on the surface of all capillaries. This canal system is covered by nonmyelinated nerve fibers and the entire structure is surrounded by a fibrous capsule. Normally the glomus is about 1 mm in diameter. However, the size varies with the location, and there may be considerable difference in size even in the same location according to Allen, Barker, and Hines.[3] Popoff in serial sections of a toe in a young adult found 64 normal glomera, with 24 of these being beneath the nail bed.

Historic Considerations

The first description of this lesion is credited to William Wood who in 1812, according to Ewing[13] described the classic, small, bluish, painful, subcutaneous tubercle of slow growth which was benign.

In 1920 Barré[5] described the signs and symptoms of the tumor in three patients and advocated surgical excision as the method of treatment.

Adair,[1] in 1934, reported 10 cases and stated that in 1929 he and Stewart[2] had reported a single case.

Masson in 1924, according to Popoff,[33] was the first to call this lesion a "glomus tumor" and indicated that it had its origin from the normal neuromyoarterial glomas.

Mason and Weil[27] in 1934, in their case report, listed all the other names by which this tumor had appeared in the literature.

Etiology

Trauma has been accused as being the etiologic factor that causes the normal neuromyoarterial glomus to become hypertrophied and produce clinical symptoms; however, Blanchard[6] has reported that it did not occur in most cases. Adair[1] stated in 1934 that patients with glomus tumors may have a tumor tendency since they were frequently associated with other tumors.

Stout[41] in a summary of 107 cases of glomus tumors found 60 men and 46 women (sex was not recorded in one case). He found that in 23 subungual tumors in the fingers, all but 3 were in women.

Grauer and Burt[17] suggested that there might be a congenital weakness in the glomera of affected persons that allowed minor trauma to trigger off the hypertropy. Kohout and Stout[22] were able to assemble 57 cases known to have started in childhood. Of these, six were congenital and 16 developed in the first five years of life.

Diagnosis

The signs and symptoms of the patient with a glomus tumor are classic. The presenting complaint is one of pain. The pain is paroxysmal in character and may be triggered off by exposure of the part to cold. The intense pain may come on after emotional upset, as when the patient becomes angry. One patient seen by the author frequently developed pain when dining out where there was emotional tension associated with eating. This same patient could produce the pain by allowing the neck to become chilled, so she wore a wool scarf about the neck constantly in cold weather.

A protective posture habit of the affected part may be assumed.

Many patients learn that once the pain develops, placing the hand in warm water will bring about relief.

The severity of the pain should lead one immediately to consider this diagnosis as a possibility. The patient frequently gives a history of long duration of pain over many years and of having seen many doctors and tried many remedies without improvement.

Grossly, as the affected finger is examined, one may or may not see the bluish discoloration beneath the fingernail or in the subcutaneous tissue.

The most important single clinical finding is the exquisite pinpoint tenderness over the tumor, which one can elicit with the blunt point of a small clamp. One will be able to localize this pinpoint area of pain to the area of the tumor just as one can localize the neuroma of a divided digital nerve (Fig. 17.3.8).

Allen, *et al.* have described the "pin test." The blunt head of a pin is used to delineate the normal surrounding skin or nail; the patient's crying out from the excruciating pain when the small diameter of the head of a pin is pressed over the lesion is seldom misleading.

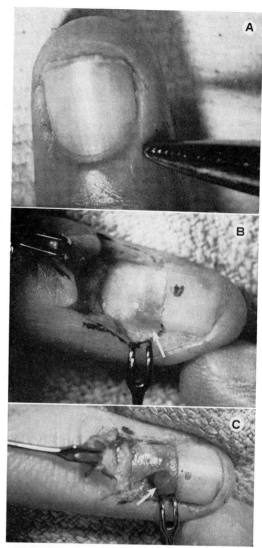

Figure 17.3.8.A. Point of small mosquito clamp indicates localized point of exquisite tenderness over glomus tumor. *B.* Portion of fingernail removed and glomus tumor is visible beneath the nail matrix. *C.* Nail matrix has been turnèd back exposing the round tumor deeper in color than the surrounding tissue. This patient, one year later, developed another glomus tumor beneath the fingernail, just distal to where this one had been excised.

The fingernail may be ridged overlying the lesion or an actual convexity of the nail may be seen at its distal margin.

While this lesion may be found anywhere in the body, about half of those reported have been in the subungual region.

Stout has emphasized that while the majority of these tumors are found at the junction of the corium and the subcutaneous tissue they are occasionally found in muscle, periosteum, and even joint capsule.

Vasomotor disturbances in the extremity may be associated with the tumor. In one personal case a true sympathetic dystrophy of the entire hand, with stiffness of all the finger joints, was present due to a glomus tumor 1 cm in diameter in the web space between two fingers. Excision of the lesion gave a complete cure.

Roentgenogram of the finger, particularly in the lateral plane, may reveal an erosion of the phalanx caused by pressure of the tumor.

In a case reported by Ley and Roca de Vinals,[25] the tumor was associated with such an erosion of the phalanx, with cyst formation and a Horner's syndrome.

Differential Diagnosis

The other tumors which might be encountered in this subungual area, such as exostosis, mucous cyst, ganglion, or melanoma, verruca, papilloma, or fibroma do not as a rule present the clinical, painful lesion seen with the glomus. This is also true of the neurofibroma, the angioma fibroma or painful lipomas which might be seen in the subcutaneous tissue in other areas of the hand. Only the tenderness of a neuroma might be confusing. Here the difference is that percussion over the neuroma gives the classical pins-and-needle or "shock-like" sensation not found with the glomus tumor. Microscopically, one must differentiate the glomus tumor from the hemangiopericytoma.

Grossly, the tumor, as a rule, is deep red or purple in color, more deeply colored than the surrounding tissue. When emptied of blood, as under tourniquet, it will appear slightly darker in color than the surrounding tissue and will shell out of the surrounding tissue.

Treatment

Complete surgical excision is the only method of treatment. Radiation therapy is not successful.

It is rare to see more than a single tumor in a given patient, but one must remember that multiple tumors may be encountered in a patient.[32] In one personal case, five separate glomus tumors all linked together were found in the subcutaneous tissue of a terminal phalanx (Fig. 17.3.9).

It is doubtful that recurrence ever occurs. However in one personal case, one lesion was removed, subungually, to be followed approximately two years later by a recurrence of symptoms, and another tumor was found subungually, just distal to the previously excised one. I felt that this represented not a recurrence but another tumor developing in another normal neuromyoarterial glomus.

When the tumor lies beneath the fingernail, the fingernail is removed in its entirety and the matrix overlying the lesion opened and reflected. The lesion can easily be shelled out and the matrix then closed with 6-0 plain catgut sutures to aid in the regrowth of a normal nail.

The lesion is best excised under tourniquet technique but one should remember that with all the blood expressed from the part, the tumor may not have the classic red or purple appearance.

Prognosis

The result after surgery is in general excellent. However, Allen et al.[3] report that several of their patients did not have complete pain relief. This, they think, may be related to the pain pathway to the consciousness having been so indelibly established through years of pain.

Stout has recorded a recurrence after eight years. He sited a similar case of recurrence in a case reported by Loutchitch. Allen et al.[3] had one case in which there seemed to be a recurrence.

Experience with a personal case in which there was a return of complaints approximately two years after excision revealed that the new glomus tumor was in the same general area, but just distal to the one previously excised.

Another case reported here, in which there was five separate glomus tumors, leads me to believe that most so-called recurrences are due to inadequate excision, the surgeon having missed other tumors at the first operation, or to other normal glomera in the general area undergoing hypertrophy.

Shugart et al.[39] in a study of 74 patients with glomus tumors, found none with more than one lesion; 47 patients were men, but of the 20 subungual tumors, 15 were in women. All tumors were painful. Surgery relieved this pain in all but 11 patients. The results were poor in five of the 20 subungual tumors.

HEMANGIOPERICYTOMA

This is a vascular tumor described by Stout[43] in which the pericyte is the dominant cell. It may be benign or malignant. The benign form resembles the glomus tumor, except that it does not structurally resemble the normal neuromyoarterial glomus. Stout prefers to say that the hemangiopericytoma is nonorganoid as compared to the organoid character of the glomus. Most of the tumors have developed in the soft tissues of the body.

The treatment of the tumor is surgical excision.

Stout reports that of the 258 tumors, 40, or 14 per cent, are known to have metastasized. There has been local recurrence if the excision has not been adequate.

MALIGNANT TUMORS OF BLOOD VESSELS AND LYMPH VESSELS

The malignant tumors of blood and lymph vessels are extremely rare in the hand and upper extremity. They are occasionally seen, however, and must be considered in the differential diagnosis of tumors in this region.

The tumors themselves are classified differently by various authors. Stout[45] prefers to classify them on the basis of the cell from which they originate. On this basis one has hemangioendotheliomas arising from the endothelial cells, hemangiopericytomas which arise from the pericytes found on the external surface of capillaries, Kaposi's sarcoma whose microscopic picture is a mixture of vascular and fibrosarcomatous tissue, the lymphangiosarcomas in which lymph vessels predominate, and hemangiosarcomas where the vascular tissue predominates.

Hemangioendothelioma

Those tumors which result from a malignant proliferation of endothelial cells have been called endotheliomas, whereas, when the microscopic picture is one of involvement of both fibroblastic connective tissue and vascular tissue, the tumor is called hemangiosarcoma.

The degree of malignancy of these tumors varies from slow growing to those which grow rapidly and metastasize early. Pack and Ariel[30] feel that all hemangioendotheliomas should be considered malig-

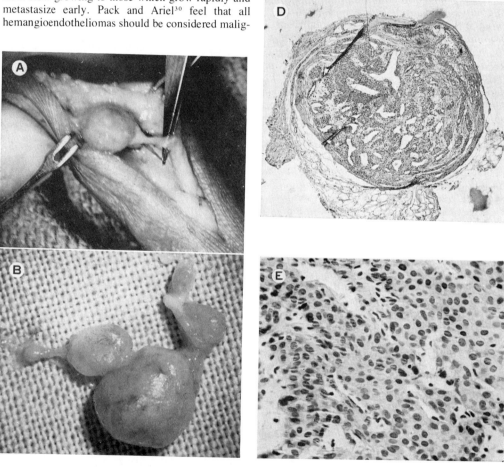

Figure 17.3.9. Patient caught finger in car door 15 years ago and has had pain in finger since then. *A.* Glomus tumor in subcutaneous tissue of the flexor surface of the terminal phalanx of finger. Point of scissors isolates branch of digital nerve to tumor. *B.* Gross specimen demonstrates that there are five separate glomus tumors. *C.* Cross-section photomicrograph though two of glomus tumors with nerve and blood vessels. × 20. *D.* Photomicrograph of one of the glomus tumors reveals organoid character. × 60. *E.* Photomicrograph shows the epithelial-like glomal cells or pericytes about small tumor vessels. × 400.

nant from the clinical standpoint for it is impossible to predict their behavior on a histologic basis.

Allen *et al.*[3] and Stout recommend radical surgical excision and in some instances amputation should be resorted too. Stout found that most of these tumors arising in the hand and fingers had not metastasized when the diagnosis was made which was not the case of those of other parts of the body.

Radiation therapy, Pack and Ariel[30] believe, may be palliative but should not be the primary form of therapy.

Hemangiosarcoma

These extremely malignant vascular tumors are papidly growing and metastazie early. Even though one carries out a radical resection or even amputation, the tumor may have metastasized before surgery. McCarthy and Pack[28] reported only 9 per cent five-year cure rate. The average survival time was 2½ years in their series. The authors recommend early radical amputation as the treatment of choice. Roentgen radiation may be palliative.

KAPOSI'S SARCOMA

Introduction

This rare, malignant vascular tumor which involves the skin has been called multiple idiopathic hemorrhagic sarcoma, or idiopathic pigment sarcoma.

Historic Considerations

This disease was first described by Kaposi in 1872. Later reports have appeared by Becher and Thatcher, as well as by Dorffel. Both authors feel that this is a disease of the reticuloendothelial system. The origin of this disease is unknown. Stout feels it has the same ambiguous position as Hodgkins disease.

Diagnosis

The disease is characterized by a lesion that frequently begins on the hands or feet, but may start on any part of the body. The onset is that of small pinhead size to larger, discrete or grouped lesions, which are flat nodules in the beginning and reddish brown or bluish red. These lesions later seem almost to coalesce and form larger plaques. Some lesions may appear to involute and leave atropic pigmented scars.

The diagnosis is best confirmed by biopsy of the lesions. In a single specimen one may see, microsopically, all stages of the disease, as described by Allen *et al.*[3] from the dilatation of blood vessels and deposits of hemosiderin to the stage of proliferation of lymphocytoid cells and infiltration of the cutis, to the later stage of endothelial proliferation resembling a hemangioendothelioma. The fourth stage is that of a nodular sarcomatous tumor, with many mitotic figures.

Treatment

The treatment is that of repeated, carefully control-led roentgen therapy, given in small doses of low voltage.

Pack and Ariel[30] state that occasionally wide surgical excision of the early solitary tumor may yield gratifying results.

The prognosis in this disease is poor. A five-year survival rate of 19 per cent has been reported by McCarthy and Pack.[28] Death may occur as soon as eight months after the onset although there have been reports of patients living as long as 25 years. The usual course is a downhill one, with death in two to ten years after onset. Since the disease may involve the viscera, this may the cause of death or intercurrent infection may be responsible for death.

LYMPHANGIOSARCOMA

This tumor of the upper extremity is seen in the chronic lymphedematous extremity which follows radial mastectomy and in the extremity with lymphangiomatosis. Scott *et al.*[38] have reported a lymphosarcoma in the hand and report three others they collected from the literature.[40]

Treatment is radical amputation (Pack, Miller, and Ariel[30, 31]) and (Dembrow and Adair[11]).

PYOGENIC GRANULOMA

Introduction

This is a common tumor on the hand and is seen most commonly after chronic infections about the fingernail. It may appear spontaneously, however, with no previous infection or wound. Michelson,[29] in a series of 29 cases, reported 11 of these occurring on the hands.

Historic Considerations

This lesion has been recognized since 1902 as a pyogenic granuloma.

Etiology

Chronic infection is believed by most authors to be the cause of this lesion. For this reason when there has been trauma with an open wound, in which secondary infection is present, one frequently finds such an overgrowth of granulation tissue developing. This overgrowth seems to be aided and abetted by a moist wound in which considerable exudate is present. Stout, on the other hand, prefers to call these lesions capillary hemangiomas of granuloma type; and he feels suppuration is not responsible for the lesion.

Diagnosis

Grossly the tumor is a raised, red, friable, lesion. The growth may be pedunculated. The granulation tissue of which it is composed bleeds easily. It may be as small as 1 mm in diameter to as large as 1 cm.

Microscopic examination of the specimen shows it

to be composed of granulation tissue and inflammatory cells. Stout[45] describes the capillaries as having a lobular arrangement, with each lobule springing from a feeding vessel.

As a rule, the diagnosis can be made by the presence of the raised, red, mushroom-like lesion. There may be a history of a wound, with secondary infection. With a history of a puncture wound by a foreign body, such as a splinter, with drainage and development of the granuloma, one must suspect that a portion of the foreign body remains in the hand.

Treatment

Since the *Staphylococcus aureus* is frequently cultured from the exudate about this lesion, one may be successful in curing the small granuloma by local treatment with an ointment containing 2 per cent nitrofurazone (Furacin soluble dressing) (Fig. 17.3.10), which is drying in character yet bacteriocidal. By combating the local infection, and at the same time obtaining a dry covering of thin epithelial cells over the surface of the granuloma, the lesion will frequently, when small, disappear.

Treatment has consisted of surgical excision, with fulguration of the base with a high frequency electric current or with silver nitrate. When these procedures fail, roentgen therapy may be indicated.

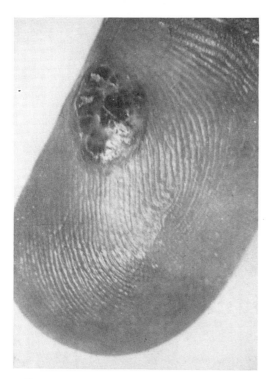

Figure 17.3.10. Pyogenic granuloma of finger which was cured by excision and 2 per cent nitrofurazone ointment (Furacin soluble dressing).

REFERENCES

1. Adair, F. E. Glomus tumor: A clinical study with a report of ten cases. Am. J. Surg., *25:* 1-6, 1934.
2. Adair, F., and Stewart, F. W. A tumor of the glomus. Bull. Mem. Hosp. New York, *1:* 42-45, 1929.
3. Allen, E. V., Barker, N. W., and Hines, E. A. *Peripheral Vascular Diseases.* Philadelphia, Saunders, 1946.
4. Allen, E. V., and Camp, J. B. Arteriography. A roentgenographic study of the peripheral arteries of the living subject following their injection with a radiopaque substance. J. A. M. A., *104:* 618-624, 1935.
5. Barré, J. A. Sur certaines; sympathalgies de la pérepherie des membres. Leur traitement chirurgical simple. Paris Méd., *45:* 311-315, 1922.
6. Blanchard, A. J. The pathology of glomus tumors. Can. Med. Assoc. J., ××: 357-360, 1941.
7. Byars, L. T. *Congenital Surface Vascular Disorders in Children.* Advances in Surgery, Johns Hopkins Hospital, 75th Anniversary, May 15, 1964.
8. Chamberlain, R. H., and Pendergrass, E. P. Some considerations regarding the treatment of hemangiomas. Pa. Med., *51:* 867-869, 1948.
9. Coursley, G., Ivins, J. C., and Baker, N. W. Congenital arteriovenous fistulas in the extremities: An analysis of sixty-nine cases. Angiology, *7:* 201, 1956.
10. Curtis, R. M. Congenital arteriovenous fistulae of the hand. J. Bone Joint Surg., *35A:* 917-928, 1953.
11. Dembrow, V. D., and Adair, F. E. Lymphangiosarcoma in the postmastectomy lymphedematous arm: Case report of a ten-year survivor treated by interscapulothoracic amputation and excision of local recurrence. Cancer, *14:* 210, 1961.
12. Elkins, D. C., and Cooper, F. W., Jr. Extensive hemangioma; report of cases. Surg. Gynecol. Obstet. *84:* 897-902, 1947.
13. Ewing, J. *Neoplastic Diseases: A Treatise on Tumors,* Ed. 4. Philadelphia, Saunders, 1940.
14. Geschickter, C. F., and Keasby, L. E. Tumors of blood vessels. Am. J. Cancer, *23:* 568-591, 1935.
15. Gherini (Abstract). Société Impériale de Chirurgie. Séance du 12 Juin, 1867. Gaz. d. Hôp., *40:* 303, 1867.
16. Goidanich, I. F., and Campanacci, M. Vascular hamartomata and infantile osteohyperplasia of the extremities. J. Bone Joint Surg., *44A:* 815-842, 1962.
17. Grauer, R. C., and Burt, J. C. Unusual location of glomus tumor; report of two cases. J. A. M. A., *112:* 1806-1810, 1939.
18. Harkins, G. A., and Sabiston, D. C., Jr. Lymphangioma in infancy and childhood. Surgery, *17:* 811, 1960.
19. Harkins, H. N. Hemangioma of a tendon or tendon sheath. Report of a case with a study of twenty-four cases from the literature. Arch. Surg., *34:* 12, 1937.
20. Horton, B. T., and Ghormley, R. K. Congenital arteriovenous fistulae of the extremities visualized by arteriography. Surg. Gynecol. Obstet., *60:* 978-983, 1935.
21. Hoyer, H. Quoted by Popoff.[33]
22. Kohout, E., and Stout, A. P. The glomus tumor in

children. Cancer, *14:* 555, 1961.

23. LaSorte, A. F. Cavernous hemangioma of striated muscle; review of literature and report of a case. Am. J. Surg., *100:* 593, 1960.

24. Lewis, D. W. Congenital arteriovenous fistulae. Lancet, *2:* 621-628; 680-686, 1930.

26. Losli, E. J. Intrinsic hemangiomas of the peripheral nerves. A report of two cases and a review of the literature. Arch. Pathol., *53:* 226,1952.

27. Mason, M. L., and Weil, A. Tumor of a subcutaneous glomus: tumeur glomique; tumeur du glomus neuromyo-artériel; subcutaneous painful tubercle; angiomyoneurome; subcutaneous glomal tumor. Surg. Gynecol. Obstet., *58:* 807-816, 1934.

28. McCarthy, W. D., and Pack, G. T. Malignant blood vessel tumors: A report of fifty-six cases of angiosarcoma and Kaposi's sarcoma. Surg. Gynecol. Obstet., *91:* 465, 1950.

29. Michelson, H. E. Granuloma pyogenicum. Arch. Dermat., *2:* 492-505, 1925.

30. Pack, G. T., and Ariel, I. M. *Tumors of the Soft Somatic Tissues,* Ed. 2. New York, Hoeber, 1964.

31. Pack, G. T., and Miller, T. R. Hemangioma classification, diagnosis, and treatment. Angiology, *1:* 405, 1950.

32. Plewes, B. Multiple glomus tumors; four in one finger tip. Can. Med. Assoc. J., *44:* 364-365, 1941.

33. Popoff, N. W. The digital vascular system with reference to the state of the glomus in inflammation, arteriosclerotic gangrene, diabetic gangrene, thrombo-angiitis obliterans, and supernumerary digits in man. Arch. Pathol., *18:* 295-330, 1934.

34. Ravitch, M. M. Radical treatment of massive mixed angiomas (hemolymphangiomas) in infants and children. Ann. Surg., *134:* 228, 1951.

35. Russo, P. E., and Dewar, J. P. Congenital lymphangioma. Am. J. Roentgenol., *85:* 726, 1961.

36. Sabin, F. R. Origin and development of the primitive vessels of the chick and of the pig. Contrib. Embryol. (Carnegie Inst.), *6:* 61-124, 1917-1918.

37. Schatten, W. E., Kramer, W. M., and Thomas, L. B. Multiple cavernous hemangiomas involving veins of an upper extremity. Report of a case treated by extensive local resection. Ann. Surg., *148:* 104-110, 1958.

38. Scott, R. B., Nydich, I., and Conway, H. Lymphangiosarcoma arising in lymphedema. Am. J. Med., *28:* 1008, 1960.

39. Shugart, R. R., Soule, E. H., and Johnson, E. W., Jr. Management of glomus tumors. Surg. Gynecol. Obstet., *117:* 334-340, 1963.

40. Stewart, F. W., and Treves, H. Lymphangiosarcoma in post-mastectomy lymphedema; a report of six cases in elephantiasis chirurgica. Cancer, *1:* 64, 1948.

41. Stout, A. P. Tumors of the neuromyo-arterial glomus. Am. J. Cancer, *24:* 255-272, 1935.

42. Stout, A. P. Hemangioendothlioma: A tumor of blood vessels featuring vascular endothelial cells. Ann. Surg., *118:* 445, 1945.

43. Stout, A. P. Hemangiopericytoma. A study of twenty-five new cases. Cancer, *2:* 1027, 1949.

44. Stout, A. P. Tumors featuring pericytes. Glomus tumor and hemangiopericytoma. Lab. Invest., *5:* 217, 1956.

45. Stout, A. P. Tumors of the soft tissues. In *Armed Forces Institute of Pathology Atlas of Tumor Pathology,* Washington, D. C., 1953.

46. Sucquet. Quoted by Popoff.[33]

47. Veal, J. R., and McCord, W. M. Congenital abnormal arteriovenous anastomoses of the extremities with special reference to diagnosis by arteriography and by the oxygen saturation test. Arch. Surg., *33:* 848-866, 1936.

48. Watson, W. L., and McCarthy, W. D. Blood and lymph vessel tumors; a report of 1,056 cases. Surg. Gynecol. Obstet. *71:* 569-588, 1940.

49. Willard, H. H. The development of the principal arterial stems in the forelimb of the pig. Contrib. Embroyol. (Carnegie Inst.), *14:* 139-154, 1922.

D.

Nerve Tumors

John J. Byrne, M.D.

Peripheral nerves are derived from ectoderm, the ventral roots from the neural tube, and the dorsal roots from the neural crests. From these ectodermal elements two cell types arise, the neuroblasts or embryonic nerve cells and the supporting elements or sheath of Schwann's cells. At the end of the fourth week of development the ventral roots grow out of the spinal cord and soon thereafter the primitive dorsal root ganglia develop from the neural crest and send dorsal fibers to the spinal cord and peripheral fibers to join the ventral root fibers. The nerves then grow into the arm bud forming the normal adult arrangement as the bud differentiates into its various components. The nerve fibers end in their predestined pattern, the efferent fibers in motor end plates and the afferent fibers in a host of specialized sense organs: free nerve endings, tactile discs, Pacinian corpuscles, and neuromuscular spindles. Melanoblasts also derive from the primitive neural crest tissue.

As the nerves leave the spinal cord they acquire a connective tissue covering of mesenchymal origin which closely invests the nerve as epi-, peri-, and endoneurium. In addition, it acquires its own blood supply.

The mature nerve consists of numerous fascicles of nerve fibers surrounded by various layers of connective tissue. The fibers consist of the axons and their associated sheath of Schwann. This sheath is composed of cells with flat oval nuclei which wrap themselves around the axons and connect with each other by cell processes at the nodes of Ranvier. Myelin develops in the Schwann's cells as a "highly ordered lamellar system of membranes."[2] The outer layer of connective tissue is called the *epineurium* and is composed of longitudinally arranged connective tissue cells and collagenous fibers. The nerve fascicles are surrounded by *peri-neurium* from which fine strands of connective tissue pass through and around the individual nerve fibers as *endoneurium* (sheath of Henle). Blood vessels follow the connective tissue.

Tumors may thus be derived from ectodermal Schwann's cells and specialized nerve endings, mesodermal connective tissue, and blood vessels or metastases from distant organs. Axons do not form true neoplasms but contribute to the development of amputation neuromas.

AMPUTATION "NEUROMAS"

An amputation "neuroma" is a nonneoplastic tumor which occurs at the central end of a cut nerve as nerve fibrils or axons grow out from the cut end and become incorporated in a mass of scar tissue derived from the supporting tissue of the nerve. It may also occur as a lateral neuroma or a neuroma in continuity if the nerve is partially injured. Particularly liable nerves are the sensory digital nerves and the sensory nerves at the level of the wrist (dorsal ulnar nerve, palmar cutaneous branch of the median nerve, and the terminal branches of the superficial radial nerve). These may be injured in operations for ganglia and DeQuervain's disease. When stimulated, such a neuroma may produce painful paresthesias consisting of "pins-and-needles" sensation or "shooting" pains along the course of the nerve's normal skin distribution or at the site of the neuroma itself. The pain may become very severe and may eventually spread up the entire extremity. The fiber interaction of injured nerves may explain this diffuse involvement.[9, 24] Another explanation is Head's theory involving increased excitement in the internuncial pool of the spinal cord or in higher sensory centers so that normal impulses in the area are interpreted as painful.

Neuromas occurring at amputation sites become painful when stimulated by touching or grasping the amputated stump. If the neuroma is adherent to the terminal scar or bone end, there may be pain on mere motion of the affected digit.

Infection in the amputation stump may stimulate the development of the neuroma. Petropoulos and Stefanko[21] recently studied the growth of amputation neuromas in dogs under various physiologic conditions. The found that inflammatory processes produced much larger and more irregular neuromas than the controls. There was more mixing of the supporting cells and nerve elements in the inflammatory neuromas as compared to a more regular and orderly arrangement in the controls. The neuromas in malnourished animals were smaller than in controls.

Suspicious lesions should be carefully searched for with a small palpating area such as a blunt pencil end. The "neuroma" will be found as a sharp localized area which, when palpated, produces painful paresthesiae. Large "neuromas" can be palpated.

The pain of most neuromas usually disappears months after the injury by some process unexplainable at the present time. Perhaps it is similar to the disappearance of Tinel's sign in an injured nerve as the nerve fibers become insulated by the sheath of Schwann. The new fibrils may become encased in fibrous tissue and stop growing and then become ensheathed by the Schwann's cells making them insensitive to painful stimuli.

Russell and Spalding[26] believe that regenerating nerve fibers are more vulnerable to trauma than normal nerves and applied their theory to the treatment of amputation neuromas by repeated percussion performed with a mallet and wooden applicator, consisting of a wooden shaft with a smooth metal dome on the end place over the neuroma, and a crutch rubber on the other to deaden the sound of the tapping. Percussion is performed for 20 min or so and is repeated three or four times daily. If the neuroma is exquisitely tender, anesthesia is obtained for the first few minutes by applying a tourniquet proximally at a pressure sufficient to occlude the arterial circulation. After a short period of time, the occlusive tourniquet is not needed and the patient can be trained to perform his own percussion. In 33 cases, the results were good to excellent in 19, improved in five, and unchanged in nine.

I have had no experience with this method but have had occasional success from advising patients to massage the neuroma vigorously using lanolin or Vaseline petroleum jelly as a lubricating agent. When such conservative methods fail, however, a surgical approach is usually necessary.

Surgical Treatment

When the discomfort is severe, the amputation neuroma should be surgically treated. Blind excision of scar tissue or reamputation is of little avail since the newly cut nerve merely reincorporates itself in the new amputation stump.

After the nerve has been explored and the neuroma uncovered, a decision has to be made concerning prevention of future neuromas. Many procedures have been proposed for this and recently Petropoulos and Stefanko[22] tested most of them in dogs. Nerve stumps treated with cauterization, electrocoagulation, and freezing showed smaller neuromas than the controls. Ligation of the nerve trunk above the site of resection produced a small neuroma. Implantation of the nerve into muscle produced no neuromas nor were any found in trunks treated with 5 per cent formalin, HCl, and pepsin, alcohol, or phenol. Best results were obtained with local application or general administration of nitrogen mustard.

My preference has been for the method described so well by Munro and Mallory[17] wherein the nerve is lightly crushed (to destroy the axons but keep the sheath intact) 0.5 cm proximal to the site of nerve division. A silk ligature of appropriate size for the nerve diameter (No. 1 for median nerve and 3-0 for digital nerve) is tied firmly around this crushed area (Fig. 17.4.1).

It is essential that the nerve end so treated be placed in a position away from scar, tendon, or cut bone surface. An ideal site is muscle if it is available for not only is the nerve end cushioned from tactile and grasping forces but, as Petropoulos and Stefanko[22] have shown, the nerve ends grow in an isomorphic pattern resembling normal nerve and may even terminate in spiral nerve terminals. When treating amputation neuromas in the hand, such transfer is possible only when the neuromas occur near an interosseous muscle (Fig. 17.4.2).

When the amputation neuroma occurs in the fingers, the crushed and ligated nerve end may be placed in bone (Fig. 17.4.3) or transplanted to lie on the dorsum of the finger away from the tactile volar surface (Fig. 17.4.4). If the nerve end is placed in a phalanx, it is essential that the nerve lie loosely in its bed so that it is not affected by motion of the finger. If the nerve is

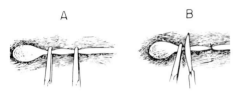

Figure 17.4.1. Treatment of amputation neuroma to prevent recurrence. A. Nerve is lightly crushed 0.5 cm proximal to site of nerve division. B. Crushed nerve is ligated firmly with nonabsorbable ligature and amputation neuroma excised.

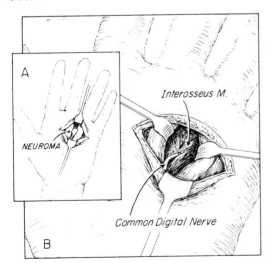

Figure 17.4.2. A. Amputation neuroma in common digital nerve to ring and long fingers. Neuroma had regrown at site of previous catgut ligature. B. Amputation neuroma excised according to method shown in Figure 17.4.1 and nerve transplanted in interosseous muscles.

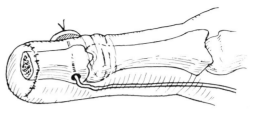

Figure 17.4.3. Amputation neuroma treated as shown in Figure 17.4.1 and digital nerve placed in phalanx, care being taken that nerve is not taut.

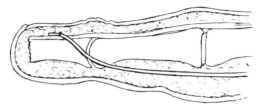

Figure 17.4.4. Amputation neuroma treated as shown in Figure 17.4.1 and nerve transplanted to dorsal subcutaneous space.

taut after such bone implantation, motion may stimulate pain similar to that found in the original neuroma.

Prevention of Amputation "Neuromas"

Such painful neuromas may be prevented by careful attention to details at the time of the original amputation repair. If the nerve end is obviously visible or redundant, it should be freed up for a short distance into the proximal subcutaneous tissue. The most proximal portion should be lightly crushed with a hemostat and ligated with 3-0 silk. The nerve should be incised about 0.5 cm distal to the ligature and allowed to retract into the subcutaneous tissue which should serve as a cushion against tactile pressures. If no such subcutaneous fat pad is available, it should probably be transferred to the dorsal subcutaneous tissue. The amputation should be closed by whatever means is suitable.

If the nerve ends are not obviously visible and seem unlikely to become involved in the amputation scar, no special effort is needed to locate them before completing the amputation repair.

NERVE SHEATH TUMORS

The origin of these tumors has been the subject of much debate with some (Nageotte,[19] Masson[14]) believing they have the histologic attributes of the sheath of Schwann and others that they are of mesodermal or fibroblastic origin (Mallory,[12] Penfield,[20] Tarlov[28]). Tissue culture studies by Murray and Stout[18] appear to favor a Schwannian origin. Experimental studies may also amplify this view. Causey[5] experimentally produced peripheral nerve tumors by injecting dimethyl benzanthracene under the perineurium and just inside the epineurium in crushed and noncrushed nerves. Tumors arising inside the nerve showed rounded nuclei with a lack of longitudinal orientation and a tendency to form rosettes. Tumors arising outside the nerve resembled fibrosarcomas. He also found a higher incidence of such tumors inside the nerve when the injection was made in crushed nerves. Since the sheath of Schwann is more active in such areas of trauma, the addition of a carcinogen should be more apt to produce a tumor.

The *benign encapsulated neurilemoma* is the most common variety of nerve tumor and usually forms a round or fusiform mass located in connection with smaller nerve twigs or within the sheath of a major nerve. The tumors are firm and white although occasionally they may be cystic and of a jelly-like consistency. The tumor is made up of long slender cells with the nuclei arranged in a palisade fashion, the so-called Verocay body or Antoni A areas (Fig. 17.4.5). Thorsrud[29] reviewed 452 cases and correlated various pathologic criteria with prognosis. Tumors made up predominately of Antoni A areas would be Type II in his classification, and this made up 35.2 per cent of the total series. In other parts of the same tumor the tissue may appear to be a loose reticulum of cells with small nuclei and radiating fibrils with minute areas of cystic degeneration, the so-called Antoni B areas which are most prominent in the acoustic nerve tumors (Fig. 17.4.6). This would be Thorsrud Type I, which was found in 6.2 per cent of the series. A combination of Types I and II resulted in Type III which made up 4.4 per cent of the series and which was usually found in the skin of von Recklinghausen's disease.

These tumors are usually solitary but may be multiple. Due to the long controversey concerning their site of origin, there have been many pseudonyms for this tumor: acoustic nerve tumor, neurilemoma, acoustic neuroma, angioneurofibroma, false neuroma, fibroglioma, fibromyxoma, glioma, myoschwannoma, neurilemoblastoma, neurinoma, neurofibromyxoma, perineural fibroblastoma, Schwannoma, peripheral glioma, perineural glioma.

These tumors are usually well encapsulated and can be shelled out of the involved nerve with ease. Surgical treatment of Types I, II, and III revealed only one death from tumor in Thorsrud's series of 122 patients who could be accurately traced, and this tumor was not a peripheral lesion. Other recent series of such cases confirm their benignity.[8] [11]

The *neurofibroma* is a tumor associated with von Recklinghausen's disease wherein there is a great thickening of the nerve sheath elements which separates the individual nerve fibrils (Fig. 17.4.7), sometimes producing a pressure atrophy. These changes may be found in the autonomic as well as in the peripheral and cranial nerves. Extensive involvement may produce a marked tortuosity of the nerve or plexus known as a plexiform neuroma. Proximal growth may extend through the intervertebral foramina to involve the spinal cord. Other stigmas of von Recklinghausen's disease may be present such as fibroma mollusca, cafe-au-lait spots, sebaceous adenomas, lipomas, intestinal tumors, bone deformities, and meningiomas. Patients with this disease may also have neurilemomas, usually of the Antoni B type (Thorsrud I).

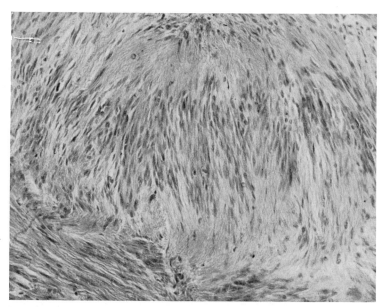

Figure 17.4.5. Benign neurilemoma showing palisading of nuclei (Verocay body, Antoni A area, Thorsrud Type II). (Reprinted by permission of the authors[3] and the *American Journal of Surgery.*)

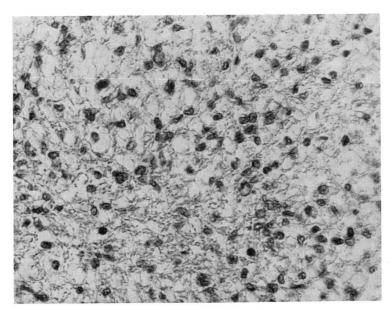

Figure 17.4.6. Benign neurilemoma showing loose reticulum of cells (Antoni B area, Thorsrud Type I). (Reprinted by permission of the authors[3] and the *American Journal of Surgery*.)

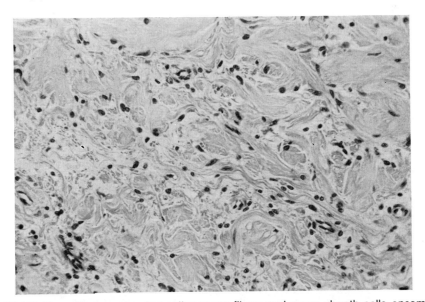

Figure 17.4.7. Neurofibroma showing collagenous fibers and nerve sheath cells encompassing nerve fibrils. (Reprinted by permision of the authors[3] and the *American Journal of Surgery*.)

Over the years, these tumors have acquired numerous pseudonyms such as plexiform neuroma, dumbbell tumor, elephantiasis neuromatosa, fibroma molluscum, hour glass tumors of the spine, multiple neurofibromatosis, multiple neuroma, neurinomatosis, neuroblastomatosis, neurofibromatosis, neuromatosis, von Recklinghausen's disease.

These tumors are usually multiple. Patients with multiple tumors and neurofibromatosis in Thorsrud's series were younger than those with solid neurinoma. Since such patients had predominately a Type I tumor, this has suggested that patients with multiple neurinomas may be looked upon as subclinical or abortive instances of neurofibromatosis.

According to the literature these tumors have a high potential for malignancy. Inadequate excision may stimulate their growth either along the nerve or as a metastasizing malignancy. Spontaneous transformation has been estimated to occur in 13 per cent of von

Recklinghausen's disease.[10] Removal of these tumors has been followed by sarcomatous changes in distant neurofibromas or by the development of neurofibromas elsewhere in the body.

The relative hopelessness of this group of patients usually dictates that surgery only be done for tumors undergoing rapid growth or presenting cosmetic or functional disabilities. Surgery consists of wide nerve excision and not enucleation.

In deference toward surgery in this group one must remember, however, that people with von Recklinghausen's disease may develop tumors in other organs.

A *malignant neurilemoma* consists of sheath cells growing in cords often in a whorling design resembling a fibrosarcoma (Fig. 17.4.8). In addition there may be capsule invasion (Fig. 17.4.9), pleomorphism of cells, mitoses (Fig. 17.4.10), and bizarre giant cells in the more advanced malignancies. Approximately half the malignant neurilemomas are associated with von Recklinghausen's disease.

Thorsrud has classified the malignancies in a manner similar to Quick and Cutler.[23] Type IV has abundant intercellular substance with a scarcity of cells forming the interlacing bundles. This is a low grade malignancy, since there were deaths from tumor in only 5 per cent of cases and only 11.7 per cent recurred.

Type V has a medium amount of cells and intercellular substance with interlacing bundles and a few mitoses. This is a medium grade malignancy since 21 per cent of such patients died from their tumor and 43 per cent had recurrences.

Type VI showed densely packed cells with very little intercellular substance, pleomorphism and many mitoses. There was some interlacing of cells but usually the cells showed a loss of polarity. This is a high grade malignancy and 40 per cent of such patients died of their tumor and 44 per cent had recurrence.

Ten patients in Thorsrud's series had metastases to lungs: eight were Type VI and two Type V tumors. Size also correlated with the cellular classifications. Small tumors (less than 1.5 cm) and medium tumors (1.5 to 7 cm in width) showed the different cell types in equal distribution. Among large tumors (greater than 7 cm in width), however, Types IV, V, and VI were predominent (87.6 per cent). This was interesting in the light of Woyke's[32] work on experimental tumors. In the early stages they looked like Schwannomas, but with added growth they resembled anablastic sarcomas.

These tumors grow proximally along the nerve trunks into adjacent tissue or metastasize by blood stream. Synonyms for these tumors are neurogenic sarcoma, neurofibrosarcoma, malignant neurinoma, malignant peripheral glioma.

At the present time, the therapy for malignant neurilemomas is not good. It involves wide excision of the nerve for 6 to 8 inches proximal to the tumor site. If there is a spread to adjacent tissue or if one is operating on a recurrent nerve tumor, an amputation will usually be necessary, with care being taken that the involved nerve is dissected for about 12 to 15 inches proximal to the tumor, if possible, since there is a great tendency for these malignancies to grow along the nerve trunk.

A rare variant of malignant nerve sheath tumors is the neuroepithelioma, which according to Stout[27] is

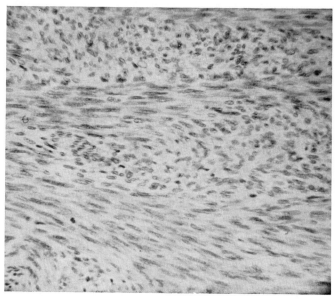

Figure 17.4.8. Malignant neurilemoma demonstrating cords of cells with elongated nuceli, little intercellular substance, and growing in interlacing bundles.

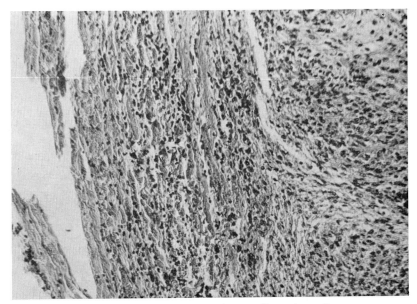

Figure 17.4.9. Capsule invasion in a malignant neurilemoma

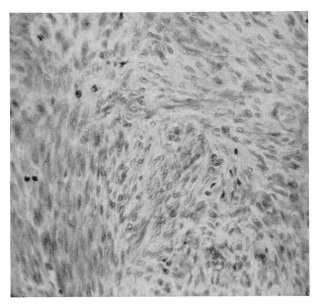

Figure 17.4.10. Malignant neurilemoma showing mitoses

derived from cells of the neurocrest and produces lesions which histologically resemble tumors of the central nervous system. However, they differ in one important aspect; they may metastasize via the blood stream. They are composed of neuroepithelial cells in sheets (neuroepithelioma) or with rosettes or structures which resemble embryonal medullary canal (medulloepithelioma). Mannarino and Watts[13] described such a tumor of the sciatic nerve which after radical block dissection spread to both lungs resulting in death in four months. Michel[15] reviewed 18 cases of

such tumors including one of his patients and emphasized their malignant potential. He believes they should be classified as "malignant neurilemoma with epithelial elements."

MISCELLANEOUS TUMORS

Mesodermal Tumors

Although fibroma and fibrosarcomas could develop from nerve peri- and epineurium, they are almost nonexistent. Stout[27] has never seen one in his experience.

Ganglia have been reported in numerous peripheral nerves: median, tibial, peroneal, and ulnar. However, it appears that these do not arise in the epi-or perineurium but invade the nerve from neighboring structures.[31] It is probably not necessary to resect these lesions since simple decompression of the nerve can be performed by longitudinal incision. In such a case involving the peroneal nerve, Tupman[30] had a complete return of function.

Vascular tumors may arise in a peripheral nerve but only one such case was seen by Stout[27] in the Surgical Pathology Laboratory of Columbia University. Usually, local hemangiomas invade the nerves from outside and become intimately intertwined in them making surgical excision difficult.

There is a rare lipofibroma of the median nerve which occurs in the palm of children. Rowland[25] reported such a case and reviewed these tumors. They appear to be benign and do not require resection which may result in loss of median nerve function. Transection of the carpal tunnel relieved his patient's complaints and no further growth was noted in three years. In fact, the tumor seemed to get smaller. These tumors feel fatty in the gross specimen, but microscopically one finds hypertrophied perineurial and endoneurial connective tissue about the nerve bundles which are separated by fibrofatty tissue.

I have seen one tumor attached to the lateral antibrachial cutaneous nerve which was a pure lipoma.

Metastatic Nerve Lesions

These are extremely rare in peripheral nerves and have been reported from the lungs.[6] Diffuse involvement with lymphoma may produce a dense infiltration with lymphoma cells.[16]

Tumor of Tactile End Organs

A tumor that appeared to be composed of tactile end organs was reported by Cammermyer.[4] It occurred on a finger of a 50-year-old man and it was not painful. Since it had been present at birth, however, one wonders whether it was a congenital anomaly rather than a true neoplasm.

SURGICAL PLAN OF ACTION

Since the great majority of nerve tumors are of nerve sheath origin, this discussion will concern itself with them alone.

What Should the Surgeon Do When He Faces a Tumor in a Peripheral Nerve?

The first decision that will have to be made is whether it is encapsulated, and can it easily be dissected from the nerve. If so, it is probably a benign neurilemoma, and there should be no resultant nerve palsy and no likelihood of recurrence. However, the dissection should be completely free and easy, and no sharp dissection should be necessary.

If the tumor cannot be easily shelled out from its nerve bed, it should be excised *in toto* with a generous margin of nerve on either side, providing a reanastomosis is possible, or if not, a suitable tendon transfer is possible.

If these conditions are not met, then a generous biopsy should be performed and subsequent surgery await the pathologic diagnosis. The size may help here some since we have seen that tumors over 7 cm in width are usually malignancies of various grades. A frozen section should be done since an experienced pathologist can usually tell a benign neurilemoma (Thorsrud Types I to III) from the varying degrees of malignancies (Thorsrud Types IV to VI). If he is even suspicious, the tumor should be resected. If the diagnosis is a malignancy, a generous nerve excision should be done even if repair is impossible. Large gaps in nerves can be overcome in many ways: mobilization of the proximal and distal nerves, flexing of adjacent joints, or by nerve rerouting.[17] If the diagnosis is neurofibroma, however, probably no further surgery is indicated in the case where a nerve repair or tendon transfer is not possible.

Necessary Amputation

An amputation is necessary when the disease has transgressed the nerve boundary.

Is any further treatment of value?

X-ray offers nothing since these tumors are notably radioresistant. No chemotherapy is available.

REFERENCES

1. Babcock, W. W. A standard technique for operations on peripheral nerves. Surg. Gynecol. Obstet., 45: 364, 1927.
2. Bloom, W., and Fawcett, D. W. A Textbook of Histology, Ed. 8. Philadelphia, Saunders, 1962.
3. Byrne, J. J., and Cahill, J. M. Tumors of major peripheral nerves. Am. J. Surg., 102: 724, 1961.
4. Cammermyer, J. Tumor of the tactile end organs. Arch. Pathol., 42: 1, 1946.
5. Causey, G. Experimental tumors of peripheral nerve in mice Acta Union Internat. Contra Cancrum, 15: 142, 1959.
6. Cohn, J. Epithelial neoplasms of the peripheral and cranial nerves. Arch. Surg., 17: 117, 1928.
7. Cutler, E. C., and Gross, R. E. The surgical treatment of tumors of the peripheral nerves. Ann. Surg., 104: 436, 1936.
8. Dinakar, I., and Rao, S. B. Neurilemomas of peripheral nerves. Int. Surg., 55: 15, 1970.
9. Granit, R., Leksell, L., and Skoglund, C. R. Fiber interaction in injured or compressed region of nerve. Brain, 67: 125, 1944.
10. Hosoi, K. Multiple neurofibromatosis (von Recklinghausen's disease). Arch. Surg., 22: 258, 1931.

11. Jacobs, R. L., and Barncada, R. Neurilemoma. Arch. Surg., *102:* 181, 1971.
12. Mallory, F. B. The type cell of the so-called dural endothelioma J. Med. Res., *41:* 349, 1920.
13. Mannarino, E., and Watts, J. W. Malignant tumors arising from peripheral nerves. J. Int. Coll. Surg., *37:* 550, 1962.
14. Masson, P. Experimental and spontaneous schwannomas. Am. J. Pathol., *8:* 367, 1932.
15. Michel, S. L. Epithelial elements in malignant neurogenic tumor of the tibial nerve. Am. J. Surg., *113:* 404, 1967.
16. Moore, R. Y., and Oda, Y. Malignant lymphoma with diffuse involvement of the peripheral nervous system. Neurology, *12:* 186, 1962.
17. Munro, D., and Mallory, G. K. Elimination of the so-called amputation neuromas of divided peripheral nerves. N. Engl. J. Med., *260:* 358, 1959.
18. Murray, M. R., and Stout, A. P. Schwann cell versus fibroblast as the origin of the specific nerve sheath tumor. Am. J. Pathol., *16:* 41, 1940.
19. Nageotte, J. Sheaths of the peripheral nerves: Nerve degeneration and regeneration. In *Cytology and Cellular Pathology of the Nervous System,* Vol. I, Section 5. Edited by W. Penfield. New York, Hoeber, 1932, p. 191.
20. Penfield, W. Tumors of the sheaths of the nervous system. In *Cytology and Cellular Pathology of the Nervous System,* Vol. 3, Section 19, edited by W. Penfield. New York, Hoeber, 1932, p. 955.
21. Petropoulos, P. C., and Stefanko, S. Experimental studies of post-traumatic neuromas under various physiological conditions. J. Surg. Res., *1:* 235, 1961.
22. Petropoulos, P. C., and Stefanko, S. Experimental observations on the prevention of neuroma formation. J. Surg. Res., *1:* 241, 1961.
23. Quick, D., and Cutler, M. Neurogenic sarcoma. Ann. Surg., *86:* 810, 1927.
24. Rosenblueth, A. The stimulation of myelinated axons by nerve impulses in adjacent myelinated axons. Am. J. Physiol., *132:* 119, 1941.
25. Rowland, S. A. Lipofibroma of the median nerve in the palm. J. Bone Joint Surg., *49A:* 1309, 1967.
26. Russell, W. R., and Spalding, J. M. K. Treatment of painful amputation stumps. Br. Med. J., *2:* 68, 1950.
27. Stout, A. P. Tumors of the peripheral nervous system, In: *Atlas of Tumor Pathology,* Section II, Fascicle 6. Washington, U.S. Armed Forces Institute of Pathology, 1953.
28. Tarlov, I. M. Origin of perineural fibroblastoma. Am. J. Pathol., *16:* 33, 1940.
29. Thorsrud, G. Neurinoma. Acta chir. Scandi. (Suppl.), *252:* 16, 1960.
30. Tupman, G. S. Axonotmesis of anterior tibial branch of lateral popliteal nerve due to ganglion of the nerve sheath. Br. J. Surg., *45:* 23, 1957.
31. Warren, R. Ganglion of the common peroneal nerve. Ann. Surg., *124:* 152, 1946.
32. Woyk, S. Experimental tumors in rats produced by a carcinogenic agent (methylcholantrene) in partly isolated nerve trunks. Acta Unio Internat. Contra Cancrum, *18:* 30, 1962.

INDEX